ATLAS OF VASCULAR SURGERY AND ENDOVASCULAR THERAPY:
Anatomy and Technique

CO-EDITORS

Ronald M. Fairman, MD
The Clyde F. Barker – William Maul Measey Professor of Surgery
Chief, Division of Vascular Surgery and Endovascular Therapy
Vice-Chairman for Clinical Affairs, Department of Surgery
Professor of Surgery in Radiology
Hospital of the University of Pennsylvania
Philadelphia, Pennsylvania

Peter Gloviczki, MD
Joe M. and Ruth Roberts Professor of Surgery
Chair Emeritus, Division of Vascular and Endovascular Surgery
Director Emeritus, Gonda Vascular Center
Mayo Clinic
Rochester, Minnesota

Kimberley J. Hansen, MD
Professor of Surgery
Department of Vascular and Endovascular Surgery
Wake Forest University School of Medicine
Winston-Salem, North Carolina

Glenn M. LaMuraglia, MD
Associate Professor of Surgery
Harvard Medical School
Division of Vascular and Endovascular Surgery
Massachusetts General Hospital
Boston, Massachusetts

George H. Meier, MD, RVT, FACS
Professor and Chief
Department of Vascular Surgery
University of Cincinnati College of Medicine
Cincinnati, Ohio

Mark D. Morasch, MD, FACS
Department of Cardiovascular Surgery
St. Vincent Healthcare
Billings, Montana

Marc L. Schermerhorn, MD
Chief, Division of Vascular and Endovascular Surgery
Beth Israel Deaconess Medical Center
Associate Professor of Surgery
Harvard Medical School
Boston, Massachusetts

ATLAS OF VASCULAR SURGERY AND ENDOVASCULAR THERAPY:
Anatomy and Technique

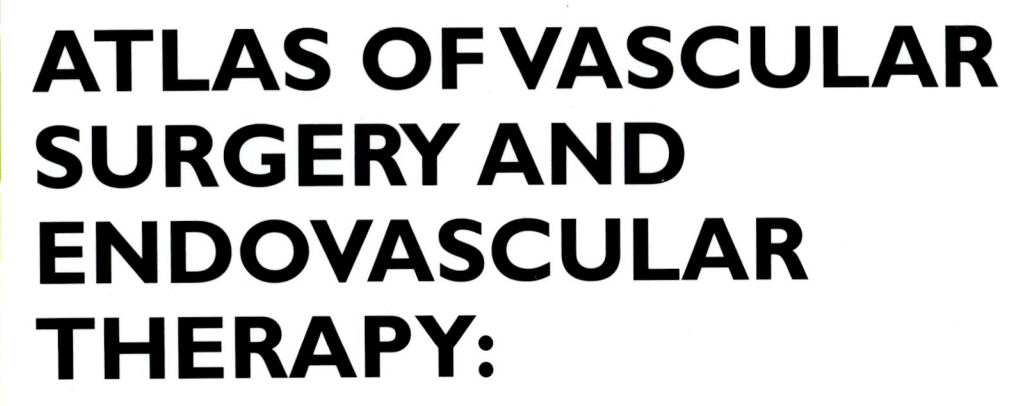

Elliot L. Chaikof, MD, PhD
Johnson and Johnson Professor of Surgery
Harvard Medical School
Chairman, Roberta and Stephen R. Weiner Department of Surgery
Surgeon-in-Chief
Beth Israel Deaconess Medical Center
Boston, Massachusetts

Richard P. Cambria, MD
The Robert R. Linton MD Professor of Vascular and Endovascular Surgery
Harvard Medical School
Chief, Division of Vascular and Endovascular Surgery
Department of Surgery
Massachusetts General Hospital
Boston, Massachusetts

ELSEVIER
SAUNDERS

ELSEVIER
SAUNDERS

1600 John F. Kennedy Blvd.
Ste. 1800
Philadelphia, PA 19103-2899

Atlas of Vascular Surgery and Endovascular Therapy:　　　ISBN: 978-1-4160-6841-9
Anatomy and Technique
Copyright © 2014 by Saunders, an imprint of Elsevier Inc.

No part of this publication may be reproduced or transmitted in any form or by any means, electronic or mechanical, including photocopying, recording, or any information storage and retrieval system, without permission in writing from the publisher. Details on how to seek permission, further information about the Publisher's permissions policies and our arrangements with organizations such as the Copyright Clearance Center and the Copyright Licensing Agency, can be found at our website: www.elsevier.com/permissions.

This book and the individual contributions contained in it are protected under copyright by the Publisher (other than as may be noted herein).

Notices

Knowledge and best practice in this field are constantly changing. As new research and experience broaden our understanding, changes in research methods, professional practices, or medical treatment may become necessary.

Practitioners and researchers must always rely on their own experience and knowledge in evaluating and using any information, methods, compounds, or experiments described herein. In using such information or methods they should be mindful of their own safety and the safety of others, including parties for whom they have a professional responsibility.

With respect to any drug or pharmaceutical products identified, readers are advised to check the most current information provided (i) on procedures featured or (ii) by the manufacturer of each product to be administered, to verify the recommended dose or formula, the method and duration of administration, and contraindications. It is the responsibility of practitioners, relying on their own experience and knowledge of their patients, to make diagnoses, to determine dosages and the best treatment for each individual patient, and to take all appropriate safety precautions.

To the fullest extent of the law, neither the Publisher nor the authors, contributors, or editors assume any liability for any injury and/or damage to persons or property as a matter of products liability, negligence or otherwise, or from any use or operation of any methods, products, instructions, or ideas contained in the material herein.

Library of Congress Cataloging-in-Publication Data

Atlas of vascular surgery and endovascular therapy : anatomy and technique / [edited by] Elliot L. Chaikof, Richard P. Cambria.
   p. ; cm.
  Includes bibliographical references and index.
  ISBN 978-1-4160-6841-9 (hardcover : alk. paper)
  I. Chaikof, Elliot L., editor of compilation. II. Cambria, Richard P., editor of compilation.
  [DNLM: 1. Vascular Surgical Procedures--methods--Atlases. 2. Intraoperative Complications--prevention & control--Atlases. WG 17]
  RD598.6
  617.4'13--dc23
　　　　　　　　　　　　　　　　　　　　　　　　　　　　　　2013045756

Executive Content Strategist: Michael Houston
Content Development Specialist: Laura Schmidt
Publishing Services Manager: Anne Altepeter
Project Manager: Louise King
Design Manager: Ellen Zanolle

Printed in China

Last digit is the print number:　9　8　7　6　5　4　3　2

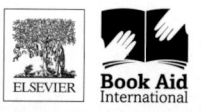

Working together to grow libraries in developing countries

www.elsevier.com • www.bookaid.org

To our patients, families, students, and teachers,
who have inspired us and provided us with
the privilege of being able to serve

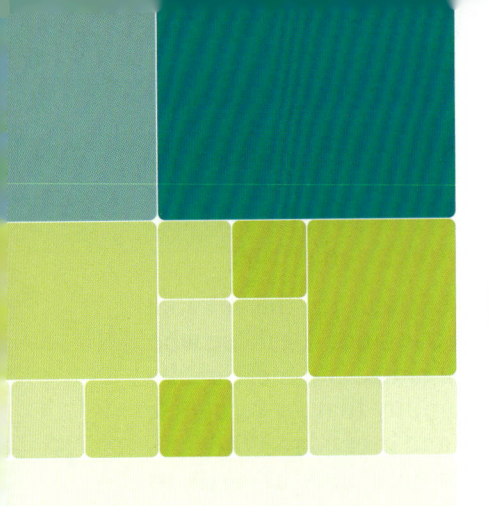

Preface

The grammar of all medicine consists not in its tools but in its method: to effectively treat clinical problems based on fundamental principles and an ordered framework. Those principles require detailed knowledge not only of a patient's complaint and physical findings, but also through effective communication, intimate familiarity with the patient as a person, as well as the patient's family and unique circumstances. A framework is necessary for the care of the surgical patient. That framework is derived from an organized and structured approach that considers all options in formulating a therapeutic plan. Above all, it requires humility in the face of the existing limits inherent in the recommended treatment, so that the patient and the patient's family are provided with an understanding of the nature of the problem and recommended course of treatment with compassion, composure, and calm.

It has been difficult for surgeons living in the first decades of the twenty-first century to accurately measure the relative significance of what our age is contributing to the history of medicine. Our contributions can only be weighed from a single vantage point—a perspective based on the past. However, with the past as our reference, it appears that we have now entered a third era in vascular surgery, witnessing a revolutionary change that has made it necessary to rewrite our textbooks and profoundly alter our approach to the care of patients with vascular disease. Our field has evolved over the past 100 years, from one that focused largely on the applications of fundamental anatomic principles that rendered the entire vascular system surgically accessible, but with limited capability for repair, to a specialty capable of heroic feats of reconstruction and replacement. This third era in which we find ourselves today is defined by a focus on achieving these goals in a manner that seeks to limit the trace of our footprint.

An atlas provides a guide that allows us to trace our way through highly diverse pathways of surgical care. Although it is inevitable that during periods of rapid technical change, when new advances continue to afford changes in care, fundamental principles of surgical techniques and methods of teaching surgical techniques will remain unchanged. The proficient surgeon often performs many sophisticated surgical procedures automatically or intuitively through a process that has evolved over decades of experience. Nevertheless, effective teaching in the operating room requires a detailed understanding of the evolution of each clinical situation as a rational system of logical rules that can be communicated, demonstrated, and applied. To conduct an operation is to orchestrate a team in the interpretation of a score of anatomic findings and physiologic principles using an existing set of instruments. The strategic plan for each patient dictates that the surgeon select a pathway that is as safe and efficient as possible, based on an appreciation of all relevant pitfalls and danger points.

This atlas emphasizes operative and interventional strategy based on anatomic and physiologic principles, critical intraoperative decision making, and technique. In several instances, the technique described in print is supplemented by a video presentation. Each description is preceded by a review of the rationale guiding the underlying approach, preoperative care, intraoperative pitfalls and errors, and techniques to achieve an effective result, including postoperative care.

In Greek mythology, Atlas was the primordial Titan who held up the celestial sphere, carrying the burden of this task in the service of mankind. For those who pursue a career in surgery, this chosen mission serves to organize and measure the best of our energies and skills as clinicians. It is with humility that we recognize that to be a surgeon is not easy, for surgery tests us each and every day. When patients and their families put their lives and their health in our hands, as surgeons we recognize, as represented by Atlas in an era long ago, that the burden of our duty is not light. Surgical training is not short or finite, but lifelong. We hope this atlas will be a source of both information and ideas that leads to more effective care of patients with vascular disease, easing the burden and lightening the load, so that we continue to move forward toward perfection.

Elliot L. Chaikof, MD, PhD
Richard P. Cambria, MD
Boston, Massachusetts

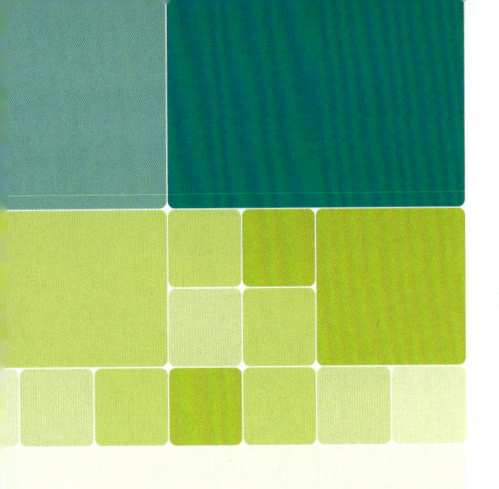

Contributors

Matthew J. Alef, MD
Clinical Fellow
Vascular and Endovascular Surgery
Division of the Cardiovascular
 Institute
Beth Israel Deaconess Medical Center
Boston, Massachusetts
Chapter 48: Endovascular Treatment of Femoral-Popliteal Arterial Occlusive Disease

Javier E. Anaya-Ayala, MD
Vascular Research Fellow
Cardiovascular Surgery
Houston Methodist DeBakey Heart &
 Vascular Center
Houston, Texas
Chapter 43: Endovascular Treatment of Hepatic, Gastroduodenal, Pancreaticoduodenal, and Splenic Artery Aneurysms

George Andros, MD
Medical Director
Amputation Prevention Center
Valley Presbyterian Hospital
Los Angeles, California
Chapter 52: Amputations of the Forefoot

Frank R. Arko III, MD
Vascular and Endovascular Surgery
Sanger Heart and Vascular Institute
Carolinas Medical Center
Charlotte, North Carolina
Chapter 58: Endovascular Treatment of Iliofemoral and Femoral-Popliteal Deep Vein Thrombosis

George J. Arnaoutakis, MD
Resident in General Surgery
Department of Surgery
The Johns Hopkins Hospital
Baltimore, Maryland
Chapter 16: Transaxillary Rib Resection for Thoracic Outlet Syndrome

Jeffrey L. Ballard, MD, FACS
Clinical Professor of Surgery
Department of Surgery
University of California, Irvine
Staff, Vascular Surgeon
Vascular Institute
St. Joseph Hospital
Orange, California
Chapter 32: Spine Exposure

Adam W. Beck, MD
Assistant Professor of Surgery
Division of Vascular Surgery
University of Florida College of
 Medicine
Gainesville, Florida
Chapter 4: General Principles of Endovascular Therapy: Guidewire and Catheter Manipulation

Michael Belkin, MD
Professor of Surgery
Harvard Medical School
Chief of Vascular and Endovascular
 Surgery
Brigham and Women's Hospital
Boston, Massachusetts
Chapter 23: Direct Surgical Repair of Aneurysms of the Infrarenal Abdominal Aorta and Iliac Arteries

Nicholas J. Bevilacqua, DPM
Associate, Foot and Ankle Surgery
North Jersey Orthopaedic
 Specialists, P.A.
Teaneck, New Jersey
Chapter 52: Amputations of the Forefoot

James H. Black III, MD
Bertram M. Bernheim MD Associate Professor of Surgery
Johns Hopkins University School of Medicine
Attending Vascular and Endovascular Surgeon
The Johns Hopkins Hospital
Baltimore, Maryland
Chapter 24: Direct Surgical Repair of Juxtarenal and Suprarenal Aneurysms of the Abdominal Aorta

Arash Bornak, MD
Assistant Professor of Surgery
Vascular and Endovascular Surgery
University of Miami Miller School of Medicine
Miami, Florida
Chapter 41: Endovascular Treatment of Occlusive Superior Mesenteric Artery Disease

Thomas C. Bower, MD
Professor of Surgery
Mayo College of Graduate Medical Education
Chair, Division of Vascular and Endovascular Surgery
Mayo Clinic
Rochester, Minnesota
Chapter 56: Surgical Reconstruction of the Inferior Vena Cava and Iliofemoral Venous System

Peter B. Brant-Zawadzki, MB, BCh
Vascular Surgery Fellow
Department of Surgery
University of Wisconsin School of Medicine and Public Health
Madison, Wisconsin
Chapter 5: General Principles of Endovascular Therapy: Angioplasty, Stenting, Recanalization, and Embolization

David C. Brewster, MD
Clinical Professor of Surgery
Harvard Medical School
Division of Vascular and Endovascular Surgery
Massachusetts General Hospital
Boston, Massachusetts
Chapter 28: Direct Surgical Repair of Aortoiliac Occlusive Disease

W. John Byrne, MCh, FRCSI (Gen)
Vascular Surgeon
The Institute for Vascular Health and Disease
Albany, New York
Chapter 7: Eversion Endarterectomy and Special Problems in Carotid Surgery

Keith D. Calligaro, MD
Clinical Professor of Surgery
Chief, Section of Vascular Surgery
University of Pennsylvania School of Medicine
Chief, Section of Vascular Surgery and Endovascular Therapy
Pennsylvania Hospital
Philadelphia, Pennsylvania
Chapter 63: Radial Artery–Cephalic Vein and Brachial Artery–Cephalic Vein Arteriovenous Fistula

Marc A. Camacho, BS, MD
Resident Physician
Division of Vascular Surgery
University of North Carolina
Chapel Hill, North Carolina
Chapter 22: Endovascular Treatment of Traumatic Thoracic Aortic Disruption

Richard P. Cambria, MD
The Robert R. Linton MD Professor of Vascular and Endovascular Surgery
Harvard Medical School
Chief, Division of Vascular and Endovascular Surgery
Department of Surgery
Massachusetts General Hospital
Boston, Massachusetts
Chapter 6: Carotid Endarterectomy

Elliot L. Chaikof, MD, PhD
Johnson and Johnson Professor of Surgery
Harvard Medical School
Chairman, Roberta and Stephen R. Weiner Department of Surgery
Surgeon-in-Chief
Beth Israel Deaconess Medical Center
Boston, Massachusetts
Chapter 6: Carotid Endarterectomy

Kenneth J. Cherry, MD
Edwin P. Lehman Professor of Surgery
Vascular and Endovascular Surgery
University of Virginia
Charlottesville, Virginia
Chapter 11: Direct Surgical Repair of Aortic Arch Vessels

Timothy A.M. Chuter, BM, BS, DM
Professor in Residence
University of California at San Francisco
Director, Endovascular Surgery
University of California at San Francisco Medical Center
San Francisco, California
Chapter 19: Endovascular Repair of the Aortic Arch and Thoracoabdominal Aorta

Daniel G. Clair, MD
Professor and Chairman
Department of Vascular Surgery
Cleveland Clinic
Lerner College of Medicine of Case Western Reserve University
Cleveland, Ohio
Chapter 31: Special Problems in the Endovascular Treatment of Aortoiliac Occlusive Disease

Thomas Conlee, MD
Vascular Surgery Fellow
Department of Vascular and Endovascular Surgery
Wake Forest Baptist Medical Center
Winston-Salem, North Carolina
Chapter 38: Endovascular Treatment of Renal Artery Stenosis

Mark F. Conrad, MD
Assistant Professor of Surgery
Massachusetts General Hospital
Boston, Massachusetts
Chapter 37: Extraanatomic Repair for Renovascular Disease

Robert S. Crawford, MD
Assistant Professor
Division of Vascular Surgery
University of Maryland Medical Center
Baltimore, Maryland
Chapter 28: Direct Surgical Repair of Aortoiliac Occlusive Disease

David L. Cull, MD
Department of Surgery
University of South Carolina School of Medicine – Greenville
Greenville, South Carolina
Chapter 66: Unconventional Venous Access Procedures for Chronic Hemodialysis

R. Clement Darling III, MD
Professor of Surgery
Department of Surgery
Albany Medical College
Chief, Division of Vascular Surgery
Albany Medical Center Hospital
Director, The Institute for Vascular Health and Disease
Albany, New York
Chapter 7: Eversion Endarterectomy and Special Problems in Carotid Surgery

Mark G. Davies, MD, PhD, MBA
Professor and Vice Chairman
Cardiovascular Surgery
Houston Methodist Hospital
Houston, Texas
Weill Cornell Medical College
New York, New York
Chapter 43: Endovascular Treatment of Hepatic, Gastroduodenal, Pancreaticoduodenal, and Splenic Artery Aneurysms

Christopher A. DeMaioribus, MD
Division of Vascular and Endovascular Surgery
St. Mary's Duluth Clinic Medical Center
Duluth, Minnesota
Chapter 34: Neoaortoiliac System Procedure for Treatment of an Aortic Graft Infection

Joel K. Deonanan, MD
Vascular and Endovascular Surgery
Wake Forest Baptist Medical Center
Winston Salem, North Carolina
Chapter 38: Endovascular Treatment of Renal Artery Stenosis

Hasan H. Dosluoglu, MD
Associate Professor of Surgery
State University at Buffalo
Chief, Department of Surgery
Chief, Division of Vascular Surgery
Veterans Affairs Western New York Healthcare System
Buffalo, New York
Chapter 67: Distal Revascularization Interval Ligation Procedure

Matthew J. Dougherty, MD
Clinical Professor of Surgery
Section of Vascular Surgery
Pennsylvania Hospital
University of Pennsylvania
Philadelphia, Pennsylvania
Chapter 63: Radial Artery–Cephalic Vein and Brachial Artery–Cephalic Vein Arteriovenous Fistula

Adam J. Doyle, MD
Vascular Surgery Resident
Division of Vascular Surgery
University of Rochester Medical Center
Rochester, New York
Chapter 17: Endovascular Therapy for Subclavian-Axillary Vein Thrombosis

Yazan M. Duwayri, MD
Assistant Professor of Surgery
Division of Vascular Surgery and Endovascular Therapy
Emory University School of Medicine
Atlanta, Georgia
Chapter 15: Supraclavicular Approach for Surgical Treatment of Thoracic Outlet Syndrome

Matthew S. Edwards, MD, MS, RVT, FACS
Associate Professor of Surgery and Public Health Sciences
Chairman, Department of Vascular and Endovascular Surgery
Wake Forest Baptist Medical Center
Winston Salem, North Carolina
Chapter 38: Endovascular Treatment of Renal Artery Stenosis

John F. Eidt, MD
Vascular Surgery
Greenville Health System University Medical Center
Greenville, South Carolina
Chapter 51: Above- and Below-Knee Amputation

Mark K. Eskandari, MD
James S.T. Yao, MD Professor of Education in Vascular Surgery
Professor of Surgery, Radiology, and Medicine
Chief and Program Director, Division of Vascular Surgery
Northwestern University Feinberg School of Medicine
Chicago, Illinois
Chapter 13: Endovascular Treatment of Aortic Arch Vessels—Innominate, Carotid, and Subclavian Arteries

Anthony L. Estrera, MD
Professor
Cardiothoracic and Vascular Surgery
The University of Texas Health Science Center
Houston, Texas
Chapter 18: Direct Surgical Repair of Aneurysms of the Thoracic and Thoracoabdominal Aorta

Ronald M. Fairman, MD
The Clyde F. Barker – William Maul Measey Professor of Surgery
Chief, Division of Vascular Surgery and Endovascular Therapy
Vice-Chairman for Clinical Affairs, Department of Surgery
Professor of Surgery in Radiology
Hospital of the University of Pennsylvania
Philadelphia, Pennsylvania
Chapter 27: Endovascular Treatment of Aneurysms of the Juxtarenal and Pararenal Aorta

Mark A. Farber, MD
Associate Professor
Director, University of North Carolina Aortic Center
Department of Surgery and Radiology
University of North Carolina
Chapel Hill, North Carolina
Chapter 22: Endovascular Treatment of Traumatic Thoracic Aortic Disruption

CONTRIBUTORS

Peter L. Faries, MD, FACS
Professor of Surgery
Chief, Division of Vascular Surgery
Mount Sinai School of Medicine
New York, New York
Chapter 49: Endovascular Treatment of Tibial-Peroneal Arterial Occlusive Disease

Thomas L. Forbes, MD, FRCSC, FACS
Professor of Surgery and Chair
Division of Vascular Surgery
London Health Sciences Centre
The University of Western Ontario
London, Ontario, Canada
Chapter 47: Direct Surgical Repair of Popliteal Entrapment

Julie Ann Freischlag, MD
William Steward Halsted Professor
Chair, Department of Surgery
Johns Hopkins Medical Institutions
Baltimore, Maryland
Chapter 16: Transaxillary Rib Resection for Thoracic Outlet Syndrome

Michael J. Gaffud, MD
Fellow, Section of Vascular Surgery and Endovascular Therapy
University of Alabama
Birmingham, Alabama
Chapter 35: Surgical Treatment of Pseudoaneurysm of the Femoral Artery

Shawn M. Gage, PA-C
Senior Vascular Physician Assistant
Division of Vascular Surgery
Duke University Medical Center
Durham, North Carolina
Chapter 64: Forearm Loop Graft and Brachial Artery–Axillary Vein Interposition Graft

Manuel Garcia-Toca, MD
Assistant Professor of Surgery
Alpert Medical School of Brown University
Providence, Rhode Island
Chapter 13: Endovascular Treatment of Aortic Arch Vessels—Innominate, Carotid, and Subclavian Arteries

Patrick J. Geraghty, MD
Associate Professor of Surgery and Radiology
Department of Surgery
Section of Vascular Surgery
Washington University School of Medicine
Saint Louis, Missouri
Chapter 50: Endovascular Treatment of Popliteal Aneurysm

Sidney Glazer, MD
Clinical Associate Professor
Department of Surgery
University of California at Irvine
Orange, California
Chapter 65: Basilic and Femoral Vein Transposition

Peter Gloviczki, MD
Joe M. and Ruth Roberts Professor of Surgery
Chair Emeritus, Division of Vascular and Endovascular Surgery
Director Emeritus, Gonda Vascular Center
Mayo Clinic
Rochester, Minnesota
Chapter 55: Surgical Reconstruction for Superior Vena Cava Syndrome

Christopher J. Godshall, MD
Assistant Professor of Surgery
Wake Forest University
Winston-Salem, North Carolina
Chapter 36: Direct Surgical Repair of Renovascular Disease

Kaoru R. Goshima, MD
Assistant Professor of Surgery
Department of Vascular and Endovascular Surgery
The University of Arizona Medical Center
Tucson, Arizona
Chapter 44: Open Surgical Bypass of Femoral-Popliteal Arterial Occlusive Disease

Wayne S. Gradman, MD
Attending
Department of Surgery
Cedars Sinai Medical Center
Los Angeles, California
Chapter 65: Basilic and Femoral Vein Transposition

Ryan T. Hagino, MD, FACS
Section Head, Vascular and Endovascular Surgery
Essentia Health Duluth Clinic
Duluth, Minnesota
Chapter 34: Neoaortoiliac System Procedure for Treatment of an Aortic Graft Infection

Eugene Hagiwara, MD
Interventional Radiology
University of California – San Francisco
San Francisco, California
Chapter 57: Transjugular Intrahepatic Portosystemic Shunt Procedure

Kimberley J. Hansen, MD
Professor of Surgery
Department of Vascular and Endovascular Surgery
Wake Forest University School of Medicine
Winston-Salem, North Carolina
Chapter 36: Direct Surgical Repair of Renovascular Disease

Jeremy R. Harris, MD, FRCSC
Assistant Professor of Surgery
Division of Vascular Surgery
London Health Sciences Center
London, Ontario, Canada
Chapter 47: Direct Surgical Repair of Popliteal Entrapment

Linda M. Harris, MD, FACS
Associate Professor of Surgery
Chief, Division of Vascular Surgery
Program Director, Vascular Surgery Residency and Fellowship
State University of New York at Buffalo
Medical Director, Noninvasive Vascular Lab
University at Buffalo Surgeons, Inc.
Buffalo, New York
Chapter 67: Distal Revascularization Interval Ligation Procedure

Ravishankar Hasanadka, MD
Vascular and Endovascular Surgery
OSF/HeartCare Midwest
Peoria, Illinois
Chapter 3: General Principles of Endovascular Therapy: Access Site Management

Mounir J. Haurani, MD
Assistant Professor of Surgery
Division of Vascular Diseases and Surgery
The Ohio State University Medical Center
Columbus, Ohio
Chapter 37: Extraanatomic Repair for Renovascular Disease
Chapter 39: Endovascular Treatment of Renal Artery Aneurysms

Daniel J. Hayes, Jr., MD
Vascular Fellow
Section of Vascular Surgery
Pennsylvania Hospital
University of Pennsylvania
Philadelphia, Pennsylvania
Chapter 63: Radial Artery–Cephalic Vein and Brachial Artery–Cephalic Vein Arteriovenous Fistula

Thomas S. Huber, MD, PhD
Professor of Surgery
Chief, Division of Vascular and Endovascular Surgery
University of Florida College of Medicine
Attending Surgeon
Shands Hospital at the Unversity of Florida
Gainesville, Florida
Chapter 40: Direct Surgical Repair for Celiac Axis and Superior Mesenteric Artery Occlusive Disease

Zhen S. Huang, MD
Fellow
New York-Presbyterian Hospital/Weill Cornell Medical Center
New York, New York
Chapter 48: Endovascular Treatment of Femoral-Popliteal Arterial Occlusive Disease

Mark D. Iafrati, MD
Associate Professor of Surgery
Tufts University School of Medicine
Chief, Division of Vascular Surgery
Tufts Medical Center
Boston, Massachusetts
Chapter 59: Varicose Vein Stripping and Ambulatory Phlebectomy

Karl A. Illig, MD
Professor of Surgery
Director, Division of Vascular
 Surgery
Department of Surgery
University of South Florida
Tampa, Florida
Chapter 17: Endovascular Therapy for Subclavian-Axillary Vein Thrombosis

Mihaiela Ilves, MD
Research Assistant
Department of Vascular and
 Endovascular Surgery
The University of Texas Southwestern
 Medical Center
Dallas, Texas
Chapter 58: Endovascular Treatment of Iliofemoral and Femoral-Popliteal Deep Vein Thrombosis

William D. Jordan, Jr., MD
Professor and Chief
Section of Vascular Surgery and
 Endovascular Therapy
University of Alabama at Birmingham
Birmingham, Alabama
Chapter 35: Surgical Treatment of Pseudoaneurysm of the Femoral Artery

Venkat R. Kalapatapu, MD, FRCS, FACS
Assistant Professor
Department of Vascular Surgery
University of Pennsylvania Health
 Sysytem
Philadelphia, Pennsylvania
Chapter 51: Above- and Below-Knee Amputation

Manju Kalra, MBBS
Associate Professor of Surgery
Division of Vascular and Endovascular
 Surgery
Mayo Clinic
Rochester, Minnesota
Chapter 55: Surgical Reconstruction for Superior Vena Cava Syndrome

Vikram S. Kashyap, MD, FACS
Professor of Surgery
Case Western Reserve University
Chief, Division of Vascular Surgery
 and Endovascular Therapy
Co-Director, Harrington Heart and
 Vascular Institute
University Hospitals Case Medical
 Center
Cleveland, Ohio
Chapter 2: General Principles of Sedation, Angiography, and Intravascular Ultrasound

Karthikeshwar Kasirajan, MD
Division of Vascular Surgery
Department of Surgery
Emory University School of Medicine
Atlanta, Georgia
Chapter 21: Endovascular Treatment of Aortic Dissection

Rebecca Kelso, MD
Department of Vascular Surgery
Cleveland Clinic Foundation
Cleveland, Ohio
Chapter 2: General Principles of Sedation, Angiography, and Intravascular Ultrasound

Ali Khoobehi, MD
Vascular Surgery Fellow
Department of Surgery
Vanderbilt University Medical Center
Nashville, Tennessee
Chapter 9: Carotid Body Tumor

Alexander Kulik, MD, MPH, FRCSC, FACC, FAHA
Cardiovascular Surgeon
Christine E. Lynn Heart and Vascular
 Institute
Boca Raton Regional Hospital
Affiliate Associate Professor
Charles E. Schmidt College of Medicine
Florida Atlantic University
Boca Raton, Florida
Chapter 20: Endovascular Treatment of Thoracic Aneurysms

Christopher J. Kwolek, MD
Director, Vascular and Endovascular
 Surgery Training Program
Department of Surgery
Massachusetts General Hospital
Associate Professor of Surgery
Harvard Medical School
Boston, Massachusetts
*Chapter 39: Endovascular Treatment of
 Renal Artery Aneurysms*

Jeffrey H. Lawson, MD, PhD
Professor of Surgery
Vascular Division
Department of Surgery
Duke University Medical Center
Durham, North Carolina
*Chapter 64: Forearm Loop Graft
 and Brachial Artery-Axillary Vein
 Interposition Graft*

W. Anthony Lee, MD, FACS
Director, Endovascular Program
Christine E. Lynn Heart and Vascular
 Institute
Boca Raton, Florida
*Chapter 4: General Principles of
 Endovascular Therapy: Guidewire and
 Catheter Manipulation*

Layla C. Lucas, MD
Attending Vascular Surgeon
Tucson Medical Center
Tucson, Arizona
*Chapter 44: Open Surgical Bypass of
 Femoral-Popliteal Arterial Occlusive
 Disease*

Alan B. Lumsden, MD
Professor of Cardiovascular Surgery
Chairman, Department of
 Cardiovascular Surgery
Houston Methodist Hospital
Houston, Texas
*Chapter 43: Endovascular Treatment
 of Hepatic, Gastroduodenal,
 Pancreaticoduodenal, and Splenic
 Artery Aneurysms*

Harry Ma, MD, PhD
Assistant Professor of Surgery
Department of Surgery
Division of Vascular and Endovascular
 Surgery
University of Oklahoma
Tulsa, Oklahoma
*Chapter 59: Varicose Vein Stripping and
 Ambulatory Phlebectomy*

Michel S. Makaroun, MD
Professor and Chief
Division of Vascular Surgery
University of Pittsburgh School of
 Medicine
Chief, Vascular Surgery
University of Pittsburgh Medical Center
Pittsburgh, Pennsylvania
*Chapter 25: Endovascular Treatment of
 Aneurysms of the Infrarenal Aorta*

Thomas S. Maldonado, MD
Associate Professor of Surgery
Vascular Surgery
New York University
Chief of Vascular Surgery
Department of Surgery
Bellevue Hospital
New York, New York
*Chapter 42: Direct Surgical Repair of
 Visceral Artery Aneurysms*

Jon S. Matsumura, MD
Professor of Surgery
Chair, Division of Vascular Surgery
University of Wisconsin School of
 Medicine and Public Health
Madison, Wisconsin
*Chapter 5: General Principles of
 Endovascular Therapy: Angioplasty,
 Stenting, Recanalization, and
 Embolization*

Robert B. McLafferty
Chief of Surgery
Department of Surgery
Portland Veterans Affairs Medical
 Center
Professor of Surgery
Division of Vascular Surgery
Department of Surgery
Oregon Health Sciences University
Portland, Oregon
*Chapter 3: General Principles of
 Endovascular Therapy: Access Site
 Management*

George H. Meier, MD, RVT, FACS
Professor and Chief
Department of Vascular Surgery
University of Cincinnati College of
 Medicine
Cincinnati, Ohio
*Chapter 68: Surgical and Endovascular
 Intervention for Arteriovenous Graft
 Thrombosis*

Joseph L. Mills, Sr., MD
Professor of Surgery and Chief
Vascular and Endovascular Surgery
Co-Director, Southern Arizona Limb Salvage Alliance
Tucson, Arizona
Chapter 44: Open Surgical Bypass of Femoral-Popliteal Arterial Occlusive Disease

Ross Milner, MD
Associate Professor of Surgery
The University of Chicago School of Medicine
Chicago, Illinois
Chapter 41: Endovascular Treatment of Occlusive Superior Mesenteric Artery Disease

Renee C. Minjarez, MD
Fellow, Vascular and Endovascular Surgery
Division of Vascular Surgery
Oregon Health and Science University
Portland, Oregon
Chapter 45: Direct Surgical Repair of Tibial-Peroneal Arterial Occlusive Disease

Gregory L. Moneta, MD
Professor and Chief
Division of Vascular Surgery
Department of Surgery
Oregon Health and Science University
Portland, Oregon
Chapter 45: Direct Surgical Repair of Tibial-Peroneal Arterial Occlusive Disease

Mark D. Morasch, MD, FACS
Department of Cardiovascular Surgery
St. Vincent Healthcare
Billings, Montana
Chapter 10: Surgical Treatment of the Vertebral Artery
Chapter 12: Extraanatomic Repair of Aortic Arch Vessels

Eric Mowatt-Larssen, MD
Assistant Professor, Phlebology
Department of Vascular Surgery
Duke University
Durham, North Carolina
Chapter 62: Sclerotherapy

Erin H. Murphy, MD
Assistant Professor of Clinical Surgery
Division of Vascular Surgery and Endovascular Interventions
New York-Presbyterian Hospital/Columbia University Medical Center
New York, New York
Chapter 58: Endovascular Treatment of Iliofemoral and Femoral-Popliteal Deep Vein Thrombosis

Thomas C. Naslund, MD
Professor of Surgery
Division of Vascular Surgery
Vanderbilt University School of Medicine
Nashville, Tennessee
Chapter 9: Carotid Body Tumor

Peter Naughton, MD
Beaumont Hospital
Dublin, Ireland
Chapter 13: Endovascular Treatment of Aortic Arch Vessels—Innominate, Carotid, and Subclavian Arteries

James L. Netterville, MD
Professor of Otolaryngology
Mark C. Smith Chair in Head and Neck Surgery
Vanderbilt University Medical Center
Nashville, Tennessee
Chapter 9: Carotid Body Tumor

Marc A. Passman, MD
Professor of Surgery
Section of Vascular Surgery and Endovascular Therapy
University of Alabama at Birmingham
Birmingham, Alabama
Chapter 54: Placement of Vena Cava Filter

David A. Peterson, MD
Fellow in Vascular Surgery
Department of Surgery
Duke University
Durham, North Carolina
Instructor, Department of Surgery
Stanford University
Stanford, California
Chapter 64: Forearm Loop Graft and Brachial Artery-Axillary Vein Interposition Graft

Amani D. Politano, MD, MS
Resident, Department of Surgery
University of Virginia
Charlottesville, Virginia
Chapter 11: Direct Surgical Repair of Aortic Arch Vessels

Frank B. Pomposelli, MD
Professor of Surgery
Tuft's University School of Medicine
Chairman, Department of Surgery
St. Elizabeth's Medical Center
Boston, Massachusetts
Chapter 46: Direct Surgical Repair of Popliteal Artery Aneurysm

Richard J. Powell, MD
Chief, Section of Vascular Surgery
Heart and Vascular Center
Dartmouth-Hitchcock Medical Center
Lebanon, New Hampshire
Chapter 30: Endovascular Treatment of Aortoiliac Occlusive Disease

Alessandra Puggioni, MD
Vascular Surgeon
Scottsdale Healthcare System
Scottsdale, Arizona
Chapter 61: Surgical Treatment of Lower Extremity Deep and Perforator Vein Incompetence

Brenton E. Quinney, MD
Fellow, Department of Surgery
Section of Vascular Surgery and Endovascular Therapy
The University of Alabama at Birmingham
Birmingham, Alabama
Chapter 54: Placement of Vena Cava Filter

Venkatesh G. Ramaiah, MD, FACS
Director, Peripheral Vascular and Endovascular Research
Department of Vascular Surgery
Arizona Heart Institute
Medical Director, Arizona Heart Hospital
Phoenix, Arizona
Chapter 20: Endovascular Treatment of Thoracic Aneurysms

Atul S. Rao, MD
Attending Vascular Surgeon
Maimonides Medical Center
Brooklyn, New York
Chapter 25: Endovascular Treatment of Aneurysms of the Infrarenal Aorta

Todd E. Rasmussen, MD
Associate Professor of Surgery
Uniformed Services University of the Health Sciences
Bethesda, Maryland
Chief, Vascular Surgery Services
San Antonio Military Vascular Surgery
San Antonio, Texas
Deputy Commander
U.S. Army Institute of Surgical Research
Fort Sam Houston
Houston, Texas
Chapter 53: Upper and Lower Extremity Fasciotomy

Thomas Reifsnyder, MD
Assistant Professor
Chief, Vascular Laboratory
Department of Surgery
Johns Hopkins Bayview Medical Center
Baltimore, Maryland
Chapter 16: Transaxillary Rib Resection for Thoracic Outlet Syndrome

Thomas S. Riles, MD
Frank C. Spencer Professor of Surgery
Associate Dean, Medical Education and Technology
New York University Langone Medical Center
New York, New York
Chapter 1: General Principles of Vascular Surgery

Caron B. Rockman, MD
Associate Professor of Surgery
Director of Clinical Research
Division of Vascular Surgery
New York University Medical School
New York, New York
Chapter 42: Direct Surgical Repair of Visceral Artery Aneurysms

Lee C. Rogers, DPM
Associate Director
Amputation Prevention Center
Valley Presbyterian Hospital
Los Angeles, California
Chapter 52: Amputations of the Forefoot

Wael Saad, MD
Associate Professor
Department of Radiology
University of Virginia
Charlottesville, Virginia
Chapter 43: Endovascular Treatment of Hepatic, Gastroduodenal, Pancreaticoduodenal, and Splenic Artery Aneurysms

Hazim J. Safi, MD
Professor and Chairman
Department of Cardiothoracic and Vascular Surgery
The University of Texas Medical School at Houston
Chief, Cardiothoracic and Vascular Surgery
Heart and Vascular Institute
Memorial Hermann Hospital
Houston, Texas
Chapter 18: Direct Surgical Repair of Aneurysms of the Thoracic and Thoracoabdominal Aorta

Luis A. Sanchez, MD
Gregorio Sicard Professor of Vascular Surgery
Chief, Vascular Surgery Section
Washington University School of Medicine
Saint Louis, Missouri
Chapter 50: Endovascular Treatment of Popliteal Aneurysm

Andres Schanzer, MD, FACS
Associate Professor of Surgery and Quantitative Health Sciences
Program Director, Vascular Surgery Residency
University of Massachusetts Medical School
Worcester, Massachusetts
Chapter 23: Direct Surgical Repair of Aneurysms of the Infrarenal Abdominal Aorta and Iliac Arteries

Marc L. Schermerhorn, MD
Chief, Division of Vascular and Endovascular Surgery
Beth Israel Deaconess Medical Center
Associate Professor of Surgery
Harvard Medical School
Boston, Massachusetts
Chapter 48: Endovascular Treatment of Femoral-Popliteal Arterial Occlusive Disease

Darren B. Schneider, MD
Associate Professor of Surgery
Chief, Vascular and Endovascular Surgery
Weill Cornell Medical College
New York-Presbyterian Hospital/Weill Cornell Medical Center
New York, New York
Chapter 57: Transjugular Intrahepatic Portosystemic Shunt Procedure

Joseph R. Schneider, MD, PhD
Professor of Surgery
Northwestern University Feinberg School of Medicine
Chicago, Illinois
Vascular and Interventional Program
Cadence Health
Winfield, Illinois
Geneva, Illinois
Chapter 29: Extraanatomic Repair of Aortoiliac Occlusive Disease

Peter A. Schneider, MD
Chief, Vascular Therapy
Hawaii Permanente Medical Group and Kaiser Foundation Hospital
Honolulu, Hawaii
Chapter 8: Carotid Angioplasty and Stenting

Dhiraj M. Shah, MD
Professor of Surgery
Albany Medical College
The Institute for Vascular Health and Disease
Albany, New York
Chapter 7: Eversion Endarterectomy and Special Problems in Carotid Surgery

Tejas R. Shah, MD
Vascular Fellow
Division of Vascular and Endovascular Surgery
Department of Surgery
New York University Medical Center
New York, New York
Chapter 49: Endovascular Treatment of Tibial-Peroneal Arterial Occlusive Disease

Cynthia Shortell, MD
Professor of Surgery
Chief of Vascular Surgery
Department of Surgery
Duke University Medical Center
Durham, North Carolina
Chapter 62: Sclerotherapy

Sunita Srivastava, MD
Assistant Professor of Surgery
Department of Vascular Surgery
Cleveland Clinic
Lerner College of Medicine of Case Western Reserve University
Cleveland, Ohio
Chapter 33: Total Graft Excision and Extraanatomic Repair for Aortic Graft Infection

W. Charles Sternbergh III, MD
Professor and Chief
Section of Vascular and Endovascular Surgery
Vice Chair for Research, Department of Surgery
Ochsner Clinic Foundation
New Orleans, Louisiana
Chapter 26: Special Problems in the Endovascular Treatment of the Infrarenal Aorta

Julianne Stoughton, MD, FACS
Instructor in Surgery
Department of Vascular Surgery
Massachusetts General Hospital
Harvard Medical School
Boston, Massachusetts
Chapter 60: Endovenous Thermal Ablation of Saphenous and Perforating Veins

Robert W. Thompson, MD
Professor
Departments of Surgery, Radiology, and Cell Biology and Physiology
Section of Vascular Surgery
Washington University School of Medicine and Barnes-Jewish Hospital
Saint Louis, Missouri
Chapter 15: Supraclavicular Approach for Surgical Treatment of Thoracic Outlet Syndrome

Jessica M. Titus, MD
Resident Physician
Department of Vascular Surgery
Cleveland Clinic Foundation
Cleveland, Ohio
Chapter 31: Special Problems in the Endovascular Treatment of Aortoiliac Occlusive Disease

R. James Valentine, MD
Chair, Division of Vascular and Endovascular Surgery
Alvin Baldwin, Jr. Chair in Surgery
The University of Texas Southwestern Medical Center
Dallas, Texas
Chapter 14: Surgical Treatment of the Subclavian and Axillary Artery

Raghuveer Vallabhaneni, MD
Assistant Professor of Surgery
Division of Vascular Surgery
Department of Surgery
University of North Carolina School of Medicine
Chapel Hill, North Carolina
Chapter 50: Endovascular Treatment of Popliteal Aneurysm

Grace J. Wang, MD
Assistant Professor of Surgery
Department of Surgery
Hospital of the University of Pennsylvania
Philadelphia, Pennsylvania
Chapter 27: Endovascular Treatment of Aneurysms of the Juxtarenal and Pararenal Aorta

Joseph M. White, MD
Vascular Surgery Fellow
Walter Reed National Military Medical Center
Bethesda, Maryland
Chapter 53: Upper and Lower Extremity Fasciotomy

Mark C. Wyers, MD
Assistant Professor
Department of Vascular and Endovascular Surgery
Beth Israel Deaconess Medical Center
Boston, Massachusetts
Chapter 46: Direct Surgical Repair of Popliteal Artery Aneurysm

Contents

Section 1 — SURGICAL AND ENDOVASCULAR TECHNIQUES

1 General Principles of Vascular Surgery — 2
THOMAS S. RILES

2 General Principles of Sedation, Angiography, and Intravascular Ultrasound — 17
REBECCA KELSO • VIKRAM S. KASHYAP

3 General Principles of Endovascular Therapy: Access Site Management — 29
RAVISHANKAR HASANADKA • ROBERT B. McLAFFERTY

4 General Principles of Endovascular Therapy: Guidewire and Catheter Manipulation — 41
ADAM W. BECK • W. ANTHONY LEE

5 General Principles of Endovascular Therapy: Angioplasty, Stenting, Recanalization, and Embolization — 50
PETER B. BRANT-ZAWADZKI • JON S. MATSUMURA

Section 2 — EXTRACRANIAL CEREBROVASCULAR DISEASE

6 Carotid Endarterectomy — 64
ELLIOT L. CHAIKOF • RICHARD P. CAMBRIA

7 Eversion Endarterectomy and Special Problems in Carotid Surgery — 77
R. CLEMENT DARLING III • W. JOHN BYRNE • DHIRAJ M. SHAH

8 Carotid Angioplasty and Stenting — 86
PETER A. SCHNEIDER

9 Carotid Body Tumor — 102
ALI KHOOBEHI • JAMES L. NETTERVILLE • THOMAS C. NASLUND

10 Surgical Treatment of the Vertebral Artery — 111
MARK D. MORASCH

Section 3 — AORTIC ARCH VESSELS

11 Direct Surgical Repair of Aortic Arch Vessels — 126
AMANI D. POLITANO • KENNETH J. CHERRY

12 Extraanatomic Repair of Aortic Arch Vessels — 139
MARK D. MORASCH

13 Endovascular Treatment of Aortic Arch Vessels—Innominate, Carotid, and Subclavian Arteries — 148
PETER NAUGHTON • MANUEL GARCIA-TOCA • MARK K. ESKANDARI

14 Surgical Treatment of the Subclavian and Axillary Artery — 157
R. JAMES VALENTINE

Section 4 — UPPER EXTREMITY VASCULAR DISEASE

15 Supraclavicular Approach for Surgical Treatment of Thoracic Outlet Syndrome — 172
YAZAN M. DUWAYRI • ROBERT W. THOMPSON

16 Transaxillary Rib Resection for Thoracic Outlet Syndrome — 193
GEORGE J. ARNAOUTAKIS • JULIE ANN FREISCHLAG • THOMAS REIFSNYDER

17 Endovascular Therapy for Subclavian-Axillary Vein Thrombosis — 204
KARL A. ILLIG • ADAM J. DOYLE

Section 5 — THE THORACIC AORTA

18 Direct Surgical Repair of Aneurysms of the Thoracic and Thoracoabdominal Aorta — 216
HAZIM J. SAFI • ANTHONY L. ESTRERA

19 Endovascular Repair of the Aortic Arch and Thoracoabdominal Aorta — 232
TIMOTHY A.M. CHUTER

20 Endovascular Treatment of Thoracic Aneurysms — 251
VENKATESH G. RAMAIAH • ALEXANDER KULIK

21 Endovascular Treatment of Aortic Dissection — 274
KARTHIKESHWAR KASIRAJAN

22 Endovascular Treatment of Traumatic Thoracic Aortic Disruption — 289
MARK A. FARBER • MARC A. CAMACHO

Section 6 — THE ABDOMINAL AORTA AND ILIAC ARTERIES

23 Direct Surgical Repair of Aneurysms of the Infrarenal Abdominal Aorta and Iliac Arteries — 296
ANDRES SCHANZER • MICHAEL BELKIN

24 Direct Surgical Repair of Juxtarenal and Suprarenal Aneurysms of the Abdominal Aorta — 309
JAMES H. BLACK III

25 Endovascular Treatment of Aneurysms of the Infrarenal Aorta — 321
ATUL S. RAO • MICHEL S. MAKAROUN

26 Special Problems in the Endovascular Treatment of the Infrarenal Aorta — 336
W. CHARLES STERNBERGH III

27 Endovascular Treatment of Aneurysms of the Juxtarenal and Pararenal Aorta — 343
RONALD M. FAIRMAN • GRACE J. WANG

28 Direct Surgical Repair of Aortoiliac Occlusive Disease — 350
ROBERT S. CRAWFORD • DAVID C. BREWSTER

29 Extraanatomic Repair of Aortoiliac Occlusive Disease — 362
JOSEPH R. SCHNEIDER

30 Endovascular Treatment of Aortoiliac Occlusive Disease — 373
RICHARD J. POWELL

31 Special Problems in the Endovascular Treatment of Aortoiliac Occlusive Disease — 383
DANIEL G. CLAIR • JESSICA M. TITUS

32 Spine Exposure — 392
JEFFREY L. BALLARD

Section 7 — LATE AORTIC GRAFT COMPLICATIONS

33 Total Graft Excision and Extraanatomic Repair for Aortic Graft Infection — 404
SUNITA SRIVASTAVA

34 Neoaortoiliac System Procedure for Treatment of an Aortic Graft Infection — 419
RYAN T. HAGINO • CHRISTOPHER A. DeMAIORIBUS

35 Surgical Treatment of Pseudoaneurysm of the Femoral Artery — 427
WILLIAM D. JORDAN, JR. • MICHAEL J. GAFFUD

Section 8 — RENAL ARTERY DISEASE

36 Direct Surgical Repair of Renovascular Disease — 436
KIMBERLEY J. HANSEN • CHRISTOPHER J. GODSHALL

37 Extraanatomic Repair for Renovascular Disease — 449
MOUNIR J. HAURANI • MARK F. CONRAD

38 Endovascular Treatment of Renal Artery Stenosis — 456
MATTHEW S. EDWARDS • JOEL K. DEONANAN • THOMAS CONLEE

39 Endovascular Treatment of Renal Artery Aneurysms — 466
CHRISTOPHER J. KWOLEK • MOUNIR J. HAURANI

Section 9 — SUPERIOR MESENTERIC AND CELIAC ARTERY DISEASE

40 Direct Surgical Repair for Celiac Axis and Superior Mesenteric Artery Occlusive Disease — 476
THOMAS S. HUBER

41 Endovascular Treatment of Occlusive Superior Mesenteric Artery Disease — 491
ARASH BORNAK • ROSS MILNER

42 Direct Surgical Repair of Visceral Artery Aneurysms — 500
CARON B. ROCKMAN • THOMAS S. MALDONADO

43 Endovascular Treatment of Hepatic, Gastroduodenal, Pancreaticoduodenal, and Splenic Artery Aneurysms — 513
JAVIER E. ANAYA-AYALA • WAEL SAAD • MARK G. DAVIES • ALAN B. LUMSDEN

Section 10 — LOWER EXTREMITY ARTERIAL DISEASE

44 Open Surgical Bypass of Femoral-Popliteal Arterial Occlusive Disease — 526
LAYLA C. LUCAS • KAORU R. GOSHIMA • JOSEPH L. MILLS, SR.

45 Direct Surgical Repair of Tibial-Peroneal Arterial Occlusive Disease — 543
RENEE C. MINJAREZ • GREGORY L. MONETA

46 Direct Surgical Repair of Popliteal Artery Aneurysm — 561
FRANK B. POMPOSELLI • MARK C. WYERS

47 Direct Surgical Repair of Popliteal Entrapment — 572
JEREMY R. HARRIS • THOMAS L. FORBES

48 Endovascular Treatment of Femoral-Popliteal Arterial Occlusive Disease — 578
MATTHEW J. ALEF • ZHEN S. HUANG • MARC L. SCHERMERHORN

49 Endovascular Treatment of Tibial-Peroneal Arterial Occlusive Disease — 590
TEJAS R. SHAH • PETER L. FARIES

CONTENTS

50 Endovascular Treatment of Popliteal Aneurysm — 598
RAGHUVEER VALLABHANENI • LUIS A. SANCHEZ • PATRICK J. GERAGHTY

51 Above- and Below-Knee Amputation — 604
JOHN F. EIDT • VENKAT R. KALAPATAPU

52 Amputations of the Forefoot — 610
NICHOLAS J. BEVILACQUA • LEE C. ROGERS • GEORGE ANDROS

53 Upper and Lower Extremity Fasciotomy — 617
TODD E. RASMUSSEN • JOSEPH M. WHITE

Section 11 VENOUS DISEASE

54 Placement of Vena Cava Filter — 628
BRENTON E. QUINNEY • MARC A. PASSMAN

55 Surgical Reconstruction for Superior Vena Cava Syndrome — 641
PETER GLOVICZKI • MANJU KALRA

56 Surgical Reconstruction of the Inferior Vena Cava and Iliofemoral Venous System — 650
THOMAS C. BOWER

57 Transjugular Intrahepatic Portosystemic Shunt Procedure — 664
EUGENE HAGIWARA • DARREN B. SCHNEIDER

58 Endovascular Treatment of Iliofemoral and Femoral-Popliteal Deep Vein Thrombosis — 672
ERIN H. MURPHY • MIHAIELA ILVES • FRANK R. ARKO III

59 Varicose Vein Stripping and Ambulatory Phlebectomy — 684
HARRY MA • MARK D. IAFRATI

60 Endovenous Thermal Ablation of Saphenous and Perforating Veins — 694
JULIANNE STOUGHTON

61 Surgical Treatment of Lower Extremity Deep and Perforator Vein Incompetence — 708
ALESSANDRA PUGGIONI

62 Sclerotherapy — 721
ERIC MOWATT-LARSSEN • CYNTHIA SHORTELL

Section 12 ARTERIOVENOUS ACCESS FOR HEMODIALYSIS

63 Radial Artery–Cephalic Vein and Brachial Artery–Cephalic Vein Arteriovenous Fistula — 730
MATTHEW J. DOUGHERTY • DANIEL J. HAYES, JR. • KEITH D. CALLIGARO

64 Forearm Loop Graft and Brachial Artery–Axillary Vein Interposition Graft — 739
SHAWN M. GAGE • DAVID A. PETERSON • JEFFREY H. LAWSON

65 Basilic and Femoral Vein Transposition — 747
WAYNE S. GRADMAN • SIDNEY GLAZER

66 Unconventional Venous Access Procedures for Chronic Hemodialysis — 758
DAVID L. CULL

67 Distal Revascularization Interval Ligation Procedure — 772
LINDA M. HARRIS • HASAN H. DOSLUOGLU

68 Surgical and Endovascular Intervention for Arteriovenous Graft Thrombosis — 781
GEORGE H. MEIER

Video Contents

Section 1 — SURGICAL AND ENDOVASCULAR TECHNIQUES

Video Demonstrations

- **2-1** Ultrasound-guided arterial puncture
- **3-1** Brachial artery access

Section 2 — EXTRACRANIAL CEREBROVASCULAR DISEASE

Video Demonstrations

- **7-1** Eversion endarterectomy
- **8-1** Carotid angioplasty and stenting
- **10-1** Vertebral to carotid artery transposition

Section 3 — AORTIC ARCH VESSELS

Video Demonstrations

- **12-1** Subclavian to carotid artery transposition

Chapter 13 Endovascular treatment of subclavian artery occlusive disease

- **13-1** Diagnostic angiogram of a left subclavian artery occlusion
- **13-2** Crossing a left subclavian artery occlusion
- **13-3** Balloon angioplasty of a left subclavian artery occlusion
- **13-4** Stenting of a left subclavian artery occlusion
- **13-5** Diagnostic angiogram of a right subclavian artery stenosis
- **13-6** Stenting of a right subclavian artery stenosis

Section 4 — UPPER EXTREMITY VASCULAR DISEASE

Video Demonstrations

- **16-1** Axillary approach for treatment of thoracic outlet syndrome

Section 5 — THE THORACIC AORTA

Video Demonstrations

- **18-1** Surgical repair of thoracoabdominal aortic aneurysm

Section 6 — THE ABDOMINAL AORTA AND ILIAC ARTERIES

Video Demonstrations

- **24-1** Surgical repair of a suprarenal aortic aneurysm

Chapter 27 Endovascular repair of a pararenal aortic aneurysm

- **27-1** Positioning a fenestrated graft in the pararenal aorta of a juxtrarenal aneurysm
- **27-2** Alignment of the fenestrations of an aortic endograft
- **27-3** Canulation of the left fenestration and corresponding renal artery
- **27-4** Canulation of the right fenestration and corresponding renal artery
- **27-5** Wire access to both renal arteries
- **27-6** Deployment of a right renal artery stent and flaring of the proximal end of the stent
- **27-7** Deployment of a left renal artery stent and flaring of the proximal end of the stent
- **27-8** Angiogram after bilateral renal artery stent deployment
- **27-9** Balloon apposition of the endograft to the aortic neck
- **27-10** Delivery and deployment of the infrarenal bifurcated component of the endograft
- **27-11** Completion angiogram of the proximal portion of a deployed fenestrated endograft
- **27-12** Completion angiogram of the distal portion of a deployed fenestrated endograft

Section 7 — LATE AORTIC GRAFT COMPLICATIONS

Video Demonstrations

- **34-1** Surgical exposure and harvest of the femoropopliteal vein

Section 8 — RENAL ARTERY DISEASE

Video Demonstrations

- **36-1** Ex vivo surgical repair of a right renal artery aneurysm
- **38-1** Renal artery angioplasty and stenting

Section 9 — SUPERIOR MESENTERIC AND CELIAC ARTERY DISEASE

Video Demonstrations

- **43-1** Endovascular treatment of a splenic artery aneurysm

Section 10 — LOWER EXTREMITY ARTERIAL DISEASE

Video Demonstrations

- **50-1** Endovascular treatment of a popliteal artery aneurysm

Section 11 — VENOUS DISEASE

Video Demonstrations

Chapter 62 Sclerotherapy

62-1 Tessari method for foaming detergent sclerosants

62-2 Technique of injection sclerotherapy

Section 12 — ARTERIOVENOUS ACCESS FOR HEMODIALYSIS

Video Demonstrations

66-1 Femoral vein transposition

Section I

SURGICAL AND ENDOVASCULAR TECHNIQUES

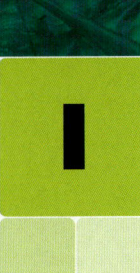

1 General Principles of Vascular Surgery

THOMAS S. RILES

As most vascular surgeons will attest, among the many attractions to our discipline are the vast array of instruments and procedures available to address some of the most severe medical problems known to mankind and the opportunity to apply our surgical skills to virtually every portion of the human body. Because of the many presentations of vascular disease, the vascular surgeon must have extensive knowledge, sound judgment, and in many cases exceptional technical skill to choose and then apply the best treatment for an individual. This chapter discusses some general principles in vascular surgery with a focus on open surgical procedures. The basic principles specific to endovascular repair are discussed in Chapter 2.

Presentation and Natural History of Vascular Diseases

Essential to effective management is a thorough understanding of the anatomy, pathology, and physiologic manifestations of vascular diseases. Some conditions, such as an embolus to the popliteal artery, can cause devastation in hours if not properly diagnosed and treated. Other conditions, such as a chronic occlusion of a subclavian artery, may be tolerated for decades without causing symptoms or posing a risk to an individual.

The mechanism of causing symptoms also varies from one condition to another. Superficial femoral artery disease may cause pain to a lower extremity by reducing blood flow to the limb. However, an atherosclerotic plaque in the carotid artery is more likely to cause symptoms by showering emboli to the distal circulation than by reducing blood flow. The major risk of an aneurysm of the aorta is rupture and bleeding, whereas in other locations it may be thrombosis and ischemia. A vascular surgeon must have a thorough understanding of the pathophysiologic mechanisms of vascular disease, the natural history for various clinical conditions, the risks associate with surgical procedures, and the expected course after successful intervention. Equally important, the surgeon must have the ability to explain what are often complex issues to patients and referring physicians.

Diagnosis

Patients in their seventh decade and beyond, particularly those with heart disease, hypertension, diabetes, smoking, hypercholesterolemia, or a family history of vascular disease, are at greatest risk for atherosclerotic vascular disease. Less common conditions such as carotid dissection, fibromuscular dysplasia, entrapment syndrome, thoracic outlet syndrome, Marfan syndrome, and Ehlers-Danlos syndrome occur more often in younger adults than older ones. Congenital arteriovenous malformations and hemangiomas may be diagnosed at birth. Assessment of the patient's general condition, family history, and social background is the first step in formulating a differential diagnosis and in reaching a definitive diagnosis.

Most vascular conditions can be diagnosed with a careful history and physical examination. A complaint of pain in the calf with walking, relieved by rest, almost always leads to the diagnosis of a chronic superficial femoral artery occlusion.

A history of sudden swelling and discoloration of an upper extremity after strenuous physical activity is caused by subclavian vein thrombosis until proven otherwise. Transient loss of vision in one eye invariably leads to the diagnosis of an atherosclerotic plaque in the ipsilateral carotid artery. The physical findings for patients with arterial and venous occlusive disease, aneurysm disease, and a host of congenital vascular conditions are often striking: absence of pulses in occlusive disease, pulsating masses with aneurysmal disease, varicose veins and reflux with incompetent venous valves, and mottling of the skin with athroemboli to the extremities, to name a few.

Confirmation of a diagnosis usually begins with noninvasive laboratory tests. Ultrasound is the workhorse of every vascular laboratory. It is used to assess the size of an abdominal aorta, the severity of a carotid artery stenosis, the presence of thrombus in a femoral vein, pressure in an artery in an extremity, and many other conditions. For planning interventions, more detailed information can be obtained with magnetic resonance angiography, computed tomography, computed tomography angiography, and conventional catheter-directed angiograms. Knowing the advantages and disadvantages of each, as well as how to make the most effective use of these tests to assist in making a diagnosis, is part of the clinical skill of the vascular surgeon.

Planning a Treatment

After making the diagnosis, the first question is, "Does the patient need to be treated?" Many vascular conditions are self-limited, produce minor or no symptoms, or pose little risk during the remaining life of the individual. Good examples are the moderate asymptomatic carotid stenosis, the small (<4 cm) abdominal aortic aneurysm, and the patient with occasional intermittent claudication. Medical therapy to minimize the risk of symptoms or progression may be all that is needed. Common medications include aspirin and clopidogrel to prevent thrombus formation, statins to minimize plaque progression and instability, and antihypertensive agents for blood pressure control. Counseling to stop smoking, lose weight, and exercise are equally important. Because of the unpredictability of vascular disease, the surgeon or referring physician should set up a program for periodic evaluation.

If a condition exists that may be a risk to the patient's life or health, such as an aneurysm that exceeds 5.4 cm in diameter or an ischemic limb resulting in pain, then the specific risks and benefits of possible treatments must be weighed against the risks of medical therapy alone. The permutations of conditions, as well as the risks and benefits of a specific treatment, are many, and the choice for one patient may often be inappropriate for another. For example, a sedentary older male with an aortic occlusion but only symptoms of moderate claudication may be best managed by medical therapy. In a younger male with a job that requires extensive walking and impotence, aortic occlusion may best be treated with open aortoiliac bypass with preservation of hypogastric artery flow. For an elderly woman with heart disease and an ischemic ulcer on her foot, the surgeon might advise treatment with an axillofemoral bypass graft. Assessment of associated medical illnesses, the expected longevity of the patient, and the prognosis for the underlying vascular condition are essential in selecting the best treatment for any given patient.

Once a choice is made, the options, the surgeon's recommendation, and the potential risks and benefits should be clearly explained to the patient, the family if indicated, and the referring physician. In addition, it is wise to record the assessment of the situation and the particulars of the conversations, including the risks and benefits of the proposed treatment, in a letter to the referring doctor with a copy to the patient. Sending the copy to the patient eliminates misunderstanding and supplements formal informed consent.

Preoperative Assessment

Because of the association of aneurysm and occlusive disease with coronary artery disease, preoperative consideration of the cardiac status of the patient is essential. For a younger patient or someone who will undergo a relatively minor procedure, a careful history and a preoperative electrocardiogram (EKG) may be all that is necessary. For older patients who have risk factors for coronary artery disease or who are to undergo more extensive operations, the workup may include a cardiac echo to assess cardiac function, a nuclear stress test looking for foci of myocardial ischemia, or even cardiac catheterization. In some cases the planned surgery needs to be deferred until the patient first undergoes coronary revascularization. For complex cases, it is wise to have the patient evaluated by a cardiologist preoperatively and to engage the cardiologist's help in the postoperative management.

Renal and pulmonary dysfunction can be a cause of significant morbidity for major vascular procedures, and both require careful intraoperative and postoperative management. Preoperative assessment of coagulation parameters is essential for every vascular case. The surgeon must be aware of the patient's medications. Steroids, beta-blockers, antiplatelet agents, and medications for the management of diabetes are a few medications that may significantly affect the events in the operating room, as well as the patient's recovery. Finally, the surgeon must pay attention to the patient's mental state and functional capacity, as well as family support and the patient's home situation. All are important in setting expectations and planning for disposition after the hospitalization.

Preparation in the Operating Room

Once in the operating room, a number of issues must be addressed before the surgery commences. Foremost is assuring all in the room that they are working with the correct patient, the correct side, and the correct procedure. The Universal Protocol for Preventing Wrong Site, Wrong Procedure and Wrong Person Surgery became effective July 1, 2004, for all accredited hospitals, ambulatory care, and office-based surgery facilities as mandated by the Joint Commission. The three principal components of the protocol include a preprocedure verification, site marking, and a time-out. Although this may seem trite, every experienced surgeon knows of a wrong-side surgery story, sometimes resulting in an injury to the patient, a lawsuit, and irreparable damage to a surgeon's reputation and career. Assuring the correct operation is being performed cannot be delegated to a subordinate; it is always the responsibility of the surgeon.

Almost every major vascular surgery, open and endovascular, requires an arterial monitoring line and venous access for possible blood transfusion. Subclavian artery occlusions are not uncommon in patients with vascular disease. The anesthesiologist must be sure to monitor the arterial blood pressure from the nonaffected limb. If the anesthesia staff is having difficulty obtaining arterial access, the surgical staff should be ready to assist with a cut down on an artery or placement of a femoral artery catheter. In addition to the EKG and O_2 saturation, longer cases require monitoring of urine output and body temperature. Warming blankets may be necessary to prevent hypothermia.

The surgeon should be attentive to the placement of grounding pads, because they may obstruct the view if imaging is to be used. If the patient has a pacemaker, particularly an older model, the surgeon may need to use bipolar cautery. Defibrillators must be turned off.

Depending on the operation to be performed, other preparatory measures may include an epidural catheter for control of postoperative pain, a lumbar drain for spinal fluid drainage for thoracic aneurysmectomy, and a double lumen Carling endotracheal tube to isolate the right lung should the surgeon plan a left thoracotomy. Depending on the surgeon's practice, an electroencephalogram or evoked potential monitoring may be desired for carotid surgery.

Positioning and Prepping the Patient

As in any surgery, the patient must be padded to assure adequate ventilation and to avoid pressure on critical areas, particularly for operations performed in the oblique, lateral, or prone position. In addition, special care must be taken for patients with lower limb ischemia to avoid contact between the heels and the operating table pad and prevent pressure sores. In the case of transaxillary first rib resection for thoracic outlet syndrome, lateral positioning of the patient and support of the arm during the operation are crucial to the ability of the surgeon to safely remove the rib without injury to the vessels or the brachial plexus.

With prepping and draping, it is important to prepare to extend the surgical field should the disease broaden beyond what was expected or should there be a need to emergently obtain proximal control of a vessel. To minimize the risk of infection, covering exposed skin with adherent antiseptic drapes is wise.

Lastly, prophylactic antibiotics are routinely given just before the incision in vascular cases. The surgical staff should be aware of the institutional directives for prophylactic antibiotics and make an explanatory note in the chart if the surgeon intends to deviate from the protocol.

Surgical Exposure

Perhaps one of the most pleasurable aspects of doing vascular surgery is the myriad of operations needed to reach most major blood vessels in the body. For many medical students, the most memorable experience of surgical clerkship is being in the operating room with a vascular surgery team and watching the team members perform surgery on the aorta, the carotid artery, a tibial artery, or a femoral artery—sometimes all in the same day. In addition to being able to operate in every part of the body, a skilled vascular surgeon needs to know multiple approaches to vessels to address various situations. For example, the posterior approach may be ideal for a popliteal aneurysm, whereas the medial approach may be better for a bypass or embolectomy. Details of the operations, including the pros and cons of surgical approaches, are discussed in subsequent chapters.

Vascular Reconstructions

For open surgery for arterial disease, most conditions can be managed with a bypass procedure, a resection with an interposition graft, or a patch repair, with or without an endarterectomy. Endarterectomy is primarily used for short segment occlusive disease, as seen at the carotid bifurcation, although endarterectomy has been used for aortoiliac and femoral artery disease. The plane for doing the endarterectomy can either be between the media and the intima or, more commonly, between the adventitia and the media.

Patch angioplasty is also useful for short segment stenoses when the focus is simply to enlarge the lumen of the vessel. Patches can be constructed from veins, synthetic materials such as Dacron or polytetrafluoroethylene (PTFE), and even the adventitia harvested from an occluded artery. Patches may be helpful in closing an arteriotomy in a severely diseased artery, a situation often encountered after an embolectomy or after passing an endograft through the femoral artery.

For long segment occlusive disease, a bypass procedure is the preferred means of reconstruction. A saphenous vein is the best conduit for lower extremity occlusive disease. If a vein is not available, PTFE grafts can be used—but not with the same expected durability. Synthetics are commonly used for bypass procedures involving the aorta and its major branches, including the arch vessels, the mesenteric and renal arteries, and the iliac arteries, because the diameter requirements are greater. For aneurysmal disease, repair with an interposition graft composed of synthetic material is performed for larger vessels and repair with a vein graft is performed for disease of smaller arteries, such as a popliteal artery aneurysm.

For bypass procedures, an end-to-side reconstruction is commonly used to preserve circulation distal to the anastomosis. A longitudinal arteriotomy is made in the native artery, and the graft is typically beveled to make an obtuse angle with the inflow or outflow tract. The suture is a fine monofilament typically beginning at the "heel" and meeting a second suture from the "toe" midway between the two. Vessels are commonly unclamped momentarily before completing the suture line for prograde flushing and retrograde backbleeding and, thus, to assure there is no thrombus proximal or distal to the clamps.

End-to-end anastomoses are commonly used in the reconstruction of aneurysmal disease and for trauma. For an aortic anastomosis, a Dacron tube is sewn in place with a heavy 2-0 or 3-0 polypropylene suture. For repair of small arteries with end-to-end anastomoses, the surgeon may choose to bevel the ends of both vessels to avoid a stenosis.

Basic Principles of Vascular Surgery

VISUALIZATION OF THE OPERATIVE FIELD

Accurate visualization of the operative field is essential for successful vascular exposure and repair. Vision is enhanced by use of ×2.5 to ×3.5 magnification operating loupes. Although peripheral vision may be compromised, magnification is advisable for those components of the operation when accurate dissection and reconstruction are required. The use of fiberoptic headlamps to provide intense, focused light greatly facilitates illumination of deep or unusual exposures. Intravenous administration of heparin is necessary to achieve systemic anticoagulation for nearly all operations on blood vessels.

EXPOSURE AND CONTROL OF BLOOD VESSELS

The principle of traction and countertraction on tissue to expose the dissection plane is useful for exposure of blood vessels (Fig. 1-1). Atraumatic DeBakey vascular forceps are used to grip the vessel on the adventitial surface only and to distract the vessel to expose surrounding connective tissue fibers that are divided by scissors. Opening the scissors perpendicular to the vessel assists in exposing perpendicularly oriented branch vessels, rather than tearing these vessels should the scissors be opened longitudinal to the blood vessel. Large vessels such as the aorta are better retracted using a lap pad technique, in which manual traction is distributed over a wider area while minimizing trauma to the vessel wall (Fig. 1-2). Once a vessel is mobilized sufficiently, a vessel tape or loop can be passed around and used for retraction. Occasionally, retraction of two tapes or loops can enhance exposure of an intervening vascular segment, such as in the dissection of the origin of the profunda femoris artery while retracting the common femoral and superficial femoral arteries.

VASCULAR OCCLUSION

Vascular occlusion can be achieved using a relatively small number of atraumatic vascular clamps. For example, occlusion of the aorta can be performed using a 10.5-inch DeBakey curved clamp. Most other arteries can be occluded with a DeBakey 7-inch straight jaw 35-degree angled peripheral vascular clamp. Partial occluding clamps are available in a variety of sizes and shapes. Atherosclerotic plaque forms eccentrically, most often on the posterior wall of the artery. To avoid inadvertent embolization of atherosclerotic plaque, arterial dissection, or puncturing of the vessel wall by the plaque, it is best to apply the clamp in an orientation that compresses the nondiseased, soft portion of the vessel wall against the

GENERAL PRINCIPLES OF VASCULAR SURGERY 7

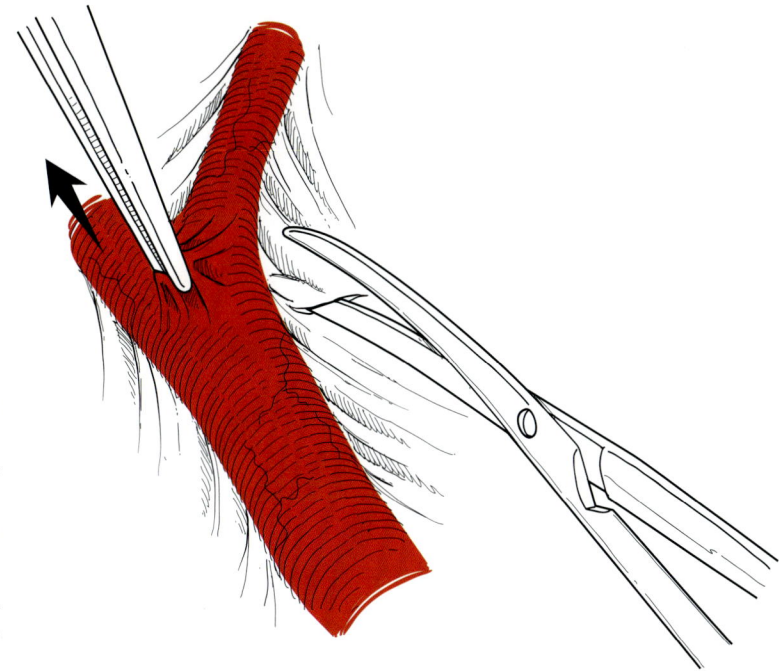

Figure 1-1. Exposure of small and medium-sized blood vessels. The principle of traction and countertraction to expose the dissection plane is useful for exposure of blood vessels. An atraumatic DeBakey vascular forceps is used to grip the vessel in the adventitial surface and to distract the vessel to expose surrounding connective tissue fibers that are divided by scissors. Opening the scissors perpendicular to the vessel helps expose perpendicularly oriented branch vessels.

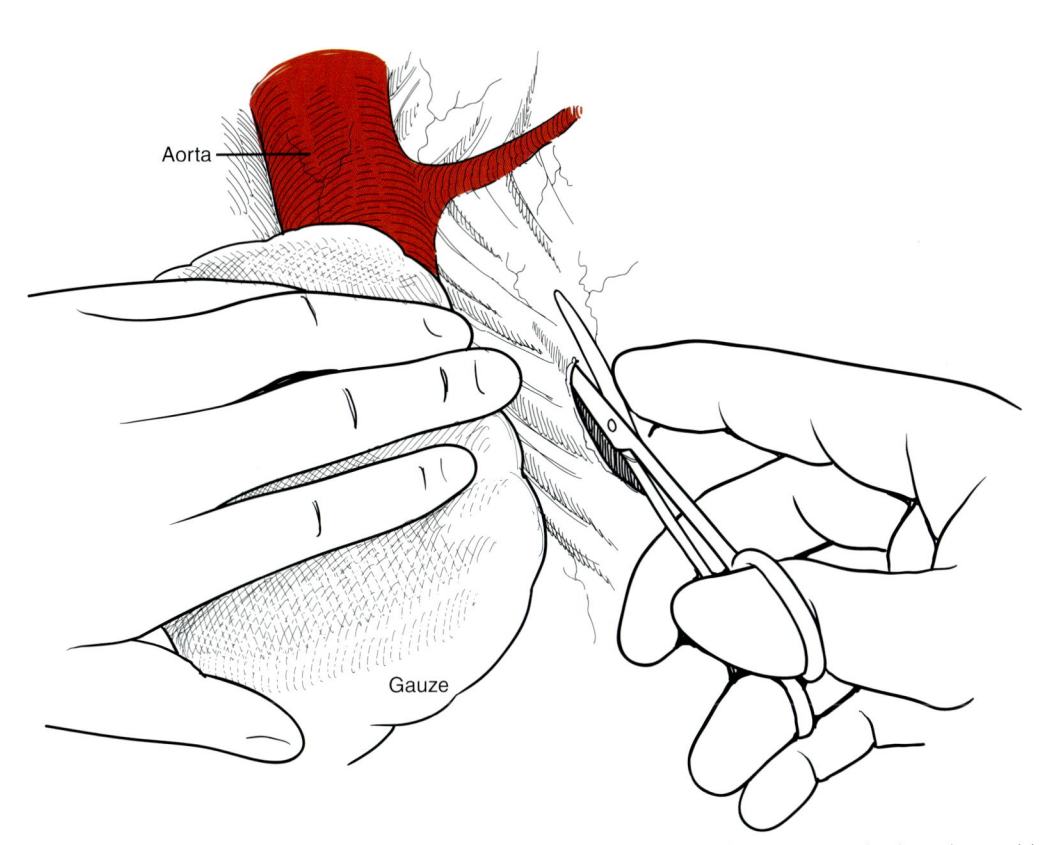

Figure 1-2. Exposure of large vessels. Large vessels, such as the aortic aneurysm, are best retracted using a lap pad, in which manual traction is distributed over a wider area to gently displace the vessel in gaining exposure while minimizing trauma to the vessel wall.

plaque (Fig. 1-3). Multiple grooves in the closure mechanism of the clamp allow the surgeon to apply graded closure to a point sufficient to occlude the vessel without inducing plaque rupture. Occlusion of small vessels requires a device that can exert gentle compression without damaging the intima. Typically, bulldog clamps of a variety of shapes and sizes are available. A dose of heparin at 100 units per kilogram is sufficient to prevent coagulation of blood during most procedures requiring vascular occlusion, but redosing with 1000 units may be required at hourly intervals should the procedure extend over a prolonged period.

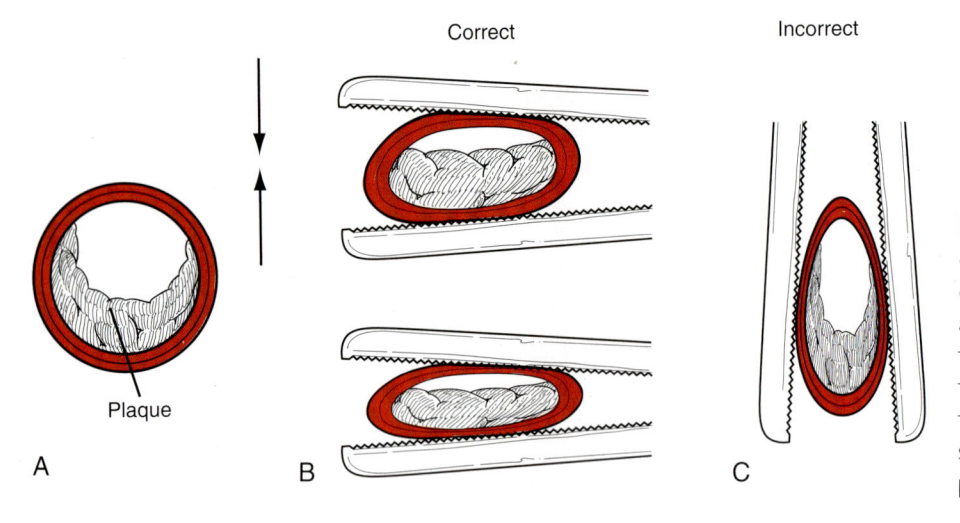

Figure 1-3. Vascular occlusion. Atherosclerotic plaque forms most often on the posterior wall of the artery. To avoid inadvertent embolization, dissection, or puncturing of the vessel wall by the plaque, apply the clamp in an orientation that compresses the nondiseased, soft portion of the vessel wall against the plaque.

PERFORMING AN ARTERIOTOMY

Several approaches have been described for performing an arteriotomy (Fig. 1-4). Sequential incision of the layers of the vessel wall with a No. 15 blade until intraluminal entry is confirmed by the escape of blood, which minimizes the risk of injury to the back wall. Stab incision with a No. 11 or No. 12 blade may be performed for convenience, but care should be taken to avoid injury to the back wall of the vessel or disruption of the plaque. For use on tibial or pedal arteries, miniature Beaver-type blades and handles are available. The arteriotomy can be extended using Potts vascular scissors. Scissors of varying sizes and tip angles are available to facilitate performing the arteriotomy.

TECHNIQUES OF ANASTOMOSIS

Most anastomoses can be performed using a continuous, simple, over-and-over suture technique with the exception of small vessels, for which interrupted and continuous suture techniques can be combined to reduce the risk of a flow-limiting stenosis. A basic principle of vascular anastomosis is passage of the needle from "inside out" through the intimal to the adventitial surface of the host vessel to minimize the risk of the intima being separated from the underlying media. However, when the arterial wall has minimal or no atherosclerotic plaque, an "outside in" technique can be safely used to avoid awkward body positioning or unnecessary torque against the curve of the needle that would disrupt the intimal surface. A variety of vascular needle holders and drivers exist in a range of sizes, shapes, and weights appropriate to surgeon preference and anastomosis type. Creation of a precise vascular anastomosis in small blood vessels may be enhanced by use of a 5.5- or 7-inch Castroviejo-type needle driver.

Beveled End-to-Side Anastomosis

The most common anastomosis is the joining of a beveled graft to a longitudinal arteriotomy (Fig. 1-5). When performing a vein-to-artery, end-to-side anastomosis, the surgeon should be careful to avoid large bites of the vein when securing the heel of the anastomosis, which in turn avoids narrowing the vein graft and producing an "hourglass" stenosis. Lateral traction on the free end of the suture pulls apart the edges of the vessel incision and enhances exposure of the rest of the anastomosis.

A number of acceptable variations on this technique describe different approaches to the heel and toe of the anastomosis. For example, a "two-suture" technique can be used, in which one suture secures the heel that is subsequently run up on both sides of the anastomosis to a point midway to the toe and a second suture used to secure the toe of the graft, which is then run down to the free ends of the first suture. Proponents of this approach note the ability to precisely match the size of the beveled end of the graft to the length vessel opening. In the instance of an anastomosis

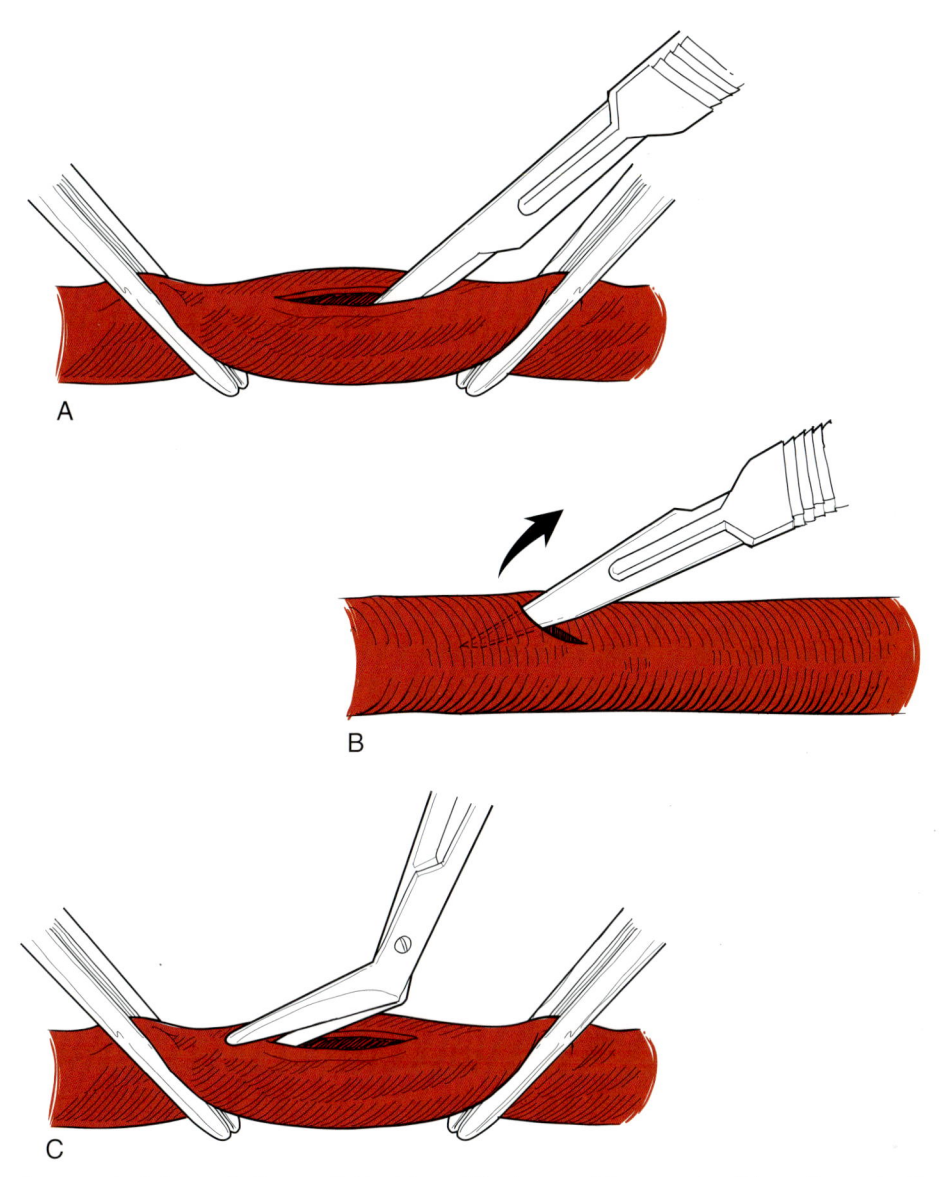

Figure 1-4. Performing an arteriotomy. **A,** Sequential incision of the layers of the vessel wall is performed with a No. 15 blade until intraluminal entry is confirmed by the escape of blood, minimizing the risk of injury to the back wall. **B,** Stab incision with a No. 11 or No. 12 blade may be performed, but care should be taken to avoid injury to the back wall of the vessel. **C,** The arteriotomy can be extended using Potts vascular scissors.

to a small vessel, three to five sutures can be individually placed at the toe and only tied down after all have been placed. One suture is first placed at the apex, and additional sutures are placed in equal number on either side of the apex stitch. A single needle is left on each of the last stitches to be placed and used to run the remainder of the anastomosis on each side. The advantage of this approach for small vessel anastomosis is the ability to precisely visualize the placement of each stitch at the critical distal outflow site of the anastomosis. A third alternative involves a "parachuting" technique, in which a series of approximately five suture loops are placed between the heel of the graft and the host vessel while the graft is held apart from the vessel to provide exposure. The initial two loops are placed on the side opposite the operator, the third loop is at the apex of the heel, and the remaining two loops are placed on the side of the operator. The sutures are then gently pulled up to parachute the graft onto the vessel, and the anastomosis completed as described earlier.

Prograde and retrograde flushing should be performed before the completion of anastomosis. In select circumstances, before the completion of the anastomosis, careful passage of a vascular dilator or dilators can be performed through the toe of the anastomosis through the clamp site to ensure complete expansion of the vessel lumen. Because only a few stitches remain to complete the anastomosis, the

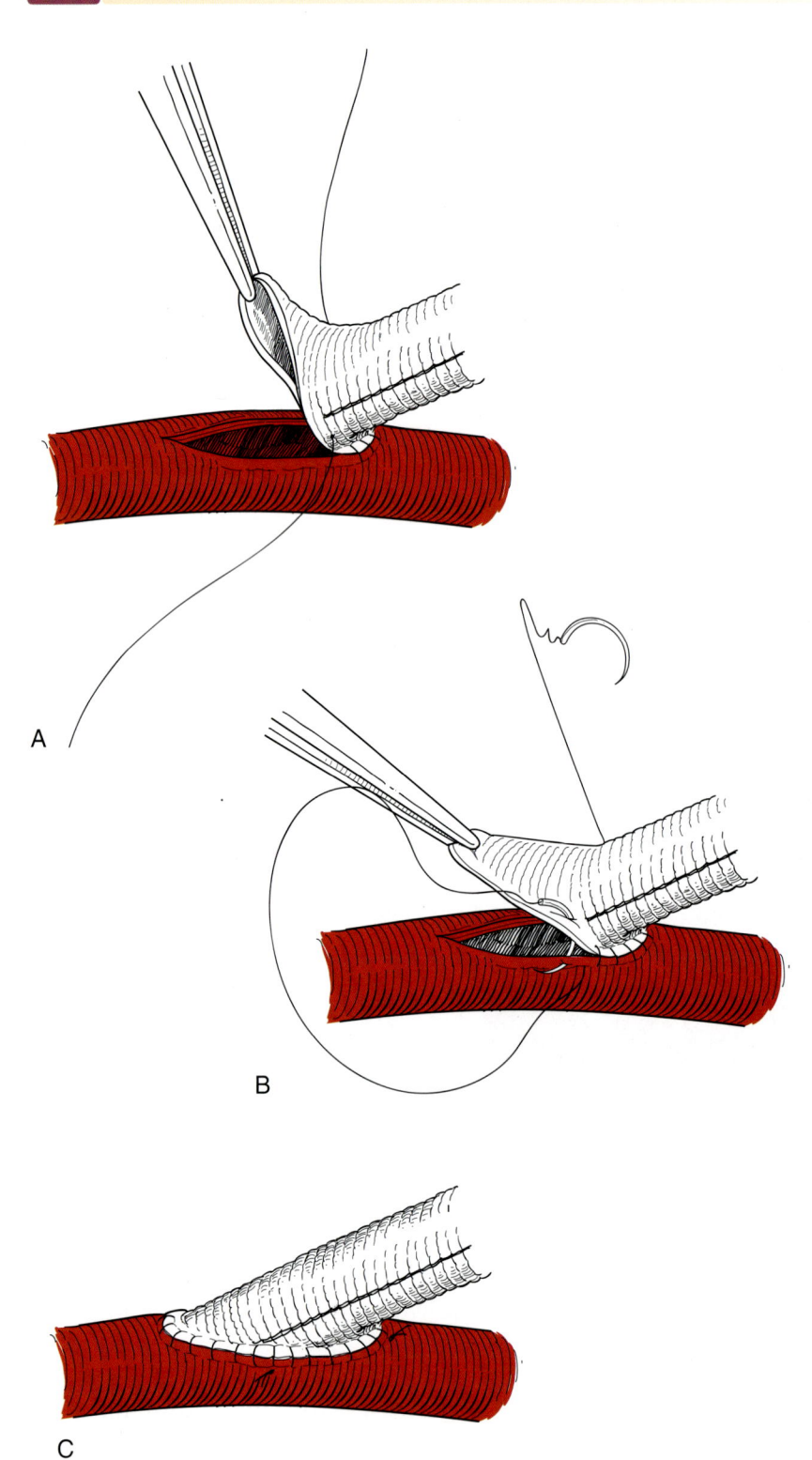

Figure 1-5. Beveled end-to-side anastomosis. **A,** A suture is typically placed at the heel of the graft and secured in place with three throws of a knot. Stitches are first placed to the side opposite of the operator, running up to approximately the midpoint between the heel and the toe of the graft. **B,** Subsequently, stitches are run up along the side of the operator to a position approximately midway between the heel and the toe of the graft. **C,** Completion of the anastomosis involves running the suture, opposite the operator, around the toe of the anastomosis. Prograde and retrograde flushing are performed before completion of the anastomosis at a point midway between the heel and the toe of the anastomosis.

distal clamp does not need to be reapplied. Pulling up on both free ends of the suture approximates edges of the graft and vessel wall with limited or no loss of blood through that portion of anastomosis remaining to be sutured.

Nonbeveled End-to-Side Anastomosis

A nonbeveled end-to-side anastomosis is typically required between the end of a graft and the subclavian or axillary artery, as in the case of a carotid-subclavian or axillofemoral bypass, respectively (Fig. 1-6). This type of anastomosis is performed by beginning in the midpoint of the back row. The suture is secured in place with three throws of the knot, and each end of the suture is run up along either side of the back row through the vessel in an inside-out

GENERAL PRINCIPLES OF VASCULAR SURGERY   11

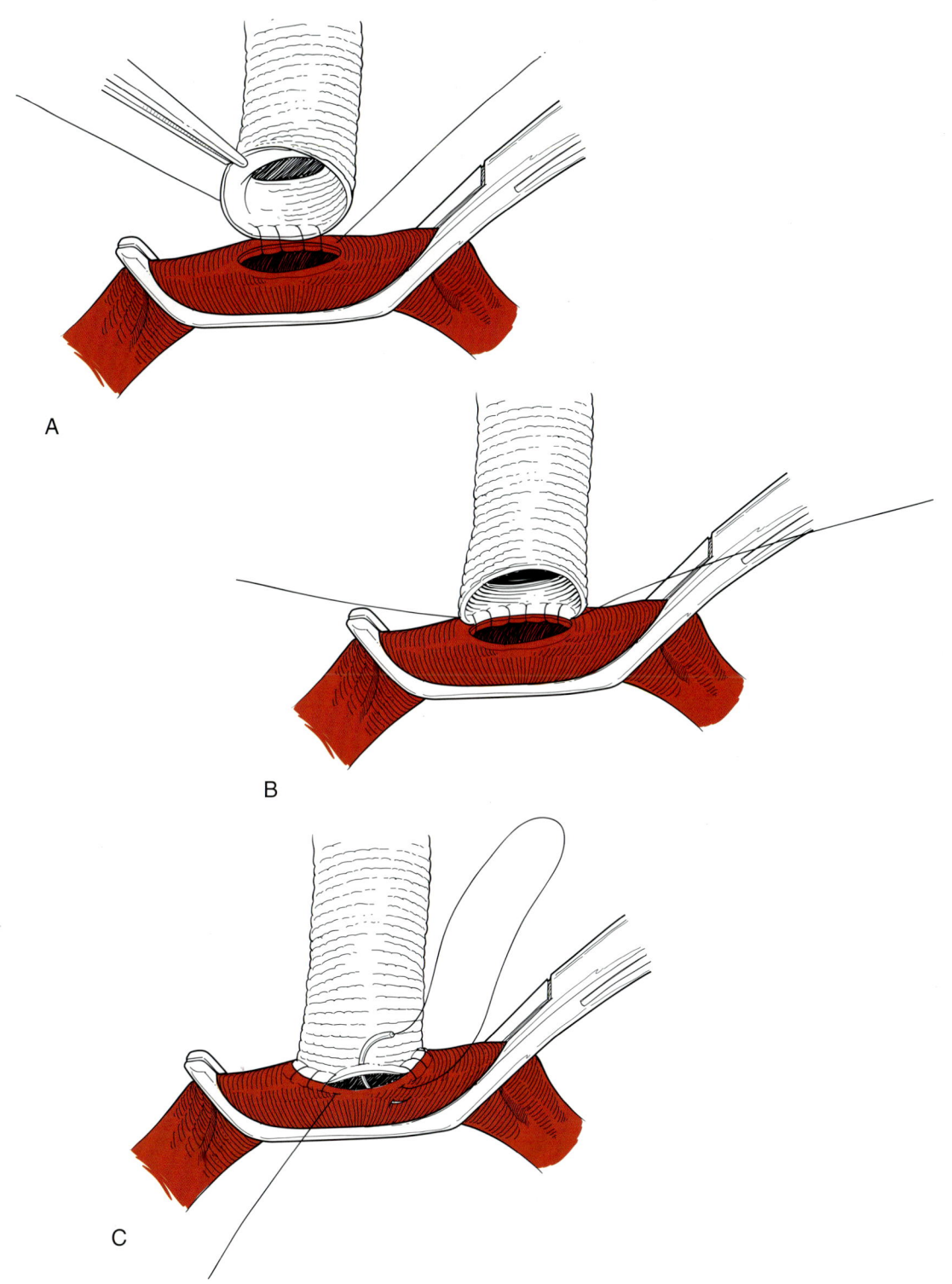

Figure 1-6. Nonbeveled end-to-side anastomosis. **A,** Begin the suture line in the midpoint of the back row. **B,** Continue the suture in both directions around each apex of the anastomosis to the proximal row. **C,** After flushing, complete the front row and tie the two ends of the suture to one another.

fashion. The suture is brought continuously around each apex of the anastomosis to the front row. Appropriate flushing is performed before completion of the anastomosis.

End-to-End Anastomosis

A simple continuous suture technique is used to perform an end-to-end anastomosis of a graft to a large vessel. The back row is completed first. Although a "parachute" technique can be performed as described earlier, the most common approach is to secure the initial stitch at the 4-, 6-, or 8-o'clock position, depending on the surgeon's position and preference. Offsetting the initial stitch

TABLE 1-1 Topical Hemostatic Agents and Suture Line Sealants

Agent	Trade name	Mechanism of Action	Comments
Gelatin foam	Gelfoam	Matrix for clot initiation	Recommended as hemostatic plug wrapped in oxidized cellulose with or without thrombin Adsorbed within 4 to 6 weeks
Oxidized cellulose	Surgicel	Matrix for clot initiation	Adsorbed within 2 to 6 weeks
Microfibrillar collagen	Avitene Flour Avitene Sheet	Platelet adhesion and activation	Adsorbed within 8 weeks Sticks to gloves
Thrombin	Recombinant human thrombin (Recothrom) Human thrombin (Evithrom)	Converts local fibrinogen to fibrin	Most effective when used to soak a gelatin foam plug wrapped in a sheet of oxidized cellulose
Thrombin with gelatin	Floseal	Gelatin granules crosslinked into matrix	Better control of moderate bleeding than fibrin sealants Single syringe
Fibrin sealants	Tisseel	Thrombin and exogenous fibrinogen	Double barrel syringe Adsorbed within 2 weeks
Polyethylene glycol (PEG) hydrogel	Coseal	Thiol-PEG and succinimide-PEG	Double barrel syringe Swells up to four times initial volume Polymerized within 60 seconds
Glutaraldehyde crosslinked albumin	Bioglue	Glutaraldehyde crosslinks bovine albumin	Double barrel syringe Full strength in 2 minutes

from the midline allows the surgeon to forehand a longer length of the back row without awkward positioning of the body and elbow around the operating table. Three loops to secure a knot are sufficient for the initial stitch of a continuous anastomosis, which may be performed over a small felt pledget if desired. Typically, the suture is given an outside-in placement through the graft so that the needle passes through the intimal surface of the vessel. The anterior row of sutures is run to complete the anastomosis. In the case of an end-to-end anastomosis to a large vein, which often is collapsed, placement of two initial sutures at 4 and 8 o'clock may help to line up the lumens of the graft and vein to avoid a size mismatch.

In the case of tenuous host tissue, the suture line can be run over a felt strip. In this instance the felt can both buttress the anastomosis and limit bleeding at the anastomosis that may have incurred because of suture holes in the host tissue. An aortic anastomosis is infrequently buttressed by placement of a circumferential external Dacron strip around the anastomosis. The strip is secured in place by a horizontal mattress stitch just beneath a vascular clamp, which secures the tightened ends of the strip around the anastomosis. Although the presence of pulsatile bleeding after the completion of a vascular anastomosis always warrants placement of a repair suture, diffuse oozing at a suture line can be managed using a range of topical hemostatic agents (Table 1-1).[1]

Small Vessel End-to-End Anastomosis

End-to-end anastomosis of small vessels, such as most often required in the creation of a composite, spliced vein graft, may be accomplished by spatulating the ends of the vein grafts and using a two-suture technique (Fig. 1-7). Each suture is placed through the heel and toe of each vein graft, secured in place with a knot, and then run up to a midpoint along each side of the anastomosis. Use of fine bulldogs for traction on free sutures can help to stabilize the ends of the vein grafts while performing the anastomosis. In addition, careful placement of fine vascular forceps, such as Gerald forceps, within the opening of the anastomosis can facilitate visualization of the edge of the vein graft and precise placement of each stitch. Common instruments used in open vascular reconstruction are illustrated in Figure 1-8.

GENERAL PRINCIPLES OF VASCULAR SURGERY 13

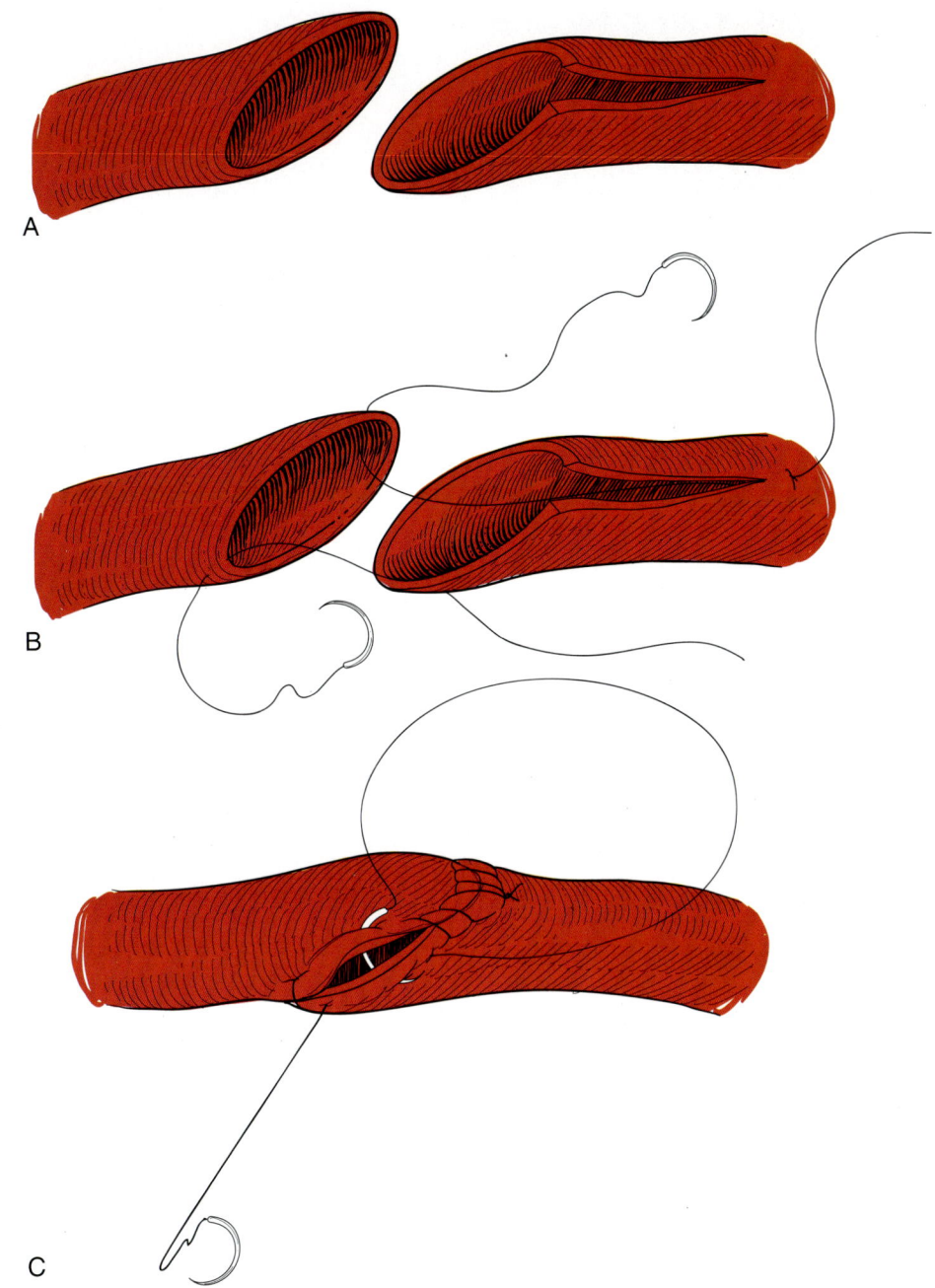

Figure 1-7. Small vessel end-to-end anastomosis. **A,** End-to-end anastomosis in the creation of a composite, spliced vein graft may be accomplished by spatulating the ends of the vein grafts and using a two-suture technique. **B,** Each suture is placed through the heel and toe of each vein graft, secured in place with a knot, and then run up to a midpoint along each side of the anastomosis. Use of small, plastic bulldog clamps for traction on free sutures can help to stabilize the ends of the vein grafts while performing the anastomosis. **C,** Completion of the anastomosis involves running each pair of sutures to a point midway between the heel and the toe of the anastomosis.

Common Problems Associated With Vascular Surgery

Success comes from understanding the causes of early failure of a vascular operation and knowledge of the technical maneuvers to avoid failures. The following are some common problems associated with arterial reconstructions and measures to avoid each.

INJURY TO ADJACENT STRUCTURES

Except in the thorax and abdomen, the arteries and veins are always close to nerves. The first step in dissection is to identify nerves or at least be aware of their locations to avoid injury from a clamp, the electrocautery, a retractor, or forceps. Trauma to any motor or sensory nerve can be devastating, particularly in the neck, where injury to the cranial nerves and brachial plexus can cause major disabilities. In abdominal aortic

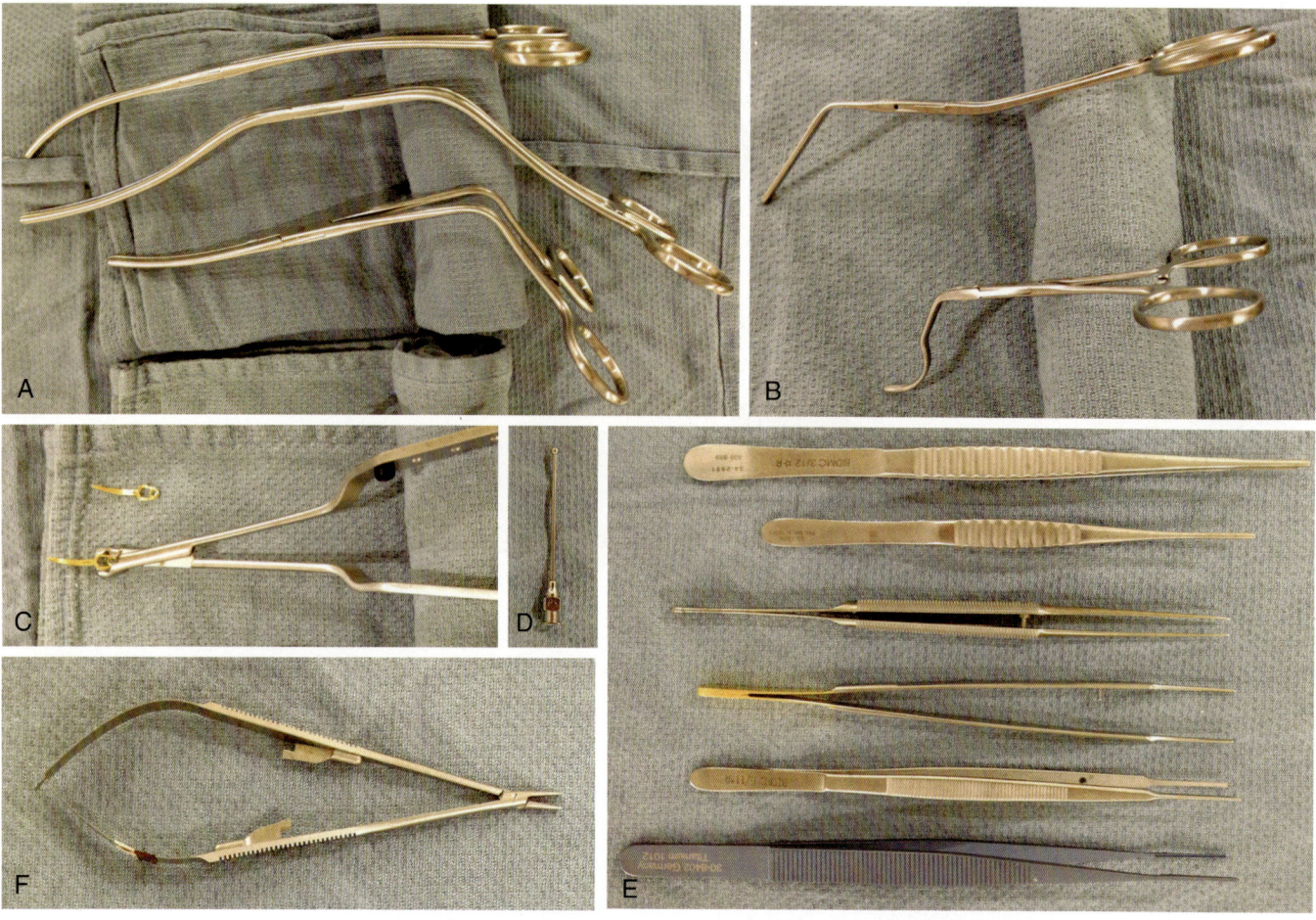

Figure 1-8. Instruments used in vascular reconstruction. **A,** Coarctation (top), Cherry (middle), and Zanger (bottom) clamps used to cross-clamp large vessels. **B,** Impra (top) and profunda (bottom) clamps used to cross-clamp medium-sized vessels. **C,** Yasargil clips to clamp small vessels. **D,** Webster tip needle for infusion of vein grafts with heparinized saline. **E,** DeBakey, Gerald, and other fine vascular forceps. **F,** Castroviejo needle holders.

surgery the surgeon must be aware to avoid injury to the duodenum and ureters, both close to major vessels. Retraction injuries to the spleen and liver are also potential risks.

Injury to adjacent structures is more common in reoperative surgery and procedures when there is inflammation or scarring. Good assistance, good lighting, sharp dissection, and patience are essential for these operations. The surgeon should not hesitate to ask for help from colleagues, particularly if an injury is suspected.

EMBOLIZATION OF ATHEROMA, THROMBUS, OR BOTH

Irretrievable damage can come from embolization of plaque or thrombus to a distal vascular bed. This can occur during the time of the dissection, at the time of unclamping and restoring flow, and postoperatively if fresh thrombus forms at the site of the reconstruction. If working on a vessel known to have loose atheromas or thrombus, the distal and proximal vessels should be dissected and clamped before manipulating the diseased segment of the vessel. This is especially important in the neck, where the dislodging of a particle from a plaque can result in a stroke.

When placing a vascular clamp, it is wise to palpate the vessel first to be sure it is soft and collapsible in order to avoid dislodging plaque or thrombus with the clamp. When operating on an abdominal aorta with intraluminal thrombus near the renal arteries, it may be necessary to first clamp above the renals, open the infrarenal aorta to remove thrombus, and then move the clamp to the infrarenal position. Another common problem in aortic surgery is a calcified iliac artery. If there is concern that a vascular clamp will fracture a plaque, the surgeon may choose to open the aorta without first clamping distally and then control backflow with a temporary balloon catheter in the iliac artery. This same maneuver can be used in the internal carotid and superficial femoral arteries and even tibial vessels using small balloon or probes. Before restoring flow, vessels are briefly unclamped to permit backbleeding and ensure there is no particulate material on the other side of the clamp.

END-ORGAN ISCHEMIA

The consequences of interruption of the blood supply vary according to the end organ, the collateral blood flow, and the duration of ischemia. The brain cannot tolerate anoxia for more than 4 minutes. Under normothermic conditions, a kidney, without renal preservation fluid, may tolerate ischemia for 30 to 60 minutes. The muscles of the leg can tolerate up to 6 hours of ischemia. Whatever the end organ, the surgeon must be aware of the limits of ischemia and provide protection should the time limit be exceeded. In carotid surgery, if the patient does not have adequate collateral circulation, a temporary shunt must be used.

In the lower extremity, patients with an acute arterial occlusion because of either embolus or trauma are at particular risk because they, unlike those with chronic disease, have poor collateral circulation. In these cases the surgeon must remember that ischemia began at the time of the injury or embolization. If surgery has been delayed, the distal muscle and nerves may already have suffered damage. Depending on the extent of the ischemia to the muscle tissue, restoration of flow may be associated with muscle swelling. If a fasciotomy to release the muscle compartments is not performed, further injury may occur from a rise in compartment pressures leading to continued ischemia. In more prolonged ischemia, muscle cells may already have died. Restoration of blood flow to necrotic tissue may cause a release of potassium and myoglobin into the circulation, resulting in cardiac and renal failure.

ARTERIAL THROMBOSIS AFTER A VASCULAR RECONSTRUCTION

Perhaps the major cause of failure in vascular surgery is postoperative thrombosis. Although inadequate outflow may be the cause, more often it is because of a technical failure. Common technical problems that lead to thrombosis include injury to the artery from a vascular clamp resulting in an intimal flap, residual stenosis, retained plaque, kinking of a vessel or graft, and inadequate inflow. Any configuration that leads to turbulent blood flow can cause deposition of platelets, embolization, and thrombosis. The success of a vascular operation is related to the reconstruction of the vessel. Careful assessment after restoring flow, in some cases with ultrasound or angiography, should be performed if there is any question regarding the quality of the reconstruction. The role of postoperative anticoagulation in the prevention of early thrombosis is not clear, but many surgeons choose to have those patients at high risk of thrombosis continue taking heparin postoperatively, accepting the increased risk of bleeding.

BLEEDING, HEMATOMAS, AND LYMPHOCELES

Preventing postoperative bleeding is part of the basic skill of vascular surgery. Special care must be used for patients taking antiplatelet medications and those who will require heparin anticoagulation postoperatively. Because postoperative bleeding can occur in the best of hands, a surgeon must be prepared to return to the operating room for the earliest signs of a hematoma, drop in hematocrit, or instability that could result from internal hemorrhage.

A potentially serious complication, particularly with groin incisions, is lymphatic secretions, either as a lymph fistula or as a lymphocele. These can be prevented by taking care to cauterize or ligate lymphatics with dissection and by careful closure of the wound. Should a lymphocele develop, it often resolves over time, but the patient should be examined frequently and reassured. If the lymphocele continues to grow or shows signs of infection, reoperation is necessary, with the focus on ligating the feeding lymph channels.

INFECTION

Infection can be devastating for any vascular procedure, particularly if it is close to a prosthetic material. Every effort should be made to avoid contamination of the graft or wound. Important measures include prophylactic antibiotics, careful preparation of the skin with antiseptic agents, covering the skin with sterile adhesive antimicrobial dressings, sharp clean incisions to minimize dissection, special care to prevent postoperative hematoma and lymphocele, meticulous wound closure, and attention to postoperative dressings and wound care.

Once the graft is seeded, it is nearly impossible to sterilize and therefore almost always must be removed. If the graft is still providing vital blood flow to a distal organ, vascular reconstruction may be part of the plan to remove the graft. The choices for reconstruction may include in-line reconstruction with autologous tissue or reconstruction with a bypass graft, synthetic or autologous, placed in a fresh tissue bed. The consequences of each must be carefully weighed, taking into consideration the general health of the individual and the risk of further infection. In some cases, such as an infected lower extremity graft, an amputation without reconstruction may be the wiser choice.

REFERENCES

1. Achneck HE, Sileshi B, Jamiolkowski RM, et al: A comprehensive review of topical hemostatic agents: Efficacy and recommendations for use. *Ann Surg* 251:217-228, 2010.

2 General Principles of Sedation, Angiography, and Intravascular Ultrasound

REBECCA KELSO • VIKRAM S. KASHYAP

Historical Background

In 1927 Moniz at the University of Lisbon was the first to demonstrate the clinical utility of angiography by performing the first cerebral angiogram using sodium iodide. In 1929 dos Santos performed the first aortogram.[1] Swick in 1928 reported the initial experience with water-soluble iodinated organic compounds as intravenous contrast agents for urography.[2] By 1956 a less toxic, triiodinated, fully substituted benzene derivative, diatrizoic acid (Hypaque, iodine content 300 mgI/mL, 1550 mosm/kg H_2O) was introduced, and in 1968 Almén began to develop lower-osmolar (400-800 mosm/kg H_2O) nonionic compounds to limit hemodynamic alterations, which had been attributed to the high osmolality of prior ionic agents. Low-osmolar ionic compounds such as ioxaglate (Hexabrix, iodine content 320 mgI/mL, 580 mosm/kg H_2O) and nonionic contrast media such as iohexol (Omnipaque, iodine content 350 mgI/mL, 884 mosm/kg H_2O) and iopamidol (Isovue, iodine content 370 mgI/mL, 796 mosm/kg H_2O) were introduced to the United States in the late 1980s. This was followed by the introduction of an iso-osmolar contrast agent, iodixanol (Visipaque, iodine content 320 mgI/mL, 290 mosm/kg H_2O), with an osmolality similar to blood but with considerably increased viscosity.

Intravascular ultrasound (IVUS) supplements the two-dimensional (2D) and three-dimensional (3D) images obtained by angiography and computed tomography scanning with cross-sectional ultrasound images of the vessel and its wall. Early studies of intracardiac ultrasound and IVUS by Cieszynski in the 1950s, as well as by Eggleton and Carelton in the 1960s, led to the first report of IVUS applied as an alternative to transthoracic echocardiography in 1972.[3] In the late 1980s Yock at Stanford University introduced the first IVUS catheter designed for clinical use, which was quickly adapted for use in coronary and peripheral circulation.

Sedation, Analgesia, and Anesthesia

Pain associated with percutaneous or limited surgical procedures for arterial access can be managed in the majority of patients with local infiltration of an anesthetic, such as 1% lidocaine. In most angiography suites or operating rooms, hemodynamic monitoring is readily available and procedural sedation can be administered by appropriately privileged nurses and physicians. Sedation improves patient tolerance of the procedure by reducing symptoms of anxiety and claustrophobia while decreasing the discomfort associated with manipulation of devices or balloon angioplasty. General recommendations include monitoring for arrhythmias with an electrocardiogram, as well as monitoring blood pressure, pulse, respiratory rate, oxygen saturation, and pain level. Sedation should be administered in accordance with the American Society of Anesthesia guidelines for nonanesthesiologists and the Joint Commission standards.[4,5]

Sedation is usually achieved by a combination of a narcotic opioid and benzodiazepine. Shorter-acting drugs, such as fentanyl and midazolam (e.g., Versed), are preferred. Each drug is given as a slow intravenous injection, with typical initial dosing for fentanyl at 0.5 mcg/kg (e.g., 25 mcg) and for midazolam at 0.02 mg/kg (e.g., 1 mg). The initial dose and all subsequent doses should always be titrated slowly, administered over at least 2 minutes, and monitored over 2 minutes or longer to fully evaluate the sedative effect. Smaller, incremental doses are recommended for elderly patients and those with renal or hepatic failure. The initial dose of midazolam should not exceed 2.5 mg in a normal healthy adult. Oversedation may limit the patient's ability to follow directions and may paradoxically produce a disinhibited, agitated state; it may also limit the physician's ability to identify changes in a neurologic examination. Monitoring of vital signs and patient responsiveness to verbal or tactile stimulation is critical to recognizing oversedation from which the patient may exhibit depressed cardiac function and hypoxia that may progress to airway compromise and apnea. Oversedation and disinhibition are treated similarly, although disinhibition is related to only benzodiazepines. In both cases the procedure needs to be stopped to allow proper assessment of the patient, cessation of medication, and continuation of supportive care. Both opioids and benzodiazepines can be treated by administration of an opioid antagonist, such as naloxone hydrochloride (e.g., Narcan), or flumazenil (Romazicon), a benzodiazepine receptor antagonist. The intravenous dose of naloxone hydrochloride should be titrated according to the patient's response at increments of 0.2 mg given intravenously at 2- to 3-minute intervals to the desired degree of reversal. Likewise, flumazenil is administered at 200 mcg every 1 to 2 minutes until the effect is seen, to a maximum of 1 mg in 10 minutes or 3 mg in 1 hour. Both medications are short-lived, and sedation or agitation may return.

The use of anesthesiologist-directed sedation, spinal anesthesia, or general anesthesia may be dictated by the complexity and length of the procedure and the necessity for an associated surgical procedure. Other relative indications for the involvement of an anesthesiologist include the need for deep sedation in a patient with a difficult airway; cardiopulmonary, renal, or hepatic comorbidities (American Society of Anesthesiologists level > 2); or a high anxiety level. As an example, general anesthesia is usually required in hybrid cases that involve both an endovascular and an open surgical procedure when concerns exist over the patient's ability to maintain an airway or when deployment of a thoracic endograft may require cardiac overdrive pacing or medical asystole with adenosine. Spinal anesthesia provides complete analgesia of the lower abdomen, groin, and legs, which can allow a hybrid procedure in a patient with severe chronic obstructive pulmonary disease. Likewise, complex catheter-based procedures that are better tolerated under general anesthesia or monitored anesthesia care (MAC) include recanalization of an occluded superior vena cava or removal of a malpositioned inferior vena cava filter. The extended duration of such procedures and requirement for a large sheath in the neck increase patient anxiety and discomfort despite optimal sedation and local pain control.[6] In general, MAC should also be considered for interventions lasting more than 2 hours and for patients with low tolerance such as those with movement disorders or chronic back pain.

Fluoroscopic Principles

The performance of endovascular procedures requires a thorough understanding of image acquisition, contrast injection techniques, radiation safety, and ultrasound-guided puncture.

IMAGE ACQUISITION

Digital angiography is required for optimal diagnosis and therapy using 2D imaging. In selective circumstances, rotational angiography with 3D image reconstruction is used. Digital subtraction angiography (DSA) removes background structures with computer-based subtraction to create a high-fidelity image with lower amounts of iodinated contrast material. In the usual acquisition sequence the mask image is obtained, contrast is injected, and the computer subtracts the opacified vessels from the native mask image. Postprocessing can improve image quality in the presence of slight motion artifact, but patient movement should be avoided having the patient hold his or her breath or using other maneuvers. *Road mapping* is a term that refers to use of an image selected from DSA that is overlaid on the monitor during live fluoroscopy to limit the number of angiographic runs and facilitate vessel access during interventions. Intravenous DSA is now used infrequently for angiography with the advent of low-profile, high-flow, multihole flush arterial catheters.

CONTRAST INJECTION TECHNIQUES

Despite the convenience of manual contrast injection, use of a power injector allows precise selection of the rate, total volume, maximum pressure, and rate of rise or time to peak flow of administered contrast. In general, the rate and total volume of contrast administered are increased when imaging larger vessels. Some general guidelines can be found in Table 2-1. Whereas flush multihole catheters can accommodate higher delivery pressures and are often rated up to 1200 psi, end-hole catheters require lower pressures. General settings for pressure are 900 psi for a flush catheter and 300 to 500 psi for an end-hole catheter. Likewise, reducing the maximum injection pressure to 100 to 200 psi, as well as the rate of rise, should be considered when a catheter could be easily dislodged from the orifice of a vessel. Power injection also allows all personnel to move away from the x-ray source, thus decreasing radiation exposure.

RADIATION EXPOSURE AND SAFETY

Increasing complexity of endovascular cases has increased fluoroscopy times, with an attendant risk of radiation injury leading to increased lifetime cancer risk, cataracts, bone marrow suppression, and sterility, as well as local injury progressing from dermatitis to a full-thickness dermal ulcer or cancer. Increased awareness has led to consensus statements regarding best practices[7] and an initiative by the U.S. Food and Drug Administration in 2010 focused on modifying fluoroscopy use and reducing radiation scatter and exposure consistent with as low as reasonably achievable (ALARA) radiation exposure guidelines (Box 2-1). In general, fluoroscopy should be avoided unless acquiring an image or actively performing a task that requires visualization. For example, fluoroscopy should not be performed during a catheter exchange.

Several techniques can also be used to minimize scatter and exposure. Because the radiation source is below the table and the image intensifier is above the patient, raising the table height and bringing the image intensifier as close to the patient as feasible provides a larger field of view and decreases x-ray scatter. Most modern imaging systems use an automatic dose rate control that modulates the radiation dose for denser objects to allow x-ray penetration and image sharpness. Thus removing metal objects such as clamps from the field of view avoids an automatic

TABLE 2-1 Guidelines for Contrast Power Injection by Vascular Bed

	Type of Catheter	Pressure (psi)	Rate of Rise (sec)	Rate (mL/sec)	Total Volume (mL)
Aortic arch	Flush	900-1200	0.1	15	30
Carotid	End hole	300	0.7	3-5	6-10
Subclavian/brachial segments*	End hole	300	0.7	3-5	6-10†
Abdominal aorta	Flush	900	0.1	15	30
Superior mesenteric/celiac artery	End hole	200	1.0	3	6-20†
Renal	End hole	200	1.0	3	6
Pelvic vessels	Flush	900	0.1	10	20
Infrainguinal segments*	End hole	300	0.7	3-5	6-10

*Contrast rate and volume increase with distal extremity imaging and increasing vessel disease.
†Use larger volumes to fill distal and/or venous vasculature.

> **Box 2-1 STRATEGIES TO MINIMIZE RADIATION EXPOSURE**
>
> Ensure that all medical personnel are wearing leaded aprons, thyroid shields, and leaded glasses.
>
> Modifications to image acquisition technique:
> - Minimize the number of angiographic runs.
> - Use DSA.
> - Decrease the frame rate during routine pulsed fluoroscopy.
> - Minimize fluoroscopy.
> - Use road map or fluorofade and reference imaging.
> - Increase kilovolt and lower milliampere settings.
>
> Reduce radiation scatter and exposure:
> - Use leaded shields.
> - Move the table far from the radiation source and closer to the image intensifier.
> - Remove all metal objects from the field of view.
> - Use collimation to confine x-rays to the area of interest.
> - Use filters.
> - Avoid routine magnification or extreme angulation.
>
> Other measures:
> - Use information from other imaging studies such as computed tomography angiography or magnetic resonance angiography to improve preprocedural planning.
> - Monitor fluoroscopy times and consider staging long, complex endovascular procedures.

increase in radiation dose. In addition, use of collimators to confine the x-rays and focus on the anatomic area of interest reduces radiation exposure to the patient and minimizes scatter. Filters decrease scatter and improve image clarity. Minimizing radiation exposure can also be achieved by minimizing magnification and angulation of the radiation source.

Reducing radiation exposure can be achieved by use of leaded shielding and fluoroscopy table skirts, as well as personal protection equipment, including circumferential leaded aprons, thyroid shields, and lead-containing eyeglasses. Dosimeters should also be worn by personnel to monitor their exposure levels. The maximum allowable whole-body exposure to medical personnel from all sources is 5 rem/yr.[8]

PRINCIPLES OF ULTRASOUND-GUIDED ARTERIAL PUNCTURE

Ultrasound-guided arterial puncture (UGAP) should be used routinely, because it reduces access site–related complications both for routine procedures and for those procedures in which large sheaths are used (Video 2-1).[9] Device requirements for UGAP include a portable ultrasound device with a 5- to 10-MHz probe that allows both B-mode and color flow imaging. Access is usually obtained by using a micropuncture set with a microneedle, short 0.018-inch guidewire, and microsheath of normal flexibility—or stiffened, should access be required through significantly scarred regions.

Ultrasound imaging of the common femoral, superficial femoral, and profunda femoris arteries, as well as the adjacent femoral vein, documents the location, patency, and extent of calcification (Fig. 2-1). A typical radiographic landmark

GENERAL PRINCIPLES OF SEDATION, ANGIOGRAPHY, AND INTRAVASCULAR ULTRASOUND   21

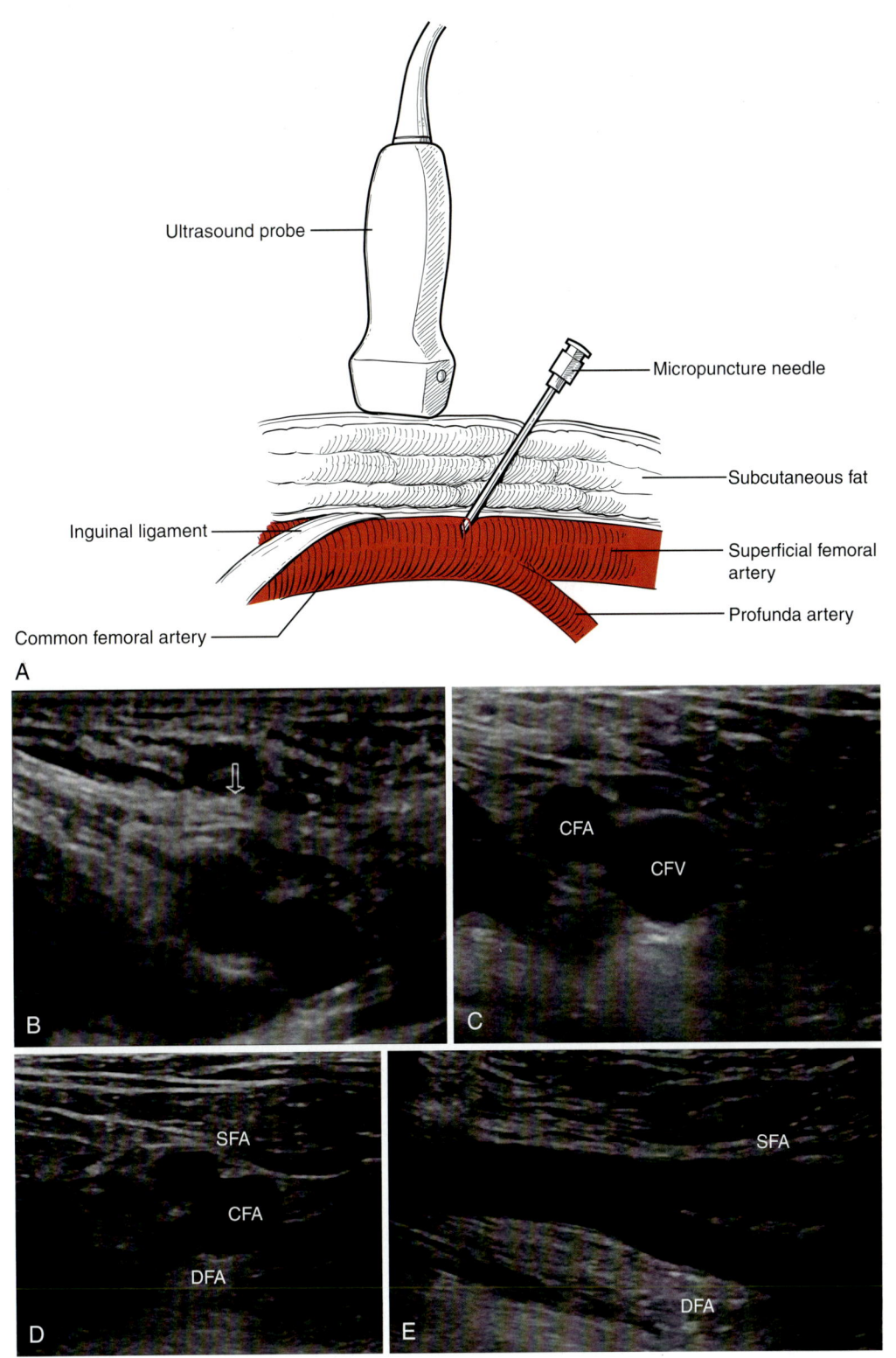

Figure 2-1. **A**, Ultrasound-guided arterial puncture. Transverse images of the femoral artery from cranial to caudal identifying (**B**) the inguinal ligament *(arrow)*, (**C**) common femoral artery (CFA) and common femoral vein (CFV), and (**D** and **E**) bifurcation of the superficial femoral artery (SFA) and deep femoral artery (DFA).

for common femoral artery puncture is the middle third of the femoral head. To maximize the transverse diameter of the vessel, the puncture is performed while holding the ultrasound probe in one hand and the needle in the other. It is often necessary to adjust the positioning of the ultrasound to optimize images of the needle tip entering the anterior wall of the vessel. After a single anterior wall puncture, arterial flow is noted at the hub of the needle, allowing wire passage and placement of a microsheath. The microdilator is removed, allowing placement of a 0.035-inch wire. The standard Seldinger technique allows placement of a regular, short, or long interventional sheath.

> **Box 2-2 MINIMIZING THE RISK OF CONTRAST-INDUCED NEPHROPATHY**
>
> Use low-osmolar or iso-osmolar, nonionic contrast.
>
> Renal protection:
> - Provide hydration with saline.
> - Administer N-acetylcysteine.
>
> Reduce contrast volume:
> - Decrease contrast strength (1:1 dilution with saline).
> - Minimize repetitive contrast runs through use of road map or fluorofade with reference imaging.
> - Use information from other imaging studies such as computed tomography angiography or magnetic resonance angiography to improve preprocedural planning.
>
> Noniodinated contrast imaging modalities:
> - Take pressure gradient measurements.
> - Perform CO_2 angiography.
> - IVUS

Performing arterial puncture in this manner not only improves success and efficiency in cases of potentially difficult access but also ensures that the puncture is on the anterior surface of the vessel. This minimizes vessel injury, enhances successful use of closure devices, and decreases access complications during thrombolysis.

Angiographic Contrast Media

The most common contrast media used in the United States are the low-osmolar, nonionic contrast media iohexol (Omnipaque, iodine content 350 mgI/mL, 884 mosm/kg H_2O) and the iso-osmolar but higher-viscosity contrast agent iodixanol (Visipaque, iodine content 320 mgI/mL, 290 mosm/kg H_2O).

SPECIAL CONSIDERATIONS: PATIENTS WITH RENAL DYSFUNCTION

The risk for contrast-induced nephropathy (CIN) increases in the elderly (age older than 70 years), as well as in those patients with a history of renal dysfunction, previous renal impairment after contrast administration, diabetes, dehydration, and congestive heart failure.[10] Iodinated contrast agents appear to cause direct tubular toxicity and decrease the glomerular filtration rate as a result of increased osmolality, induced diuresis, and release of vasoactive mediators. All efforts should be undertaken to provide renal protection and minimize the contrast load (Box 2-2). The oral hypoglycemic metformin should be not be taken 48 hours before or after the administration of contrast because of increased risk of CIN.[10]

Renal protective measures that can be instituted before the procedure include intravenous hydration and administration of N-acetylcysteine (Mucomyst). Intravenous hydration with isotonic fluids such as normal saline has been shown as the most effective method to prevent CIN.[11] A single randomized controlled trial also found that bicarbonate infusion may further reduce this risk from 13.6% to 1.7% when compared with normal saline.[12] Oral hydration is also effective, because many procedures are performed on an outpatient basis. N-acetylcysteine has antioxidant properties and may be protective against CIN.[13,14] If the patient is tolerating oral medications, 600- to 1200-mg capsules in two oral doses every

GENERAL PRINCIPLES OF SEDATION, ANGIOGRAPHY, AND INTRAVASCULAR ULTRASOUND

TABLE 2-2A Recommended Strategies for Preserving Renal Function

eGFR* (mL/min)	Recommendation
≥60	No preventive measures required.
With risk factors†	Periprocedure oral hydration is suggested.
45-59	Oral hydration is suggested.
With risk factors†	Oral hydration is necessary.
30-44	Oral hydration is necessary; IV hydration should be considered.
With risk factors†	IV hydration is necessary.
15-29	IV hydration is necessary; consider alternative studies.
<15	Contrast only if the patient is receiving dialysis and can undergo dialysis within 48 hr.

IV, Intravenous.
*Estimated glomerular filtration rate (eGFR) less than 60: Dye use should not exceed 60 g of iodine or ~200 mL of a low-osmolar, nonionic agent within a 72-hour period.
†Diabetes, congestive heart failure, age older than 70, or taking diuretics.

TABLE 2-2B Recommended Hydration Regimens

Fluid options	0.9% normal saline solution or bicarbonate solution consisting of 3 ampules of sodium bicarbonate in 500-mL solution of 5% dextrose in water
Inpatient	1 mL/kg/hr for 12 hr before and after procedure for total of 2 L Adjustments should be based on cardiac status, with monitoring for volume overload or pulmonary edema; for example, 6 hr of fluid can be provided before the procedure if a history of congestive heart failure or volume restrictions for chronic renal disease
Outpatient	150 mL/hr for 2 or 3 hr before examination Oral fluids recommended after procedure
Oral	500-1000 mL of salty fluids before contrast load

12 hours before and after contrast administration is appropriate. Alternatively, N-acetylcysteine may be given as a 600- to 1200-mg intravenous dose more than 15 minutes before the procedure. The patient should avoid diuretics on the day of contrast administration. A general strategy for renal protective measures based upon patients' GFR can be seen in Table 2-2A. In addition, Table 2-2B outlines a recommended hydration regimen adapted from the literature.[15-17] Although image quality may be reduced, renal toxicity can also be minimized by dilution of contrast with normal saline at a 1:1 ratio. Iodixanol has also been suggested for patients with an estimated glomerular filtration rate (eGFR) of less than 60 mL/min, but its benefit remains controversial.[18,19]

Additional approaches to minimize contrast load include use of road mapping, IVUS, and carbon dioxide (CO_2) angiography. Likewise, measuring the systolic pressure gradient at rest (>10 mm Hg) or following intraarterial administration of 30 mg of papaverine (>20 mm Hg) may be used to determine whether a hemodynamically significant stenosis is present.

SPECIAL CONSIDERATION: PATIENTS WITH CONTRAST MEDIA REACTIONS

Contrast media reactions are related to histamine release from basophils and eosinophils rather than an immunoglobulin E–mediated reaction. Patients with contrast or iodine allergy have a fivefold increased risk of reaction upon repeat exposure. A history of shellfish allergy, previously thought to predict contrast reaction, is now recognized to be unreliable.[15]

Premedication with prednisone, 50 mg given orally, 13, 7, and 1 hour before the procedure with 50 mg of diphenhydramine given 1 hour before the procedure reduces the risk of a contrast-induced allergic reaction.[20] For an emergent procedure, intravenous regimens have been used, but they are not as effective when given less than 4 hours before contrast administration. The most widely accepted intravenous regimen includes 50 mg of diphenhydramine given 1 hour before contrast loading and either 40 mg of methylprednisolone or 200 mg of hydrocortisone given every 4 hours during contrast administration.[21]

TABLE 2-3 Treatment of Allergic Reactions to Contrast Media

Urticaria	1. No treatment needed in most cases
	2. Diphenhydramine 25-50 mg PO/IM/IV
	If severe or widely disseminated: Epinephrine 0.1-0.3 mg SC (if no cardiac contraindications)
Facial or laryngeal edema	1. Epinephrine 0.1-0.3 mg SC or IM or if hypotensive, administer IV and repeat as needed up to 1 mg
	2. Consider corticosteroids, e.g., hydrocortisone 100 mg IV
Bronchospasm	1. Treat as for facial or laryngeal edema
	2. Albuterol 2-3 puffs and repeat as necessary or, if unresponsive to inhalers, give epinephrine SC, IM, or IV
	3. For persistent bronchospasm or persist hypoxia (oxygen saturation < 88%), consider ICU and possible intubation
Hypotension and tachycardia	1. Place patient in Trendelenburg position
	2. Secure airway based on patient's level of consciousness
	3. Rapidly administer lactate Ringer solution or normal saline
	If unresponsive to fluid resuscitation and persistently tachycardic: Administer epinephrine 0.1 mg IV and repeat as needed up to 1 mg
	If bradycardic: Administer atropine 0.6-1 mg IV and slowly and repeat as needed up to total dose of 0.04 mg/kg (2-3 mg) in adults
Severe hypertension	1. Nitroglycerin 0.4 mg sublingual (may repeat 3×) or topical 2% ointment applied as 1-inch strip
	2. If unresponsive, consider labetalol 20 mg IV and then 20-80 mg IV every 10 minutes up to 300 mg
Seizures	1. Diazepam 5 mg IV or midazolam 0.5-1 mg IV
	2. Consider phenytoin infusion 15-18 mg/kg at 50 mg/min
Pulmonary edema	1. Furosemide 20-40 mg IV with slow push
	2. Cautiously consider morphine 1-3 mg IV

From American College of Radiology. Manual on contrast media. Version 7.0 2010. Available at http://www.acr.org. (Accessed February 22, 2011.)
IM, Intramuscularly; *IV,* intravenously; *PO,* orally; *SC,* subcutaneously.

TREATMENT FOR CONTRAST MEDIA REACTIONS

With the development and increasing use of low-osmolar, nonionic contrast agents, the incidence of contrast-related reactions has decreased. Prompt identification and proper treatment of reactions is important, because most are dose independent and unpredictable. Histamine-related allergic reactions range from a warm or flushed sensation to hives, bronchospasm, and anaphylaxis. Initial treatment includes oxygenation and antihistamines, as well as steroids, adrenergic inhalers, or epinephrine as the severity of the reaction increases. Patients who develop an anaphylactic reaction may require cardiopulmonary support, including mechanical ventilation and vasopressors. Treatment should be tailored to the type of reaction and the accompanying symptoms (Table 2-3). All patients with cardiopulmonary compromise require continuous monitoring, consideration of intubation, and if symptoms persist or worsen, admission to an intensive care unit (ICU).

CIN may range from a transient rise in creatinine to renal failure. Depending on the definition used for CIN, serum creatinine rises 20% to 50% above baseline, with an increase of 0.5 to 2 mg/dl. Although CIN usually occurs within the first 72 hours, the onset of renal dysfunction may occur up to 5 days after exposure. Should CIN develop, medications known to affect kidney function should be discontinued and intravenous fluids should be administered based on volume status and severity of renal failure. Dialysis should be initiated as needed to control hyperkalemia, pulmonary edema, metabolic acidosis, and uremic symptoms. Treatment is primarily supportive, with the continuation of hemodialysis until recovery is complete.

CO_2 ANGIOGRAPHY

CO_2 angiography is an underused imaging modality that is ideal for patients with renal dysfunction. Nonetheless, it is not recommended for imaging procedures above the diaphragm or for patients with intracardiac septal defects, because embolization to coronary and cerebral arteries can be lethal.

CO_2 displaces blood from vessels, causing a variation in density detected by DSA, particularly with recent advancements in imaging enhancement software that has improved image quality (Box 2-3). CO_2 is a colorless gas, which requires the use of a

GENERAL PRINCIPLES OF SEDATION, ANGIOGRAPHY, AND INTRAVASCULAR ULTRASOUND

> **Box 2-3 STRATEGIES TO IMPROVE IMAGE QUALITY OF CO_2 ANGIOGRAPHY**
>
> Ensure tight connections.
> Use a self-contained system.
> Flush the system three times to remove air.
> Elevate vessels of interest above the catheter.
> Prime the catheter with CO_2 prior to injection.
> Compress CO_2 for good bolus delivery.
> Allow time between injections to prevent gas trapping.
> Acquire images at a rate of 4-6 frame/sec.
> Manipulate images after the procedure.
> Use small aliquots of iodinated contrast to improve detail.

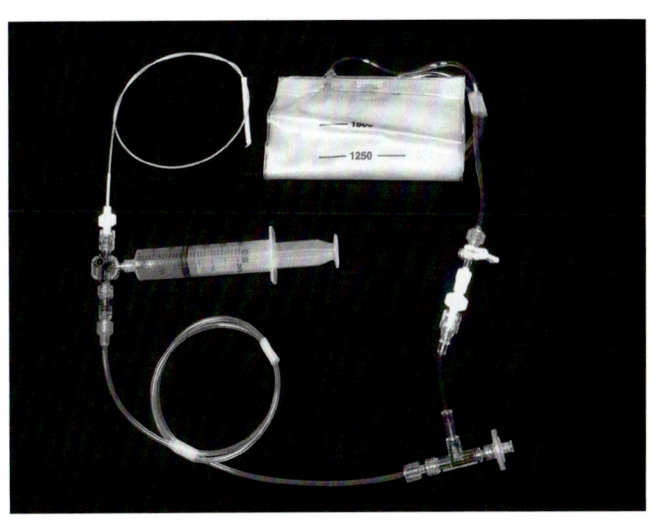

Figure 2-2. CO_2 delivery system connected to a diagnostic catheter. The delivery system uses a three-way stopcock, one-way check valves, and a filter port connected to a gas tank (not shown). A 1500-mL bag is attached to the delivery system with low-pressure tubing and a two-way stopcock. A 60-mL Luer-Lok syringe is required for hand injection. The three-port fitting is connected by 100 cm of connecting tubing to a second three-port fitting and a 3-mL purge syringe. Once the gas bag is filled with CO_2 directly from the gas tank, the syringe is pulled back to fill with gas from the gas bag. Because of a one-way valve distal to the syringe, only gas from the bag can be withdrawn. Another reversed one-way valve proximal to the syringe forces gas to travel only to the patient on injection. After assembly of the system, purging of the tubing with three syringe volumes (180 mL) of gas prevents the possibility of accidental injection of air. *(From Cronenwett JL, Johnston KW, editors. Rutherford's vascular surgery, ed 7, Philadelphia, 2010, Saunders, p 390, Fig. 18-5.)*

contained delivery system (e.g., Angioflush III fluid collection bag, AngioDynamics, Queensbury, N.Y.) that is flushed at least three times to remove room air in order to eliminate the risk of gas embolization (Fig. 2-2). Typically, the CO_2 delivery system consists of a 1500-mL plastic bag reservoir that is kept flaccid and has extension tubing, one-way check valves, and delivery and purge syringes. After the plastic bag reservoir is filled with CO_2 gas, the delivery syringe can be filled with noncompressed CO_2 so that a known volume of CO_2 can be injected. The purge syringe (3 mL) is used to completely fill the angiographic catheter with CO_2 and remove residual blood or saline. Proper positioning of stopcocks and functioning of check valves to maintain a closed system are necessary to limit room air contamination before delivery.

CO_2 is converted to bicarbonate when exposed to H_2O and is excreted by the lungs. There is no risk of allergic reaction or renal toxicity, and there is no maximum dose limit. The rate of dissolution of CO_2 is greater than that of oxygen, and clearance occurs after 2 to 3 minutes. Enough time should be allowed between injections to allow for complete elimination. One of the rare complications of CO_2 occurs when rapid repetitive injections cause "gas trapping" such that a CO_2 gas bubble prevents blood flow and causes distal ischemia. Vulnerable vessel beds

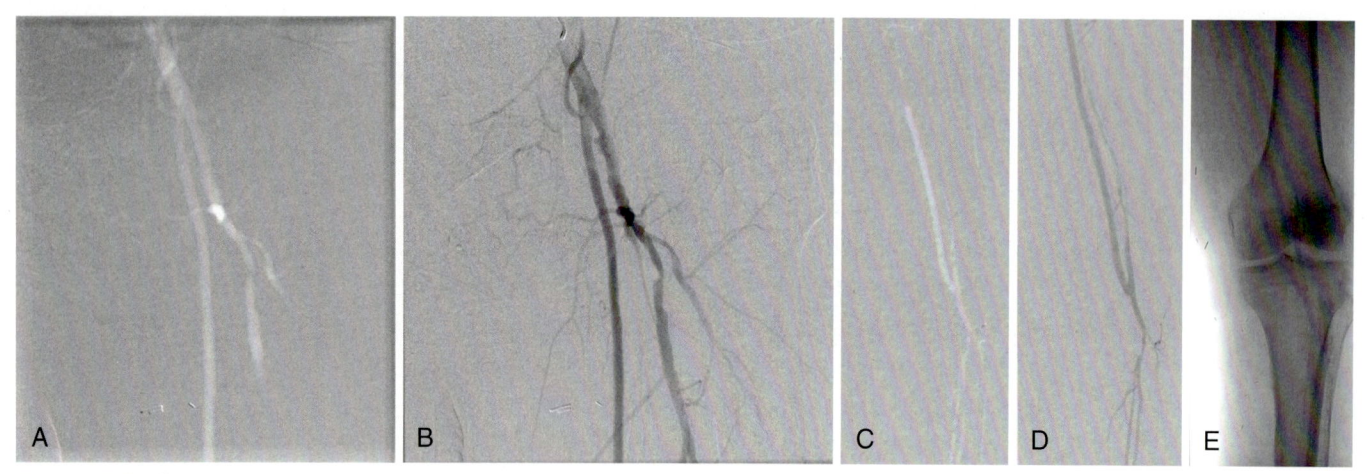

Figure 2-3. Selective lower extremity runoff with CO_2 angiography. A 55-year-old male with a renal transplant and serum creatinine of 3.5 mg/dl required an angiogram for a graft-threatening lesion identified by duplex ultrasound. **A**, A glide catheter is placed at the common femoral artery for imaging of the proximal anastomosis. CO_2 displacement generates fluoroscopic images that display vessel outlines as white. This can be digitally converted to grayscale and is usually depicted as black for filming purposes. **B**, An angiogram obtained with iodinated contrast diluted with saline (1:1). **C**, The distal anastomosis is visualized with CO_2 imaging. Some bubble artifact, as seen in the proximal vein graft and tibial outflow, may be observed with CO_2 administration. Computer stacking of an angiographic run overcomes this limitation. **D**, Subtracted angiogram of the distal anastomosis obtained with iodinated contrast diluted with saline (1:1) with (**E**) a corresponding nonsubtracted image.

are the inferior mesenteric artery and pulmonary artery, with gas trapping causing colonic ischemia and hypotension, respectively.

Two additional properties that affect the quality of imaging are compressibility and buoyancy. CO_2 is often compressed in the delivery syringe before injection because it improves the bolus of the injection. Priming catheters with CO_2 before injection may limit the tendency of the gas to rapidly expand as it exits the catheter in the form of an "explosive delivery," which may cause pain. Patient discomfort also occurs when CO_2 is injected in the lower extremities or visceral vessels and can be decreased by reducing both the volume of CO_2 and the number of injections (Fig. 2-3).

Buoyancy is also a characteristic that can be used to improve images. Because CO_2 is lighter than air, supine abdominal images provide good angiograms of the celiac and superior mesenteric artery anatomy. Lateral decubitus or 15- to 25-degree Trendelenburg positioning can also help improve flow to the renal and lower extremity arteries, respectively. Locally injected nitroglycerin is also useful because it causes vasodilation and improves CO_2 flow to the distal vessels. For vessels larger than 10 mm, such as the aorta or vena cava, buoyancy is a limitation that can cause incomplete luminal filling (Fig. 2-4).

CO_2 image quality can be improved by increasing the fluoroscopic data acquisition rate to 4 to 6 frame/sec and by using a 1024 × 1024 image intensifier. DSA can also be used to remove artifacts caused by movement, respiration, and bowel gas peristalsis. Administration of simethicone (125-mg oral tablet) before the procedure or glucagon (0.1 mg intravenously) during the procedure can also reduce bowel gas artifact. Stacking software that combines sequential image frames and adjusts image brightness and contrast may further improve images (see Box 2-3).

Intravascular Ultrasound

IVUS imaging permits tomographic visualization of a cross section through the vessel wall with a spatial resolution of 80 to 100 μm radially and 150 to 200 μm circumferentially. Current IVUS catheters, which are as small as 0.9 mm in diameter, permit the interrogation of vessels as small as 2 to 3 mm. Three-dimensional

GENERAL PRINCIPLES OF SEDATION, ANGIOGRAPHY, AND INTRAVASCULAR ULTRASOUND   27

Figure 2-4. **A**, Diagnostic CO_2 angiogram identifying a right renal artery stenosis in a patient, with serum creatinine of 4.6 mg/dl enabling renal artery access and placement of a sheath. **B**, Selective right renal artery angiogram with iodinated contrast, which allows for precise stent placement while minimizing contrast volume.

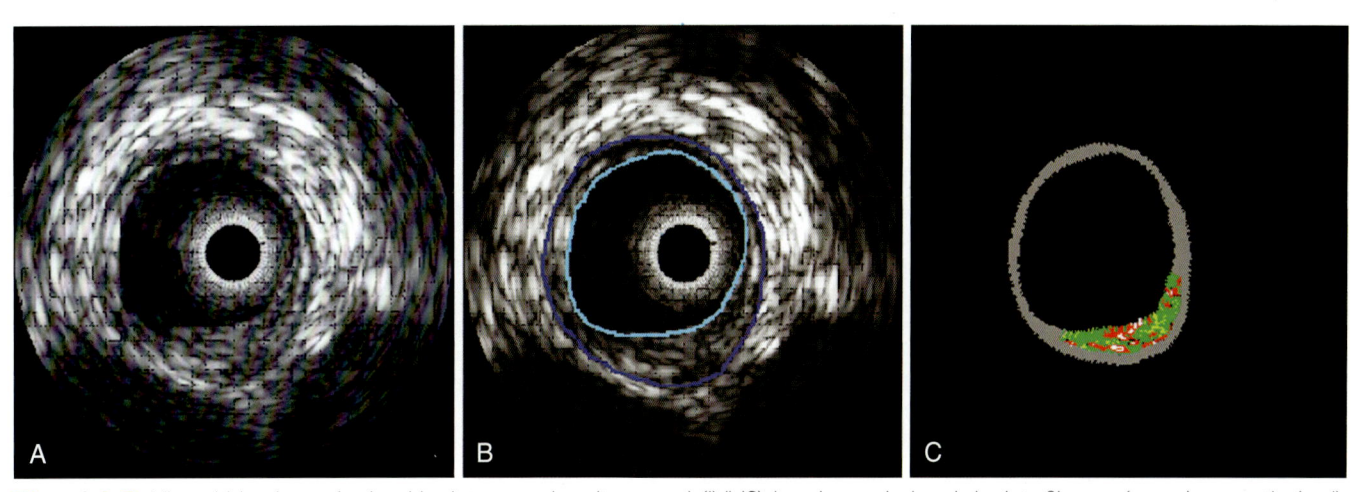

Figure 2-5. Virtual histology obtained by intravascular ultrasound (IVUS) is color-coded and depicts fibrous (green), necrotic (red), and calcific (white) areas based on a radiofrequency algorithm. **A**, IVUS image. **B**, Border analysis. **C**, Virtual histology.

information can be obtained during a pullback maneuver, while acquiring cross-sectional images along the length of the vessel.[22] The extent of atherosclerotic plaque is defined as the region between the medial-adventitial border and the luminal border.

As an example, the In-Vision Gold IVUS console (Volcano Corp., Rancho Cordova, Calif.) and the 3.5-Fr Eagle Eye phased array IVUS catheter tracks over a 0.014-inch guidewire and has a 20-MHz ultrasound probe that produces a 20-mm diameter image. The IVUS catheter is advanced beyond the lesion, and then imaging data are collected at 1 frame/sec using a Trak Back II pullback device at a motorized pullback rate of 0.5 mm/sec. Spectral profiles yield "virtual histology" with classification of atherosclerotic plaque morphology as fibrous, calcific, or necrotic (Fig. 2-5). IVUS has proved to be an important adjunct in the treatment of thoracic aortic dissection.

REFERENCES

1. dos Santos R, Lama A: Clada P: L'artériographie des membres, de l'aorte et des ses branches abdominales, *Bull Mem Soc Natl Chir* 55:587-601, 1929.
2. McClennan BL: Ionic and nonionic iodinated contrast media: Evolution and strategies for use, *Am J Roentgenol* 155:225-233, 1990.
3. Bom N, Lancee CT, van Egmond FC: An ultrasonic intracardiac scanner, *Ultrasonics* 10:72-76, 1972.
4. Gross JB, Bailey PL, Connis RT, et al: Practice guidelines for sedation and analgesia by non-anesthesiologists, *Anesthesiology* 96:1004-1017, 2002.

5. Standards and Intents for Sedation and Anesthesia Care. In Joint Commission on Accreditation of Healthcare Organizations, editor: *Revisions to Anesthesia Care Standards*, Oakbrook Terrace, Ill, 2001, Comprehensive Accreditation Manual for Hospitals. Available at http://www.jointcommission.org.
6. Beddoes L, Botti M, Duke MM: Patients' experiences of cardiology procedures using minimal conscious sedation, *Heart Lung* 37:196-204, 2008.
7. Bashore TM, Bates ER, Berger PB, et al: American College of Cardiology/Society for Cardiac Angiography and Interventions Clinical Expert Consensus Document on cardiac catheterization laboratory standards. A report of the American College of Cardiology Task Force on Clinical Expert Consensus Documents, *J Am Coll Cardiol* 37:2170-2214, 2001.
8. Limacher MC, Douglas PS, Germano G, et al: ACC expert consensus document: Radiation safety in the practice of cardiology. American College of Cardiology, *J Am Coll Cardiol* 31:892-913, 1998.
9. Arthurs ZM, Starnes BW, Sohn VY, et al: Ultrasound-guided access improves rate of access-related complications for totally percutaneous aortic aneurysm repair, *Ann Vasc Surg* 22:736-741, 2008.
10. Thomsen HS: Guidelines for contrast media from the European Society of Urogenital Radiology, *Am J Roentgenol* 181:1463-1471, 2003.
11. Morcos SK, Thomsen HS, Webb JA: Contrast-media-induced nephrotoxicity: A consensus report. Contrast Media Safety Committee, European Society of Urogenital Radiology (ESUR), *Eur Radiol* 9:1602-1613, 1999.
12. Merten GJ, Burgess WP, Gray LV, et al: Prevention of contrast-induced nephropathy with sodium bicarbonate: A randomized controlled trial, *JAMA* 291:2328-2334, 2004.
13. Birck R, Krzossok S, Markowetz F, et al: Acetylcysteine for prevention of contrast nephropathy: Meta-analysis, *Lancet* 362:598-603, 2003.
14. Trivedi H, Nadella R, Szabo A: Hydration with sodium bicarbonate for the prevention of contrast-induced nephropathy: A meta-analysis of randomized controlled trials, *Clin Nephrol* 74:288-296, 2010.
15. American College of Radiology: *Manual on contrast media*. Version 7.0 2010. Available at http://www.acr.org. Accessed February 22, 2011.
16. Levey AS, Coresh J, Balk E, et al: National Kidney Foundation practice guidelines for chronic kidney disease: Evaluation, classification, and stratification, *Ann Intern Med* 139:137-147, 2003.
17. Weisbord SD, Palevsky PM: Acute kidney injury: Intravenous fluid to prevent contrast-induced AKI, *Nat Rev Nephrol* 5:256-257, 2009.
18. Aspelin P, Aubry P, Fransson SG, et al: Nephrotoxic effects in high-risk patients undergoing angiography, *N Engl J Med* 348:491-499, 2003.
19. Heinrich MC, Haberle L, Muller V, et al: Nephrotoxicity of iso-osmolar iodixanol compared with nonionic low-osmolar contrast media: Meta-analysis of randomized controlled trials, *Radiology* 250:68-86, 2009.
20. Lasser EC, Berry CC, Talner LB, et al: Pretreatment with corticosteroids to alleviate reactions to intravenous contrast material, *N Engl J Med* 317:845-849, 1987.
21. Greenberger PA, Halwig JM, Patterson R, et al: Emergency administration of radiocontrast media in high-risk patients, *J Allergy Clin Immunol* 77:630-634, 1986.
22. Arthurs ZM, Bishop PD, Feiten LE, et al: Evaluation of peripheral atherosclerosis: A comparative analysis of angiography and intravascular ultrasound imaging, *J Vasc Surg* 51:933-938, 2010.

3 General Principles of Endovascular Therapy: Access Site Management

RAVISHANKAR HASANADKA • ROBERT B. McLAFFERTY

Historical Background

Throughout the 1940s and early 1950s, angiographic procedures required surgical exposure with placement of a blunt metal trocar and were often cumbersome and dangerous. A percutaneous approach was first described by Jönsson in 1949 with passage of a blunt trocar into the thoracic aorta via the common carotid artery.[1] Seldinger's report in 1953[2] was the first description of a soft, polyethylene catheter rather than a rigid metal trocar to achieve percutaneous access, which made the technique safer and, as a consequence, was widely adopted. With use of an introducer needle, followed by a "leader" or guidewire, a flexible catheter could be easily inserted into the artery or vein over a wire. This technique facilitated supine positioning of the patient, allowed repetitive contrast injections, and minimized bleeding at the access site. Subsequent development of catheters of different shapes allowed a range of angiographic imaging via the common femoral artery.

Indications

The common femoral artery is the most common axial vessel used to gain intravascular access for catheter-based procedures. This site allows wires and catheters to be placed in the aorta, as well as branch vessels to lower and upper extremities, renal and visceral vessels, and cerebral arteries. For atherosclerotic occlusive and aneurysmal disease, angiography is usually reserved for patients in whom delineation of the arterial anatomy and related vascular pathology is required for evaluation and treatment.

Although atherosclerotic occlusive disease remains the most common problem treated in the endovascular suite, less common indications for angiography via a common femoral artery access site include treatment of gastrointestinal bleeding, traumatic arterial injuries, arteriovenous fistulas, pseudoaneurysms and true aneurysms, arteriovenous malformations, tumor chemoembolization, and symptomatic uterine fibroids.

Although less common since the advent of duplex ultrasonography, historically, axial veins had been used as access sites for ascending and descending phlebography to evaluate lower extremity venous insufficiency and deep venous thrombosis. With the development of a growing array of catheter-based approaches for disorders of the venous system, the site for venous access is selected based on the task. For example, selected access points may include the common femoral, femoral, popliteal, posterior tibial, great saphenous, small saphenous, dorsal pedal, median antecubital, brachial, basilic, axillary, subclavian, and internal jugular veins. Common indications for percutaneous access via an axial vein includes placement and retrieval of inferior vena cava filters, as well as treatment of acute thrombosis of the femoral-popliteal, iliofemoral, and axillary-subclavian veins.

Somewhat less common indications include treatment of chronic venous obstruction with angioplasty and stenting, pelvic congestion treated with sclerotherapy and embolization, pulmonary arteriography for diagnostic and therapeutic intervention, portal vein hypertension with transjugular intrahepatic portosystemic shunting, and venous blood sampling of adrenal and renal veins.

General Considerations for Access

ACCESS SITE

The location of the planned diagnostic or therapeutic intervention dictates the selection of left- or right-sided access sites, as well as the choice of an antegrade or retrograde approach in which access is obtained with the intent of passing a catheter in the same direction as or opposite to blood flow, respectively. The farther the planned task is from the access site, the less responsive catheters and wires may be in performing the procedure. This factor, as well as characteristics of the vascular pathway, including the presence of tortuosity, dilated or aneurysmal regions, and stenotic, calcified, compressed, or thrombosed segments, may also influence the selected access site. Other considerations include vessel diameter in relation to the diameter of the catheter required for the procedure, local vascular disease, scarring around the access site, and body habitus.

COAGULATION

Review of the patient's history, including use of medications, should be performed to assess risk of bleeding or thrombosis. For example, patients with renal failure, liver insufficiency, or other bleeding diatheses may need ultrasound guidance or use of a micropuncture needle. Likewise, repletion with appropriate blood products or use of a closure or compression device may be required upon completing the procedure.

The American College of Chest Physicians proposed guidelines for antithrombotic prophylaxis in patients receiving warfarin therapy with different risk factors (Tables 3-1 and 3-2). If the annual risk for thromboembolism is low, warfarin therapy can be withheld for 4 to 5 days before a procedure without "bridging" with therapeutic subcutaneous low-molecular-weight heparin or intravenous unfractionated heparin. Bridging anticoagulation is recommended in patients with a history of a mechanical heart valve, atrial fibrillation, or venous thromboembolism who are at high risk for thromboembolism (e.g., known thrombophilia or hypercoagulable state, rheumatic atrial fibrillation, or arterial or venous thromboembolism within preceding 1-3 months) or moderate risk for thromboembolism (e.g., thromboembolism within preceding 6 months or atrial fibrillation with ejection fraction of less than 40% and valvular heart disease). Bridging therapy with low-molecular-weight heparin would need to be stopped 24 hours before the procedure. Bridging therapy has been associated with an increased risk of bleeding, including pseudoaneurysm formation after arterial puncture.[3]

Patients who have had placement of a bare metal coronary stent within 6 weeks should have aspirin and clopidogrel continued during the periprocedural period. Likewise, continuing aspirin and clopidogrel is recommended if a drug-eluting coronary stent has been placed within the previous 12 months. Indeed, patients may be loaded with antiplatelet medications to minimize the risk of platelet thrombus formation if femoral, renal, or carotid angioplasty and stenting are anticipated.

LABORATORY TESTING

Basic testing should include an international normalized ratio (INR), a complete blood count to assess hemoglobin level and platelet count, and a serum creatinine to assess overall renal function.

TABLE 3-1 Patients Who Should Receive Bridging Heparin: Risk for Thromboembolism

High	Moderate	Low
Inherited thrombophilia	Arterial or venous thromboembolism within 3-6 mo	Arterial or venous thromboembolism after >6 mo
Unknown hypercoagulable state	Atrial fibrillation with multiple risk factors for embolism (e.g., ejection fraction less than 40%, diabetes, hypertension, valvular heart disease)	Atrial fibrillation without multiple risk factors for embolism
Arterial or venous thromboembolism within 3 mo	Mechanical heart valve in aortic position	
Rheumatic atrial fibrillation		
Atrial fibrillation with history of embolism		
Mechanical heart valve in mitral position		
Intracardiac thrombus		

Adapted from Jaffer AK, Brotman DJ, Chukwumerije N: When patients on warfarin need surgery. *Cleveland Clinic J Med* 70:973-984, 2003.

TABLE 3-2 Protocol for Low-Molecular-Weight Heparin as a Bridge for Patients on Warfarin

Before Procedure	After Procedure
If preoperative INR is 2-3:	
Stop warfarin 5 days before procedure	Restart low-molecular-weight heparin 24 hr after procedure
If preoperative INR is 3-4.5:	
Stop warfarin 6 days before procedure	Restart warfarin 24 hr after procedure
Start low-molecular-weight heparin 36 hr after last warfarin as follows:	Daily PT and INR until INR is in therapeutic range
Enoxaparin (Lovenox) 1 mg/kg SC q12h *or*	Discontinue low-molecular-weight heparin when INR is between 2 and 3
Enoxaparin (Lovenox) 1.5 mg/kg q24h	
Dalteparin (Fragmin) 120 unit/kg SC q12h *or*	
Dalteparin (Fragmin) 200 unit/kg SC q24h	
Give last dose of low-molecular-weight heparin 24 hr before procedure	
Ensure that INR is <1.8 prior to initiating procedure	

Adapted from Jaffer AK, Brotman DJ, Chukwumerije N: When patients on warfarin need surgery. *Cleveland Clinic J Med* 70:973-984, 2003.
INR, International normalized ratio; *PT*, prothrombin time; *SC*, subcutaneously.

PATIENT POSITIONING

Each area of the body that needs to be accessed percutaneously requires specific positioning to optimize success. Access to vessels in the femoral region requires the patient be in the supine position with arms to the side. A large abdominal panniculus should be taped so that it pulls the abdominal skin and adipose tissue superiorly to expose the groin area. Access in the popliteal fossa requires the patient be in the prone position. Access to the posterior tibial vessels requires the patient be in the supine position with the knee slightly flexed and externally rotated. Access to the brachial region requires the arm to be positioned perpendicular to the body. For access to the axillary region, the patient is best positioned by putting the hand behind the head. Access to the jugular vein is facilitated by elevating the patient's shoulders to extend the neck, placing the patient in the Trendelenburg position, and turning the patient's head away from the intended puncture site.

ANESTHESIA

The large majority of patients undergoing catheter-based procedures require short-acting intravenous sedatives, pain management with small doses of short-acting narcotics, and administration of local anesthesia at the access site. The importance of managing these three regimens cannot be underestimated in obtaining safe percutaneous access. With the exception of initial pain from injection of local anesthesia, obtaining access to axial vessels should be anxiety and pain free. Patients not meeting these criteria are more difficult to access because they may move suddenly and the potential for incomplete diagnosis, treatment, or avoidable errors is increased as a result of the operator's desire to then rush through the procedure. A small minority of patients require general anesthesia as a result of overwhelming anxiety, prolonged procedure time, inability to remain immobile during the procedure, or anticipated pain that may be difficult to tolerate. Conversely, the rare patient who may not be able to tolerate intravenous sedation, such as a frail elderly patient or one with sleep apnea, may be better served with local anesthesia alone.

ULTRASOUND GUIDANCE

Ultrasound guidance is a common adjunct to percutaneous access of axial vessels and is mandatory for accessing vessels that cannot be easily palpated. These include virtually all commonly accessed veins in the extremities. Other indications include obesity and edema or when accessing the jugular vein or an axillary or proximal brachial artery, where there may be an increased risk of injury to adjacent structures.

Direct visualization of the needle entering an axial vessel using ultrasound requires anticipation and timing of where the needle will be in relation to the depth of the vessel. When the transverse view is used for access, the point of skin puncture varies in terms of its distance from the ultrasound probe. This means that as the vessel becomes deeper, the distance between the needle puncture and where the ultrasound probe lay on the skin increases (Fig. 3-1). Conversely, use of the longitudinal view of the ultrasound probe requires meticulous attention to maintaining the needle constantly in a single plane of view for direct visualization. Central to both techniques is the need for slow hand adjustments when using the ultrasound probe.

Basic Strategies for Commonly Accessed Vessels

COMMON FEMORAL ARTERY

Access to the common femoral artery serves as a model for many other arterial access points. Although retrograde or antegrade access to the common femoral artery may be obtained, most commonly, retrograde access is used to assess arterial inflow to both lower extremities and to facilitate crossing over the aortic bifurcation to assess and treat any pathologic conditions in the contralateral leg.

The anatomic landmarks of the pubic tubercle and the anterior superior iliac spine mark the line of the inguinal ligament. The common femoral artery traverses inferiorly and deep to the ligament and is located one third the distance from the pubic tubercle to the anterior superior iliac spine. Palpation of the pulse can often be significantly distal to the common femoral artery in that the groin skinfold is often located more inferior to the inguinal ligament. The femoral head of the femur represents a landmark for locating the point where the common femoral artery should be punctured (Fig. 3-2). By placing a hemostat clamp on the skin over the center of the femoral head using fluoroscopy, the physician can then palpate the common femoral artery pulse in the correct position for arterial access.

For patients with a normal pulse and no previous surgery in the groin, a standard 18-gauge needle is commonly used for puncturing the artery (Fig. 3-3). A standard 0.035-inch J wire is advanced through the needle into the artery under direct fluoroscopic view. Occasionally, if the wire will not pass, very small changes in angulation or turning the needle slightly to change the position of the bevel facilitates wire passage. If difficulty persists but pulsatile flow from the needle is present, then a straight wire with a floppy tip may better traverse the artery than a J wire. Wires should always pass freely and never be forced or buckled, and constant visualization using fluoroscopy remains paramount to preventing iatrogenic injury. After the wire is in its proper position, the needle is removed and a sheath placed under fluoroscopic visualization while the wire is pinned.

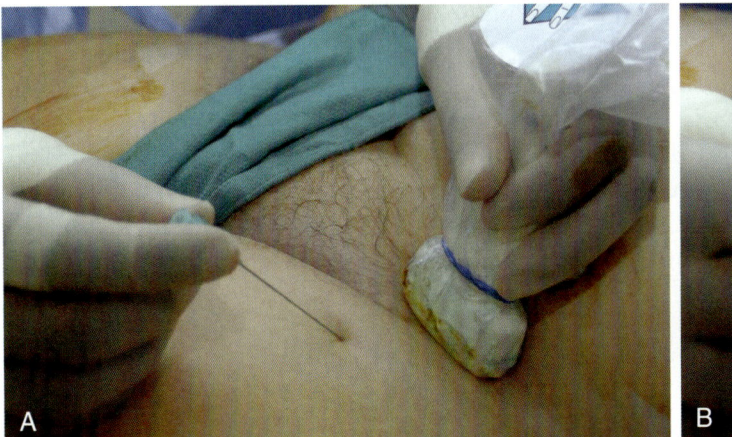

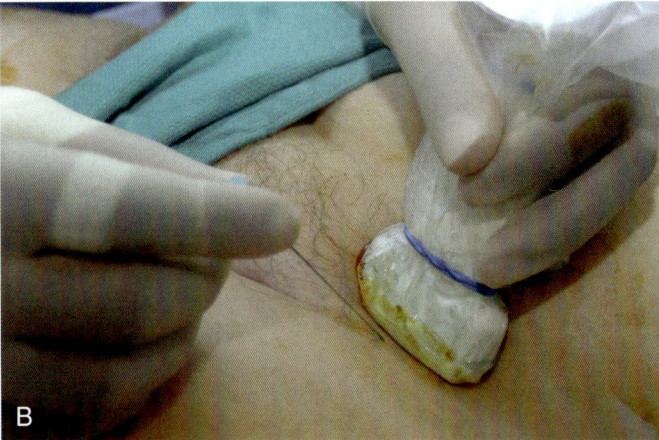

Figure 3-1. Relative positioning of the ultrasound probe and arterial entry needle. **A,** Retrograde access of the left common femoral artery is achieved by positioning the entry needle several centimeters away from the ultrasound probe. The path of visualization of the ultrasound probe should intersect with the trajectory of the needle and the common femoral artery. **B,** If the entry needle is placed too close to the ultrasound probe, access requires the needle to be positioned almost 90 degrees to the skin, which is not favorable for passing either subsequent guidewires or sheaths.

Figure 3-2. Position of the common femoral arteries over the femoral heads. The femoral artery should be punctured 1 cm lateral to the most medial cortex of the femoral head for either retrograde or antegrade femoral artery catheterizations. To avoid parallax, the femoral head should be centered in the field of view and rotation of the patient's pelvis on the angiography table avoided. Visualization of a calcific blood vessel can also help guide successful puncture when the femoral pulse is weak or absent. *(From Cronenwett JL, Johnston KW, editors: Rutherford's vascular surgery, ed 7, Philadelphia, 2010, Saunders, p 1270, Fig. 84-9.)*

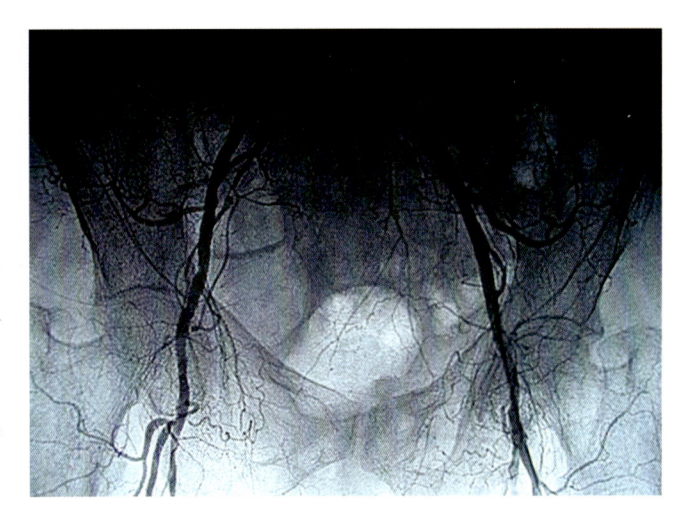

Figure 3-3. Double-wall and single-wall puncture techniques. A double-wall puncture needle (left) and three single-wall puncture needles (right) are shown. Double-wall puncture needles are two-component systems that combine a blunt-tipped hollow needle with a bevel-tipped stylet, which projects slightly from the end of the needle. The double-wall puncture technique involves the intentional passage of the needle-stylet assembly through both walls of the vessel until it contacts the underlying bone. The stylet is removed, and the outer needle is slowly withdrawn until blood return is noted. Single-wall needles are single-component systems in which the needle is advanced toward the target vessel until the anterior wall of the vessel is punctured and pulsatile blood flow is noted. For venous punctures, gentle aspiration of an attached syringe may be necessary to confirm entry into the target vein. Once blood return is confirmed, the needle is stabilized, and a guidewire advanced through the needle. *(From Cronenwett JL, Johnston KW, editors: Rutherford's vascular surgery, ed 7, Philadelphia, 2010, Saunders, p 1270, Fig. 84-1.)*

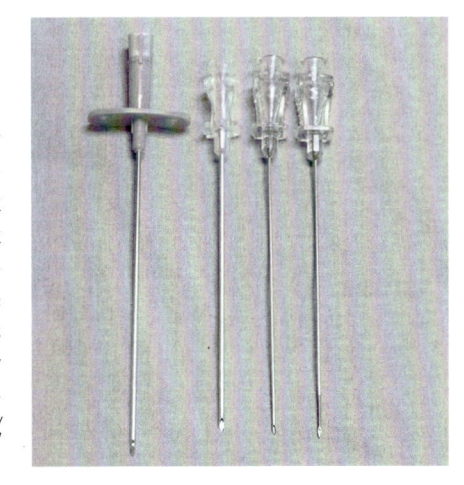

BRACHIAL ARTERY

Although either brachial artery can be accessed depending on the endovascular task at hand, most often the left brachial artery is used to avoid the risk of cerebral embolization that might exist by the presence of guidewire, sheaths, or catheters crossing the orifices of the innominate and left common carotid arteries. Given the smaller size of a brachial artery, a micropuncture needle kit should be used

(Fig. 3-4). With the arm abducted 60 to 90 degrees, the pulse is palpated in the antecubital fossa and access is obtained just proximal to the crease of the elbow. Following blood return through the needle, a 0.018-inch curved wire with a floppy tip is advanced retrograde under fluoroscopic imaging. Flow through a 21-gauge needle is often not pulsatile, and if the wire will not easily advance, subtle movements with the needle to redirect the wire tip may be helpful. With the wire tip in the axillary artery, the needle is exchanged for a transition introducer sheath. The inner dilator is removed along with the 0.018-inch wire, which is exchanged for a 0.035-inch guidewire. The outer transition introducer can then be exchanged for the desired sheath.

AXILLARY ARTERY

Unlike the brachial artery, the axillary artery allows placement of a sheath of up to 7 to 8 Fr, and as this access site is closer to the central circulation, its use may assist in the treatment of remote target lesions, such as those in the popliteal artery. The arm needs to be abducted at 90 degrees and externally rotated, with a towel roll placed under the axilla. Alternatively, the axillary region may be exposed by flexing the arm at the elbow and placing the hand behind or just above the head. A micropuncture needle access kit is recommended for access.

ARTERIAL BYPASS GRAFTS

The configuration of an arterial bypass graft can limit whether a retrograde or an antegrade access approach can be achieved and may dictate contralateral access or access from the left arm. For example, at the level of the common femoral artery, bypass grafts may include aortofemoral, axillofemoral, and femoral-femoral grafts, as well as grafts between the femoral and a distal artery in the lower extremity. An axillofemoral bypass is best accessed over the chest wall or the iliac crest to allow for manual compression of the puncture site against these bony landmarks. Similarly, a femoral-femoral bypass can be accessed over the common femoral hood or in the midline over the pubic bone.

INTERNAL JUGULAR VEIN

The internal jugular vein can be accessed using an anterior or posterior approach. In the anterior approach, the patient is supine and in a slight Trendelenburg position, with the neck extended and the head turned toward the opposite side of access. The area to access begins at the apex of a triangle formed by the two heads of the sternocleidomastoid muscle, with the vein medial to the carotid artery pulse. Ultrasound is used to identify the site of puncture, and the position, angle, and depth of the jugular vein are defined using a 22-gauge, 1.5-inch "finder" needle attached to a syringe for gentle aspiration. This vein is then accessed with a larger 18-gauge, 2-inch needle followed by passage of a guidewire. Patients with a history of multiple catheter placements should undergo duplex ultrasonography to exclude the presence of a diminutive or thrombosed vein.

Patient positioning is identical when accessing the internal jugular vein using the posterior approach. Anatomic landmarks include the course of the sternocleidomastoid muscle and the external jugular vein. When ultrasound guidance is used, a 22-gauge finder needle is directed just superior to where the external jugular vein crosses the posterior edge of the sternocleidomastoid muscle, typically one third the distance cephalad from the clavicular insertion of the sternocleidomastoid muscle. The needle is directed to the sternal notch.

COMMON FEMORAL VEIN

Positioning and anatomic landmarks to access the common femoral vein are identical to those used to access the common femoral artery, with the needle positioned medial to the arterial pulse. Because of the supine position and variance in volume status, the access needle may puncture both the anterior and posterior

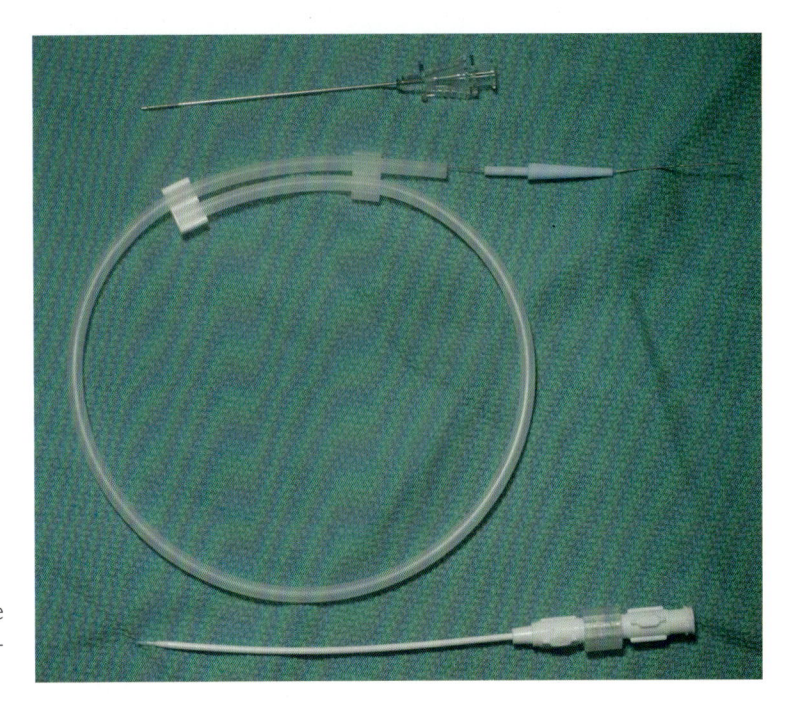

Figure 3-4. Micropuncture kit. Components include a 21-gauge needle, a 0.018-inch wire, and a microintroducer sheath (AngioDynamics, Latham, N.Y.).

walls of the vein. Gentle aspiration using a syringe on withdrawal of the needle confirms intraluminal positioning by a flash of venous blood.

BRACHIAL AND BASILIC VEINS

Access to either the brachial or the basilic veins requires 90-degree abduction of the upper extremity (Video 3-1). One or two towels placed under the triceps displace the posteromedial portion of the upper arm anteriorly for ease of access. The brachial vein runs parallel to the brachial artery. The basilic vein is more superficial and located within the posteromedial aspect of the upper arm. Access of the brachial or basilic veins requires ultrasound guidance and the use of a micropuncture needle access kit. Use of an aspiration syringe is not helpful given the veins' small diameter and collapsible thin walls.

POPLITEAL AND POSTERIOR TIBIAL VEINS

Access to the popliteal vein between the two heads of the gastrocnemius muscle requires prone positioning of the patient with use of a micropuncture needle. Two popliteal veins often course medial and lateral to the popliteal artery.

Access to the posterior tibial vein requires the patient be supine with the leg externally rotated and the knee slightly flexed. Access can occur along any point of the posterior tibial vein from the calf to the ankle. Paired tibial veins can be present on either side of the posterior tibial artery; therefore visualization of needle entry by ultrasound is an essential step in gaining access.

Strategies for the Difficult Groin

OBESITY

The groin crease in obese patients is often distal to the inguinal ligament and lies over the superficial femoral and profunda femoral arteries. Retracting the panniculus superiorly using adhesive tape, along with fluoroscopy to locate the center of the femoral head, can assist in locating the common femoral artery. The patulous nature of the skin and fatty tissue can also increase the difficulty of passing a sheath over a standard J wire. Use of a stiffened wire, such as an Amplatz Super Stiff Guidewire (Boston Scientific, Natick, Mass.), along with a longer sheath, can help relieve this problem. Personnel performing compression after removal of the sheath should be made aware of where to specifically compress the artery.

SCARRED GROIN

Patients who have had recent surgery in the groin should not undergo percutaneous access in the vicinity of the incision, and those with scarring from remote surgery often require modification of the standard technique. Because scarring can make it difficult to push a sheath over the wire, use of a stiff wire and serial dilation of the scar tissue is often helpful. A 2- to 3-mm incision should be made around the wire, followed by dilation of the outer portion of the tract with a hemostatic clamp and then serial exchanges over an Amplatz wire of introducers from 4- and 5-Fr sheaths. A twisting motion of the introducers close to the skin may help dilate the tract but should not be used once the sheath is in the vessel because of the risk of intimal dissection.

CALCIFICATION

Fluoroscopy may reveal one of two calcification patterns. Calcification of the medial arterial layer, which is observed in chronic end-stage renal failure, outlines the vessel and is not typically associated with significant stenosis. A second pattern is characterized by large, calcified irregularities in the intimal region of femoral and popliteal arteries and may be associated with significant stenosis. When the latter is suspected, percutaneous access to the affected common femoral artery should be avoided or, if necessary, accessed with a micropuncture needle access kit using ultrasound guidance.

PULSELESSNESS

Access of the pulseless femoral artery may be required to recanalize an occluded or stenotic iliac artery. Ultrasound guidance can be used, and angiography from the contralateral common femoral artery can be used to create a road map of the vessel.

Compression and Closure Devices

MANUAL COMPRESSION TECHNIQUE

Using a single piece of folded gauze held against the skin, two to three fingers apply firm point pressure, with the other hand placed on top applying equivalent pressure, for at least 15 minutes without interruption. Early inspection only increases the chances of hemorrhage from quick dissolution of the forming platelet plug. Focal pressure for up to 30 minutes may be required after removal of 7-Fr or larger sheaths or in the presence of a heavily calcified vessel. Manual compression after venous access usually requires 5 to 10 minutes of pressure.

BLOOD PRESSURE

Systolic blood pressure should be less than 160 mm Hg before removing a sheath. If necessary, intravenous administration of labetalol, hydralazine, or nitroglycerin—or rarely, sodium nitroprusside—can be administered (Table 3-3).

ANTICOAGULATION

If intravenous heparin has been administered, the anticoagulant effect may be reversed with protamine sulfate, with dosing dependent on the time of planned catheter removal. An activated clotting time (ACT) of less than 150 to 200 seconds

TABLE 3-3 Intravenous Medications for Periprocedural Blood Pressure Control

Medications	Dose	Comments
Labetalol hydrochloride	10 mg IV (0.25 mg/kg)	May repeat every 10 min
Hydralazine hydrochloride	10-20 mg IV	Repeat every 6 hr
Nitroglycerin	5 mcg/min	May increase by 5 mcg/min every 3-5 min
Sodium nitroprusside	0.3 mcg/kg/min	May increase every 1-3 min

IV, Intravenously.

is often reported in protocols for sheath removal, but ACT levels may depend on the instrument type, how it has been calibrated, and whether venous or arterial blood has been used.

ACTIVITY RESTRICTIONS

After manual compression of a common femoral artery puncture, bed rest for 6 hours with minimal hip and knee flexion is recommended. If a closure device is used, bed rest requirements range from 2 to 4 hours, depending on the nature of the procedure and the diameter of the sheath. After a brachial artery puncture, the arm should be immobilized on an arm board with a simple pressure dressing for 4 to 6 hours. After sheath removal from large axial veins, immobilization for 1 to 2 hours before resuming activity is sufficient. Patients should be restricted to light activity for the next 24 hours.

EXTERNAL COMPRESSION DEVICES

A C-clamp type device (CompressAR StrongArm, Advanced Vascular Dynamics, Portland, Ore.) can be used as an alternative to manual compression (Fig. 3-5, *A*). The device has a focal clamp that slides down onto the groin, with counterforce applied by the larger side of the device, which is placed under the ipsilateral hip. A compression assist device (FemoStop Gold, St. Jude Medical, St. Paul, Minn.) applies femoral artery compression by wrapping a belt around the body and inflating a dome to provide moderate focal pressure at 60 to 80 mm Hg (Fig. 3-5, *B*). The sheath is then removed, and the device is inflated to 20 mm Hg above systolic blood pressure for up to 3 minutes. Pressure is then lowered until a palpable distal pulse is noted. The pressure is reduced by 20 mm Hg at 2 hours and again at 4 hours, followed by a reduction to 30 mm Hg for the last 2 hours of bed rest. Close surveillance is necessary to ensure that the device is not inadvertently dislodged.

ARTERIAL CLOSURE DEVICES

The intent of percutaneous closure devices is to minimize manual compression time and allow earlier return to ambulation. In all instances, location of the puncture site should be assessed fluoroscopically before the deployment of the device. Significant arterial calcification or the presence of an exceedingly small common femoral artery should preclude the use of arterial closure devices. Common devices used for closure of the common femoral artery are described.

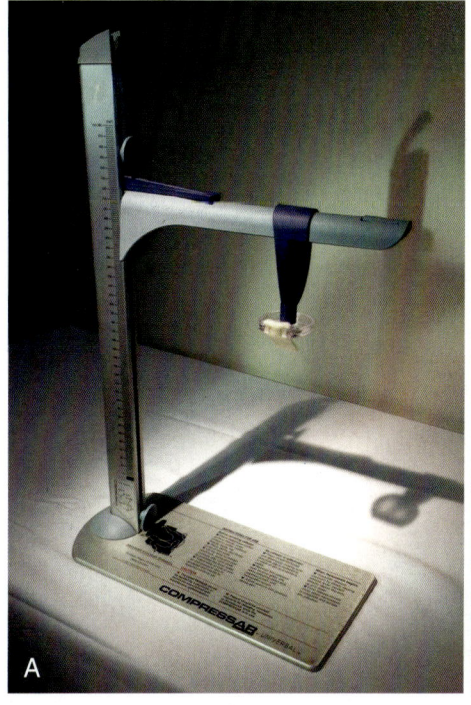

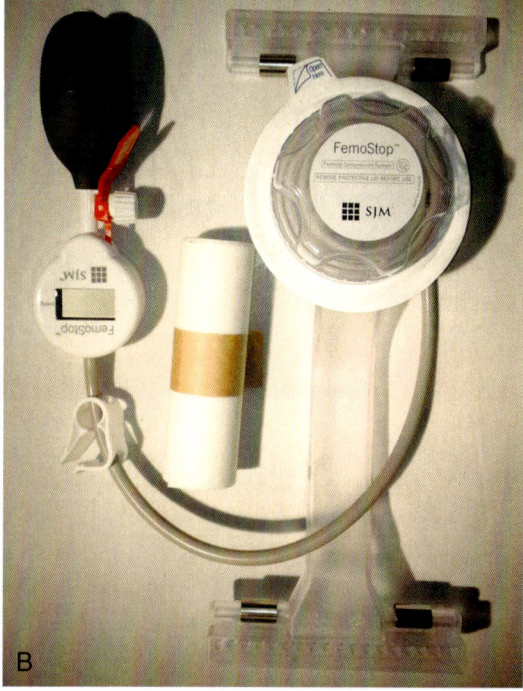

Figure 3-5. External compression devices. **A**, The CompressAR StrongArm device. A disc is positioned over the femoral artery for constant pressure. **B**, The FemoStop Gold compression assist device. The transparent, inflatable dome is positioned over the femoral artery with pressure adjusted using a digital manometer.

The Angio-Seal device (St. Jude Medical) is designed for closure of puncture sites produced by a 6- to 8-Fr sheath (Fig. 3-6). Deployed over a J wire, the device sandwiches the arterial wall with an absorbable copolymer plate on the inside of the artery and a collagen plug on the outside of the vessel wall. The device can cause an inflammatory response, which may increase the difficulty of subsequent dissection, if surgery is performed within 6 to 12 weeks of use.

The StarClose device (Abbott Vascular, Abbott Park, Ill.) is designed for closure of puncture sites produced by 5- to 6-Fr sheaths (Fig. 3-7). The device is placed into a specifically designed interlocking 6-Fr sheath, and a nitinol clip closes the adventitia and a portion of the media wall.

The Perclose device (Abbott Vascular) can be used for closure of arterial punctures ranging from 5 to 8 Fr (Fig. 3-8). The device places an absorbable polyester suture within the arterial wall, using two needles that access the artery on either side of the arteriotomy. A knot pusher then cinches the knot through the puncture site.

Vascular Complications

Local vascular complications resulting from percutaneous access may result in hematoma, pseudoaneurysm, dissection, thrombosis, and arteriovenous fistula.[3] Although most hematomas do not require intervention, even small collections of blood several centimeters in diameter can cause pain as a result of stretching the skin or compressing the femoral nerve.[4] Hematomas may also appear small when, in fact, they are quite large. If the external iliac artery is punctured and hemorrhage ensues, a very large retroperitoneal hematoma that tracks along the psoas muscle may result. Patients may have persistent hypotension without evidence of a groin hematoma. Palpation of the lower lateral abdominal wall often elicits tenderness, and a discernible fullness is present. If suspicion is high, immediate resuscitation and intervention are recommended. Otherwise, computed tomography confirms the diagnosis. Large groin hematomas, which produce substantial pain or threaten skin viability, require surgical decompression. Femoral mononeuropathy from compression by a hematoma may manifest as medial leg and calf numbness and

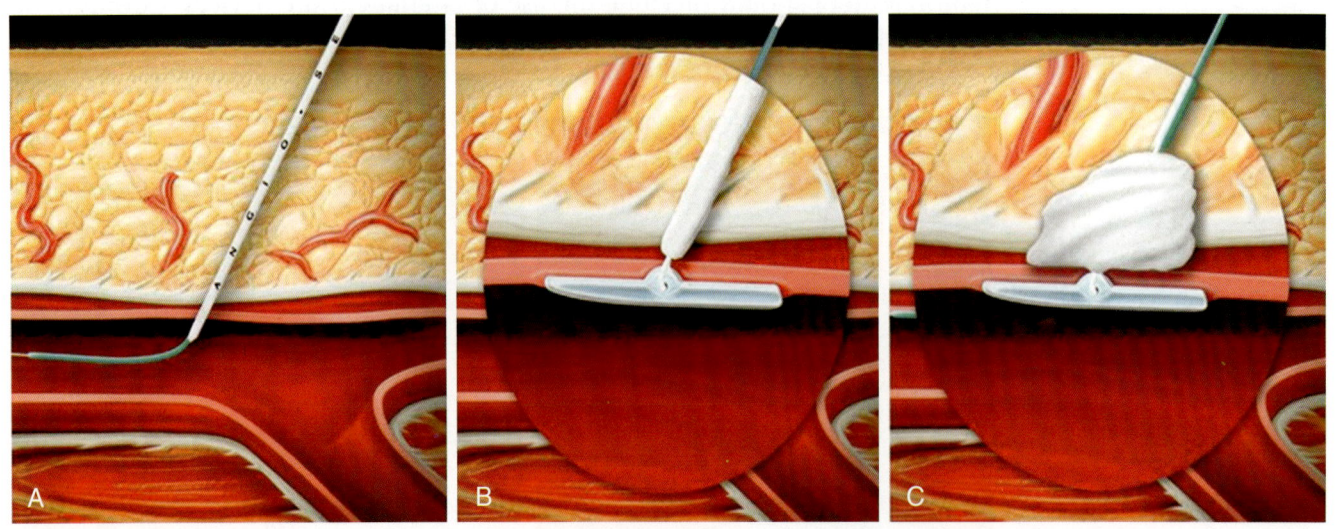

Figure 3-6. Deployment of the Angio-Seal closure device. **A**, The Angio-Seal sheath is placed within the vessel via the existing guidewire. It is advanced until blood flows out through the exit hole in the dilator, as shown. It is then withdrawn until blood flow ceases and is again advanced until the blood flow restarts. **B**, The locator and guidewire are removed. The Angio-Seal is inserted fully into the sheath with the two arrows on the sheath and the device assembly meeting. The anchor is then released beyond the sheath tip. The barrel of the device is retracted with a double "click," and the whole assembly is then withdrawn. The anchor is fixed against the inside of the vessel by gentle traction. A tamper becomes visible on the suture as the sheath is removed. **C**, Once fully visible, the tamper is advanced forward to tie a knot over the collagen plug, which becomes compressed against the puncture site. The suture is then cut above the tamper, and the tamper is removed. *(From Bechara CF, Annambhotla S, Lin PH: Access site management with vascular closure devices for percutaneous transarterial procedures. J Vasc Surg 52:1682-1696, 2010, Fig. 1.)*

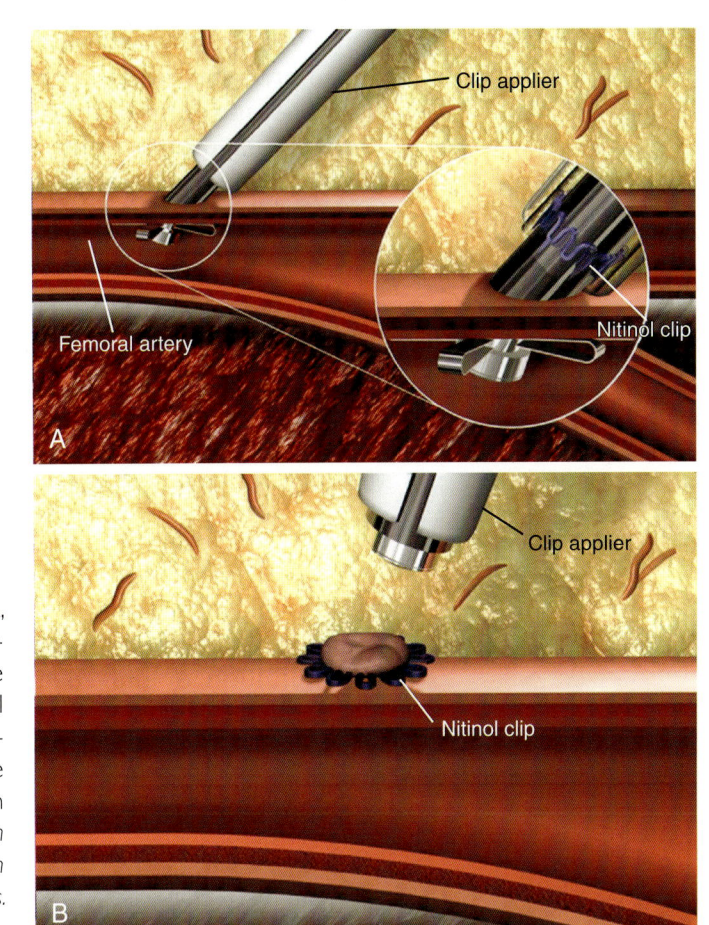

Figure 3-7. Deployment of the StarClose closure device. **A**, The sheath is introduced first over a wire, and then the StarClose device is inserted into the sheath after wire removal. The vessel locator button is depressed. The device is pulled out until resistance is felt. The advancement of the thumb advancer completes the splitting of the sheath. The device is raised to an angle of slightly less than 90 degrees. **B**, The clip is deployed to catch adventitia for hemostasis, and the device is retracted. *(From Bechara CF, Annambhotla S, Lin PH: Access site management with vascular closure devices for percutaneous transarterial procedures. J Vasc Surg 52:1682-1696, 2010, Fig. 7.)*

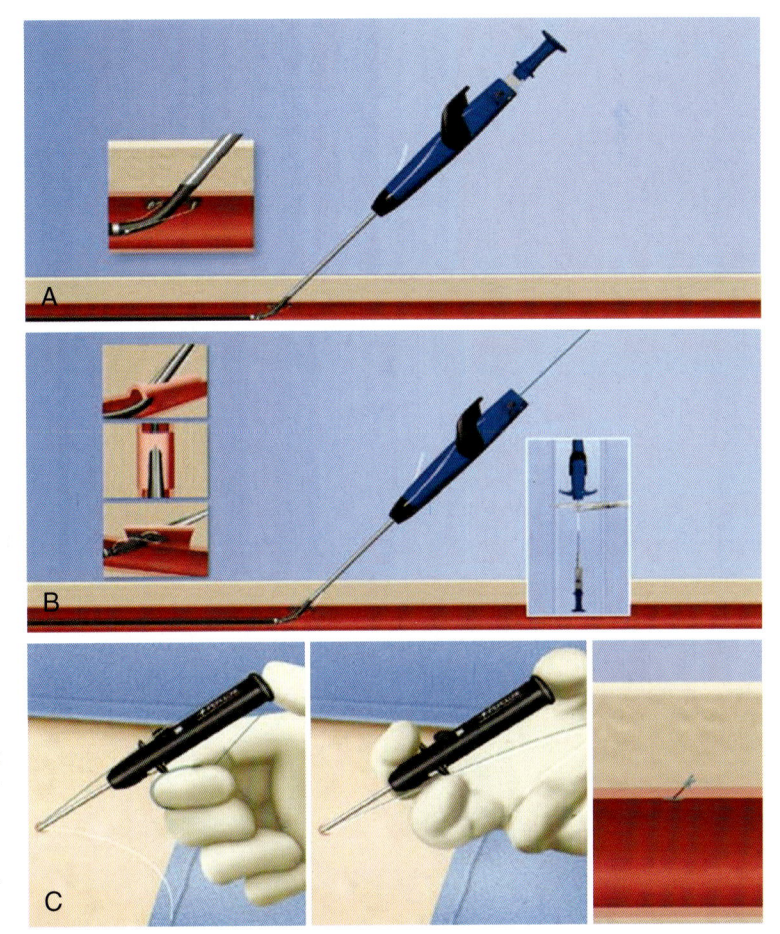

Figure 3-8. Deployment of the Perclose closure device. **A**, Insertion and positioning of the 6-Fr Perclose device over the wire into the femoral access site until pulsatile flow through the marker lumen is seen, indicating an adequate intraluminal device position. **B**, Deployment of the foot and positioning against the arterial wall by pulling the device upward in preparation for needle deployment. Sutures are deployed around the arteriotomy and are pulled from the device outside the skin. **C**, The pretied knot is pushed down using the knot pusher that comes with the device. Once hemostasis is achieved, the suture is cut using a knot cutter. The final suture lies securely around the arteriotomy to achieve hemostasis. *(From Bechara CF, Annambhotla S, Lin PH: Access site management with vascular closure devices for percutaneous transarterial procedures. J Vasc Surg 52:1682-1696, 2010, Fig. 5.)*

weakness of the quadriceps muscle. A hematoma after brachial artery access can compress the median nerve, causing weakness of the forearm flexors and the first and second lumbrical muscles of the hand, as well as numbness on the palmar side of the thumb, index, and middle fingers and lateral portion of the hand.[5]

A pseudoaneurysm should be suspected if a hematoma is "pulsatile" or continued expansion and persistent pain are noted. Independent risk factors for pseudoaneurysm include hypertension and obesity.[6-8]

Changes in distal perfusion status, along with new-onset limb pain, paresthesias, claudication, or change in pulse status, should suggest the possibility of dissection, thrombosis, or embolization. Delay in the evaluation even in the presence of a Doppler signal could contribute to eventual limb loss. Thrombosis of a major axial vein can manifest as local limb swelling, pain, or pulmonary embolism. Prompt evaluation and treatment are necessary.

An arteriovenous fistula is identified by the presence of a bruit and thrill on physical examination but may not be recognized until well after the procedure. Although most arteriovenous fistulas are asymptomatic and do not necessarily require treatment, a large arteriovenous fistula can lead to congestive heart failure, claudication, or limb edema. Ipsilateral distal pulses may be diminished or absent on examination.

REFERENCES

1. Jönsson G: Thoracic aortography by means of a cannula inserted percutaneously into the common carotid artery, *Acta Radiol* 31:376, 1949.
2. Seldinger SI: Catheter replacement of the needle in percutaneous arteriography: A new technique, *Acta Radiol* 39:368-376, 1953.
3. Waksman R, King SB, Douglas JS, et al: Predictors of groin complications after balloon and new-device coronary intervention, *Am J Cardiol* 75:886-889, 1995.
4. Kent KC, Moscucci M, Mansour KA, et al: Retroperitoneal hematoma after cardiac catheterization: Prevalence, risk factors, and optimal management, *J Vasc Surg* 20:905-910, 1994.
5. Kennedy AM, Grocott M, Schwartz MS, et al: Median nerve injury: An underrecognized complication of brachial artery cardiac catheterization? *J Neurol Neurosurg Psychiatry* 63:542-546, 1997.
6. Knight CG, Healy DA, Thomas RL: Femoral artery pseudoaneurysms: Risk factors, prevalence, and treatment options, *Ann Vasc Surg* 17:503-508, 2003.
7. Ates M, Sahin S, Konuralp C, et al: Evaluation of risk factors associated with femoral pseudoaneurysms after cardiac catheterization, *J Vasc Surg* 43:520-524, 2006.
8. Gabriel M, Pawlaczyk K, Waliszewski K, et al: Location of femoral artery puncture site and the risk of postcatheterization pseudoaneurysm formation, *Inter J Card* 120:167-171, 2007.

4 General Principles of Endovascular Therapy: Guidewire and Catheter Manipulation

ADAM W. BECK • W. ANTHONY LEE

Historical Background

The age of endovascular therapy began with Dr. Sven Seldinger's publication in 1953 of his technique for vascular access over a wire.[1] The field expanded rapidly with subsequent seminal publications, including those by Dr. Charles Dotter, an American radiologist, in 1964[2] that demonstrated a technique to cross an atherosclerotic lesion. Indeed, Dotter was the first to describe flow-directed balloon catheterization, the double-lumen balloon catheter, the safety guidewire, and the "J" tipped guidewire. In his angiography laboratory in Oregon, Dotter and his technicians were the first to make wire guides and produced Teflon catheters using a blowtorch. These pioneering endeavors set the stage for Andreas Gruntzig, who developed the technique of balloon angioplasty,[3] as well as Julio Palmaz, who designed the first balloon expandable stent in 1985.[4]

Without first obtaining the basic skills of wire and catheter selection and manipulation, the interventionist cannot be successful with endoluminal therapies. To that end, the following text describes the basic concepts of selecting and utilizing various catheters and guidewires.

Guidewire Selection

Guidewires are available in many sizes, shapes, and compositions, which are dictated by their intended purpose (Table 4-1). Their diameters are measured in inches, with standard sizes on which current endovascular platforms are based, including 0.035-, 0.018-, and 0.014-inch guidewires. Guidewire length is chosen based on the sum of the distance from the site of vascular entry to the site of intervention and the device platform, such as an over-the-wire or monorail system.

Guidewires are composed of a nonhydrophilic metal but may be coated with a hydrophilic polymer film that once moistened affords a low friction surface. The hydrophilic coating can be on a portion of the tip or on the entire guidewire shaft. Hydrophilic guidewires should not be used for initial arterial entry because of the risk of shearing off the film coating with the beveled edge of the entry needle, as well as an increased risk of subintimal dissection. Aside from the guidewire type and diameter, other important characteristics include radiopacity; flexibility; "torquability" or "steerability," which reflects the capacity to turn the guidewire tip; "trackability," or the ability to pass the wire into the target vessel once the tip is engaged within the vessel orifice; and tip shape, which may be straight, angled, or J shaped (Fig. 4-1).

TABLE 4-1 Common Wires

Guidewire	Manufacturer	Tip Style	Features	Function
0.035 inch				
Storq	Cordis	Straight, angled, modified J	Various stiffnesses, SLX (proprietary) coating, stainless steel core	Initial access, vessel selection, stable access for device delivery
Advantage	Terumo	Angled	Hydrophilic tip	Initial access, vessel selection, stable access for device delivery
Bentson	Boston Scientific		Long soft tip	Initial access, working wire for device delivery
ZIPwire	Boston Scientific	Straight, angled, J	Hydrophilic polyurethane coating, nitinol core	Vessel selection, traversing complex lesions
Roadrunner Nimble	Cook Medical	Angled platinum	AQ (proprietary) hydrophilic coating, nitinol core	Vessel selection, traversing complex lesions
Rosen	Cook Medical	Tight curve	Stiff stainless steel wire	Stiff working wire for stable access and device delivery
Amplatz Super Stiff	Boston Scientific	Flexible straight, J	PTFE coating, extrastiff stainless steel core, short and long soft tip	Extrastiff working wire for stable access and device delivery
Meier Wire	Boston Scientific	Flexible C and J	PTFE coating, stiff stainless steel shaft	Superstiff wire for large sheath or device delivery (e.g., endograft delivery)
Lunderquist	Cook Medical	Straight, curved	TFE coating, superstiff stainless steel core	Superstiff wire for large sheath or device delivery (e.g., endograft delivery)
0.018 inch				
ZIPwire	Boston Scientific	Straight, angled, J	Hydrophilic polyurethane coating, nitinol core	Small vessel selection (e.g., renal and tibial vessels), high-order vessel selection, traversing complex lesions
Thruway	Boston Scientific	Straight, J (shapeable)	Stainless steel core	Small vessel selection and intervention (e.g., renal and tibial vessels)
V18	Boston Scientific	Straight (shapeable)	ICE (proprietary) hydrophilic coating, stiff Scitanium (proprietary) core	Small vessel selection and intervention, subintimal entry for angioplasty (off label)
0.014 inch				
Hi-Torque Balance Middleweight	Abbott Vascular	Straight	Elastinite nitinol	Intended to facilitate placement of balloon dilatation catheters and stents
Hi-Torque Spartacore 14	Abbott Vascular			Traversing chronic total occlusions
ASAHI MiracleBros 6	Abbott Vascular			Traversing chronic total occlusions with controlled drilling technique
ASAHI Prowater	Abbott Vascular	Straight	Not specified	Traversing chronic total occlusions
ASAHI Confianza Pro 12	Abbott Vascular	Straight	Not specified	Traversing chronic total occlusions with controlled penetration technique
ChoICE PT Extra Support Guidewire	Boston Scientific	Straight, J (shapeable)	Stainless steel core	High level of support designed for easier device delivery in highly resistant lesions
ChoICE PT Floppy Guidewire	Boston Scientific	Straight, J (shapeable)	Hydrophilic coating, stainless steel core	Hydrophilic-coated polymer sleeve with intermediate tip and flexible body for tortuous anatomy and resistant lesions
Journey	Boston Scientific	Straight, J	Hydrophilic coating, nitinol distal core	High level of support designed for easier device delivery in highly resistant lesions
Victory 18 or 30	Boston Scientific	Straight	Stainless steel core	High-gram-load tip options (12-30 g) designed for cross-resistant lesions
Thruway	Boston Scientific	Straight, J (shapeable)	Stainless steel core	Small vessel selection and intervention (e.g., renal and tibial vessels), high-order vessel selection
Approach CTO Wire	Cook Medical	Straight (shapeable)	Stainless steel core, various tip weights (6, 12, 18, and 25 g)	Complex lesion crossing in large and small vessels

CTO, Chronic total occlusion; *PTFE,* Polytetrafluoroethylene; *TFE,* Tetrafluoroethylene.

Many guidewires have gradations of diameter and flexibility, and familiarity should be sought with the transition points along a given guidewire. The degree of flexibility along a guidewire has implications for both its trackability and its torquability. In addition, guidewires with various tip weights are available, with a heavier tip associated with decreased flexibility that may improve the ability of the wire to cross a dense, heavily calcified plaque.

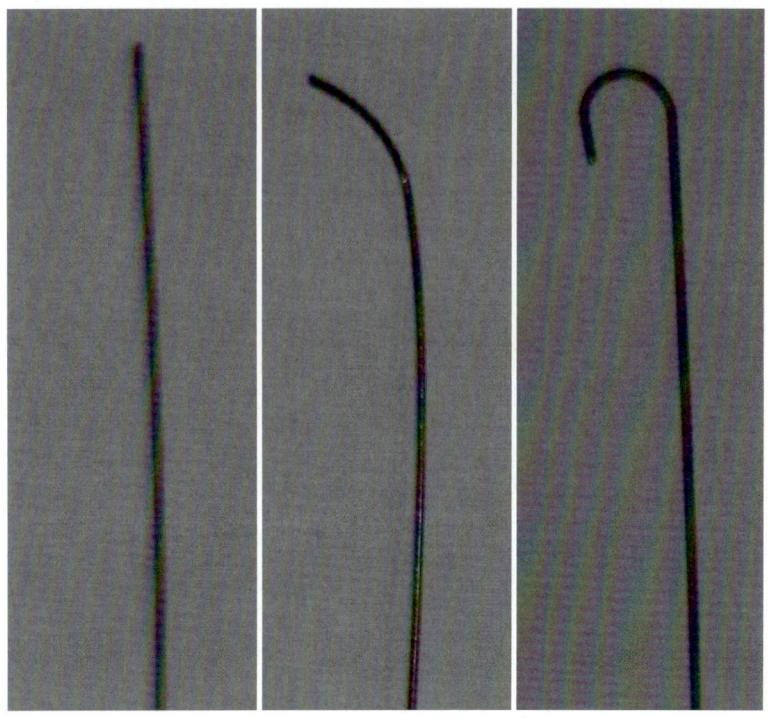

Figure 4-1. Straight, angled, and J-tip wire shapes.

Guidewire Handling

The importance of good guidewire control, both internal and external to the patient, cannot be overemphasized. Proper management of the back of the guidewire mandates constant communication between the primary operator and the assistant. Poor communication can lead to loss of access across a difficult lesion and dissection or perforation of a vessel with a device or guidewire tip. Guidewire length should be sufficient to perform the intended intervention but no longer. Unused wire length creates more difficulty with guidewire management during the procedure and can lead to tangling with other catheters and inadvertent contamination. The unused portion of the guidewire can be gently looped or, optimally, laid straight on the interventional table.

Although most guidewires come with a flexible straight tip, many have a preformed tip or can be shaped to facilitate navigation and crossing of a lesion. Shaping can be performed by using the index finger and thumb to shape the wire tip over an instrument, such as a hemostat or a needle, similar to putting a curl in a ribbon. Care should be taken not to traumatize the end of the guidewire so that it loses its integrity or creates too great a curve. Straightening a guidewire tip after shaping is difficult, if not impossible, and in general, the technique should be used sparingly. The "tightness" or radius of the curvature imparted on the tip is a function of the distance grasped from the guidewire tip and the force used to shape it.

Turning the guidewire tip within a vessel can be relatively easy in a straight vessel, but once it has traversed several angles, precise maneuvering can become quite difficult. Use of a moist sponge or a torque device can help the guidewire user grip the wire and torque it directly. There are multiple types of torque devices (Fig. 4-2), which are meant to grip the guidewire and allow one-handed manipulation.

Catheter Selection

Simultaneous maneuvering of the catheter and guidewire is often essential to traversing complex anatomy. Catheter selection depends on the intended use and ultimate destination within the vascular tree, and catheter composition can greatly affect its function (Table 4-2). Catheters are generally made from or coated

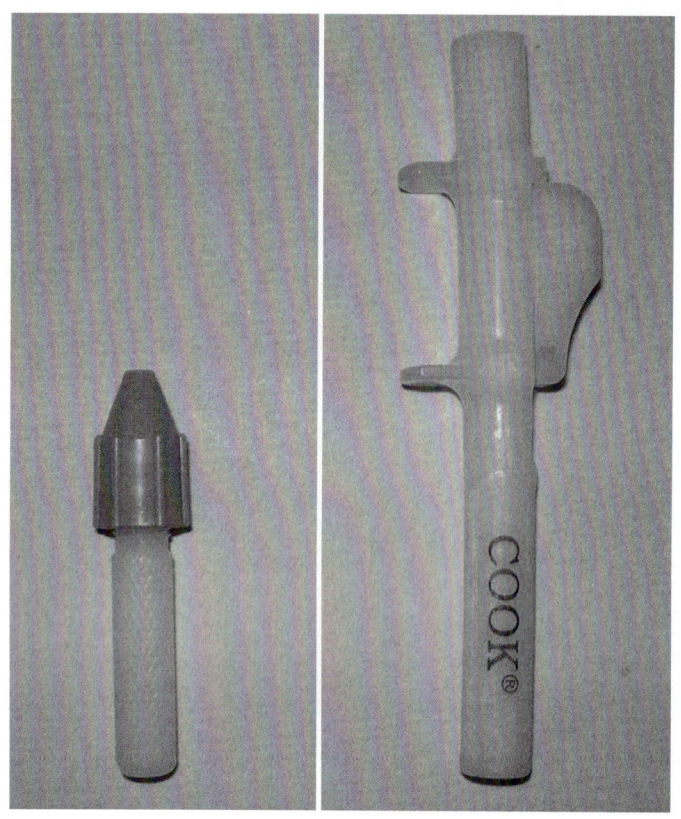

Figure 4-2. Pin vise (Terumo Medical Corp., Somerset, N.J.) and Olcott (Cook Medical, Bloomington, Ind.) torque devices.

TABLE 4-2 Common Catheters

Catheter	Manufacturer	Tip Style	Features	Function
Pigtail flush	Various	Pigtail	Multiple side holes, marker and nonmarker varieties	Flush arteriogram in large vessels, up-and-over iliac access, aortic catheterization from brachial access
Straight flush	Various	Straight	Multiple side holes, marker and nonmarker varieties	Flush arteriogram, markers can be used for device or balloon sizing
Omni Flush, SOS	Various	Complex reverse curve	Multiple side holes, marker and nonmarker varieties	Flush arteriogram in large vessels, up-and-over iliac access, visceral vessel or renal access, aortic catheterization from brachial access
Omni Select, SOS Select	Various	Complex reverse curve	End-hole catheter	Up-and-over iliac access, visceral or renal vessel selection
Berenstein	Various	Simple angled	End-hole catheter	Selective catheter, various lengths, various diameters
Kumpe	Various	Simple angled	End-hole catheter	Selective catheter, various lengths, various diameters
Cobra 1, Cobra 2	Various	Double curve	End-hole catheter	Selective catheter, visceral or renal vessel selection, aortic catheterization from brachial access
JB-1	Various	Double curve	End-hole catheter, available with hydrophilic coating	Brachiocephalic vessel selection, carotid intervention
TC, TC-BNK	Cook Medical	Rounded tight curve	Flexible tip	Selective catheter for tight angles (e.g., endograft fenestration access, severely angled visceral or renal vessels, and high-order vessel selection)
H-1	Various	Double curve	End-hole catheter, available with hydrophilic coating	Brachiocephalic vessel selection, carotid intervention
Vertebral	Various	Simple angled	End-hole catheter	Selective catheter with various uses, including brachiocephalic interventions

H-1, Headhunter 1; *TC*, tight curve; *TC-BNK*, tight curve Binkert modification.

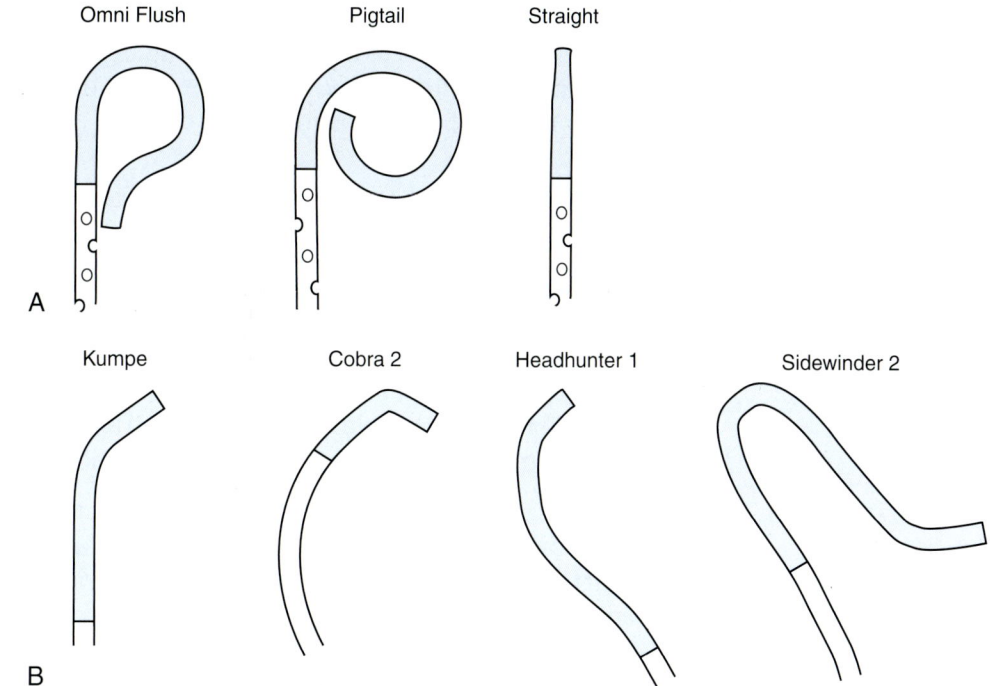

GENERAL PRINCIPLES OF ENDOVASCULAR THERAPY: GUIDEWIRE AND CATHETER MANIPULATION

Figure 4-3. Angiographic catheters are categorized as nonselective (**A**) and selective (**B**) catheters. *(Courtesy AngioDynamics, Latham, N.Y. From Cronenwett JL, Johnston KW, editors: Rutherford's vascular surgery, ed 7. Philadelphia, 2010, Saunders, p 1270, Figs. 84-2 and 84-3.)*

with various polymers, including Teflon, nylon, polyurethane, polypropylene, or polyethylene that determines their flexibility, their torquability, and the friction created upon contact with tissue or sheath. Some catheters have a woven wire or nylon skeleton that provides a stiffer shaft. Catheter fatigue refers to loss of the original shape of the catheter or an increase in catheter pliability that can occur during difficult catheterization and with prolonged exposure to body temperature. Catheter fatigue may be evident when a catheter that successfully selected a vessel at the onset of a procedure failed to do so at a later stage and suggests the need to replace the catheter.

Catheters are sized by their length in centimeters and outer diameter in French size, where 3 Fr is the equivalent of 1 mm. Most angiographic selective catheters are either 4 or 5 Fr. Larger sizes are usually "guiding" catheters used during interventions, and smaller sizes are designed for use during microcatheter techniques. Longer catheters are required for more distant lesions, such as those located in carotid or tibial vessels, and are often placed through a guiding sheath in order to allow more maneuverability at the target site. Most 4- and 5-Fr catheters are 0.035- and 0.038-inch guidewire compatible, whereas smaller catheters require 0.018- or 0.014-inch guidewires. Placing an undersized guidewire within a larger catheter lumen allows the edge of the catheter to potentially dissect the intima in a snowplow-type effect. In addition leakage around the guidewire can occur unless a valve adapter, such as a Tuohy-Borst adapter, is placed at the catheter hub.

There are two basic types of catheters: flush or angiographic nonselective and end-hole or angiographic selective (Fig. 4-3).[5] Flush catheters have multiple side holes that allow for rapid injection of contrast to image high-flow vessels, such as the aorta. End-hole catheters are available in various configurations, with their shape ultimately determining their function. Despite the variety of available catheters, in practice, most interventionists use 3 or 4 catheters in the majority of cases. Familiarity with 5 to 10 additional catheters may be required when encountering unusual or difficult anatomy. The basic types of end-hole catheters include simple or single-curved, double-curved, and reverse-curved catheters. The unique shape of a catheter determines the translational movement of the catheter tip when positioned in a side branch in response to the coaxial force applied along its shaft. Tips can move forward or backward when pushed or pulled and vice versa. Because a double- or reverse-curved catheter is initially delivered over a straight wire, its shape must be re-formed within the aorta (Fig. 4-4). The curved portions of complex catheters can be selected with the varying degrees and sizes of the radial curvature and should be calibrated to the parent vessel diameter and the location of the orifice for intended catheterization.

Catheter Handling

Successful catheter manipulation requires good hand-eye coordination, which improves with experience; knowledge of the vascular anatomy; and an appreciation of how specific guidewires and catheters move alone and in relation to one another. In general catheters should be advanced over a guidewire in order to avoid vessel injury, but certain catheter shapes are atraumatic when advanced and can be moved forward or withdrawn without a guidewire. The catheter shape can help select a vessel origin or traverse a complex lesion in conjunction with a straight or curved wire tip.

In addition to length, diameter, and tip shape, catheter flexibility, radiopacity, torquability, and trackability should be considered in catheter selection. A single catheter may not provide every necessary characteristic to complete a planned intervention. For example, in a bovine aortic arch, initial catheterization of the left carotid artery is often best performed using a reverse-curved catheter. However, the ability of that catheter to track over a guidewire and provide stable access may be limited. Careful exchange to a simple curved catheter may facilitate catheterization of the more distal target vessel and tracking of a guiding sheath into the common carotid artery. Although a complex curve catheter can facilitate engagement of a vessel origin, trackability may be compromised compared with straight or simple curved catheters.

Catheter manipulation can become increasingly difficult after traversing tortuous arterial anatomy. This can be mitigated by using coaxial systems, such as a long guiding sheath placed over the aortic bifurcation, which decreases the friction generated by interaction of the catheter to the arterial wall and allows for stable access and focused angiographic injections without loss of guidewire access. It should also be appreciated that catheter tip orientation may change once a guidewire is positioned to the end of the catheter.

Crossing a Stenosis

As a matter of principle, care should be exercised when advancing any guidewire, but especially one with a hydrophilic or weighted tip. Close attention must be paid to subtle deflections of the guidewire tip and the tactile feedback as it moves through a diseased vessel. Allowing a short loop to form at the leading end of a guidewire can facilitate passage through a lesion that otherwise would have caught the tip. Two-handed catheter and guidewire manipulation is important, and the operator should advance the catheter forward as deeper purchase of the guidewire is achieved in the target vessel. This further supports the guidewire, allows greater pushability, and helps prevent loss of guidewire access.

Avoiding and Managing a Subintimal Guidewire

Unintentional entry into a subintimal plane can easily occur with hydrophilic or weighted tip guidewires, and there may be no immediate visual indication that this event has occurred. Subintimal passage should be considered if resistance is met during guidewire advancement. One visual indication is spiraling of the guidewire along the course of the vessel. Unless intentional, the guidewire should be removed and an attempt should be made to find the true lumen of the vessel in a different location using an angled tip catheter. Once a wire has passed into a subintimal plane, it is often difficult to find a new path for the guidewire, especially in the presence of occlusive disease.

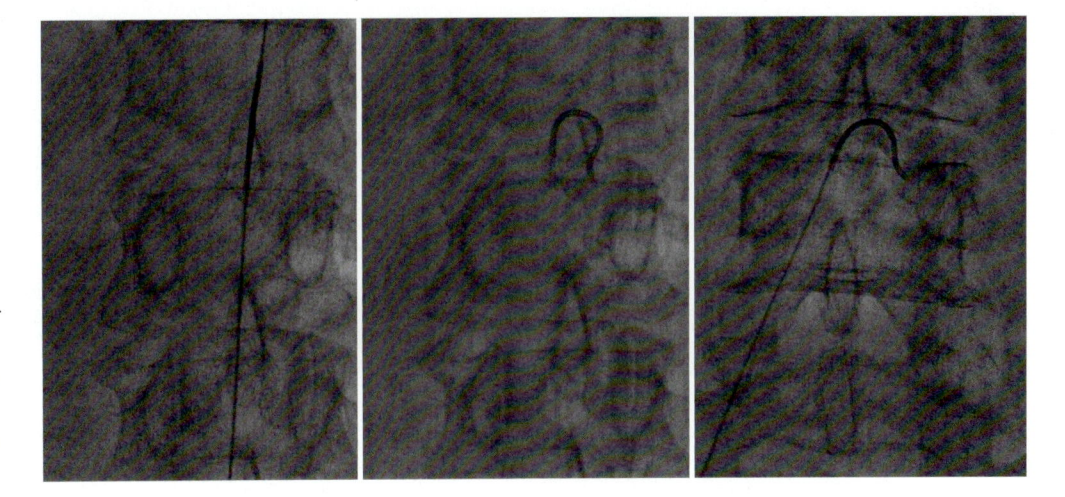

GENERAL PRINCIPLES OF ENDOVASCULAR THERAPY: GUIDEWIRE AND CATHETER MANIPULATION   47

Figure 4-4. SOS catheter straight on the guidewire, reformed with retraction of the wire, and seated on the aortic bifurcation for contralateral lower extremity access.

Figure 4-5. Looped Glidewire (Terumo Medical Corp., Somerset, N.J.) wire through a straight Quickcross catheter (Spectranetics, Colorado Springs, Colo.) traversing an occluded superficial femoral artery, with successful reentry and placement of an atraumatic J-tip Rosen wire (Cook Medical, Bloomington, Ind.) for further intervention. Reentry should be confirmed by injection of contrast through the catheter before continuing with intervention (*inset*).

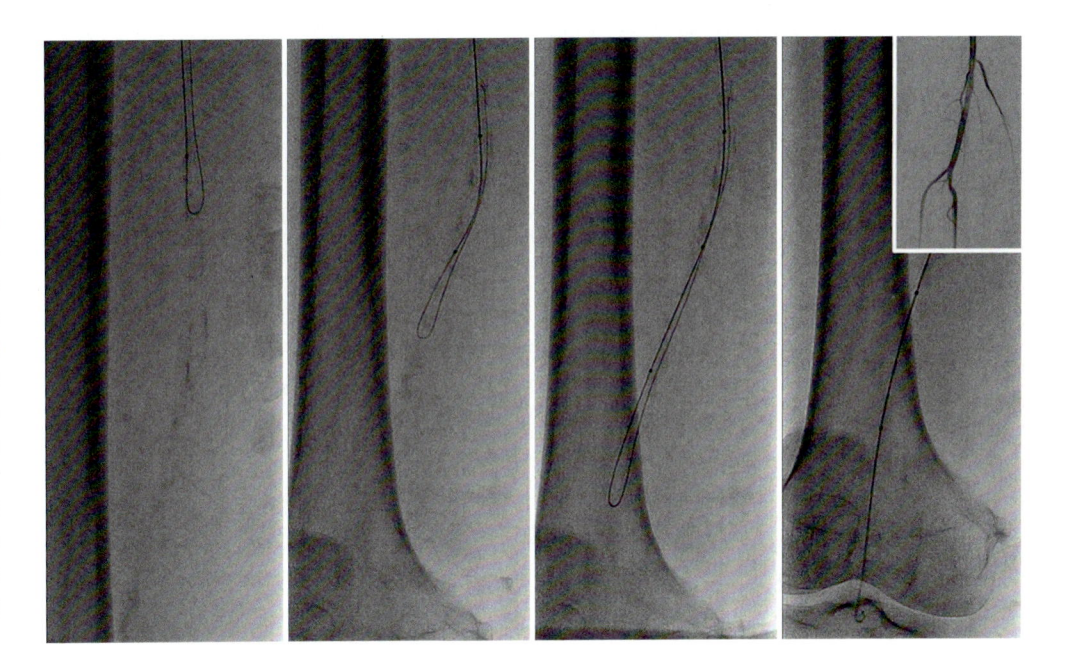

Crossing an Occlusion

Acute or subacute thrombosis of an existing atherosclerotic lesion can often be traversed despite the appearance of a complete angiographic occlusion. If the proximal aspect of the thrombus can be engaged with the guidewire, deliberate advancement through the lesion can help achieve access to the true lumen, although it is often difficult or impossible to assure true lumen access throughout the course of the guidewire. Close attention must be paid to the action of the guidewire tip while advancing. Presence of a wire loop or spiral suggests it may be within a subintimal plane.

Atherosclerotic plaques within occluded vessels often have a "cap" of calcified atheroma in the proximal vessel, which can prevent entry into the softer central portion of the plaque. Devices are available to access the cap (e.g., Frontrunner XP chronic total occlusion catheter, Cordis Corp., Bridgewater, N.J.). If entry into a subintimal dissection plane to bypass an occlusion has been intentional, care should be taken to avoid vessel perforation by allowing a loop to form at the tip of a hydrophilic guidewire and then pushing the loop forward (Fig. 4-5).[6,7] If this technique is used, the radius of loop should appear to be tight, as a broad-based loop suggests perforation.

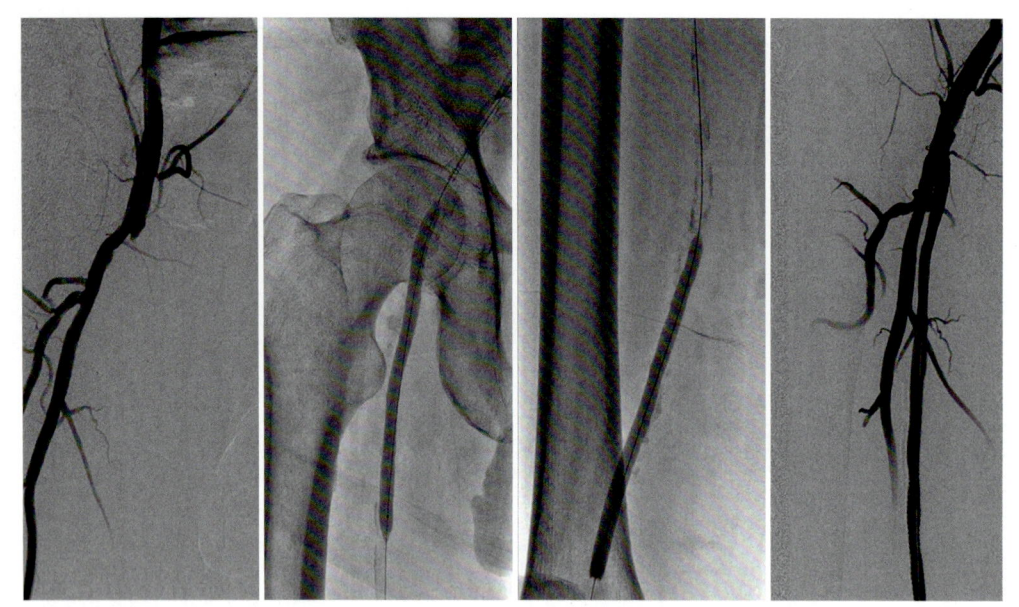

Figure 4-6. Chronic superficial femoral artery occlusion with subintimal angioplasty and selective stenting. The *far right panel* demonstrates the completion digital subtraction image.

After passage of the guidewire into the subintimal plane, access to the distal true lumen must be gained. Angiography can be used to identify the site of vessel reconstitution. An angled catheter can be used to direct the guidewire toward the lumen, and the intima can be punctured with the guidewire tip to gain entry into the true lumen. Because the intima is often diseased at the desired level of reentry, this technique may not be successful. Reentry catheters such as the Pioneer (Medtronic Vascular, Santa Rosa, Calif.)[8] or Outback (Cordis)[9] devices have been introduced to puncture the intima for true lumen reentry.

Reestablishing lower extremity flow via a subintimal angioplasty has been used to recanalize chronically occluded arteries without the need for stenting.[10] In this technique standard-sized balloons and other interventional devices will not pass through the subintimal plane because of the limited space, and predilation with a small diameter balloon can facilitate passage of catheters and devices (Fig. 4-6).

While crossing an occluded vessel, stable access must be maintained in order to prevent losing guidewire access. The catheter should be advanced periodically over the guidewire, which allows greater pushability that is often essential to traversing long dense lesions. Reentry into the true lumen distally must be accomplished in order to successfully treat the occluded vessel and must always be confirmed before the intended intervention by a gentle injection of contrast dye through the catheter.

REFERENCES

1. Seldinger SI: Catheter replacement of the needle in percutaneous arteriography; a new technique, *Acta Radiol* 39:368-376, 1953.
2. Dotter CT, Judkins MP: Transluminal treatment of arteriosclerotic obstruction. Description of a new technic and a preliminary report of its application, *Circulation* 30:654-670, 1964.
3. Grüntzig A, Hopff H: [Percutaneous recanalization after chronic arterial occlusion with a new dilator-catheter (modification of the dotter technique) (author's transl)], *Deutsche medizinische Wochenschrift (1946)* 99:2502-2511, 1974.
4. Palmaz JC, Sibbitt RR, Reuter SR, Tio FO, Rice WJ: Expandable intraluminal graft: A preliminary study. Work in progress, *Radiology* 156:73-77, 1985.
5. Cronenwett JL, Johnston KW, editors: *Rutherford's vascular surgery*, ed 7, Philadelphia, 2010, Saunders, p 1270.
6. Bolia A, Brennan J, Bell PR: Recanalisation of femoral-popliteal occlusions: Improving success rate by subintimal recanalisation, *Clinical Radiology* 40:325, 1989.

7. Bolia A, Miles KA, Brennan J, Bell PR: Percutaneous transluminal angioplasty of occlusions of the femoral and popliteal arteries by subintimal dissection, *Cardiovasc Intervent Radiol* 13:357-363, 1990.
8. Krishnamurthy VN, Eliason JL, Henke PK, Rectenwald JE: Intravascular ultrasound-guided true lumen reentry device for recanalization of unilateral chronic total occlusion of iliac arteries: Technique and follow-up, *Ann Vasc Surg* 24:487-497, 2010.
9. Hausegger KA, Georgieva B, Portugaller H, Tauss J, Stark G: The outback catheter: A new device for true lumen re-entry after dissection during recanalization of arterial occlusions, *Cardiovasc Intervent Radiol* 27:26-30, 2004.
10. Spinosa DJ, Harthun NL, Bissonette EA, et al: Subintimal arterial flossing with antegrade-retrograde intervention (SAFARI) for subintimal recanalization to treat chronic critical limb ischemia, *JVIR* 16:37-44, 2005.

5 General Principles of Endovascular Therapy: Angioplasty, Stenting, Recanalization, and Embolization

PETER B. BRANT-ZAWADZKI • JON S. MATSUMURA

Historical Background

Angioplasty was first used by Dotter and Judkins[1] in 1964 for the treatment of peripheral vascular lesions using rigid intravascular dilators. Although relatively unnoticed in the United States, this approach was used to treat large numbers of patients in Europe. Grüntzig[2] substituted a balloon-tipped catheter for the rigid dilator and performed the first peripheral balloon angioplasty in 1974. Dotter[3] also described the use of a tubular coiled wire stent graft in canines in 1969. Tillet and Garner[4] isolated streptokinase in 1933, but it was not until the 1950s that Clifton and Grunnet[5] first reported its use as a thrombolytic agent. In 1960 Luessenhop and Spence[6] first described intravascular embolization to treat a cerebral arteriovenous malformation using a handmade plastic pellet.

Indications

Indications for percutaneous transluminal angioplasty (PTA) of specific anatomic sites are detailed in later chapters but typically include an occlusive lesion that is symptomatic or at high risk for causing significant morbidity should progression to complete occlusion occur. Specific indications for stenting after an initial angioplasty include flow-limiting dissection, residual stenosis of more than 30%, or the presence of a significant pressure gradient across the treated lesion. Primary stent placement is commonly practiced for carotid and renal interventions or for a lesion that is embolizing but has not proved beneficial over selective stenting in the iliac system.[7] It is common to selectively stent infrainguinal lesions based on the postangioplasty results, and long-term outcomes for superficial femoral artery (SFA) stents, stent grafts, and drug-eluting stents are evolving.

The exact roles for adjunctive percutaneous mechanical thrombectomy and pharmacologic thrombolytic therapy are debated, but these modalities are predominantly considered in the setting of acute arterial or venous thrombosis. Atherectomy for chronic peripheral lesions is advocated by some, but its role is controversial with a paucity of randomized data.[8]

Indications for intravascular embolization include control of hemorrhage, treatment of vascular anomalies, exclusion of aneurysmal segments or vessels that have been treated with an endograft, and interruption of tumor vasculature.

ANGIOPLASTY, STENTING, RECANALIZATION, AND EMBOLIZATION 51

Preoperative Preparation

- History and physical examination, as well as noninvasive physiologic and imaging studies, establishes the location and severity of vascular disease.
- If angioplasty or stenting is planned, preprocedural administration of antiplatelet therapy with aspirin (325 mg daily) or clopidogrel (75 mg daily) is recommended for 5 days before the procedure. If patients have not received clopidogrel, an oral loading dose of 300 mg can be administered after the procedure.

Pitfalls and Danger Points

- **Inadvertent embolization.** Crossing any lesion can lead to inadvertent embolization, but irregular, ulcerated, or complex lesions, especially those that are symptomatic or aneurysmal with the presence of irregular thrombus, are at increased embolic risk. Judicious use of anticoagulation and cautious passage of atraumatic wires and intravascular devices through these lesions help minimize embolization.
- **Dissection.** Dissection may occur as a consequence of wire or catheter manipulation or after primary angioplasty. Dissection from a guidewire may be avoided by frequent "twirling" of the wire tip to ensure an intraluminal position. If the position of the catheter is in doubt, contrast angiography should be performed to identify a subintimal plane of dissection. Dissection after angioplasty occurs most frequently in the region of significant plaque burden or after overdilation of a vessel. Most iatrogenic dissections are clinically silent and are not flow limiting, but if a flow-limiting dissection is present, stenting is required.
- **Rupture.** Vessel rupture can occur with wire manipulation, balloon angioplasty, or insertion of other devices, such as a large sheath. Rupture after angioplasty is often secondary to overdilation of the lesion. Circumferentially and highly eccentric calcified lesions are at high risk of rupture and should be approached cautiously. Subintimal angioplasty may also increase the risk for perforation compared with intraluminal procedures.

Operative Strategy

All interventional procedures follow a common series of steps, beginning with vascular access and placement of an appropriate sheath. Puncture site planning and sheath sizing depend on the location of the lesion. For example, if both inflow and outflow lesions are suspected in the presence of unilateral lower extremity ischemia and diminished ipsilateral pulses, access through a retrograde puncture in the contralateral common femoral artery allows treatment of an inflow lesion using a 6-Fr sheath and 0.035-inch system, followed by treatment of the distal outflow lesion through a long 4-Fr sheath and 0.014-inch system placed within the 6-Fr sheath. An alternative strategy is treatment of the inflow lesion alone through a retrograde puncture on the affected side, followed by treatment of the outflow lesion via a separate antegrade puncture.

Operative Technique

ANESTHESIA

Most percutaneous procedures can be performed with local anesthesia and conscious sedation using a combination of narcotics and sedatives with continuous cardiovascular and respiratory monitoring. Occasionally patients are unable to tolerate a procedure because of anxiety, discomfort, or inability to lay immobile for prolonged periods in the interventional suite. In these instances a general anesthetic may be required.

ANGIOPLASTY

A stenosis may appear moderate on two-dimensional imaging yet cause no significant flow limitation. Multiple views or transduction of pressure gradients may be required when there is doubt as to a lesion's hemodynamic significance. For example, multiple oblique images of the pelvic vasculature may be required to identify posterior lesions and better visualize hypogastric and profunda vessel origins in a nonoverlapping projection. When a decision has been made to intervene, a therapeutic dose of heparin (50-100 units/kg) is administered. The activated clotting time is often measured during the procedure to ensure therapeutic anticoagulation, frequently with a goal of greater than 200 seconds and greater than 250 seconds for carotid and tibial procedures, respectively.

Intervention in the form of balloon angioplasty is accomplished by exerting a radial force, with plaque fracture and intimal injury creating a larger flow channel. Dissection is frequently visible after angioplasty, but the flow-limiting characteristics of the dissection determine whether stent placement is required.

Balloon selection can be challenging because there is a great deal of variation in available devices and selecting an appropriate size requires some experience. Balloon catheters are either coaxial, in which there exist two separate hub lumens for guidewire and balloon inflation, or monorail, in which a single hub lumen exists for balloon inflation (Fig. 5-1). Coaxial and monorail balloon catheters are typically used with 0.035- and 0.014-inch guidewires, respectively. Coaxial, or over-the-wire, balloons can be used on 0.014-inch systems for greater support. Balloons can vary in length from 2 cm to greater than 12 cm and in diameter from 1 to 40 mm (Table 5-1). Most balloons are fabricated from polyethylene or nylon, which has a combination of strength and low compliance so that the balloon profile does not change shape as the inflation pressure is increased. All balloons are rated for the nominal pressure at which they obtain their reported diameter, in addition to their burst pressure at which 5% of balloons rupture. Balloons can rupture on sharp, calcified plaques or because of overinflation. When balloon rupture occurs, it is sometimes possible to compensate for the extravasation of contrast by exerting high volumes via an inflation device. If this fails to adequately dilate the lesion, a high-pressure balloon can be used that is less prone to rupture. An additional variable in balloon selection is the profile, which determines a balloon's ability to cross a lesion. Low-profile balloons are more likely to cross tight lesions than high-profile balloons.

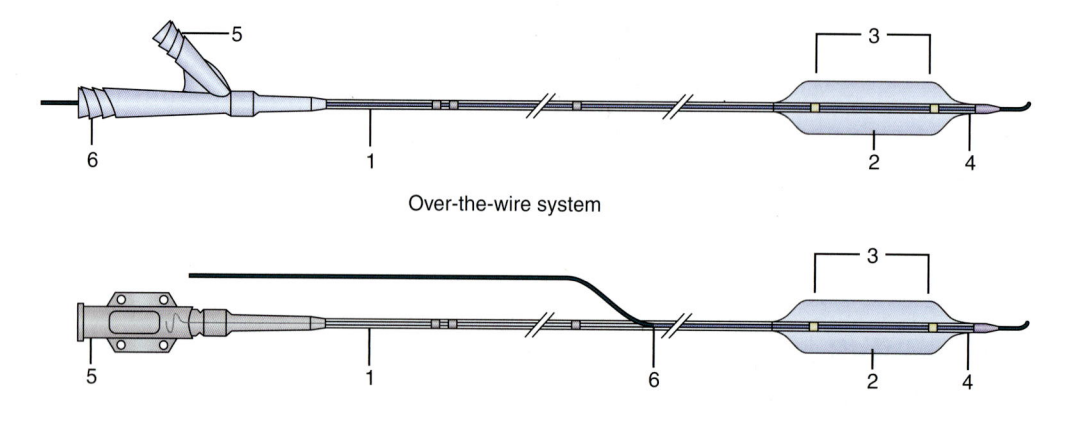

Figure 5-1. Comparison of coaxial (e.g., over-the-wire) and monorail (e.g., rapid exchange) balloons. The coaxial design has both a guidewire port and a balloon port. The monorail design has a single port for balloon inflation, but the wire exits the shaft of the catheter and allows the operator to manipulate both the wire and the balloon with greater ease. 1, catheter shaft; 2, balloon; 3, marker or balloon size; 4, tapered tip; 5, inflation port; 6, guidewire exit port. *(From Cronenwett JL, Johnston KW, editors: Rutherford's vascular surgery, ed 7, Philadelphia, 2010, Saunders, p 1278, Fig. 85-1C.)*

ANGIOPLASTY, STENTING, RECANALIZATION, AND EMBOLIZATION 53

TABLE 5-1 Toolbox

PTA Balloons (0.035 inch)			
Manufacturer Product	**Shaft Length (cm)**	**Balloon Diameters (mm)**	**Balloon Lengths (mm)**
Abbott Vascular Fox Cross	50, 80, 135	3, 4, 5, 6, 7, 8, 9, 10, 12, 14	20, 30, 40, 60, 80, 100, 120
AngioDynamics WorkHorse II	50, 75, 100	5, 6, 7, 8, 9, 10	20, 40, 60
Bard Peripheral Conquest	50, 75, 120	5, 6, 7, 8, 9, 10, 12	20, 30, 40, 60, 80
Bard Peripheral Atlas	75, 120	12, 14, 16, 18, 20, 22, 24, 26	20, 40, 60
Bard Peripheral Dorado	40, 80, 120, 135	3, 4, 5, 6, 7, 8, 9, 10	20, 40, 60, 80, 100, 120, 150, 170, 200
Boston Scientific Blue Max	40, 75, 120	4, 5, 6, 7, 8, 9, 10	20, 30, 40, 80, 100
Boston Scientific Synergy	50, 75, 90, 135, 150	3, 4, 5, 6, 7, 8, 9, 10, 12	15, 20, 30, 40, 60, 80, 100
Cook Medical ATB Advance	40, 80, 120	4, 5, 6, 7, 8, 9, 10, 12, 14	20, 30, 40, 50, 60, 70, 80
Cordis Opta Pro PTA	80, 110, 135	3, 4, 5, 6, 7, 8, 9, 10, 12	10, 15, 20, 30, 40, 60, 80, 100
Cordis Powerflex P3 PTA	40, 65, 80, 110, 135	4, 5, 6, 7, 8, 9, 10	10, 15, 20, 30, 40, 60, 80, 100
Cordis Maxi LD PTA	80, 110	14, 15	20, 40, 60, 80
ev3 EverCross 0.035	40, 80, 135	3, 4, 5, 6, 7, 8, 9, 10, 12	15, 20, 30, 40, 60, 80, 100, 120, 150, 200
Medtronic Admiral Xtreme	80, 130	3, 4, 5, 6, 7, 8, 9, 10, 12	20, 40, 60, 80, 120, 150, 200, 250, 300

PTA Balloons (0.014 and 0.018 inch)			
Manufacturer Product	**Shaft Length (cm)**	**Balloon Diameters (mm)**	**Balloon Lengths (mm)**
Abbott Vascular RX Viatrac 14	80, 135	4, 4.5, 5, 5.5, 6, 6.5, 7	15, 20, 30, 40
Abbott Vascular Fox sv 18	90, 150	2, 2.5, 3, 4, 5, 6	15, 20, 30, 40, 60, 80, 100, 120
Bard Peripheral Ultraverse 014	150	1.5, 2, 2.5, 3, 3.5, 4, 5	20, 40, 80, 120, 150, 220
Bard Peripheral VascuTrak	140	2, 2.5, 3, 3.5, 4, 5, 6, 7	20, 40, 60, 80, 100, 120, 150, 200, 250, 300
Boston Scientific Sterling Monorail	80, 135	3, 3.5, 4, 4.5, 5, 5.5, 6, 6.5, 7, 8	10, 15, 20, 30, 40, 60
Boston Scientific Sterling OTW	40, 80, 135	4, 5, 6, 7, 8, 9, 10	20, 30, 40, 60, 80, 100
Cook Medical Advance 14LP	170	2, 2.5, 3, 4	20, 40, 60, 80, 120, 160, 200
Cordis Sleek OTW PTA	150	1.25, 1.5, 2, 2.5, 3, 3.5, 4, 5	15, 20, 40, 80, 100, 120, 150, 220
Cordis Aviator Plus PTA	142	4, 4.5, 5, 5.5, 6, 7	15, 20, 30, 40
ev3 NanoCross 0.014	90, 150	1.5, 2, 2.5, 3, 3.5, 4	20, 40, 80, 120, 150, 210
Medtronic Amphirion Deep OTW	120, 150	1.5, 2, 2.5, 3, 3.5, 4	20, 40, 80, 120, 150, 210
Medtronic Sprinter OTW	Variable	1.5, 2, 2.25, 2.5, 2.75, 3, 3.25, 3.5, 3.75, 4	6, 10, 12, 15, 20, 25, 30

Specialized Balloons			
Manufacturer Product	**Shaft Length (cm)**	**Balloon Diameters (mm)**	**Balloon Lengths (mm)**
AngioScore AngioSculpt Scoring	137	2, 2.5, 3, 3.5	10, 20
Boston Scientific Peripheral Cutting (OTW and RX)	50, 90, 140	2, 2.5, 3, 3.5, 4, 5, 6, 7, 8	15, 20

Continued

TABLE 5-1 Toolbox—*cont'd*

Stents (balloon expandable)			
Manufacturer Product	**Shaft Length (cm)**	**Stent Diameters (mm)**	**Stent Lengths (mm)**
Abbott Vascular Omnilink Elite peripheral stent system	80, 15	4-10	12, 16, 19, 29, 39, 59
Boston Scientific Express LD	75, 135	6-10	17, 25, 27, 37, 57
Cook Medical Formula 418 (0.018)	80, 135	5-8	12, 16, 20, 24, 30
Cordis Palmaz iliac and renal stents (unmounted)	N/A	4-8	10, 15, 20, 29
Cordis Palmaz iliac stent (unmounted)	N/A	8-12	30
ev3 Visi-Pro (0.014, 0.018)	80, 135	5-8	12, 17, 27, 37, 57
ev3 IntraStent LD (unmounted)	N/A	9-12	16, 26, 36, 56, 76
Medtronic Bridge Assurant	80, 130	6-10	20, 30, 40, 60
Medtronic Racer	80, 130	4-7	12, 18

Stents (self-expanding)			
Manufacturer Product	**Shaft Length (cm)**	**Stent Diameters (mm)**	**Stent Lengths (mm)**
Abbott Vascular Xpert Self-Expanding	80, 80, 120, 135	3-8	20, 30, 40, 50, 60
Abbott Vascular Absolute Pro LL peripheral self-expanding	80, 135	5-8	120, 150
Bard Peripheral Eluminexx	80, 135	7-10	20, 30, 40, 50, 60, 80, 100
Bard Peripheral LifeStent (reg and XL)	80, 130	6, 7	20, 30, 40, 60, 80, 100, 120, 150, 170
Boston Scientific Wallstent Iliac	100, 160	6-10	18, 20, 23, 24, 34, 35, 36, 38, 39, 46, 47, 49, 52, 55, 59, 61, 66, 67, 69
Boston Scientific Wallstent	75, 135	5-8, 10, 12, 14, 16, 18, 20, 22, 24	20, 35, 40, 42, 45, 55, 60, 68, 70, 80, 90, 94
Boston Scientific Sentinol	75, 135	5-9, 10	20, 40, 60, 80
Cook Medical Zilver 518 and 635	125	6-10	20, 30, 40, 60, 80
Cordis SMART Control Iliac	80, 120	6-10	20, 30, 40, 60, 80, 100
ev3 Protégé EverFlex	80, 120	5-8	20, 30, 40, 60, 80, 100, 120, 150
ev3 Protégé GPS	80, 120, 135	6-10, 12, 14	20, 30, 40, 60, 80
Medtronic Complete self-expanding	80, 130	4-10	20-150

Stent Grafts			
Manufacturer Product	**Shaft Length (cm)**	**Stent Diameters (mm)**	**Stent Lengths (mm)**
Atrium Medical iCast covered stent	80, 120	5-12	16, 22, 38, 59
Bard Peripheral Flair endovascular stent	80	6-9	30, 40, 50
Gore & Associates Viabahn	75, 110, 120	7-12	25, 50, 100, 150
LeMaitre Vascular aSpire	50	6-9	20, 30, 50, 100

TABLE 5-1 Toolbox—cont'd

Embolization Tools				
Manufacturer Product	**Delivery Catheter Sizes (ID)**	**Coil Diameter (mm)**	**Coil Length (mm)**
AGA Amplatzer plugs (Table 5-3)	4- to 7-Fr sheath	3-22	6-18
Boston Scientific VortX-18 diamond coils	0.021 inch	2/3, 2/4, 2/5, 2/6	2.3, 4.1, 5.8, 8
Boston Scientific VortX-35 vascular coils	0.038 inch	2/4, 3/5, 3/6, 3/7	3, 3.5, 5.3, 6.7
Cook Medical Tornado microcoils	0.018 inch	3/2, 4/2, 5/2, 6/2, 7/3, 8/4, 10/4	2-14.2
Cook Medical Tornado coils	0.035 inch	5/3, 6/3, 7/3, 8/4, 8/5, 10/5	4.1-12.5
Cordis Trufill n-BCA liquid embolic system		N/A	N/A
ev3 Onyx liquid embolic system		N/A	N/A
Terumo Interventional Azur HydroCoil Detachable	0.022-0.025 inch	3, 4, 6, 8, 10, 12, 15, 20	5, 10, 15, 20, 30
Terumo Interventional Azur HydroCoil Detachable	0.038 inch	4, 6, 8, 10, 12, 15, 20	5, 10, 15, 20, 30

Therapeutic Infusion Catheters		
Manufacturer Product	**Guidewire Size (inches)**	**Working Length (cm)**
AngioDynamics Unifuse infusion catheter	0.035	45, 90, 135
ev3 ProStream infusion wire	0.035	145, 175
Merit Medical Systems Mistique infusion catheter	0.035	45, 90, 135

n-BCA, n-Butyl cyanoacrylate; *ID,* inner diameter; *N/A,* not applicable; *OTW,* over the wire; *RX,* rapid exchange.

Several specialized balloons have been introduced for treatment of complicated lesions, such as restenotic lesions after angioplasty. A cutting balloon incorporates several microrazors onto the balloon surface in either a longitudinal or a spiral orientation to sharply cut through areas of myointimal hyperplasia when inflated (Fig. 5-2). A cryoplasty balloon incorporates a small liquid nitrogen canister to cool the balloon to −40°C in hopes of limiting postangioplasty dissection and vessel recoil. More recently, drug-coated balloons have been used to deliver antiproliferative agents, such as paclitaxel, directly to the lesion, with promising short-term results in SFA and popliteal arteries. There is a lack of long-term data to suggest superiority of any of these modalities over conventional angioplasty. Postangioplasty stent placement is discussed in a later section in the chapter.

When a decision has been made to perform balloon angioplasty, the insufflation lumen of the balloon catheter is aspirated and a dilute mixture of contrast is prepared for use with an insufflation device, which allows continuous measurement of balloon pressure during balloon inflation. The ratio of contrast to saline for balloon insufflation varies with the size of the balloon. Typically a 50:50 ratio is appropriate for angioplasty balloons used for peripheral interventions. For large balloons used in the aorta and vena cava, contrast may be diluted down to about 20%, because the balloons are easily identified radiographically and the less viscous mixture allows for more rapid filling and deflation.

Balloon sizing is based on the diameter of the vessel and target lesion so as to dilate the lesion while avoiding vessel rupture. The length of the balloon should not significantly extend beyond the lesion in order to avoid damaging the normal vessel wall. Inflation of the balloon within a lesion typically identifies an atherosclerotic "waist," which dilates with progressive pressure (Fig. 5-3). Balloon

56 SURGICAL AND ENDOVASCULAR TECHNIQUES

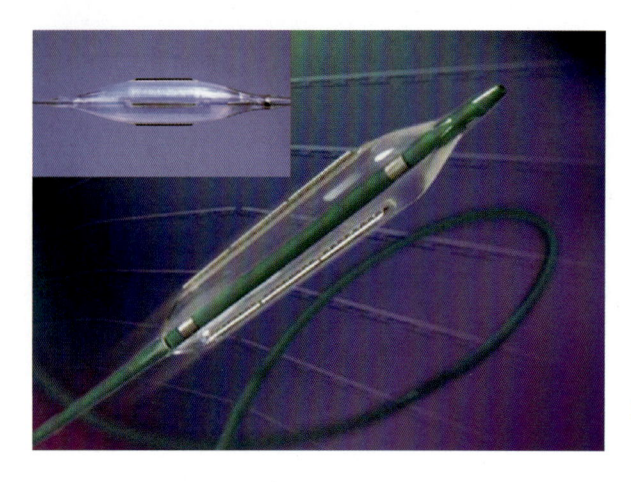

Figure 5-2. Cutting balloons have razors implanted in the balloon. *(Courtesy Boston Scientific Corp., Natick, Mass.)*

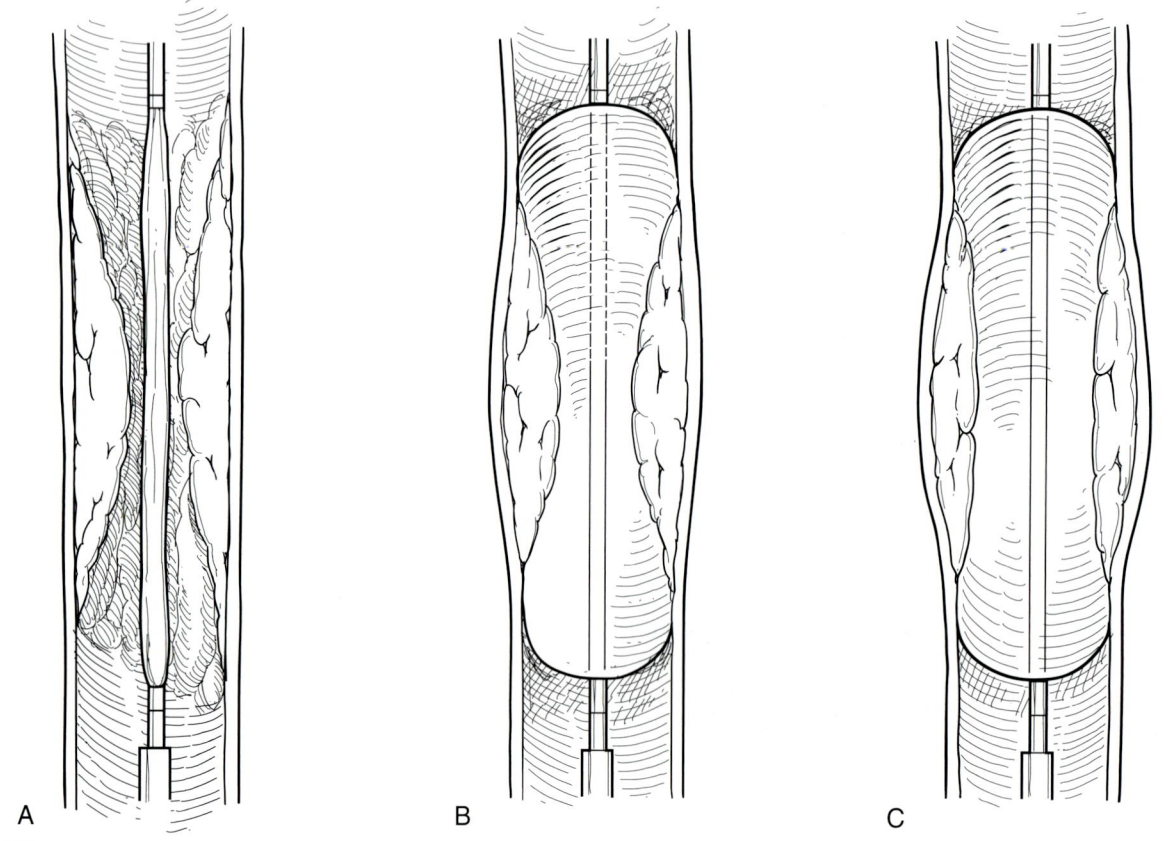

A   B   C

Figure 5-3. An atherosclerotic waist is identified using angiography. **A,** An appropriately sized balloon catheter is selected and positioned to straddle the stenosis. **B,** The balloon is inflated while monitoring the pressure and watching it take shape. **C,** The atherosclerotic waist is visualized and ultimately dilated with increasing pressure to the diameter of the surrounding vessel.

inflation commonly causes the patient to experience pain because of stretching of the vessel adventitia, which should resolve after balloon deflation. Continued pain after angioplasty is a concerning sign and mandates immediate repeat arteriography to evaluate the potential of rupture or dissection.

When multiple lesions require treatment, sequential dilatation of the most distal to proximal lesion is recommended while maintaining guidewire access across all lesions. If the proximal lesions are too narrow to allow passage of a balloon, the order of treatment may need to be reversed. Some experts advocate sequential angioplasty from proximal to distal lesions in order to maintain adequate inflow to the next downstream lesion. The presumption is that this approach minimizes the risk of thrombosis during the interval in which the presence of untreated proximal lesions may limit flow across the thrombogenic surface of a distal angioplastied segment. If postangioplasty stents are necessary, stent deployment from distal to proximal sites is advocated in order to minimize manipulation through

TABLE 5-2 Average Arterial Diameters

Vessel	Diameter (mm)
External carotid	3-5
Internal carotid	4-7
Common carotid	5-9
Vertebral	3-5
Brachiocephalic	8-12
Subclavian	6-10
Axillary	6-8
Brachial	5-7
Radial or ulnar	2-4
Thoracic aorta	20-28
Abdominal aorta	10-24
Celiac trunk	6-9
Splenic	4-7
Hepatic	4-6
Superior mesenteric	4-7
Renal	4-6
Common iliac	6-12
External iliac	5-9
Internal iliac	5-7
Common femoral	5-8
Profunda	4-5
SFA	4-6
Popliteal	3-5
Tibials	1-4

a freshly placed stent that would otherwise be required with the passage of each new sequentially placed distal stent.

STENTING

When a decision is made to stent a lesion, selection of the appropriate dimensions and appropriate type of stent is paramount. Stent size is related to the specific vessel and lesion being treated, but rules of thumb based on usual vessel dimension should recognize the inherent variability among patients' arterial diameters (Table 5-2). If a lesion is predilated with a balloon catheter, diameter and length of the stent can usually be inferred. Predilation of a lesion in anticipation of stent placement is used if the stent is not able to cross the lesion or if the risk of embolization from an entrapped stent deployment system would have devastating consequences, such as a stroke. A catheter or device can also serve as a reference in the calibration of vessel diameter. This technique, known as vessel analysis, allows automated measurement of the diameter and length of the lesion and the surrounding unaffected vessel.

The two major subsets of stents are self-expanding and balloon expandable (Fig. 5-4; see also Table 5-1). Balloon-expandable stents can be simply and precisely deployed, whereas self-expanding stents require a greater degree of operator stabilization to maintain stent position during the period of unsheathing the stent. Balloon-expandable stents can be dilated beyond their reported diameter, but with a correspondent shortening of the stent. Self-expanding stents cannot be postdilated beyond their nominal or unsheathed diameter and therefore must be oversized by 1 to 3 mm in order to exert continuous outward radial force and thus avoid stent migration. Self-expanding stents are more flexible than balloon-expandable stents and thus better situated for use in mobile or tortuous vessels, such as the SFA. Balloon-expandable stents have higher hoop strength ratings and are better used in orificial lesions, such as those commonly observed with renal artery stenosis. In some instances self-expanding stents may display residual collapse because of insufficient hoop strength. In these instances a balloon-expandable stent can be placed off label within the self-expanding stent.

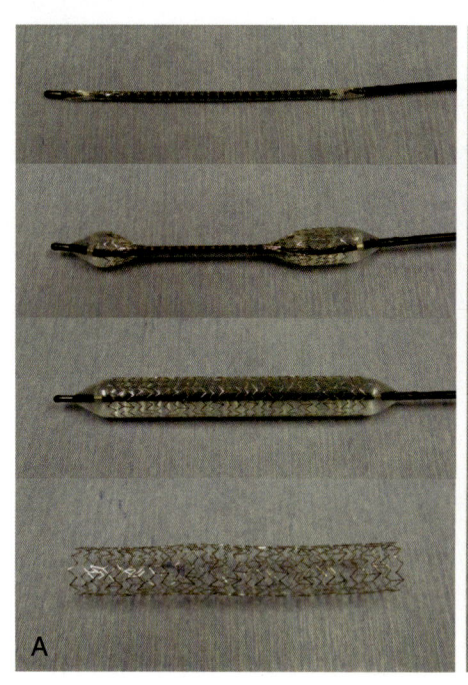

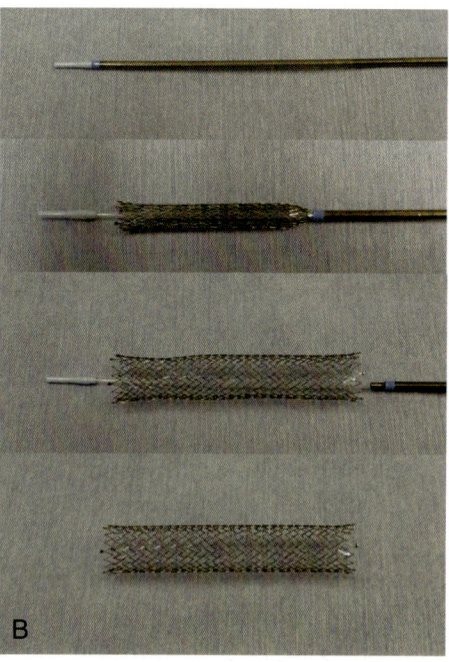

Figure 5-4. Stents vary in size, composition, delivery system, and characteristics. **A,** Balloon-expandable stents are more rigid than self-expanding stents and are deployed by balloon inflation using either a premounted or a self-mounted technique. **B,** Self-expanding stents are more flexible than balloon-expandable stents and frequently made of nickel-titanium alloy. *(From Cronenwett JL, Johnston KW, editors: Rutherford's vascular surgery, ed 7, Philadelphia, 2010, Saunders, p 1278, Fig. 85-1C.)*

Most balloon-expandable stents are premounted on a balloon, but separate stents, such as the large-diameter Palmaz stent (Cordis Corp., Bridgewater, N.J.) can be crimped onto a balloon for delivery and deployment. Self-mounted stents are at increased risk for becoming dislodged from their balloon during advancement and balloon insufflation. Drug-eluting stents are commonly used in coronary vessels, but their usefulness in the peripheral circulation remains under investigation.[9]

RECANALIZATION

Three randomized trials of thrombolytic therapy for acute limb ischemia were performed in the 1990s, with subgroup analysis of the Surgery versus Thrombolysis for Ischemia of the Lower Extremity (STILE) trial data suggesting a beneficial effect of thrombolysis among patients presenting with an occluded prosthetic bypass graft or an acute arterial occlusion of less than 14 days duration.[10-12] Recombinant tissue plasminogen activator (tPA) is the most widely used of the thrombolytic agents, which include alteplase (Activase, Genentech, South San Francisco), derived from cloned human tissue plasminogen activator (tPA); and two engineered tPA mutants, reteplase (Retevase, Centocor, St. Louis), a deletion mutant lacking two domains at the amino terminus, and tenecteplase (TNKase, Genentech), containing three point mutations. The thrombolytic agent is delivered by an infusion catheter to the specific site of the thrombus either alone or in conjunction with mechanical therapy to accelerate the process of thrombus resolution. A variety of devices have been designed to facilitate clot dissolution, and some have the capacity to "spray" a clot with heparinized saline or tPA. After 10 to 30 minutes of infusion for initial clot dissolution, the clot can be mechanically emulsified and aspirated.

In general, an acute thrombus is more amenable to lytic therapy as it is softer and less organized than a chronic thrombus. After vascular access has been obtained and an appropriately sized sheath has been placed, a guidewire is used to cross the thrombus. Specialized lytic catheters are available in varying sizes that are designed to infuse long lengths of the thrombus with a lytic agent using a soaker-hose configuration with an infusion wire. Various regimens exist for dosing of tPA, but in general, more aggressive infusions are used early when the clot burden is highest. Many practitioners lace the clot with bolus injections of tPA before infusing at a rate of 1 to 2 mg/hr for the first 4 to 6 hours before decreasing the rate by one half. Frequent repeat angiography is needed to monitor the progression of the lysis. Different institutional protocols exist for monitoring a patient undergoing lytic therapy, including the measurement of hematocrit, platelet count, prothrombin

ANGIOPLASTY, STENTING, RECANALIZATION, AND EMBOLIZATION

> **Box 5-1**   **ATHERECTOMY DEVICES**
>
> - Diamondback (Cardiovascular Systems, St. Paul, Minn.)
> - TurboHawk and SilverHawk (ev3 Endovascular, Plymouth, Minn.)
> - Jetstream (Pathway Medical Technologies, Kirkland, Wash.)
> - Laser atherectomy (The Spectranetics Corp., Colorado Springs, Colo.)

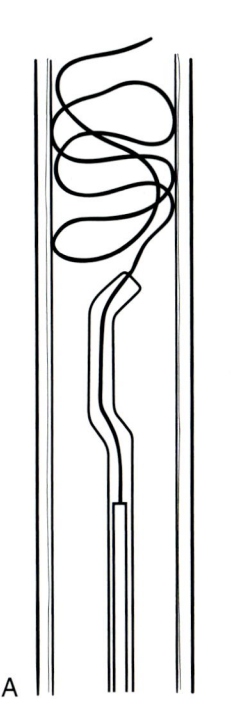

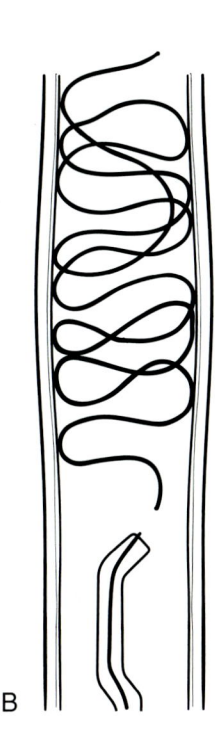

Figure 5-5. A, Coil embolization of peripheral artery by positioning a catheter in the desired vessel and pushing the coil through until it deploys in the vessel and assumes its shape. **B,** Multiple coils can be placed to "pack" the vessel and induce thrombosis.

time, partial thromboplastin time, and fibrinogen levels every 6 hours. Patients must be monitored for bleeding at the sheath site or at other distant sites, and a low threshold for terminating lytic therapy should be maintained.

Directional atherectomy devices have been designed to recanalize chronic occlusive lesions by removing intraluminal atheroma using a cutting device in which atheromatous material, collected within the catheter tip, is periodically removed by the operator. Recurrent stenosis rates continue to be high after atherectomy, and there is a risk of distal embolization during the procedure. Newer atherectomy devices have combined an element of aspiration with the cutting process or laser ablation to minimize embolic risk (Box 5-1).

THERAPEUTIC EMBOLIZATION

The rich collateral network of arterial blood supply to many organs and tissues allows sacrifice of an injured, aneurysmal, or bleeding vessel in the treatment of traumatic vascular injuries, gastrointestinal bleeding, visceral aneurysm or pseudoaneurysm formation, and pulmonary arteriovenous malformations. Embolization of tumor vasculature has also been used for various conditions, including uterine fibroids.[13] Embolization of distant vessels that would be difficult to approach in an open surgical fashion has dramatically altered the treatment of conditions, such as traumatic hemorrhage from pelvic fractures.[14]

There are a variety of embolic materials and devices (see Table 5-1). Perhaps the most common method uses steel coils that are prepackaged in their straightened conformation and are available in a variety of sizes. A delivery catheter is positioned at the desired site of embolization, and the coil is pushed out of the catheter using a pusher or guidewire assuming its coiled shape (Fig. 5-5). The key to accurate coil deployment is to maintain delivery catheter position as the coil is pushed out in order to prevent the entire system from backing out

TABLE 5-3 Amplatzer II Vascular Plugs (AGA Medical Corp.)*

Diameter (mm)	Length (mm)	Minimum Sheath Size (Fr)	Minimum Guide Catheter Size (Fr)
3	6	4	5
4	6	4	5
6	6	4	5
8	7	4	5
10	7	5	6
12	9	5	6
14	10	6	8
16	12	6	8
18	14	7	9
20	16	7	9
22	18	7	9

*All are mounted on a 100-cm-long delivery wire.

of the desired location. Telescoping with multiple coaxial catheters to improve support can facilitate accurate deployment in challenging locations. Initially a larger stainless steel coil is often used to prevent migration and to provide a scaffold for smaller, more flexible platinum coils to occlude the vessel.

Alternate embolization devices are also available, which are packaged in a delivery sheath and deployed to act as a large plug in a vessel of interest. These devices come in a variety of sizes and are typically oversized by 30% to 50% to avoid migration (Table 5-3). Variant clamshell shapes were initially used as closure devices to treat congenital cardiac defects, such as a patent foramen ovale or atrial septal defect. These devices have an attached delivery wire that screws into the base, allowing them to be recaptured into the sheath and repositioned.

Postoperative Care

- **Antiplatelet therapy is initiated after angioplasty or stent placement.** For many patients, 81 mg of aspirin daily is sufficient. The use of clopidogrel depends on the vascular bed that was treated and whether or not a stent was placed. Generally, clopidogrel is used for carotid and tibial interventions for a minimum of 4 weeks. For iliac, SFA, and popliteal lesions, either aspirin or clopidogrel is acceptable.
- **Objective assessment of post-procedural outcome.** Non-invasive vascular studies are typically obtained within 4 weeks of the intervention. Treatment that impacts the lower extremity is assessed by pulse volume recordings (PVR) of segmental waveforms and related segmental blood pressures, ankle-brachial index (ABI), duplex imaging, and velocity measurements. Likewise, interventions that influence the circulation of the upper extremity can be assessed by measurement of segmental waveforms and blood pressures, as well as duplex measurements. Procedures that impact the carotid and visceral vessels are assessed by duplex examination.
- Patients should be monitored for disease progression and failure of the initial intervention at regular intervals.

Postoperative Complications

Angioplasty specific complications include flow-limiting dissection, embolization, thrombosis, perforation, and arterial spasm.

- **Dissection** is a frequent finding after angioplasty but does not require treatment unless flow limiting, in which case stenting is required.
- **Embolization** is infrequent but can cause limb or end-organ ischemia. The diagnosis is established by demonstrating compromised flow in an area that

was previously patent. Management includes heparinization with attempts to remove the thrombus with specialized aspiration catheters or an over-the-wire embolectomy balloon. Infusion of tPA with or without mechanical thrombolysis can also be attempted. Failure to reestablish flow may require open surgical revascularization.

- **Arterial perforation** secondary to angioplasty is uncommon, especially if judicious balloon sizing and inflation are practiced. Perforation must be suspected in instances of unexplained hypotension, and immediate angiography should be used to confirm the diagnosis. Perforation of smaller vessels, such as tibial vessels, is usually self-limiting. Large vessel hemorrhage can be controlled rapidly by carefully reinflating the balloon at the site of injury. Reversal of heparin should be considered, and blood products can be ordered. Bleeding may be controlled with gentle pressure from the inflated balloon, but if extravasation persists, a covered stent can be placed at the injury site. To facilitate this without losing the tamponade affect of the balloon, it may be necessary to gain intravascular access at a separate location. An example is an inadvertent external iliac artery puncture that is not easily accessible for covered stent placement through an ipsilateral retrograde femoral puncture. In this situation a balloon can control bleeding from the ipsilateral groin, whereas the contralateral groin can be accessed and a covered stent can be precisely delivered. If a suitable covered stent is unavailable and hemorrhage continues, open surgical repair is necessary.

Acute complications of stent placement include dislodgment, incomplete expansion, and misplacement.

- **Stent dislodgment.** When a stent becomes partially dislodged from a delivery device, it can often be salvaged by repositioning a balloon through the stent and deploying it fully. It can be difficult to visualize a dislodged stent, and it may be useful to magnify the image, increase resolution by using a higher number of frames per second, and use filters to minimize scatter. In addition filming in various projections may be necessary to identify the optimal position for stent visualization.
- **Incomplete stent expansion**. Incomplete stent expansion can usually be treated with angioplasty, but it is occasionally necessary to reline the area with another stent.
- **Malpositioned stents.** Malpositioned stents usually occur during deployment of self-expanding stents, which have a tendency to jump forward during unsheathing. Stent deployment precision can be improved by ensuring there is no buildup of energy in the system through wire buckling or twisting, elimination of wire slack, and controlled deployment. If the malpositioned stent does not treat the lesion, a second overlapping stent can be placed.
- **Stent migration.** If a stent migrates because it is incorrectly sized, then the original lesion should be treated and the migrated stent may be snared or "jailed" at a site distal to the lesion by placement of an overlapping stent. In cases of stent fracture or embolization leading to an intravascular foreign body, options include snare retrieval; disposal of the debris into a noncritical artery, such as a hypogastric artery; or stenting to trap the debris against the wall of the vessel. Open surgical retrieval is an option, if necessary.

REFERENCES

1. Dotter CT, Judkins MP: Transluminal treatment of arteriosclerotic obstruction. Description of a new technic and a preliminary report of its application, *Circulation* 30:654-670, 1964.
2. Grüntzig A, Kumpe DA: Technique of percutaneous transluminal angioplasty with the Grüntzig balloon catheter, *Am J Roentgenol* 132:547-552, 1979.
3. Dotter CT: Transluminally placed coilspring endarterial tube grafts: Long-term patency in canine popliteal artery, *Invest Radiol* 4:329-332, 1969.
4. Tillet WS, Garner RL: The fibrinolytic activity of hemolytic streptococci, *J Exp Med* 58:485, 1933.

5. Clifton EE, Grunnet M: Investigations of intravenous plasmin (fibrinolysin) in humans, *Circulation* 14:919, 1956.
6. Luessenhop AJ, Spence WT: Artificial embolization of cerebral arteries. Report of use in a case of arteriovenous malformation, *J Am Med Assoc* 12(172):1153-1155, 1960.
7. Tetteroo E, van der Graaf Y, Bosch JL, et al: Randomised comparison of primary stent placement versus primary angioplasty followed by selective stent placement in patients with iliac-artery occlusive disease. Dutch Iliac Stent Trial Study Group, *Lancet* 351:1153-1159, 1998.
8. Tielbeek AV, Vroegindeweij D, Buth J, et al: Comparison of balloon angioplasty and Simpson atherectomy for lesions in the femoropopliteal artery: Angiographic and clinical results of a prospective randomized trial, *J Vasc Interv Radiol* 7:837-844, 1996.
9. Duda SH, Bosiers M, Lammer J, et al: Drug-eluting and bare nitinol stents for the treatment of atherosclerotic lesions in the superficial femoral artery: Long-term results from the SIROCCO trial, *J Endovasc Ther* 13:701-710, 2006.
10. Ouriel K, Shortell CK, DeWeese JA, et al: A comparison of thrombolytic therapy with operative revascularization in the initial treatment of acute peripheral arterial ischemia, *J Vasc Surg* 19:1021-1030, 1994.
11. Surgery versus Thrombolysis for Ischemia of the Lower Extremity investigators: Results of a prospective randomized trial evaluating surgery versus thrombolysis for ischemia of the lower extremity. The STILE trial, *Ann Surg* 220:251-266, 1994.
12. Ouriel K, Veith FJ, Sasahara AA: A comparison of recombinant urokinase with vascular surgery as initial treatment for acute arterial occlusion of the legs. Thrombolysis or Peripheral Arterial Surgery (TOPAS) Investigators, *N Engl J Med* 338:1105-1111, 1998.
13. Goodwin SC, Spies JB, Worthington-Kirsch R, et al: Uterine artery embolization for treatment of leiomyomata: Long-term outcomes from the FIBROID Registry, *Obstet Gynecol* 111:22-33, 2008.
14. Agolini SF, Shah K, Jaffe J, et al: Arterial embolization is a rapid and effective technique for controlling pelvic fracture hemorrhage, *J Trauma* 43:395-399, 1997.

Section 2

EXTRACRANIAL CEREBROVASCULAR DISEASE

6 Carotid Endarterectomy

ELLIOT L. CHAIKOF • RICHARD P. CAMBRIA

Historical Background

Although Carrea, Molins, and Murphy[1] performed a successful carotid resection in 1951 and DeBakey[2] completed a successful carotid endarterectomy (CEA) in 1953, the potential benefit of surgical treatment for symptomatic carotid occlusive disease was first highlighted by Eastcott, Pickering, and Rob in 1954.[3] Use of a carotid shunt was then described by Al-Naaman, Carton, and Cooley in 1956.[4] Two large multicenter randomized trials, the North American Symptomatic Carotid Endarterectomy Trial[5,6] and the European Carotid Surgery Trial,[7] have since demonstrated that CEA reduces the risk of stroke in patients with ipsilateral symptomatic carotid stenosis. The efficacy of CEA in asymptomatic patients has also been confirmed in three randomized clinical trials that included patients with moderate to severe stenosis.[8-10]

Indications

CEA is indicated to prevent stroke in patients with carotid bifurcation occlusive disease.[11] Multiple randomized prospective studies support CEA for: (1) asymptomatic patients with carotid stenosis of more than 60%, and (2) symptomatic patients with a history of recent transient ischemic attack (TIA) or amaurosis fugax and ipsilateral carotid stenosis of more than 50%.

Additional indications for CEA have been reported. Given limited available evidence, the decision to recommend treatment should be based upon the surgeon's complication rate and patient preference. Specifically, the benefits of CEA are less established for: (1) patients with carotid stenosis of more than 50% and nonhemispheric symptoms, vertebrobasilar symptoms, stroke in evolution, or a completed acute stroke, and (2) symptomatic patients with an ulcerated carotid plaque and ipsilateral carotid stenosis of less than 50%.

Preoperative Preparation

- The use of aspirin (81-325 mg/day) or clopidogrel (75 mg/day) during the preoperative and postoperative periods is an evidence-based adjunct to diminish perioperative complications.[12,13]
- Several studies attest to the protective effect of perioperative statins.[14]
- Perioperative imaging may consist of a duplex scan alone, provided that the quality control aspects of the noninvasive vascular laboratory have been verified and the surgeon can evaluate both the technical adequacy and the original data of the study. Additional imaging may consist of magnetic resonance angiography, computed tomography (CT) angiography, or conventional catheter-based angiography. However, the inherent risk of the latter and the current reliability of CT angiography means invasive angiography is rarely needed.
- Evaluation of cardiac risk is recommended by clinical profiling or in select patients through use of noninvasive stress testing.
- Evaluation of vocal cord function should be performed in patients with a history of prior CEA.

- Prophylactic antibiotics are advisable.
- Nasotracheal intubation and mandibular subluxation should be considered for exposure of the distal internal carotid artery (ICA).
- Intraoperative arterial line monitoring of blood pressure is recommended.
- Intraoperative cerebral monitoring may be used to indicate a need for a carotid shunt.

Pitfalls and Danger Points

- Stroke
  - The performance of a technically perfect operation is the most important variable in stroke prevention.
  - Perioperative antiplatelet therapy is an evidence-based adjunct to diminish risk of stroke.
- Cranial nerve (CN) injury
- Hematoma
- Restenosis
  - Recurrence of stenosis is more common in women and small arteries.
  - Patch angioplasty is an evidence-based adjunct to diminish risk of restenosis.

Operative Strategy

AVOIDING INTRAOPERATIVE STROKE

The perioperative combined mortality and major stroke risk for CEA in all patient subgroups ranges between 2% and 5%.[12,15] This risk is less for asymptomatic patients (<3%), increases for those who have had a recent TIA, and is greatest for patients who present with a stroke in evolution or recent stroke.

The following considerations should be parts of the operative strategy to reduce the risk of intraoperative stroke:

1. *Timing of intervention in the symptomatic patient.* Patients with moderate to severe (>50%) stenosis and symptoms should have "urgent" endarterectomy within 2 weeks. Timing of CEA in patients with an established stroke is a matter of clinical judgment, with the size of the infarct on brain imaging an important variable. Most patients with minor stroke can have an indicated CEA performed during the same hospital admission. In the rare case of a patient requiring bilateral endarterectomies the second procedure can be performed 2 weeks after the initial operation.

2. *Operative technique.* Manipulation of the carotid bifurcation should be avoided, and a "no-touch" technique should be applied to the lesion.

3. *Intraoperative hypotension and arrhythmias.* Lidocaine can be injected into the area of the carotid sinus nerve to prevent bradyarrhythmias and hypotension during exposure of the carotid bifurcation. However, this maneuver may be associated with postoperative reflex hypertension.

4. *Carotid shunts.* Some surgeons advocate routine carotid shunting, whereas others prefer the selective use of a shunt, noting that fewer than 10% of patients display ischemic symptoms during intraoperative occlusion of the carotid artery. In the awake patient symptoms of ischemia may manifest as the inability to follow verbal commands or as on-table seizure activity. Under general anesthesia, a change in cerebral monitoring (e.g., electroencephalogram, cerebral oximetry, or transcranial Doppler) can be used as an indication for shunting. Systolic blood pressure should be maintained between 120 and 180 mm Hg.

5. *Securing the endarterectomy endpoint.* If the transition at the distal endpoint of the endarterectomy is not smooth, a distal intimal flap may be present

that should be secured with 7-0 polypropylene tacking sutures. Careful visualization of the endpoint may require additional exposure of the distal ICA and extension of the arteriotomy. Saline irrigation confirms that the flap is adequately secured. An important technical principle is to remove all disease so that the endarterectomy "endpoint" occurs in the anatomically normal distal ICA.

6. *Avoidance of residual stenosis.* Routine patch closure is supported by randomized prospective trials and should be performed to minimize the risk of residual distal stenosis. This risk is accentuated in women with small arteries. Although we do not routinely perform completion intraoperative imaging, Duplex ultrasound has been advocated in some centers to exclude the presence of an intimal flap or residual stenosis.

7. *Management of carotid kinks and coils.* Excessive length of the ICA may be associated with a coil or kink at or distal to the site of occlusive disease. After removal of the plaque, redundancy of the ICA may lead to an accentuated bend or narrowing at the distal endpoint of the arteriotomy. This may be treated by resection and shortening of either the common carotid artery or the ICA. Shortening of the common carotid artery requires the presence of redundancy in both the ICA and the external carotid artery (ECA). Alternatively, eversion CEA is a convenient way to deal with such redundancy.

AVOIDING CRANIAL NERVE INJURIES

The incidence of nerve injury as a result of CEA that persists beyond hospital discharge is approximately 4%, with most deficits resolving over the subsequent few months.[16] Injury may occur because of transection, excessive traction, or electrocauterization. Injuries to the hypoglossal (CN XII), vagus (CN X), and marginal mandibular branch of the facial nerve (CN VII) are most common, whereas the spinal accessory nerve (CN XI) and glossopharyngeal nerves (CN IX) are rarely injured.[17-20] Several factors contribute to a failure to identify and properly protect the CNs:

1. *Anatomic variability.* The vagus nerve usually lies posterior to the common carotid artery but occasionally may be found anterior to the artery. It should be distinguished from the ansa hypoglossi nerve upon opening of the carotid sheath and exposure of the common carotid artery. An anterior vagus nerve needs to be mobilized laterally.

2. *Short, fat neck.* The hypoglossal nerve crosses the ICA at a variable distance from the bifurcation. A low-lying hypoglossal may be injured during division of the common facial vein. Otherwise, the nerve is at risk for injury during dissection through lymphovascular tissue in the upper medial portion of the operative field. Identification of the hypoglossal nerve is facilitated by following the ansa hypoglossi nerve to its junction with the hypoglossal trunk.

3. *High carotid bifurcation.* The glossopharyngeal nerve courses between the ICA and the internal jugular vein, lying deep to the styloid process and attached muscles. It is at risk for injury during removal of the styloid process to expose the distal ICA.[21,22] Confining dissection to the periadventitial tissue of the ICA minimizes the risk of injury. The spinal accessory nerve exits the skull with the glossopharyngeal and vagus nerves and pierces the sternocleidomastoid (SCM) muscle superiorly before continuing inferiorly until it reaches the trapezius muscle. The nerve is at risk of injury during distal dissections or with excessive traction on the upper extent of the SCM muscle.

4. *Excessive dissection.* The superior laryngeal nerve courses behind the ECA. Encircling the artery at its most proximal point lessens the risk of injury.

5. *Placement of the skin incision.* The marginal mandibular branch of the facial nerve may be injured if the incision is placed less than one fingerbreadth from the angle of the jaw. Traction or retractors at the superior extent of the incision should be

directed superior and lateral, rather than hooking the mandible, which increases the risk of injury to the marginal mandibular branch. The greater auricular nerve may be injured during superior extension of the skin incision.

Operative Technique

CHOICE OF ANESTHESIA

CEA can be performed under local, regional, or general anesthesia. General anesthesia is recommended for patients who may be anxious or have difficult anatomy. Randomized trials have shown no evidence that a specific anesthetic technique is associated with reduced operative morbidity or mortality.[23]

INCISION AND POSITION

The patient is positioned at the edge of the table of the affected side. The neck is extended, and the head is turned to opposite the side of the intended incision and placed upon a soft rubber ring (Fig. 6-1, A). Elevation of the shoulders with a rolled sheet or "thyroid bag" enhances neck extension, especially in patients with short, broad necks. The upper chest, lower face, and lower ear are prepped and draped. An incision paralleling the anterior margin of the SCM muscle affords maximum exposure of the entire cervical course of the carotid artery. A common error is to carry the inferior aspect of the incision too medially, allowing the larynx to interfere with exposure. The incision should be curved slightly along a skin crease, should be extended just inferior to the lobe of the ear at its distal end, and may need to be extended to the mastoid in distal, difficult lesions. This posterior displacement of the incision, one fingerbreadth below the angle of the jaw, helps avoid injury to the marginal mandibular branch of the facial nerve.

MOBILIZATION OF THE STERNOCLEIDOMASTOID MUSCLE

The incision is deepened through the platysma muscle, and the investing layer of the deep cervical fascia is opened on the anterior border of the SCM muscle (Fig. 6-1, B). The anterior edge of the SCM muscle is mobilized, and the muscle is separated from the underlying vascular sheath by a sharp dissection on its medial border. The small sternomastoid branch of the superior thyroid artery requires ligation during this maneuver; this and other perforating vessels supplying the SCM muscle signal that the SCM has been sufficiently mobilized laterally. The spinal accessory nerve, which may cross from beneath the SCM at the superior aspect of the wound, is at risk of injury if the SCM is subjected to excessive traction.

MOBILIZATION OF THE JUGULAR VEIN AND DIVISION OF THE COMMON FACIAL VEIN

By retracting the freed SCM muscle posteriorly, the carotid sheath is identified; often the anterior surface of the internal jugular vein is visible at this point, but this depends on the degree of overlying lymphatic and adipose tissue. The sheath is opened superior to the omohyoid muscle with more proximal exposure necessitating division of the muscle. The internal jugular vein is dissected along its medial border in the central part of the field and retracted posteriorly with the SCM muscle. This maneuver requires division of the common facial vein (Fig. 6-2). The common facial vein is divided, as well as other medially coursing branches, and the internal jugular vein is mobilized laterally. The ansa hypoglossi lies over the carotid artery and can be divided with impunity.

EXPOSURE OF THE COMMON CAROTID ARTERY

The common carotid artery is isolated using sharp dissection before manipulation of the atherosclerotic bifurcation (Fig. 6-3). The vagus nerve should be identified and protected. Once the common carotid artery is freed from the surrounding tissue, it is encircled with tape away from the bifurcation area. Clearance of tissues from the anterior surface of the common carotid artery may be facilitated by transection of the ansa hypoglossi nerve.

68 EXTRACRANIAL CEREBROVASCULAR DISEASE

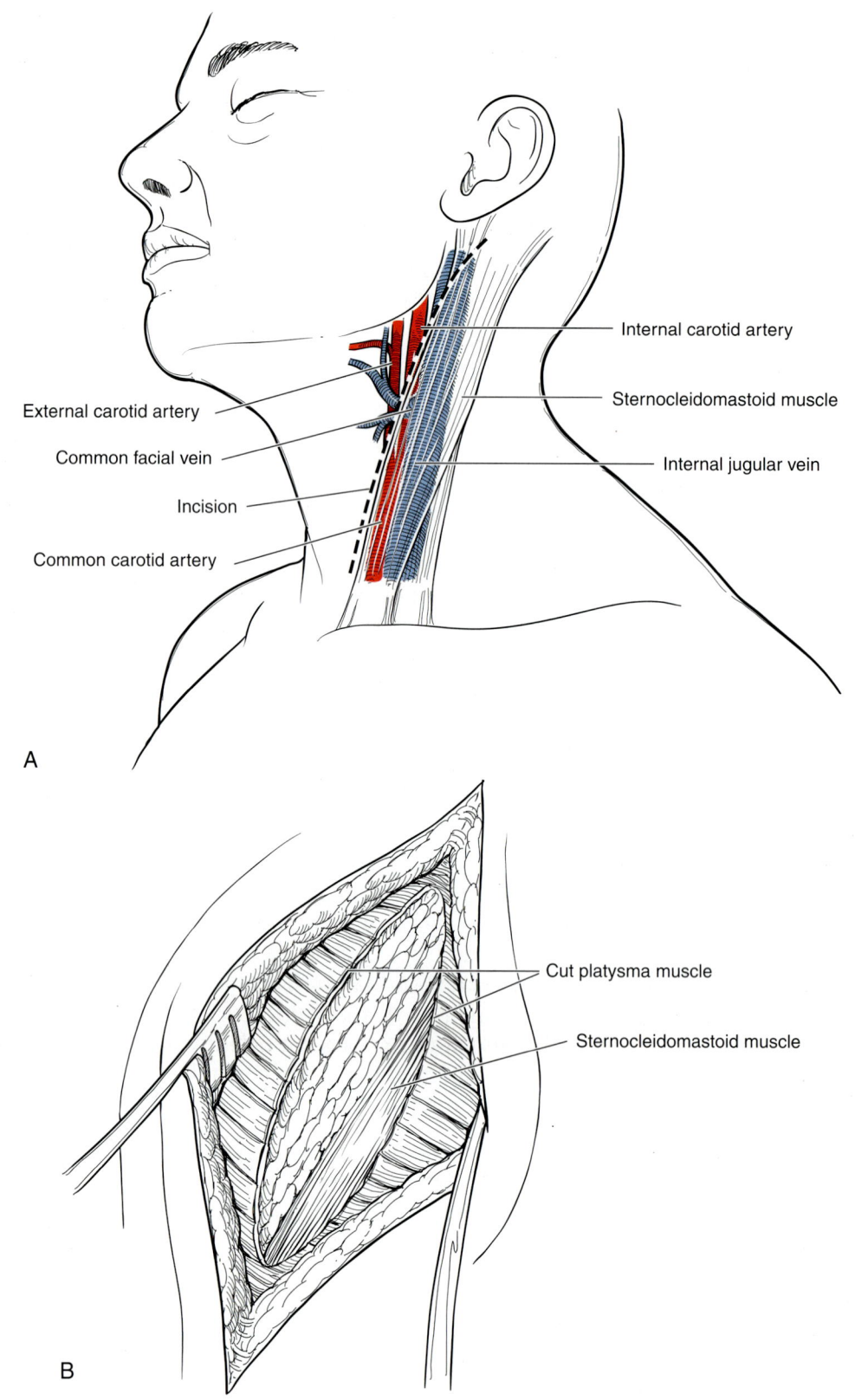

Figure 6-1. A, The neck is extended, and the head is turned to opposite the side of the intended incision and placed upon a soft rubber ring. Elevation of the shoulders with a rolled sheet or "thyroid bag" enhances neck extension, especially in patients with short, broad necks. **B,** An incision paralleling the anterior margin of the sternocleidomastoid muscle affords maximum exposure of the entire cervical course of the carotid artery. The incision is deepened through the platysma muscle.

ISOLATION OF THE EXTERNAL CAROTID ARTERY

The ECA is isolated just above the bifurcation, which is never grasped, and encircled with tape. Care should be taken to minimize manipulation of the carotid bifurcation and thus avoid atheroembolization. The superior thyroid artery requires isolation when it branches directly from the common carotid artery. Once

CAROTID ENDARTERECTOMY   69

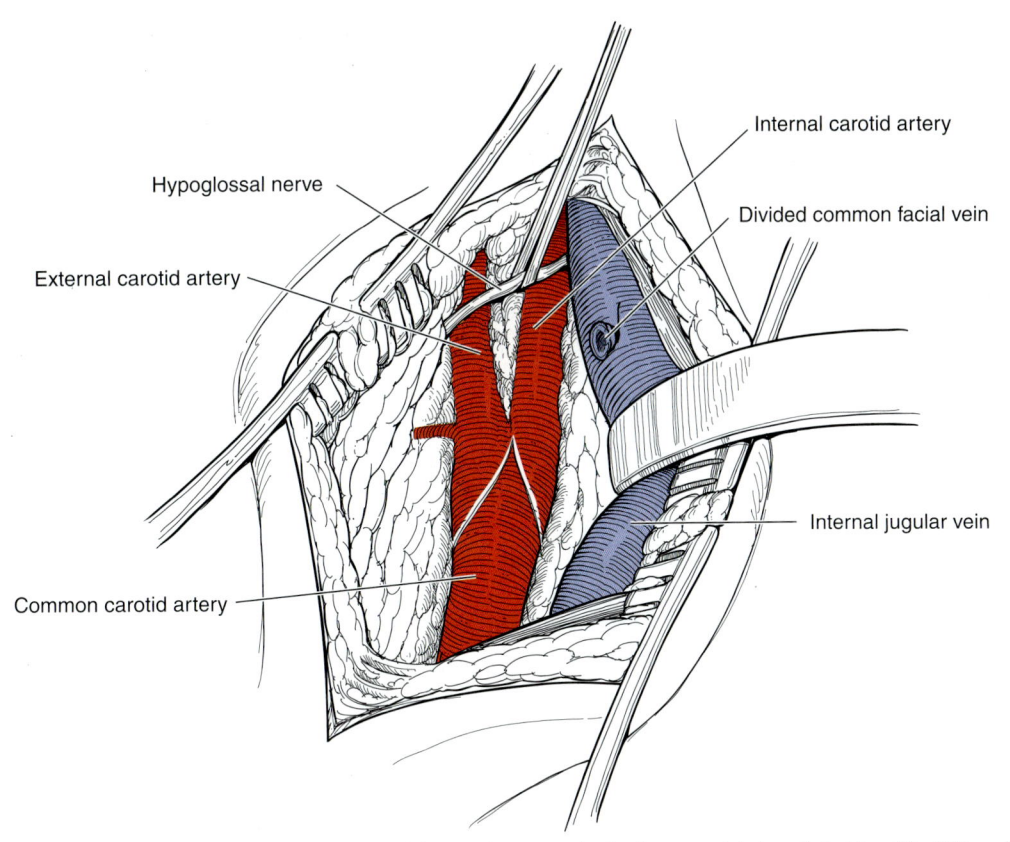

Figure 6-2. By retracting the freed sternocleidomastoid muscle posteriorly, the carotid sheath is identified. The sheath is opened superior to the omohyoid muscle. The internal jugular vein is dissected along its medial border in the central part of the field and retracted posteriorly. This maneuver requires division of the common facial vein. The ansa hypoglossi lies over the carotid artery, and a search for an anterior vagus nerve is conducted.

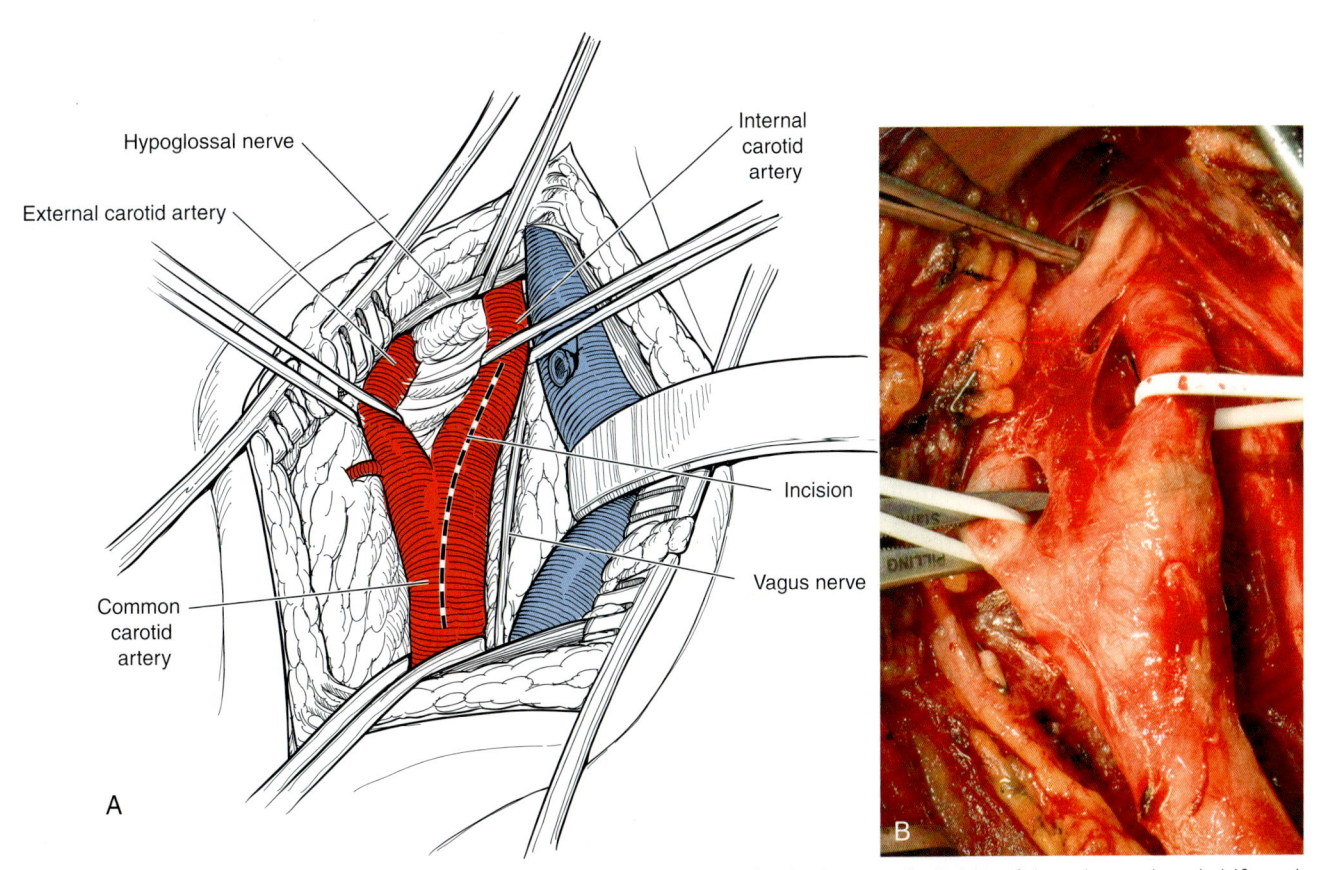

Figure 6-3. A, The common carotid artery is isolated using sharp dissection before manipulation of the atherosclerotic bifurcation. The vagus nerve usually lies posterior to the common carotid artery and should be identified and protected. **B,** Once the common carotid artery is freed from the surrounding tissue, it is encircled with tape away from the bifurcation.

dissection progresses cephalad to the bifurcation, grasping the neural tissue between the ECA and the ICA, rather than the diseased ICA, facilitates distal dissection of the ICA.

ISOLATION OF THE INTERNAL CAROTID ARTERY

The ICA is isolated next. It is often located posterior to the ECA and found deep to the internal jugular vein. Dissection along the medial border of the internal jugular vein in the superior wound allows exposure of the ICA away from the bifurcation. Lymphatic tissue overlying the vein requires division. Small venous branches above the level of the common facial vein should be identified and ligated to prevent bleeding. The hypoglossal nerve trunk crosses the ICA at a variable distance from the bifurcation and often courses medial enough such that the ICA can be thoroughly exposed without having to manipulate the nerve. However, mobilization of the hypoglossal nerve from lateral to medial is sometimes required, necessitating division of the occipital artery at the lateral border of the field. The ICA should be controlled 1 cm beyond the visible extent of atheromatous disease and encircled with tape.

EXPOSURE OF THE DISTAL INTERNAL CAROTID ARTERY

In the case of distal disease, exposure of the upper cervical segment of the ICA can be achieved by mandibular subluxation.[24] General anesthesia with nasotracheal intubation is required for this approach. The mandibular condyle on the side to be operated is subluxed and transfixed with transnasal or oral wiring. Exposure of the common carotid artery and the ICA and mobilization of the hypoglossal nerve proceed as described earlier. Division of the posteriorly belly of the digastric muscle allows exposure of the ICA within 2 cm of the skull base (Fig. 6-4). Care should be taken to ligate small branches of the jugular vein that cross the anterior surface of the ICA. The lower edge of the parotid gland is retracted superiorly during this maneuver. Higher exposure of the ICA is obtainable by dividing the stylohyoid ligament, as well as stylohyoid, stylopharyngeus, and styloglossus muscles to permit removal of the styloid process. Confining dissection to the periadventitial tissue of the ICA minimizes risk of injury to the glossopharyngeal nerve.

ARTERIOTOMY AND SHUNT PLACEMENT

Heparin (75-100 units/kg) is administered intravenously. The ICA is clamped with a bulldog clamp where it is visibly normal, followed by clamping of the common carotid artery and the ECA using angled vascular clamps. An arteriotomy is made on the anterolateral surface on the common carotid artery and extended to the ICA beyond the atheromatous plaque with Potts scissors.

The shunt is advanced into the ICA, and free retrograde flow is confirmed (Fig. 6-5). The shunt is then temporally occluded to prevent continued blood loss, and the proximal end is placed into the lumen of the common carotid artery. The shunt should be placed under direct vision after aspiration of blood in order to minimize the risk of inadvertent embolization of debris from the operative field through the lumen of the shunt. The angled vascular clamp is removed, the shunt advanced into the common carotid artery, and tapes with rubber tourniquets are made snug around the shunt. The average size of a shunt that fits into the distal ICA is 10 Fr (2.5-mm lumen). An 8- or 12-Fr shunt can be used for smaller or larger vessels, respectively. As shunts may occasionally malfunction because of abutment of the distal end of the shunt against the wall of ICA (e.g., at a coil or kink), flow through the shunt should be assessed after placement with a Doppler flow probe.

ENDARTERECTOMY

The atheromatous plaque is separated from the carotid artery by dissection in the layer between media and adventitia, revealing the distinct pinkish color of the limiting adventitia. A Freer or Penfield elevator is the most useful instrument (Fig. 6-6). Optical magnification (×2.5-×3.5) provides accurate visualization.

CAROTID ENDARTERECTOMY | 71

Forceps are used to retract the vessel wall as the plaque is pushed away. The dissection is started in the common carotid artery. The plaque is completely divided just proximal to the lowest extent to the arteriotomy. Scissors are used to cut the plaque at the point of separation, leaving a smooth proximal edge in the common carotid artery. The plaque is then separated from the ECA by an eversion technique. Separation of the plaque from the ICA is the most critical maneuver. As the end of the plaque is approached, a transition is made to a more superficial layer in the intima media so that the plaque comes away and leaves a firm attachment of the intima layer. Microscissors may be used to cut into the

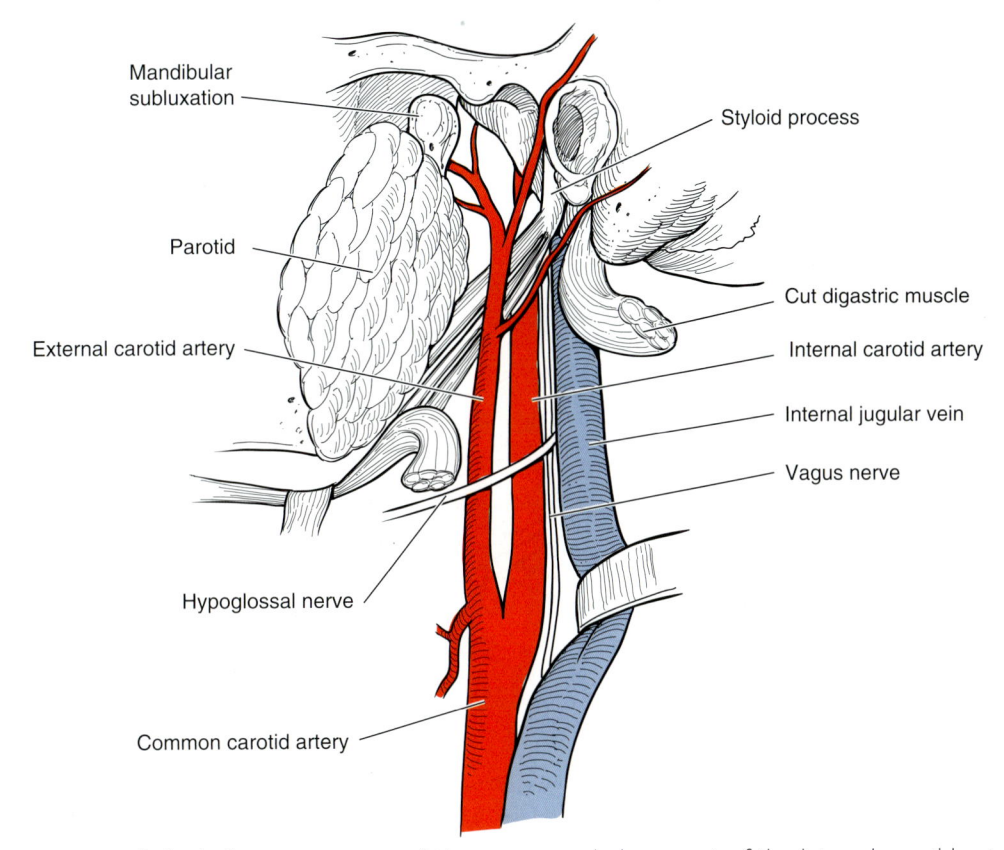

Figure 6-4. In the case of distal disease, exposure of the upper cervical segment of the internal carotid artery (ICA) can be achieved by mandibular subluxation. Division of the posterior belly of the digastric muscle allows exposure of the ICA within 2 cm of the skull base. Care should be taken to ligate small branches of the jugular vein that cross the anterior surface of the ICA. Higher exposure of the ICA is obtainable by dividing the stylohyoid ligament, as well as stylohyoid, stylopharyngeus, and styloglossus muscles to permit removal of the styloid process.

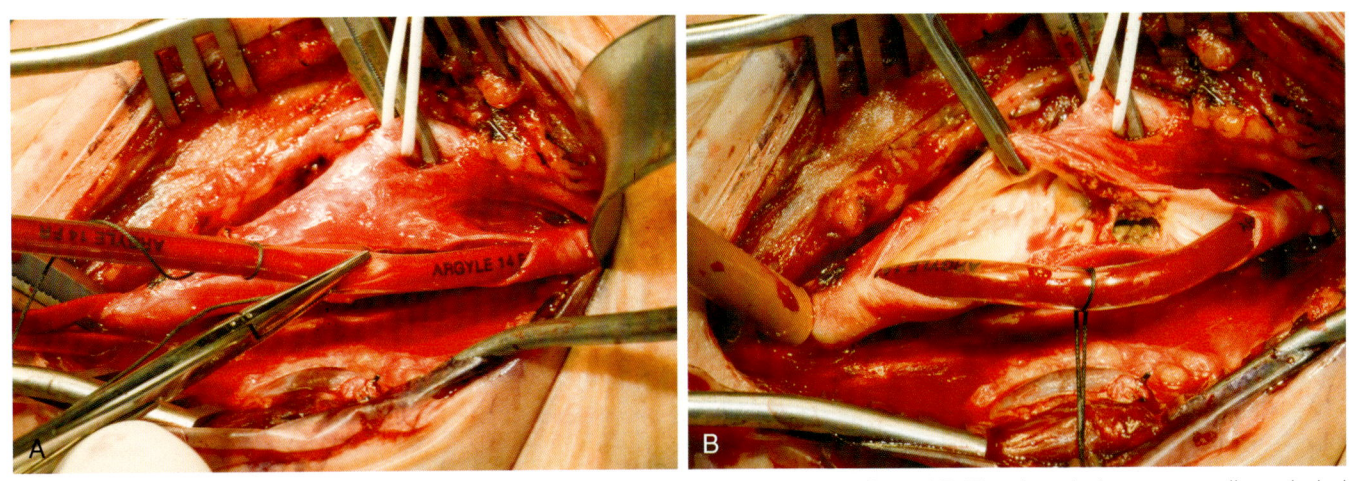

Figure 6-5. **A,** The shunt is advanced into the ICA, and free retrograde flow is confirmed. **B,** The shunt is then temporally occluded to prevent continued blood loss, and the proximal end is placed into the lumen of the common carotid artery. The average size of a shunt that fits into the distal ICA is 10 Fr (2.5-mm lumen). An 8- or 12-Fr shunt can be used for smaller or larger vessels, respectively.

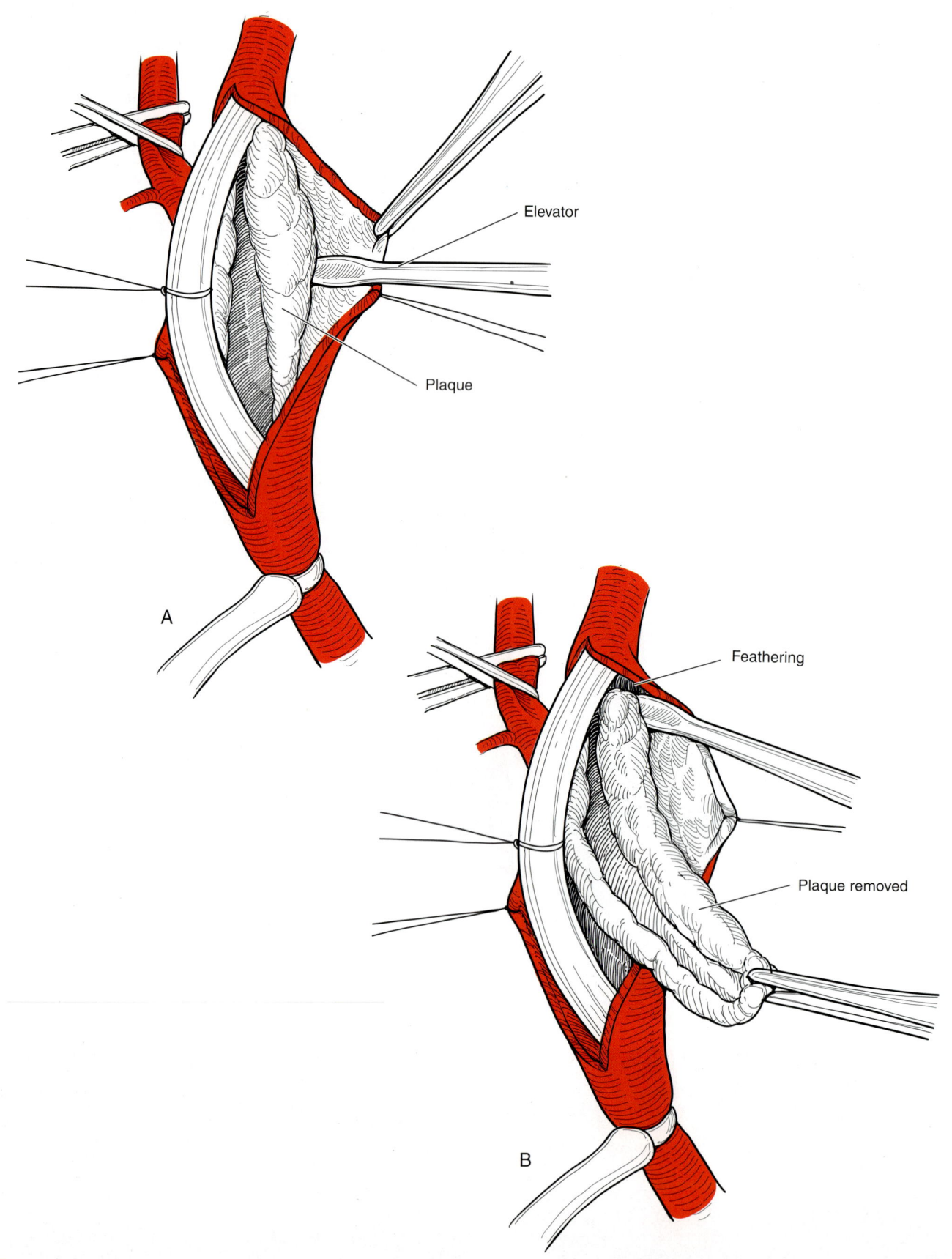

Figure 6-6. A, The atheromatous plaque is separated from the carotid artery by dissection in the layer between the media and adventitia, revealing the distinct pinkish color of the limiting adventitia. Forceps are used to retract the vessel wall as the plaque is pushed away by a Freer or Penfield elevator or mosquito forceps. **B,** The dissection is started in the common carotid artery and completed distally in the ICA. **C,** Operative photo demonstrating pinkish colored, deep medial plane between the atheromatous plaque and the outer wall of the carotid artery.

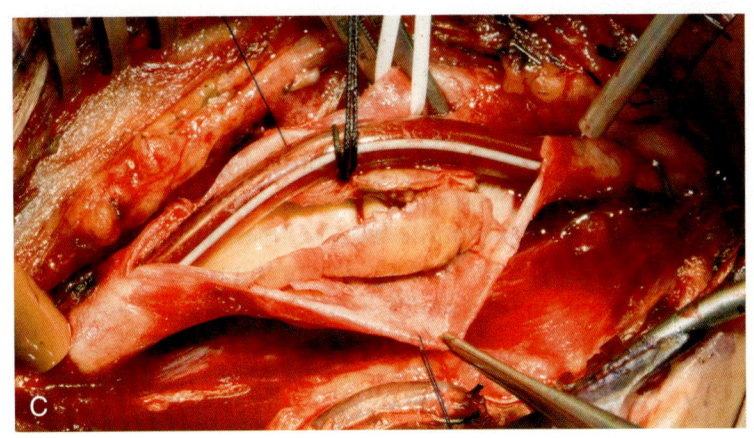

Figure 6-6, cont'd

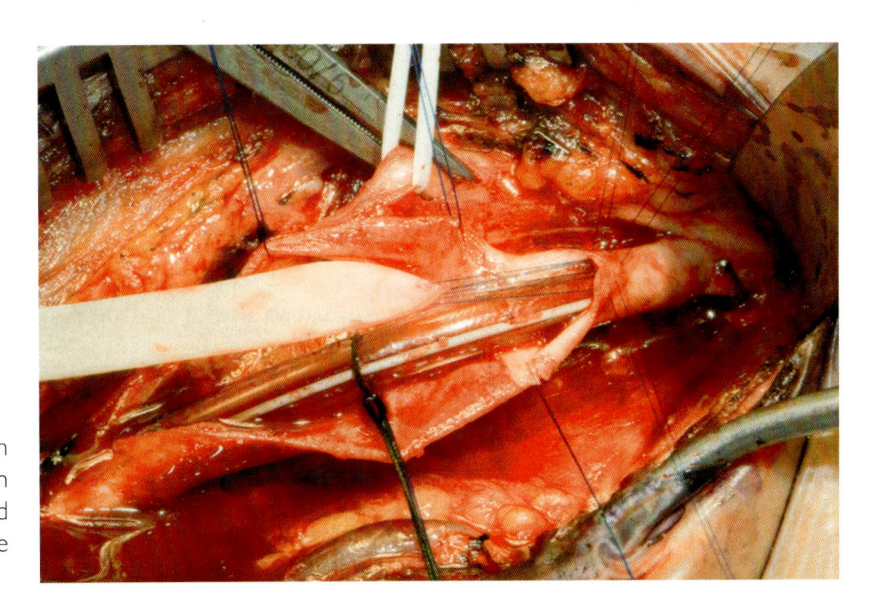

Figure 6-7. Routine use of a prosthetic or vein patch is recommended to close the arteriotomy in order to reduce the risk of perioperative stroke and restenosis. Interrupted 6-0 or 7-0 polypropylene sutures afford precision and optimal visualization.

edge of the most distal end of plaque to assist in feathering of the plaque. If the transition at the distal endpoint is not smooth, the distal intima can be secured by use of 7-0 polypropylene tacking sutures. Flooding the artery with saline irrigation exposes remaining loose fragments, which can be removed with forceps.

PATCH ANGIOPLASTY

Routine use of a prosthetic (e.g., Dacron, pericardium, or polytetrafluoroethylene) or vein patch is recommended to close the arteriotomy in order to reduce the risk of perioperative stroke and restenosis. Interrupted 6-0 or 7-0 polypropylene sutures secure the patch at the distal end, with initial sutures carefully placed in the ICA using the smallest possible amount of the vessel wall, which is consistent with security of the arteriotomy closure (Fig. 6-7). An alternative method is to use three interrupted mattress sutures, which affords precise visualization. A 5-0 polypropylene suture can be used to close the proximal end of the patch.

Before final closure of the arteriotomy, the shunt is removed, the common carotid artery and ICA are clamped, and all three vessels are flushed to remove debris from the arteriotomy site. The common carotid artery can be digitally occluded after the shunt is removed and before clamp placement. The arteriotomy closure is completed, and flow is restored first to the ECA and subsequently to the ICA. The flow dynamics of the completed repair are evaluated by Doppler ultrasound.

CLOSURE

Hemostasis should be assessed, including the patch anastomosis, jugular vein, ligated common facial vein, and SCM muscle. A Valsalva maneuver can be performed to assess the integrity of the jugular vein. Protamine administration is controversial, because some reports have associated this with increased risk of perioperative stroke. A Society for Vascular Surgery guidelines document on carotid disease could not reach consensus on this point.[11] A 7-Fr Jackson-Pratt drain may be placed and removed the next day. The platysma is closed with a 3-0 absorbable suture, and the skin is approximated with a 4-0 subcuticular suture. If the patient received general anesthesia, the surgical nurse and instrument table should remain sterile and the patient should remain in the operating room until the presence of any neurologic finding that might warrant reexploration is excluded.

Postoperative Care

- Patients are usually discharged the day after their operation, but at home blood pressure monitoring is advised.
- Patients are monitored with an arterial line to assess fluctuations in blood pressure in the postanesthesia care unit for a period of at least 2 hours. If medications are required to maintain normal blood pressure, the patient should be transferred to the intensive care unit for overnight monitoring. Avoidance of significant hypertension is important.
- Patients are usually kept on bed rest on the day of operation and encouraged to ambulate the next day.
- Clear liquids are recommended the day of operation in the unlikely event of a need to return to the operating room. Patients are allowed to resume a regular diet the next day.
- One dose of a cephalosporin or, in the case of a penicillin allergy, vancomycin is given before the operation and continued for 24 hours (e.g., Cefazolin 1 gm IV q8h; Vancomycin 1 gm IV q12h).
- Discomfort from the neck incision is usually minimal, and patients often discontinue narcotics in favor of over-the-counter analgesics after the first day.
- Life-long aspirin (81-325 mg/day) is recommended. Additional intraoperative and postoperative antiplatelet agents (e.g., low-molecular-weight dextran) may be added at the surgeon's discretion, particularly in patients who have not received preoperative aspirin or clopidogrel.
- A postoperative duplex scan at 1 month and repeated at an annual interval is an appropriate follow-up strategy.
- Patients should be referred for atherosclerotic risk reduction therapy—including administration of an angiotensin-converting enzyme inhibitor, angiotensin receptor blocker, or both and a statin agent—and where appropriate for antihypertensive therapy.

Complications

CARDIAC COMPLICATIONS

Although the stress of CEA is low, most patients have evidence of cardiovascular disease and are at risk for myocardial ischemia or cardiovascular-related death. Whereas a postoperative electrocardiogram is appropriate, routine assessment of cardiac isoenzymes is not.

STROKE

Although CEA is intended to prevent stroke, stroke is a recognized complication. A patient who presents with a neurologic deficit upon emergence from anesthesia or soon thereafter should be promptly reexplored. The most common cause of this event is thrombosis at the operative site. A minor, transient, or both types of deficits should prompt urgent duplex or CT angiography. Embolization of platelet debris with a patent reconstruction is the most common cause.

CEREBRAL HYPERPERFUSION SYNDROME

The complication of cerebral hyperfusion syndrome occurs in less than 1% of cases but carries a mortality rate of more than 30%. Hyperperfusion syndrome can cause severe headaches, seizures, neurologic deficits, and ultimately death from cerebral hemorrhage. It may manifest 3 to 6 days after CEA. Risk factors include high-grade ipsilateral stenosis (>90%), contralateral carotid occlusion, recent history of stroke, and severe postoperative hypertension. Of these risk factors, only postoperative hypertension can be controlled. Therefore large fluctuations in blood pressure are best managed in the intensive care unit with appropriate vasopressors or vasodilators. Complaints of headache should not be dismissed.

NERVE INJURY

Transient deviation of the tongue toward the side of operation may result from injury or traction on the hypoglossal nerve. Transection of the hypoglossal is rare and may require urgent repair. In this instance patients may have difficulty swallowing and with speech articulation. Aspiration precautions may be appropriate. In most patients with postoperative tongue deviation resolution occurs within 48 hours, because edema rather than frank nerve injury is the usual mechanism. A brief course of steroids and elevating the head of the bed often facilitates resolution.

Injury to the vagus nerve may result in either temporary or permanent hoarseness. Trauma to the marginal mandibular branch of the facial nerve results in drooping at the corner of the mouth. Injury to the superior laryngeal nerve may cause fatigability of the voice and impairment in phonation. Damage to the spinal accessory nerve is uncommon but may result in shoulder dysfunction and neck weakness. Suspicion of a CN injury warrants consultation with an otolaryngologist.

BRADYCARDIA

Bradyarrhythmia is a common event attributed to manipulation of the carotid sinus. Atropine is administered if bradycardia is persistent or is associated with hypotension. Lidocaine may be administered into the area of the carotid sinus nerve at the time of operation but may be associated with reflex hypertension.

HEMATOMA

Postoperative wound hematomas occur in about 5% of patients. Of these, a small fraction requires evacuation. An expanding hematoma in the neck must be treated expeditiously to avoid airway compromise.

PERIINCISIONAL HYPESTHESIA

Patients may complain of numbness of the ear lobe if the greater auricular nerve has been injured. More frequently, patients experience diminished sensation in the region of the neck incision because of interruption of cutaneous cervical nerves. Typically, this resolves over several months.

CAROTID RESTENOSIS

Most restenoses are asymptomatic and occur within 2 years of primary surgery because of intimal hyperplasia. The risk can be minimized by routine use of patch angioplasty. Additional recommendations include smoking cessation and atherosclerotic risk factor reduction. Reoperation is undertaken for the same indications as primary operation.

REFERENCES

1. Carrea R, Molins M, Murphy G: Surgery of spontaneous thrombosis of the internal carotid in the neck; carotido-carotid anastomosis; case report and analysis of the literature on surgical cases, *Medicina (B Aires)* 15:20-29, 1955.
2. DeBakey ME: Successful carotid endarterectomy for cerebrovascular insufficiency. Nineteen-year follow-up, *JAMA* 233:1083-1085, 1975.

3. Eastcott HH, Pickering GW, Rob CG: Reconstruction of internal carotid artery in a patient with intermittent attacks of hemiplegia, *Lancet* 267:994-996, 1954.
4. Al-Naaman YD, Carton CA, Cooley DA: Surgical treatment of arteriosclerotic occlusion of common carotid artery, *J Neurosurg* 13:500-506, 1956.
5. North American Symptomatic Carotid Endarterectomy Trial Collaborators: Beneficial effect of carotid endarterectomy in symptomatic patients with high-grade carotid stenosis, *N Engl J Med* 325:445-453, 1991.
6. Barnett HJ, Taylor DW, Eliasziw M, et al: Benefit of carotid endarterectomy in patients with symptomatic moderate or severe stenosis. North American Symptomatic Carotid Endarterectomy Trial Collaborators, *N Engl J Med* 339:1415-1425, 1998.
7. European Carotid Surgery Trialists' Collaborative Group: MRC European Carotid Surgery Trial: Interim results for symptomatic patients with severe (70%-99%) or with mild (0%-29%) carotid stenosis, *Lancet* 337:1235-1243, 1991.
8. Role of carotid endarterectomy in asymptomatic carotid stenosis: A Veterans Administration Cooperative Study, *Stroke* 17:534-539, 1986.
9. Executive Committee for the Asymptomatic Carotid Atherosclerosis Study: Endarterectomy for asymptomatic carotid artery stenosis, *Jama* 273:1421-1428, 1995.
10. Halliday A, Mansfield A, Marro J, et al: Prevention of disabling and fatal strokes by successful carotid endarterectomy in patients without recent neurological symptoms: Randomised controlled trial, *Lancet* 363:1491-1502, 2004.
11. Hobson RW 2nd, Mackey WC, Ascher E, et al: Management of atherosclerotic carotid artery disease: Clinical practice guidelines of the Society for Vascular Surgery, *J Vasc Surg* 48:480-486, 2008.
12. Kresowik TF, Bratzler D, Karp HR, et al: Multistate utilization, processes, and outcomes of carotid endarterectomy, *J Vasc Surg* 33:227-234, 2001.
13. Goodney PP, Likosky DS, Cronenwett JL: Factors associated with stroke or death after carotid endarterectomy in Northern New England, *J Vasc Surg* 48:1139-1145, 2008.
14. McGirt MJ, Perler BA, Brooke BS, et al: 3-hydroxy-3-methylglutaryl coenzyme A reductase inhibitors reduce the risk of perioperative stroke and mortality after carotid endarterectomy, *J Vasc Surg* 42:829-836, 2005.
15. Kang JL, Chung TK, Lancaster RT, et al: Outcomes after carotid endarterectomy: Is there a high-risk population? A National Surgical Quality Improvement Program report, *J Vasc Surg* 49:331-338, 2009.
16. Cunningham EJ, Bond R, Mayberg MR, Warlow CP, Rothwell PM: Risk of persistent cranial nerve injury after carotid endarterectomy, *J Neurosurg* 101:445-448, 2004.
17. Hertzer NR, Feldman BJ, Beven EG, Tucker HM: A prospective study of the incidence of injury to the cranial nerves during carotid endarterectomy, *Surg Gynecol Obstet* 151:781-784, 1980.
18. Massey EW, Heyman A, Utley C, Haynes C, Fuchs J: Cranial nerve paralysis following carotid endarterectomy, *Stroke* 15:157-159, 1984.
19. Schauber MD, Fontenelle LJ, Solomon JW, Hanson TL: Cranial/cervical nerve dysfunction after carotid endarterectomy, *J Vasc Surg* 25:481-487, 1997.
20. Tucker JA, Gee W, Nicholas GG, McDonald KM, Goodreau JJ: Accessory nerve injury during carotid endarterectomy, *J Vasc Surg* 5:440-444, 1987.
21. Rosenbloom M, Friedman SG, Lamparello PJ, Riles TS, Imparato AM: Glossopharyngeal nerve injury complicating carotid endarterectomy, *J Vasc Surg* 5:469-471, 1987.
22. Shaha A, Phillips T, Scalea T, et al: Exposure of the internal carotid artery near the skull base: The posterolateral anatomic approach, *J Vasc Surg* 8:618-622, 1988.
23. Lewis SC, Warlow CP, Bodenham AR, et al: General anaesthesia versus local anaesthesia for carotid surgery (GALA): A multicentre, randomised controlled trial, *Lancet* 372:2132-2142, 2008.
24. Fisher DF Jr, Clagett GP, Parker JI, et al: Mandibular subluxation for high carotid exposure, *J Vasc Surg* 1:727-733, 1984.

7 Eversion Endarterectomy and Special Problems in Carotid Surgery

R. CLEMENT DARLING III • W. JOHN BYRNE • DHIRAJ M. SHAH

Historical Background

Conventional carotid endarterectomy (CEA) is an excellent and time-tested technique; however, eversion CEA is quicker to perform, avoids insertion of prosthetic material, and is associated with postoperative morbidity and restenosis rates that are comparable with those for conventional CEA.[1,2] Because it is faster to perform, it is ideal for carotid surgery under regional anesthesia.

Eversion CEA was first performed by Kieny and associates[3] in 1985, improving upon the technique described by DeBakey[4] from 1959 and Etheredge[5] in 1970. The DeBakey-Etheredge technique involved transecting the common carotid artery and the everting internal carotid artery (ICA) and external carotid artery (ECA) as one. The Kieny technique confines eversion to the ICA.

Until recently, eversion CEA has been slow to gain widespread acceptance. Many surgeons found it a difficult technique to master, some had concerns about adequate visualization of the distal endpoint, and many were worried about inserting a shunt expeditiously when needed. This chapter reviews the technique of eversion CEA, paying special attention to commonly perceived problems and related strategies that may need to be applied to achieve an optimal outcome.

Indications

CEA is indicated to prevent stoke in patients with carotid bifurcation occlusive disease.[6] Multiple randomized prospective studies support CEA for (1) asymptomatic patients with a carotid stenosis of at least 60% and (2) symptomatic patients with a history of recent transient ischemic attack (TIA) or amaurosis fugax and an ipsilateral carotid stenosis of at least 50%.

Additional indications for CEA have been reported. Given the limited available evidence, the decision to recommend treatment should be based upon the surgeon's complication rate and the patient's preference. Specifically, the benefits of CEA are less established for (1) patients with a carotid stenosis of at least 50% and nonhemispheric symptoms, vertebrobasilar symptoms, stroke in evolution, or a completed acute stroke and (2) symptomatic patients with an ulcerated carotid plaque and an ipsilateral carotid stenosis of less than 50%.

Preoperative Preparation

- All patients should have a preoperative duplex ultrasound. Computed tomography (CT) angiography may be considered to confirm the presence of a significant stenosis. Magnetic resonance angiography has few advantages over CT angiography yet has a potentially higher false-positive rate for the detection of a hemodynamically significant carotid lesion. Conventional contrast angiography is rarely needed.

- Patients should have preoperative cardiac clearance.
- Patients who are on aspirin and clopidogrel should have both medications continued through the perioperative period. All patients should be on at least one antiplatelet agent.
- Nearly all patients may undergo eversion CEA under a regional block consisting of a combined deep and superficial cervical plexus block or a superficial cervical plexus block only. Sedation in the form of remifentanil (Ultiva), a very short-acting narcotic, is used to allow strict control of the patient's sedation score. General anesthesia is required in fewer than 1% of their patients.
- Cerebral function is assessed clinically by noting changes in the patient's ability to converse or recall simple facts. A more objective measure is to ask the patient to squeeze a pressure bag attached to a pressure transducer when the ICA is clamped.
- Perioperative systolic blood pressure is maintained between 120 and 170 mm Hg, especially during carotid clamping, to allow adequate cerebral perfusion. Beta-blockers, such as labetalol (Trandate) administered intravenously in 5-mg increments, is used as a first-line agent, and hydralazine, administered intravenously in 10-mg aliquots, is often a second-line agent.

Operative Strategy

Surgeons adopting eversion CEA need not alter their basic technique for exposure of the carotid arteries (Video 7-1). The anesthetic, as well as the methods of cerebral monitoring and protection, are similar for both eversion and standard CEA. Eversion CEA under cervical block anesthesia is preferred, with selective shunting for patients who develop neurologic changes during carotid artery clamping.

Eversion CEA can be used to treat almost all cases of primary carotid bifurcation disease and select cases of recurrent stenosis. It is ideal for treatment of carotid arteries with kinks or loops, because shortening of the artery can be incorporated within the process of eversion. The use of shunts is straightforward and safe, and in some cases, a shunt can facilitate the procedure. Once inserted, the shunt can be used as a mandrel to evert the ICA and adequately remove the atherosclerotic plaque. The extent of disease at the carotid bifurcation may affect the ease of performing CEA by any method. Disease limited to or near the bifurcation is easier to treat than disease that extends distally. Inspection of the ICA guides the surgeon on the extent of the plaque before division of the ICA. Treatment of extensive disease in the ICA up to or beyond the level of the anterior digastric muscle can be challenging. Such cases should be treated by conventional CEA until ample experience with eversion CEA is gained on arteries with focal bifurcation disease.

Although the eversion technique can be used for treatment of recurrent carotid stenosis after an initial eversion procedure, it is contraindicated in patients who underwent conventional CEA with prosthetic patch angioplasty. A carotid artery patched with autogenous vein may be suitable for treatment using the eversion technique, but failure rates are higher than recurrent disease in vessels without a patch angioplasty. Radiation-induced carotid artery stenosis may also impose limitations on the eversion technique because of the difficulty in defining an endpoint and may be better served by patch angioplasty.

Operative Technique

EXPOSURE OF THE CAROTID ARTERY

Exposure of the carotid artery for eversion CEA is similar to that for conventional CEA. However, several points deserve emphasis. In the eversion technique, moreso than in conventional CEA, it is essential to mobilize the distal ICA circumferentially, well beyond the plaque, to the level where the uninvolved artery achieves a bluish hue. The clamp should be placed on the normal ICA beyond the endpoint or transition zone of the plaque to facilitate eversion and allow examination of the endpoint of the endarterectomy. It is also important to clear all periadventitial tissue away from the ICA to allow adequate eversion of the ICA. This can be performed after transection of the ICA and allows much of the dissection to be done with the ICA "out of the wound," thus minimizing the risk of cranial nerve injury.

After administration of heparin (30 units/kg, average 2500 units per patient), the ICA is clamped using Yasargil neurosurgical clips. Then the ECA and common carotid artery are dissected and clamped. The ICA is then transected obliquely at its origin using an 11 blade and dissecting scissors and is freed from remaining periadventitial tissue. The ICA should be divided at the bifurcation or carotid bulb, not in the proximal ICA (Fig. 7-1). If the proximal ICA is divided, it makes the subsequent anastomosis more technically challenging. The arteriotomy is

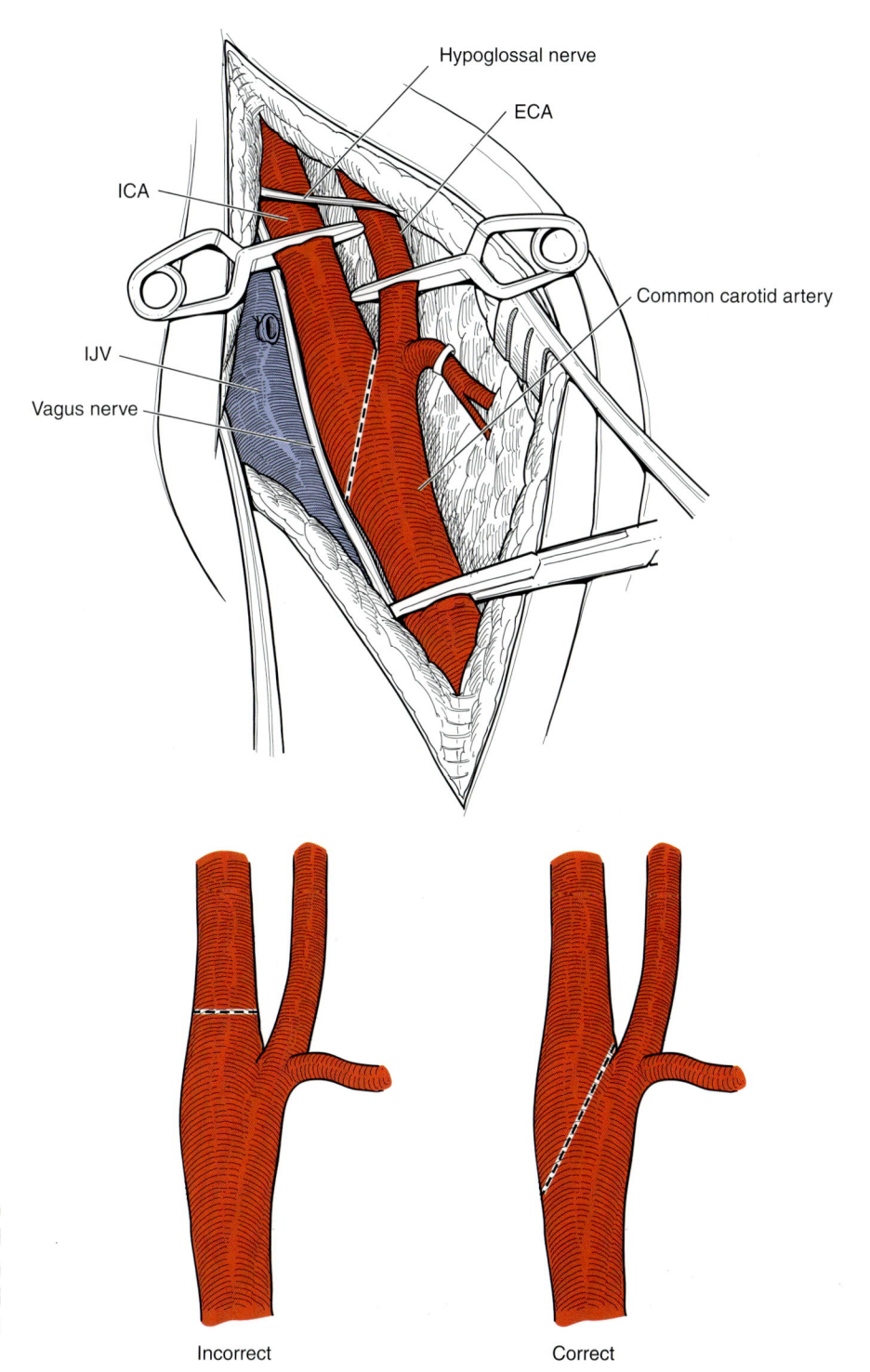

Figure 7-1. Position of Yasargil clamps on carotid arteries. Incorrect (*bottom left*) and correct (*bottom right*) oblique transaction of the internal carotid artery at the carotid bulb. *ECA*, External carotid artery; *ICA*, internal carotid artery; *IJV*, internal jugular vein.

extended along the medial side of the ICA for 1 to 2 cm (Fig. 7-2). The arteriotomy in the common carotid artery is extended for a similar distance. At this stage, the ICA should be fully mobilized and anchored only by the distal ICA Yasargil clip.

ENDARTERECTOMY OF THE INTERNAL CAROTID ARTERY

Eversion CEA of the ICA is then performed. A dissection plane is first identified on the proximal ICA. The adventitia is then peeled off the plaque (Fig. 7-3). As the eversion proceeds, fragments of plaque that remain on the arterial side of the adventitia are removed. The plaque is not extracted from the artery; rather the adventitia is peeled off the stationary plaque, much like peeling a glove from a hand. As the adventitia is peeled off, the plaque begins to "feather out" where it ends before separating from the adventitia. A small rim of residual plaque may be seen after removal of the bulk of the plaque, which is removed as a spiral to minimize the risk of dissection plane of the distal normal intima. Irrigation with heparinized saline removes residual debris and provides a clearer view of residual strands on the intimal surface of the ICA. A critical part of this operation is good visualization of the distal endpoint of the endarterectomy. If not clearly visible, the Yasargil clamp should be moved more cephalad on the ICA.

Two technical problems are possibly encountered at this stage:

- *Lack of a distal end point.* When the ICA is inverted, the plaque may not "feather out" but instead may become continuous with the distal intima. This is analogous to endarterectomy of the superficial femoral or iliac arteries. The surgeon must stop the endarterectomy before the ICA is out of reach at the skull base. The ICA with its plaque may be transected, and often the distal endpoint is secure. If this does not occur, the plaque may be tacked with 7-0 or 8-0 polypropylene sutures or a common carotid artery to ICA bypass may be performed.
- *Unstable distal endpoint.* After successful endarterectomy, there may be concern that the intima is separating from the distal ICA, which could dissect after reestablishing flow. Tacking (Kunlin) sutures, made with 7-0 or 8-0 polypropylene, may be used to secure the distal intima.

ENDARTERECTOMY OF THE COMMON CAROTID ARTERY

Endarterectomy of the common carotid artery is performed using an endarterectomy spatula or elevator. A plane is identified between the plaque and the adventitia. The plaque is transected proximally with either Metzenbaum or Potts scissors or a No. 15 blade just beyond the ECA origin and, if required, the ECA is everted in a similar fashion to that used for the ICA. In rare cases, the plaque is confined within the ICA or does not involve the common carotid artery. However, in our experience, failure to endarterectomize the common carotid artery predisposes the patient to a higher incidence of restenosis, usually in the common carotid artery. It is also easier to suture to an endarterectomized common carotid artery.

The technical problem possibly encountered at this stage is extensive plaque in the common carotid artery. With such situations, it may be necessary to extend the arteriotomy proximally on the common carotid artery to perform a more extensive endarterectomy. This results in a size mismatch between the common carotid artery arteriotomy and the ICA origin. Because the common carotid artery is wide enough to accommodate primary closure without undue narrowing of its lumen, primary closure of the common carotid artery arteriotomy can be performed with 6-0 polypropylene. The ICA can then be sewn to its origin, which results in a Y-shaped suture line.

ANASTOMOSIS OF THE INTERNAL TO THE COMMON CAROTID ARTERY

The ICA is reanastomosed to its origin on the common carotid artery with a continuous 6-0 polypropylene suture using a parachute technique (Fig. 7-4). The anastomosis

EVERSION ENDARTERECTOMY AND SPECIAL PROBLEMS IN CAROTID SURGERY

Figure 7-2. Placement of internal carotid artery (*ICA*) and common carotid artery arteriotomies. *ECA*, External carotid artery.

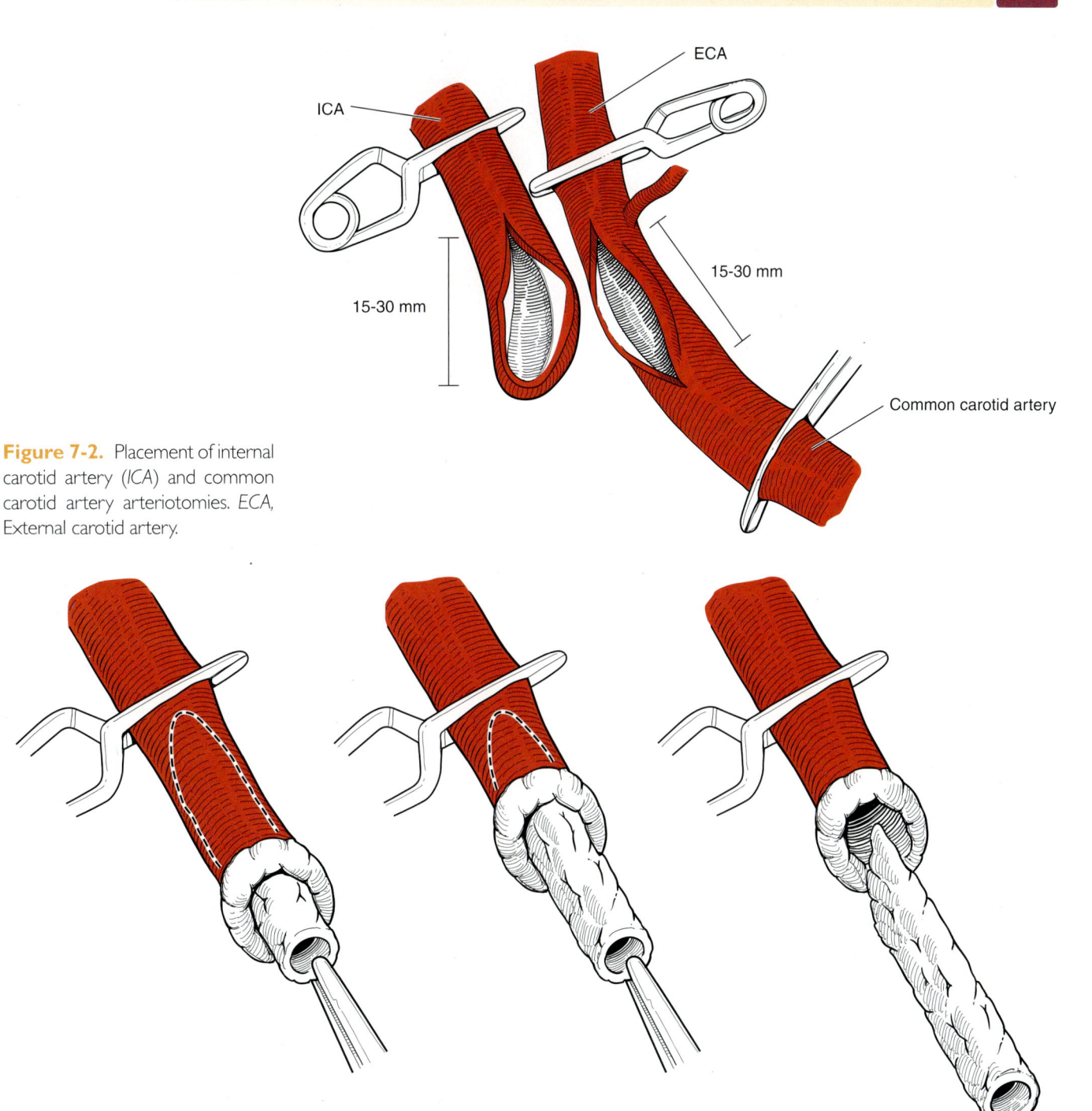

Figure 7-3. Eversion of the internal carotid artery with visualization of the endpoint. The dashed line indicates the extent of atherosclerotic plaque.

has the advantage of being performed in the center of the incision, not at its most cephalad extent. It is difficult to narrow the lumen. Before completion of the anastomosis, the clamps are released and the artery is irrigated with heparinized saline. After release of the clamps, flow is confirmed by Doppler insonation or Duplex imaging of both the ICA and the ECA.

Technical problems may be encountered at this stage:

- *No flow in the ECA.* Lack of ECA flow implies a problem with the endpoint of the dissection and likely occlusion of the ECA, which in some patients may result in jaw or masseter muscle claudication. The "counsel of perfection" is to reexplore the ECA. However, if the operation has been difficult and a shunt required, wiser counsel suggests matters be left alone.

- *No flow in the ICA.* Reexploration is mandated when there is no ICA flow, even if the patient is not experiencing a neurologic deficit.

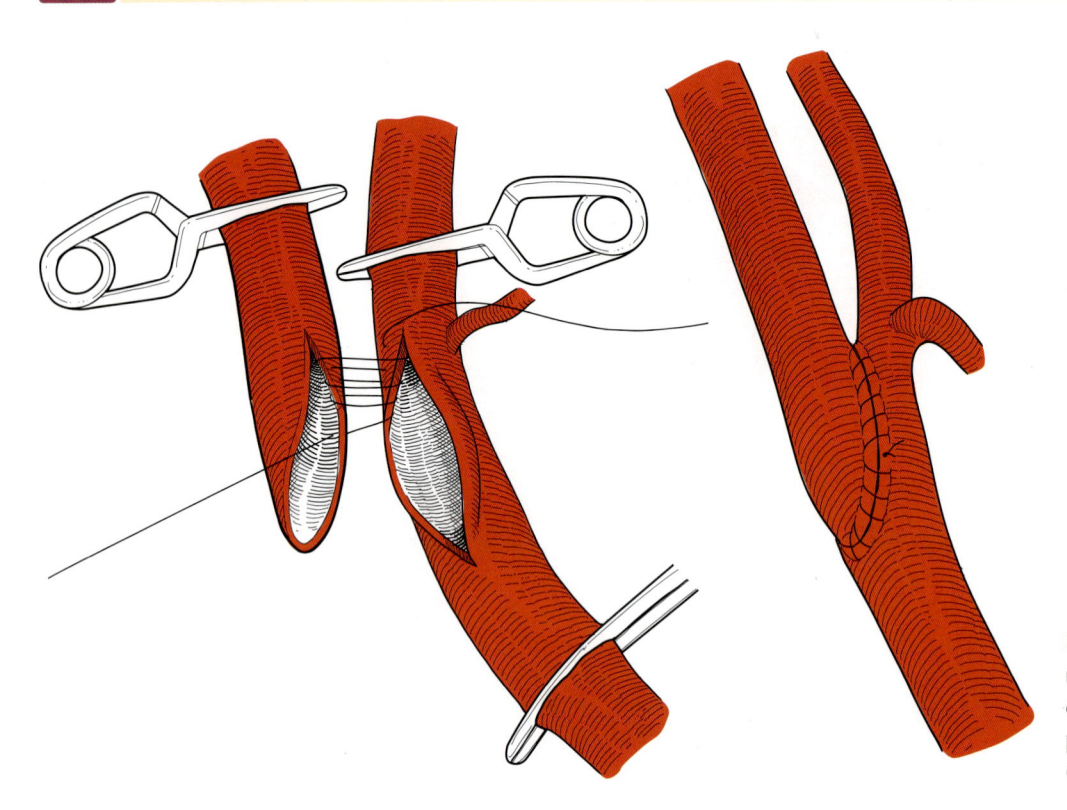

Figure 7-4. End-to-side internal carotid artery to common carotid artery anastomosis. The posterior row is run first with 6-0 polypropylene.

- *ICA thrombosis.* An emergent situation is thrombosis, and reexploration is mandated. "Red" thrombus usually results from thrombosis of the ICA and the endpoint must be evaluated and revised, as needed. A No. 2 or No. 3 Fogarty embolectomy catheter may be used to carefully retrieve a thrombus, but catheter length should be measured to avoid causing a carotid-cavernous sinus fistula. In most circumstances retrograde flow from the ICA flushes the thrombus out, and catheter extraction is not necessary. If "white" thrombus is found, aberrant platelet aggregation may be the cause and a technical issue often may not be identified. Replacement of the endarterectomized ICA with a vein interposition graft may be considered along with use of a more potent antiplatelet agent, such as low-molecular-weight dextran. Heparin-induced thrombocytopenia should be excluded.

SHUNTING DURING EVERSION CAROTID ENDARTERECTOMY

The placement of shunt during eversion CEA is not more difficult than when performed during a conventional CEA, and any conventional shunt may be used, such as a Javid, Sundt, or Pruitt-Inahara shunt. The ICA is transected and an eversion CEA is performed expeditiously. The shunt is then inserted and secured with a shunt clamp or balloon (Fig. 7-5). The distal end of the shunt can also be inserted before endarterectomy in the rare circumstance that the ICA plaque is so short that transection of the ICA and performance of an arteriotomy along the medial aspect of the ICA allows easy access to the distal ICA. The proximal end is then inserted into the common carotid artery and secured, usually before performing an endarterectomy. When the shunt has been inserted, flow is confirmed by Doppler insonation. Endarterectomy of the common carotid artery can then be performed. Finally, the ICA is anastomosed to its origin on the common carotid artery around the shunt and the shunt is removed before completion of the anastomosis.

Postoperative Care

- Patients are usually discharged the day after the operation, but at-home blood pressure monitoring is advised.

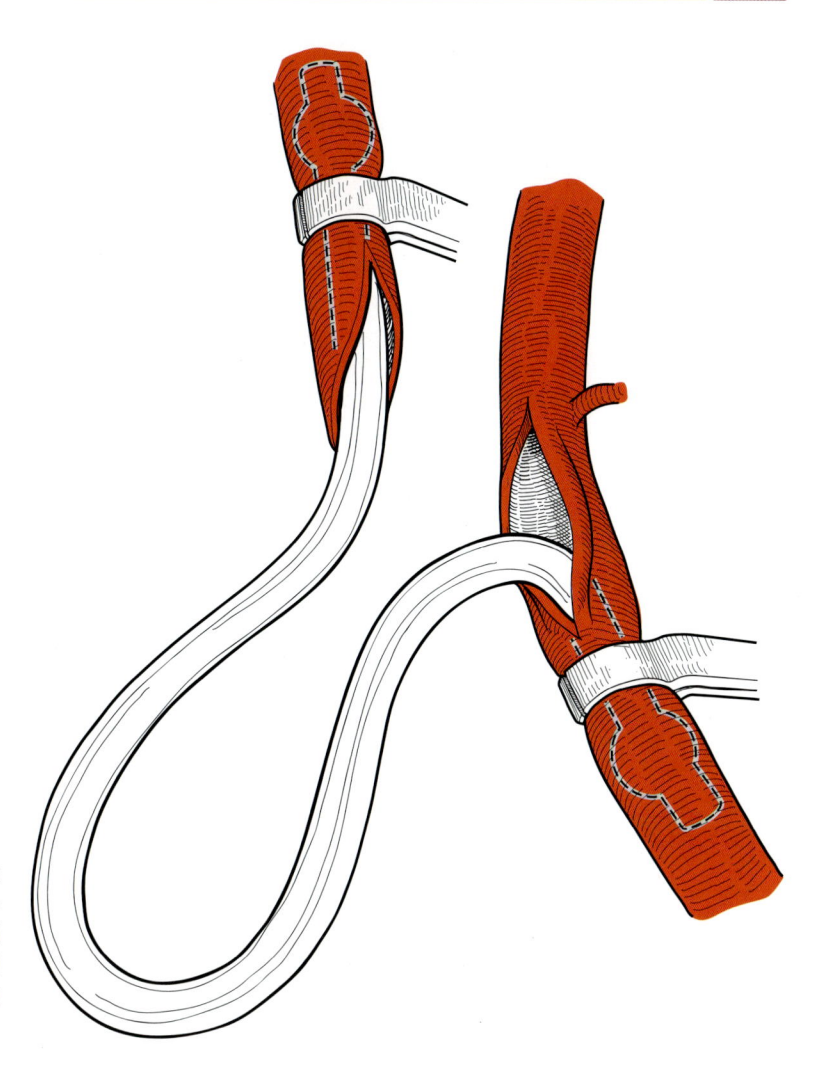

EVERSION ENDARTERECTOMY AND SPECIAL PROBLEMS IN CAROTID SURGERY | 83

Figure 7-5. Technique of shunt insertion during eversion conventional carotid endarterectomy. Plaque removal is completed before shunt insertion. The distal end of the shunt is placed into the internal carotid artery first, followed by placement of the proximal end of the shunt into the common carotid artery.

- Patients are monitored with an arterial line to assess fluctuations in blood pressure in the postanesthesia care unit for at least 2 hours. If medications are required to maintain normal blood pressure, the patient should be transferred to the intensive care unit for overnight monitoring. Avoidance of significant hypertension is important.
- Patients are usually kept on bedrest the day of the operation and encouraged to ambulate the next day.
- Clear liquids are recommended the day of the operation in the unlikely event of a need to return to the operating room. Patients are allowed to resume a regular diet the following day.
- One dose of a cephalosporin or, in the case of a penicillin allergy, vancomycin is given before the operation and continued for 24 hours.
- Discomfort from the neck incision is usually minimal, and patients often discontinue narcotics in favor of over-the-counter analgesics after the first day.
- Lifelong aspirin (81-325 mg/day) is recommended. Additional intraoperative and postoperative antiplatelet agents (e.g., low molecular weight dextran) may be added at the surgeon's discretion, particularly for patients who have not received preoperative aspirin or clopidogrel.
- A postoperative duplex scan at 1 month and repeated at an annual interval is the recommended postoperative surveillance protocol.
- Patients should be referred for atherosclerotic risk reduction therapy, including administration of an angiotensin-converting enzyme inhibitor, an angiotensin receptor blocker, or both; a statin agent; and where appropriate, antihypertensive therapy.

Complications

RECURRENT STENOSIS

Restenosis can be classified as either early or late. Early restenosis, perhaps better characterized as persistent restenosis, is seen on the first postoperative duplex scan. This usually indicates technical error and failure to fully endarterectomize the distal ICA or common carotid artery. If the stenosis is severe (>80%), there is a role for carotid angioplasty and stenting. Late restenosis because of neointimal hyperplasia usually appears in the first 12 to 18 months after surgery, typically after an initial normal duplex scan at an annual incidence of 1%.[7] Management depends on the degree of stenosis, symptoms, and other medical factors. Restenosis many years after surgery most often occurs because of recurrent atherosclerosis.

INFECTION

Wound infection occurs infrequently; however, the absence of prosthetic material with eversion CEA makes serious infections less likely than after standard CEA and patch angioplasty. However, on rare occasions, an arterial infection may occur, manifesting as a postoperative pseudoaneurysm with a "herald bleed" or catastrophic hemorrhage. Management is excision of infected tissue and replacement with autologous saphenous vein.

Eversion Carotid Endarterectomy in Special Circumstances

KINKS AND COILS IN THE INTERNAL CAROTID ARTERY

The redundant ICA lends itself to the eversion technique and may be the primary indication for eversion CEA. Because the entire ICA is mobilized in the eversion technique, after division of the ICA from its origin, it is a simple matter to tailor the appropriate length of redundant ICA so that the ICA lies in a gentle, nonredundant orientation.

Isolated symptomatic kinks and coils without associated stenosis are rarely encountered. Patients may present with TIAs in association with head motion. The management is similar to that for a redundant carotid artery. The ICA is fully mobilized, transected from its origin, and anastomosed after the excision of excess artery.

FIBROMUSCULAR DYSPLASIA

Patients with fibromuscular dysplasia (FMD) of the ICA differ from patients with atheromatous disease in that they are predominantly young, female, and rarely symptomatic. FMD of the ICA is a relatively recent discovery, first reported in 1964.[8] It is frequently bilateral (65%),[9] and up to 30% of patients have intracranial aneurysms.[9] Before the advent of balloon angioplasty, management consisted of clamping the common carotid artery and the ECA, followed by a vertical arteriotomy in the common carotid artery and passage of serial dilators into the ICA, analogous to the Dotter angioplasty technique of the 1960s. Current management is usually angioplasty. Surgical treatment for those not amenable to endovascular therapy is interposition bypass with a reversed vein graft.

REDO CAROTID SURGERY

Recurrent Carotid Stenosis

Patients with high-grade recurrent stenoses and symptoms of stroke, TIA, or amaurosis fugax warrant treatment. Many patients may be managed by stenting because of the perceived increased risk of reoperation. However, the results of open surgery for recurrent carotid stenosis are good and show it to be a durable operation. Concerns about difficult dissection and excessive nerve injuries may be exaggerated.[6] Both eversion carotid endarterectomy or conventional patch angioplasty of the common carotid artery and ICA may be used. More than three fourths of the patients presenting with recurrent carotid stenosis can undergo redo eversion CEA.[12] In patients with persistent or recurrent disease that is extensive, patch angioplasty or interposition bypass is preferred.

Carotid Patch Aneurysm

Patch aneurysm is a late complication of conventional carotid patch angioplasty, affecting 0.4% of Dacron or Gore-Tex patches. It manifests either as a pulsatile neck mass or occasionally with embolic symptoms. Surgery is performed under general anesthesia with the aneurysmal portion of the carotid artery replaced with an interposition graft. Care is taken with dissection to prevent distal embolization, and risk of cranial nerve injury is increased.

Infected Carotid Patch

In a recent review[10] the risk of Dacron patch infection was as high as 0.5% and was associated with a history of postoperative hematoma after CEA. Patients present with neck swelling or a draining local sinus, and cultures often grow *Staphylococcus epidermidis* or *Staphylococcus aureus*. A duplex scan is diagnostic, although CT angiography is critical for operative planning. The principles of management include excision of the synthetic patch and all grossly infected tissue, appropriate antibiotic coverage, and carotid reconstruction with a vein graft.

REFERENCES

1. Raithel D: Carotid eversion endarterectomy: A better technique than the standard operation? *Cardiovasc Surg* 5:471-472, 1997.
2. Cao P, Giordano G, De Rango P, Zannetti S, et al: A randomized study on eversion versus standard carotid endarterectomy. Study design and preliminary results: The Everest Trial, *J Vasc Surg* 27:595-605, 1998.
3. Kieny R, Hirsch D, Seiller C, et al: Does carotid eversion endarterectomy and reimplantation reduce the risk of restenosis? *Ann Vasc Surg* 7:407-413, 1993.
4. DeBakey ME: Regarding "A randomized study on eversion versus standard carotid endarterectomy. Study design and preliminary results: The Everest trial," *J Vasc Surg* 28:753, 1998.
5. Etheredge SN: A simple technic for carotid endarterectomy, *Am J Surg* 120:275-278, 1970.
6. Coscas R, Rhissassi B, Gruet-Coquet N, et al: Open surgery remains a valid option for the treatment of recurrent carotid stenosis, *J Vasc Surg* 51:1124-1132, 2010.
7. Black JH 3rd, Ricotta JJ, Jones CE: Long-term results of eversion carotid endarterectomy, *Ann Vasc Surg* 24:92-99, 2010.
8. Palubiskas AJ, Ripley HR: Fibromuscular dysplasia in extrarenal arteries, *Radiology* 82:451-455, 1964.
9. Osborn AG, Anderson RE: Angiographic spectrum of cervical and intracranial fibromuscular dysplasia, *Stroke* 8:617-626, 1977.
10. Knight BC, Tait WF: Dacron patch infection following carotid endarterectomy: A systematic review of the literature, *Eur J Vasc Endovasc Surg* 37:140-148, 2009.
12. Shah DM, Darling RC 3rd, Chang BB, Paty PS, Kreienberg PB, Lloyd WE, Leather RP: Carotid endarterectomy by eversion technique: Its safety and durability, *Ann Surg* 228:471-478, 1998.

8 Carotid Angioplasty and Stenting

PETER A. SCHNEIDER

Historical Background

Balloon angioplasty of the carotid artery was first described in the late 1970s as an intervention for carotid artery stenosis.[1] It was proposed as an alternative to carotid endarterectomy (CEA) in medically high-risk patients and those with hostile neck anatomy. Early trials demonstrated the feasibility of the technique but were not widely accepted because of small study size, high complication rates, and only occasional use of stenting.[2-4] Carotid angioplasty and stenting (CAS) has evolved to its current form with improvements in equipment and technique, increased operator experience, and standard use of cerebral protection during carotid stent placement.

Indications

Key trials have helped to determine which patients are best treated with CAS, but this issue is not yet resolved.[5-8] The current indication for CAS is high anatomic or physiologic risk for CEA (Table 8-1).

Preoperative Care

- Obtain an understanding of the arch, carotid, and cerebral arterial anatomy before the procedure by arteriogram, computed tomography (CT) angiography, or magnetic resonance angiography. This enhances patient selection and procedural planning.
- A CT or magnetic resonance imaging (MRI) scan of the brain is obtained in symptomatic patients and in those older than 80 years to evaluate for preprocedural cerebral pathology. Patients older than 80 years are at higher risk for stroke after CAS.[9]
- Antiplatelet therapy is initiated with aspirin at 325 mg/day and clopidogrel at 75 mg/day for 5 days before the procedure. In all cases patients should have received clopidogrel (total dose of 300 mg) before the intervention. Patients are asked to discontinue beta-blockers on the day of the stent procedure to help avoid poststent bradycardia.
- A neurologic examination is performed and a stroke scale is completed.
- The procedure is performed under local anesthesia with minimal or no sedation to facilitate patient cooperation and neurologic monitoring. An arterial line is placed for continuous blood pressure monitoring. External pacer pads should be readily available. Patients with severe aortic stenosis undergo placement of a temporary venous pacemaker. Because of the minimal use of sedation, patients may be apprehensive and hypertensive. Avoid acutely reducing the blood pressure during the intervention with pharmacologic agents because poststent hypotension or bradycardia is not uncommon. If antihypertensive medication is required, it is best to use a short-acting agent.

TABLE 8-1 Indications for Carotid Angioplasty and Stenting in Patients at High Risk for Carotid Endarterectomy

Physiologic Criteria	Anatomic Criteria
Unstable angina	Lesion above C2 or below the clavicle
MI within 30 days	Tandem carotid lesions requiring treatment
NYHA class 3 or 4 CHF	Restenosis with prior CEA
Multivessel coronary artery disease (nonrevascularizable)	Radical neck dissection
Left ventricular ejection fraction < 30%	Tracheostomy
Cardiac surgery within 30 days	Cervical radiation
COPD (FEV1 < 30% of predicted)	Contralateral carotid occlusion
Age > 80 years	Contralateral CEA with cranial nerve injury

CHF, Congestive heart failure; *COPD,* chronic obstructive pulmonary disease; *FEV1,* forced expiratory volume in 1 sec; *NYHA,* New York Heart Association.

Pitfalls and Danger Points

- **Stroke.** Stroke may occur with CAS. The perioperative risk of stroke, ipsilateral postprocedural stroke, and death in the Carotid Revascularization Endarterectomy versus Stenting Trial (CREST) was 2.5% for asymptomatic patients and 6.0% for symptomatic patients.[8] Although minor stroke was higher with CAS than with CEA, the incidence of major stroke and death was similar between the two procedures.

- **Difficult access of the carotid artery.** Tortuous aortic arch or great vessel anatomy must be analyzed and the appropriate steps must be taken to achieve access safely. A reverse-curved catheter may be required for common carotid artery cannulation. A variety of stiff exchange wires may be used to support a carotid access sheath. In some patients with a diseased arch CAS should be avoided.[10]

- **Unable to cross the lesion.** The curve at the tip of the guidewire may be altered or the crossing wire may be supported with a directional catheter. The patient's neck position may be changed to make the course into the lesion less angulated. The residual lumen of a complex lesion is most likely to be just posterior to the flow divider. A buddy wire may also be used to facilitate crossing of the lesion.

- **Spasm of the distal internal carotid artery (ICA).** If ICA spasm is identified during the CAS procedure, small doses of nitroglycerine may be administered into the carotid sheath. Spasm resolves after the filter and wire are removed.

- **No flow after stenting.** The filter may be full of obstructive debris and should be aspirated before removal.

- **Hypotension, bradycardia, or both.** Hypotension and bradycardia occur regularly with CAS but are rarely sustained. They are supported with the appropriate pharmacologic agent.

- **In-stent restenosis.** Recurrent in-stent stenosis appears to occur with a similar frequency after CAS as it does after CEA.[11] It is usually treated with repeat balloon angioplasty and occasionally with repeat stenting. It is rare for carotid stent patients to require arterial replacement.

Endovascular Strategy

ANGIOGRAPHIC ANATOMY

Study the anatomy of the arch, carotid, and cerebral arteries before the procedure. A view may be obtained by arteriogram, CT angiography, or magnetic resonance angiography and permits patient selection and procedural planning (Table 8-2). Several anatomic factors may be considered relative contraindications to CAS, including severe arch atherosclerosis or tortuosity, diffuse common carotid artery disease or tortuosity, severe angulation of the bifurcation, kinking of the distal ICA, and lack of a filter landing zone in the distal ICA.

TABLE 8-2 Anatomic and Pathologic Conditions That Enhance the Difficulty of Carotid Angioplasty and Stenting

Anatomy or Pathology	Arch	Common Carotid Artery	Bifurcation	Distal ICA
Tortuosity	More challenging sheath placement	Potential for less stability of the sheath during the procedure	More challenging lesion crossing	No filter landing zone
Calcification	Increased stroke risk with cannulation in the calcified arch		Greater likelihood of embolization with stenting	
Both tortuosity and calcification	Greater likelihood of sheath placement to be a prohibitive risk	More risk of injury to the common carotid artery	Potential inability to deliver the stent	
Complex carotid plaque morphology			Echogenic plaque; large plaque burdens are at higher risk for embolization during stent placement	
Thrombus			Free floating thrombus; use proximal protection	
Extra lesions in inconvenient locations		Possible requirement of a separate balloon-expandable stent at the origin of the common carotid artery	Occluded external carotid artery; this branch cannot be used to anchor the exchange guidewire for sheath placement	
Anatomic variants	Identification and management of well-described arch variants			Cerebral collaterals, isolated hemisphere

FAVORABLE VERSUS UNFAVORABLE AORTIC ARCH ANATOMY

Arch tortuosity is a significant deterrent to safe and simple access sheath placement.[12] The arch is considered type I if the branches originate at the top of the arch, type II if the arch vessels arise between the parallel planes delineated by the outer and the inner curves of the arch (moderate angulation), and type III if the branches originate along the upslope of the arch, proximal or caudal to the lesser curvature of the arch, or off the ascending aorta (severe angulation; Fig. 8-1).

CAROTID LESIONS AT RISK FOR EMBOLIZATION

Risky lesions for CAS include those with circumferential calcification, heavy plaque burden, or echolucent plaque and those that are symptomatic, especially if there has been a recent stroke or a series of transient ischemic attacks.[13]

KINKS AND COILS OF THE CAROTID ARTERY

Tortuous carotid arteries can make crossing the lesion challenging, may make the landing zone for the filter too short, or may present a situation in which stenting is not possible because the stent is unable to conform to the tortuous bifurcation and distal ICA. Tortuosity of the artery is not alleviated by stent placement and may be worsened by propagating the tortuosity to another segment of nonstented artery.

OCCLUDED EXTERNAL CAROTID ARTERY

The external carotid artery is used as a location to anchor the exchange wire so that sheath insertion is stable. When the external carotid artery is occluded, or when the carotid bifurcation lesion involves the distal common carotid artery, this is not possible and other maneuvers are required to achieve sheath access, such as telescoping the sheath into the common carotid artery (Fig. 8-2).

SEVERE STENOSIS AND STRING SIGN

When there is little residual lumen, there may be slow flow or thrombus accumulation, and flow may stop when the wire is placed across the lesion. With a string

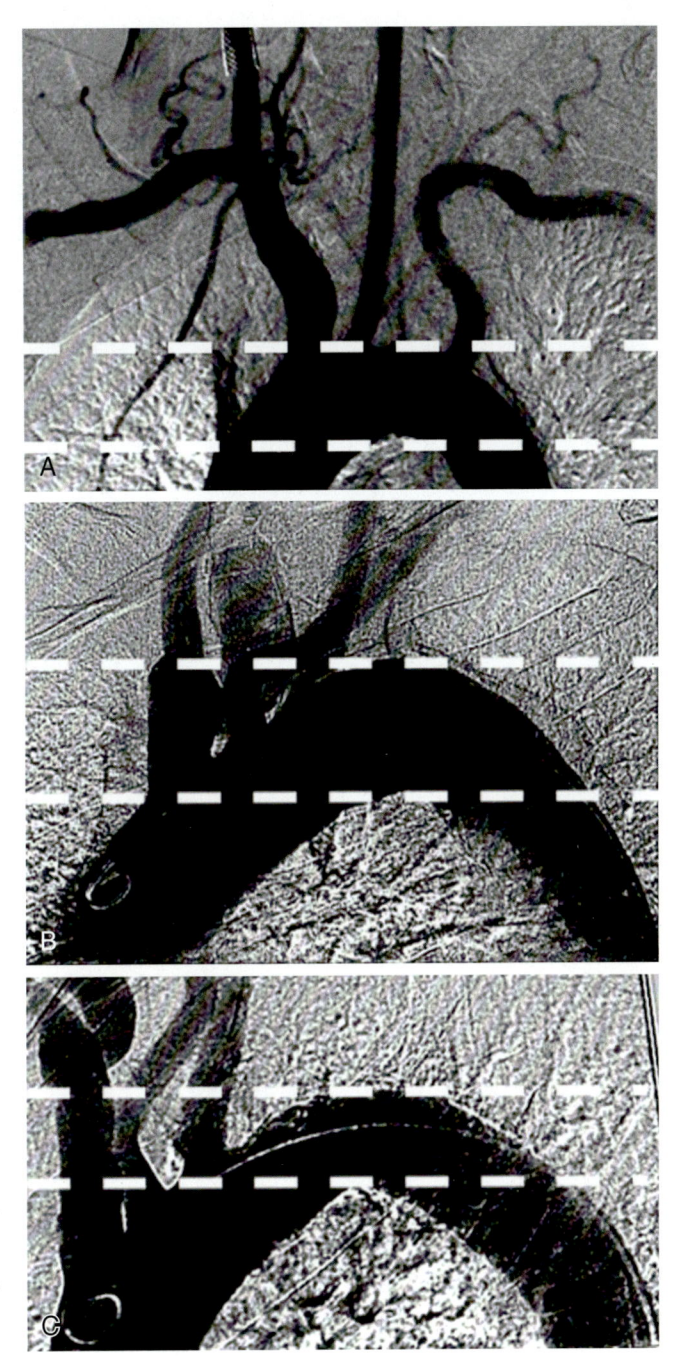

Figure 8-1. Aortic arch classification. **A,** Type I: The great vessels arise above or in the same horizontal plane as the outer curvature of the arch. **B,** Type II: The origin of the innominate artery lies between the horizontal planes of the outer and the inner curvatures of the aortic arch. **C,** Type III: The innominate artery lies below the horizontal plane of the inner curvature of the arch. (From Cronenwett JL, Johnston KW, editors: Rutherford's vascular surgery, ed 7, Philadelphia, 2010, Saunders, p 1472, Fig. 96-1.)

sign (severe stenosis with collapse of the distal lumen), sizing of distal filters is difficult because the distal lumen may or may not expand after angioplasty of the bifurcation lesion.

TANDEM LESIONS IN THE COMMON CAROTID ARTERY

Occasionally, a lesion occurs in the proximal common carotid artery (especially at its origin from the arch) and at the bifurcation and both lesions require treatment. Balloon angioplasty of the arch lesion is required to create space for the sheath. The bifurcation lesion is treated with a stent using distal protection in the usual manner, and the common carotid artery origin is stented before fully withdrawing the sheath.

FIBROMUSCULAR DYSPLASIA

The pathology of fibromuscular dysplasia responds well to balloon angioplasty. A stent may be required if the residual surface is highly irregular or mobile. Because the process extends to the base of the skull, there is usually an inadequate landing zone for a filter, and proximal occlusion with reversed flow may be used for

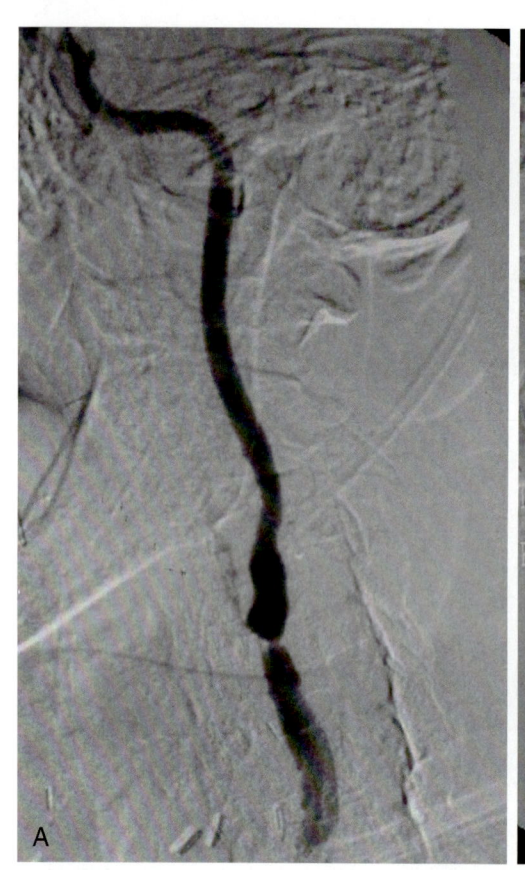

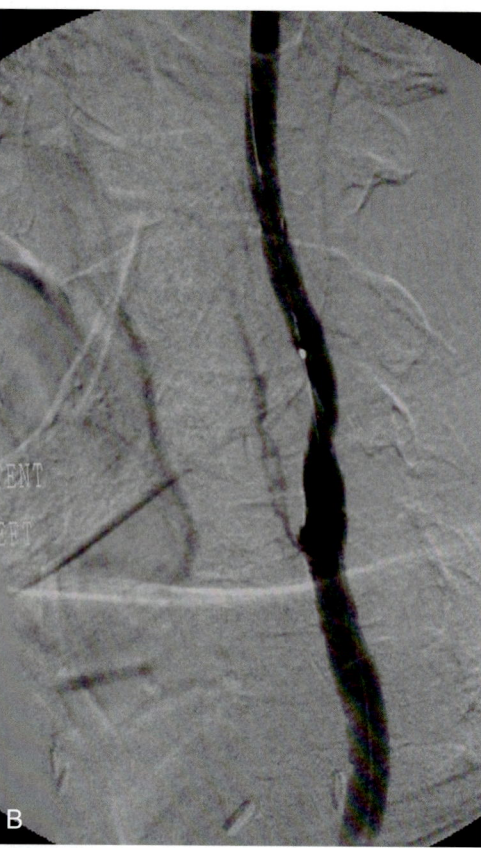

Figure 8-2. In this example the external carotid artery is occluded. The external carotid artery is commonly used to anchor the exchange guidewire and stabilize sheath insertion. When the external carotid artery is occluded, or when the carotid bifurcation lesion involves the distal common carotid artery, sheath insertion is accomplished by telescoping the sheath into the common carotid artery. This patient had a recurrent stenosis after a previous CEA. The pretreatment (**A**) and completion (**B**) arteriograms are shown.

cerebral protection. Do not perform angioplasty if the artery is aneurysmal or there is evidence of dissection.[14]

SELECTION OF A STENT: OPEN- VERSUS CLOSED-CELL DESIGNS

Open-cell stents are more flexible and more appropriate for tortuous carotid arteries. Closed-cell stents have smaller cells and better outward radial force. They may result in a lower rate of stroke, but are less conformable.[15]

CEREBRAL PROTECTION DEVICES

Currently, the choice for cerebral protection is between filters and occlusion devices (with or without reversed flow). Most stents are placed with filters, but data are developing on proximal occlusion using a variety of techniques. Filter technology continues to improve, but filtration is not complete.[16,17]

REDO CAROTID ANGIOPLASTY

Repeat balloon angioplasty is usually adequate to restore the lumen of a restenotic carotid stent, but occasionally an additional stent is required.

Endovascular Technique

ACCESS

The common femoral artery is the access site in most cases, although CAS has also been performed using upper extremity access or direct common carotid artery access. The access site with the simplest and safest path to the bifurcation should be selected. Occasionally, brachial or radial access may be used in the case of a bovine arch or tortuous great vessels. A micropuncture set (21-Ga needle) may be used for the initial access; this has significantly reduced the number of femoral access complications. Following guidewire access, an introducer sheath is placed in the common femoral artery that is the same size as that intended for the carotid

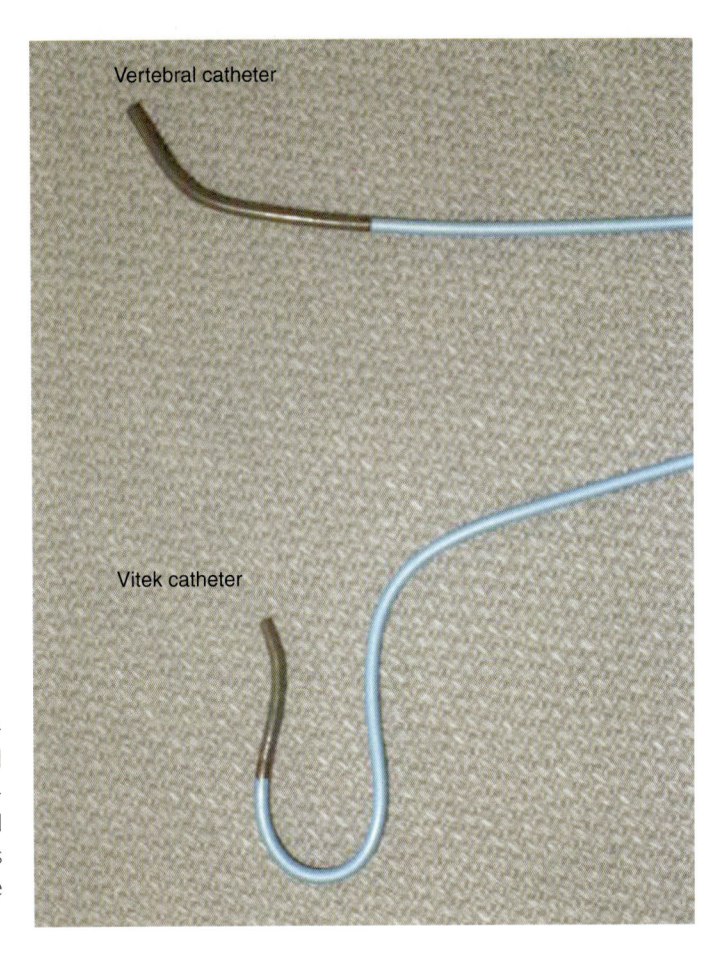

Figure 8-3. Catheterization of arch branches can be performed with either a simple curve catheter, like the vertebral catheter (top), or a complex curve catheter, like the Vitek catheter (bottom). The vertebral catheter has a single, simple bend at the catheter tip. The Vitek catheter has a series of bends that provide a reverse curve so that tortuous pathways can be navigated.

stent placement, usually 6 or 7 Fr. When the arch or proximal great vessels are too tortuous or there is significant arch disease, another option is to perform a short transverse neck incision, clamp the common carotid artery, and insert the stent directly through a short sheath. Cerebral protection may be performed using reversed flow or a filter.

CATHETERIZATION OF THE COMMON CAROTID ARTERY

Catheterization can almost always be accomplished using one of two preshaped catheters: a simple curve catheter such as a vertebral catheter or a complex curve catheter such as the reversed angle Vitek catheter (Fig. 8-3). The image intensifier is maintained in its fixed left anterior oblique (LAO) position, and bony landmarks or a road map may be used to guide vessel cannulation. The catheter of first choice in most cases is a simple curve catheter. The angle formed by the vertebral catheter, along with the tip angle on an angled Glidewire, is adequate to cannulate most common carotid arteries. Once the Glidewire has accessed the common carotid artery, the catheter is advanced over the wire for selective angiograms of the common carotid artery. Do not pass the guidewire into the carotid artery bifurcation without doing an arteriogram. As the cerebral catheter rounds the turn from the arch into the common carotid artery, it tends to straighten out and the guidewire may "jump" forward. This catheter advancement should be visualized under fluoroscopy and carefully controlled. If the catheter catches during advancement, apply only gentle forward pressure so that excessive tension does not build up in the system. Sometimes, having the patient take a deep breath or cough aids catheter passage.

Reversed angle catheters are usually required when the aortic arch is tortuous (type III arch) or the common carotid arteries are retroflexed toward the patient's left or there is a bovine configuration (Fig. 8-4). The VTK is best reformed in the proximal descending aorta and then pushed proximally into the arch. The most challenging are those branches that originate from the upslope of the ascending aorta.

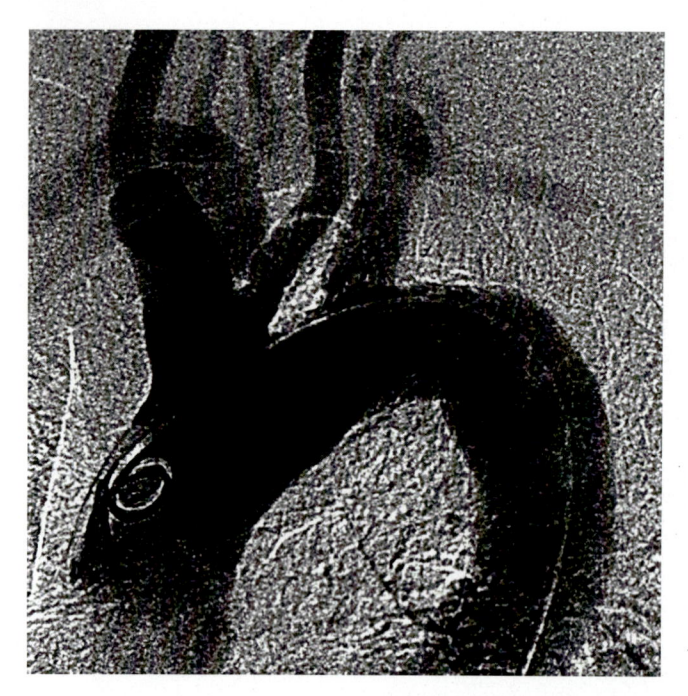

Figure 8-4. A common anatomic variant of the arch is the bovine configuration. The right and left common carotid arteries originate from the innominate artery. When treating a left carotid artery originating from a bovine arch, a complex curve catheter is required, such as a Vitek, JB2, or Simmons 2. *(From Cronenwett JL, Johnston KW, editors: Rutherford's vascular surgery, ed 7, Philadelphia, 2010, Saunders, p 1472, Fig. 96-2.)*

ANGIOGRAPHY OF THE AORTIC ARCH, CAROTID, AND CEREBRAL CIRCULATION

Arch manipulations with guidewires, catheters, and sheaths carry a risk of neurologic events. In several studies of CAS, especially early in the experience, up to 1% of patients sustained a stroke in the contralateral hemisphere, suggesting that carotid access may be a contributor to morbidity.[18] Better patient selection that avoids some of the riskiest anatomic pitfalls has helped to reduce these adverse events. Administer systemic heparin before aortic arch manipulation. An initial arch angiogram is performed through a pigtail catheter with the image intensifier in the LAO position. The head of the pigtail catheter is placed in the midascending aorta. The LAO position is maintained, the pigtail is exchanged for the cerebral catheter of choice, and the common carotid artery is cannulated, as described earlier. Selective carotid and cerebral arteriography is performed with the catheter in the midcommon carotid artery. The catheter tip is placed at least a few centimeters proximal to the carotid bifurcation. Contrast is administered at 3 or 4 mL/sec for 2 seconds. The rate of rise is usually set at 0.5 second so that injection pressure at the tip of the catheter peaks over about 0.5 second through the tip of the end-hole catheter. In performing a complete carotid arteriogram each carotid bifurcation is evaluated with two views, usually an oblique and a lateral, and sometimes with more views if needed. Cerebral arteries are evaluated using a lateral view and a craniocaudal anteroposterior view. If pathology is discovered, additional views are required. Usually, a complete carotid arteriogram is not performed as part of the stent procedure; instead it is performed before stenting or the information is derived from CT or MRI.

SHEATH PLACEMENT FOR PLANNED INTERVENTION

During CAS, it is optimal to select the appropriate catheter, access sheath, filter, predilatation balloon, postdilatation balloon, stent, and filter retrieval catheter and prepare all selections before cannulating the common carotid artery.

Carotid sheath access requires placement of an adequate length of exchange guidewire into the common carotid artery. This sometimes can be accomplished by placing the tip of the exchange guidewire in the distal common carotid artery but usually requires cannulation of the external carotid artery and use of this vessel to anchor the stiff guidewire (Fig. 8-5). Blind guidewire and catheter manipulation in the carotid artery is avoided. Selective external carotid cannulation can be accomplished with a 260-cm angled Glidewire and the cerebral diagnostic catheter. Choose a safe branch of the external carotid artery that permits several

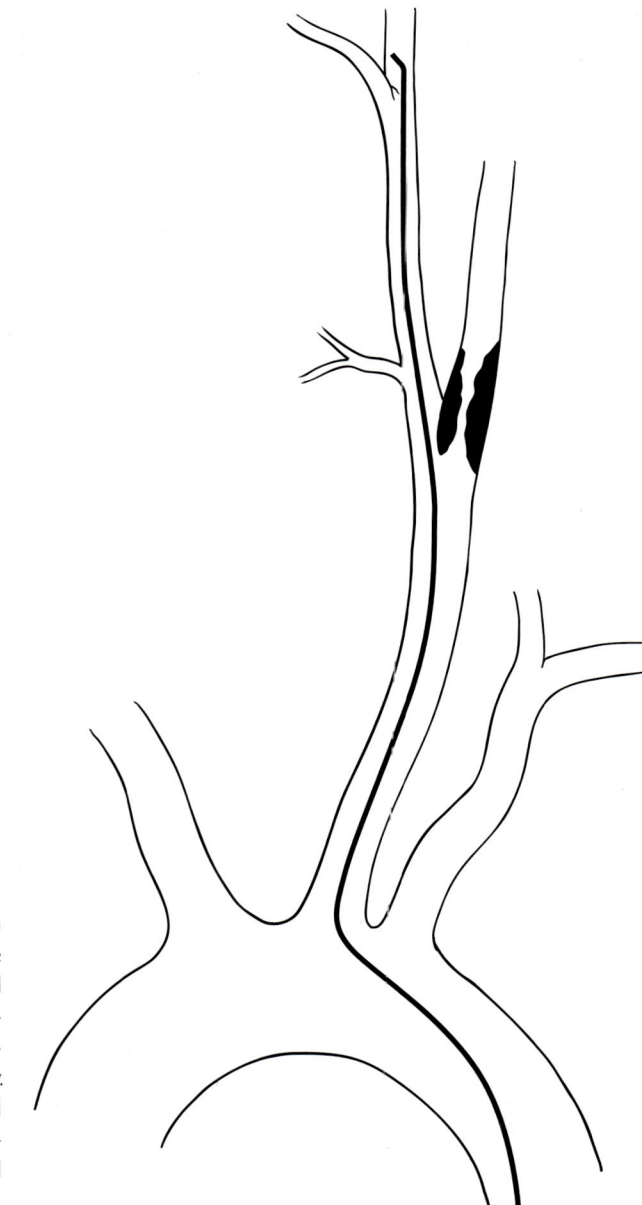

Figure 8-5. Carotid sheath access is simplest if an adequate length of exchange guidewire is placed into the common carotid artery. The cerebral catheter of choice is used to cannulate the common carotid artery. A road map of the carotid bifurcation is performed. The Glidewire is advanced into the external carotid artery. The cerebral catheter is advanced over the Glidewire into the external carotid artery. The catheter is advanced into the longest, safe branch of the external carotid artery. The superior thyroid artery is not adequate for anchoring. The stiff exchange guidewire is advanced through the cerebral catheter into the external carotid artery.

centimeters of clearance distal to the bifurcation. The superior thyroid artery is not adequate because it is too short, and the lingual artery should be avoided because a rupture of this artery resulting from wire trauma could cause airway obstruction. Passage of the stiff exchange guidewire into the small external carotid artery branches must be performed with caution to avoid perforation of these small branches. CAS can usually be accomplished with a 6- or 7-Fr sheath. The Glidewire is then withdrawn from the vertebral catheter and a 260-cm Amplatz superstiff or other exchange guidewire is passed into the external carotid artery. This allows an adequate guidewire length to be placed beyond the carotid bifurcation for subsequent placement of the carotid sheath. If it is necessary to evaluate the external carotid artery with an arteriogram, contrast injections into the carotid system should not be done unless free backflow of blood is present at the hub of the diagnostic catheter. Otherwise there is a risk of pushing microbubbles into the system. In the external carotid artery, backbleeding may be diminished by the tight fit of the catheter in the small external carotid artery branches. In this event the cerebral catheter is slowly withdrawn until adequate backflow is noted.

The catheter is withdrawn, leaving the Amplatz guidewire in the external carotid artery. The groin sheath is removed. A 90-cm-long carotid access sheath is advanced over the Amplatz guidewire into the common carotid artery (Fig. 8-6).

94 EXTRACRANIAL CEREBROVASCULAR DISEASE

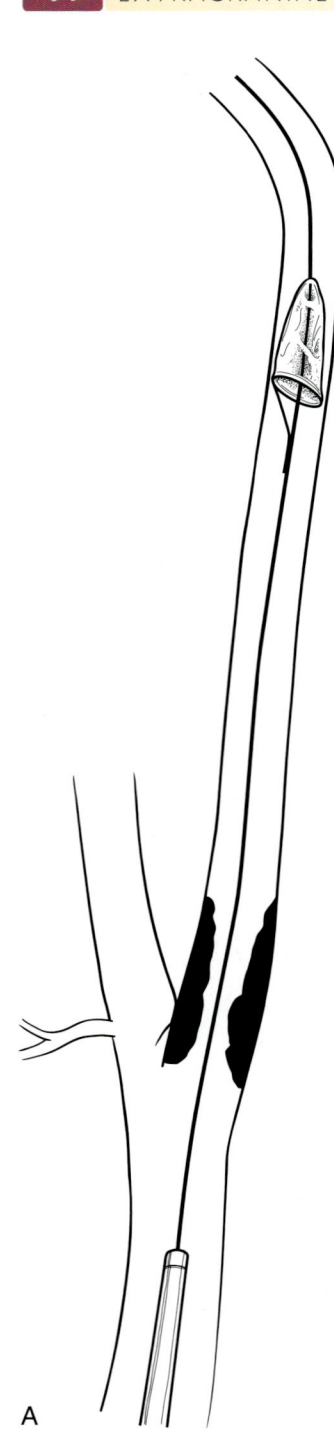

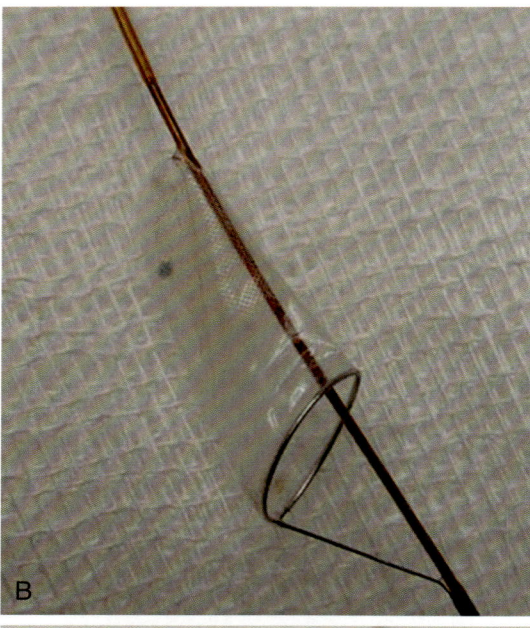

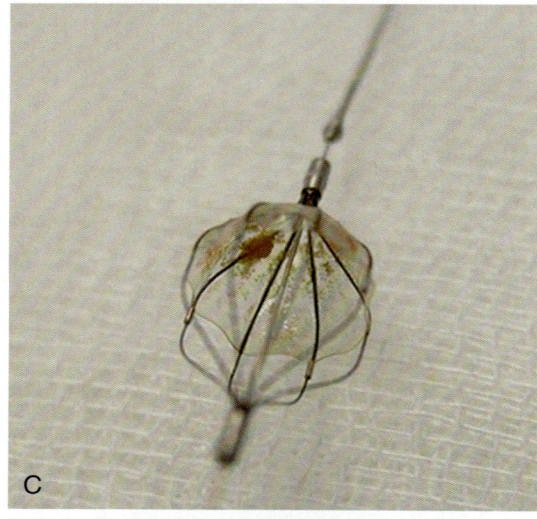

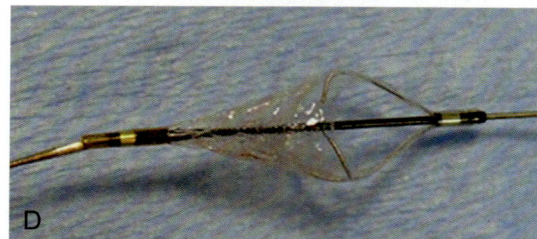

Figure 8-6. A, The carotid sheath, 6 or 7 Fr, is advanced over the stiff exchange guidewire. The tip of the sheath is placed in the middle or distal common carotid artery. Care is taken to avoid advancing the dilator tip into the bifurcation. After sheath placement, the exchange guidewire and introducer are removed. A new road map is performed. The prepared distal filter is advanced across the lesion and into the ICA. The filter is deployed a few centimeters distal to the lesion in a relatively straight segment of the ICA. **B** to **D,** Alternate filters are depicted. (**B,** Courtesy Boston Scientific, Natick, Mass.; **C,** Courtesy Cordis, Somerville, N.J.; **D,** Courtesy Abbott Vascular, Redwood City, Calif. From Cronenwett JL, Johnston KW, editors: Rutherford's vascular surgery, ed 7, Philadelphia, 2010, Saunders, p 1478, Fig. 96-4.)

Image the tip of the Amplatz guidewire in the external carotid artery and the last turn from the arch into the common carotid artery during sheath passage. If the tip of the advancing sheath hangs up at the turn into the common carotid artery or the tip of the guidewire moves back, it indicates that the sheath is not advancing appropriately over the guidewire. Reassess the curvature in the system and make sure that an adequate length of stiff exchange guidewire is present. Occasionally, it is helpful to have the patient take a deep breath as the sheath tip is rounding the corner out of the arch and into the common carotid artery. This maneuver alters the configuration of the branch origin a bit and can offer a more favorable anatomic trajectory for sheath placement.

The dilator tip for the 90-cm carotid sheath is long and not well visualized during fluoroscopy. After the dilator and sheath are advanced into the common carotid artery, if a position closer to the bifurcation is needed, the dilator is held steady

CAROTID ANGIOPLASTY AND STENTING

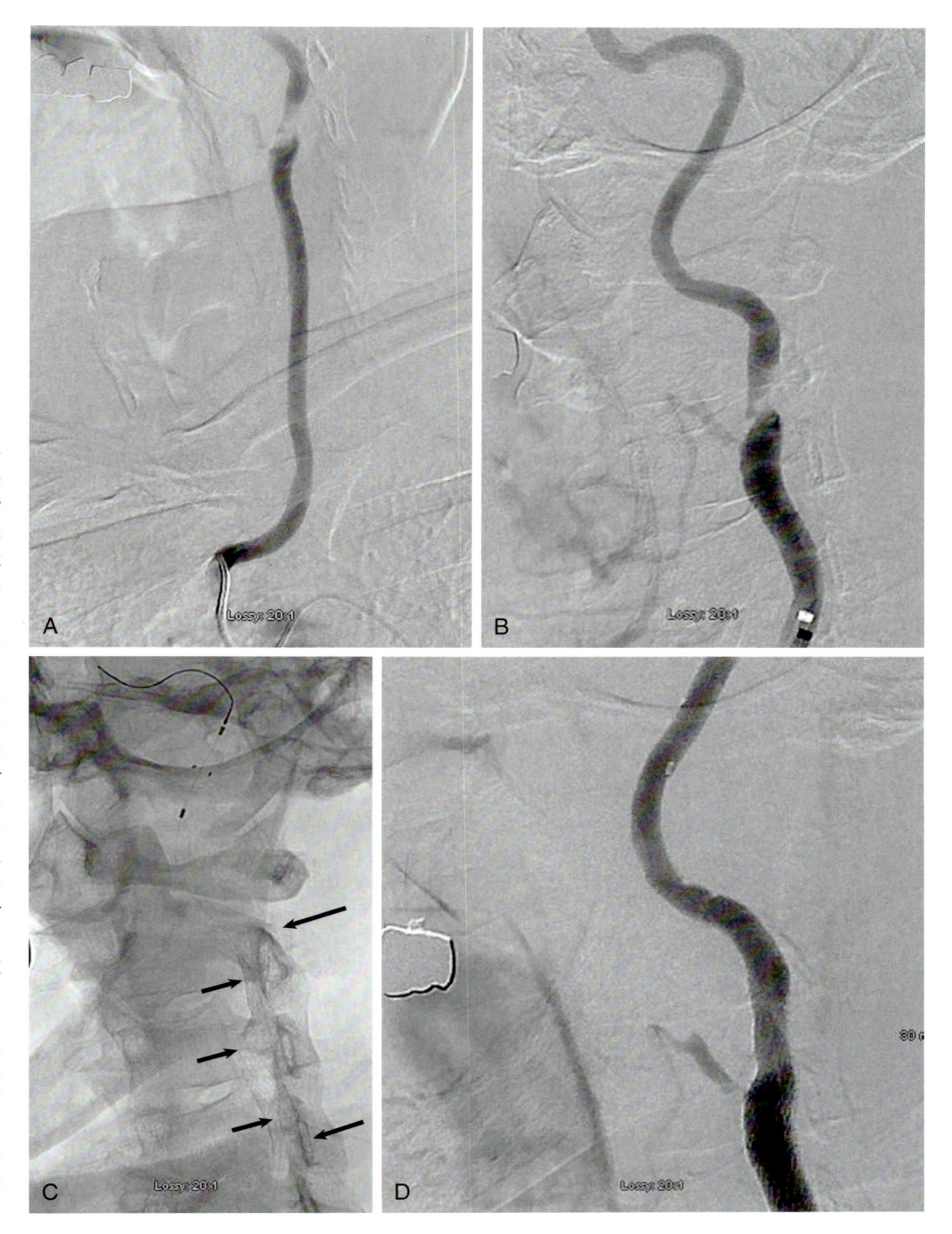

Figure 8-7. A, A Vitek catheter is used to cannulate the left common carotid artery and a carotid arteriogram is performed. **B,** Because the left external carotid artery was occluded, an exchange guidewire was advanced through the catheter and placed with its tip in the distal common carotid artery. A 6-Fr catheter was advanced over the exchange guidewire. A 6-Fr sheath was advanced over the combination of the exchange guidewire and the catheter in a telescoping maneuver. The tip of the sheath is in the inferior aspect of the image. The distal ICA, where the filter landing zone is located, is in the superior aspect of the image. **C,** The distal filter is deployed in the ICA. The stent has been deployed across the carotid bifurcation lesion (arrows indicate the stent). **D,** A completion arteriogram demonstrates a patent stent.

while the sheath is advanced over it. Anatomic landmarks or a road map may be used to be sure that the sheath tip is not advanced into the bifurcation. The stiff exchange guidewire and the dilator are withdrawn, and the carotid angiogram is repeated through the long 6- or 7-Fr sheath with a road map of the carotid bifurcation stenosis in preparation for crossing the lesion.

CROSSING A LESION AND CEREBRAL PROTECTION

A lesion may be crossed and cerebral protection may be performed with one of a variety of cerebral protection devices that are available. Filter devices are designed to maintain flow in the distal ICA during the course of intervention. Movement of the sheath after filter placement could also move the filter to ensure that the sheath is in a stable position before filter placement. The image intensifier is positioned such that the tip of the sheath is visible on the inferior aspect of the monitor screen and the filter landing zone is visible on the superior aspect. This position is maintained for the remainder of the CAS procedure (Fig. 8-7). The landing zone for the filter is assessed in advance; it must be reachable with the proposed filter and be long enough and straight enough to accommodate the filter. Placing the filter into a tortuous segment could impede filter function by causing spasm or making wall apposition poor. An activated clotting time (ACT) of 250 seconds or higher is required before placing filter devices. After each step of the intervention, flow of contrast through the filter is observed using arteriography.

The filter system may be a free-wire or a fixed-wire system. With a free-wire system, the wire is separate from the filter and is passed across the lesion, and the filter is placed over the wire. There is a knob on the wire to act as a stop so that the filter cannot slip off the end of the wire. The fixed-wire system has the filter mounted on the wire so that the entire apparatus is advanced across the lesion. There is a transition from the wire tip to the portion of the filter delivery catheter that houses the filter, and this transition sometimes hangs up when advancing across a tight or tortuous lesion. If there is any wire movement after placement, the filter also moves. The tip of the leading guidewire is hand shaped with a curve to provide directionality for crossing the lesion. Most lesions that are isolated to the proximal ICA are posterior wall plaques. In passing the guidewire tip to cross the lesion, the best pathway is usually anterior in the proximal ICA, just behind the flow divider. Bifurcation lesions that involve the distal common carotid artery are usually more complex and less predictable. The key is to lead with the guidewire tip; do not make a loop and probe the lesion as little as possible.

The crossing profile of the filter delivery catheter may be larger than the residual lumen in a tight stenosis. It may be difficult to cross extremely stenotic, tortuous, or calcified lesions. A "buddy wire" (0.010 or 0.014 inches) is occasionally used to provide extra support during filter placement. A slightly larger sheath is needed to accommodate a buddy wire. Tortuosity may also be improved by changing the patient's neck position. When a tight lesion cannot be crossed with a filter, occasionally (<5%) balloon predilatation with a 2.5-mm-diameter angioplasty balloon is required. When critically stenotic carotid lesions or highly tortuous carotid bifurcations are involved, the use of a free-wire filter system (e.g., Emboshield or Spider) has advantages over a fixed-wire system (e.g., Accunet or FilterWire). This permits guidewire crossing and placement and optimization of position before the filter is advanced. The usual tendency during the procedure is for tension on the guidewire to result in partial withdrawal of the filter, in the direction of the stent. This may induce spasm, spill debris that the filter holds, or entangle the filter with the stent, making it difficult to withdraw the filter.

Another cerebral protection option is proximal occlusion with reversed flow (Gore Neuro Protection System) or with aspiration (MO.MA). The sheath is larger than for filtered CAS. Flow in the common carotid artery is stopped by inflating an occlusion balloon surrounding the sheath tip and then placing an occlusion balloon in the external carotid artery. The common carotid artery sheath may be connected to the femoral vein, producing an arteriovenous fistula and reversal of flow in the ICA. At this point, intervention can be performed under complete protection, because antegrade flow in the ICA does not occur until after the procedure is completed. Alternatively, in the case of the MO.MA device, flow is stopped and the area is aspirated before restoring flow. In each situation there is still no way to protect the brain during sheath insertion before proximal occlusion. There are also a small number of patients who cannot tolerate proximal occlusion or flow reversal, usually because of poor cerebral collateral circulation or even an isolated hemisphere (Figs. 8-8 and 8-9).

Surgeons experienced with CEA know the potential for dislodging the friable material present in carotid bifurcation plaques. Studies of CAS with transcranial Doppler monitoring have demonstrated frequent embolic signals prevalent during several stages of the procedure, including lesion crossing, predilation, stent placement, and postdilation.[19] Diffusion-weighted MRI scans performed after

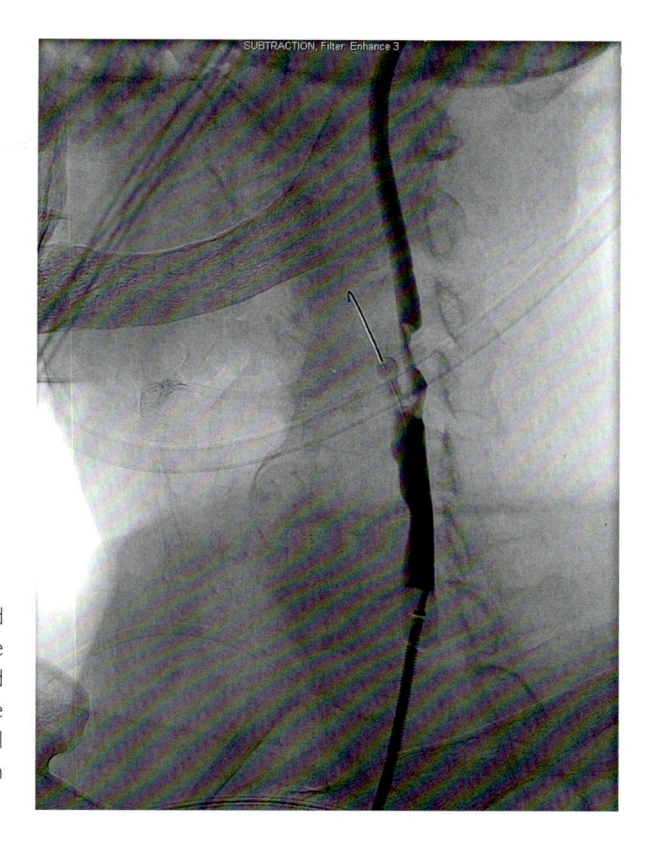

Figure 8-8. Carotid stenting using flow reversal. The common carotid sheath has an occlusive balloon preventing inflow. A separate balloon wire is inflated in the external carotid to prevent backflow that would send debris into the ICA territory. Through a side port on the sheath, passive retrograde flow is established, allowing blood and any debris to travel through a filter and into a femoral venous sheath. Cerebral protection with flow reversal is in place before the lesion is crossed.

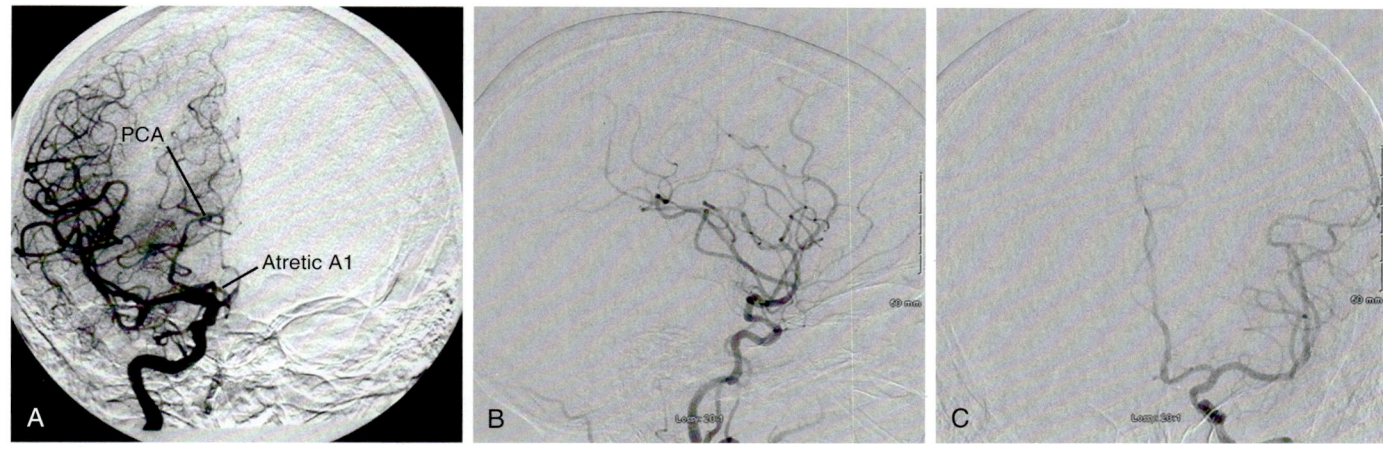

Figure 8-9. **A,** Occasionally, a carotid lesion requires treatment that also serves an isolated cerebral hemisphere. Reversed flow may not be tolerated. During stent placement, it is useful to support the blood pressure and minimize the dwell time of the catheters across the carotid lesion. In this image cross-filling from the right hemisphere to the left is absent because of an atretic A1 segment. **B** and **C,** In a second patient, absence of cross-filling is noted from the left to the right hemisphere. Normal cerebral arteriogram after the left carotid stent, lateral view (**B**) and craniocaudal view (**C**). Note the absence of the anterior communicating artery. *PCA,* Posterior cerebral artery.

CAS have shown evidence of lesions that are likely embolic. Most filters allow particles smaller than 100 μm to pass through, resulting in small, usually asymptomatic, cerebral lesions detected by diffusion-weighted MRI studies of the brain.[20,21] This type of distal microembolization, although not immediately associated with gross neurologic deficits, may lead to late cognitive impairment. Flow reversal permits CAS with the opportunity to diminish microembolization.[22]

ANGIOPLASTY (Video 8-1)

After the lesion has been crossed and the filter deployed, predilation is performed with a 3-mm-diameter rapid exchange balloon. This balloon is usually 4 cm in length to avoid slippage of the balloon during inflation. Some operators routinely administer small doses of atropine (0.25-0.5 mg) before balloon dilatation, except in patients with a recurrent stenosis. The pressure used for predilatation is the nominal pressure for that balloon, with higher pressure (14-16 atm) reserved for heavily calcified stenoses. If the balloon immediately attains its full shape, as it almost always does, the predilatation time can be short. Observe the monitor for bradycardia or even asystole. The purpose of predilatation is to create a tract for stent delivery, and most stent delivery catheters are about 2 mm in diameter.

STENTING

A variety of self-expanding stents, mostly constructed of nitinol, are available for use with the respective embolic protection devices. The self-expanding stent is deployed using a bifurcation road map. The stent is placed from the normal artery distal to the lesion to the normal artery proximal to the lesion. This usually means placing the stent across the origin of the external carotid artery (Fig. 8-10). The self-expanding stent is usually postdilated with a 5-mm rapid exchange balloon, depending on the size of the ICA. A 5-mm balloon is almost always adequate; a 6-mm balloon is rarely required after stent deployment. Overdilatation is avoided, even though lesions in multiple other vascular beds are treated this way. The carotid stent is used as scaffolding to modify the flow surface of a lesion at long-term risk for cerebral embolization. The stent provides continuous expansile energy after the procedure, and there is a desire to avoid disrupting the lesion more than necessary because this is associated with embolization during the CAS procedure. The patient may be pretreated again with a small dose of atropine to blunt the carotid sinus response to stretching. A residual stenosis of less than 30% may be accepted. Following stent deployment, shorter (2 cm) balloons are used to dilate the narrow portion of the stent, where the residual stenosis (the "waist") is visible in the stent contour using fluoroscopy. The balloon used for poststent PTA is placed within the stent to avoid dilating nonstented artery and to avoid dissection. Nominal pressure is used to fully expand the balloon and the stent.

Kinks and bends in the ICA may pose a problem with stent implants. Deploy stents across tortuous segments only if they are isolated. Avoid placing the distal end of the stent into kinks and tortuosities of the ICA if more than a single bend is noted. A tortuous ICA should be considered a relative contraindication for CAS, as acute occlusions are more common following stent placement in these tortuous vessels. In addition there may be difficulty in advancing the stent delivery catheter into place in this situation.

COMPLETION STUDIES

Reasonable prograde flow through the stented segment and the filter should be present. After poststent dilation but before the filter is removed, an arteriogram of the carotid is performed. If there is normal flow through the stent and no filling defects, the filter is removed. If the filter is filled with debris, it may manifest itself as sluggish flow or a filling defect in the filter. In this case the filter must be aspirated with an aspiration catheter. When removing a full device, it is important not to recapture it completely, as debris may be extruded from it and embolize distally. The filter retrieval catheter is passed carefully through the stent to capture the filter. Open-cell stent designs have excellent contourability but also have more open cells and diamond-shaped points in the lumen that can snag the retrieval catheter. If the filter retrieval catheter catches on the stent, withdraw the catheter and change the patient's neck position to make a straighter pathway. Most operators also obtain a completion cerebral arteriogram after the completion arteriogram of the stented segment is deemed acceptable.

MANAGEMENT OF ARTERIAL SPASM, EMBOLIZATION, AND ACUTE OCCLUSION

Attention is paid to the ICA immediately distal to the stent. Spasm in this segment may be encountered. A small dose of intraarterial nitroglycerine (50-100 mcg) is

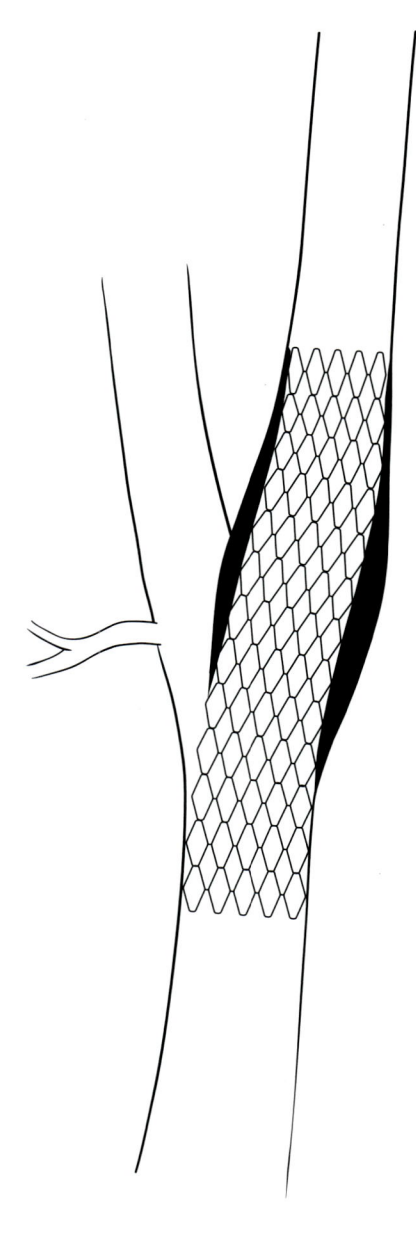

Figure 8-10. The carotid stent has been placed across the bifurcation and passes across the origin of the external carotid artery. It is desirable to place the stent from the normal artery, across the lesion, to the normal artery.

directly administered into the ICA if significant spasm is encountered. Multiple small doses are preferable to large doses. Spasm can occur anytime during the procedure and is relatively common. Sometimes it does not resolve until after the filter and wire are removed. Acute occlusion may occur because of intense spasm, a full filter, thrombosis of the filter or the stent site, or an acute dissection. If acute occlusion occurs, it is an urgent situation. Check the anticoagulation status, pass an aspiration catheter, administer a thrombolytic agent (such as tissue plasminogen activator, or tPA), and make sure the patient has oxygen and adequate systemic blood pressure. Usually there are clues along the course of the case that lead to the diagnosis of the acute occlusion. Distal dissection is rare but when present must be identified and remedied with an additional stent of appropriate size. If there is a dissection, it could occur distal to the stent or as a result of the tip of the lead wire in the distal ICA.

NEURORESCUE TECHNIQUES

When significant distal embolization occurs, make sure the patient is well supported. If the patient becomes agitated or cannot be oxygenated, place the patient under general anesthesia. Finish stenting the carotid bifurcation. Aspirate the stented segment and the artery proximal to the filter. If there is reasonable forward flow and no sign of filling defects in the stented segment, take the filter out. Pass a microcatheter though the sheath, direct it into the appropriate cerebral artery, and administer tPA.

Keep the patient well anticoagulated. Consider infusing intraarterial glycoprotein IIb/IIIa receptor inhibitors to break up platelet clumps. If the embolus does not respond to these measures, a small-caliber angioplasty balloon may be placed in a focal cerebral filling defect to dilate the artery and restore the lumen.

Postoperative Care

- **Access site management.** At present access site hemostasis is achieved in suitable patients at the end of the procedure using one of several approved arterial closure devices. If a calcified or severely diseased vessel is encountered during needle puncture, closure devices are not used. The long carotid access sheath is exchanged for a short sheath of the same caliber. This sheath is removed when the ACT is less than 180 seconds, and manual pressure is held for the appropriate period.
- **Perioperative management.** Patients are monitored in the hospital overnight. It is not uncommon for patients to respond to carotid sinus distension with bradycardia and hypotension.[23] Occasionally, vasopressor or inotropic support is required before the carotid sinus adapts to the radial force of the self-expanding stent. Avoiding extreme oversizing of the stents helps to decrease the incidence of post-CAS hypotension. The presence of significant hypotension in the absence of bradycardia is unusual in the immediate postprocedure period. Other causes (e.g., retroperitoneal bleed related to access site problems) should also be excluded as the cause. A neurologist is routinely involved in the predischarge evaluation, and a stroke scale is completed. Carotid duplex and CT angiography of the head and neck are obtained in the event that the patient sustains a neurologic event in the period before discharge. Medications include aspirin at 325 mg/day indefinitely and clopidogrel at 75 mg/day for 1 month. Follow-up includes 1-month, 6-month, and yearly clinical evaluation and duplex examination.

Postoperative Complications

- **Stroke.** Risk factors for stroke with CAS include age older than 80 years, symptomatic lesions, and high-risk anatomy. Stroke is more frequent with CAS than with CEA but tends to be minor and may be delayed from hours to days after the procedure.[8]
- **Hypotension.** CAS causes hypotension in many patients, but in less than 5% it can be a significant problem and requires continued hospitalization and medical treatment until resolved.
- **Hyperperfusion syndrome.** Hyperperfusion syndrome is associated with critical bilateral occlusive disease, previous stroke, hypertension, and advanced age.[24] It usually causes unilateral headache as the initial symptom and can be seen as focal edema by head CT scan. It is treated by aggressively lowering blood pressure. If untreated, it may progress to somnolence and coma as cerebral edema worsens.
- **Cardiac complications.** Myocardial infarction (MI) may occur, especially because many of the patients selected for CAS are physiologically poor candidates for CEA. In standard-risk patients in the CREST, the rate of MI was higher after CEA than after CAS.[8]
- **Access site complications.** The most common complications of any endovascular procedure relate to the access site and include hematoma, pseudoaneurysm, arteriovenous fistula, or retroperitoneal hematoma. Access site complications can be diminished by using ultrasound-guided puncture and a micropuncture set for access.
- **Restenosis.** Recurrent stenosis can occur in any stent and is less than 10% at 3 years. Longer-term data from the Stenting and Angioplasty with Protection in Patients at High-Risk for Endarterectomy trial show that recurrent stenosis was similar between CAS and CEA.[11]

REFERENCES

1. Mathias K: A new catheter system for percutaneous transluminal angioplasty of carotid artery stenosis, *Fortschr Med* 95:1007-1011, 1997.
2. Kastrup A, Groschel K, Krapf H, et al: Early outcome of carotid angioplasty and stenting with and without cerebral protection devices: A systematic review of the literature, *Stroke* 34:813-819, 2003.
3. Naylor AR, Bolia A, Abbott RJ, et al: Randomized study of carotid angioplasty and stenting versus carotid endarterectomy: A stopped trial, *J Vasc Surg* 28:326-334, 1998.
4. CAVATAS Investigators: Endovascular versus surgical treatment in patients with carotid stenosis in the Carotid and Vertebral Artery Transluminal Angioplasty Study (CAVATAS): A randomised trial, *Lancet* 357:1729-1737, 2001.
5. The SPACE Collaborative Group: 30-day results from the SPACE trial of stent-protected angioplasty versus carotid endarterectomy in symptomatic patients: A randomized inferiority trial, *Lancet* 368:1239-1247, 2006.
6. Mas J-L, Chatellier G, Beyssen B, et al: Endarterectomy versus stenting in patients with symptomatic severe carotid stenosis, *N Engl J Med* 355:1660-1671, 2006.
7. Yadav JS, Wholey MH, Kuntz RE, et al: Protected carotid-artery stenting versus endarterectomy in high-risk patients, *N Engl J Med* 351:1493-1501, 2004.
8. Brott TG, Hobson RW 2nd, Howard G, et al: Stenting versus endarterectomy for treatment of carotid-artery stenosis, *N Engl J Med* 363:11-23, 2010.
9. Hobson RW 2nd, Howard VJ, Roubin GS, et al: Carotid artery stenting is associated with increased complications in octogenarians: 30-day stroke and death rates in the CREST lead-in phase, *J Vasc Surg* 40:1106-1111, 2004.
10. Faggioli GL, Ferri M, Freyrie A, et al: Aortic arch anomalies are associated with increased risk of neurological events in carotid stent procedures, *Eur J Vasc Endovasc Surg* 33:436-441, 2007.
11. Gurm HS, Yadav JS, Fayad P, et al: Long-term results of carotid stenting versus endarterectomy in high-risk patients, *N Engl J Med* 358:1572-1579, 2008.
12. Bohannon WT, Schneider PA, Silva MB: Aortic arch classification into segments facilitates carotid stenting. In Schneider PA, Bohannon WT, Silva MB, editors: *Carotid interventions*, New York, 2004, Marcel Dekker, pp 15-22.
13. Biasi GM, Froio A, Dietrich EB, et al: Carotid plaque echolucency increases the risk of stroke in carotid stenting: The Imaging in Carotid Angioplasty and Risk of Stroke (ICAROS) study, *Circulation* 110:756-762, 2004.
14. Schneider PA: Carotid artery disease: Fibromuscular dysplasia. In Cronenwett JL, Johnston KW, editors: *Rutherford's vascular surgery*, Philadelphia, 2010, Saunders, pp 1487-1496.
15. Hart JP, Peeters P, Verbist J, et al: Do device characteristics impact outcome in carotid artery stenting? *J Vasc Surg* 44:725-730, 2006.
16. Kasirajan K, Schneider PA, Kent KC: Emboli protection filters during carotid angioplasty and stenting, *J Endovasc Ther* 10:1039-1045, 2003.
17. Coppi G, Moratto R, Silingardi R, et al: PRIAMUS—proximal flow blockage cerebral protection during carotid stenting: Results from a multicenter Italian registry, *J Cardiovasc Surg* 46:219-227, 2005.
18. Gray WA, Hopkins LN, Yadav S, et al: Protected carotid stenting in high-surgical-risk patients: The ARCHeR results, *J Vasc Surg* 44:258-268, 2006.
19. Garami ZF, Bismuth J, Charlton-Ouw KM, et al: Feasibility of simultaneous pre- and postfilter transcranial Doppler monitoring during carotid artery stenting, *J Vasc Surg* 49:340-344, 2006.
20. Tavares A, Caldas JG, Castro CC, et al: Changes in perfusion-weighted magnetic resonance imaging after carotid angioplasty with stent, *Interv Neuroradiol* 16:161-169, 2010.
21. Bonati LH, Jongen LM, Haller S, et al: New ischaemic brain lesions on MRI after stenting or endarterectomy for symptomatic carotid stenosis: A substudy of the International Carotid Stenting Study (ICSS), *Lancet Neurol* 9:353-362, 2010.
22. Flores A, Doblas M, Criado E: Transcervical carotid artery stenting with flow reversal eliminates emboli during stenting: Why does it work and what are the advantages with this approach, *J Cardiovasc Surg (Torino)* 50:745-749, 2009.
23. Bussière M, Lownie SP, Lee D, et al: Hemodynamic instability during carotid artery stenting: The relative contribution of stent deployment versus balloon dilation, *J Neurosurg* 110:905-912, 2009.
24. Moulakakis KG, Mylonas SN, Sfyroeras GS, Andrikopoulos V: Hyperperfusion syndrome after carotid revascularization, *J Vasc Surg* 49:1060-1068, 2009.

9 Carotid Body Tumor

ALI KHOOBEHI • JAMES L. NETTERVILLE • THOMAS C. NASLUND

Historical Background

Reigner[1] performed the first carotid body tumor (CBT) resection in 1880, though the patient did not survive. In 1889 Albert[2] became the first to excise a CBT without cranial nerve or carotid artery injury, and Scudder[3] was the first to do so in the United States in 1903. Though the days when "many of the contributions to the literature…are based upon a solitary case" have passed,[4,5] these tumors are still quite rare and most vascular surgeons encounter few in their career. Earlier diagnosis, improvements in technology and technique, and advances in intraoperative management contribute to low perioperative mortality. Despite this, morbidity because of cranial nerve dysfunction remains a concern.[6,7]

Preoperative Preparation

- Duplex ultrasound scans show a highly vascular mass that widens the carotid bifurcation. Concomitant carotid occlusive disease may be identified in patients at risk of atherosclerosis.
- Fine needle aspiration or open biopsy of a suspected CBT are contraindicated because of the risks of hemorrhage or injury to the carotid artery.
- Computed tomography (CT) and magnetic resonance imaging (MRI) scanning can be used to identify a CBT and estimate its size and extent. Proximity to other vital neck structures can be ascertained. CT scanning is particularly valuable in demonstrating the presence or absence of a plane between the internal carotid artery (ICA) and the tumor. CT may assist in the preoperative assessment as to whether the tumor can be removed without disruption of the ICA. Both CT and MRI scanning are useful in determining bilaterality, which occurs in approximately 5% of patients.
- Angiography demonstrates the tumor's blood supply and its relationship to neighboring vascular structures. CT angiography may be preferred over conventional angiography because of the lack of embolic risk. However, angiography has been used in conjunction with peroperative embolization of large tumors and balloon occlusion testing to determine whether the ICA can be ligated during resection, if required and reconstruction is not possible.
- Prophylactic antibiotics should be administered. Invasive arterial blood pressure monitoring and intraoperative cerebral monitoring are recommended.

Pitfalls and Danger Points

- Cranial nerve injury is the most common complication and occurs most often with larger tumors.[8]
- Stroke
- Hematoma
- Horner syndrome
- First bite syndrome
- Baroreflex failure

Operative Strategy

CLASSIFICATION AND SURGICAL ANATOMY OF CAROTID BODY TUMORS

The normal carotid body lies in the posterior medial adventitia of the carotid artery bifurcation. The blood supply is derived from the external carotid artery (ECA). CBTs vary from reddish brown to pink with a soft, rubbery consistency and have a thin fibrous capsule. They can grow quite large and can envelop local structures or extend to the skull base.

In 1971 Shamblin and associates[9] developed a classification system for CBTs that is still used today (Table 9-1). It is possible to classify the tumor based on preoperative imaging, but the surgeon must always be prepared to shunt or reconstruct the carotid artery. Patients should be prepared for the potential need for vein graft harvest, as well as replacement of the carotid artery at the time of tumor resection.

AVOIDING CRANIAL NERVE INJURIES

Particularly with Shamblin's Group II/III tumors, cranial nerve injury may be unavoidable and sacrifice of a cranial nerve may be required to facilitate a complete resection. However, steps should be taken to minimize injury by carefully identifying adjacent cranial nerves. To do so, comprehensive understanding of the regional anatomy is essential.

The hypoglossal nerve (cranial nerve XII) exits the skull base via the hypoglossal canal and courses caudally between the internal jugular vein and the ICA. It passes medially over the ICA and ECA and posterior to the digastric muscle. There may be significant variability in the course of the hypoglossal nerve. Although typically found crossing the ICA and ECA about 2 to 4 cm cephalad to the carotid bifurcation, it can be found as caudal as the bifurcation or sometimes adherent to the posterior surface of the common facial vein.[10] During CBT resection, the hypoglossal nerve is frequently encountered in the fascia overlying the superior aspect of the tumor.

The vagus nerve (cranial nerve X) normally lies in a posterolateral position relative to the ICA, though occasionally it may be found in an anteromedial position, putting it at greater risk for injury. During CBT resection, the vagus nerve may be identified at its junction with the hypoglossal nerve and then followed caudally. As the vagus nerve courses inferiorly, it must be carefully dissected away from its intimate association with the tumor and the carotid artery. The superior laryngeal nerve can be found in the fascia posterior to the tumor. It courses posterior to the internal carotid artery with the external branch lying posterior to the superior thyroid artery. Injury to the external branch may cause impaired phonation and easy voice fatiguability. The recurrent laryngeal nerve courses in the tracheoesophageal groove and is typically well removed from the surgical field. Vocal cord dysfunction may result from vagal trunk injury.

The marginal mandibular branch of the facial nerve (cranial nerve VII) courses along the masseter muscle parallel to the mandibular ramus. It is at risk with retraction deep to the mandible and with an incision that does not course posterior toward the mastoid process.

The spinal accessory nerve (cranial nerve XI) and glossopharyngeal nerve (cranial nerve IX) are at risk during a resection that extends near the skull base. The spinal accessory nerve lies anterior to the most distal portion of the ICA and posterior to

TABLE 9-1 Shamblin's Classification System for Carotid Body Tumor

Group I	Tumors are small and may be easily dissected from adjacent vascular structures.
Group II	The tumor partially surrounds adjacent vessels and is more adherent to the adventitia.
Group III	The tumor is densely adherent to and circumferentially surrounds adjacent vascular structures.

Modified from Shamblin WR, ReMine WH, Sheps SG, Harrison EG Jr: Carotid body tumor (chemodectoma): clinicopathologic analysis of ninety cases. *Am J Surg* 122:732-739, 1971.

the stylohyoid muscle. It should be identified as it enters the sternocleidomastoid muscle. The glossopharyngeal nerve crosses anterior to the internal jugular vein and ICA near the skull base.

The deep fascia of the tumor may be intimately associated with the sympathetic trunk. Sacrifice of this structure during resection may lead to Horner syndrome.

AVOIDING INTRAOPERATIVE STROKE

A "no touch" technique should be used in handling the carotid bifurcation, particularly when atherosclerosis is present. With large tumors, this may not be possible. Heparin is used if carotid replacement is required.

PREOPERATIVE EMBOLIZATION

Preoperative embolization may reduce intraoperative blood loss,[11] but improvement in clinical outcome has not been demonstrated.[12] With the possible exception of tumors exceeding 4 to 5 cm in size preoperative embolization is not performed because the risk of embolism outweighs the benefit of reduced intraoperative blood loss.

BIPOLAR ELECTROCAUTERY

The use of bipolar electrocautery minimizes risk of injury to adjacent cranial nerves and is of particular value while separating the tumor from cranial nerves. Combined with a meticulous dissection, bipolar electrocautery can reduce intraoperative blood loss.

Operative Technique

INCISION

A rolled sheet should be placed underneath the shoulder to facilitate neck extension. The head should be turned away from the surgical site and placed in a foam ring. The neck, mandible, ear, and upper chest should be prepped. The face anterior to the ear and the entire occipitotemporal region posterior to the ear should be prepped, as well, for the possibility of requiring higher exposure.

A transverse cervical incision is made along a neck crease. As the sternocleidomastoid muscle is approached, the incision is curved cranially toward the earlobe. If higher exposure is necessary, the incision can be extended in a curvilinear fashion posterior to the ear. For younger patients with CBT, we use a "hairline" incision that passes in a craniocaudal direction along the posterior neck (Fig. 9-1). Alternatively, an incision can be made overlying the sternocleidomastoid muscle, extending from just cranial to the clavicular head toward the earlobe as typically performed for a carotid artery exposure.

EXPOSURE OF THE CAROTID BIFURCATION

The subcutaneous tissue and platysma are sharply divided. Platysma muscle flaps are developed and reflected to expose the underlying tissues.

The sternocleidomastoid muscle is identified and reflected laterally. Because of a 5% risk of metastatic disease, a limited dissection of the level IIA lymph nodes (LNs), which typically overlie the CBT, should be performed. The LN dissection extends from posterior to the submandibular gland to the posterior border of the internal jugular vein. Once the LN mass has been freed, outward tension allows for careful dissection off of the CBT. Any abnormally enlarged LNs are also sampled.

The vagus nerve should be identified to avoid injury (Fig. 9-2). The digastric muscle should be identified separately and often must be divided for a larger CBT. Care should be taken to identify and avoid injury to the glossopharyngeal and spinal accessory nerves.

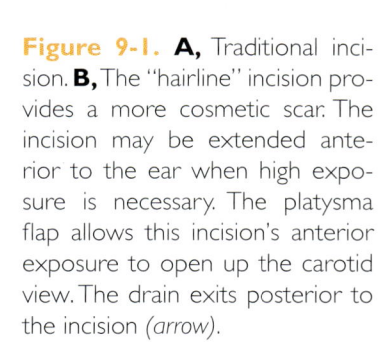

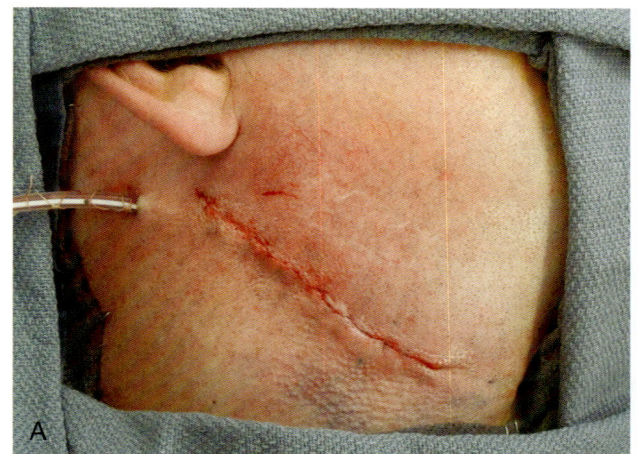

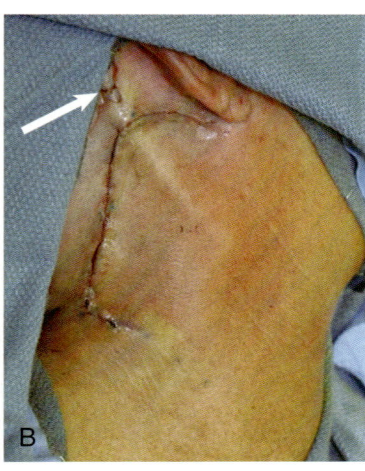

Figure 9-1. A, Traditional incision. **B,** The "hairline" incision provides a more cosmetic scar. The incision may be extended anterior to the ear when high exposure is necessary. The platysma flap allows this incision's anterior exposure to open up the carotid view. The drain exits posterior to the incision *(arrow)*.

Figure 9-2. The vagus nerve (cranial nerve X) *(arrow)* is typically found posterolateral to the internal carotid artery (ICA). It should be identified and carefully dissected away to avoid injury. The left portion of the image indicates the superior extent of the surgical field. The *dashed line* indicates carotid body tumor. The ICA is lifted anteriorly, exposing the vagus posteriorly.

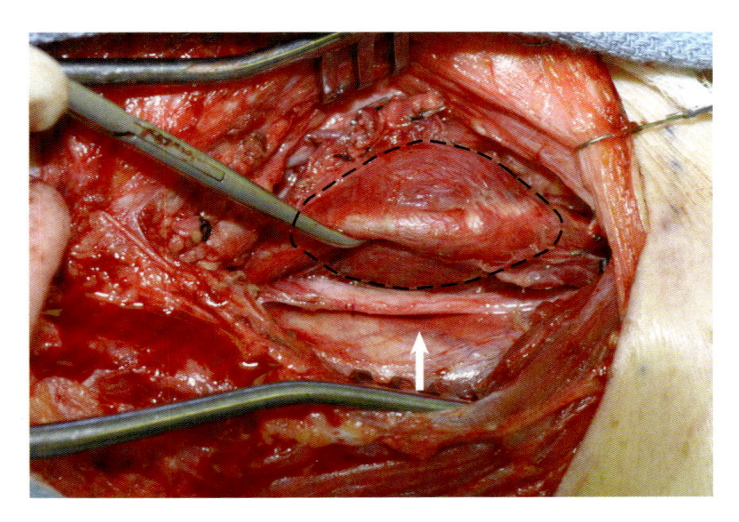

The common carotid artery, ICA, and ECA should be mobilized. The proximal branches of the ECA, particularly the ascending pharyngeal artery, may be identified as they pass deep to the CBT. Branches that appear to feed the CBT may be ligated.

Resection of the Shamblin Type I Carotid Body Tumor

The hypoglossal nerve and ansa cervicalis frequently lie on the anterior surface of the CBT. The ansa cervicalis can be divided if necessary.

The arterial dissection is initiated through the periadventitial plane through the "white line" described by Gordon-Taylor.[4] This white line can be most clearly visualized by grasping and providing countertension between the CBT and the ICA and ECA. Dissection of the CBT in a caudocranial direction is often described,[1,13] but we typically proceed with the dissection circumferentially (Fig. 9-3). When the countertension is appropriate, the strands of the white line reveal themselves and can be easily divided using bipolar electrocautery. Vessels feeding the tumor may be encountered and should be divided. There is often a small vessel at the most caudal aspect of the tumor adjacent to the carotid artery bifurcation. A single U stitch at the bifurcation may be needed to control this vessel.

Once circumferential dissection of the CBT is complete only the deep attachments remain. These should be carefully divided under tension. Care should be taken to avoid injury to the superior laryngeal nerve, which often lies on the posterior surface of the tumor with the external branch lying posterior to the superior thyroid artery (Fig. 9-4).

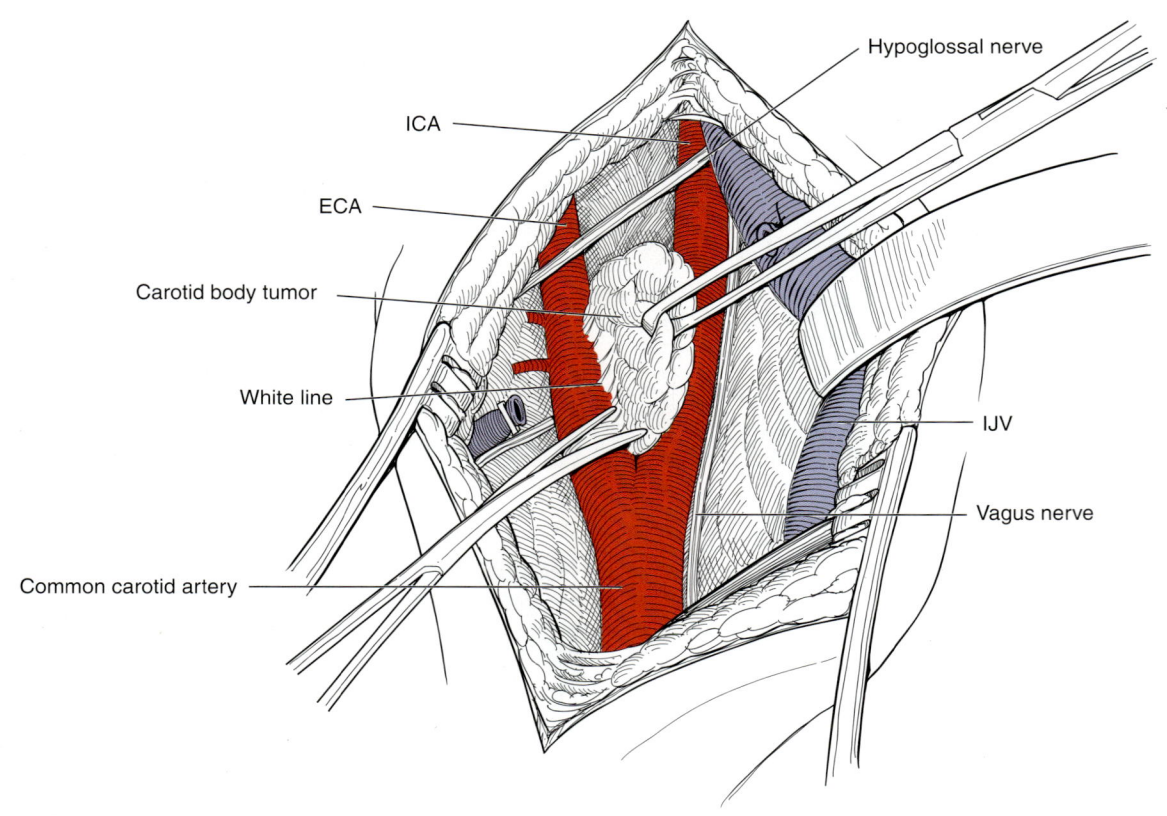

Figure 9-3. Countertension between the carotid body tumor (CBT) and the carotid bifurcation reveal the periadventitial white line, shown here as the tumor is dissected initially off the external carotid artery (*ECA*). The common facial vein is divided and ligated, and the internal jugular vein (*IJV*) has been retracted both posteriorly and laterally. The dissection proceeds circumferentially, cauterizing or ligating the vessels feeding the CBT as necessary. *ICA,* Internal carotid artery.

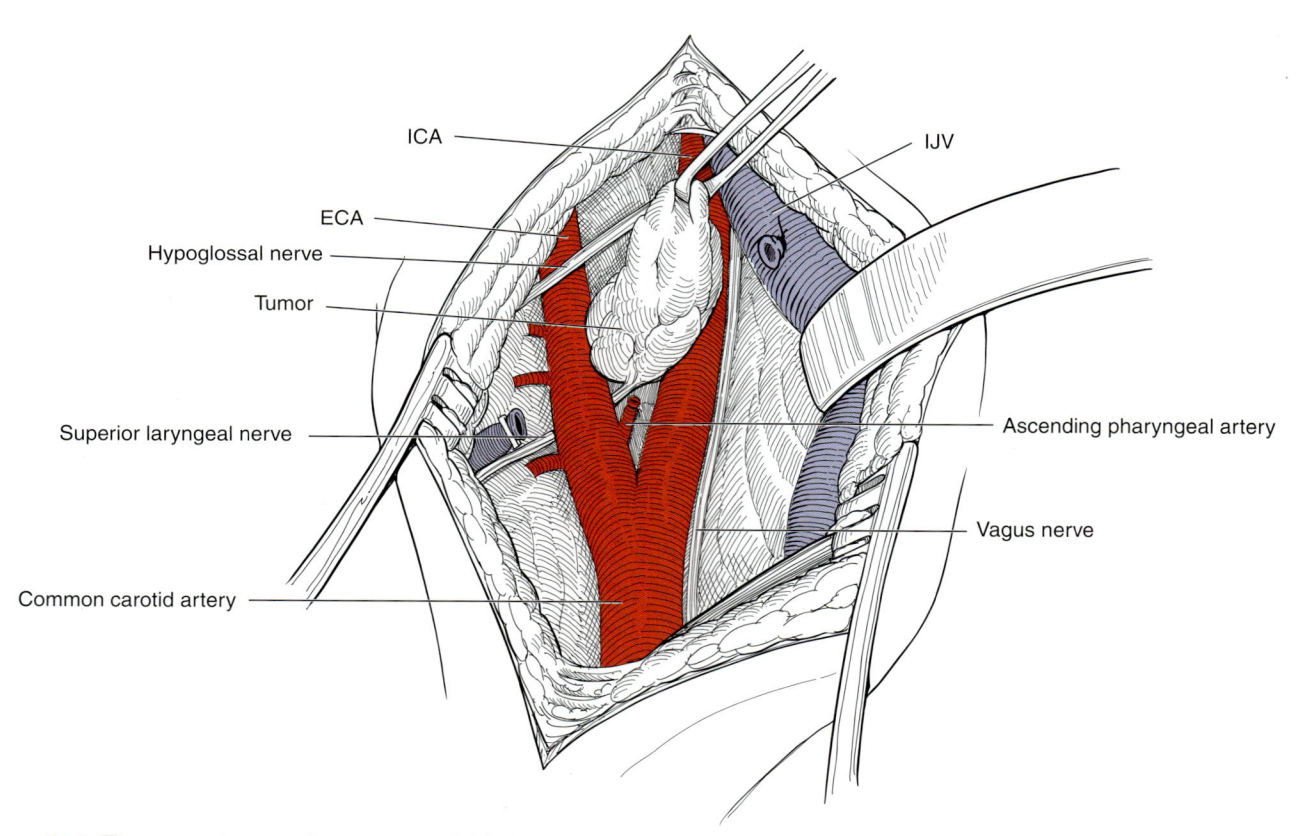

Figure 9-4. The posterior attachments are divided, and particular care is taken to avoid injury to the superior laryngeal nerve, which frequently lies just posterior to the carotid body tumor. The ascending pharyngeal artery may be encountered and can be divided. *ECA,* External carotid artery; *ICA,* internal carotid artery; *IJV,* internal jugular vein.

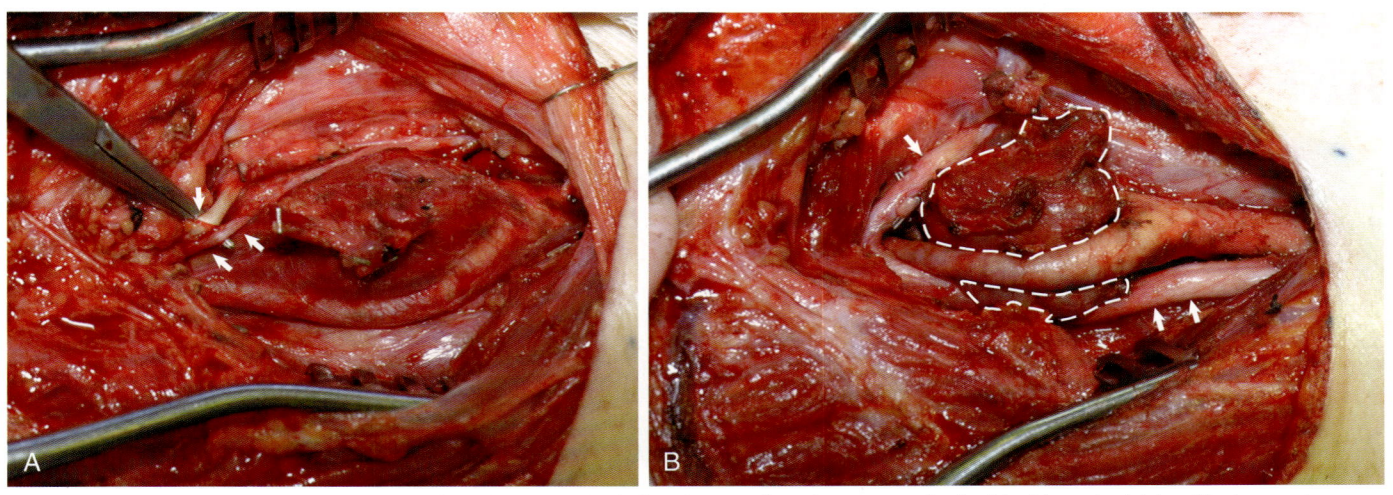

Figure 9-5. A, The hypoglossal nerve (cranial nerve XII) *(single arrow)* and ansa cervicalis *(double arrow)* identified anterior to a carotid body tumor (CBT). The left portion of the image indicates the superior extent of the surgical field. **B,** This CBT has been dissected completely free *(dashed line)* and left *in situ* to demonstrate its anatomic relationship to the surrounding tissue. The hypoglossal nerve *(single arrow)* and vagus nerve *(double arrow)* have been dissected away from the tumor.

Resection of the Shamblin Type II/III Carotid Body Tumor

As with resection of a Shamblin type I tumor, dissection is begun in the periadventitial plane and proceeds circumferentially when dealing with resection of a Shamblin type II/III tumor.

As the tumor is mobilized and can be retracted with greater ease, feeder vessels are exposed and should be divided. With large tumors, early ligation and division of the ECA may aid resection. The devascularized ECA can then be clamped to serve as a "handle" to facilitate retraction of the CBT.[1]

Resection should be limited to the periadventitial tissue and not extend through the media of the ICA. A compromised arterial wall puts the patient at risk for a postoperative carotid rupture. When the arterial wall is involved, or with a Shamblin type III tumor that envelops the ICA, dissection of the tumor should be continued, but its attachments to the ICA are preserved in anticipation of a carotid vein graft interposition.

The sacrifice of cranial nerves is often unavoidable with larger Shamblin type II/III tumors, though unnecessary cranial nerve injury should be avoided. The hypoglossal nerve is frequently on the anterior surface of the CBT and at particular risk (Fig. 9-5).

When the tumor has been mobilized save the ICA, attention is turned to performing a carotid vein interposition graft. Size mismatch should be taken into account but is generally well accommodated by either a saphenous vein or a superficial femoral vein. The saphenous vein is the preferred conduit as long as it is judged to be of acceptable quality.

The vein graft is harvested in the standard fashion, a straight carotid shunt may be placed through the graft, and systemic heparin is administered in preparation of carotid clamping. A clamp is placed on the common carotid artery caudal to the site chosen for resection, and the distal ICA is occluded with a bulldog clamp. The vessels are transected, and the specimen is submitted with the proper orientation clearly indicated for pathologic analysis.

The vein graft, with the indwelling shunt, is introduced into the open ICA. The bulldog clamp is replaced with a Rummel tourniquet, and as backbleeding is allowed through the shunt, the proximal end is introduced into the common carotid artery. The proximal clamp is then removed, and a Rummel tourniquet is used for control.

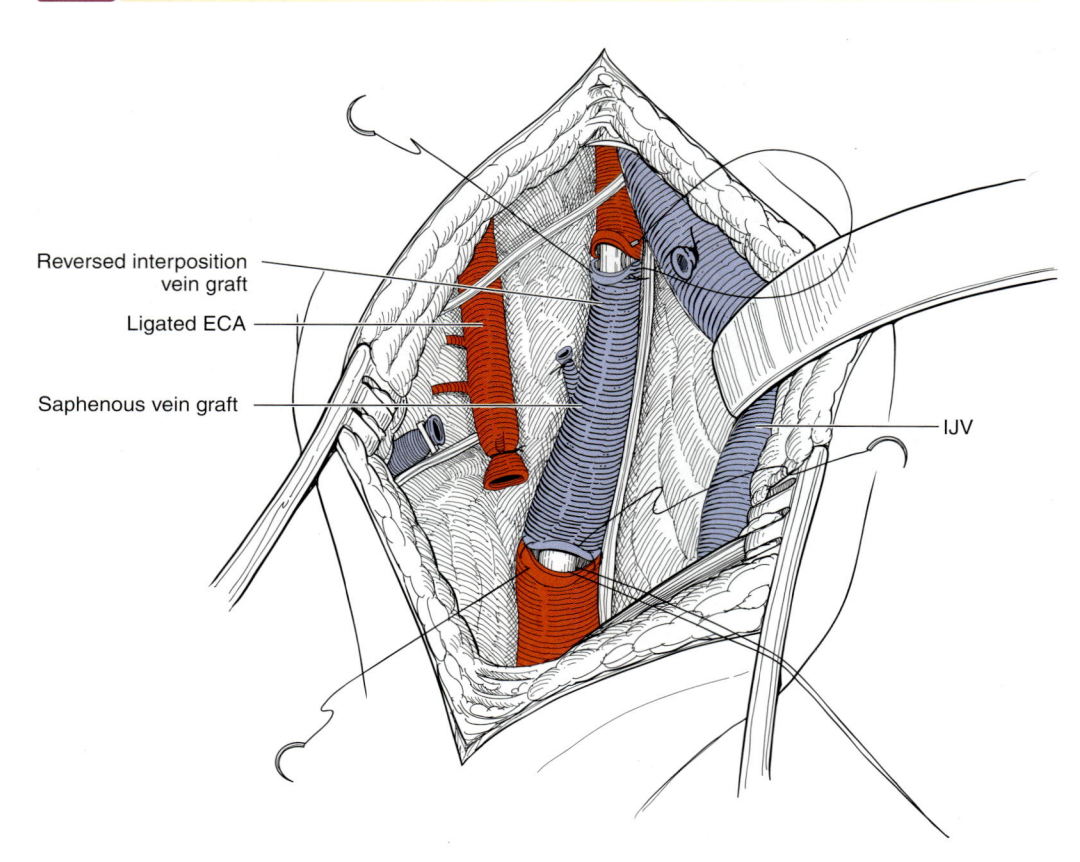

Figure 9-6. The reversed interposition vein graft is first flushed via the proximal anastomosis. The shunt is removed and the final flushing is performed before completion of the distal anastomosis. The presence of vein valves mandates that the distal anastomosis be vented last. *ECA*, External carotid artery; *IJV*, internal jugular vein.

The ICA and the adjacent end of the vein graft are both spatulated. Anastomoses are performed end to end, with the last several sutures in the anterolateral portion omitted to allow for later flushing.

The vein graft is cut to length and spatulated to allow for the proximal end-to-end anastomosis to the common carotid artery. The vein graft should be shortened and stretched to the point of some tension in order to avoid having a redundant graft upon release of the clamps.

The proximal anastomosis is subtotally completed to allow for shunt removal. The shunt is removed and the ICA and common carotid artery are again clamped. The proximal anastomosis is completed and the vein graft is flushed. The ICA is vented via the incomplete distal anastomosis, which is then completed (Fig. 9-6). Because the saphenous vein graft is reversed, the final flushing is performed through the distal anastomosis to accommodate for the presence of valves. With more extensive tumor resections, placement of a closed suction drain may be considered.

The platysma is closed with a running absorbable suture and the skin closed with a running subcuticular layer.

Postoperative Care

- The patient should be observed overnight for development of a hematoma at the surgical site. Depending on the size of the tumor resection, the patient may be hospitalized for as little as 1 day or as many as 3 days.
- The patient may resume a regular diet and is encouraged to ambulate on the first postoperative day.
- Blood pressure is typically monitored via an arterial line for several hours in the recovery room. Systemic hypertension may require management in an intensive care unit (ICU) setting.

- If the patient has had a previous CBT resection on the contralateral side, monitoring in the ICU is necessary because of the risk of baroreflex failure.

Postoperative Complications

- **Nerve injury.** When cranial nerve injury has occurred, the patient should be evaluated by otolaryngology and a swallowing study. If unable to swallow safely, placement of a gastrostomy tube may be necessary. Cranial nerve recovery is expected over time, especially if the primary insult is a traction- or stretch-related injury.
- **Stroke.** Neurologic deficits may indicate a technical problem with the interposition graft. Urgent duplex imaging or operative reexploration should be undertaken in an effort to avoid permanent neurologic sequelae.
- **Hematoma.** Any sizable hematoma requires reexploration in the operating room.
- **Horner syndrome.** Operative injury to the carotid sympathetic chain can result in an ipsilateral Horner syndrome. If portions of the sympathetic chain remain intact, symptoms may improve over time.
- **First bite syndrome.** The first bite entity is characterized by severe cramping in the parotid region after the first bite of a meal and can be particularly severe in the early postoperative period. The pain typically improves with subsequent bites. A likely mechanism is damage to the cervical sympathetics that innervate the parotid gland.[14] A diet of "bland" food may reduce symptoms. Refractory symptoms may warrant botulinum toxin injections into the parotid gland.
- **Baroreflex failure.** The carotid sinus consists of baroreceptor tissue innervated via the nerve of Hering, which is a branch of the glossopharyngeal nerve. Bilateral CBT resection may disrupt the negative feedback mechanism of the carotid baroreceptor tissue, resulting in baroreflex failure. This entity can result in a life-threatening hypertensive crisis.[15] Patients should be monitored in an ICU setting for 24 to 48 hours after bilateral CBT resection. Hypertensive episodes should be managed aggressively. In some patients continued blood pressure lability can be a significant detriment to the quality of life. Clonidine may reduce the "peaks" of the hypertensive episodes and with less of an effect during periods of normotension.[16]

REFERENCES

1. Krupski WC: Uncommon disorders affecting the carotid arteries. In Rutherford RB, editor: *Rutherford's textbook of vascular surgery*, ed 5, Philadelphia, 2000, Saunders, pp 2066-2073.
2. Albert cited by Staats EF, Brown RL, Smith RR: Carotid body tumors, benign and malignant, *Laryngoscope* 76:907, 1966.
3. Scudder CL: Tumor of the intercarotid body: A report of one case, together with all cases in literature, *Am J Med Sci* 126:1384, 1903.
4. Gordon-Taylor G: On carotid tumours, *Br J Surg* 28:163-172, 1940.
5. Peterson EW, Meeker LH: Tumors of the carotid body, *Ann Surg* 103:554-571, 1936.
6. Netterville JL, Reilly KM, Robertson D, et al: Carotid body tumors: A review of 30 patients with 46 tumors, *Laryngoscope* 105:115-126, 1995.
7. Westerband A, Hunter GC, Cintora I, et al: Current trends in the detection and management of carotid body tumors, *J Vasc Surg* 28:84-92, 1998.
8. Smith JJ, Passman MA, Dattilo JB, et al: Carotid body tumor resection: Does the need for vascular reconstruction worsen outcome? *Ann Vasc Surg* 20:435-439, 2006.
9. Shamblin WR, ReMine WH, Sheps SG, et al: Carotid body tumor (chemodectoma): Clinicopathologic analysis of ninety cases, *Am J Surg* 122:732-739, 1971.
10. Schauber MD, Fontanelle LJ, Solomon JW, et al: Cranial/cervical nerve dysfunction after carotid endarterectomy, *J Vasc Surg* 25:481-487, 1997.
11. Kafie FE, Freischlag JA: Carotid body tumors: The role of preoperative embolization, *Ann Vasc Surg* 15:237-242, 2001.

12. Litle VR, Reilly LM, Ramos TK: Preoperative embolization of carotid body tumors: When is it appropriate? *Ann Vasc Surg* 10:464-468, 1996.
13. van der Bogt KE, Vrancken Peeters MP, van Baalen JM, et al: Resection of carotid body tumors: Results of an evolving surgical technique, *Ann Surg* 247:877-884, 2008.
14. Netterville JL, Jackson CG, Miller FR, et al: Vagal paraganglioma: A review of 46 patients treated during a 20-year period, *Arch Otolaryngol Head Neck Surg* 124:1133-1140, 1998.
15. De Toma G, Nicolanti V, Plocco M, et al: Baroreflex failure syndrome after bilateral excision of carotid body tumors: An underestimated problem, *J Vasc Surg* 31:806-810, 2000.
16. Robertson D, Hollister AS, Biaggioni I, et al: The diagnosis and treatment of baroreflex failure, *N Engl J Med* 329:1449-1455, 1993.

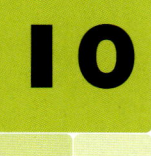

10 Surgical Treatment of the Vertebral Artery

MARK D. MORASCH

Historical Background

Reconstruction of the subclavian arteries via thromboendarterectomy was first described by Cate and Scott in 1957[1] and a year later, Crawford, DeBakey, and Fields[2] described the technique of transsubclavian endarterectomy of the vertebral artery. In 1964 Parrott[3] introduced the technique of transposition of the second portion of the subclavian artery to the common carotid artery. Transposition of the proximal vertebral artery to the common carotid artery was described by Clark and Perry in 1966 through a similar approach.[4]

During the 1970s the saphenous vein was used to bypass vertebral artery origin stenoses.[5] Eventually it was recognized that transposition techniques[6] were superior solutions for proximal subclavian and vertebral disease. These have supplanted endarterectomy and bypass as the reconstruction options of choice. The approach to the distal vertebral artery was first described by Matas[7] and later by Henry[8] and was used for the treatment of traumatic injury. During the late 1970s, venous bypass and skull base transposition procedures to revascularize the distal vertebral artery were developed using a similar approach.[9,10]

Indications

The most common disease affecting the vertebral artery is atherosclerosis. Less common pathologic processes include trauma, fibromuscular dysplasia, Takayasu disease, osteophyte compression, dissections, aneurysms and other arteritides.

Disease involving the vertebrobasilar arteries can lead to symptoms of posterior circulation ischemia. Approximately 25% of all ischemic strokes occur in the vertebrobasilar territory. One half of patients present initially with stroke, and 26% of patients present with transient ischemic symptoms rapidly followed by stroke.[11] For patients who experience vertebrobasilar transient ischemic attacks, disease in the vertebral arteries portends a 22% to 35% risk of stroke over 5 years.[12-14] The mortality associated with a posterior circulation stroke is 20% to 30%, which is higher than that for an anterior circulation event.[15-17]

Ischemia affecting the temporooccipital areas of the cerebral hemispheres or segments of the brainstem and cerebellum characteristically produces bilateral symptoms. The classic symptoms of vertebrobasilar ischemia include dizziness, vertigo, drop attacks, diplopia, perioral numbness, alternating paresthesia, tinnitus, dysphasia, dysarthria and ataxia. Box 10-1 gives a complete list of symptoms. When patients present with two or more of these symptoms, the likelihood of vertebrobasilar ischemia is high.

In general, the ischemic mechanisms can be broken down into those that are hemodynamic and those that are embolic. Hemodynamic symptoms occur as a result of transient "end organ" (brainstem, cerebellum, occipital lobes, or all a combination of these) hypoperfusion and can be precipitated by postural changes or

> **Box 10-1 SYMPTOMS ASSOCIATED WITH VERTEBROBASILAR ISCHEMIA**
>
> | | |
> |---|---|
> | Disequilibrium | Dysphagia |
> | Vertigo | Dysarthria |
> | Dizziness | Quadriplegia |
> | Diplopia | Drop attacks |
> | Cortical blindness | Ataxia |
> | Alternating paresthesia | Perioral numbness |
> | Tinnitus | |

transient reduction in cardiac output. Ischemia from hemodynamic mechanisms rarely results in infarction; rather, symptoms are short lived, repetitive, and more of a nuisance than a danger. For hemodynamic symptoms to occur in direct relation to the vertebrobasilar arteries, significant occlusive pathology must be present in both of the paired vertebral vessels or in the basilar artery. In addition compensatory contribution from the carotid circulation via the circle of Willis must be incomplete. Alternatively, hemodynamic ischemic symptoms may follow proximal subclavian artery occlusion and the syndrome of subclavian or vertebral artery steal. In the later years of life, vertebral artery stenosis is a common arteriographic finding and dizziness is a common complaint. The presence of both cannot necessarily be assumed to have a cause-effect relationship. Surgical reconstruction is not indicated in an asymptomatic patient with stenotic or occlusive vertebral lesions, because these patients are well compensated from the carotid circulation through the posterior communicating vessels. The minimal anatomic requirement to justify vertebral artery reconstruction for hemodynamic symptoms is (1) stenosis greater than 60% diameter in both vertebral arteries if both are patent and complete or (2) the same degree of stenosis in the dominant vertebral artery if the opposite vertebral artery is hypoplastic, ends in a posteroinferior cerebellar artery, or is occluded. A single, normal vertebral artery is sufficient to adequately perfuse the basilar artery, regardless of the patency status of the contralateral vertebral artery.

It is estimated that up to one third of vertebrobasilar ischemic episodes are caused by distal embolization from plaques or mural lesions of the subclavian, vertebral, or basilar arteries or some combination of them.[18] Arterial to arterial emboli can arise from atherosclerotic lesions, from intimal defects caused by extrinsic compression or repetitive trauma, and rarely from fibromuscular dysplasia, aneurysms, or dissections. Although fewer patients suffer from embolic phenomena than do those with hemodynamic mechanisms, actual infarctions in the vertebrobasilar distribution are most often the result of embolic events. Patients with embolic ischemia often develop multiple and multifocal infarcts in the brainstem, cerebellum, and occasionally, posterior cerebral artery territory. For patients with posterior circulation ischemia secondary to microembolism and appropriate lesions in a vertebral artery, the potential source of the embolus needs to be eliminated regardless of the status of the contralateral vertebral artery. Patients with symptomatic vertebrobasilar ischemia because of emboli are candidates for surgical correction of the offending lesion regardless of the condition of the contralateral vertebral artery. Surgical intervention is not indicated in asymptomatic patients who harbor suspicious radiographic findings.

Preoperative Preparation

- A number of medical conditions may mimic vertebrobasilar ischemia. A precise diagnosis of vertebrobasilar ischemia begins with an accurate assessment of the manifesting symptom complex. An important aspect of the history is identifying triggering events such as positional or postural changes. This must be followed by efforts to exclude other causes for patient symptoms (Box 10-2).

| Box 10-2 | NONVASCULAR AND CARDIAC CONDITIONS THAT CAUSE OR MIMIC VERTEBROBASILAR ISCHEMIA |

Cardiac arrhythmia
Pacemaker malfunction
Cardioemboli
Labyrinthine dysfunction
CPA tumors

Antihypertensives
Cerebellar degeneration
Myxedema
Electrolyte imbalance
Hypoglycemia

CPA, Cerebellopontine angle.

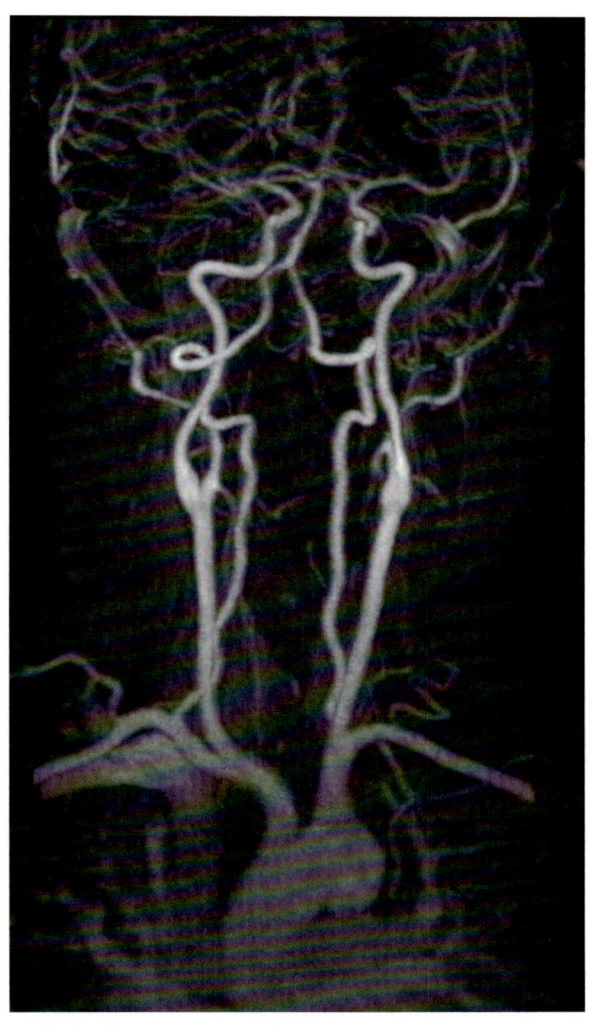

Figure 10-1. Four vessel cerebral magnetic resonance angiogram.

- Duplex ultrasound is an excellent tool for detecting lesions in the carotid artery, but it has significant limitations when used to detect vertebral artery pathology. The usefulness of duplex ultrasound lies in its ability to confirm reversal of flow within the vertebral arteries and detect flow velocity changes consistent with a proximal stenosis.[19]
- Contrast-enhanced magnetic resonance angiography with three-dimensional reconstruction and maximum image intensity techniques provide full imaging of the vessels, including the supraaortic trunks and the carotid and vertebral arteries (Fig. 10-1). Transaxial magnetic resonance images can readily diagnose both acute and chronic posterior fossa infarcts. Brainstem infarctions are often missed by computed tomography (CT) scan because they tend to be small and the resolution of the CT scan in the brainstem is poor. In patients who are candidates for vertebral artery reconstruction, magnetic resonance brain scans are

performed preoperatively to ascertain whether infarctions have taken place in the vertebrobasilar territory.
- Selective subclavian and vertebral angiography remains the gold standard for preoperative evaluation of patients with vertebrobasilar ischemia. The most common site of disease, the vertebral artery origin, may not be well imaged with ultrasound or magnetic resonance angiography and often can only be displayed with oblique projections that are not part of standard arch evaluation. Patients with suspected vertebral artery compression should undergo dynamic angiography, which incorporates provocative positioning. Lastly, delayed imaging should be performed in order to demonstrate reconstitution of the extracranial vertebral arteries through cervical collaterals, such as the occipital artery (Fig. 10-2) or via collaterals from the ipsilateral subclavian artery via branches of the thyrocervical trunk (Fig. 10-3).[20] Because of this collateral network, the distal vertebral and basilar arteries usually remain patent despite a proximal vertebral artery occlusion. A patent V3 segment can be exploited as a distal target for reconstruction.
- Preoperative aspirin is indicated.
- Evaluation of cardiac risk is recommended by clinical profiling or in select patients through use of noninvasive stress testing.
- Evaluation of vocal cord function should be performed in patients with a history of prior carotid surgery.
- Prophylactic antibiotics should be administered within an hour of surgery.
- Intraoperative arterial line monitoring of blood pressure is recommended.

Pitfalls and Danger Points

- Proximal Vertebral Reconstruction
  - Low (C7) entry to the transverse spine process
  - Horner syndrome
  - Vagus nerve injury
  - Thoracic duct or lymph leak
- Distal Vertebral Reconstruction
  - Spinal accessory nerve injury
  - Vagus nerve injury
  - Venous plexus bleeding
  - Carotid clamp injury and embolization

Operative Strategy

The location of disease dictates the type of surgical reconstruction that is required. With rare exceptions, most reconstructions of the vertebral artery are performed to relieve either an orificial stenosis (V1 segment) or a stenosis, dissection, or occlusion of its intraspinal component (V2 and V3 segments).

A number of operations have been described to treat stenosing ostial lesions in V1,[21] but transposition of the proximal vertebral artery onto the adjacent carotid artery is generally preferred. Similarly, for distal vertebral reconstruction a bypass from the common carotid artery to the vertebral artery between C1 and C2 is most easily mastered.

Surgical Anatomy of the Vertebral Artery

The surgical anatomy of the paired vertebral arteries has traditionally been divided into four segments: V1, the origin of the vertebral artery arising from the subclavian artery to the point at which it enters the C6 transverse process; V2, the segment

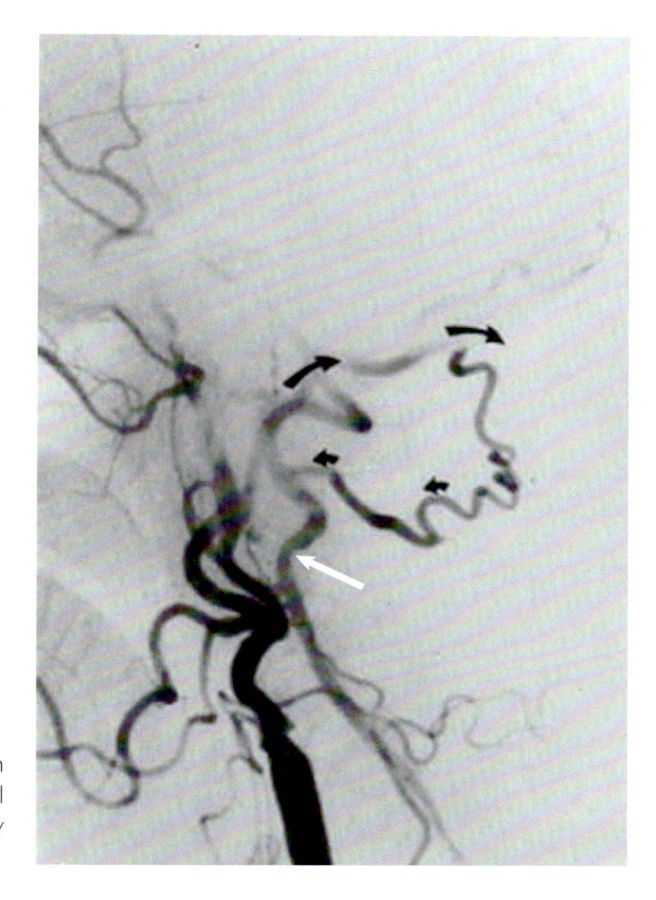

Figure 10-2. The distal vertebral artery being fed *(black arrows)* by an occipital collateral from the external carotid artery in a patient with distal vertebral artery occlusion. Retrograde filling of the distal vertebral artery is demonstrated *(white arrow)*.

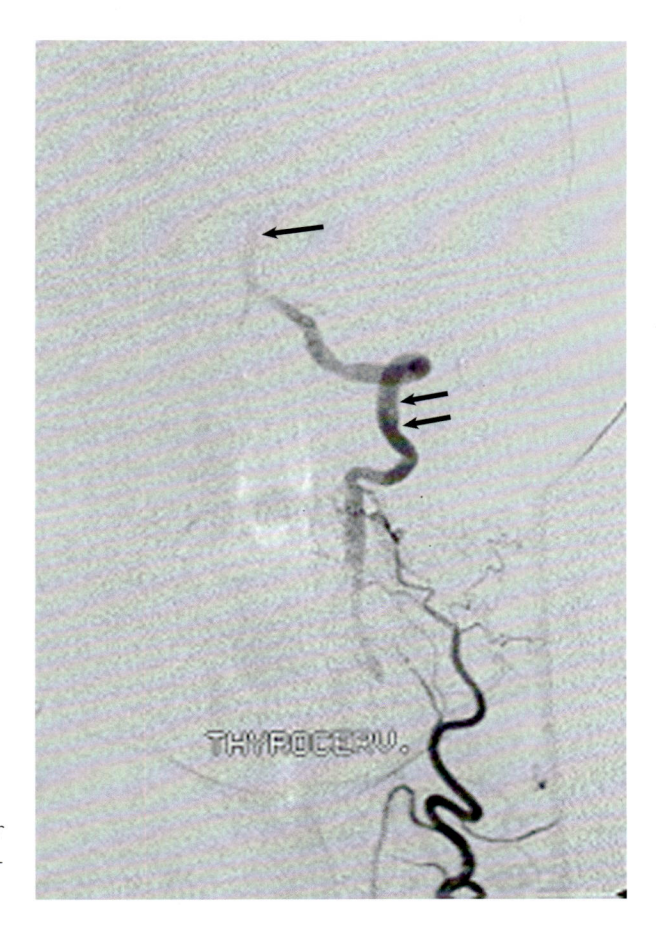

Figure 10-3. The distal vertebral artery *(double arrow)* and basilar artery *(single arrow)* fed by thyrocervical collateral in a patient with proximal vertebral artery occlusion.

116 EXTRACRANIAL CEREBROVASCULAR DISEASE

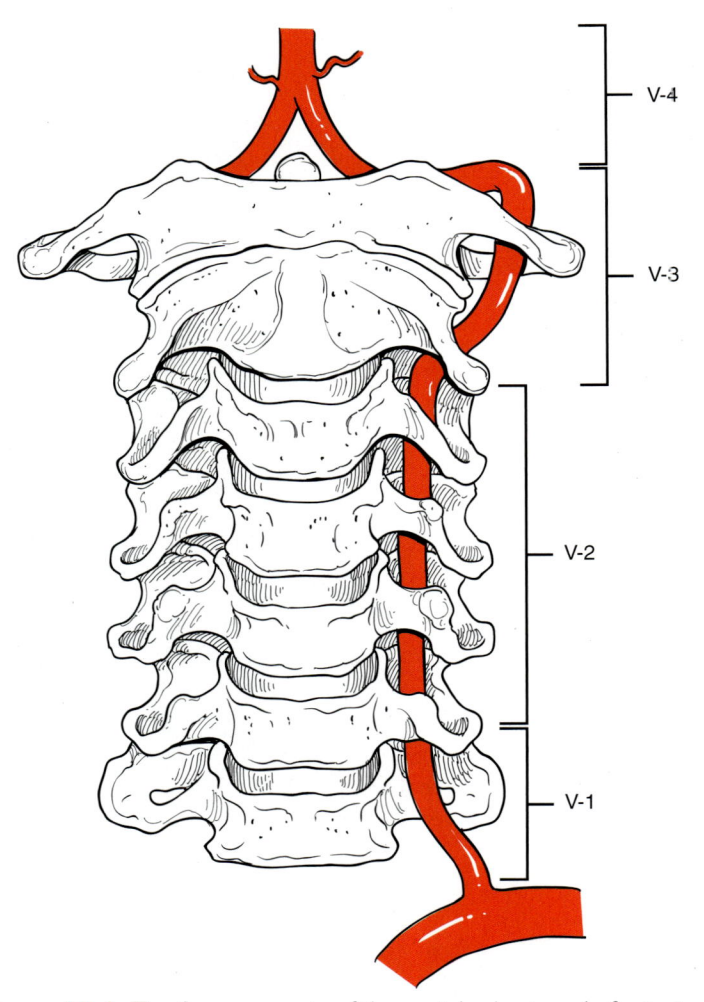

Figure 10-4. The four segments of the vertebral artery (refer to text).

of the artery buried deep within intertransversarium muscle and the cervical transverse processes of C6 to C2; V3, the extracranial segment between the transverse process of C2 and the base of the skull before it enters the foramen magnum; and V4, the intracranial portion beginning at the atlantooccipital membrane and terminating as the two vertebrals converge to form the basilar artery (Fig. 10-4).

Operative Techniques

EXPOSURE AND TRANSPOSITION OF THE VERTEBRAL ARTERY INTO THE COMMON CAROTID ARTERY

The approach to the proximal vertebral artery is similar to that used for subclavian-to-carotid transposition. The patient is positioned in a slight chair position with the table flexed and the back tilted upward approximately 30 degrees to decrease venous pressure. The incision is placed transversely about a finger's breadth above the clavicle and directly over the two heads of the sternocleidomastoid muscle. Subplatysmal skin flaps are created to provide for adequate exposure. Dissection is carried down directly between the two bellies of the sternocleidomastoid muscle, and the omohyoid muscle is divided. The jugular vein is retracted laterally, and the carotid sheath is entered. The vagus nerve is retracted medially with the common carotid artery (Fig. 10-5). The carotid should be exposed proximally as far as possible, which is facilitated if the surgeon temporarily stands at the head of the patient with a view into the mediastinum. The remainder of the dissection is carried out between the jugular vein, the subclavian vein, and the carotid artery at the base of the neck.

SURGICAL TREATMENT OF THE VERTEBRAL ARTERY

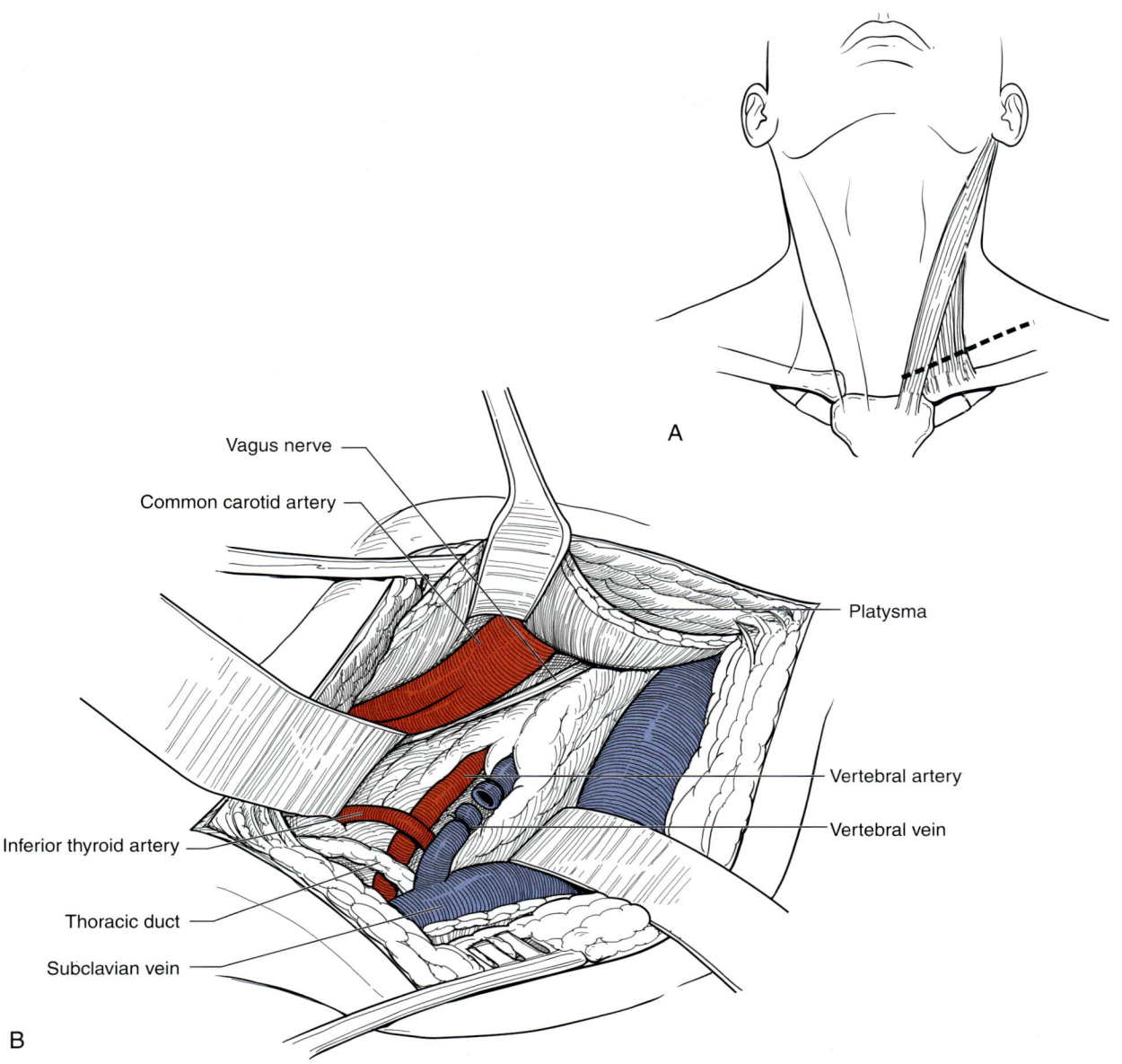

Figure 10-5. **A,** Access to the proximal vertebral artery is achieved with a supraclavicular incision between the sternocleidomastoid muscle bellies. **B,** Exposure is facilitated by retracting the common carotid artery anteriorly and the subclavian vein inferiorly and by dividing the vertebral vein that overlies the vertebral artery.

On the left side, the thoracic duct is encircled with a right-angled clamp and then divided between ligatures, avoiding transfixion sutures that may lead to a lymph leak. The proximal end of the thoracic duct is doubly ligated. Accessory lymph ducts—often seen on the right side of the neck—are identified, ligated, and divided. The entire dissection is confined medial to the prescalene fat pad that covers the anterior scalene muscle and phrenic nerve. These structures are left unexposed lateral to the field. The inferior thyroid artery runs transversely across the field, which is ligated and divided.

The vertebral vein is identified as it emerges from the angle formed by the longus colli and the anterior scalene muscles. The vein invariably overlies the proximal vertebral artery and, at the lower end of the field, the subclavian artery. It is ligated in continuity and divided, providing exposure to the vertebral and subclavian arteries. It is important to identify and avoid injury to the adjacent sympathetic chain. The vertebral artery is dissected superiorly to the tendon of the longus colli and inferiorly to its origin from the subclavian artery. The vertebral artery is freed from the sympathetic trunk, which lies behind it, without damaging the trunk or the stellate ganglion.

Once the artery is fully exposed, an appropriate site for reimplantation in the common carotid artery is selected. Systemic heparin is administered and the distal portion of the V1 segment of the vertebral artery is clamped below the edge of the longus colli with a microclip placed vertically to indicate the orientation of the artery and to avoid axial twisting during its transposition. The proximal vertebral artery is closed with a transfixion of 5-0 polypropylene immediately above the stenosis at its origin. The artery is divided at this level and its proximal stump is further secured with a hemoclip. The artery is then transposed to the common carotid artery, and its free end is spatulated for an end-to-side anastomosis.

The carotid artery is then cross-clamped and an elliptical 5- to 7-mm arteriotomy is created in the posterolateral wall of the common carotid artery with an aortic punch. The anastomosis is performed in parachute fashion with a continuous 7-0 polypropylene suture (Video 10-1), avoiding tension on the vertebral artery, which may tear easily (Fig. 10-6). Before completion of the anastomosis, the suture slack is tightened appropriately with a nerve hook, standard flushing maneuvers are performed, and the suture is tied, reestablishing flow (Fig. 10-7). A drain is placed, and the incision is closed by reapproximating the platysma and closing the skin with a subcuticular suture.

EXPOSURE OF THE V2 SEGMENT OF THE VERTEBRAL ARTERY

The second segment of the vertebral artery, the portion that ascends within the foramina of the cervical vertebrae, is the site of a variety of pathology. However, the V2 segment is rarely accessed surgically because of its mostly interosseous position. The most common indication for exposure of the V2 segment is for control of hemorrhage, which is best treated with proximal and distal ligation of the artery in the V1 and V3 segments. Alternatively, direct exposure of the V2 segment requires resection of the transverse processes at the cervical vertebrae.

V3 EXPOSURE AND DISTAL VERTEBRAL ARTERY RECONSTRUCTION

The technique most often used to reconstruct the distal vertebral artery includes great or small saphenous vein bypass from the common carotid or subclavian artery.[20] Alternatively, the radial artery can be used as conduit in the absence of suitable vein. The distal portion of the reconstruction is generally completed at the C1 through C2 spinal level.

The skin incision is placed anterior to the sternocleidomastoid muscle, the same as in a carotid operation, and is carried superiorly to immediately below the earlobe. The dissection proceeds between the jugular vein and the anterior edge of the sternocleidomastoid muscle, exposing the spinal accessory nerve (Fig. 10-8). The nerve is followed proximally as it crosses in front of the jugular vein and the transverse process of C1. The first cervical vertebrae can be easily felt by finger palpation.

The next step involves the identification of the levator scapula muscle by removal of the fibrofatty tissue overlying it. Once the anterior edge of the levator scapula is identified, the anterior ramus of C2 can be seen. With the ramus as a guide, a right-angled clamp is slid under the levator scapula and over the ramus, and the muscle is elevated. The muscle is transected from its insertion on the C1 transverse process (Fig. 10-9). The C2 ramus divides into three branches after crossing the vertebral artery. The ramus should be cut (Fig. 10-10) before it branches; underneath it, the vertebral artery can be identified. The artery is freed from the surrounding venous plexus with extreme care because hemorrhage is difficult to control at this level.

Once the vertebral artery is dissected circumferentially, the distal common carotid artery is dissected and prepared as inflow source for a saphenous vein graft. There

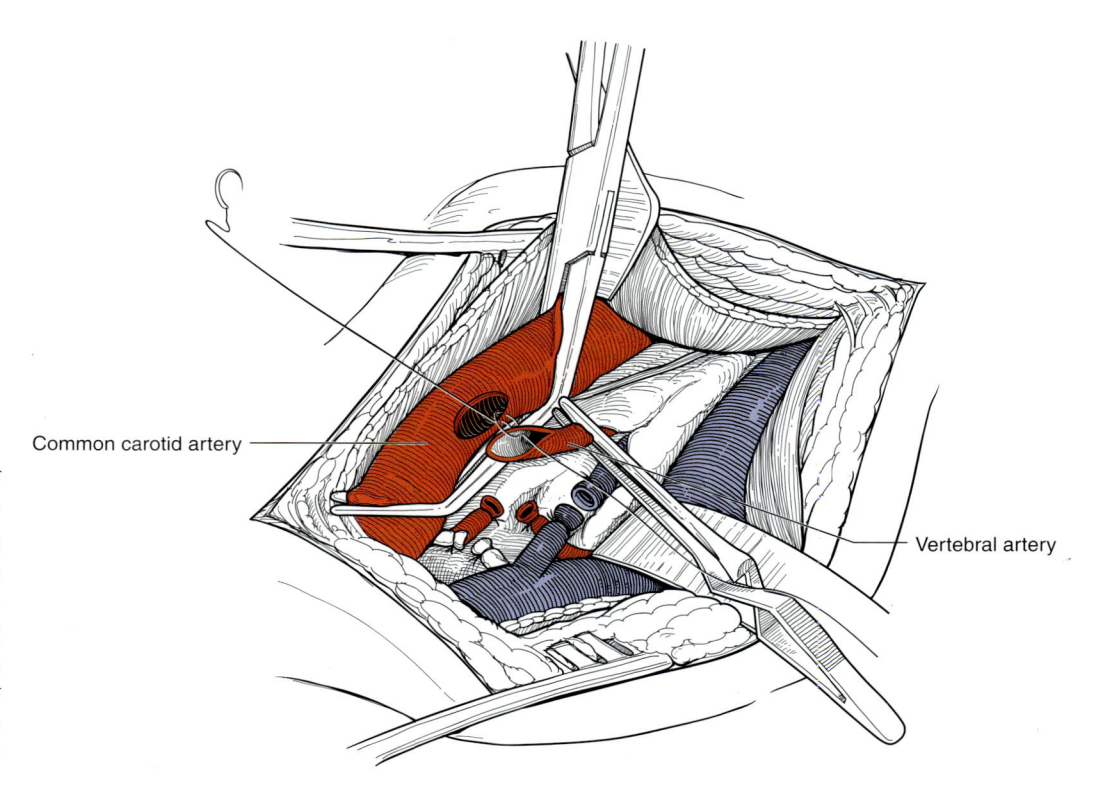

Figure 10-6. Transposition of the proximal vertebral artery to the posterior wall of the common carotid artery. The thoracic duct and inferior thyroid artery have been ligated and divided. *(Redrawn from Berguer R, Kieffer E: Surgery of the arteries to the head. New York, 1992, Springer-Verlag.)*

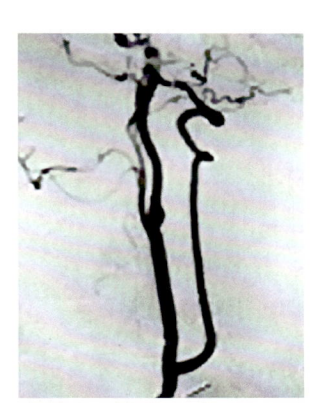

Figure 10-7. Completion angiogram of proximal vertebral to common carotid transposition.

is no need to dissect the carotid bifurcation. The location selected for the proximal anastomosis of the saphenous vein graft on the common carotid artery should not be too close to the bifurcation because cross-clamping at this level may fracture underlying atheroma.

A suitable conduit of appropriate length is harvested and prepared. A valveless segment of vein facilitates backbleeding of the vertebral artery after completion of the distal anastomosis. The patient is given intravenous heparin. The vertebral artery is elevated by gently pulling on an encircling vessel loop and is occluded with a small J clamp. This isolates a short segment for the initial end-to-side anastomosis. The vertebral artery is opened longitudinally over a short length adequate to accommodate the spatulated end of the vein graft. The end-to-side anastomosis is performed with a continuous 7-0 polypropylene suture. The distal anastomosis is assessed for backflow, and if satisfactory, a vascular clamp is placed on the vein graft proximal to the anastomosis, the J clamp is removed, and flow is reestablished through the vertebral artery.

The proximal end of the graft is passed behind the jugular vein and in close proximity to the side of the common carotid artery. The common carotid artery is then cross-clamped, an elliptical arteriotomy is made on its posterolateral wall with

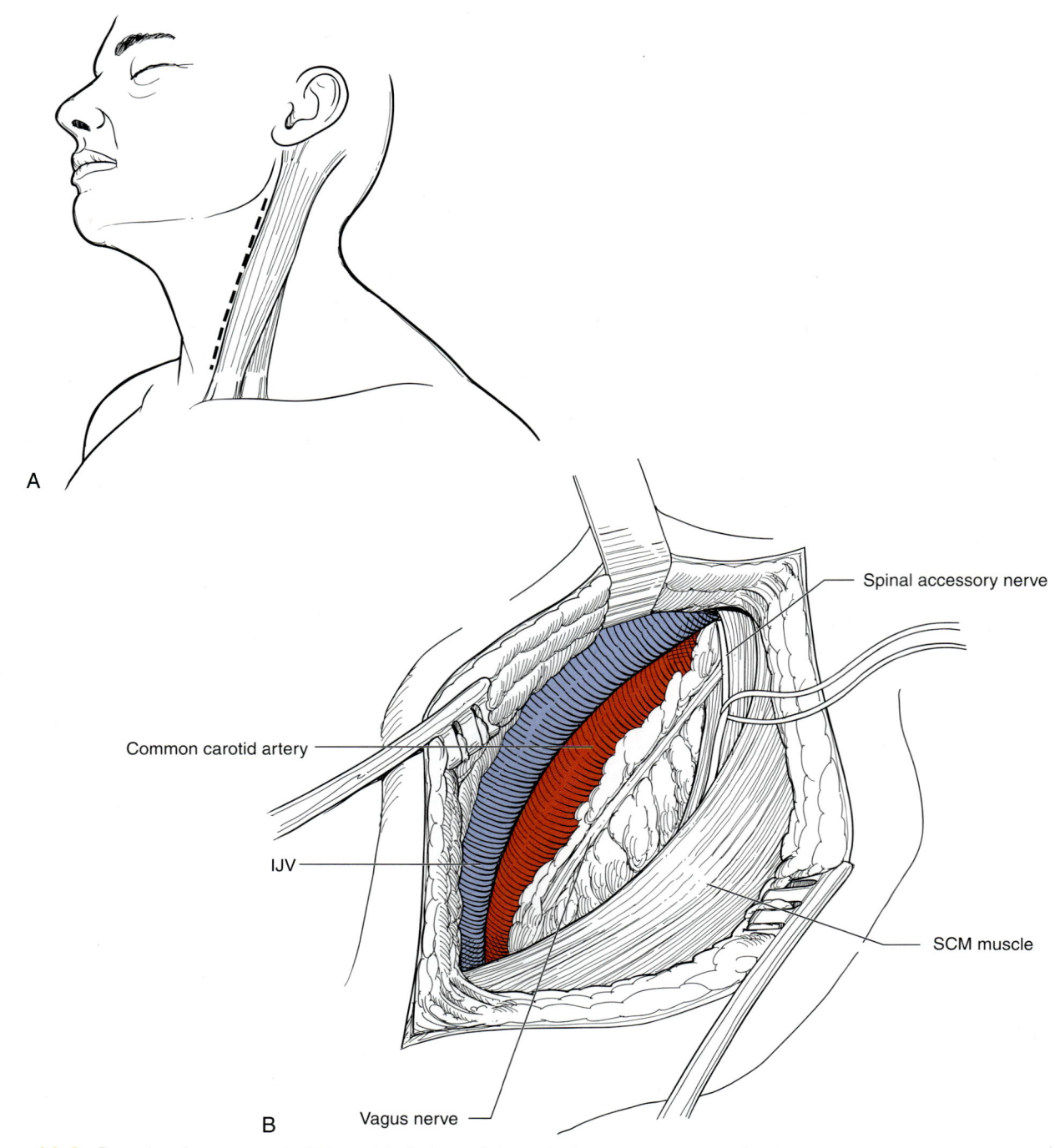

Figure 10-8. Retrojugular approach (**A**) and isolation of the spinal accessory nerve (encircled with vessel tape) (**B**). *IJV*, Internal jugular vein; *SCM*, sternocleidomastoid. *(Redrawn from Berguer R, Kieffer E:* Surgery of the arteries to the head. *New York, 1992, Springer-Verlag.)*

an aortic punch, and the proximal vein graft is anastomosed end-to-side to the common carotid artery with a continuous 6-0 polypropylene suture (Figs. 10-11 and 10-12). Before the anastomosis is completed, standard flushing maneuvers are performed, the suture is tied, and flow reestablished. The vertebral artery is occluded with a clip placed immediately below the anastomosis to create a functional end-to-end anastomosis and to avoid competitive flow or the potential for recurrent emboli. The wound is closed without a drain by reapproximating the platysma and closing the skin with a subcuticular suture.

For more distal pathology, the vertebral artery can be accessed surgically above the level of the transverse process of C1. Surgical exposure at the suboccipital segment requires resection of the C1 transverse process and part of its posterior arch. Reconstruction at this level is limited to the use of a saphenous vein bypass from

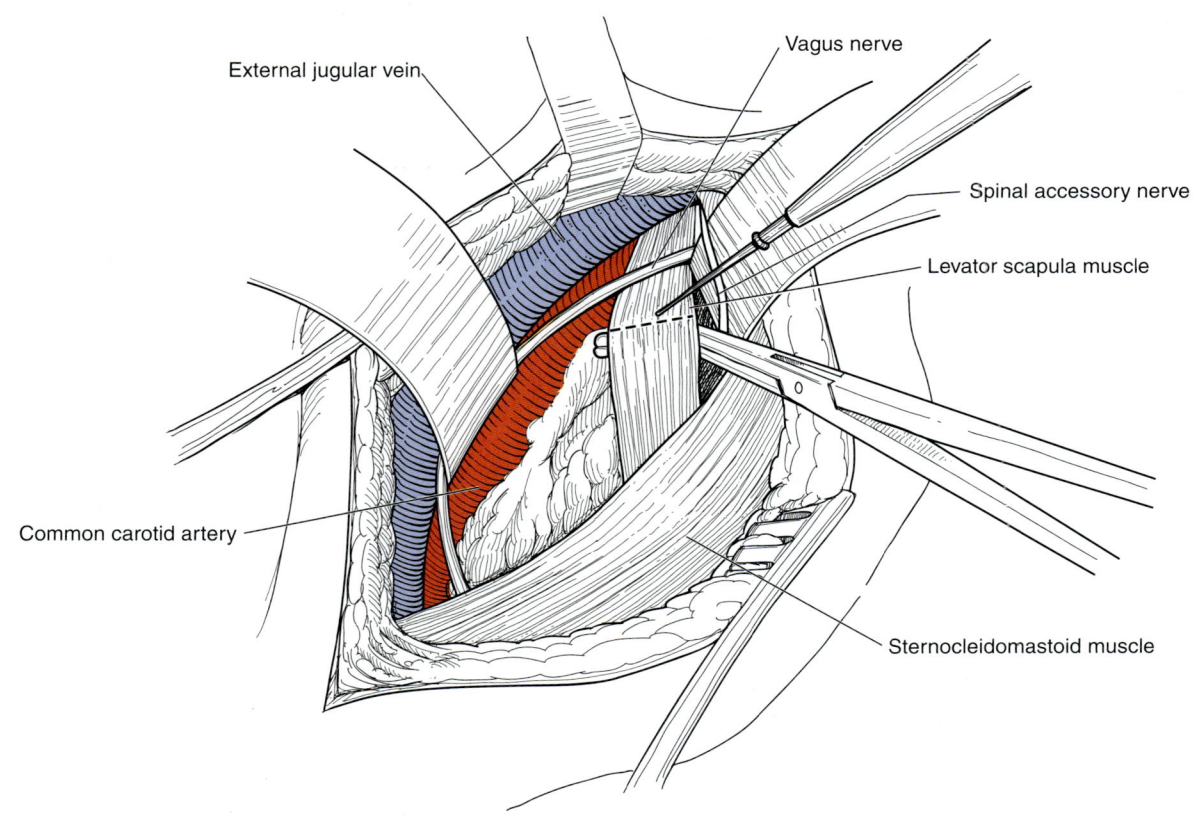

Figure 10-9. Dividing the levator scapula over the C2 ramus. The vagus and internal jugular vein are anterior to the muscle. *(Redrawn from Berguer R, Kieffer E: Surgery of the arteries to the head. New York, 1992, Springer-Verlag.)*

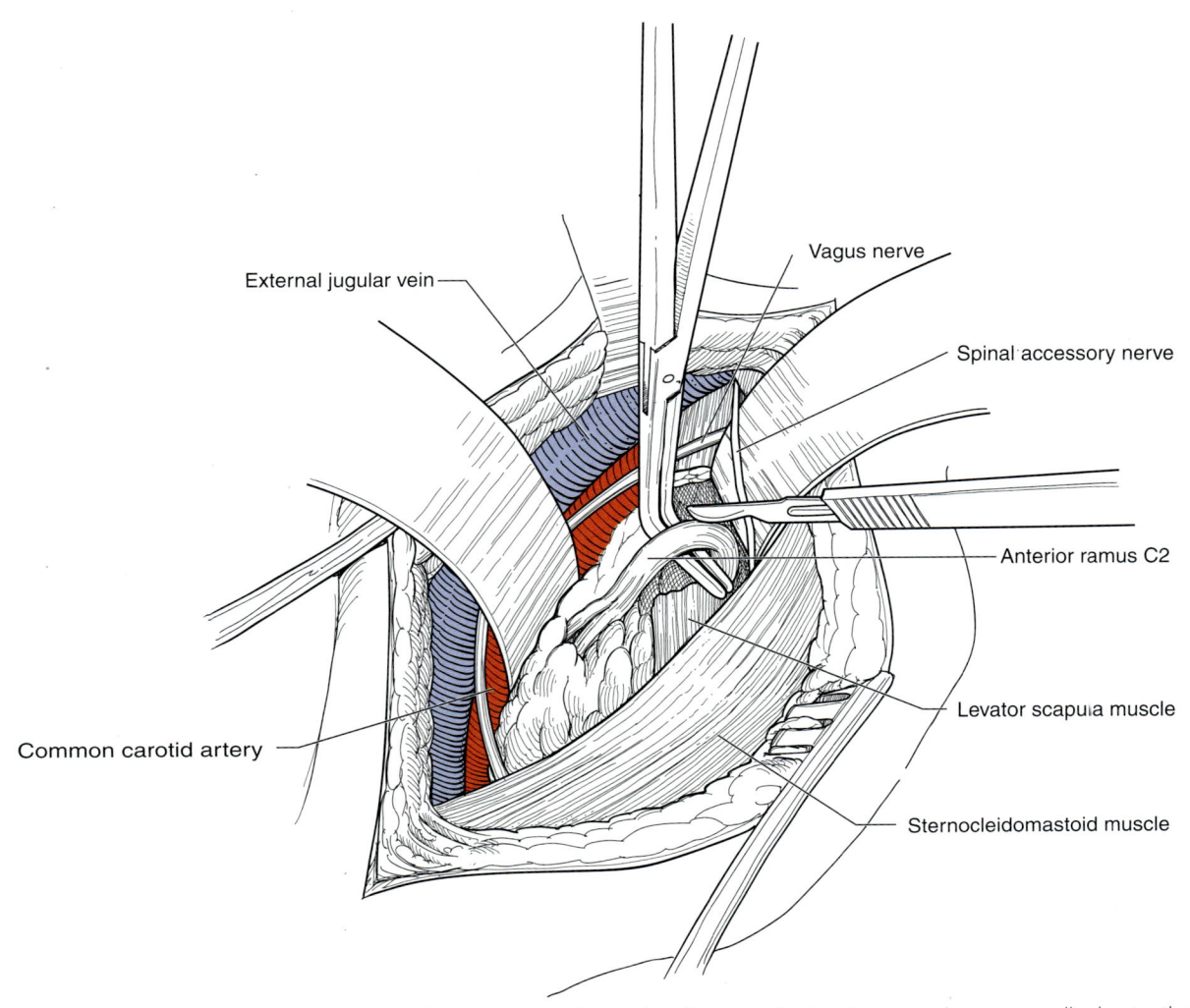

Figure 10-10. Dividing the anterior ramus of C2 to expose the underlying vertebral artery running perpendicular to the former. *(Redrawn from Berguer R, Kieffer E: Surgery of the arteries to the head. New York, 1992, Springer-Verlag.)*

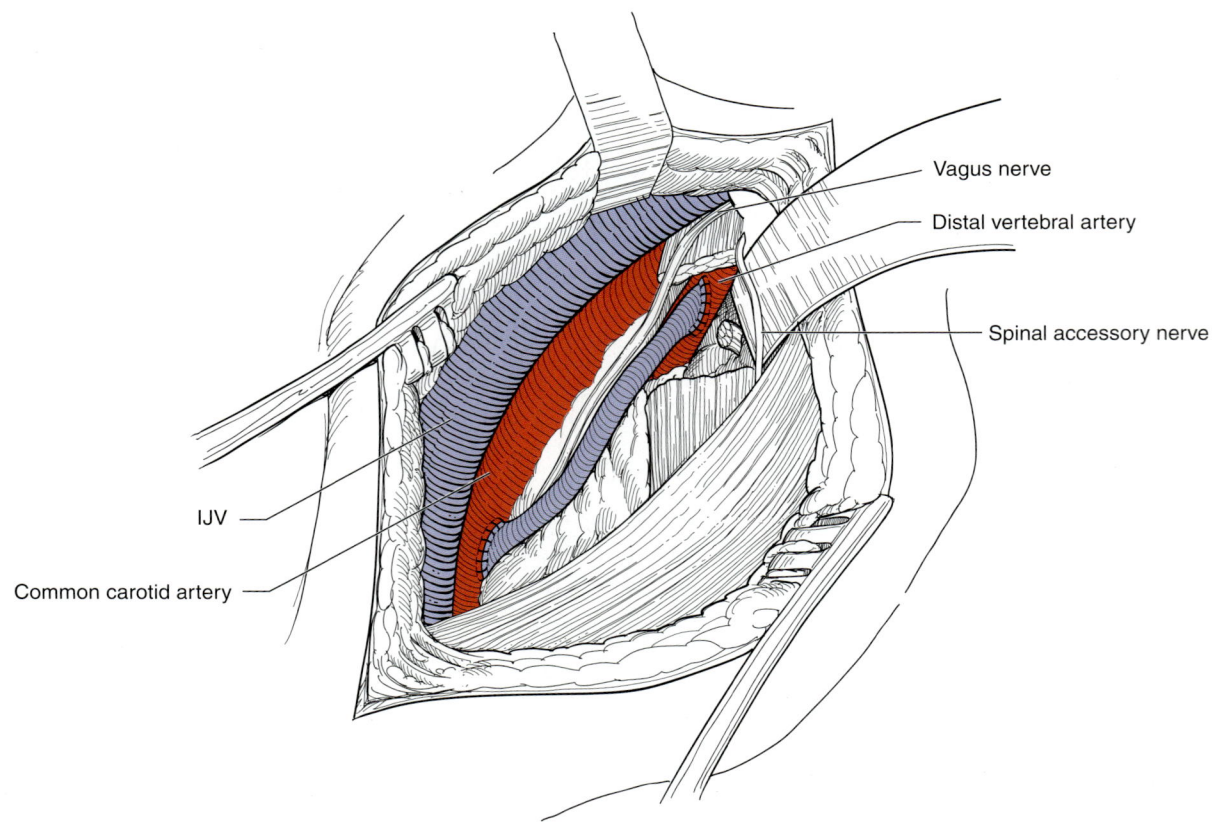

Figure 10-11. A completed common carotid artery to distal vertebral artery bypass using the saphenous vein. *IJV,* Internal jugular vein. *(Redrawn from Berguer R, Kieffer E: Surgery of the arteries to the head. New York, 1992, Springer-Verlag.)*

the distal internal carotid artery. Bypasses above the level of C1 (suboccipital) are technically demanding and have been required in only a small number of distal vertebral artery reconstructions.

Intraoperative completion imaging using digital angiography is useful and should be considered for all types of vertebral artery reconstruction. Technical flaws may be identified with repair preventing failure of the reconstruction.

Postoperative Care

- Patients spend several hours in the recovery room, where they are closely observed for airway, bleeding, or neurologic complications.
- A regular diet is provided on the day of surgery, and the patient is encouraged to get out of bed, move the ipsilateral arm, and gently rotate the neck.
- A small drain is left in place following proximal vertebral exposure until after the patient's first meal to exclude significant chylous leak. Drains can almost always be removed the morning after surgery.
- After overnight observation, the patient is discharged.
- An aspirin is given immediately after surgery.
- Postoperative discomfort is managed with acetaminophen or a nonsteroidal antiinflammatory.

Postoperative Complications

- **Stroke.** Stroke is usually the result of prolonged clamp time or immediate postoperative thrombosis of the vertebral artery or bypass conduit. Completion angiography may be helpful in preventing these complications. Distal reconstructions have a combined stroke and death rate of 3% to 4% and have higher stroke and death rates than operations on the proximal vertebral artery.[22]

SURGICAL TREATMENT OF THE VERTEBRAL ARTERY | 123

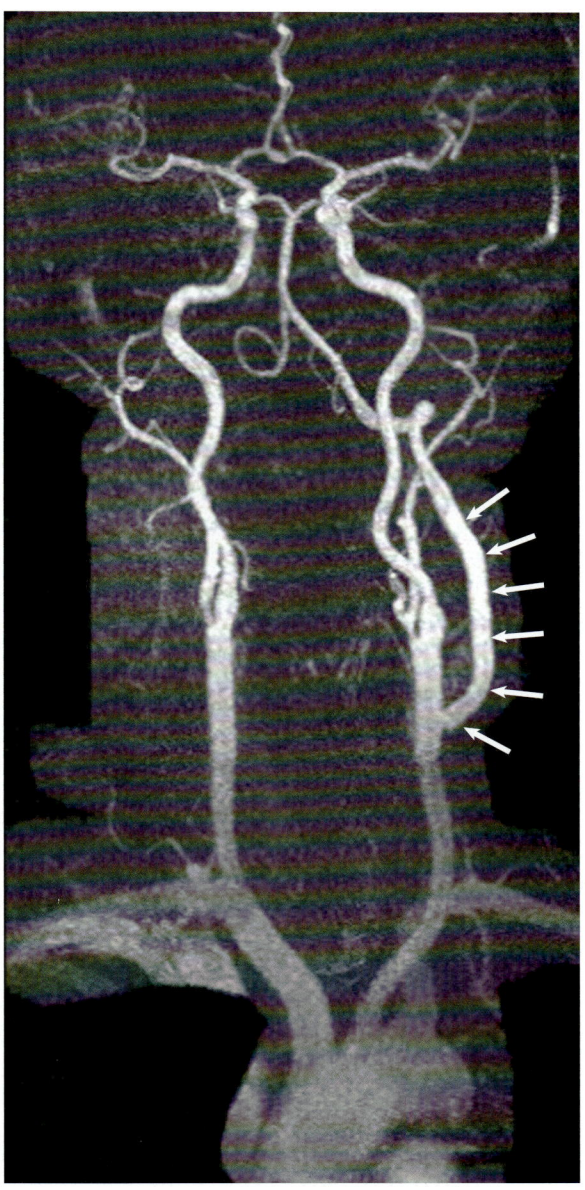

Figure 10-12. Follow-up magnetic resonance angiogram showing patent distal vertebral bypass *(arrows)*.

- **Nerve injury.** Complications unique to proximal vertebral artery reconstruction include vagus and recurrent laryngeal nerve palsy (2%) and Horner syndrome (8.4%-28%). Complications that may follow distal reconstruction include vagus (1%) and spinal accessory (2%) nerve injury.
- **Horner syndrome.** Most patients experience a short-lived Horner syndrome. The treatment is expectant. Most resolve in time.
- **Vagus nerve injury.** Injury of the vagus nerve is usually manifest as hoarseness and is most often the result of traction on the vagus during exposure of the deep neck structures or during carotid exposure more distally. Because this rarely is the result of cutting the recurrent nerve, usually time and patience are all that are required. If a vocal cord palsy persists beyond 3 months, vocal cord medialization may be warranted.
- **Spinal accessory nerve injury.** Injury to the spinal accessory nerve usually results from traction and most neuropraxia type injuries will resolve in time.
- **Chylous and lymph leak or late lymphocele and chylothorax.** Initial conservative management is appropriate for chylous or lymph leak or late lymphocele or chylothorax, because most resolve. This includes local compression, dietary manipulation, and administration of octreotide. Leaks that

persist beyond 3 days require reexploration of the surgical site with direct suture repair. Purse string placement of a small-gauge monofilament suture works best to control a large lymphatic or thoracic duct leak. If all else fails, ligation of the thoracic duct by video-assisted thoracotomy surgery can be considered.

REFERENCES

1. Cate WR Jr, Scott HW Jr: Cerebral ischemia of central origin: Relief by subclavian-vertebral artery thromboendarterectomy, *Surgery* 45:19-31, 1957.
2. Crawford ES, DeBakey ME, Fields WS: Roentgenographic diagnosis and surgical treatment of basilar artery insufficiency, *J Am Med Assoc* 168:509-514, 1958.
3. Parrott JC: The subclavian steal syndrome, *Arch Surg* 88:661-665, 1664.
4. Clark K, Perry MO: Carotid vertebral anastomosis: An alternate technic for repair of the subclavian steal syndrome, *Ann Surg* 163:414-416, 1966.
5. Berguer R, Andaya LV, Bauer RB: Vertebral artery bypass, *Arch Surg* 111:976-979, 1976.
6. Roon AJ, Ehrenfeld WK, Cooke PB, Wylie EJ: Vertebral artery reconstruction, *Am J Surg* 138: 29-36, 1979.
7. Matas R: Traumatisms and traumatic aneurysms of the vertebral artery and their surgical treatment with the report of a cured case, *Ann Surg* 18:477-521, 1893.
8. Henry A: *Extensile exposure*, London, 1945, Churchill Livingstone.
9. Carney A, Anderson E: Carotid distal vertebral bypass for carotid artery occlusion, *Clin Electroencephalogr* 9:105, 1978.
10. Corkill G, French BN, Michas C, et al: External carotid-vertebral artery anastomosis for vertebrobasilar insufficiency, *Surg Neurol* 7:109-115, 1977.
11. Wityk RJ, Chang HM, Rosengart A, et al: Proximal extracranial vertebral artery disease in the New England Medical Center Posterior Circulation Registry, *Arch Neurol* 55:470-478, 1998.
12. Cartlidge NE, Whisnant JP, Elveback LR: Carotid and vertebral-basilar transient cerebral ischemic attacks. A community study, Rochester, Minn., *Mayo Clin Proc* 52:117-120, 1977.
13. Heyman A, Wilkinson WE, Hurwitz BJ, et al: Clinical and epidemiologic aspects of vertebrobasilar and nonfocal cerebral ischemia. In Berguer R, Bauer RB, editors: *Vertebrobasilar arterial occlusive disease. Medical and surgical management*, New York, 1984, Raven Press, pp 27-36.
14. Whisnant JP, Cartlidge NE, Elveback LR: Carotid and vertebral-basilar transient ischemic attacks: Effect of anticoagulants, hypertension, and cardiac disorders on survival and stroke occurrence—a population study, *Ann Neurol* 3:107-115, 1978.
15. Jones HR Jr, Millikan CH, Sandok BA: Temporal profile (clinical course) of acute vertebrobasilar system cerebral infarction, *Stroke* 11:173-177, 1980.
16. McDowell FH, Potes J, Groch S: The natural history of internal carotid and vertebral-basilar artery occlusion, *Neurology* 11:153-157, 1961, Pt 2.
17. Patrick BK, Ramirez-Lassepas M, Synder BD: Temporal profile of vertebrobasilar territory infarction. Prognostic implications, *Stroke* 11:643-648, 1980.
18. Caplan LR, Wityk RJ, Glass TA, et al: New England Medical Center Posterior Circulation registry, *Ann Neurol* 56:389-398, 2004.
19. Berguer R, Higgins R, Nelson R: Noninvasive diagnosis of reversal of vertebral-artery blood flow, *N Engl J Med* 302:1349-1351, 1980.
20. Berguer R: Distal vertebral artery bypass: Technique, the "occipital connection," and potential uses, *J Vasc Surg* 2:621-626, 1985.
21. Edwards WH, Mulherin JL Jr: The surgical approach to significant stenosis of vertebral and subclavian arteries, *Surgery* 87:20-28, 1980.
22. Berguer R: Complex carotid and vertebral revascularizations. In Pearce WH, Matsumura JS, Yao JST, editors: *Vascular surgery in the endovascular era*, Evanston, Ill., 2008, Greenwood Academic, pp 344-352.

Section 3

AORTIC ARCH VESSELS

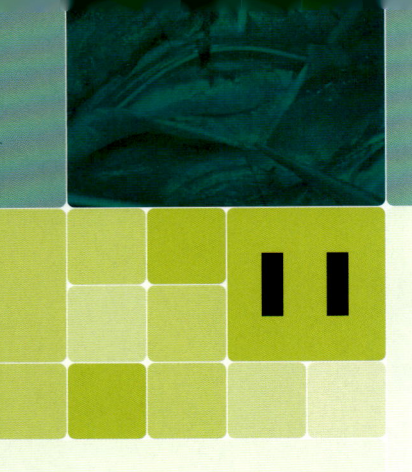

11 Direct Surgical Repair of Aortic Arch Vessels

AMANI D. POLITANO • KENNETH J. CHERRY

Historical Background

Surgical approaches to the aortic arch vessels had been described in the late nineteenth and early twentieth centuries.[1,2] In 1958 DeBakey and associates[3] described the first successful surgical reconstruction of an occluded symptomatic innominate artery using an nylon bifurcated graft from the ascending aortic arch to the left subclavian and common carotid arteries. This report was followed by a comprehensive 10-year review of the surgical treatment of occlusion of innominate common carotid and subclavian arteries in 1969.[4]

Indications

Pathologies that most commonly warrant surgical reconstruction of the great vessels include arteriosclerotic disease and inflammatory arteritides. In addition arteritis can develop in patients undergoing therapeutic radiation for cancers of the head, neck, breast, or lymph tissues.

Arteriosclerosis is by far the most common etiology.[5,6] In a series of operations involving the carotid bifurcation, vertebral arteries, or great vessels, only 7.5% of those procedures were performed for lesions of the innominate, common carotid, or subclavian vessels.[6] Although great vessel lesions are uncommon compared with carotid bifurcation disease, several larger referral centers have reported on their experience.[7-15] Arteriosclerotic disease is more prevalent in men and in younger patients, with a mean age of 50 to 61 years.

The second most common cause of great vessel disease in the United States is Takayasu arteritis. This disease is seen more frequently in younger women and those of East or South Asian descent.[16,17] This inflammatory process manifests systemically with fever, arthralgias, weight loss, and fatigue. In later stages of the disease process the central arteries develop hemodynamically significant stenosis, which can manifest as upper extremity claudication, renovascular hypertension, and focal tenderness over the involved artery. Central symptoms such as visual impairment, dizziness, headache, and stroke; cardiorespiratory findings including angina, myocardial infarction, and pulmonary hypertension can also be seen.[16]

Inflammatory markers are often elevated in the active phase of the disease but cannot be used to either confirm or eliminate the diagnosis, which is made on the basis of history and physical examination.[18] The pathologic findings associated with Takayasu arteritis include long segments of smooth-walled stenosis of the aortic arch, descending thoracic aorta, and primary branches.[16,17] The subclavian artery is most often affected. In addition to standard diagnostic imaging modalities, fluorodeoxyglucose positron emission tomography may demonstrate central vascular inflammation.[19,20]

Radiation-induced arteritis manifests with subintimal fibrosis, endothelial degeneration, and myointimal proliferation.[21] The interval between radiation therapy and vascular intervention averages 15.2 years, and patients most often present with embolic or global ischemic phenomenon.[22]

Operative intervention is indicated for symptomatic lesions manifesting as extremity or cerebral ischemia because of occlusion or severe stenosis or as distal embolization. Surgical repair of asymptomatic lesions of the common carotid artery may be indicated based on established guidelines for carotid bifurcation disease.[23] Conditions that may warrant repair of asymptomatic lesions include improving flow for existing or anticipated hemodialysis access or salvaging axillary-origin vascular grafts.[24,25] Reconstruction may be considered in patients in whom accurate blood pressure monitoring is impossible because of multiple occlusive lesions. If a patient is undergoing sternotomy for other indications, it may be preferable to treat great vessel disease at that time rather than at a later date through a reoperative field.

Preoperative Preparation

- **History.** Diagnosis and localization of brachiocephalic disease are suggested by the manifesting symptoms. Neurologic symptoms result from decreased circulation of the anterior, vertebrobasilar, or both systems. Although the frequency of patients presenting with neurologic symptoms reported in the literature is wide, from 5% to 90%,[8,9,15] several large, contemporary studies have shown a more consistent rate between 64% and 83%.[8,9,14,15] Likewise, upper extremity symptoms can be seen in 5% to 63.3%.[7,8,12,14,15] Arm ischemia often results from tight stenoses with flow limitation, although ulcerative but less stenotic lesions may manifest with microembolization. A combination of upper extremity and neurologic symptoms can be seen in 18% to 39% of patients.[14,15] Symptoms limited to a single extremity may differentiate atherosclerotic disease of the innominate or subclavian artery from systemic diseases that also manifest with upper extremity ischemia.

- **Physical examination.** Palpation and auscultation of the proximal and mid-cervical carotid arteries, the superficial temporal artery, the subclavian artery, and the brachial, radial, and ulnar vessels should be performed. Bruits or thrills noted in the proximal carotid or subclavian vessels may be indicative of stenotic lesions in the great vessels. An Allen test or its adaptations may reveal digital arterial occlusions. Blood pressure measurements should be performed in both upper extremities, and if there is concern of bilateral upper extremity stenoses, comparison should be made to the lower extremities. Evaluation of the skin and nails may reveal bluish, painful discolorations in the fingertips, splinter hemorrhages, or livedo reticularis suggestive of embolic events.

- **Imaging studies.** Patient presentation and physical examination often suggest the diagnosis, but imaging is used to confirm, characterize, and begin planning intervention for the offending lesion. Duplex ultrasound and waveform analysis of the upper extremity can aid in the diagnosis. Computed tomography angiography with intravenous contrast, and especially with the additive information obtained with volumetric three-dimensional imaging, allows assessment of the arch and four vessels with a reduced risk of stroke or access site complications. Magnetic resonance angiography with gadolinium enhancement may also be used to assess arterial anatomy in a less invasive manner.[26] Angiography may be used when other imaging modalities fail to provide the necessary information before intervention. Views of the aortic arch and subclavian, carotid, and vertebral arteries are required for accurate diagnosis, localization, characterization, and operative planning. If the offending lesions affect the carotid or vertebrobasilar system, preoperative imaging should also assess the circle of Willis.[27]

- **Management of the asymptomatic lesion.** As imaging procedures are performed for a myriad of indications, an increasing number of asymptomatic lesions involving the aortic arch vessels are being identified. Although surgical intervention has been described for asymptomatic lesions,[8,9] there is a relatively high risk of morbidity and mortality associated with the median sternotomy.

Of the patients in the series by Berguer, Morasch, and Kline, 13% were asymptomatic; there were no mortalities but one stroke.[9] They concluded that asymptomatic patients should not be offered repair in this setting. An exception would be a patient who requires another operation that involves a median sternotomy, such as a coronary artery bypass graft procedure. In this setting, it may be prudent to offer a combined repair in order to avoid the associated morbidity of a redo-sternotomy should great vessel disease become symptomatic.

- **Options for surgical repair of aortic arch vessels.** Operative repair options for patients with great vessel disease can be categorized as either direct arch or extraanatomic reconstructions. The latter were developed to reduce the morbidity and mortality associated with aortic-based reconstructions. Many patients who present with innominate artery disease requiring reconstruction have multiple supra-aortic lesions. In recent series this has varied between 61% and 84% of patients, and included both concomitant arch lesions as well as carotid bifurcation disease.[9,14,15,26] Bypass grafts can be constructed to reconstruct several areas of stenosis. Less invasive cervical or extrathoracic approaches may be more suitable for a given anatomic configuration. Examples of extraanatomic procedures include transpositions, subclavian-carotid or carotid-subclavian artery bypass, axillary-axillary artery bypass, or contralateral carotid-carotid or carotid-subclavian artery bypass. Some techniques, such as carotid-subclavian artery bypass, have remained popular and are frequently performed for more limited great vessel disease or as an adjunct to endovascular repair of the thoracic aorta. In more recent series the morbidity and mortality of direct surgical repair of great vessel occlusive disease has become more acceptable, and concerns regarding the long-term patency of extraanatomic approaches have revived interest in direct repair via median sternotomy. These techniques are the focus of this chapter.

Pitfalls and Danger Points

- **Concomitant cardiac disease.** Planned intervention for great vessel arteriosclerosis should prompt a preoperative cardiac workup to assess the need for coronary interventions that may best be performed before or concurrent with great vessel repair.[10,13] Patients with Takayasu arteritis should undergo echocardiography to assess for valvular heart disease, pulmonary hypertension, or left ventricular hypertrophy in addition to coronary lesions.[28] If radiation-induced arteritis is the etiology of occlusive disease, patients should be evaluated for cardiomyopathy and coronary artery disease.
- **Nerve injury.** Intraoperative structures of importance include the vagus nerves as they descend within the carotid sheaths and the recurrent laryngeal nerves. If more lateral dissection is required, the phrenic nerve may also be encountered.
- **Thoracic duct injury.** Meticulous dissection and ligation of lymphatics, including the thoracic duct on the left side, are also paramount.
- **Prior history of coronary artery bypass or median sternotomy.** If a patient has had previous coronary artery bypass grafting, preservation of the internal mammary circulation is also of utmost concern. A history of previous reconstructive procedures must be noted, as the anatomy may be varied and may be more difficult to discern in a reoperative field.

Operative Strategy

SURGICAL ANATOMY OF THE AORTIC ARCH AND BRANCH VESSELS

The great vessels of the aorta include the innominate, subclavian, and common carotid arteries. These vessels, in their standard configuration, begin proximally along the aorta with the origin of the innominate artery and are succeeded in order by the left common carotid artery and the left subclavian artery. Variations of this branching pattern are relatively common and include the various "bovine arch" patterns, such as a common origin of the innominate and left common carotid arteries or of the left common carotid artery arising as a branch of the innominate artery. Identification of these variations preoperatively is critical for planning surgical interventions.

AVOIDING INJURY TO ANATOMIC STRUCTURES

The vagus and recurrent laryngeal nerves are both encountered during dissection of the carotid and subclavian arteries. These should be isolated and protected during the procedure. When dissecting more laterally along the subclavian artery, the phrenic nerve may be encountered. The brachial plexus lies posterior to the subclavian vessels and may be injured if unrecognized. Although direct injury is a risk, stretch injury because of patient positioning or use of retractors is also common but can be minimized by careful planning and placement of equipment. If possible, bilateral abduction of the extremities in the operating room should be avoided.

In the left supraclavicular fossa, the thoracic duct and the junction of the subclavian and jugular veins can be found and should be appropriately ligated. Additional care to identify and similarly control smaller lymphatic vessels must be exerted. As with any operation, understanding of the anatomic location and potential variants is paramount in avoiding injury to these important structures.

AVOIDING INTRAOPERATIVE STROKE

Appropriate imaging is crucial in planning the surgical approach and may dictate the need for intraoperative cerebral shunt placement. The vertebral and carotid arteries should be assessed bilaterally to determine the dominant side, and the circle of Willis should be visualized for completeness. Use of intraoperative electroencephalographic monitoring, cerebral oximetry, or carotid stump pressure may guide the decision-making process intraoperatively. The same criteria and methods of shunting used in other carotid artery reconstructions may be considered. If multiple vessels are involved and shunting is impossible, neuroprotective anesthetic agents may be used. When both common carotid arteries are to undergo reconstruction, the more diseased artery is addressed first to maintain as much baseline cerebral blood flow as possible.

ASSESSMENT OF A SUITABLE CLAMP SITE IN THE AORTIC ARCH

The most appropriate location for the partial occlusion clamp on the aorta is determined through a combination of assessment of the preoperative imaging and intraoperative palpation of the aorta. For bypass procedures in which the graft arises from the ascending aorta, the origin of the graft should be placed as far laterally on the ascending aorta as possible to ensure optimal placement of the graft once the sternotomy is closed. An anteriorly placed graft is easily compressed by the sternum once closed. If, despite care, the sternum compresses the graft, rongeurs may be used to excise posterior elements of the sternum and sternoclavicular joint. The clamp site should avoid areas of significant plaque.

SPECIAL CONSIDERATIONS FOR PATIENTS WITH VASCULITIS

Takayasu arteritis is better treated with open bypass procedures than with either endarterectomy or stenting. Patients presenting with acute inflammation should be medically managed. Surgical intervention should be reserved for the quiescent phase of the disease or as a last resort in patients not responsive to optimal medical therapy. Proceeding with operative intervention during the acute inflammatory stage of the disease increases the risk of restenosis at the anastomoses.[29] Although patients can be treated for severe neurologic symptoms in the acute phase via endovascular approaches, the transmural nature of the disease process predisposes it to significant restenosis. This, along with the patient's youth in many cases, favors the durability seen with open repair of stenotic lesions.

Operative Technique

INCISION

Proper patient positioning aids greatly in exposure. The patient should be supine on the operating table, arms by the side, with a roll or bump placed vertically between the scapulae and the head extended, supported, and rotated slightly to the left. If bilateral carotid revascularizations are performed, the head is prepared to be rotated in either direction. The operative field should include the neck, chest, and upper abdomen. Standard methods for skin preparation and draping should be used. The initial incision is midline, with division of the entire sternum, although a partial sternotomy may be used. A hockey stick extension of this incision a short distance along the anterior border of the right sternocleidomastoid (SCM) muscle allows for exposure of the innominate artery bifurcation (Fig. 11-1). The sternal attachments of the SCM may be divided and retracted laterally to improve exposure if needed. A sternal retractor is positioned for optimal exposure.

If the planned procedure requires bypass to the carotid bifurcation, additional incisions may be required to facilitate access. On the right side, the original incision can be extended along the anterior border of the SCM as it would for a carotid endarterectomy; alternatively, a separate incision may be used. For access to the left carotid bifurcation, a separate incision may be necessary. A tunnel running just anterior to the common carotid artery is created. Anastomoses to the left common carotid artery are usually performed through the primary incision.

EXPOSURE OF THE AORTIC ARCH

Exposure of the aortic arch and great vessels requires division of the thymus gland and pericardial fat. The left innominate or, brachiocephalic, vein is identified as it traverses anterior to the arch and origins of the great vessels. This vessel can either be mobilized or ligated for further exposure (Fig. 11-2). Mobilization requires ligation and division of the tributaries to the vein. Primary division may provide enhanced exposure of the operative field but risks sequelae of venous congestion and upper extremity edema. Fortunately, these problems are usually temporary.

Preparation of the ascending aorta for the graft anastomosis may require entry into the pericardial sac. The proximal, lateral ascending aorta is more predictably free of atherocalcific disease. The ascending aorta is dissected free, particularly along the right lateral border.

The final configuration of structures in the reapproximated mediastinum should be considered for graft selection when operative intervention calls for bypass of more than one vessel. Although branched grafts are available directly from the manufacturers, the larger proximal graft body adds bulk to a confined area and may lead to graft failure, venous compression, or even tracheal compression.[7] Although some groups have had favorable results using such grafts, it appears that success is related to leaving a longer trunk of the graft than is done with infrarenal aortic grafts to prevent a high-velocity "jet stream" injury and stenosis of the graft limbs.

A single-limb graft with side arms added as necessary reduces the bulk of mediastinal contents. In order to determine the most optimal placement of a side arm, the sternal retractor can be relaxed to mimic the final position of the mediastinal contents. Other strategies to reduce mediastinal bulk include resection of the segment of the bypassed vessel and division and ligation of the left brachiocephalic vein.

DISSECTION OF THE ARCH VESSELS

Appropriate exposure of the innominate artery involves dissection past the bifurcation to the right subclavian artery and common carotid artery in order to facilitate

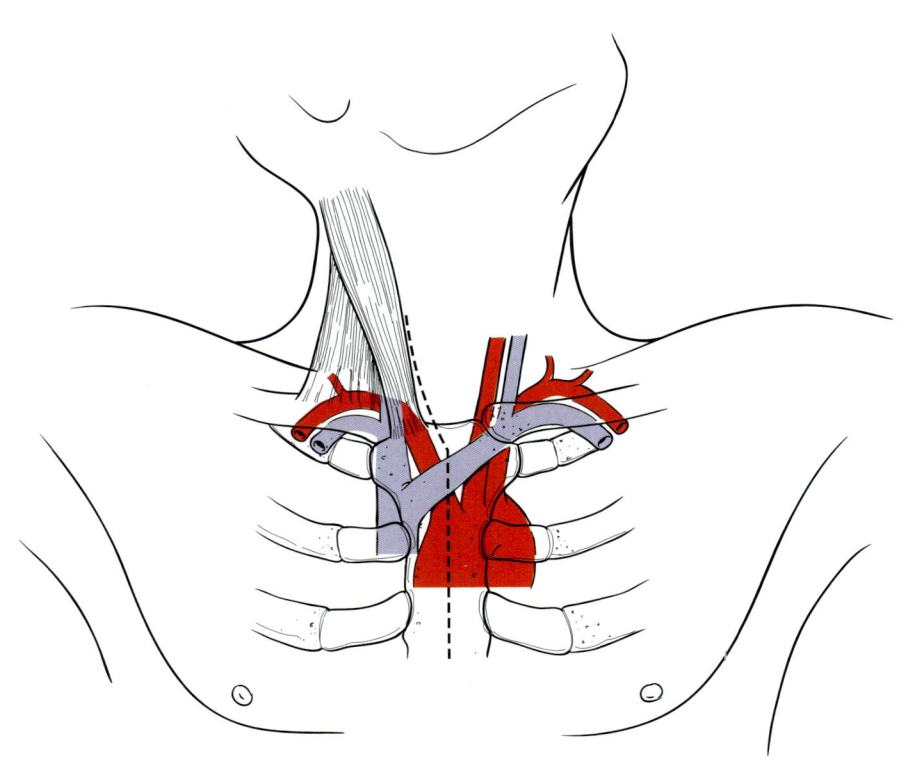

DIRECT SURGICAL REPAIR OF AORTIC ARCH VESSELS | 131

Figure 11-1. Initial incision line. The great vessels of the aorta include the innominate, left common carotid, and left subclavian arteries. Exposure of the aortic arch and great vessels requires division of the thymus gland and pericardial fat. The left innominate, or brachiocephalic, vein is identified as it traverses anterior to the arch and origins of the great vessels. Exposure is obtained by performing a median sternotomy and, if needed, a lateral extension along the anterior border of the right SCM muscle, extending to about midneck.

A — Thymus gland (divided)

B — Thymus; Left brachiocephalic vein (divided)

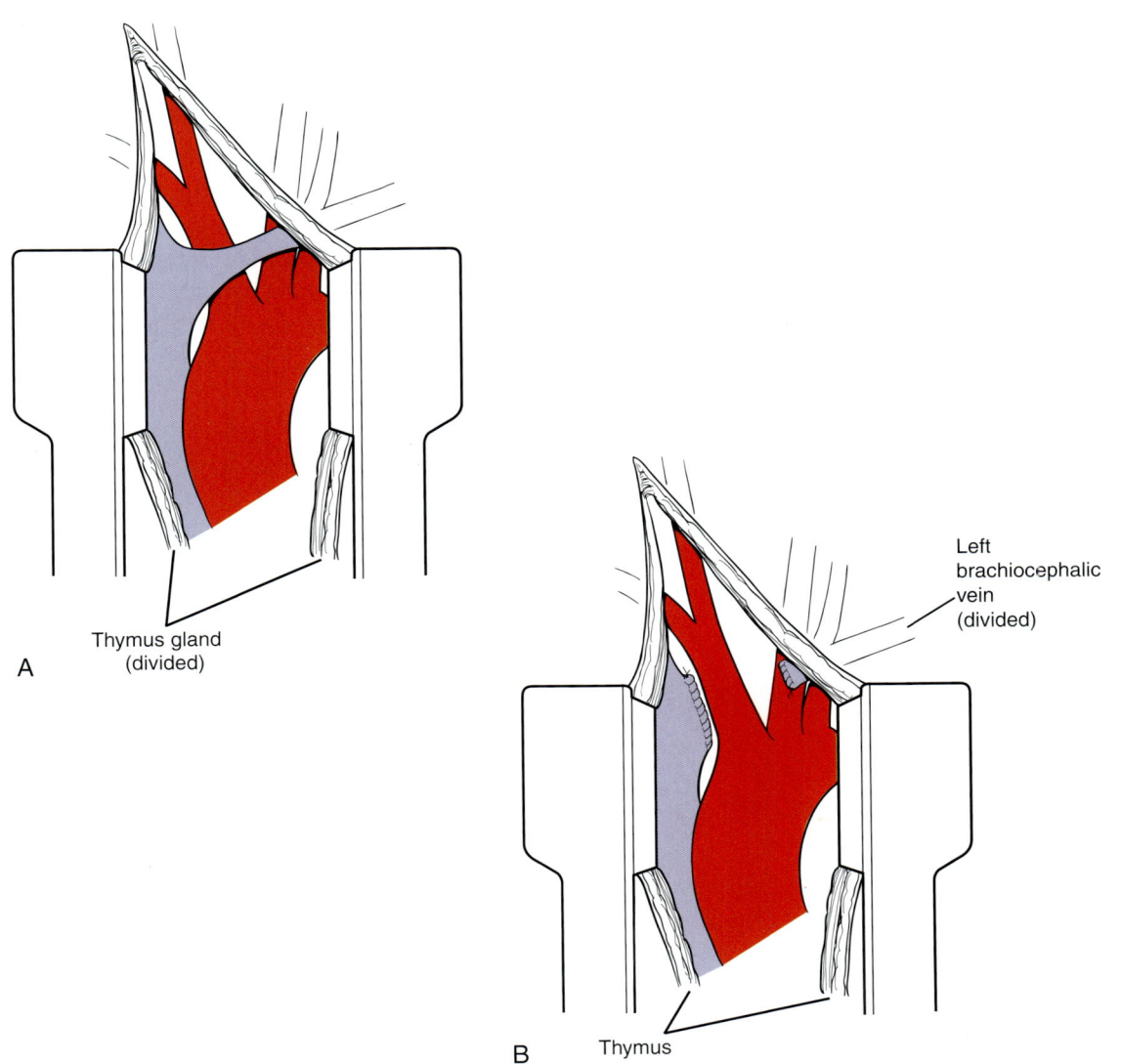

Figure 11-2. Initial dissection of the aortic arch. The thymus gland overlays the structures of interest and has been divided and reflected to either side. **A,** The left brachiocephalic vein can be encircled with a vessel loop and retracted inferiorly to reveal the arterial structures, with ligation of small branches of the vein as needed. **B,** Complete division and reflection of the left brachiocephalic vein.

distal clamp placement. The vagus nerve within the carotid sheath and the recurrent laryngeal nerve as it sweeps inferior to the subclavian artery should be identified and preserved. If the diseased portion of the subclavian artery requires further distal dissection, the phrenic nerve must also be identified and preserved.

The extent of dissection beyond the bifurcation should be predicated on the extent of the patient's underlying disease status and the optimal location for distal anastomosis, as determined by preoperative imaging studies and intraoperative assessment of the vessels. If a more distal destination on the right common carotid artery is selected, the incision may be extended to reveal the bifurcation. If the planned procedure requires bypass to the more distal portion of the left common carotid artery, a second incision is required in order to access the bifurcation of that artery.

ASCENDING AORTA-INNOMINATE ARTERY BYPASS

Once adequate exposure of the ascending aorta and the distal targets has been achieved, the proximal anastomosis is begun. The graft is selected and prepared. In general a woven Dacron graft 8 or 10 mm in diameter is appropriate for this procedure. Anticoagulation is reserved until the proximal anastomosis is complete and hemostasis at this site assured. A partial occlusion clamp such as a Cooley curved multipurpose clamp is placed on the ascending aorta in as lateral a position as possible (Fig. 11-3). A vertical aortotomy is made. The proximal end of the graft is spatulated appropriately to fit the aortotomy. Monofilament suture, generally 3-0 or 4-0 polypropylene, is used to fashion the anastomosis as a running suture. Once complete, the graft is clamped more distally and the aortic clamp is gently released to verify hemostasis. Single repair stitches are placed if needed to obtain hemostasis. In general the suture is one size smaller than that used for the primary anastomosis.

At this point, the patient is heparinized systemically, clamps are placed on the right subclavian and common carotid arteries, and finally, control of the proximal portion is obtained. This sequence of clamp placement prevents distal embolization. The innominate artery is divided distally and spatulated to accept the graft (Fig. 11-4). If the left brachiocephalic vein is intact, the graft is placed posterior to it (Fig. 11-5). The distal anastomosis is completed end to end, and both antegrade

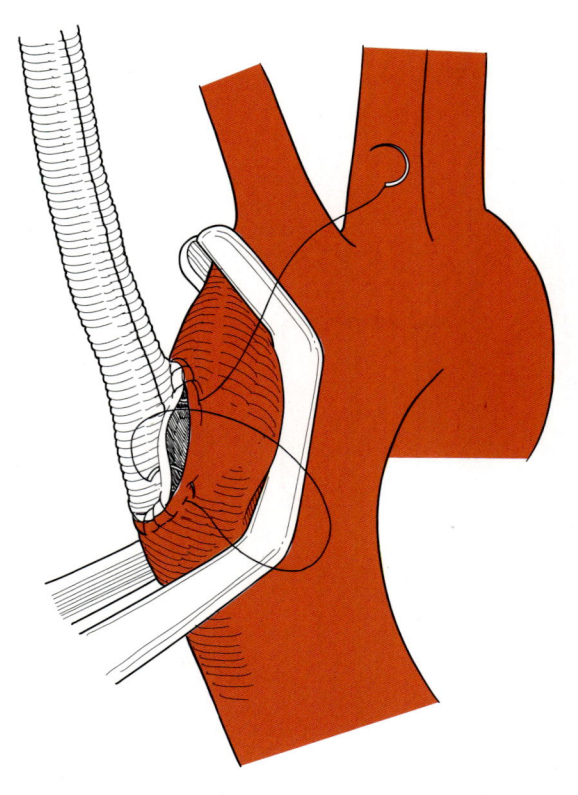

Figure 11-3. Preparing the aortic anastomosis. The left brachiocephalic vein is retracted superiorly, and the aortic arch is exposed. The pericardial sac over the right lateral aorta is opened, and a side-biting clamp is placed on the lateral portion of the aorta.

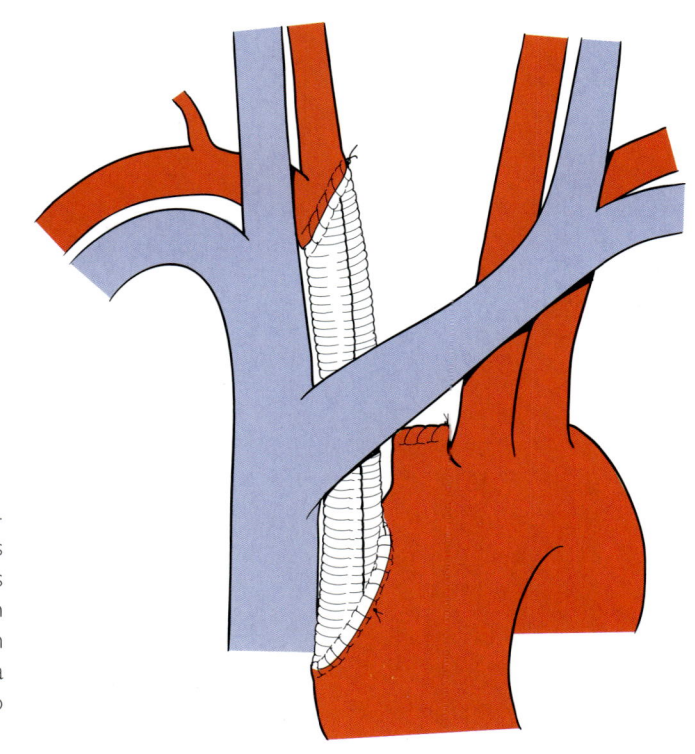

DIRECT SURGICAL REPAIR OF AORTIC ARCH VESSELS   133

Figure 11-4. Sewing the graft to the ascending aorta. A synthetic graft is anastomosed to the ascending aorta. The graft has been tunneled underneath the left brachiocephalic vein and is extending toward the right neck. The innominate artery has been oversewn proximally, just at the takeoff from the aorta. A section of innominate artery has been removed so that there is only a short portion of innominate artery proximal to the bifurcation to the left subclavian and carotid arteries.

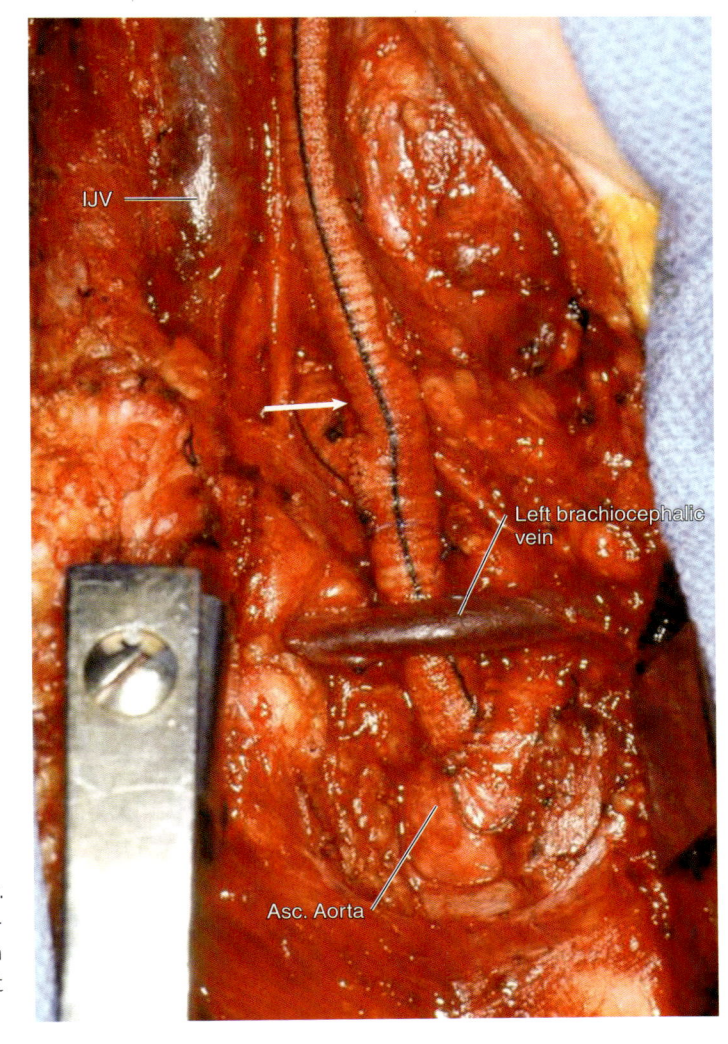

Figure 11-5. Aortocarotid-subclavian artery bypass graft. The Dacron graft from the ascending aorta to the right common carotid artery, with a side-arm graft to the right subclavian artery, demonstrates passage of the graft posterior to the left brachiocephalic vein.

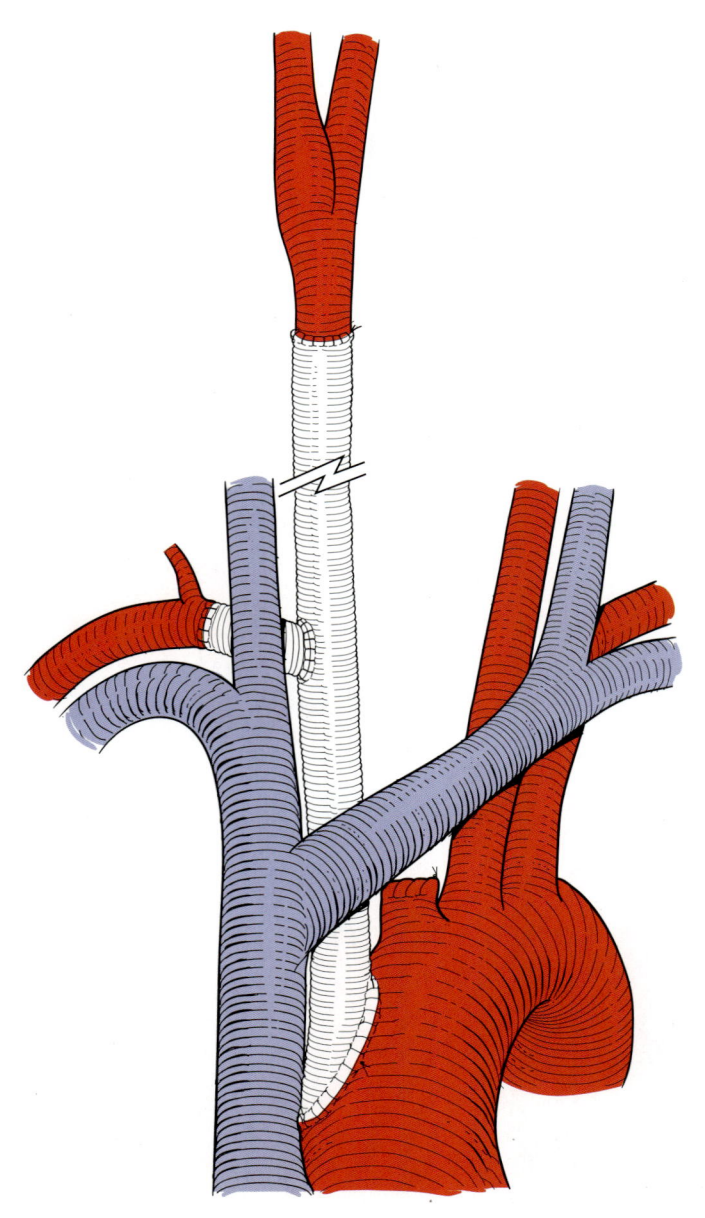

Figure 11-6. Branched graft technique to the right subclavian and carotid arteries. The graft is tunneled from its origin on the aorta posterior to the left brachiocephalic vein. A second synthetic graft of the same size is taken off of the main graft in an end-to-side manner and is sewn end to end from the lateral midportion of the first graft to the right subclavian artery.

and retrograde flushing are performed before completion of the anastomosis. Allowing retrograde bleeding from the subclavian is the safest method of checking suture line hemostasis.

Restoration of flow proceeds with release of the clamp on the subclavian artery, followed by the proximal graft and finally the carotid artery. Arterial flow should be palpable in the distal vessels. Resection of the intervening portion of the innominate artery should be performed in order to decompress the mediastinum. The proximal stump must be oversewn, with a horizontal suture followed by a running over-and-over suture of 4-0 or 3-0 polypropylene.

If the patient's disease process extends beyond the bifurcation into the subclavian artery, this can be addressed. This may be accomplished either by primary endarterectomy with tacking sutures at the distal extent or by use of a bifurcated or side-arm graft extending distally along the right subclavian artery beyond the extent of the lesion (Fig. 11-6).

ASCENDING AORTA-BILATERAL CAROTID ARTERY BYPASS

For this procedure, exposure of the aortic root is performed in the same manner as described earlier. On the right side the sternal incision may be extended superiorly along the anterior border of the SCM to reach the carotid bulb or a separate

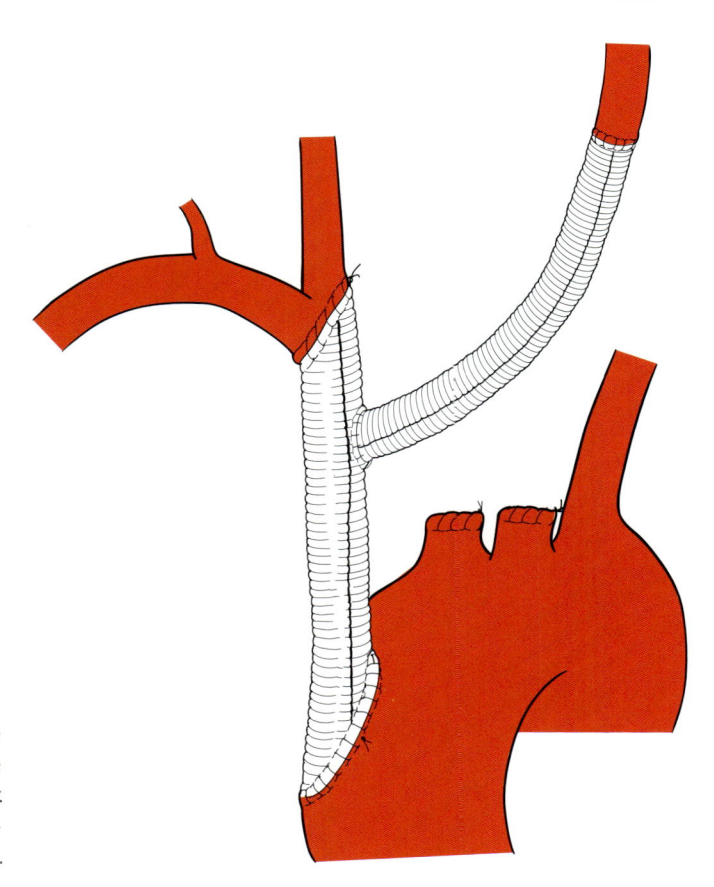

Figure 11-7. Branched graft to the innominate and left common carotid arteries. The initial graft is anastomosed to the innominate artery just proximal to the bifurcation. A side arm is taken off the left side of the graft and crosses to the left common carotid artery. This is completed end to end, and the left common carotid is oversewn close to the aorta with resection of the intervening segment.

incision may be used, and on the left side a second incision, as if for a standard endarterectomy, is performed to access the left carotid artery or bulb.

The proximal anastomosis to the ascending aorta is performed as described earlier. The more diseased of the two carotid arteries is reconstructed first to maintain as much cerebral blood flow as possible. The distal anastomosis is performed to the carotid bifurcation, either end to side or end to end. As with a branched graft to the right subclavian artery, a side arm is added on the left lateral portion of the initial bypass graft; it is carried to the left carotid artery as well (Fig. 11-7). Relaxation of the sternal retractor allows optimal placement of the side-arm anastomosis.

If necessary, standard carotid endarterectomies may be performed concurrently. Before securing the distal anastomosis, the vessels are flushed antegrade and retrograde. Restoration of flow is via the proximal graft, the external carotid artery, and then the internal carotid artery. If necessary, a trifurcated bypass graft may be performed to the right subclavian artery, the right common carotid artery, and the left common carotid artery (Figs. 11-8 and 11-9). If the patient has bilateral subclavian artery disease, the right subclavian artery is typically reconstructed, even if asymptomatic, to allow accurate assessment of blood pressure.

CLOSURE

Closure proceeds in the same fashion for either procedure. Hemostasis is confirmed throughout the operative field. Protamine is given for reversal of the effects of systemic heparin. Chest and mediastinal drains are placed. Wire reapproximation of the sternum is performed, and the subcutaneous tissue and skin are closed in layers in the standard fashion.

Postoperative Care

- **Monitoring of neurologic examination and peripheral vascular status.** In the immediate postoperative period, a complete neurologic examination should be performed, as well as assessment of pulses in the bilateral upper extremities.

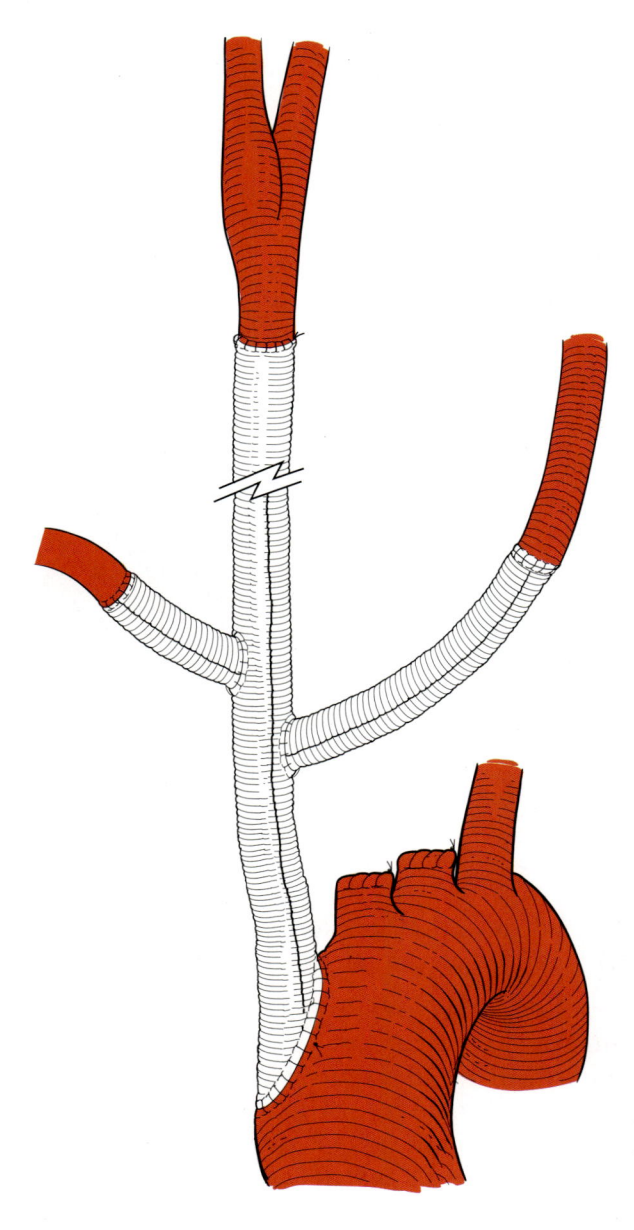

Figure 11-8. Trifurcated graft from the ascending aorta to the right subclavian, right carotid, and left carotid arteries. The main graft extends to the right common carotid artery, with two branches from either side of the main graft to the right subclavian artery and the left common carotid artery.

- **Hemodynamic monitoring.** Blood pressure should be controlled, and vasoactive agents may be used if necessary. In cases where severe bilateral carotid stenoses or obstructions are bypassed, reperfusion syndrome may be seen.

- **Chest and mediastinal tubes.** Management of chest tubes or mediastinal tubes and drains should follow standard protocols, with chest x-rays obtained postoperatively and 1 to 3 hours after removal of chest tubes, particularly in the mechanically ventilated patient. Drainage should typically not exceed 2 mL/kg/day, or 200 mL/day, before tube removal.

- **Physical activity.** Standard precautions for poststernotomy activity should be followed, and patients should be educated on these before discharge. For 5 to 8 weeks after a median sternotomy, upper extremity lifting should be restricted to 5 to 8 pounds. Range of motion and lifting of 1 to 3 pounds is permissible if there is no evidence of sternal instability such as sternal movement, pain, or popping. Progressive rehabilitation is needed after a median sternotomy to improve thoracic motion, pulmonary function, symptoms, and functional status.

- **Postoperative surveillance.** Patients should be followed at 6 weeks, 6 months, and yearly thereafter. Computed tomography angiography may be necessary, but duplex ultrasound and measurement of bilateral upper extremity blood pressure may be sufficient.

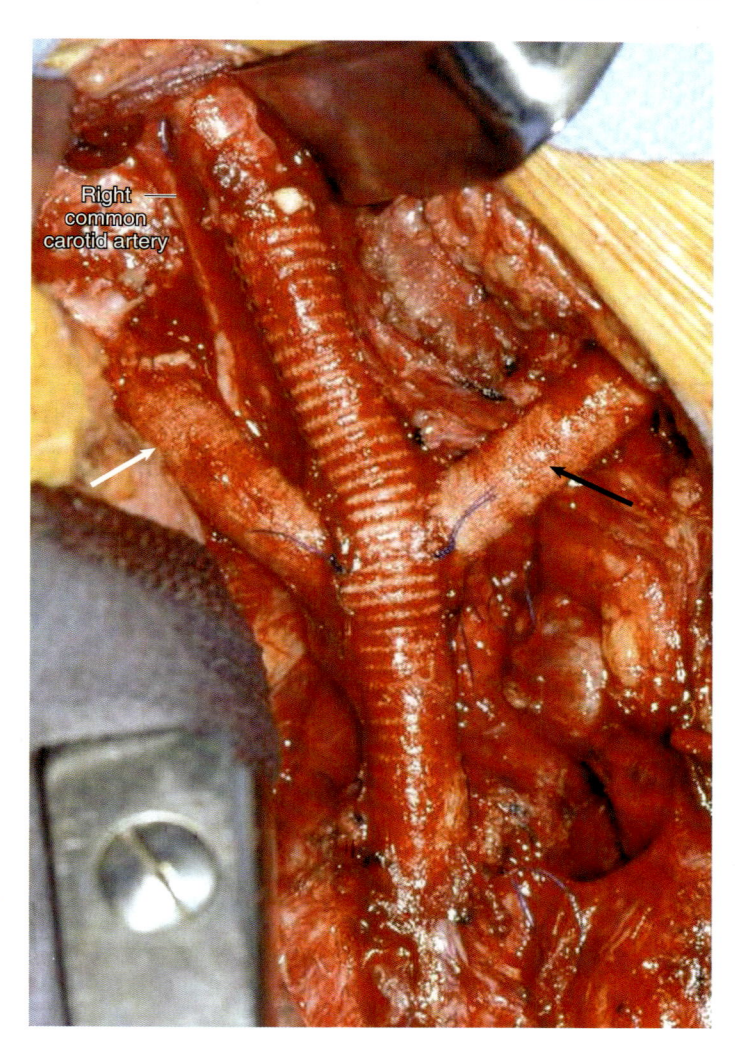

Figure 11-9. Trifurcated graft from the ascending aorta to the right subclavian, right carotid, and left carotid arteries. A Dacron bypass graft extends from the ascending aorta to the right common carotid artery, with side-arm grafts to the right subclavian artery and the left common carotid artery.

Complications

- Neurologic
  - Stroke
  - Transient ischemic attack (TIA)
  - Cerebral reperfusion syndrome
- Nerve injury
  - Horner syndrome
  - Laryngeal nerve palsy
  - Phrenic nerve palsy
  - Brachial plexus injury
- Hemorrhage
- Lymphatic leak
- Pneumothorax, hemothorax, chylothorax
  - Treatment consists of placement of chest tubes combined with control of the source of hemorrhage or lymphatic leak.

REFERENCES

1. Halsted WS: Ligation of the first portion of the left subclavian artery and excision of a subclavio-axillary aneurism, *Johns Hopkins Hospital Bulletin* 3:93-94, 1892.
2. Elkin DC: Exposure of blood vessels, *JAMA* 132:421-424, 1946.
3. DeBakey ME, Morris GC, Jordan GL, et al: Segmental thrombo-obliterative disease of branches of aortic arch: Successful surgical treatment, *JAMA* 166:998-1003, 1958.

4. Crawford ES, Debakey ME, Morris GC, et al: Surgical treatment of occlusion of innominate common carotid and subclavian arteries. A 10 year experience, *Surgery* 65:17-31, 1969.
5. Fields WS, Lemak NA: Joint Study of extracranial arterial occlusion. VII. Subclavian steal. A review of 168 cases, *JAMA* 222:1139-1143, 1972.
6. Wylie EJ, Effeney DJ: Surgery of the aortic arch branches and vertebral arteries, *Surg Clin North Am* 59:669-680, 1979.
7. Carlson RE, Ehrenfeld WK, Stoney RJ, et al: Innominate artery endarterectomy. A 16-year experience, *Arch Surg* 112:1389-1393, 1977.
8. Kieffer E, Sabatier J, Koskas F, et al: Atherosclerotic innominate artery occlusive disease: Early and long-term results of surgical reconstruction, *J Vasc Surg* 21:326-336, 1995.
9. Berguer R, Morasch MD, Kline RA: Transthoracic repair of innominate and common carotid artery disease: Immediate and long-term outcome for 100 consecutive surgical reconstructions, *J Vasc Surg* 27:34-41, 1998.
10. Vogt DP, Hertzer NR, O'Hara PJ, et al: Brachiocephalic arterial reconstruction, *Ann Surg* 196:541-552, 1982.
11. Crawford ES, Stowe CL, Powers RW Jr: Occlusion of the innominate, common carotid, and subclavian arteries: Long-term results of surgical treatment, *Surgery* 94:781-791, 1983.
12. Zelenock GB, Cronenwett JL, Graham LM, et al: Brachiocephalic arterial occlusions and stenoses. Manifestations and management of complex lesions, *Arch Surg* 120:370-376, 1985.
13. Evans WE, Williams TE, Hayes JP: Aortobrachiocephalic reconstruction, *Am J Surg* 156:100-102, 1988.
14. Cherry KJ Jr, McCllough JL, Hallett JW Jr, et al: Technical principles of direct innominate artery revascularization: A comparison of endarterectomy and bypass grafts, *J Vasc Surg* 9:718-723, 1989.
15. Reul GJ, Jacobs MJ, Gregoric ID, et al: Innominate artery occlusive disease: Surgical approach and long-term results, *J Vasc Surg* 14:405-412, 1991.
16. Schmidt WA, Gromnica-Ihle E: What is the best approach to diagnosing large-vessel vasculitis? *Best Pract Res Clin Rheumatol* 19:223-242, 2005.
17. Kerr GS, Hallahan CW, Giordano J, et al: Takayasu arteritis, *Ann Intern Med* 120:919-929, 1994.
18. Ogino H, Matsuda H, Minatoya K, et al: Overview of late outcome of medical and surgical treatment for Takayasu arteritis, *Circulation* 118:2738-2747, 2008.
19. Meave A, Soto ME, Reyes PA, et al: Pre-pulseless Takayasu's arteritis evaluated with 18F-FDG positron emission tomography and gadolinium-enhanced magnetic resonance angiography, *Tex Heart Inst J* 34:466-469, 2007.
20. Kobayashi Y, Ishii K, Oda K, et al: Aortic wall inflammation due to Takayasu arteritis imaged with 18F-FDG PET coregistered with enhanced CT, *J Nucl Med* 46:917-922, 2005.
21. Conomy JP, Kellermeyer RW: Delayed cerebrovascular consequences of therapeutic radiation. A clinicopathologic study of a stroke associated with radiation-related carotid arteriopathy, *Cancer* 36:1702-1708, 1975.
22. Hassen-Khodja R, Kieffer E: University Association for Research in Vascular Surgery. Radiotherapy-induced supra-aortic trunk disease: Early and long-term results of surgical and endovascular reconstruction, *J Vasc Surg* 40:254-261, 2004.
23. Peterson BG, Resnick SA, Morasch MD, et al: Aortic arch vessel stenting: A single-center experience using cerebral protection, *Arch Surg* 141:560-563, 2006.
24. Takach TJ, Reul GJ, Cooley DA, et al: Myocardial thievery: The coronary-subclavian steal syndrome, *Ann Thorac Surg* 81:386-392, 2006.
25. Sullivan TM, Gray BH, Bacharach JM, et al: Angioplasty and primary stenting of the subclavian, innominate, and common carotid arteries in 83 patients, *J Vasc Surg* 28:1059-1065, 1998.
26. Carpenter JP, Holland GA, Golden MA, et al: Magnetic resonance angiography of the aortic arch, *J Vasc Surg* 25:145-151, 1997.
27. Papantchev V, Hristov S, Todorova D, et al: Some variations of the circle of Willis, important for cerebral protection in aortic surgery: A study in Eastern Europeans, *Eur J Cardiothorac Surg* 31:982-989, 2007.
28. Longo MJ, Remetz MS: Cardiovascular manifestations of systemic autoimmune diseases, *Clin Chest Med* 19:793-808, 1998.
29. Fields CE, Bower TC, Cooper LT, et al: Takayasu's arteritis: Operative results and influence of disease activity, *J Vasc Surg* 43:64-71, 2006.

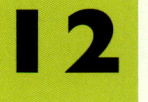

12 Extraanatomic Repair of Aortic Arch Vessels

MARK D. MORASCH

Historical Background

Savory[1] was the first to describe a patient with signs and symptoms suggesting occlusive disease involving the aortic arch vessels. Nearly 20 years later, in 1875, Broadbent[2] chronicled a patient who while living had no radial pulses and at postmortem examination was found to have brachiocephalic and left subclavian artery occlusion. In 1908 Takayasu[3] reported a patient with an ischemic retinopathy on ophthalmologic examination who later was found to have occlusive lesions in all three aortic arch vessels from a chronic inflammatory process that was later termed "pulseless disease" by Shimizu and Sano.[4] The inflammatory arteritis involving the arch branches now bears Takayasu's name. In 1960 Contorni[5] was the first to describe the anatomy of subclavian artery steal.

The first surgical procedures were performed for aneurysmal changes of the arch vessels, mostly syphilitic subclavian lesions. The first attempt at surgical correction of a proximal subclavian aneurysm, by innominate ligation, was carried out by Mott of New York City in 1818,[6] but the patient did not survive. Bahnson[7] was the first to perform a bypass from the ascending aorta to the innominate artery using an aortic homograft in a patient with occlusive lesions from syphilitic arteritis. One year later, in 1956, Davis and associates[8] described endarterectomy of an innominate artery through a right anterior thoracotomy for a symptomatic atherosclerotic occlusive lesion. Endarterectomy to reestablish flow through obliterated subclavian vessels was described by Cate and Scott[9] in 1957.

In 1956 Lyons[10] first reported a series of four subclavian to carotid artery bypasses from a cervical approach. In 1964 Parrott[11] reported two subclavian-to-carotid transpositions through a similar exposure. In 1994 Berguer and Gonzalez[12] described transcervical extraanatomic revascularization of the aortic arch vessels via a retropharyngeal route.

Indications

Atherosclerosis is, by far, the most common disease affecting the aortic arch vessels. Occlusive lesions less commonly result from inflammatory diseases such as Takayasu arteritis, or they can be the result of exposure to therapeutic radiation.

Severe disease is defined as stenosis with a diameter of more than 75%. In addition, in symptomatic patients, a deep ulcerated plaque or a thrombus within the arterial lumen is also considered a severe lesion even though the defect may be less than 75% of the diameter. When the disease is seen in multiple trunks, the occlusive process is likely an extension of disease originating within the aortic arch that has "spilled over" into the vessel ostia. Accordingly, the pathophysiology of vertebrobasilar ischemia is typically from low flow. Single trunk disease manifests more commonly as symptoms from hemispheric or upper extremity emboli. Isolated proximal disease can lead to symptomatic steal phenomenon.

Symptomatic atherosclerotic trunk disease may manifest as ocular, hemispheric, or vertebrobasilar transient ischemic attack or stroke. Patients commonly present with a combination of both anterior and posterior cerebrovascular ischemic symptoms. Cerebrovascular symptoms can be the result of emboli or low flow. Patients with subclavian steal syndrome present with posterior cerebrovascular symptoms as blood is siphoned from the basilar artery (Fig. 12-1). A similar but less common steal phenomenon can occur when the innominate artery is occluded and flow in the common carotid artery and ipsilateral vertebral artery is reversed to supply the right arm. Another rare problem is that of myocardial ischemia from the phenomenon of coronary steal, which can develop in patients with innominate or subclavian disease proximal to an internal mammary revascularization of the coronary arteries. Such patients can also present with symptoms of upper extremity ischemia. Patients may develop varying degrees of arm ischemia, ranging from the claudication observed in patients with subclavian steal to limb-threatening ischemia resulting from extensive arterial occlusion or emboli.

Over the last decade the most common indication for surgical manipulation of the aortic arch vessels has been to prepare patients with thoracic and thoracoabdominal aortic aneurysms, dissections, or traumatic tears for an endovascular stent-graft repair. Left subclavian artery and even left common carotid artery transpositions are not infrequently performed to preserve vertebral and left upper extremity flow while extending the proximal neck "landing zone" before endograft deployment (Fig. 12-2).

Preoperative Preparation

- Once a diagnosis has been established, multiplanar views of the aortic arch using digital subtraction angiography, computed tomography (CT) angiography, or magnetic resonance angiography are necessary for planning arch branch revascularization. A complete arch and four-vessel study can be performed with emphasis placed upon the vessel's origins and late views to show vascular reconstitution from steal. Magnetic resonance and CT angiography are noninvasive modalities with imaging capabilities that may equal those for invasive angiography.
- It is often useful to obtain a transesophageal echocardiogram (TEE) to assess myocardial function and rule out a cardioembolic source. In addition, like CT, TEE allows for the identification of significant calcific lesions or atheromata within the arch that would preclude aortic clamping during direct repair or contraindicate passage of wires and catheters for antegrade endolumenal therapy.
- Patients with recent brain infarcts (symptomatic or silent) should have surgery delayed, especially if multiple vessel revascularization is considered to decrease the risk of reperfusion injury.
- If a cervical approach to trunk revascularization is planned, preoperative cardiac evaluation should follow guidelines similar to those for carotid bifurcation surgery.
- Preoperative aspirin is administered before surgery based upon recommendations for carotid surgery.
- Vocal cord function should be evaluated if patients have a history of prior carotid surgery.
- A single dose of prophylactic antibiotics are administered within 1 hour of incision.
- Blood pressure monitoring by the intraoperative arterial line is advisable.

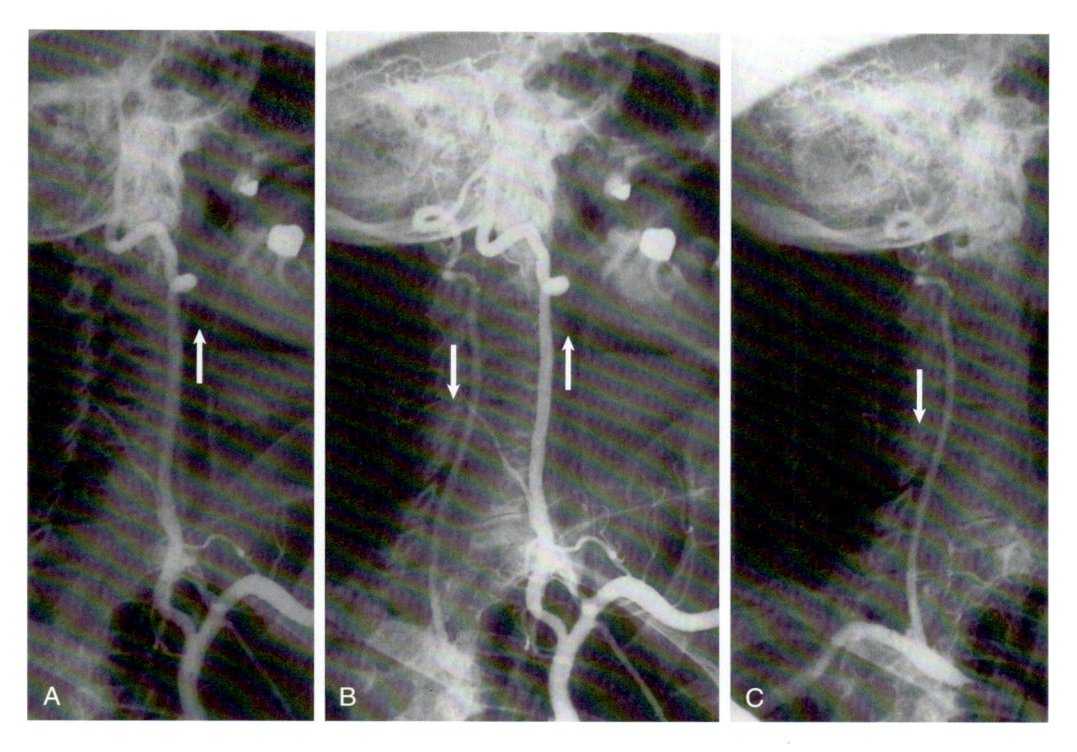

EXTRAANATOMIC REPAIR OF AORTIC ARCH VESSELS   141

Figure 12-1. Proximal right subclavian artery occlusion accounting for radiographic evidence of subclavian vertebral steal. *Arrows* depict the direction of blood flow up the left vertebral artery (**A**), down the right vertebral artery (**B**), and filling the right subclavian artery (**C**).

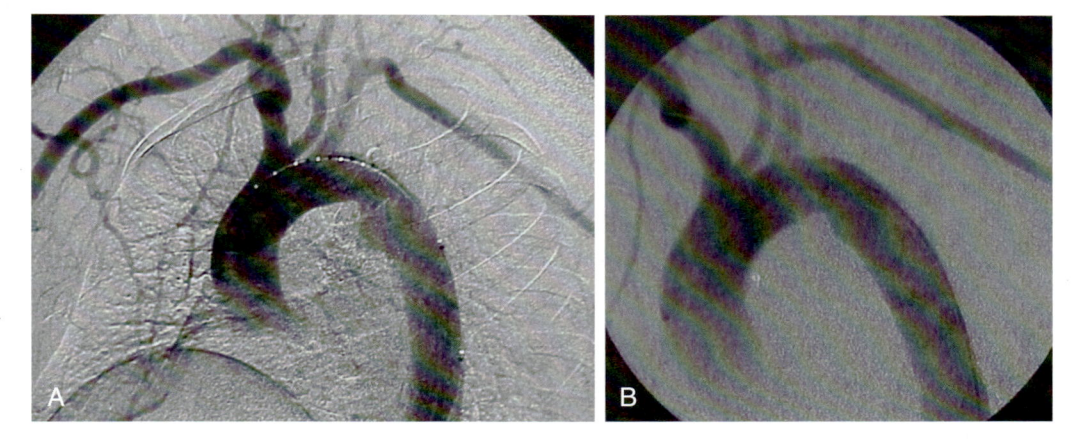

Figure 12-2. A, Angiogram showing traumatic aortic transection. **B,** Angiogram after treatment of aortic injury with endograft showing subclavian transposition.

Operative Strategy

SURGICAL ANATOMY OF THE COMMON CAROTID AND SUBCLAVIAN ARTERIES

The aortic arch vessels normally develop as three separate trunks taking origin from the arch of the aorta within the superior mediastinum. The conventional definition of the aortic arch vessels includes the innominate artery, the subclavian arteries to involve the origins of the vertebral arteries, and the common carotid arteries proximal to their bifurcations. The innominate artery and the left common carotid artery originate close to one another and ascend in the neck on either side of the trachea. The left subclavian artery is the third of three trunks, and it originates posterior to and to the left of the left common carotid artery. The vagus and right recurrent laryngeal nerves cross the anterior aspect of the right subclavian artery adjacent to the innominate bifurcation (Fig. 12-3). On the left side, the vagus nerve lies close to the left common carotid artery, and phrenic nerves cross one another between the left common carotid artery and the left subclavian artery under the cover of the pleura. On the left side, the thoracic duct drains into the venous system at the confluence of the internal jugular and subclavian veins and can clearly be seen during exposure of the proximal subclavian artery. On the right side, multiple lymphatic channels are present in a similar position.

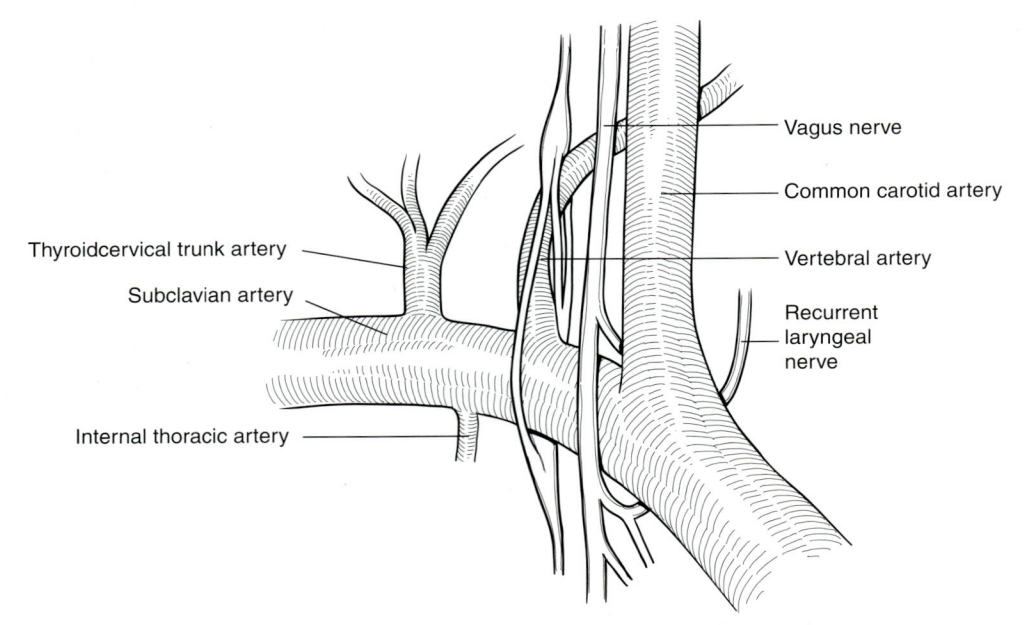

Figure 12-3. Course of the normal right recurrent laryngeal nerve.

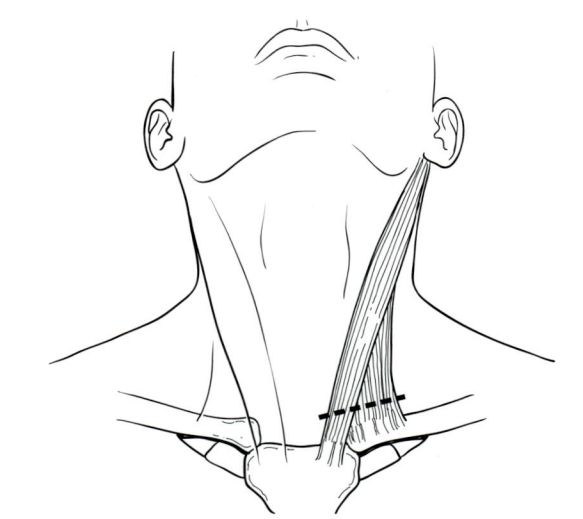

Figure 12-4. Incision for subclavian-to-carotid transposition.

CAROTID-SUBCLAVIAN ARTERY TRANSPOSITION

The subclavian artery may be transposed to the adjacent carotid artery or vice versa. Not only is preservation of the vertebral artery important, but it may be desirable to preserve the internal mammary artery when performing a subclavian transposition. In the reverse transposition from common carotid artery to subclavian artery, an adequate length of proximally narrowed common carotid artery can easily be mobilized to transpose it to the adjacent subclavian artery.

Arterial transpositions are completed through a short, medially placed transverse cervical incision above the clavicle (Fig. 12-4). Both the neck and the sternal areas should be prepped into the field. After raising subplatysmal flaps, the surgical dissection is carried out between the two heads of the sternocleidomastoid muscle. This is an important contradistinction from bypass, which is carried out lateral to the entire sternocleidomastoid muscle. After dividing the omohyoid muscle between ligatures or with electrocautery, the jugular vein is reflected laterally and the common carotid artery is reflected medially with the vagus nerve. The carotid artery is mobilized circumferentially, with the dissection carried out inferiorly toward the mediastinum. On the left side, the thoracic duct and small identifiable lymphatics

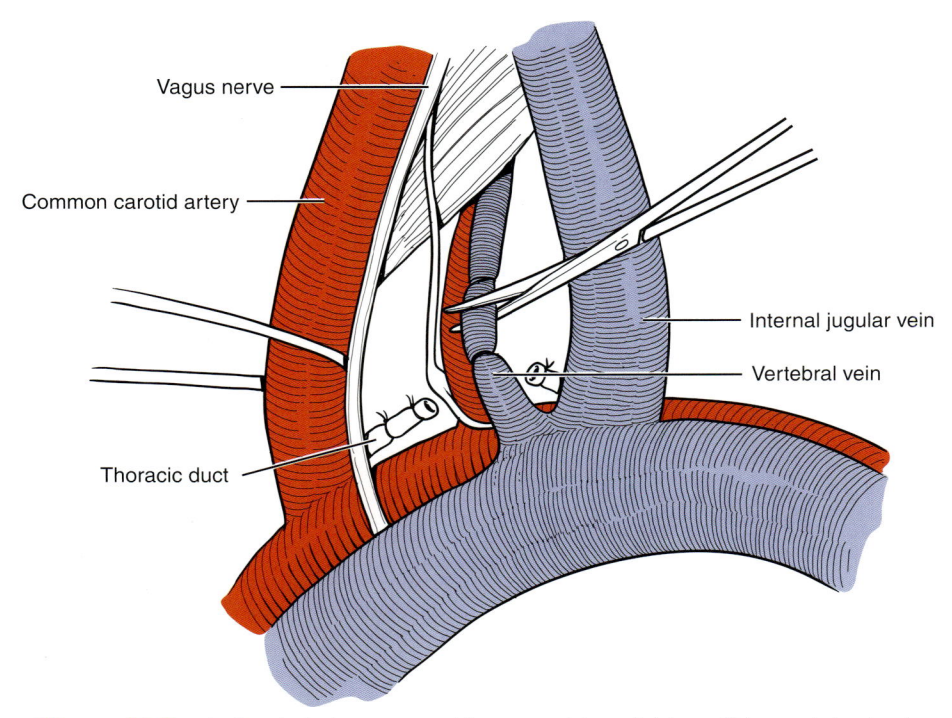

Figure 12-5. Left subclavian-to-carotid transposition: division of the vertebral vein.

are identified, ligated, and divided. On the right side, multiple cervical lymphatic channels must be tied. After dividing the vertebral vein, the subclavian artery and its proximal branches can be identified behind the clavicle (Fig. 12-5). If the vessel is patent, digital palpation can help with localization. Care must be taken when isolating and controlling the vertebral artery, because it originates from an awkward position on the posterior aspect of the subclavian artery. The medial aspect of the anterior scalene muscle may be encountered with more lateral dissection of the subclavian artery. Slight lateral reflection of this muscle may be necessary in order to obtain control of the vessel distal to the thyrocervical trunk, and there should be no hesitation to divide this muscle if needed for adequate exposure, protecting the phrenic nerve. The subclavian artery is dissected as far proximal as possible and well into the mediastinum. It is possible to enter the pleural space anteriorly. This can be avoided by keeping the dissection close to the arterial wall. Care is also taken to avoid disrupting sympathetic branches, which cross anterior to the subclavian artery and ascend in the neck alongside the vertebral artery. Once heparin has been administered, the subclavian artery and its proximal branches are controlled. The vertebral artery, mammary artery, and thryocervical trunk are temporarily occluded with microbulldog-type clamps. The distal subclavian artery can be controlled with loops or preferably with a profunda clamp. The proximal subclavian artery is then transected beyond a right-angled clamp or stapled with a vascular load stapler. It is important to secure the proximal stump immediately after the diseased artery has been divided; if control of the transected stump is lost in the chest or mediastinum, the consequences can be devastating. Control requires emergent sternotomy or thoracotomy. At this point the carotid artery is slightly rotated to expose the posterior aspect and then clamped proximally and distally. A punch arteriotomy is created in the side of the donor carotid artery and the end-to-side anastomosis is completed without tension. Occasionally some redundant subclavian artery must be resected to avoid a kink. The anastomosis is facilitated by using a parachute technique and by starting the suture line on the posterior wall (Fig. 12-6, Video 12-1). Rarely is the subclavian artery too short to reach to the side of the carotid artery. If this problem is encountered, more carotid artery can be mobilized to swing it farther lateral to the subclavian. Clamps are removed, and finally flow is reestablished into the vertebral artery. A drain is useful to collect lymphatic fluid. The wound is closed by reapproximating the platysma and closing the skin with a fine subcutaneous stitch.

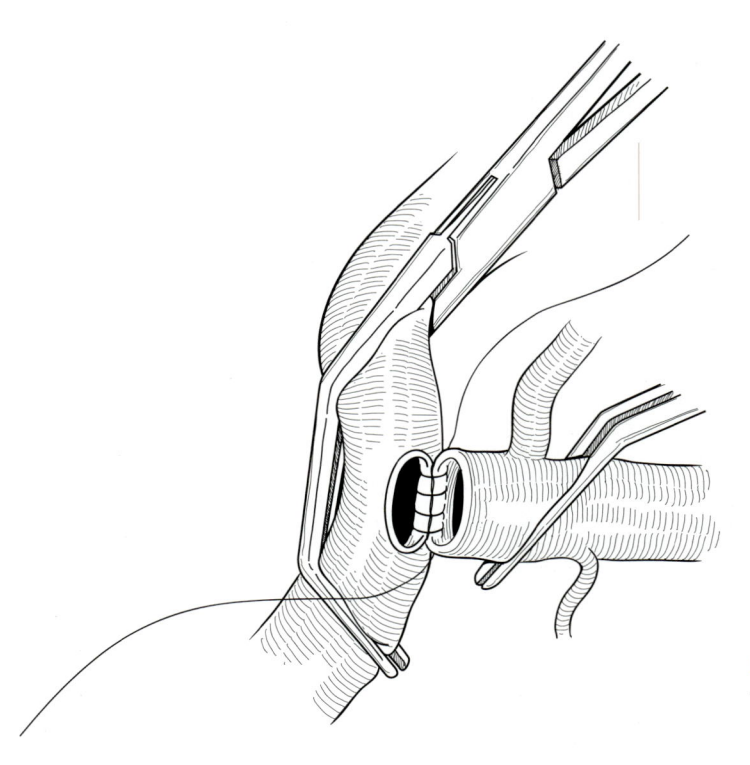

Figure 12-6. Left subclavian-to-carotid transposition: end-to-side anastomosis of the subclavian artery to the common carotid artery.

CAROTID-SUBCLAVIAN ARTERY BYPASS

Occasionally it is not feasible to do a straightforward arterial transposition, so the use of a bypass conduit becomes necessary. Arterial transposition is not possible when the vertebral artery takes off early from the subclavian artery. Another indication for carotid-subclavian bypass is proximal subclavian disease or anticipation of subclavian coverage with an endograft in a patient with symptomatic or the potential for symptomatic coronary steal and a patent internal mammary artery to coronary artery bypass graft. With the use of a cervical bypass, the arterial clamps can be placed beyond the internal mammary artery to avoid myocardial ischemia. Bypasses are performed, most expediently, through dissection just lateral to the clavicular head of the sternocleidomastoid muscle. The jugular vein is reflected medially to expose the common carotid artery. The vagus nerve is encountered during this portion of the dissection and must be protected. The scalene fat pad is divided with clamps and ligatures to prevent lymphatic leak. The subclavian artery is identified more distally than during transposition by dividing the anterior scalene muscle. Care must be taken to avoid injury to the phrenic nerve during this more lateral approach. The bypass is completed to or from the retroscalene portion of the subclavian artery, usually using a prosthetic conduit rather than a vein, by performing sequential clamping and serial anastomoses (Fig. 12-7). In this position prosthetic conduits clearly outperform autogenous vein with regard to long-term patency.[13,14]

CAROTID-CAROTID ARTERY BYPASS

If an extraanatomic approach is considered and the only inflow vessel is on the opposite side of the neck, the midline should be crossed using a retropharyngeal rather than a presternal or pretracheal path.[15] The retropharyngeal route is shorter and more direct (Fig. 12-8). A pretracheal or presternal routing of a bypass graft can result in erosion of overlying skin and is found obtrusive if the patient ever requires a sternotomy or a tracheotomy. The space can easily be indentified and a space for the graft can be created by passing a finger medial to the common carotid artery and behind the esophagus. A nasogastric tube or esophageal stethoscope helps to identify the correct plane behind the esophagus and in front of the prespinal fascia. Long subclavian-subclavian, axillary-axillary, and femoroaxillary bypasses should also be avoided unless there is no alternative because of significantly poor patency rates.

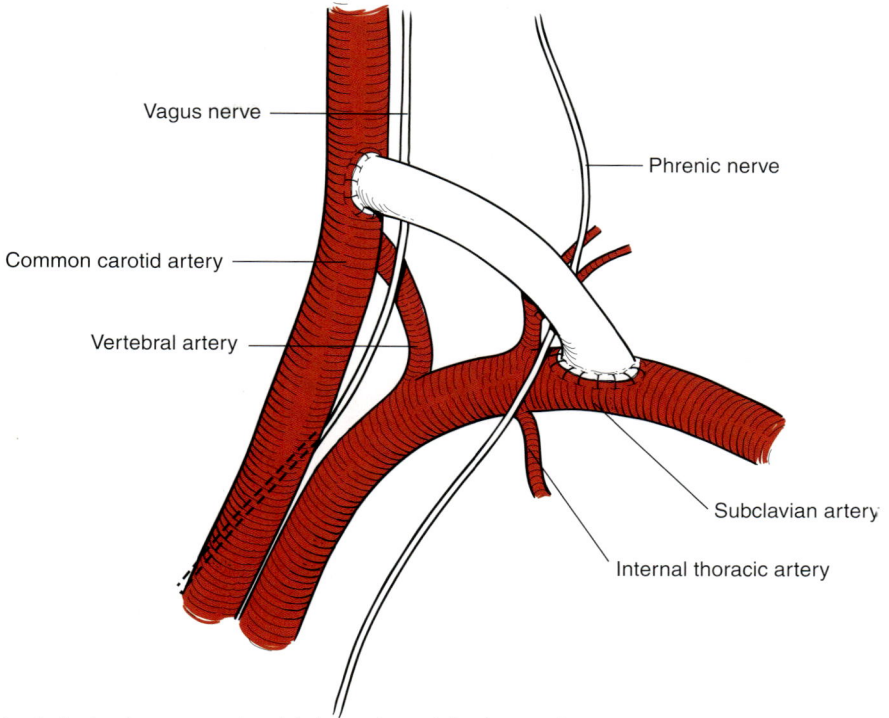

EXTRAANATOMIC REPAIR OF AORTIC ARCH VESSELS 145

Figure 12-7. Carotid subclavian bypass to the third portion of the latter: the anastomosis on the subclavian artery lies inferior to the divided scalenus anticus muscle, with preservation of the phrenic nerve.

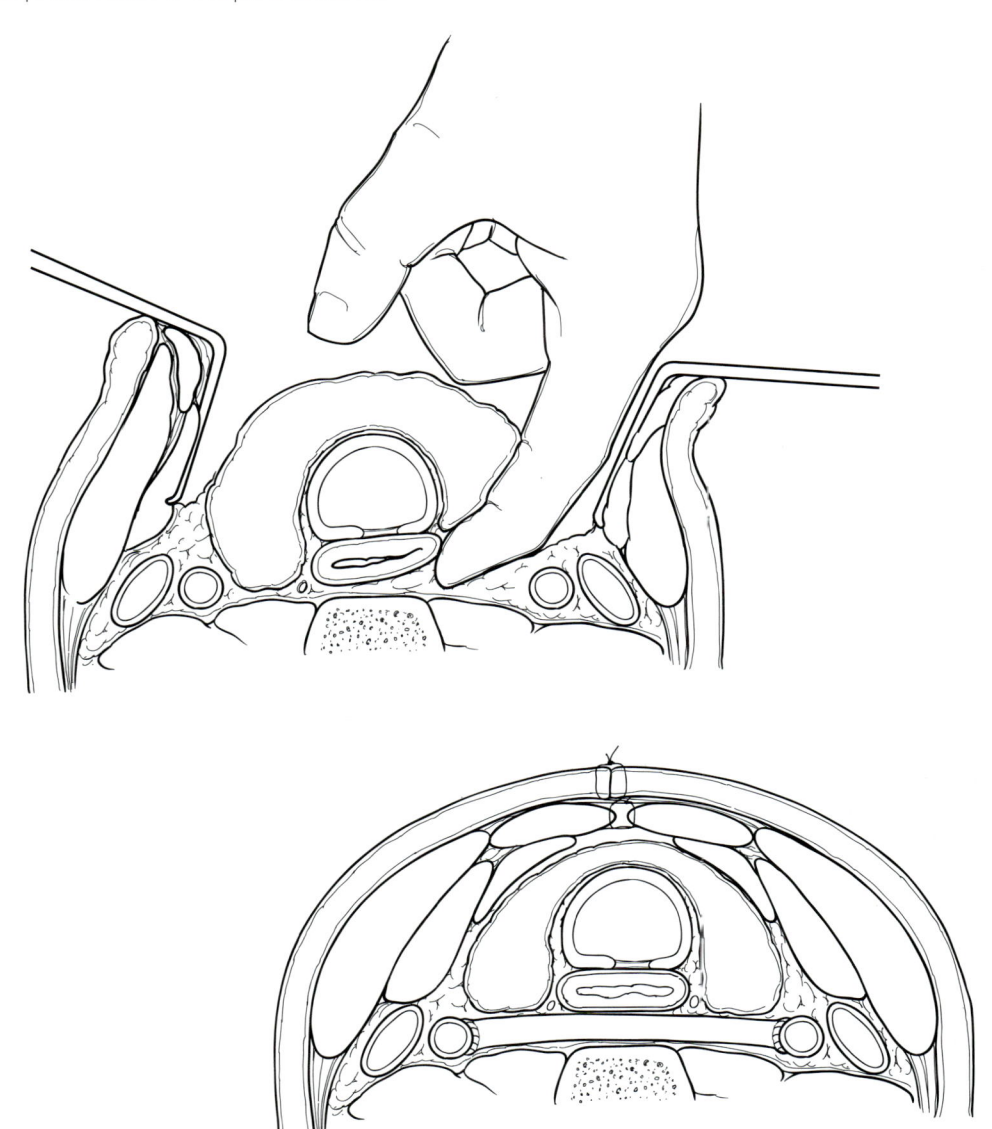

Figure 12-8. The retropharyngeal route is the shortest and most direct route for a transcervical bypass, as illustrated in this example of a right-to-left carotid-carotid bypass.

Pitfalls and Danger Points

- Vagus nerve injury
- Sympathectomy or Horner syndrome
- Thoracic duct or lymph leak
- Pneumothorax
- Loss of proximal vessel control or hemorrhage

Postoperative Care

- Patients spend 2 hours in the recovery room where they are closely observed for airway, bleeding, or neurologic complications.
- Patients are given a regular diet, encouraged to get out of bed on the day of surgery, and discharged home the following morning.
- A drain should be left in place until the first meal to exclude significant chylous leak but can almost always be removed the morning after surgery.
- Postoperative discomfort is managed with acetaminophen or a nonsteroidal antiinflammatory agent.
- An aspirin is given immediately after surgery for antiplatelet effect.
- Patency of the reconstruction can be assessed by palpating the distal radial or superficial temporal artery pulse or by measuring blood pressure.

Postoperative Complications

- **Lymph leak, lymphocele, and chylothorax.** Conservative management is appropriate initially for chylous or lymph leak, as well as late lymphocele or chylothorax, because most resolve. This includes local compression, dietary manipulation, and administration of octreotide. Leaks that persist beyond 3 days require reexploration of the surgical wound and an attempt at direct suture repair. Purse string placement of a small-gauge monofilament suture works best to control a large lymphatic or thoracic duct leak. If all else fails, ligation of the thoracic duct using video-assisted thoracotomy surgery can be considered.
- **Pneumothorax or hemothorax.** Pneumothorax can occur during proximal dissection of the subclavian artery. Entry into the pleura is easily recognized and treated at the time of occurrence. If the pneumothorax persists on a postoperative chest radiograph, it can be managed with short-term use of a small chest tube.
- **Horner syndrome.** Most patients experience at least short-lived Horner syndrome. It often is not noticeable to the patient but can be seen by observers. The treatment is expectant. Most resolve in time.
- **Vagus nerve injury.** Injury of the vagus nerve is usually manifest as hoarseness and is most often the result of traction on the vagus during exposure of the deep neck structures. Because this rarely is the result of cutting the recurrent nerve, usually time and patience are all that are required. If a vocal cord palsy persists beyond 3 months, cord medialization may be warranted.
- **Phrenic nerve injury.** Phrenic nerve palsy should not be seen with a subclavian transposition procedure and would indicate that the dissection was carried out more laterally than is necessary. It may occur during a bypass to or from the middle third of the subclavian artery when the anterior scalene is exposed and divided. Phrenic nerve palsy is manifest as shortness of breath with exertion, and a raised hemidiaphragm may be seen on a plain chest radiograph. The condition is definitively diagnosed on chest fluoroscopy. Phrenic nerve and diaphragmatic recovery usually occurs spontaneously within a few months. Alternatively, for the permanently damaged nerve, diaphragmatic pacing can be considered.

REFERENCES

1. Savory W: Case of a young woman in whom the main arteries of both upper extremities, and of the left side of the neck, were through-out completely obliterated, *Med Chir Trans* 39:205, 1856.
2. Broadbent W: Absence of pulsation in both radial arteries, the vessels being full of blood, *Trans Clin Soc (London)* 8:165, 1875.
3. Takayasu M: Case of queer changes in central blood vessels of retina, *Acta Soc Ophthalmol Jpn* 12:554, 1908.
4. Shimizu K, Sano K: Pulseless disease, *J Neurol Clin Neurol* 145:1095, 1951.
5. Contorni L: The vertebro-vertebral collateral circulation in obliteration of the subclavian artery at its origin, *Minerva Chir* 15:268-271, 1960.
6. Rutkow IM: Valentine Mott and the beginnings of vascular surgery, *Arch Surg* 136:1441, 2001.
7. Bahnson HT, Spencer FC, Quattlebaum JK Jr: Surgical treatment of occlusive disease of the carotid artery, *Ann Surg* 149:711-720, 1959.
8. Davis JB, Grove WJ, Julian OC: Thrombic occlusion of the branches of the aortic arch, Martorell's syndrome: Report of a case treated surgically, *Ann Surg* 144:124-126, 1956.
9. Cate WR Jr, Scott HW Jr: Cerebral ischemia of central origin: Relief by subclavian-vertebral artery thromboendarterectomy, *Surgery* 45:19-31, 1957.
10. Lyons C, Galbraith G: Surgical treatment of atherosclerotic occlusion of the internal carotid artery, *Ann Surg* 146:487-494, 1956.
11. Parrott JC: The subclavian steal syndrome, *Arch Surg* 88:661-665, 1964.
12. Berguer R, Gonzalez JA: Revascularization by the retropharyngeal route for extensive disease of the extracranial arteries, *J Vasc Surg* 19:217-224, 1994, discussion 225.
13. Morasch MD, Berguer R: Supra-aortic trunk revascularization. In Yao JSTP, editor: *Modern vascular surgery*, New York, 2000, McGraw-Hill, p 137.
14. Ziomek S, Quinones-Baldrich WJ, Busuttil RW, et al: The superiority of synthetic arterial grafts over autologous veins in carotid-subclavian bypass, *J Vasc Surg* 3:140-145, 1986.
15. Berguer R: Revascularization across the neck using the retropharyngeal rout. In Veith FJ, editor: *Current critical problems in vascular surgery, seventh volume*, St. Louis, 1996, Quality Medical Publishing.

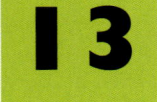

13 Endovascular Treatment of Aortic Arch Vessels—Innominate, Carotid, and Subclavian Arteries

PETER NAUGHTON • MANUEL GARCIA-TOCA • MARK K. ESKANDARI

Historical Background

Shimizu and Sano[1] first described surgical repair of an atherosclerotic aortic arch branch vessel lesion in 1951. Initially, open surgical repair was performed via a transthoracic approach, but this was replaced by the more popular extraanatomic bypass after Crawford and associates' report[2] demonstrating a mortality rate of only 5.6% for extraanatomic repair compared with 22% for those patients treated using a transthoracic approach. Their data were reinforced by a more contemporary series by Berguer and colleagues[3] that demonstrated a 10-year primary patency rate of 82% and perioperative stroke and mortality rates of 3.8% and 0.5%, respectively, among 100 consecutive cervical reconstructions for aortic arch vessel (AAV) lesions.

An endoluminal solution to atherosclerotic aortic arch branch vessel lesions is often credited to Mathias and co-workers,[4] who were the first to report a successful percutaneous transluminal angioplasty of an occlusive lesion in a supraaortic vessel in 1980. In a review of 423 subclavian and innominate artery angioplasties, a 92% initial technical success rate was achieved. However, a 19% incidence of restenosis was noted at 5 years. Subsequent reports demonstrated improved results when adjunctive stenting is used, in conjunction with angioplasty, for the treatment of stenotic lesions of branch vessels of the aortic arch.[5-7]

Indications

Atherosclerosis is the most common cause of AAV occlusive disease. Other causes include Takayasu arteritis, giant cell arteritis, and radiation-induced arteritis. As with extracranial carotid artery occlusive disease, many patients with AAV stenotic lesions do not have symptoms. Typically, the atherosclerotic process is localized to the ostium and the proximal portion of the arch vessel. Treatment is generally deemed necessary for patients presenting with symptoms referable to the involved vessel. In these instances, symptoms are due to hypoperfusion or distal embolization, which may occur either in the anterior or posterior cerebral circulation or upper extremity. In the patient with coronary revascularization based on the left internal mammary artery (LIMA), a proximal subclavian artery stenosis may lead to a coronary steal syndrome. Patients with Takayasu arteritis tend to have long, noncompliant fibrotic lesions rather than short, localized, proximal lesions and endoluminal therapy has been less durable.[8] Although firm guidelines for surgery or endoluminal therapy for aortic arch vessel lesions do not exist, most clinicians consider intervention for: (1) asymptomatic patients who present with an innominate or common carotid artery stenosis of at least

80%; or (2) symptomatic patients with an innominate, common carotid, or subclavian artery stenosis of at least 50%.

Preoperative Preparation

- Cardiovascular status should be assessed and medical management optimized. van Hattum and associates[7] observed that of 18 patients with atherosclerotic lesions of the arch vessels, 78% had coronary artery disease, 33% had carotid artery disease, and 61% were hypertensive. A history of a LIMA-based coronary artery bypass should be noted.
- Preoperative physical examination should include bilateral arm pressure measurements. Digital subtraction angiography, magnetic resonance angiography, or computed tomography angiography is advisable to identify the lesion site, length, tandem lesions, arch morphology, and preferred approach to access the lesion.
- Patients should receive clopidogrel (75 mg/day) and aspirin (325 mg/day) 5 days before the procedure. Alternatively, patients can receive a loading dose of clopidogrel (300 mg) the day prior to the planned intervention.
- Procedures may be performed under general anesthesia, monitored anesthesia care, or local anesthesia. Arterial line monitoring of blood pressure is recommended and prophylactic antibiotics should be considered.

Pitfalls and Danger Points

- Access site complications
- Inability to "seat" or position the sheath or guiding catheter
- Inability to cross the target lesion
- Stroke
- Vessel dissection or rupture
- "Jailing" the origin of the vertebral artery and internal mammary artery
- Contrast-induced nephrotoxicity
- Late stent failure

Operative Strategy

ANGIOGRAPHIC ANATOMY AND COMMON COLLATERAL PATHWAYS

The most common configuration of great vessel arch anatomy is the presence of three separate trunks, with the innominate artery giving rise to the right subclavian and common carotid arteries, the left common carotid artery nearby, and the left subclavian artery originating posterior to and to the left of the left common carotid artery. Common anatomic variants include a bovine arch configuration (16%-24%), as well as a left vertebral artery originating directly off the aortic arch (6%) and an aberrant right subclavian artery (0.5%-1%).

Collateral pathways that compensate for occlusive disease of the left subclavian artery include flow from the right subclavian artery into the right vertebral artery with retrograde flow into the left vertebral artery and subsequently into the left subclavian artery. Additional collateral pathways may arise from the external carotid artery, the ascending cervical artery, and the thyrocervical trunk.

Occlusive disease of the innominate artery will often result in retrograde flow from the right vertebral artery into the right common carotid and subclavian arteries.

ANATOMIC CONSIDERATIONS FOR AORTIC ARCH VESSELS

Long, occlusive lesions at the origin of a branch vessel or the presence of steep angulation off the aortic arch may be difficult to cross or maintain sheath access when using a femoral approach. A retrograde approach from the common carotid or brachial artery may help to overcome these problems (Fig. 13-1).

Care should be taken when treating a lesion in the subclavian artery close or innominate bifurcation to avoid jailing a major tributary such as a dominant vertebral artery or left internal mammary artery bypass to the left anterior descending coronary artery.

UNFAVORABLE ANATOMIC FEATURES

When the left common carotid artery originates from the innominate artery, there is potential for cerebral embolization.

Vessel tortuosity may be sufficiently severe to preclude endovascular intervention.

ACCESS FOR COMMON CAROTID ARTERY LESIONS

Factors influencing the decision to access a lesion using a retrograde or an antegrade approach include the presence of iliac occlusive disease, aortic arch morphology, angle of takeoff of the target vessel, lesion site and length.

If difficulty is encountered or anticipated via a transfemoral approach because of arch morphology or a tight orifice lesion, a retrograde approach may be more suitable. This approach is recommended for tandem lesions that require simultaneous carotid endarterectomy and stenting of a more proximal common carotid artery lesion.

ACCESS FOR SUBCLAVIAN AND INNOMINATE LESIONS

Lesions of the innominate artery may be treated via an antegrade (transfemoral) or retrograde (transbrachial or transcarotid) approach (Videos 13-1 through 13-4). A transbrachial approach may be performed percutaneously or via open cutdown. This approach precludes the need for selective catheterization from a remote access site.

LESION PREDILATION

Predilation with an undersized balloon is particularly useful in severely diseased lesions and lesions at the orifice in order to allow for safe passage of the stent delivery system. This technique also allows imaging of the distal extent of the lesion to assess the involvement of vertebral artery and internal mammary artery origins.

STENT SELECTION

When feasible, primary stenting has the theoretic benefit of minimizing microembolization. Short lesions close to the origin of the innominate artery or common carotid artery are best treated with a balloon-expandable stent because of their greater accuracy of placement, higher radial force, and good wall apposition. Stents should treat the target lesion and not cover excessive lengths of normal vessel.

Lesions of the mid-common carotid, subclavian, and axillary arteries, are relatively mobile, and frequently the best option is to use a self-expanding nitinol stent. Stents should not be used in the distal subclavian and proximal axillary artery because of the risk of impingement between the clavicle and the first rib. Although uncommon, late stent fracture has been observed after stenting of heavily calcified lesions of arch vessels (Fig. 13-2).

EMBOLIC PROTECTION DEVICES

When treating lesions of the common carotid, innominate, and proximal subclavian arteries via an antegrade approach, an embolic protection device should be used whenever feasible.[9] In treating a lesion of the common carotid or innominate artery through a transcarotid approach, cerebral protection can be achieved by distal clamping of the carotid artery during stent deployment, followed by aspiration of blood from the sheath before removal of the clamp.

PROTECTION OF THE VERTEBRAL ARTERY

It may be important to protect the vertebral artery when a lesion is close to the origin of this vessel. This can be achieved by inserting a second wire into the origin

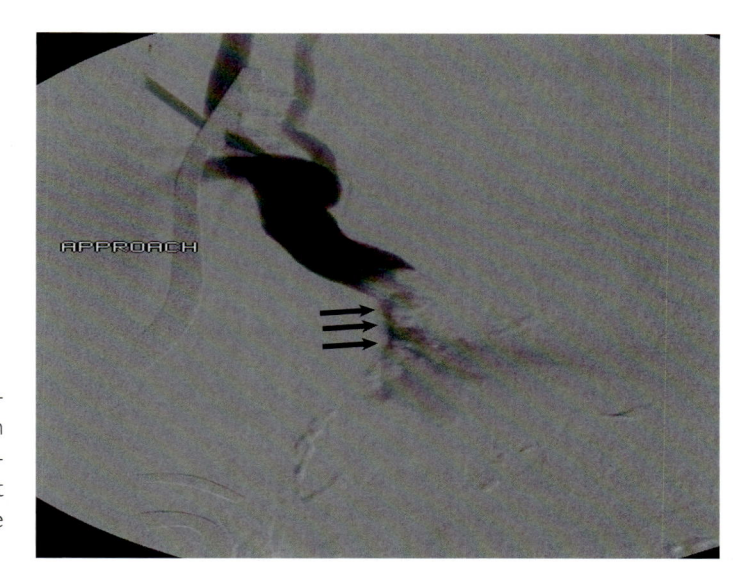

ENDOVASCULAR TREATMENT OF AORTIC ARCH VESSELS—INNOMINATE, CAROTID, AND SUBCLAVIAN ARTERIES 151

Figure 13-1. A retrograde angiogram using an open cervical approach provides an alternative strategy for visualizing an innominate lesion that may be difficult to cross using an antegrade approach. A bulky, calcific, tight lesion (arrows) is noted at the origin of the innominate artery with a blush of dye in the aortic arch.

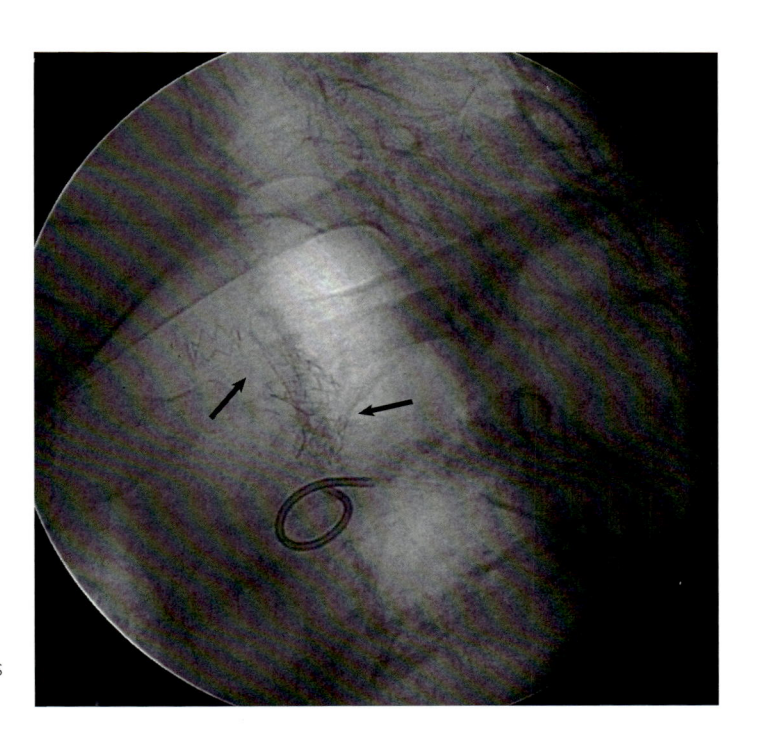

Figure 13-2. Radiographic film showing multiple stent fractures (arrows) are present in a stent placed in an innominate artery.

of the vertebral artery. If an 0.014-inch wire is used, a self-expanding stent on a 0.035-inch guidewire platform can be placed over both wires, ensuring that the origin of the vertebral artery is protected.

Operative Technique

ACCESS

Access to lesions of the aortic arch branch vessels includes percutaneous transfemoral or transbrachial approaches, as well as open or percutaneous transcarotid methods. In the transfemoral approach, a 6-Fr sheath is delivered proximal to the target lesion, thereby enabling an embolic protection device to cross the lesion. Alternatively, an angled 8-Fr guiding catheter can be used. Percutaneous transbrachial access is achieved just above the antecubital fossa using a micropuncture technique (21-Ga needle, 0.018-inch wire, and 4-Fr sheath) under ultrasound guidance (Fig. 13-3).[10] The axillary approach is used less often because of risks of hematoma and brachial plexus injury.

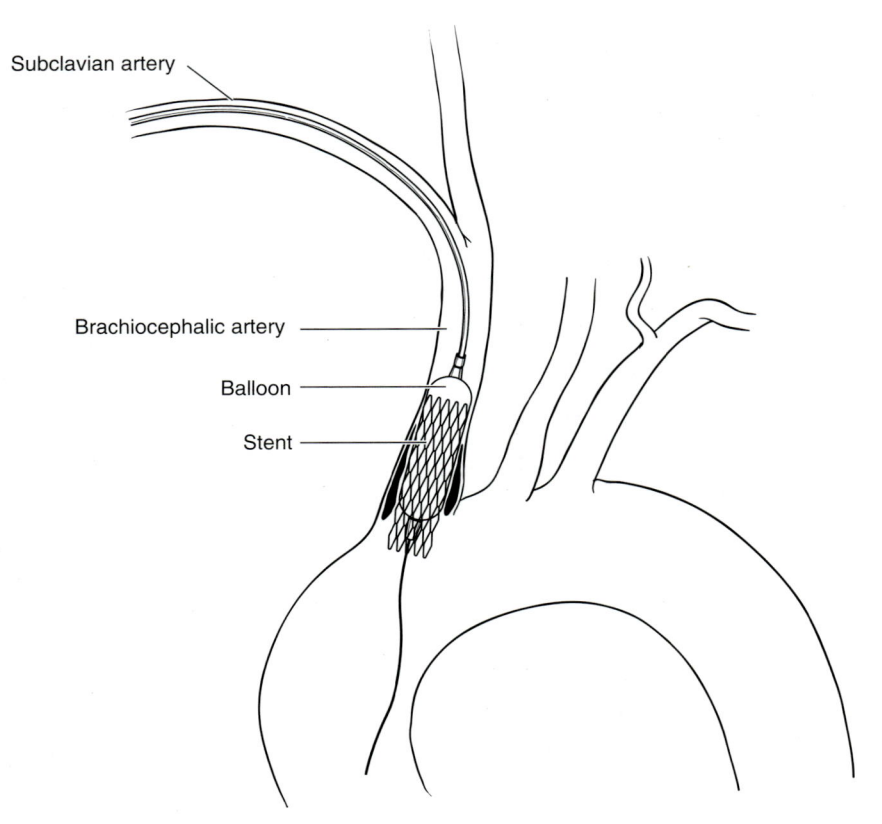

Figure 13-3. Stent deployment in the right innominate artery via brachial access. Note the stent overlap into the aortic arch.

The transcarotid approach may be performed percutaneously or by using an open cutdown. Generally, a small (2-3 cm) vertical incision at the base of the neck along the anterior border of the sternocleidomastoid muscle is used (Fig. 13-4). Cerebral protection may be achieved during the procedure by placing a vascular clamp across the common carotid artery distal to the entry site of the sheath. A pigtail catheter may also be passed transfemorally into the arch to optimize imaging during a transcarotid intervention.

ARCH VESSEL IMAGING AND SELECTIVE CATHETERIZATION

Minimizing catheter and guidewire manipulation is essential in limiting the risk of distal embolization. Similarly, great care must be taken not to introduce air bubbles into the system during the procedure, with some interventionalists recommending the use of a manifold. A left anterior oblique (30-45 degrees) projection is used to adequately visualize the origin of each of the arch vessels. A right anterior oblique (30-45 degrees) projection is helpful in visualizing the innominate bifurcation and the origins of the right subclavian and common carotid arteries. A variety of 4- and 5-Fr selective catheters may be used to cannulate arch vessels from the femoral approach, including simple curve (Davis, angled Glide, or vertebral) or complex curve (Vitek, Headhunter, or Simmons) catheters. The simple curve catheters are passed over a guidewire into the ascending aorta. The wire is then withdrawn and the catheter tip takes shape. These catheters are then gently pulled back across the aortic arch, slowly rotating in a counterclockwise direction in order to engage the vessel. Complex catheters are either self-forming (i.e., Vitek or Headhunter) or require forming within the aorta (i.e., Simmons). The Vitek catheter is generally formed in the proximal descending aorta and pushed retrograde across the aortic arch, allowing the tip to engage each of the arch vessels sequentially. The others are shaped in the ascending aorta or off the aortic valve and pulled antegrade across the arch into the appropriate vessel. When the selected vessel is cannulated a gentle injection of contrast is helpful to confirm position. These techniques are useful for selective catheterization and imaging, as well as subsequent placement of a long sheath into the origin of the vessel. Alternatively, an appropriately shaped guiding catheter (i.e., JR4) can be

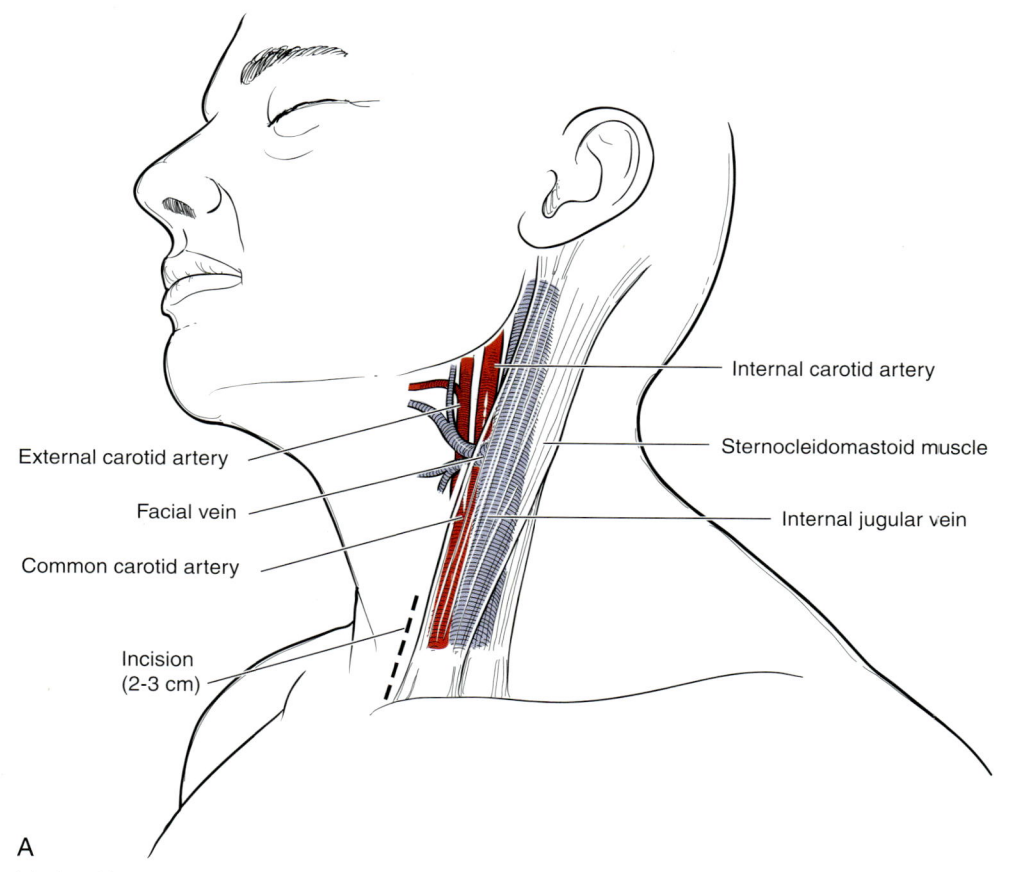

Figure 13-4. A, Neck with outlined incision in the base of the neck along the anterior border of the sternocleidomastoid muscle.
Continued

manipulated into the origin of the target vessel, particularly if the disease is proximal or if significant tortuosity is present.

INNOMINATE ARTERY STENTING

Most innominate artery atherosclerotic occlusive lesions are in the proximal portion of this short, large-diameter vessel. As such the vessel is often best approached retrograde from the right common carotid artery. Alternatively, a diagnostic aortic catheter can be placed from the femoral artery with the intervention performed through an open carotid approach under local or general anesthesia. After the common carotid artery is exposed, it is punctured under direct vision and a retrograde short 6-Fr sheath is placed. After systemic heparin has been administered, the lesion is crossed and predilated if necessary. This allows for easy passage of the stent delivery system (Videos 13-5 and 13-6). An appropriately sized short balloon-expandable stent is then placed with 2 to 3 mm of proximal extension into the aorta to avoid ostial restenosis (see Fig. 13-3). It is important not to dilate the vessel using a balloon diameter based on the more distal segment of the innominate artery, which typically has a poststenotic dilation. During each phase of the lesion manipulation, the common carotid artery distal to the sheath may be clamped and the stagnant column of blood may be aspirated from the side port of the sheath.

VERTEBRAL ARTERY ANGIOPLASTY AND STENTING

Most cases requiring vertebral artery angioplasty with stenting are performed from a femoral approach, although the brachial route has also been used. The stenotic lesion is crossed and treated with a 0.014- or 0.018-inch wire platform and small coronary-diameter balloon and stent. In contrast to intervention on the extracranial carotid artery, vertebral artery angioplasty is not usually performed with embolic protection. Balloon-expandable bare-metal stents are recommended for lesions of the V1 vertebral artery segment.

154 AORTIC ARCH VESSELS

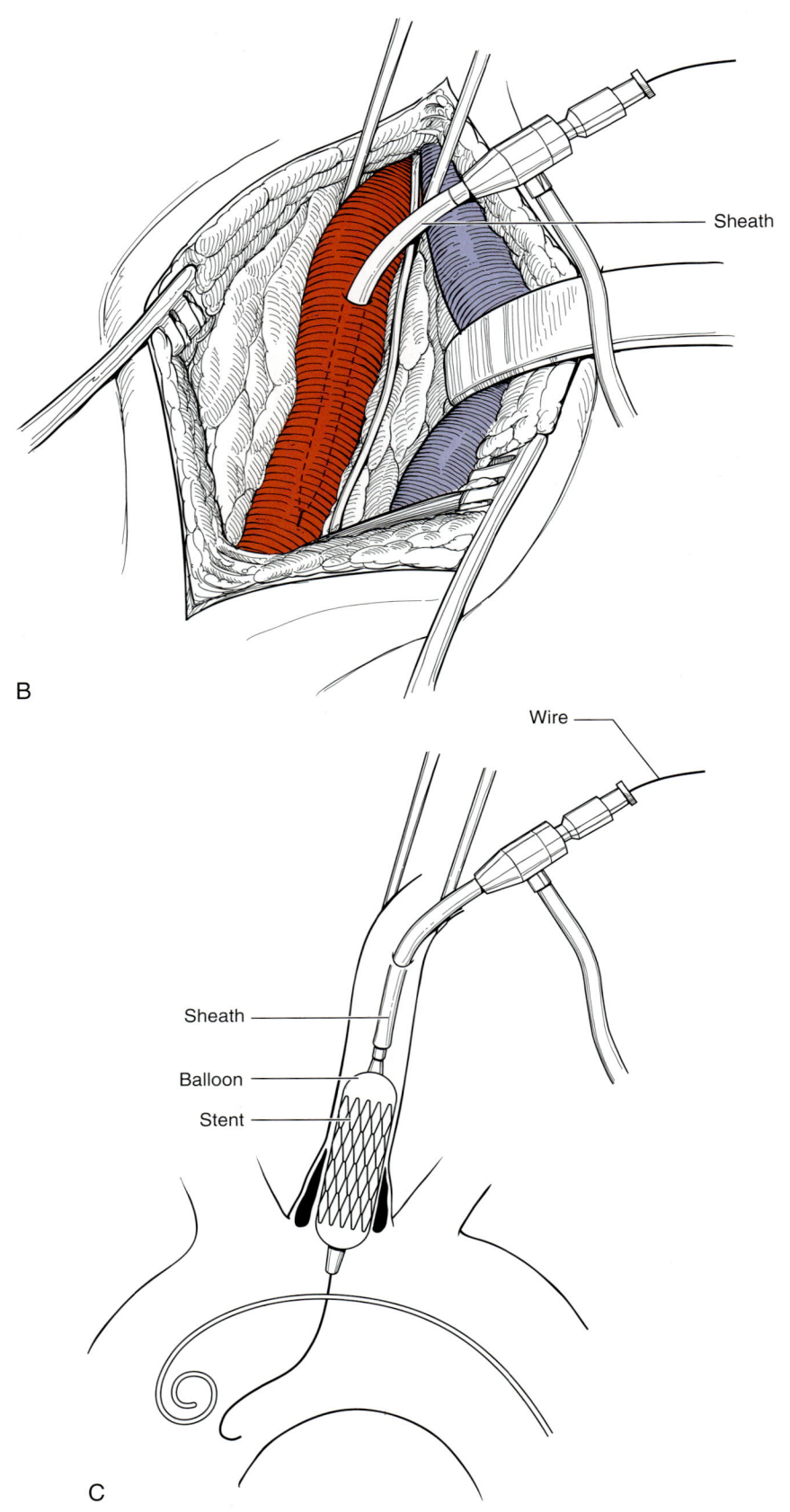

Figure 13-4, cont'd B, A 6-Fr sheath placed into the common carotid artery. **C,** Retrograde stent deployment within a lesion at the origin of the common carotid artery. The carotid artery may be clamped distal to the sheath to minimize the risk of cerebral embolization. The sheath should be aspirated before restoring flow in the distal carotid circulation.

SUBCLAVIAN AND AXILLARY ARTERY STENTING

Subclavian and axillary arteries are treated from a standard transfemoral approach either using a long 6-Fr sheath or 8-Fr shaped guiding catheter. On the left side, an origin stenosis is best treated with a short balloon-expandable stent, taking care not to jail the internal mammary or vertebral arteries. Diseased segments in the middle and distal subclavian arteries should not be stented because of the risk of stent deformity between the clavicle and the first rib. On occasion, the axillary artery may be treated using an endoluminal technique. However, open surgical reconstruction remains the most durable option. On the right side, the short segment of proximal subclavian artery before the origin of the vertebral artery can be treated endoluminally, but this is fraught with difficulty because of the proximity of the vertebral artery and common carotid artery. In addition, this segment has a higher restenosis rate than in other locations. Both the right and left subclavian artery can be approached from the brachial artery with a long 6-Fr sheath.

COMMON CAROTID ARTERY STENTING

Proximal common carotid artery lesions are best approached from the femoral or common carotid artery. Techniques are analogous to those outlined for innominate artery or internal carotid artery stenting. Cerebral protection from the femoral approach uses an embolic protection device, whereas the approach from the common carotid artery is performed with direct carotid clamping.

KOMMERELL DIVERTICULUM

An aneurysm in association with aberrant right subclavian arteries, referred to as a Kommerell diverticulum, exhibits a marked propensity toward rupture. The use of a hybrid approach offers an appealing alternative to higher-risk open repair.[10] The hybrid approach can be performed concurrently or as staged procedures. First, a right carotid-subclavian bypass or transposition is performed via a supraclavicular incision. A stent graft is then inserted to seal the origin of the aberrant right subclavian artery. If a carotid-subclavian bypass was initially performed, the right subclavian artery should be excluded with an occlusion device or coils to prevent a type II endoleak.

Postoperative Care

- Serial neurologic examinations over the next 12 to 24 hours are required following the conclusion of the procedure.
- Bed rest for 4 hours after percutaneous groin access is advised with regular checks for distal perfusion and local hematoma or pseudoaneurysm formation.
- Blood pressure is monitored with a target systolic pressure of 100 to 140 mm Hg.
- Dual antiplatelet agents are continued for at least 1 month.
- Duplex scanning and physical examination with arm pressure measurements should be obtained after the procedure and annually thereafter. Annual two-view chest radiographs are obtained to evaluate stent integrity. CT angiography may be helpful to assess for in-stent stenosis.

Complications

- **Stroke.** The risk of a permanent neurologic deficit after cerebral angiography is 0.2%.[11] Noninvasive preoperative imaging and minimizing arch manipulation diminish this risk.
- **Arterial dissection and thrombosis.** Additional stenting or thrombolysis may be needed if arterial dissection or thrombosis are noted on completion angiography.

- **Access site complications.** Access site complications include hematoma, arterial dissection, and pseudoaneurysm. Hematoma after brachial puncture is of particular concern because of the risk of median nerve compression.
- **Vagal nerve injury.** Patients undergoing exposure of the common carotid artery should be informed of the risk of vocal cord palsy.
- **Restenosis.** Restenosis occurs in approximately 20% of cases at 5 years.
- **Stent fractures.** Late stent fractures can occur but are generaly clinically asymptomatic. In a retrospective review of 27 ostial aortic arch vessel lesions managed with balloon-expandable stents, 3 stent fractures were detected in the innominate artery and 2 fractures were detected in the innominate and common carotid artery at a mean follow-up of 34 months.[12]

REFERENCES

1. Shimizu K, Sano K: Pulseless disease, *J Neuropath Clin Neurol* 1:37–46, 1951.
2. Crawford ES, DeBakey ME, Morris GC Jr, et al: Surgical treatment of occlusion of the innominate, common carotid, and subclavian arteries: A 10 year experience, *Surgery* 65:17–31, 1969.
3. Berguer R, Morasch MD, Kline RA, et al: Cervical reconstruction of the supra-aortic trunks: A 16-year experience, *J Vasc Surg* 29:239–246, 1999.
4. Mathias K, Gospos C, Thron A, et al: Percutaneous transluminal treatment of supraaortic artery obstruction, *Ann Radiol (Paris)* 23:281–282, 1980.
5. Sullivan TM, Gray BH, Bacharach JM, et al: Angioplasty and primary stenting of the subclavian, innominate, and common carotid arteries in 83 patients, *J Vasc Surg* 28:1059–1065, 1998.
6. Brountzos EN, Petersen B, Binkert C, et al: Primary stenting of subclavian and innominate artery occlusive disease: A single center's experience, *Cardiovasc Intervent Radiol* 27:616–623, 2004.
7. van Hattum ES, de Vries JP, Lalezari F, et al: Angioplasty with or without stent placement in the brachiocephalic artery: Feasible and durable? A retrospective cohort study, *J Vasc Interv Radiol* 18:1088–1093, 2007.
8. Liang P, Tan-Ong M, Hoffman GS: Takayasu's arteritis: Vascular interventions and outcomes, *J Rheumatol* 31:102–106, 2004.
9. Peterson BG, Resnick SA, Morasch MD, et al: Aortic arch vessel stenting: A single-center experience using cerebral protection, *Arch Surg* 141:560–563, 2006.
10. Shennib H, Diethrich EB: Novel approaches for the treatment of the aberrant right subclavian artery and its aneurysms, *J Vasc Surg* 47:1066–1070, 2008.
11. Schneider PA, Silva MB Jr, Bohannon WT: Safety and efficacy of carotid arteriography in vascular surgery practice, *J Vasc Surg* 41:238–245, 2005.
12. Usman AA, Resnick SA, Benzuly KH, et al: Late stent fractures following endoluminal treatment of ostial supra-aortic trunk arterial occlusive lesions, *JVIR* 21:1364–1369, 2010.

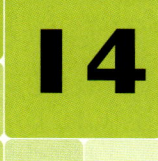

14 Surgical Treatment of the Subclavian and Axillary Artery

R. JAMES VALENTINE

Historical Background

Although arterial compression represents the least common type of thoracic outlet syndrome, developmental anomalies of the thoracic outlet were probably first recognized in patients with arterial complications. As early as the second century Galen and Vesalius[1] described arterial compression because of a cervical rib. Mayo[2] is credited with the first description of subclavian artery abnormality associated with bony compression in the thoracic outlet. In 1861 Coote[3] was the first to report successful resection of a bony abnormality causing a subclavian aneurysm. Peet and associates[4] are credited with coining the term thoracic outlet syndrome in 1956 to describe the pathology that leads to arterial occlusion.

The history of dysphagia lusoria dates back more than three centuries. The anatomy of an aberrant right subclavian artery was described as early as 1735 by Hunauld,[5] but its potential for causing dysphagia from esophageal compression was first recognized by Bayford in 1794.[6] Bayford is credited with coining the term dysphagia lusoria after *lusus naturae* (meaning "jest of nature"). In 1946 Gross[7] performed the first successful operation to correct dysphagia lusoria by simple division of the aberrant artery through a left thoracotomy. Orvalt and associates[8] are credited with performing the first extrathoracic approach for ligation, division, and reimplantation of an aberrant subclavian artery in 1972.

Preoperative Preparation

- In a patient with subclavian artery compression syndrome, preoperative imaging should begin with a duplex scan to verify the presence of a subclavian artery aneurysm or ulcerated plaque. Plain films of the chest and neck may reveal an associated cervical rib. Additional imaging should consist of magnetic resonance angiography, computed tomography (CT) angiography, or conventional catheter angiography with compression maneuvers (Fig. 14-1).
- The decision to resect the subclavian artery at the time of thoracic outlet decompression depends on the condition of the involved artery. Extrinsic compression of the subclavian artery is not always associated with aneurysmal degeneration. In some cases poststenotic dilatation may be expected to resolve spontaneously after the compression is relieved. Although the definition of subclavian artery aneurysm remains controversial, the Scher classification system[9] provides guidelines for treatment of arterial thoracic outlet syndrome based on the condition of the affected artery. These aneurysms are often modest in size, yet embolic complications are common.
- Consider catheter-directed thrombolysis in a patient with hand ischemia because of emboli from a subclavian artery aneurysm.

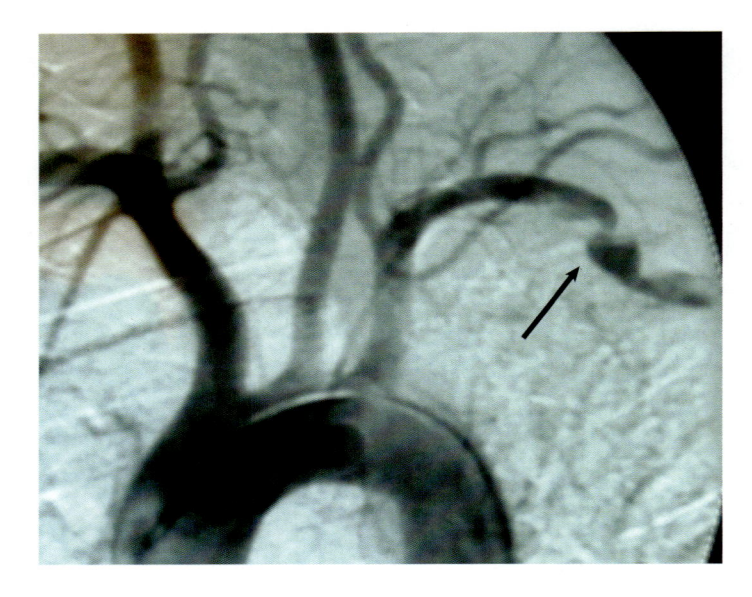

Figure 14-1. Arch aortogram showing a left subclavian artery aneurysm with a thrombus *(arrow)*.

- A patient with dysphagia and an aberrant right subclavian artery should have a barium esophagogram to document the location of external compression. Additional imaging should consist of magnetic resonance, CT, or conventional catheter angiography. Thoracic views should be included to evaluate for the presence of Kommerell diverticulum.
- Prophylactic antibiotics should be considered.

Pitfalls and Danger Points

- Phrenic nerve injury
- Thoracic duct injury
- Brachial plexus injury
- Vertebral artery injury
- Pneumothorax

Operative Strategy

SURGICAL ANATOMY OF THE SUBCLAVIAN AND AXILLARY ARTERY

In most cases, the right subclavian artery branches from the brachiocephalic trunk and the left subclavian artery arises as the most distal branch of the aortic arch. Each artery emerges from the mediastinum and arches over the ipsilateral cervical pleura and pulmonary apex to pass between the clavicle and the first rib. In this trajectory the arteries pass behind the respective anterior scalene muscle and between the clavicle and the first rib. Before passing behind the anterior scalene muscle, each artery gives off three branches. The vertebral arteries originate first on the superoposterior aspect of each subclavian artery and ascend to enter the transverse foramina of C6. Next, the internal thoracic arteries originate on the inferior aspect of each subclavian artery and descend along the anterior chest wall behind the costal cartilages. The short thyrocervical trunk originates anteriorly as the third branch near the medial border of the anterior scalene muscle and quickly divides into three or four smaller branches. As the subclavian arteries pass behind the anterior scalene muscle, each gives off a costocervical branch on the posterior aspect and a dorsal scapular branch on the lateral aspect.

Key anatomic features in the thoracic outlet include the tightly packed neurovascular structures of the superior thoracic aperture and the proximity of the phrenic nerve, thoracic duct, and subclavian vein. The nerves of the brachial plexus emerge between the anterior and the middle scalene muscles, descend posterior to the

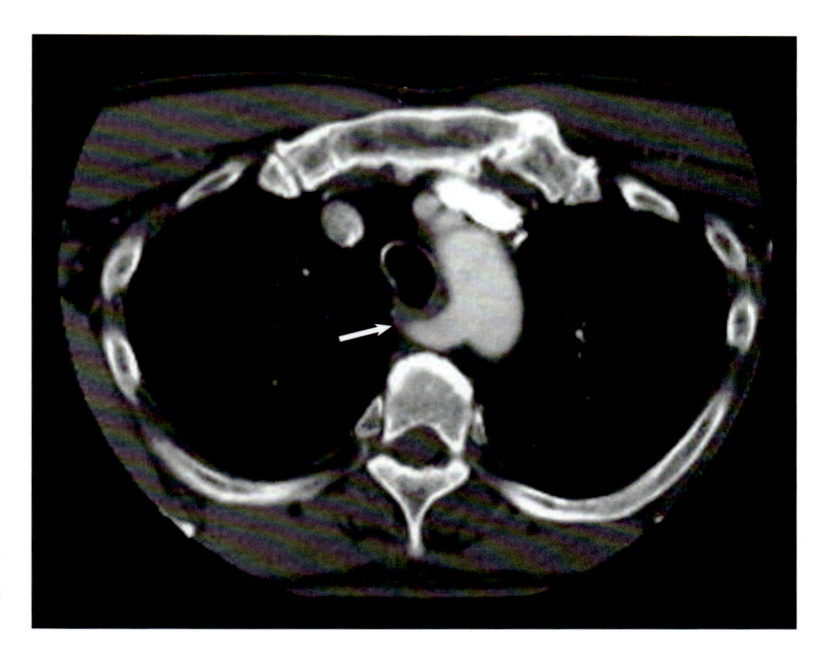

Figure 14-2. Computed tomography angiogram demonstrating an aberrant right subclavian artery in the retroesophageal position (arrow).

subclavian artery, and enter the axillary passage close to the artery at the lateral border of the first rib. The phrenic nerve runs from lateral to medial as it descends on the surface of the anterior scalene muscle. It descends into the chest between the subclavian artery and the subclavian vein, just medial to the point where the anterior scalene muscle attaches to the scalene tubercle of the first rib. The subclavian vein enters the axillary passage behind the subclavius muscle, courses anterior to the anterior scalene muscle, and joins the internal jugular vein to enter the mediastinum as a single brachiocephalic vein. On the left side, the thoracic duct arches over the subclavian artery and terminates at the junction of the internal jugular and subclavian veins.

The axillary artery extends from the lateral border of the first rib to the lateral edge of the teres major muscle. The artery is divided anatomically into three parts by the pectoralis minor muscle. The first segment, medial to the muscle, has one branch: the supreme thoracic artery. The second segment, behind the muscle, has two branches: the thoracoacromial and lateral thoracic arteries. The third segment, lateral to the muscle, has three branches: the subscapular artery and the medial and lateral humeral circumflex arteries.

The divisions and cords of the brachial plexus interdigitate around the axillary artery and form a complex array that risks injury during axillary artery dissection. The cords of the brachial plexus assume their final configuration as nerves around the third segment of the axillary artery. The truncal origins of the median nerve cross anterior to the artery at this level and are particularly prone to injury during dissection in this area.

ANATOMIC CONSIDERATIONS IN AN ABERRANT RIGHT SUBCLAVIAN ARTERY

An aberrant right subclavian artery arises as the fourth branch of the aortic arch in about 1% of the population, and the prevalence is higher in individuals with other cardiovascular anomalies, such as right-sided aortic arch.[10] The aberrant artery most often tracks across the mediastinum posterior to the esophagus and right common carotid artery to reach the right arm (Fig. 14-2). Less commonly, the artery may course between the esophagus and the trachea or anterior to the trachea.[6] A number of anatomic anomalies associated with an aberrant right subclavian artery should be considered in operative planning[11]:

- **Esophageal compression.** A small percentage of individuals with the anomaly develop symptoms associated with posterior compression of the esophagus (dysphagia lusoria) (Fig. 14-3). The true incidence of dysphagia lusoria and the

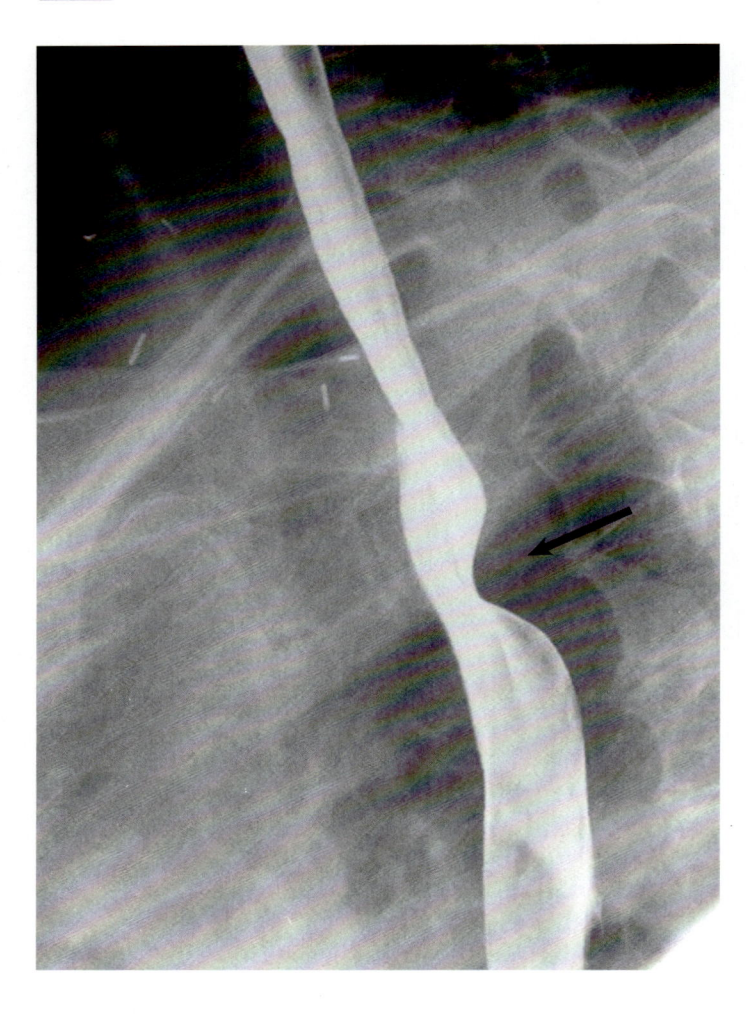

Figure 14-3. Barium esophagogram showing extrinsic compression from an aberrant right subclavian artery *(arrow)* in a patient with dysphagia lusoria.

reasons underlying late development of symptoms remain unknown. In such patients transposition of the aberrant artery can be curative and definitive in the absence of the other considerations given here.

- **Kommerell diverticulum.** Approximately 60% of individuals who have an aberrant right subclavian artery have dilation at the aortic origin known as Kommerell diverticulum.[12] This segment is prone to aneurysmal degeneration that may result in compression of surrounding structures or catastrophic rupture. Therefore the presence of Kommerell diverticulum is an indication for repair. Typically this requires a staged approach with initial transposition of the subclavian artery, followed by open or endovascular repair of the diverticulum.
- **Nonrecurrent right laryngeal nerve.** The associated anomaly of a nonrecurrent laryngeal nerve should always be considered in the patient with an aberrant right subclavian artery. Although a nonrecurrent laryngeal nerve has been reported on the left side, the anomaly is more common on the right. The nerve branches directly from the vagus nerve at the level of the carotid bifurcation and is at risk of injury during dissection of the carotid bulb, especially on the posterior or medial aspect.[13] Fortunately, carotid exposure is not required at this level during modern operations to correct dysphagia lusoria (described later).
- **Thoracic duct anomalies.** A right-sided thoracic duct may arch over the aberrant right subclavian artery to join the confluence of the internal jugular and subclavian veins.

AVOIDING INJURIES TO THE THORACIC DUCT

Chylous leak is a morbid complication of subclavian artery exposure. The complication is best avoided by meticulous ligation of lymphatics in the scalene fat pad and early identification of the thoracic duct during exposure of the left subclavian artery. The duct courses on the medial side of the fat pad and arches over the subclavian artery to reach the confluence of the subclavian and internal jugular veins. The duct should be carefully ligated and divided near its point of entry into the posterior vein wall. There may be multiple ducts that may enter the subclavian or internal jugular veins directly. A right-sided thoracic duct may be associated with an aberrant right subclavian artery.

AVOIDING INJURIES TO THE BRACHIAL PLEXUS

Most brachial plexus injuries arise as a consequence of undue traction, especially during resection of cervical ribs. During exposure of the proximal subclavian artery, self-retaining retractors should be carefully placed in the posterior incision to avoid contact with nerve roots and trunks as they course downward from their cervical origins behind the anterior scalene muscle. In the lateral wound the nerve divisions descend to join the subclavian artery as it crosses under the clavicle; nerve injury can occur from misplaced arterial clamps in this area. Nerve injury can also occur during first rib resection if the nerves are not well identified and gently retracted from the cutting instrument. The nerves course over anomalous cervical ribs, and overzealous traction must be carefully avoided during rib excision.

AVOIDING INJURIES TO THE VERTEBRAL ARTERY

The vertebral artery arises on the superoposterior aspect of the subclavian artery and may be at risk for injury from excessive traction or inadvertent entry during proximal exposure of the subclavian artery. To avoid these complications, the vertebral artery should be carefully identified during medial dissection. The vertebral artery can be identified in the center of the angle formed by the anterior scalene and longus coli muscles. It lies adjacent to the vertebral vein and sympathetic chain and is crossed by the inferior thyroid artery.

In patients with an aberrant right subclavian artery, the right vertebral artery is at risk of kinking as the aberrant subclavian artery is transposed anteriorly for anastomosis to the common carotid artery. This complication is avoided by ensuring that there is an adequate length of the subclavian artery that allows laxity as it is brought anteriorly to join the carotid artery.

AVOIDING INJURIES BEHIND THE CLAVICLE

Although exposure of the subclavian vein is rarely necessary during arterial dissection, the proximity of the vein makes it prone to injury at three points. The first is near the clavicular head, where excessive traction on the confluence with the internal jugular vein may result in a tear that is difficult to control. The second is the point at which the clavicle crosses over the first rib: the vein is prone to injury during first rib resection and should therefore be carefully identified and protected during medial rib transection. The third point of potential injury is in the thoracic outlet as the vein crosses over the first rib. During arterial reconstruction, the tunnel between the supraclavicular and the infraclavicular incisions should be created under direct vision to avoid venous injury (described later).

SELECTION OF A CONDUIT

Direct transposition and anastomosis of the subclavian artery onto the common carotid artery is associated with the highest 5-year patency and is preferred over free grafts whenever feasible. Direct transposition can usually be accomplished in patients with dysphagia lusoria (described later).

In patients who require repair of a subclavian artery aneurysm, short interposition grafts using prosthetic material such as ringed polytetrafluoroethylene represent a durable option after the aneurysm has been resected.[14] Autogenous saphenous vein grafts have also been used in this position and have the theoretical advantage of resistance to infection. However, the prosthetic graft often carries the advantage of better size match, and external ring support helps prevent graft kinking in its position beneath the clavicle.

A prosthetic graft such as ringed polytetrafluoroethylene is associated with superior patency rates compared with the autogenous saphenous vein for carotid-subclavian bypass.[15,16] The small caliber of the saphenous vein and the potential for kinking from neck mobility in multiple axes appear to limit its durability in this position.[15]

The superficial femoral vein is a durable alternative to prosthetic grafts in this location and carries the advantages of resistance to infection and superior size match. This large graft also appears to resist kinking.[17]

Operative Technique for Repair of a Subclavian Artery Aneurysm

POSITION AND INCISION

The patient is positioned supine with the arms tucked in and the head turned to the opposite side. A rolled towel may be placed between the scapulae to extend the shoulder slightly and flatten the supraclavicular fossa. Two incisions are often used to repair a subclavian artery aneurysm. A supraclavicular incision is made 1 to 2 cm above and parallel to the clavicle, and a horizontal, infraclavicular incision is made 2 cm below the middle third of the clavicle and extended laterally about 8 cm.

EXPOSURE OF THE SUPRACLAVICULAR SUBCLAVIAN ARTERY

The supraclavicular incision is deepened through the subcutaneous tissue and platysma muscle, and the external jugular vein and omohyoid muscle are divided. Medial exposure is enhanced by dividing the clavicular head of the sternocleidomastoid muscle, but this is not always necessary. The underlying internal jugular vein should be mobilized on its lateral border and retracted medially. This exposes the underlying scalene fat pad. By carefully ligating and dividing the associated lymphatic tissue, the fat pad can be mobilized on its medial, superior, and inferior borders and reflected as a pedicle into the lateral wound. On the left side, the thoracic duct should be identified and carefully ligated during dissection of the fat pad on its inferomedial corner.

The anterior scalene muscle lies directly underneath the fat pad, and the phrenic nerve is easily identified as it courses across the muscle (Fig. 14-4). The nerve should be carefully preserved as the muscle is transected near its insertion on the first rib. The subclavian artery lies directly underneath the muscle and can be easily isolated in this position.

Subclavian artery aneurysms are often associated with cervical ribs. These bony anomalies are usually embedded within the fibers of the middle scalene muscle, and partial resection of the middle scalene may be required. As noted earlier the brachial plexus courses between the anterior and the middle scalene muscles; nerve traction injuries in this area may be disastrous. After dissection of the cervical rib away from the brachial plexus, the location of subclavian artery compression should be determined. Although the artery may be compressed as it crosses over the cervical rib, it is usually pinched by anomalous fibrous bands extending between the cervical rib and the underlying first rib. Careful dissection is required to free the subclavian artery in this area. The nerves of the brachial plexus course over the cervical rib and must be protected during rib resection (Fig. 14-5).

EXPOSURE OF THE AXILLARY ARTERY

The infraclavicular incision is deepened through the subcutaneous tissue and the pectoral fascia. The underlying pectoralis major muscle is split in the direction of its fibers to expose the underlying clavipectoral fascia (Fig. 14-6). The neurovascular

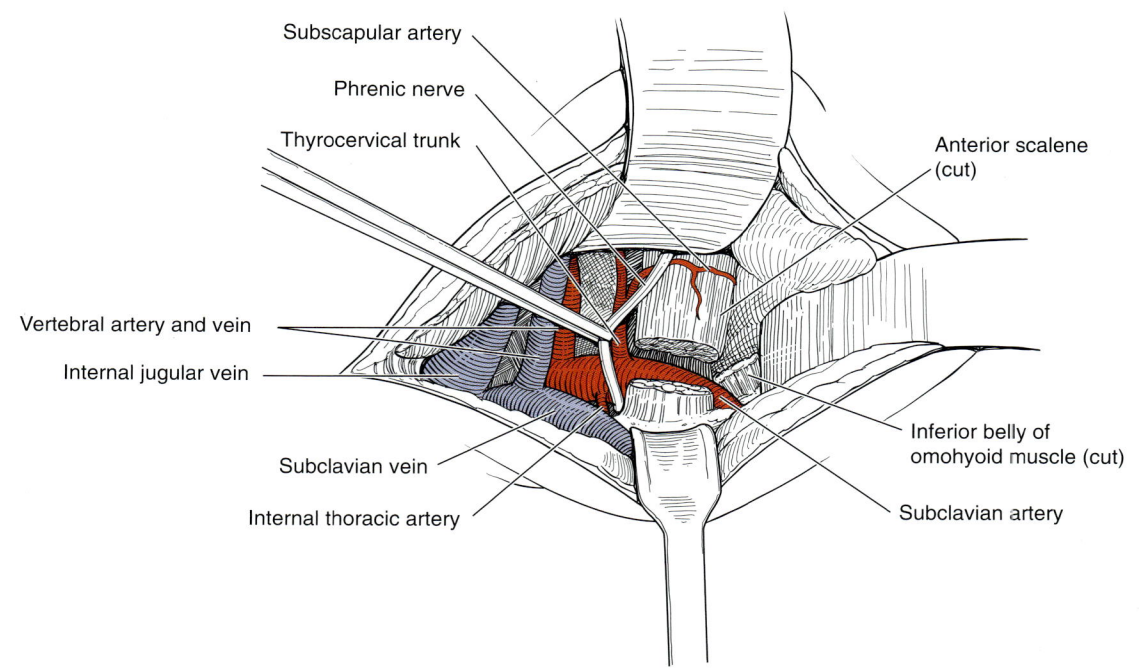

Figure 14-4. The subclavian artery is exposed by dividing the anterior scalene muscle, taking care to preserve the phrenic nerve on the muscle's medial border.

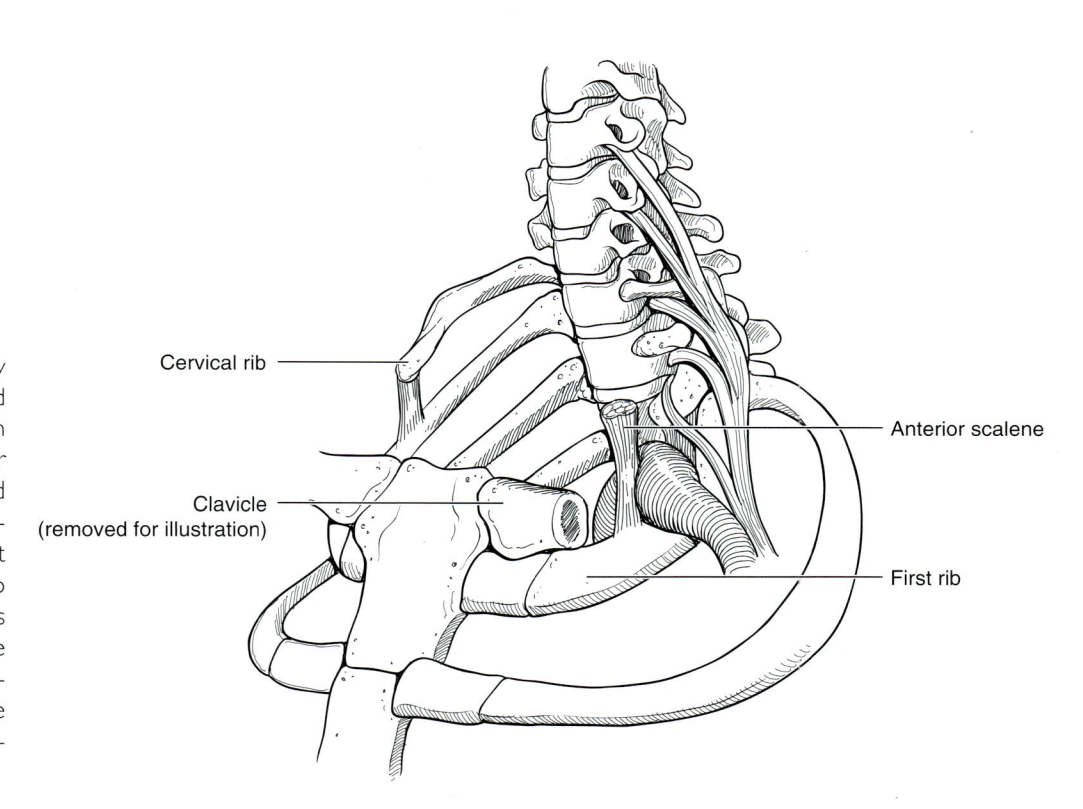

Figure 14-5. Subclavian artery aneurysms are often associated with cervical ribs. Compression of the artery may be due either to anomalous bands that extend between the end of the cervical rib and the underlying first rib or to compression related to the anterior scalene muscle, as shown on the right side of the figure. During cervical rib resection, the overlying nerves of the brachial plexus should be carefully protected.

bundle and the enveloping axillary sheath are located deep to the clavipectoral fascia. The axillary vein is the first structure to be encountered. The vein should be mobilized by carefully ligating and dividing major tributaries. The artery is most easily identified by retracting the vein caudally. The large thoracoacromial artery should be identified at its origin from the axillary artery just proximal to the pectoralis minor muscle (Fig. 14-7). This branch can usually be preserved but may require ligation if more distal exposure is required. The supreme thoracic artery is located near the chest wall and may require ligation during resection of the subclavian-axillary aneurysm.

SUBCLAVIAN-AXILLARY ARTERY BYPASS

The aneurysmal segment of the subclavian artery should be resected after all compressing structures in the thoracic outlet are removed. A tunnel should be created under the clavicle between the supraclavicular and the infraclavicular incisions, taking care to avoid injury to the adjacent vein. After the tunnel is carefully enlarged to admit two of the surgeon's fingers, the graft should be brought through the tunnel and anastomosed end to end to the transected arterial ends in both incisions.

CAROTID-BRACHIAL ARTERY BYPASS

We have occasionally found it necessary to create a more distal bypass in patients with more extensive pathology of the axillary and subclavian arteries. This has

Figure 14-6. The axillary artery is exposed through an infraclavicular incision by splitting the muscle fibers of the pectoralis major and opening the underlying clavipectoral fascia.

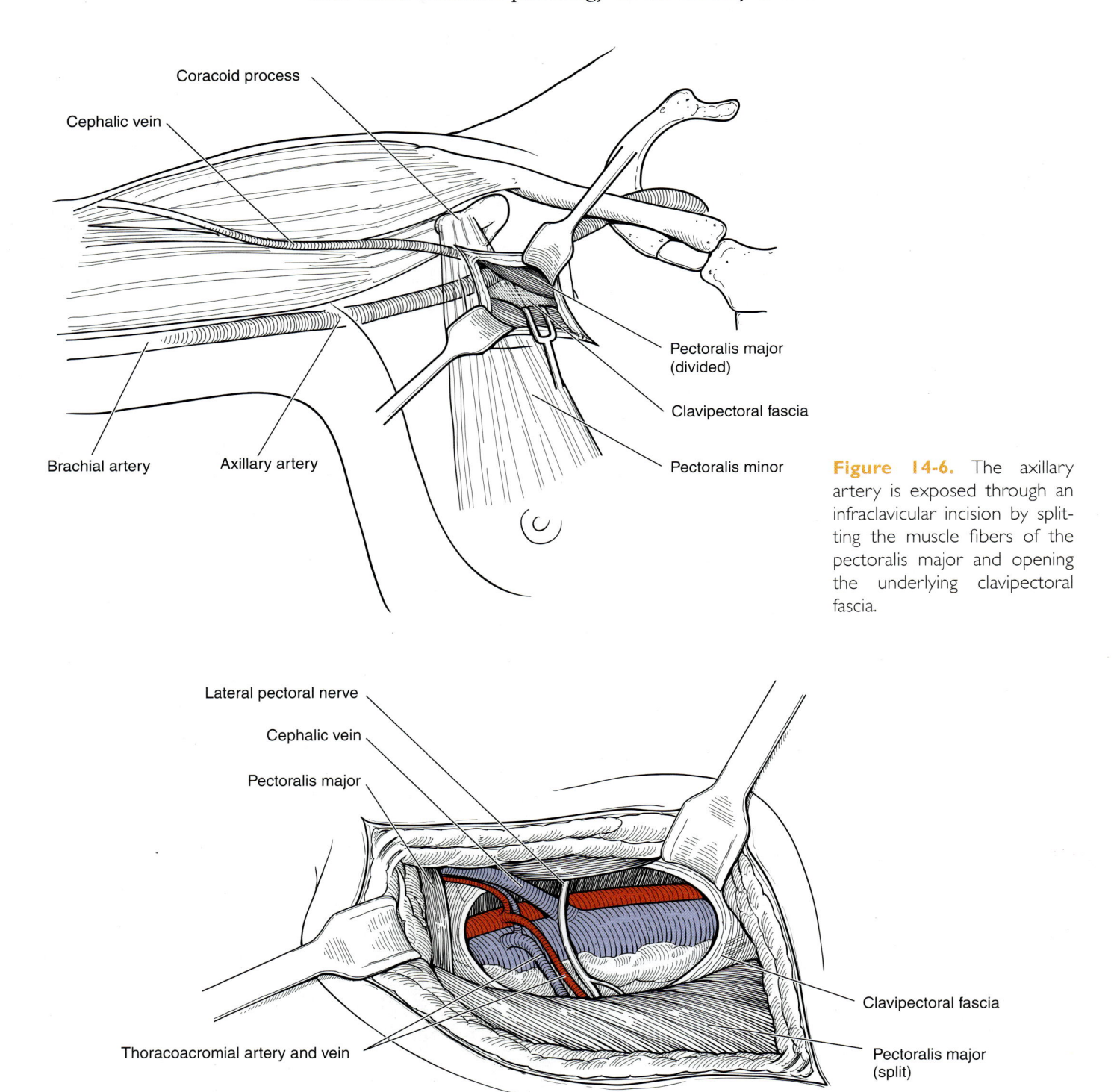

Figure 14-7. The first part of the axillary artery is located medial to the pectoralis minor muscle and has only one branch.

also been the case in patients who develop graft occlusions after subclavian artery bypass and in whom redo bypasses outside of the original operative area are desirable. In these cases we have found it advantageous to tunnel a bypass from the common carotid artery, over the distal third of the clavicle, and down the deltopectoral groove to reach the brachial artery. This option avoids repeat dissection in scarred areas and avoids kinking because the graft is positioned over the portion of the clavicle that curves posteriorly.

CLOSURE

After ensuring that there is no entry into the pleural space, the supraclavicular wound is closed by returning the scalene fat pad to its normal anatomic position. This helps to protect the graft and improve the cosmetic appearance of the supraclavicular fossa. The platysma, subcutaneous tissue, and skin are closed in layers. Drains are not routinely placed.

In the infraclavicular incision, the subclavian vein is returned to its normal anatomic position, and the split fibers of the pectoralis major muscle are reapproximated. The pectoralis fascia, subcutaneous tissues, and skin are closed in layers.

Operative Technique for Repair of an Aberrant Right Subclavian Artery

POSITION AND INCISION

Surgical correction of an aberrant right subclavian artery is most easily accomplished through a modified extrathoracic approach.[18] The operation involves division of the aberrant artery, reimplantation into the right common carotid artery, and ligation of the proximal subclavian artery segment (Fig. 14-8). These maneuvers can be accomplished through a right supraclavicular incision. As described earlier the patient is supine, arms are tucked in, and the head is turned to the opposite side. A rolled towel placed between the scapulae flattens the supraclavicular fossa and slightly extends the shoulder. The incision is made 1 to 2 cm above and parallel to the right clavicle, extending medially to the border of the sternocleidomastoid muscle.

EXPOSURE OF THE ABERRANT SUBCLAVIAN ARTERY

The aberrant right subclavian artery is more posterior than usual as it tracks across the mediastinum behind the esophagus. On the right side of the esophagus,

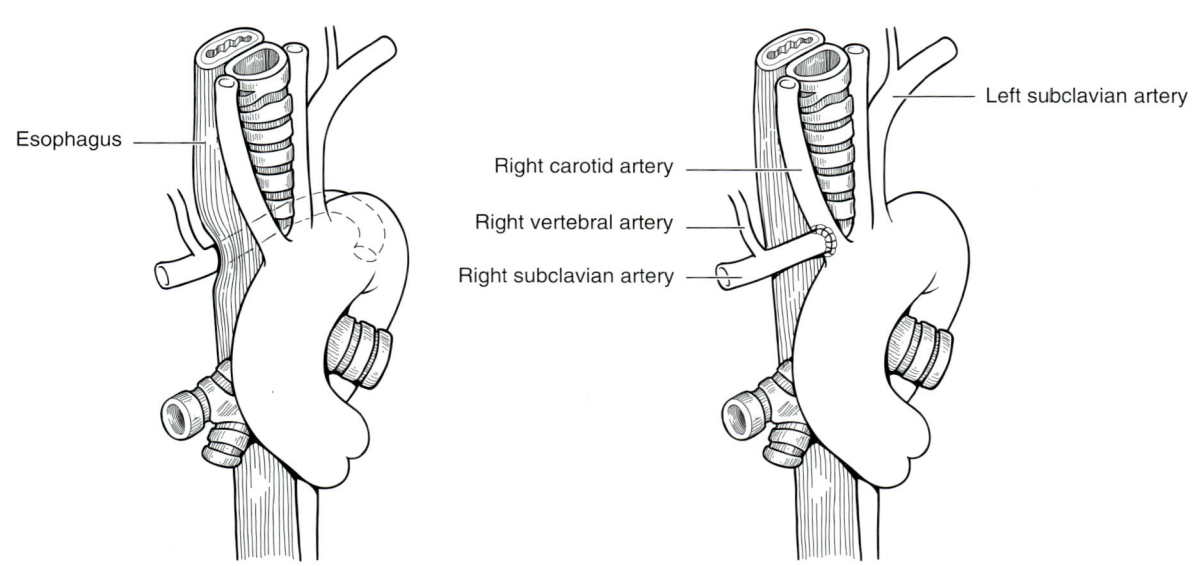

Figure 14-8. In the absence of Kommerell diverticulum, operative treatment of dysphagia lusoria can be performed through a right supraclavicular incision. Subclavian-carotid transposition, ligation of the compressing arterial segment, and esophageal dilation can be performed in the same operation.

the artery arches slightly anteriorly to assume a normal position behind the right anterior scalene muscle. The artery is exposed by dividing the platysma muscle, reflecting the scalene fat pad, and dividing the anterior scalene muscle in the manner described earlier. The artery should be isolated beneath the divided anterior scalene muscle and exposed as far medially as possible. This can be accomplished by dividing the clavicular head of the sternocleidomastoid muscle and retracting the underlying internal jugular vein along its lateral border. The vertebral artery should be carefully identified and controlled with an elastic loop.

EXPOSURE OF THE RETROESOPHAGEAL SUBCLAVIAN ARTERY

Minimal dissection is required to mobilize the subclavian artery behind the esophagus, and we have found that anterior retraction of the esophagus affords access to the subclavian artery near its aortic origin, far to the left of the esophagus.

DIVISION AND LIGATION OF THE RETROESOPHAGEAL SUBCLAVIAN ARTERY

After systemic anticoagulation, the artery should be divided as far to the left of the esophagus as possible. We have found that a long, curved clamp such as a narrow C clamp can be placed deep in the medial incision for proximal control. After the vertebral artery and distal subclavian artery are occluded, the artery is divided and the proximal stump is oversewn with permanent sutures. The distal segment can then be delivered into the incision for transposition to the carotid artery.

SUBCLAVIAN ARTERY TO CAROTID ARTERY TRANSPOSITION

The common carotid artery should be exposed in the medial incision behind the previously mobilized internal jugular vein. Care should be taken to identify the vagus nerve on the medial side of the artery. A nonrecurrent laryngeal nerve is often associated with the aberrant right subclavian artery but is not likely to be injured: the nerve branches directly from the vagus nerve at the level of the carotid bifurcation and is therefore unlikely to be encountered during dissection of the common carotid artery in the lower neck.

Once an adequate length of common carotid artery is isolated, redundant portions of an aberrant subclavian artery should be resected to allow a tension-free, end-to-side anastomosis with the common carotid artery. Interposition grafting is not needed unless the residual subclavian segment shows aneurysmal degeneration. As the distal subclavian artery is transposed anteriorly to reach the common carotid, care should be taken to ensure that the vertebral artery is not tented or kinked. This rarely requires mobilization of the proximal vertebral artery. A carotid shunt is not routinely used during this procedure.

CLOSURE

After the subclavian-carotid transposition is complete, the esophagus should be dilated under direct vision within the surgical wound. Although some have advocated balloon dilatation, we prefer to use progressive dilatation with Maloney dilators to 40 Fr (13.2 mm). Before closure, the wound should be checked for unintended entry into the pleural space. This can be accomplished by filling the incision with sterile saline and asking the anesthesiologist to hyperinflate the lungs. If there is no evidence of an air leak, then the wound is closed by returning the scalene fat pad to its normal anatomic position. The platysma, subcutaneous tissues, and skin are then closed in layers. Drains are not routinely required.

Operative Technique for Repair of Kommerell Diverticulum

POSITION AND INCISION

The optimal repair method for Kommerell diverticulum must be individualized because of the known association with other aortic abnormalities including right-sided aortic arch and aneurysms of the aortic arch or descending thoracic aorta.[19,20] A two-stage approach involving subclavian-carotid transposition followed by thoracotomy to repair Kommerell diverticulum has been advocated for most patients. Patients with left-sided arches are best approached through a left thoracotomy; patients with right-sided arches should undergo right thoracotomy. At least one recent report suggests that coverage of Kommerell diverticulum with a thoracic endograft is an excellent alternative to thoracotomy.[21] Although this procedure may require bilateral subclavian-carotid transposition, it is an attractive option because it avoids thoracotomy. However, the long-term durability of a thoracic endograft to treat Kommerell diverticulum remains unknown, and its use for this indication is not approved by the U.S. Food and Drug Administration.

For left thoracotomy, the patient should be positioned in a true lateral position, with the right side down and a roll placed beneath the right axilla. The right arm should be placed on an arm board perpendicular to the patient, and the left arm should be supported on a padded armrest. The skin incision begins between the scapula and the spine and then curves downward 1 cm below the tip of the scapula to a point just below the left nipple.

THORACIC EXPOSURE FOR PROXIMAL CONTROL OF KOMMERELL DIVERTICULUM

The proximal segment of the descending thoracic aorta is best exposed through the fourth interspace (Fig. 14-9). After verifying the location of the fourth interspace, the pleural cavity is entered by dividing the intercostal muscles along the superior border of the fifth rib. Rib spreaders should be placed and opened slowly to prevent rib fractures. After the left lung is allowed to collapse, the aortic arch and proximal descending thoracic aorta can be identified anterior to the spine. To ensure complete resection of Kommerell diverticulum, proximal aortic control may require exposure between the left common carotid artery and the left subclavian artery, as well as control of the proximal left subclavian artery. To help protect the vagus and phrenic nerves as they cross the aortic arch, a vertical incision should be made in the mediastinal pleura posterior to the vagus nerve. The left vagus nerve should be carefully swept forward until an adequate segment of aorta is cleared for placement of a clamp.

DISTAL EXPOSURE FOR CONTROL OF KOMMERELL DIVERTICULUM

After incising the mediastinal pleura directly over the descending thoracic aorta below the diverticulum, the aorta should be encircled with a heavy tape, taking care to preserve intercostals arteries.

REPAIR OF KOMMERELL DIVERTICULUM

The extent of Kommerell diverticulum repair depends on the size of the diverticular neck and the presence of associated aneurysmal deterioration of the surrounding aorta. Diverticula that involve less than one third of the circumference of the aorta can be resected using partial occlusion of the aorta with a Satinski clamp. After resection, the aortic defect is patched with prosthetic material such as Dacron. Larger diverticula and those associated with aneurysmal degeneration usually require aortic replacement. If aortic replacement is anticipated, most authors recommend using distal circulatory support such as atriofemoral bypass to reduce the incidence of paraplegia.[19]

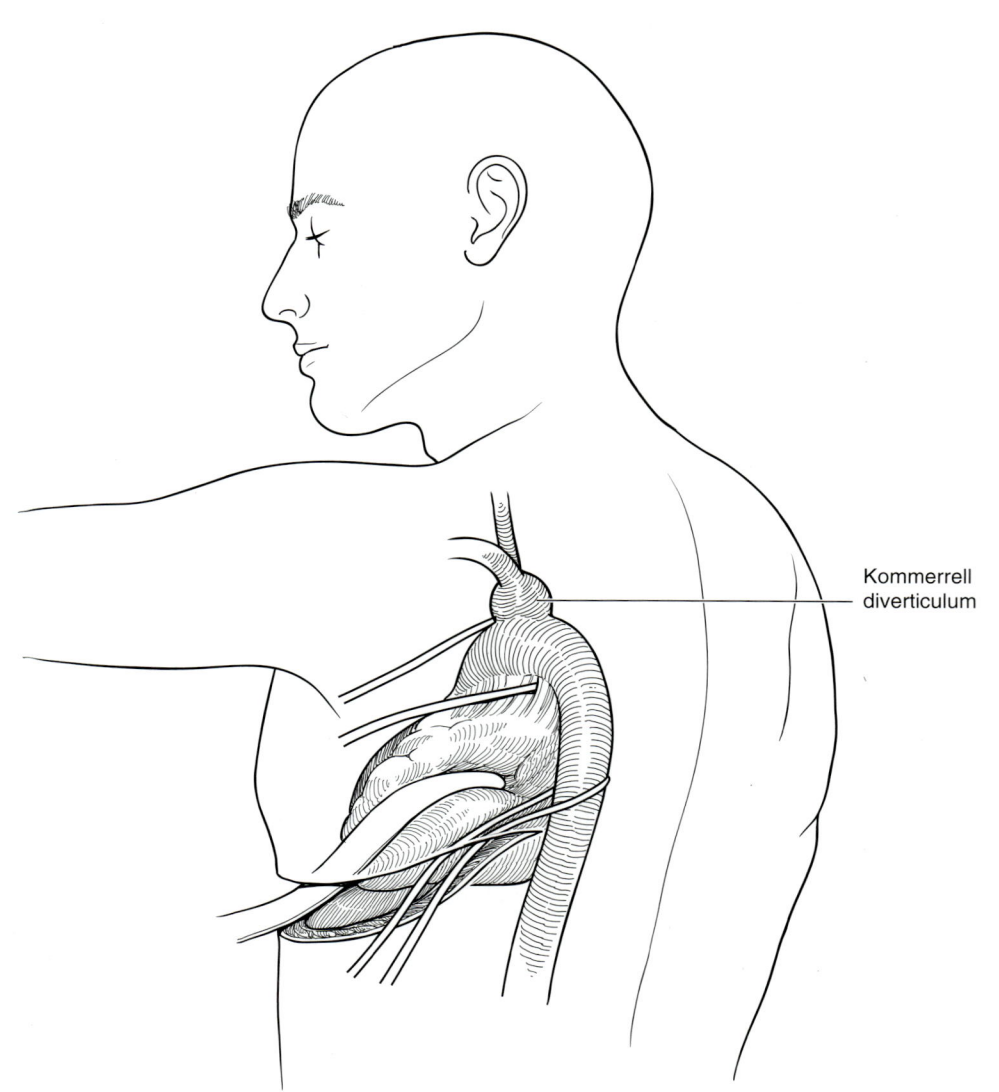

Figure 14-9. Open repair of Kommerell diverticulum is most commonly performed through a left fourth interspace thoracotomy. The diverticulum often originates on the right side of the aorta but is readily controlled through this approach.

CLOSURE

After hemostasis is assured, two large thoracostomy tubes are placed in the pleural cavity, and the lung is reexpanded. The chest incision is closed by reapproximating the ribs with large interrupted sutures. The muscle fascia, subcutaneous tissue, and ribs are closed in layers.

Postoperative Care

SUBCLAVIAN ARTERY REPAIR

- Patients are usually admitted for overnight observation and discharged 1 or 2 days after the operation.
- Patients are started on a regular diet and encouraged to ambulate on the day of surgery.
- Shoulder range-of-motion exercises should be started on the day after surgery. In some cases a course of outpatient physical therapy may be appropriate.
- One dose of a cephalosporin or vancomycin is given within 1 hour of the operation and continued for 24 hours after operation.
- Incisional pain is usually well controlled with oral narcotic medications.
- Aspirin at 81 mg may be added at the surgeon's discretion.
- Postoperative blood pressure checks in both arms should be performed to assess graft patency.

- An appropriate follow-up strategy is a postoperative duplex scan to assess graft patency and flow rates at 1 month, repeated annually.

KOMMERELL DIVERTICULUM REPAIR

- Patients are usually admitted to an intensive care unit for overnight monitoring and are transferred to the floor the day after surgery.
- Most patients are extubated in the operating room and can be started on a clear liquid diet on the day of surgery.
- After transfer to the floor, patients are encouraged to ambulate in the hall with assistance.
- The chest tubes are left on suction until there is minimal drainage and no evidence of air leak. The tubes are then placed on a water seal and removed if no recurrent pneumothorax is seen on a chest radiographic examination.
- In the absence of associated aortic abnormalities, routine imaging studies are not needed in long-term follow-up in patients who had open repair.

Postoperative Complications

- **Lymph leak.** The troublesome complication of lymph leak often represents injury to the thoracic duct or large accessory ducts in the supraclavicular region. Unless there is an associated chylothorax, treatment should begin with conservative management, including local compression, dietary manipulation, and administration of octreotide. Uncontained leaks that persist beyond 3 days require intervention. Although it is reasonable to reopen the surgical wound and attempt direct suture repair, most patients ultimately require ligation of the thoracic duct using video-assisted thoracotomy surgery.
- **Pneumothorax or hemothorax.** Findings of pneumothorax or hemothorax usually represent unintentional entry into the pleural space during subclavian artery exposure. The lung parenchyma is rarely injured. Most patients can be treated with short-term thoracostomy tube drainage.
- **Brachial plexus injury.** Fortunately, injuries to the brachial plexus are rare complications of subclavian artery or axillary artery exposure. Most are transient and presumed to be associated with excessive traction. The location and degree of the neural deficit should be documented, and the patient should be started on aggressive physical therapy.
- **Phrenic nerve injury.** Phrenic nerve palsy is a rare complication of subclavian artery exposure and can be seen after dissection of the aortic arch. The condition is diagnosed by demonstrating paralysis of the ipsilateral hemidiaphragm on chest fluoroscopy. Most patients are minimally symptomatic, and full recovery of phrenic nerve function can be expected within several months.
- **Recurrent dysphagia.** In the rare case when a patient develops recurrent dysphagia after subclavian transposition and esophageal dilatation, repeat dilatation is curative. Persistent symptoms should be investigated with esophagoscopy and esophageal motility studies to rule out other pathologic causes.

REFERENCES

1. Murphy JB: The clinical significance of cervical ribs, *Surg Gynecol Obstet* 3:514-520, 1906.
2. Mayo H: Exostosis of the first rib with strong pulsations of the subclavian artery, *Lon Med Phy J* 11:40, 1831.
3. Coote H: Exostosis of the transverse process of the seventh cervical vertebra, surrounded by blood vessels and nerves: Successful removal, *Lancet* 1:360-361, 1961.
4. Peet RM, Hendriksen JD, Anderson TP, Martin GM: Thoracic outlet syndrome: Evaluation of a therapeutic exercise program, *Proc Mayo Clin* 31:281-287, 1956.
5. Hunauld M: Examen de quelques parties d'un singe, *Hist Acad Roy Sci* 2:516-523, 1735.
6. Bayford D: An account of singular case of obstructional deglutition, *Mera Med Soc London* 2:275, 1794.

7. Gross RE: Surgical treatment of dysphagia lusoria in the adult, *Ann Surg* 124:532-534, 1946.
8. Orvalt TO, Sheerer R, Jude JR: A single cervical approach to aberrant right subclavian artery, *Surgery* 71:227-230, 1972.
9. Scher LA, Veith FJ, Haimovichi H, et al: Staging of arterial complications of cervical rib: Guidelines for surgical management, *Surgery* 95:664-669, 1984.
10. Ramaswamy P, Lytrivi ID, Thanjan MT, et al: Frequency of aberrant right subclavian artery, arch laterality, and associated intracardiac anomalies detected by echocardiography, *Am J Cardiol* 101:677-682, 2008.
11. Epstein DA, DeBord JR: Abnormalities associated with aberrant right subclavian arteries. A case report, *Vasc Endovasc Surg* 36:297-303, 2002.
12. Ota T, Okada K, Takanashi S, et al: Surgical treatment for Kommerell's diverticulum, *J Thorac Cardiovasc Surg* 131:574-578, 2006.
13. Valentine RJ, Wind GG: Carotid arteries. In Valentine RJ, Wind GG, editors: *Anatomic exposures in vascular surgery*, 2nd ed. Philadelphia, 2003, Lippincott Williams & Wilkins, pp 23-50.
14. Davidovic LB, Koncar IB, Kuzmanovic IB: Arterial complications of thoracic outlet syndrome, *Am Surg* 75:235-239, 2009.
15. Ziomek S, Quinones-Baldrich WJ, Busuttil RW, et al: The superiority of synthetic arterial grafts over autologous veins in carotid-subclavian bypass, *J Vasc Surg* 3:140-145, 1986.
16. AbuRahma AF, Robinson PA, Jennings TG: Carotid-subclavian bypass grafting with polytetrafluoroethylene grafts for symptomatic subclavian artery stenosis or occlusion: A 20-year experience, *J Vasc Surg* 32:411-419, 2000.
17. Modrall JG, Joiner DR, Seidel SA, et al: Superficial femoral-popliteal vein as a conduit for brachiocephalic arterial reconstructions, *Ann Vasc Surg* 16:17-23, 2002.
18. Valentine RJ, Carter DJ, Clagett GP: A modified extrathoracic approach to the treatment of dysphagia lusoria, *J Vasc Surg* 5:498-500, 1987.
19. Cinà CS, Althani H, Pasenau J, et al: Kommerell's diverticulum and right-sided aortic arch: A cohort study and review of the literature, *J Vasc Surg* 39:131-139, 2004.
20. Keiffer E, Bahnini A, Koskas F: Aberrant subclavian artery: Surgical treatment in thirty-three adult patients, *J Vasc Surg* 19:100-111, 1994.
21. Shennib H, Diethrich EB: Novel approaches for the treatment of the aberrant right subclavian artery and its aneurysms, *J Vasc Surg* 47:1066-1070, 2008.

Section 4

UPPER EXTREMITY VASCULAR DISEASE

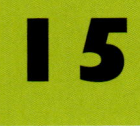

15 Supraclavicular Approach for Surgical Treatment of Thoracic Outlet Syndrome

YAZAN M. DUWAYRI • ROBERT W. THOMPSON

Historical Background

Thoracic outlet syndrome (TOS) is recognized to encompass three conditions: (1) neurogenic TOS, caused by compression of the brachial plexus nerve roots within the scalene triangle, subcoracoid space, or both; (2) venous TOS, caused by compression of the axillary, subclavian, or both veins and leading to the effort thrombosis syndrome; and (3) arterial TOS, caused by compression of the subclavian artery and leading to arterial stenosis, aneurysm formation, and thromboembolism. The early history of surgical treatment for TOS is dominated by supraclavicular operations for cervical rib resection in the treatment of subclavian artery aneurysms.[1,2] Operations initially developed for neurogenic TOS also used supraclavicular approaches, including first rib resection, scalenotomy, and anterior scalenectomy.[3-6] Transaxillary first rib resection was introduced in 1966 and became widely used, particularly with the recognition of frequent anatomic variations and scalene muscle pathology contributing to neurogenic TOS, but its popularity waned in the 1980s with reports of significant morbidity because of brachial plexus nerve injury.[7-11] Use of the supraclavicular approach was reintroduced in 1979, initially as a technique for recurrent neurogenic TOS, and was soon followed by descriptions of combined transaxillary or supraclavicular approaches and more refined techniques for supraclavicular decompression in primary operations.[12-15] Subsequent reports have emphasized the usefulness of supraclavicular decompression for all forms of TOS, exemplified by several particularly large clinical series.[16,17] The techniques described in this chapter are therefore built on rich and varied experience, with additional modifications that have enhanced the usefulness of the supraclavicular approach for all three forms of TOS.

Preoperative Preparation

- The diagnosis of neurogenic TOS is based on clinical evaluation according to the criteria listed in Box 15-1 and supplemented by relevant testing procedures to exclude alternative conditions.[18] The extent of brachial plexus compression attributable to either the scalene triangle or the subcoracoid space is also characterized by physical examination.
- A chest radiograph is obtained to determine the presence or absence of a cervical rib, but other imaging studies of the brachial plexus are usually not helpful.
- Conventional electromyography and nerve conduction studies (EMG/NCS) may be performed to exclude peripheral nerve compression disorders or cervical radiculopathy, but these tests are usually negative or nonspecific in neurogenic TOS.

> **Box 15-1 DIAGNOSTIC FEATURES OF NEUROGENIC THORACIC OUTLET SYNDROME**
>
> Unilateral or bilateral upper extremity symptoms present for at least 12 weeks that meet at least one criterion in each of the following three categories yet are not satisfactorily explained by another condition:
>
> - Manifesting symptoms
>   - Pain in the neck, anterolateral chest, medial upper back, shoulder, arm, and/or hand
>   - Complaint of numbness or paresthesias in the hand, especially in digits 4 and 5
>   - Complaint of weakness in the arm or hand
>   - Paresthesias that radiate from the supraclavicular or infraclavicular space to the arm and/or hand
> - Clinical history
>   - Symptoms that began after head, neck, or upper extremity injury (occupational or recreational)
>   - Symptoms exacerbated by overhead or work-related activities, including repetitive strain
>   - Presence of a cervical rib or previous fracture of the clavicle or first rib
> - Physical examination
>   - Local tenderness on palpation over the scalene triangle and/or subcoracoid space
>   - Reproduction of hand or digit paresthesias on palpation over the scalene triangle and/or subcoracoid space
>   - Weak handgrip, intrinsic muscles, digit 5, or thenar or hypothenar atrophy
>   - Positive upper limb tension test or 3-minute elevated arm stress test
>
> Exclusion of other conditions typically includes nonspecific or negative findings on physical examination (Spurling's test, axial compression test, Tinel's sign over the carpal tunnel or cubital tunnel, and Phalen's test), imaging studies (magnetic resonance imaging of the cervical spine and shoulder), and conventional electrophysiologic tests (upper extremity electromyography and nerve conduction studies). Adapted from the preliminary consensus diagnostic criteria developed by the Consortium for Research and Education on Thoracic Outlet Syndrome.

Thompson RW: Development of consensus-based diagnostic criteria for NTOS. In Illig KA, Thompson RW, Freischlag JA, Donahue DM, Jordan SE, Edgelow PI, editors: *Thoracic outlet syndrome*, London, 2013, Springer, pp 143-155.

- After clinical diagnosis, almost all patients should undergo an anterior scalene or pectoralis minor muscle block with a short-acting local anesthetic to support the clinical diagnosis of neurogenic TOS and to help predict the reversibility of symptoms with treatment.[18]
- After an appropriate course of physical therapy that has been directed by a therapist with specific expertise of neurogenic TOS, surgical treatment is recommended for patients with substantial disability who have not made significant improvement. Surgical treatment may also be recommended in selected patients with persistent or recurrent symptoms of neurogenic TOS after a previous operation, when there has been no response to appropriate conservative measures. In each of these situations we find that supraclavicular decompression, with or without pectoralis minor tenotomy, provides the most definitive approach for surgical treatment.
- Angiography with magnetic resonance imaging or computed tomography is performed to determine the presence or absence of a subclavian artery aneurysm

in patients with a cervical rib or first rib anomaly suspected of having arterial TOS. Similar imaging studies are performed in patients who have presented with upper extremity arterial thromboembolism to detect a proximal source of embolism in the subclavian artery or the axillary artery. Surgical treatment based on supraclavicular decompression is recommended for all patients with subclavian artery aneurysms. This should include arterial reconstruction for subclavian aneurysms that have already produced distal emboli, those associated with imaging evidence of intimal ulceration or mural thrombus, or those greater than twice the normal diameter of the subclavian artery.

- Upper extremity venography is the initial diagnostic step for patients with venous TOS who most frequently present with the axillary-subclavian vein "effort thrombosis" syndrome. Duplex imaging of the subclavian vein is usually inaccurate in this setting because of a high false-negative rate. Contrast venography is immediately followed by thrombolytic therapy, preferably with current pharmacomechanical approaches. Completion venograms typically reveal a focal area of residual subclavian vein stenosis or occlusion at the level of the first rib, often with enhancement by positional maneuvers. Balloon angioplasty of these residual stenoses is usually not helpful, and placement of stents in the subclavian vein is strongly discouraged.

- First rib resection is recommended for patients with previous axillary-subclavian vein thrombosis who remain symptomatic despite anticoagulation and restricted activity, as well as for asymptomatic individuals in whom long-term anticoagulation and restrictions on upper extremity activity are undesirable. The addition of an infraclavicular incision can be used, if needed, along with the supraclavicular approach to ensure complete medial first rib resection and to facilitate direct subclavian vein reconstruction.[19]

Pitfalls and Danger Points

- Inadequate decompression and recurrence
  - Incomplete scalenectomy
  - Incomplete brachial plexus neurolysis
  - Incomplete first rib resection
  - Insufficient methods to prevent perineural fibrosis
  - Residual subclavian vein stenosis or occlusion
- Nerve injury
  - Brachial plexus nerve roots
  - Phrenic nerve
  - Long thoracic nerve
  - First intercostal nerve
- Vascular and lymphatic injury
  - Subclavian artery
  - Subclavian vein
  - Thoracic duct

Operative Strategy

SURGICAL ANATOMY OF THE THORACIC OUTLET

Successful surgical treatment for all three types of TOS depends on a sound understanding of the relationships between musculoskeletal and neurovascular structures in this region, as well as the many anatomic variations likely to be encountered (Fig. 15-1). One of the principal advantages of the supraclavicular approach is excellent exposure of the relevant anatomy, allowing more complete decompression compared with alternative approaches. To accomplish this with

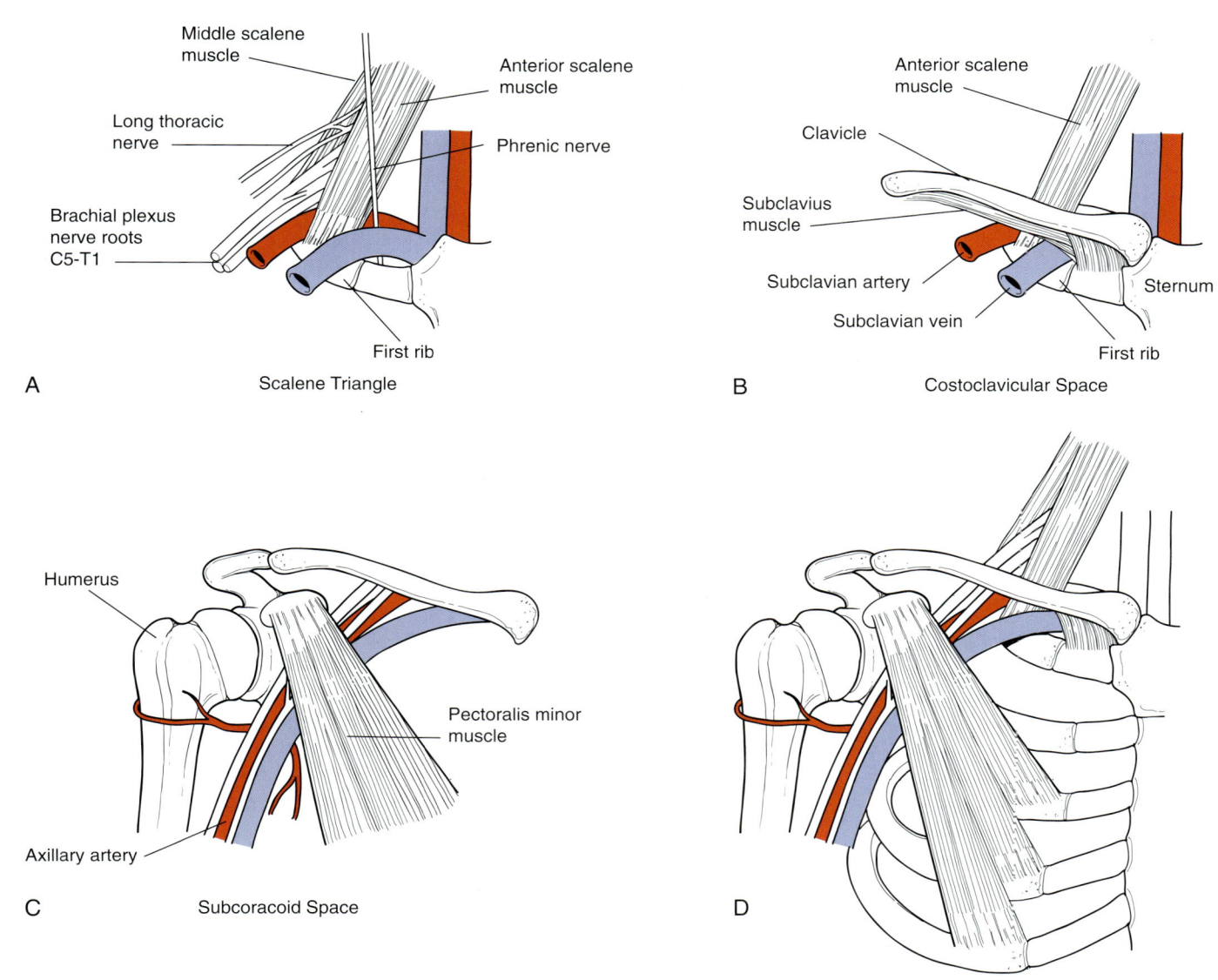

Figure 15-1. Anatomy of the thoracic outlet, focusing on the scalene triangle, the costoclavicular space, and the subcoracoid space. **A,** The scalene triangle is bounded by the anterior scalene muscle, the middle scalene muscle, and the first rib. The brachial plexus and subclavian artery pass through this space and over the first rib, whereas the subclavian vein passes over the first rib immediately in front of the scalene triangle. **B,** The costoclavicular space lies between the clavicle and the first rib and is bordered superiorly by the subclavius muscle, medially by the costoclavicular ligament, and posteriorly by the insertion of the anterior scalene muscle tendon on the first rib. The brachial plexus and subclavian artery pass over the first rib behind the costoclavicular space, whereas the subclavian vein passes over the first rib through the front part of the costoclavicular space. **C,** The subcoracoid space lies inferior to the clavicle and underneath the pectoralis minor muscle tendon, just below its insertion on the coracoid process. All of the structures of the neurovascular bundle pass through this space before reaching the axilla. **D,** Overview of the anatomy of the thoracic outlet.

the greatest margin of safety, we have defined six "critical views" of the surgical anatomy that should be sequentially obtained during the course of supraclavicular decompression (Box 15-2).

AVOIDING INADEQUATE DECOMPRESSION AND RECURRENCE

The potential for persistent or recurrent symptoms of brachial plexus compression remains one of the most challenging aspects of surgical treatment for neurogenic TOS. The supraclavicular approach is designed to avoid the most frequent causes of recurrence by addressing the following issues:

- **Extent of scalene muscle resection.** Reattachment of the anterior scalene muscle is a well-documented cause of recurrent neurogenic TOS after simple scalenotomy, partial scalenectomy, or transaxillary first rib resection.[20] In these circumstances the anterior scalene muscle may reattach to remaining portions

> **Box 15-2** **SIX CRITICAL VIEWS DURING SUPRACLAVICULAR THORACIC OUTLET DECOMPRESSION**
>
> 1. View of the operative field after lateral reflection of the scalene fat pad, with visualization of the anterior scalene muscle, phrenic nerve, brachial plexus, subclavian artery, middle scalene muscle, and long thoracic nerve.
> 2. View of the lower part of the anterior scalene muscle where it attaches to the first rib, with space sufficient to allow a finger to pass behind the anterior scalene muscle and in front of the brachial plexus and subclavian artery, before division of the anterior scalene muscle insertion from the top of the first rib.
> 3. View of the upper part of the anterior scalene muscle at the level of the transverse process of the cervical spine, in relation to the C5 and C6 nerve roots, before division of the origin of the anterior scalene muscle.
> 4. View of the insertion of the middle scalene muscle on the first rib, with each of the five nerve roots of the brachial plexus and the subclavian artery retracted medially and the long thoracic nerve retracted posteriorly, before division of the insertion of the middle scalene muscle from the top of the lateral first rib.
> 5. View of the posterior neck of the first rib, with the T1 nerve root passing from underneath the rib to join the C8 nerve root and form the inferior trunk of the brachial plexus, before division of the posterior first rib.
> 6. View of the anterior portion of the first rib, with placement of the rib shears medial to the scalene tubercle, before division of the anterior first rib.

of the first rib, to the bed of the resected first rib, to the extrapleural fascia, or directly to the brachial plexus nerve roots. Anomalous scalene muscles and fibrofascial bands may also persist as a source of brachial plexus compression if not removed. It is therefore recommended that both the anterior and the middle scalene muscles be resected, along with the anomalous scalene muscle and the fibrofascial bands that might be encountered, during supraclavicular thoracic outlet decompression.

- **Brachial plexus neurolysis.** Most patients undergoing surgery for neurogenic TOS exhibit visual evidence of fibrous scar tissue surrounding the brachial plexus nerve roots, a reflection of previous injury and inflammatory tissue healing. This fibrous tissue may contribute to nerve fixation and irritation and when retained may be a cause for residual neurogenic symptoms. It is therefore recommended that perineural fibrous scar tissue be meticulously removed from around each of the brachial plexus nerve roots during the course of thoracic outlet decompression (external neurolysis).

- **First rib and cervical rib resection.** There remains some room for debate regarding the necessity for first rib resection during supraclavicular thoracic outlet decompression, with some advocating routine first rib resection and others encouraging a more selective approach based on intraoperative findings after scalenectomy and brachial plexus neurolysis.[21] It remains unclear whether there are distinct advantages attributable to retaining the first rib, and incomplete first rib resection is often cited as a factor contributing to recurrent neurogenic TOS.[22] It is therefore recommended that first rib resection be included in supraclavicular decompression for neurogenic TOS, extending posteriorly as far as the level of the T1 nerve root and anteriorly to the costochondral junction (just medial to the scalene tubercle). The first rib is often abnormal in patients with a cervical rib and may serve as a source of persistent or recurrent nerve compression after isolated cervical rib resection. Thus first rib resection is also advocated in patients with cervical ribs, along with resection of the cervical rib, in order to ensure the most complete decompression feasible.[23] In venous TOS, the subclavian vein is typically compressed at the point where it passes over the first rib and directly underneath the clavicle. Resection of the anteriormost portion of the first rib is therefore considered important in operations for venous TOS to prevent persistent or recurrent subclavian vein obstruction, but this cannot be achieved through the supraclavicular approach alone. For this reason, and to provide more complete access to the axillary-subclavian vein (in the event that direct venous reconstruction is warranted), a medial infraclavicular incision is added to the supraclavicular approach in operations for venous TOS.[19]

- **Pectoralis minor tenotomy.** Brachial plexus compression by the pectoralis minor muscle has become increasingly appreciated as a factor contributing to neurogenic TOS.[24] In our experience up to 20% of patients with neurogenic TOS exhibit physical findings isolated to the subcoracoid space and another 30% to 40% have findings that colocalize to both the scalene triangle and the subcoracoid space. Even in patients with findings predominantly localized to the scalene triangle, residual nerve compression at the site of the pectoralis minor muscle may be a source of persistent or recurrent neurogenic TOS. Simple division of the pectoralis minor muscle tendon immediately below the coracoid process can provide substantial relief of brachial plexus compression while adding little to the operative procedure; thus pectoralis minor tenotomy should be included with supraclavicular decompression whenever suggested by preoperative clinical findings.

- **Hemostasis and fluid accumulations.** Postoperative accumulation of blood and serum may enhance local wound healing responses that promote fibrosis, thereby contributing to the potential for late neural compression and recurrent symptoms after thoracic outlet decompression. Common local sources of bleeding include the ends of the divided first rib and the edges of the resected scalene or intercostal muscles. Although bleeding from these sites is typically minimal and self-limited, effort should be made to diminish fluid accumulation in the operative field. To this end, a topical hemostatic agent is placed along the edges of the resected muscles and the scalene fat pad is closely reapproximated over the brachial plexus to reduce potential space in the wound. The pleural apex is also purposefully opened to promote dependent drainage away from the operative field, and a closed-suction drain is placed within the supraclavicular space upon completion of the procedure.

- **Absorbable film barriers.** Postoperative scarring around the brachial plexus nerve roots is inevitable after an operation for TOS, and dense perineural fibrosis is a potential cause of recurrent nerve entrapment and irritation. As in other operations involving direct nerve exposure, it is recommended that the brachial plexus nerve roots be covered with an absorbable antiadhesion film barrier, using one of several materials that have been developed for this purpose, to decrease the potential for later nerve encasement.[25]

AVOIDING NERVE INJURY

The potential for nerve injury is a primary concern in operation for TOS and may occur because of transection, electrocautery, or excessive traction. The incidence of these complications should be negligible in experienced hands, but several factors may elevate the risk of nerve injury during supraclavicular thoracic outlet decompression, including unexpected anatomic variations, pathologic findings, intraoperative bleeding, and reoperative procedures.

- **Brachial plexus nerve roots.** Meticulous operative technique is critical to avoid injury to the brachial plexus nerve roots by minimizing handling of the nerves, dissecting the perineural tissues under direct vision, and maintaining constant awareness of the extent of retraction being placed on individual nerve roots. The presence of a cervical rib or ligamentous band may displace the brachial plexus more forward than usually expected, and scalene muscle anomalies (e.g., a scalene minimus muscle) and fibrofascial bands may obscure the lower nerve roots. Division of the anterior scalene muscle from the first rib should be done with a finger placed between the muscle and the underlying brachial plexus and subclavian artery, using scissors rather than electrocautery. Before resection of the middle scalene muscle, the brachial plexus should be mobilized such that all five nerve roots are visible and gently retracted medially. Full visualization of the T1 nerve root should also be obtained, where it passes from underneath the first rib to join the C8 nerve root, before dividing the posterior neck of the first rib.

- **Phrenic nerve.** The phrenic nerve lies on the surface of the anterior scalene muscle, passing from its lateral to its medial edge before descending behind the subclavian vein into the mediastinum. Even with the gentle mobilization of the phrenic nerve necessary to complete resection of the anterior scalene muscle, intraoperative traction or postoperative inflammation around the nerve may result in temporary neuropraxia and ipsilateral diaphragmatic paralysis. Because phrenic nerve palsy may be asymptomatic and compensated by the other side, it is important to verify normal phrenic nerve function on the side of the previous operation for TOS before undertaking a contralateral procedure. An accessory phrenic nerve often arises from the edge of the brachial plexus, where it passes medially to join the primary phrenic nerve near the lower aspect of the anterior scalene muscle. In some cases the primary or accessory phrenic nerve passes anterior to the subclavian vein, known as a "prevenous" phrenic nerve. This anomaly can serve as a potential cause of subclavian vein obstruction in venous TOS and is only observed with supraclavicular or infraclavicular exposure.

- **Long thoracic nerve.** The long thoracic nerve forms within the body of the middle scalene muscle from three separate branches and then emerges from the muscle to pass over the lateral aspect of the first rib. Protection of the long thoracic nerve is achieved by direct visualization and gentle posterior retraction during middle scalenectomy.

- **First intercostal nerve.** Injury to the first intercostal nerve branch during resection of the rib may result in a painful postoperative neuroma. This can be avoided by displacing the nerve away from the neck of the posterior first rib before dividing the bone. Blunt dissection of the posterior surface of the anterior rib, maintaining a plane immediately under the bone to further displace the intercostal nerve, is also helpful to avoid injury.

AVOIDING VASCULAR AND LYMPHATIC INJURY

- **Subclavian artery.** The subclavian artery is directly exposed during supraclavicular decompression and must be protected from injury throughout the procedure. Complete mobilization of the subclavian artery, with ligation and division of small arterial branches that commonly arise from its superior aspect (i.e., the thyrocervical trunk), is helpful to avoid traction or avulsion injuries that can extend onto the main vessel.

- **Subclavian vein.** Although the subclavian vein is usually not exposed during supraclavicular decompression for neurogenic TOS, it is susceptible to injury underneath the medial clavicle and where it joins the internal jugular vein. In venous TOS an increased network of collateral veins is usually encountered throughout the supraclavicular space. Although larger collateral vessels are preserved, such as the external jugular vein, small venous collaterals should be ligated and divided to minimize intraoperative bleeding. Any localized bleeding that may occur during the course of supraclavicular decompression should be meticulously identified and controlled so that blood does not obscure the operative field and elevate the risk of nerve injury.

- **Thoracic duct.** The thoracic duct joins the venous system on the left side near the junction of the internal jugular and subclavian veins. It is susceptible to injury during mobilization of the scalene fat pad and should therefore be sought and directly divided between silk ligatures during the early stages of the operation.

SUPRACLAVICULAR APPROACH FOR SURGICAL TREATMENT OF THORACIC OUTLET SYNDROME 179

When a lymphatic leak is observed during the course of the procedure, the site of the leak is identified and oversewn with a pledgeted polypropylene suture, and a topical hemostatic or fibrin tissue sealant is applied to the site before wound closure.

Operative Technique

POSITION AND INCISION

Under general anesthesia, the patient is positioned supine with the head of the bed elevated 30 degrees. The hips and knees are flexed, and the neck is extended and turned to the opposite side. An inflatable thyroid pillow is placed between the shoulders to help extend the neck. The neck, upper chest, and affected upper extremity are prepped into the field, with the arm wrapped in a stockinette and held comfortably across the abdomen (Fig. 15-2).

A transverse neck incision is made parallel to and just above the clavicle, beginning at the lateral border of the sternocleidomastoid muscle and extending to the anterior border of the trapezius muscle (see Fig. 15-2). The incision is carried through the platysma muscle, the edge of the sternocleidomastoid muscle is lifted and retracted medially, and the scalene fat pad is mobilized, beginning by separating its medial portion from the lateral edge of the internal jugular vein. A short segment of the omohyoid muscle is resected, and the ends are allowed to retract. The scalene fat pad is mobilized from its inferior and superior attachments. Deliberate division and ligation is the preferred method because lymphatic leak is a potential complication. On the left side, the thoracic duct is usually identified

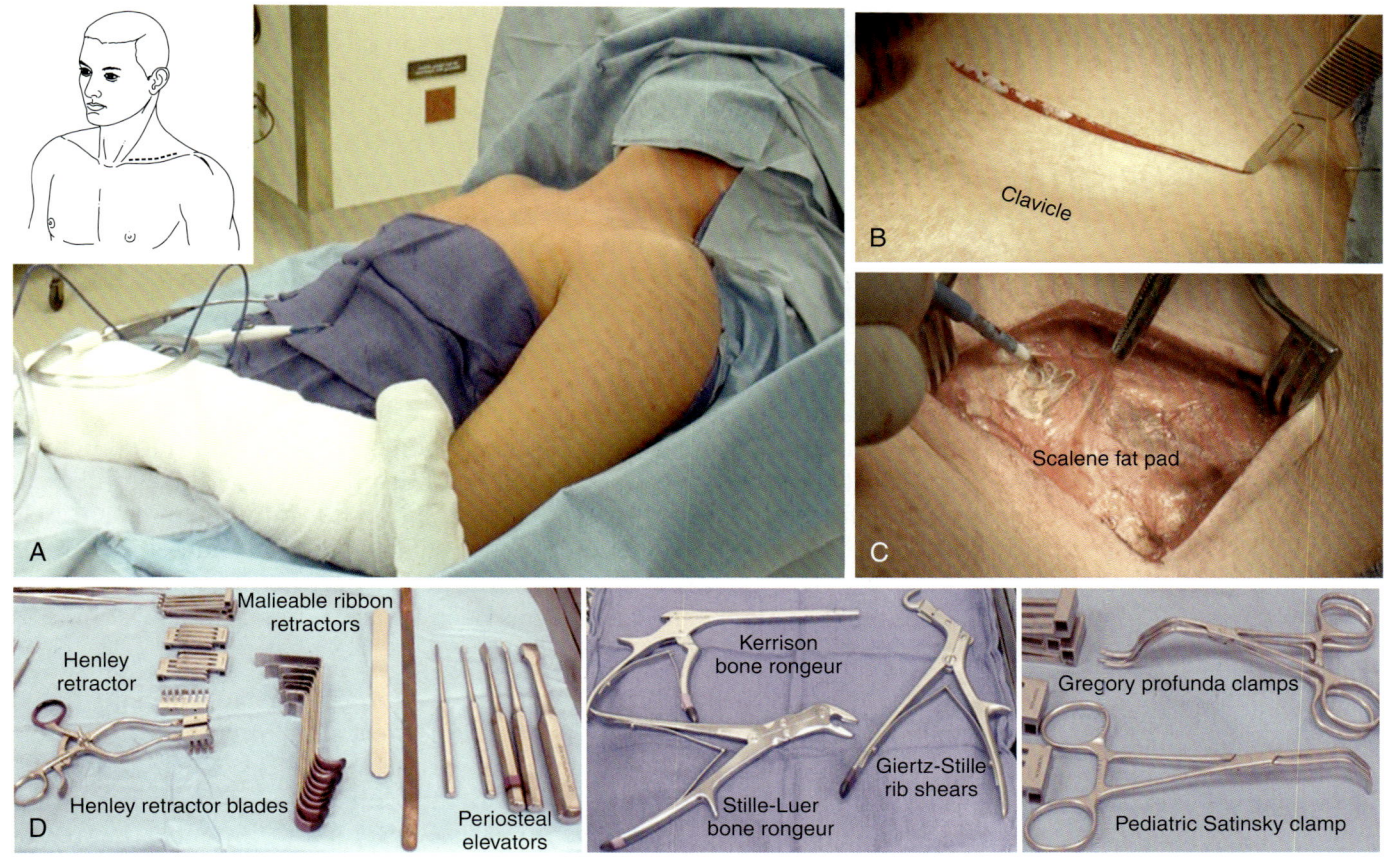

Figure 15-2. Position, incision, and instruments used for supraclavicular thoracic outlet decompression. **A,** Patient position and planned incision for supraclavicular thoracic outlet decompression (left side). **B,** The skin incision is made just above and parallel to the clavicle, extending from the lateral border of the sternocleidomastoid muscle to the anterior border of the trapezius muscle. **C,** Initial mobilization of the scalene fat pad. **D,** Instruments commonly used during supraclavicular decompression.

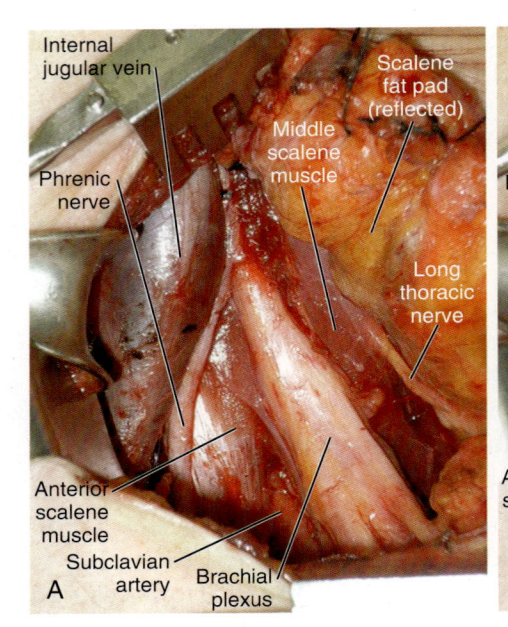

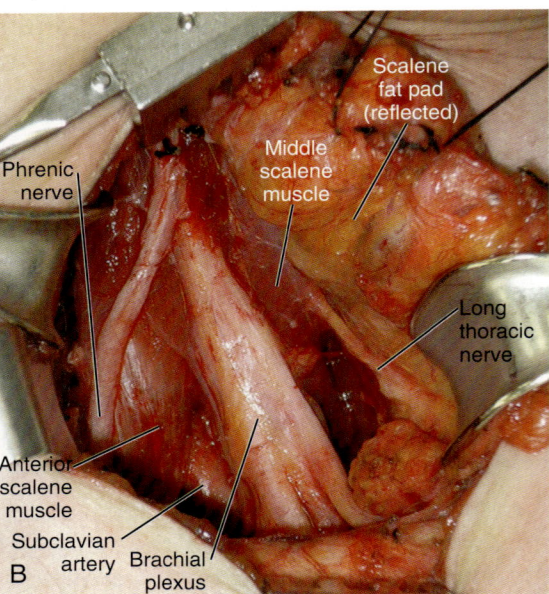

Figure 15-3. Initial exposure (critical view 1). After mobilization and lateral reflection of the scalene fat pad, direct visualization is obtained of the internal jugular vein (**A**) and the anterior scalene muscle, phrenic nerve, subclavian artery, brachial plexus, middle scalene muscle, and long thoracic nerve (**A** and **B**). Satisfactory exposure of all of these structures is crucial before beginning the next steps in the decompression procedure. Photographs depict the left side, with the head at the top of the figures.

entering the venous system near the inferomedial aspect of the scalene fat pad, where it is divided between silk ligatures.

EXPOSURE

The scalene fat pad is lifted and the underlying tissue plane is gently dissected with the tip of a finger. The fat pad is progressively reflected laterally, exposing the underlying anterior scalene muscle and phrenic nerve. Further mobilization of the scalene fat pad reveals the brachial plexus along the lateral edge of the anterior scalene muscle, followed by the middle scalene muscle behind the brachial plexus, where it attaches to the upper surface of the lateral first rib. The long thoracic nerve is observed as it emerges from the middle scalene muscle to pass across the lateral aspect of the first rib. During this dissection a small nerve stimulator may be used to verify the identity of specific nerves, but this is usually not necessary. Having all preceding structures under direct vision represents the first critical view to be obtained during supraclavicular decompression (Fig. 15-3). The scalene fat pad is subsequently held in position with several silk retraction sutures, and the exposure is maintained with a three-arm Henley self-retaining retractor, using the third arm to hold the edge of the sternocleidomastoid muscle.

SCALENECTOMY

The brachial plexus and subclavian artery are dissected away from the lower lateral edge of the anterior scalene muscle, allowing a fingertip to be introduced behind the muscle just above the first rib. With posterior displacement of the neurovascular structures, fingertip dissection is continued behind the anterior scalene muscle toward its medial edge, where the proximal subclavian artery and the phrenic nerve must also be well visualized and protected. Once the insertion of the anterior scalene muscle onto the first rib has been isolated under direct vision (Fig. 15-4), it is sharply divided using curved scissors.

By elevating the end of the divided anterior scalene muscle, additional slips of muscle, fascia, or tendon are divided, including direct attachments of the muscle to the subclavian artery and the thickened extrapleural fascia. The anterior scalene muscle is passed underneath to the medial side of the phrenic nerve and progressively lifted farther, with division of its posterior attachments and protection of the upper brachial plexus nerve roots, until it is held on a pedicle from its origin on the transverse process of the cervical spine (Fig. 15-5). The anterior scalene muscle is then sharply divided from its origin, and the entire muscle is removed.

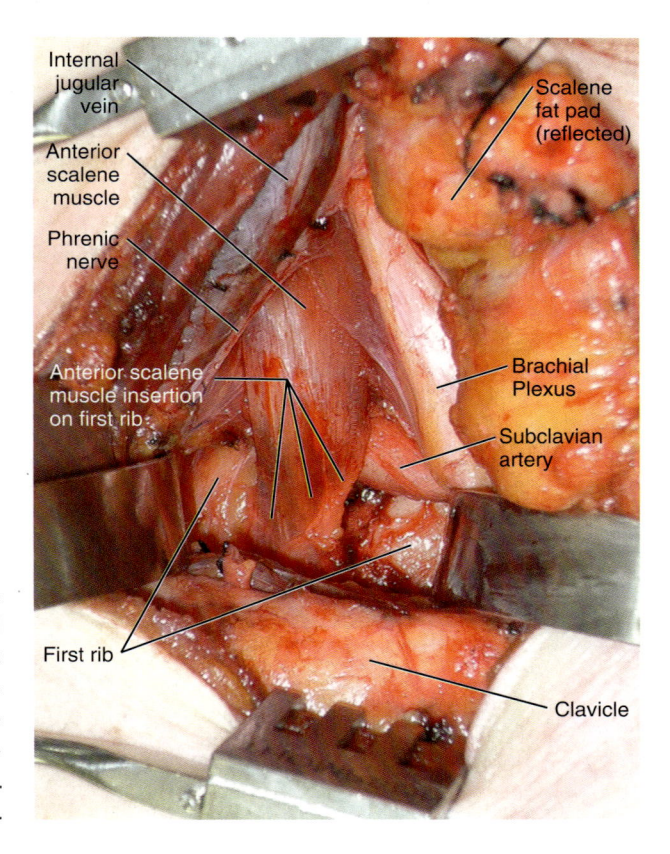

SUPRACLAVICULAR APPROACH FOR SURGICAL TREATMENT OF THORACIC OUTLET SYNDROME

Figure 15-4. Anterior scalenectomy, insertion (critical view 2). The lower part of the anterior scalene muscle is circumferentially mobilized from the underlying subclavian artery and roots of the brachial plexus to isolate the muscle insertion on the top of the first rib. Once a fingertip can be passed behind the anterior scalene muscle to protect the subclavian artery and brachial plexus, the insertion of the anterior scalene muscle is sharply divided with scissors from the top of the first rib. The photograph depicts the left side, with the head at top of the figure.

Scalene minimus muscle anomalies are usually identified during resection of the anterior scalene muscle. These are represented by additional muscle fibers that originate in the plane of the middle scalene muscle and pass between the brachial plexus nerve roots before inserting on the extrapleural fascia or first rib (either along with or independently of the anterior scalene muscle) (Fig. 15-6). Any scalene minimus muscle identified during anterior scalenectomy is therefore resected at this stage in the procedure. A number of different anomalous fibrofascial bands may also be observed after anterior scalene muscle resection, typically passing in front of the lower brachial plexus nerve roots (see Fig. 15-6). These structures are also resected as they are encountered to ensure thorough decompression and full mobility of the nerve roots.

The brachial plexus nerve roots are separated from the front edge of the middle scalene muscle, sequentially identifying each nerve root from C5 to T1, until a small malleable retractor can be placed behind the brachial plexus. The attachment of the middle scalene muscle to the lateral first rib is then exposed by medial retraction of the brachial plexus and posterolateral reflection of the long thoracic nerve (Fig. 15-7). The anterior portion of the middle scalene muscle is initially divided on the top of the rib using electrocautery. Moving posteriorly along the top of the first rib, the middle scalene muscle is further detached using electrocautery and a periosteal elevator, extending to a point parallel with the T1 nerve root. The plane separating the middle and posterior scalene muscles is defined by the oblique course of the long thoracic nerve, which is represented by two or three branches that pass through the muscle at this level. Any muscle tissue lying anterior to this nerve is considered to be the middle scalene muscle; this muscle is divided, leaving the long thoracic nerve intact, and the middle scalene muscle is thereby removed.

FIRST RIB RESECTION

After complete anterior and middle scalenectomy, the intercostal muscle attachments to the lateral edge of the first rib are divided under direct vision using electrocautery or a periosteal elevator. A fingertip is placed between the brachial plexus and the inner side of the first rib, and with blunt dissection the extrapleural tissues

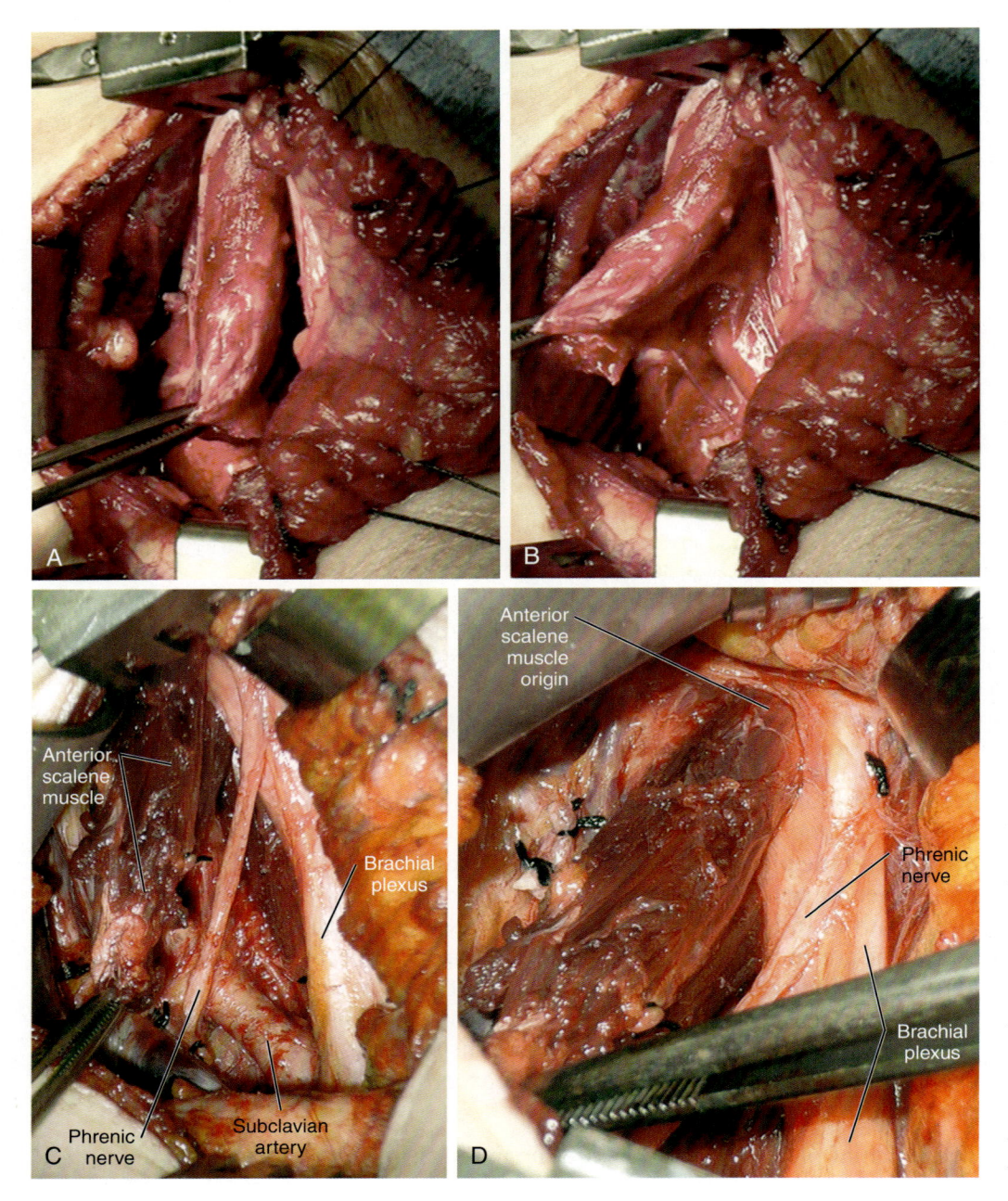

Figure 15-5. Anterior scalenectomy, origin (critical view 3). **A** and **B,** The divided distal end of the anterior scalene muscle is lifted, and the muscle is dissected free of underlying structures to the level of its origin on the transverse process of the cervical vertebra. The underlying subclavian artery and brachial plexus are both well protected during the dissection. Photographs depict the left side, with the head to the right of the figures. **C,** The anterior scalene muscle is passed underneath and to the medial side of the phrenic nerve to facilitate dissection of the upper part of the muscle. **D,** The origin of the anterior scalene muscle on the transverse process of the cervical spine is isolated, along with the upper part of the brachial plexus, after which the anterior scalene muscle may be safely divided. Photographs depict the left side, with the head at the top of the figures.

are swept away from the undersurface of the bone. The posterior neck of the first rib is exposed to the level where the T1 nerve root emerges from underneath the rib to join the C8 nerve root above the rib, thereby forming the lower trunk of the brachial plexus. A right-angled clamp is passed underneath the rib to separate remaining intercostal muscle and to displace the first intercostal nerve. With the C8 and T1 nerve roots under direct vision, modified Giertz-Stille rib shears are inserted around the neck of the first rib (Fig. 15-8). Mobility of the nerve roots is verified and the bone is divided. A Kerrison bone rongeur is used to remove additional bone needed to ensure that the remaining posterior stump of the first rib does not impinge upon the lower nerve roots, and the end of the bone is sealed with bone wax.

Using sharp and blunt dissection, the remaining intercostal muscle and fascial attachments to the anterior first rib are divided up to the level of the scalene tubercle. The clavicle is elevated with a small Richardson retractor, and the proximal portion of the rib is displaced inferiorly if necessary, with fingertip pressure on the free posterior end of the rib, to open the anterior costoclavicular space. The Giertz-Stille rib shears are inserted around the anterior first rib and positioned immediately medial to the scalene tubercle under direct vision (Fig. 15-9). The

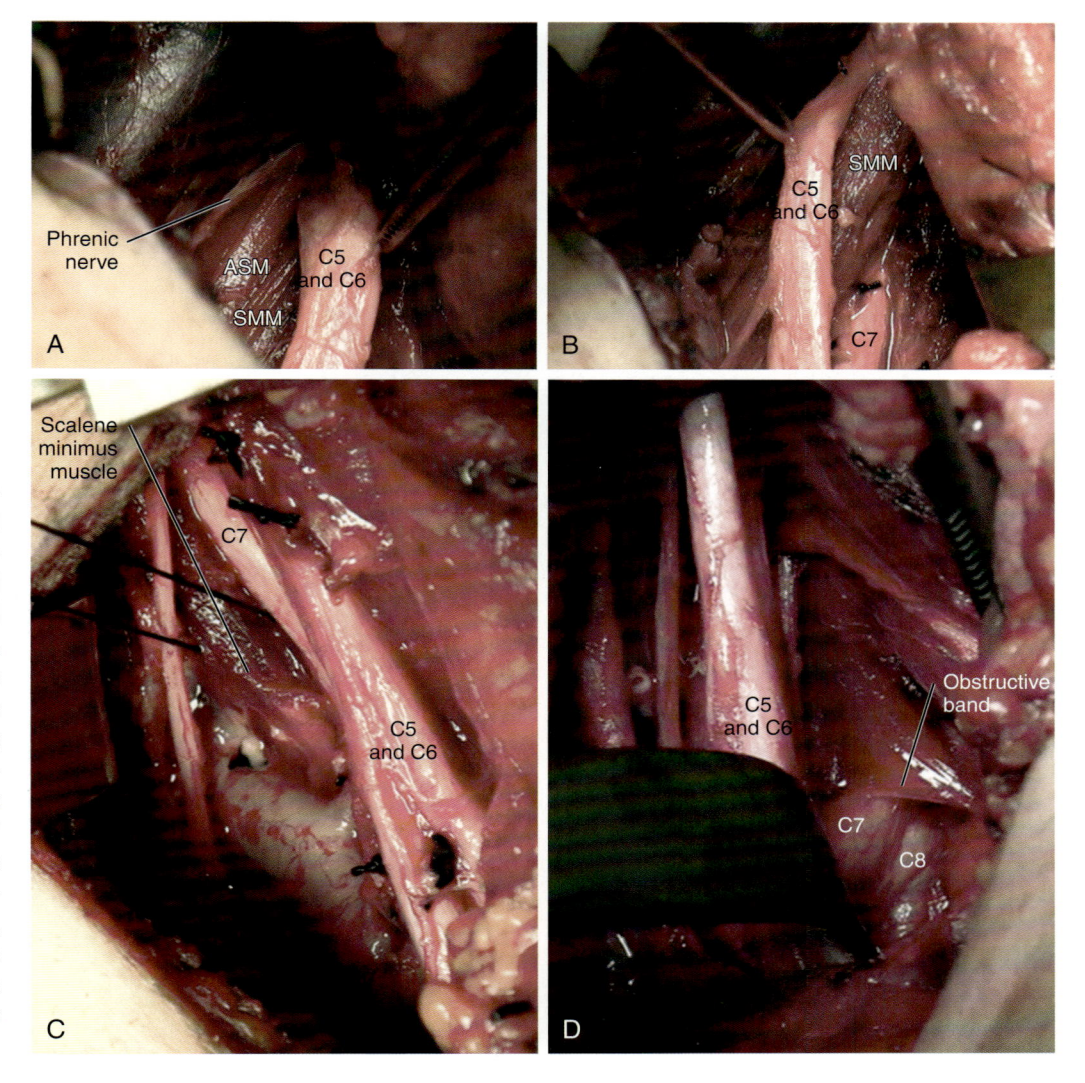

SUPRACLAVICULAR APPROACH FOR SURGICAL TREATMENT OF THORACIC OUTLET SYNDROME 183

Figure 15-6. Scalene muscle anomalies and fibrofascial bands. **A** and **B,** A large scalene minimus muscle is found passing between the C6 and C7 brachial plexus nerve roots. **C,** A scalene minimus muscle is found crossing anterior to the C7 nerve root and attaching to the extrapleural fascia posterior to the subclavian artery. **D,** An aberrant fibrofascial band is found obstructing the C7 and C8 nerve roots. Photographs depict the left side, with the head at the top of the figures. *ASM,* Anterior scalene muscle; *SMM,* Scalene minimus muscle.

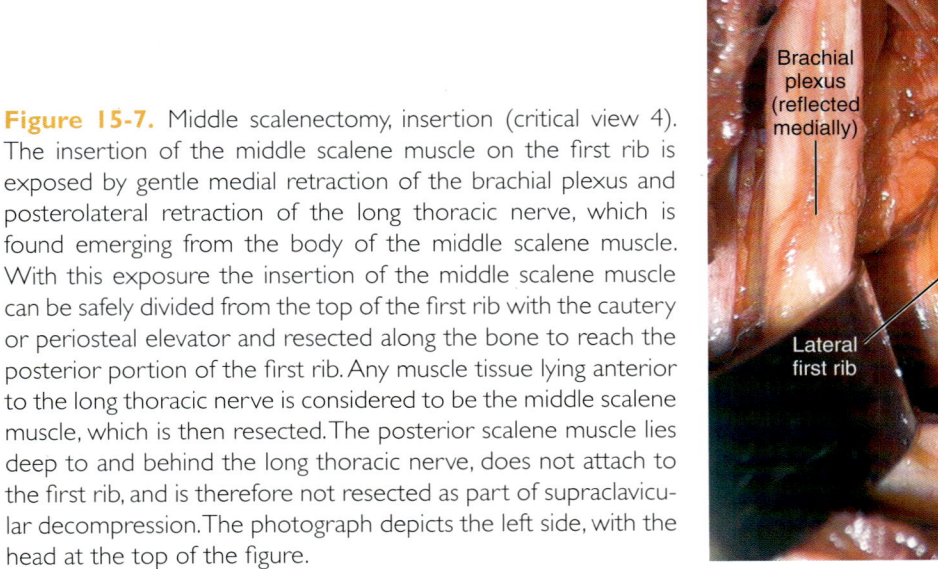

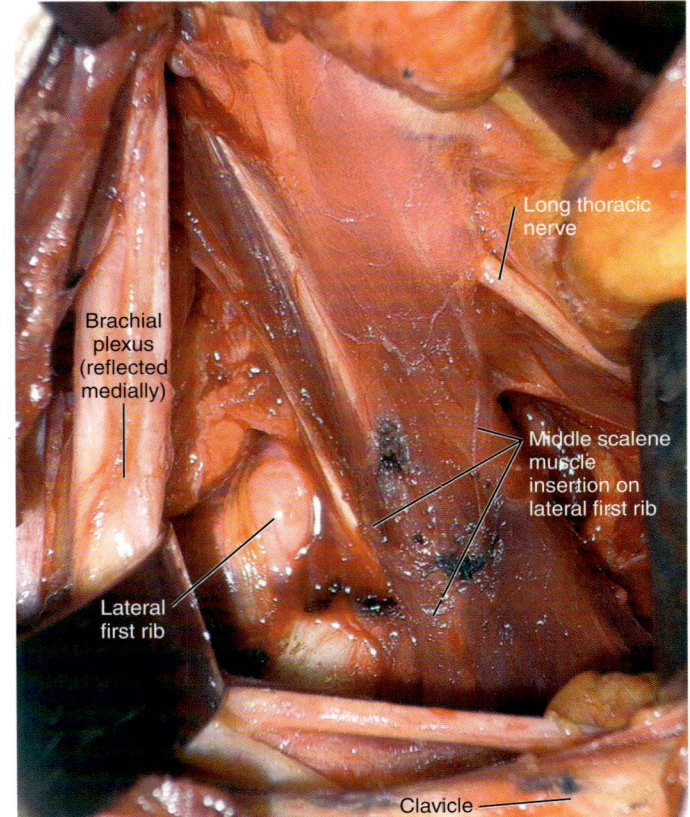

Figure 15-7. Middle scalenectomy, insertion (critical view 4). The insertion of the middle scalene muscle on the first rib is exposed by gentle medial retraction of the brachial plexus and posterolateral retraction of the long thoracic nerve, which is found emerging from the body of the middle scalene muscle. With this exposure the insertion of the middle scalene muscle can be safely divided from the top of the first rib with the cautery or periosteal elevator and resected along the bone to reach the posterior portion of the first rib. Any muscle tissue lying anterior to the long thoracic nerve is considered to be the middle scalene muscle, which is then resected. The posterior scalene muscle lies deep to and behind the long thoracic nerve, does not attach to the first rib, and is therefore not resected as part of supraclavicular decompression. The photograph depicts the left side, with the head at the top of the figure.

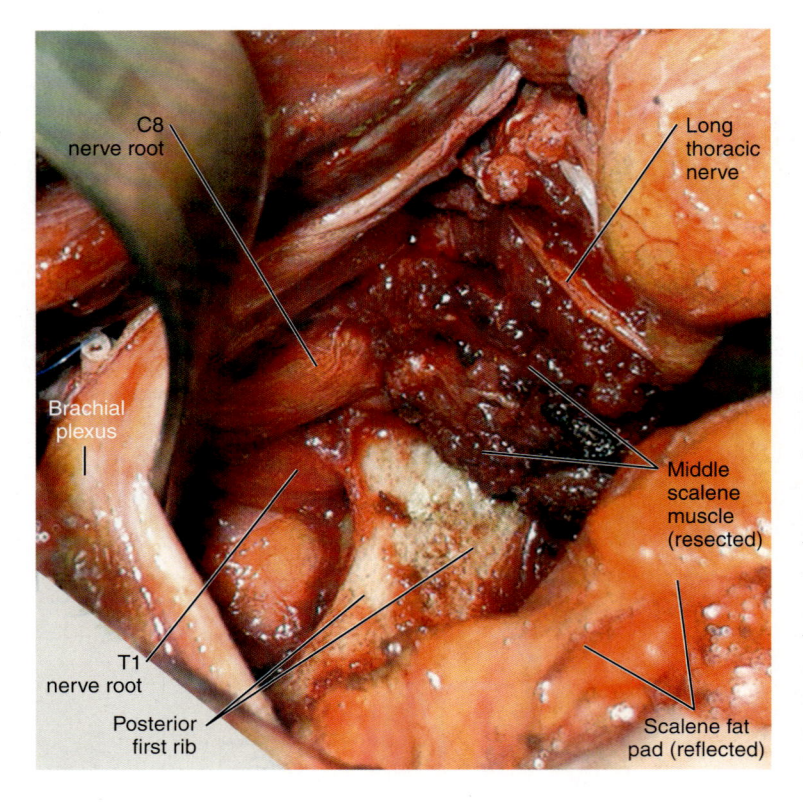

Figure 15-8. First rib resection, posterior (critical view 5). The posterior portion of the first rib is exposed after removal of the middle scalene muscle, with visualization of the entire brachial plexus. The C8 nerve root is visualized immediately above the posterior first rib, and the T1 nerve root is visualized emerging from immediately below the first rib. Once this exposure has been achieved, modified Giertz-Stille rib shears are placed around the posterior portion of the first rib in preparation for division of the bone. After application of the rib shears, the remaining posterior first rib is further remodeled with a Kerrison rongeur to obtain a smooth edge at a level immediately medial to the T1 nerve root. The photograph depicts the left side, with the head at the top of the figure.

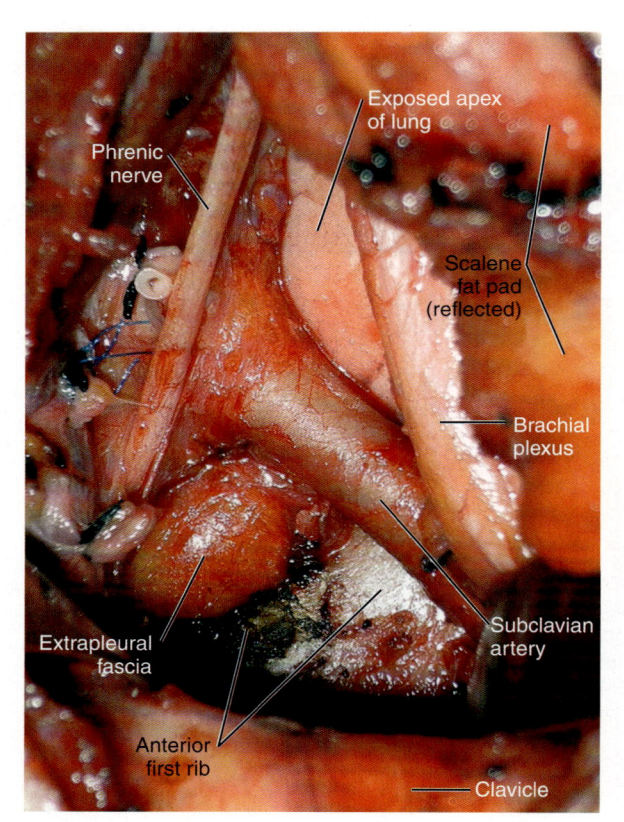

Figure 15-9. First rib resection, anterior (critical view 6). The anterior portion of the first rib is exposed underneath the clavicle and subclavian vein, where it is divided immediately medial to the scalene tubercle. The underside of the rib is bluntly dissected from the adherent extrapleural fascia, often with entry into the pleural space and exposure of the apex of the lung. Once satisfactory exposure has been obtained, modified Giertz-Stille rib shears are placed around the anterior portion of the first rib in preparation for division of the bone. After application of the rib shears, the first rib specimen is removed and the remaining anterior first rib is remodeled with a rongeur to obtain a smooth edge well underneath the clavicle. The photograph depicts the left side, with the head at the top of the figure.

proximal first rib is then divided, and the specimen is extracted from the operative field (Fig. 15-10). The remaining anterior end of the first rib is remodeled to a smooth surface with a Kerrison and Stille-Luer duckbill bone rongeur and sealed with bone wax.

When a cervical rib is present, it is first encountered within the plane of the middle scalene muscle during the course of scalene muscle resection, where it lies behind the brachial plexus and subclavian artery. The anterior end of the cervical

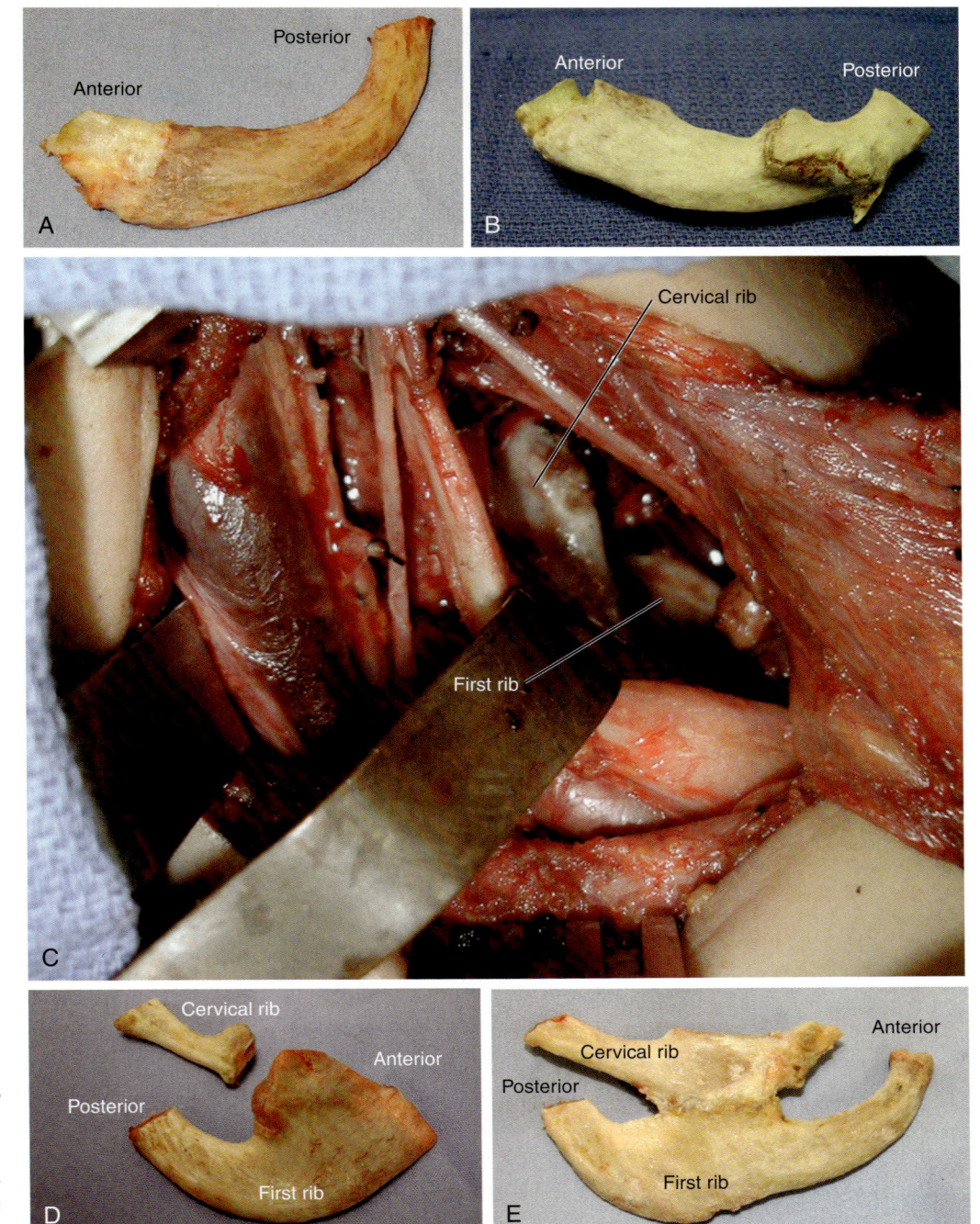

SUPRACLAVICULAR APPROACH FOR SURGICAL TREATMENT OF THORACIC OUTLET SYNDROME

Figure 15-10. First rib and cervical rib specimens. **A,** Resected specimen of the first rib. **B,** Resected specimen of the first rib, illustrating the site of a previous posterior fracture. **C,** Operative photograph demonstrating exposure of the cervical and first ribs with the brachial plexus retracted medially. The photograph depicts the left side, with the head to the right of the figure. **D,** Resected specimen of the cervical and first ribs, with an incomplete (fibrous) connection. **E,** Resected specimen of the cervical and first ribs connected by a complete bony fusion.

rib may be free, with a ligamentous extension that attaches to the first rib, or it may terminate in a junction with the first rib, often forming a true joint. The cervical rib is carefully exposed along its course to protect the brachial plexus nerves, much as described for the middle scalene muscle and the first rib. In most cases the posterior cervical rib is divided or resected before proceeding to first rib resection, with exposure and division of its posterior aspect in the same manner. The anterior cervical rib is then divided and the bone is removed. When the cervical rib forms a true joint with the first rib, the anterior portion is left attached while the first rib resection is completed, and the two are removed together as a single specimen (see Fig. 15-10, *E*).

BRACHIAL PLEXUS NEUROLYSIS

After scalenectomy and removal of the first rib, attention is returned to the brachial plexus to ensure that each of the contributing nerve roots is meticulously dissected free of perineural fibrous scar tissue. This aspect of the operation is not

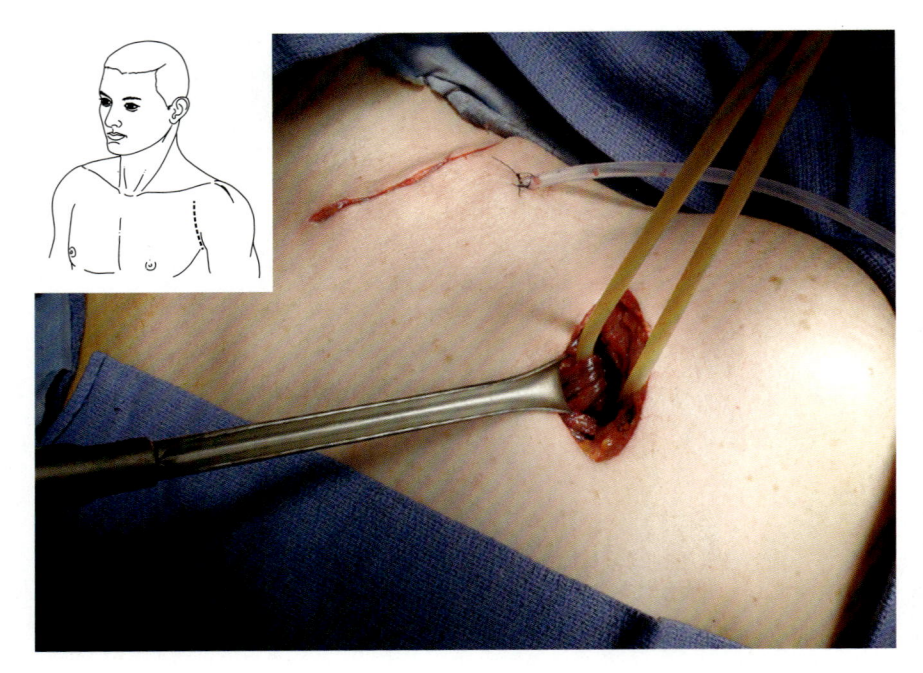

Figure 15-11. Pectoralis minor tenotomy. The pectoralis minor muscle is approached through a vertical incision in the deltopectoral groove (inset) and isolated after medial retraction of the pectoralis major muscle. The pectoralis minor muscle is divided with electrocautery immediately below its insertion on the coracoid process. The photograph depicts the left side, with the pectoralis minor tenotomy performed after completing supraclavicular thoracic outlet decompression.

complete until each nerve root from C5 to T1 is dissected throughout its course in the operative field to ensure full mobility.

PECTORALIS MINOR TENOTOMY

To ensure thorough relief of brachial plexus nerve compression for neurogenic TOS, pectoralis minor tenotomy is performed as an addition to supraclavicular thoracic outlet decompression when indicated by previous clinical findings or as an isolated procedure when this site is the dominant location of nerve compression symptoms. In the presence of distinct localizing findings, pectoralis minor tenotomy may also be performed in patients with persistent or recurrent neurogenic TOS who have previously undergone thoracic outlet decompression by other approaches.

A short, vertical infraclavicular incision is made in the deltopectoral groove, beginning just below the coracoid process (Fig. 15-11). The fascia between the deltoid and the pectoralis major muscles is divided medial to the cephalic vein and separated with a self-retaining retractor. The lateral edge of the pectoralis major muscle is gently retracted medially and lifted to expose the underlying fascia. The pectoralis minor muscle is exposed and encircled near its insertion on the coracoid process, taking care to protect the underlying neurovascular bundle (see Fig. 15-11). The pectoralis minor tendon is then divided under direct vision, within 2 cm of the coracoid, using electrocautery. The medial edge of the divided muscle is oversewn to ensure hemostasis, and the remaining clavipectoral fascia is opened to the level of the clavicle. No further dissection of the brachial plexus or axillary vessels is performed once the pectoralis minor muscle has been divided.

MANAGEMENT OF AN ASSOCIATED SUBCLAVIAN ARTERY ANEURYSM

Patients with arterial TOS are characterized by formation of poststenotic subclavian artery aneurysms, which typically arise within several centimeters of the scalene triangle where the subclavian artery crosses over the first rib and underneath the clavicle. Subclavian artery aneurysms almost always occur in association with a cervical rib or anomalous first rib. Regardless of size or potential for rupture, these lesions are frequently complicated by intimal ulceration, mural thrombus, and distal thromboembolism. Surgical treatment may initially require treatment of distal arterial occlusions because of emboli to the brachial, radial, ulnar, or a combination of these arteries. Definitive imaging assessment of the subclavian artery may be accomplished by intraoperative catheter-based arteriography, intravascular ultrasound, or both to identify intimal ulceration, mural thrombus, or wall thickening. For small aneurysms without evidence of ulceration or mural thrombus, thoracic outlet decompression alone may suffice; however, even small aneurysms with evidence of ulceration or previous thromboembolism should be repaired.

After supraclavicular decompression, as described earlier for neurogenic TOS (including removal of the cervical and first ribs), the subclavian artery is mobilized in preparation for interposition graft repair of the aneurysmal segment. In the event that satisfactory distal control of the nonaneurysmal subclavian artery cannot be obtained from the supraclavicular exposure alone, a transverse infraclavicular incision is made with division of the pectoralis minor muscle tendon, and the axillary artery is isolated for distal vascular control. The proximal subclavian artery is clamped immediately distal to the vertebral artery, and the distal subclavian artery is clamped immediately beyond the aneurysm. The intervening segment of subclavian artery is excised, and the artery is replaced with an interposition bypass graft using beveled end-to-end anastomoses. Although reversed saphenous vein grafts are typically too small in caliber for subclavian artery replacement, conduits more suitable for this type of reconstruction include Dacron or polytetrafluoroethylene prosthetic grafts, cryopreserved femoral artery allografts, and autologous deep vein (e.g., superficial femoral) or artery (e.g., iliac) grafts. In most cases a completion arteriogram is performed to evaluate the subclavian artery reconstruction in different positions of the arm and to reassess the distal circulation.

MANAGEMENT OF ASSOCIATED SUBCLAVIAN VEIN STENOSIS OR OCCLUSION

Operative management for venous TOS begins with supraclavicular decompression, as described earlier for neurogenic TOS, except that the anterior first rib is not yet divided. To accomplish complete resection of the anteromedial portion of the first rib, a second transverse skin incision is made one fingerbreadth below the medial clavicle. The upper and middle portions of the pectoralis major muscle are spread, and the anteromedial cartilaginous portion of the first rib is identified. This is facilitated by applying downward fingertip pressure to the divided posterior segment of the first rib from within the supraclavicular incision, which places the attachments between the medial first rib and the clavicle under tension and allows the superior edge of the first rib to be dissected from its soft tissue attachments through the infraclavicular incision. The subclavius muscle tendon, the costoclavicular ligament, and the muscles of the first intercostal space are all divided under direct vision without entering the subclavian vein, and the first rib is divided adjacent to the sternum with Giertz-Stille rib shears. The entire first rib is then withdrawn from the operative field as a single specimen.

The axillary-subclavian vein is identified underneath the clavicle through the lateral portion of the infraclavicular exposure and carefully separated from the subclavius muscle. Collateral vein branches that enter the subclavian vein are ligated and divided, and the subclavius muscle is resected. Further exposure of the subclavian vein is undertaken through the supraclavicular exposure and continued medially toward the junction of the subclavian and internal jugular veins to form the innominate vein. The internal jugular vein is fully exposed several centimeters superior to its junction with the subclavian vein, and the innominate vein is exposed for several centimeters into the upper mediastinum. A significant collateral branch of the subclavian vein is usually present underneath the medial clavicle, which must be ligated and divided to permit the subclavian vein to fall away from the clavicle. The course of the phrenic nerve into the upper mediastinum is also noted, and the nerve is protected where it passes underneath the subclavian vein.

Pathologic changes in the central portion of the subclavian vein are assessed both visually and by digital palpation. Because the subclavian vein is typically found to harbor a focal area of fibrous wall thickening resulting from chronic repetitive injury, residual scar tissue surrounding the vein is excised (circumferential external venolysis). In up to 50% of patients with venous TOS, this results in reexpansion of the previously constricted segment of the vein; if the underlying vein is soft to palpation and easily compressible, with evidence of rapid filling and emptying during respiratory variation, it is likely that no further venous reconstruction is necessary. When external venolysis does not alleviate subclavian vein obstruction, or when intraoperative venography demonstrates a residual stenosis despite the apparent success of external venolysis, additional venous reconstruction is performed. After systemic anticoagulation (dextran and heparin), clamp control is obtained of the distal subclavian and internal jugular veins and a pediatric Satinsky clamp is passed around the upper portion of the innominate vein. A longitudinal venotomy is created along the superior aspect of the subclavian vein, and the lumen is thoroughly inspected. If the luminal surface is smooth and free of thrombus, a vein patch angioplasty is performed using a segment of the great saphenous vein or a cryopreserved femoral vein allograft. When performing this step it is important to construct the patch angioplasty along the entire length of the affected vessel, both proximal and distal to the stenotic segment, including extension into the anteromedial aspect of the innominate vein.

When dense fibrosis remains within the wall of the subclavian vein despite external venolysis, or if there is ulceration and mural thrombus present upon inspecting the lumen, the affected segment of the subclavian vein is excised and replaced by interposition bypass. The distal portion of the interposition graft is constructed using a widely beveled end-to-end anastomosis to the unaffected axillary-subclavian vein. The proximal anastomosis is constructed in a wide end-to-side anastomosis, extending the graft into the anteromedial innominate vein. Because the caliber of the saphenous vein is usually too small to match the subclavian vein, use of the saphenous vein requires creation of a panel graft to increase the diameter to twice that of the native saphenous vein. Alternatively, subclavian vein interposition bypass can be performed with a cryopreserved femoral vein allograft, which can be readily obtained in a suitable size without the need for panel graft construction.

Finally, intraoperative venography is used to confirm satisfactory subclavian vein reconstruction, typically performed through the cephalic vein in the distal forearm. Our operative approach also includes frequent construction of a temporary radiocephalic arteriovenous (AV) fistula between the end of the distal cephalic vein and the side of the radial artery at the wrist, used as an adjunct to increase upper extremity venous blood flow during the first several months after the operation. The AV fistula is maintained until 12 weeks after surgical treatment, at which time it is ligated under local anesthesia at 12 weeks and a follow-up contrast venogram is performed.

CLOSURE

The apex of the pleural membrane is purposefully opened, and a round 19-Fr fluted silicone closed-suction Blake drain (Ethicon, Somerville, New Jersey) is placed into the supraclavicular field with a trocar through a separate stab wound, where it is placed behind the brachial plexus with its end lying within the upper posterior aspect of the pleural space (Fig. 15-12). Two small 12.5-cm multihole catheters are placed within the wound, one adjacent to the brachial plexus and one within the bed of the resected first rib. These catheters exit the skin adjacent to the wound and are connected to a sustained-infusion delivery system for postoperative administration of 0.25% to 0.5% bupivacaine (On-Q PainBuster system, I-Flow/Kimberly Clark, 400 mL at 2 mL/hr through each catheter, catalog No. PM028-A). A 100 × 130 × 0.02 mm sheet of bioresorbable polylactide film (SurgiWrap, Mast Biosurgery, catalog No. 27202-05) is placed around the brachial plexus nerve roots to limit the potential for postoperative perineural fibrosis. The

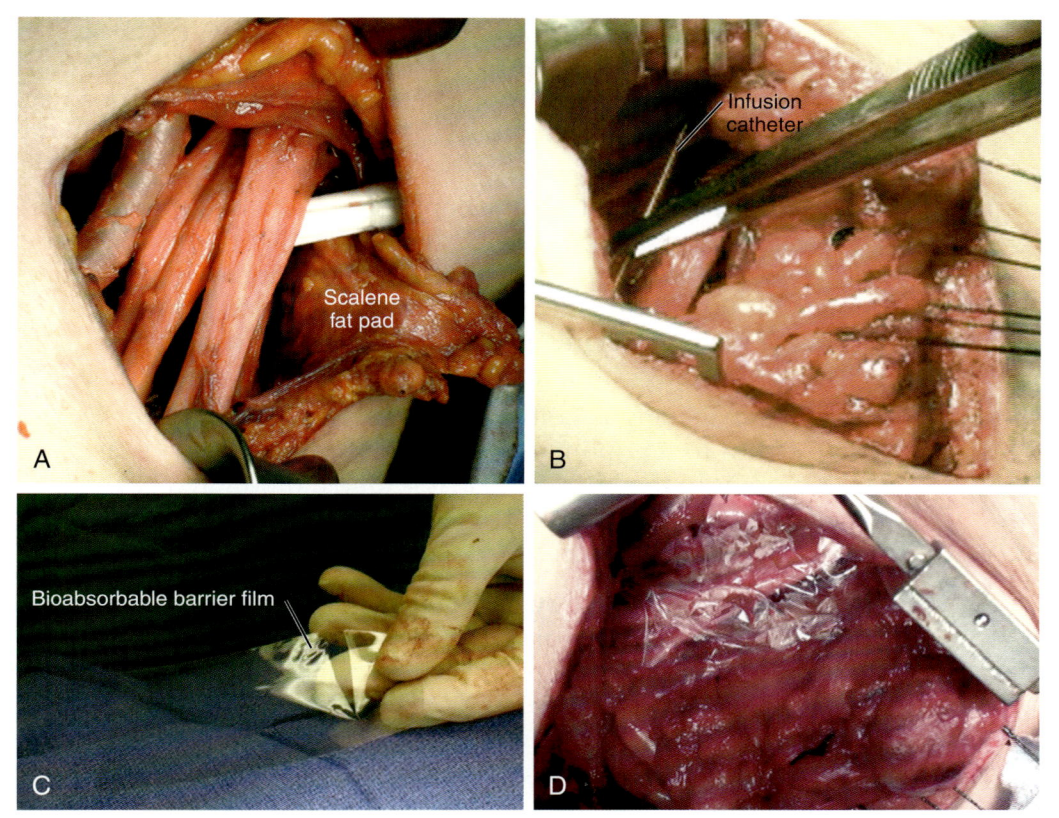

SUPRACLAVICULAR APPROACH FOR SURGICAL TREATMENT OF THORACIC OUTLET SYNDROME

Figure 15-12. Brachial plexus neurolysis and wound closure. **A,** Complete dissection of the brachial plexus nerve roots (C5 to T1) is accomplished by resection of all perineural scar tissue, ensuring complete mobility throughout the supraclavicular space. A closed-suction drain is placed behind the brachial plexus, with its tip lying within the opened pleural space. **B,** A percutaneous multihole infusion catheter is placed alongside the brachial plexus nerves for continuous postoperative infusion of local anesthetic. **C** and **D,** A sheet of bioabsorbable polymer film is prepared and wrapped around the brachial plexus nerve roots, to diminish postoperative perineural fibrosis, before reattaching the scalene fat pad. Photographs depict the left side, with the head at the tops of the figures.

film is held together with several 5-0 polydioxanone sutures (Ethicon) and attached to the base of the scalene fat pad. The scalene fat pad is reapproximated over the brachial plexus and held in position with interrupted 3-0 silk sutures to the back of the sternocleidomastoid muscle and the periclavicular fascia. The edges of the platysma muscle are reapproximated with interrupted sutures, and the skin is closed with a subcuticular stitch.

Postoperative Care

- An upright chest radiographic examination is performed in the recovery room and each day after surgery. Small air or pleural fluid collections are observed with the expectation of spontaneous resolution.
- Postoperative pain medication is provided by intravenous opiates (patient-controlled analgesia) until adequate control can be achieved by oral medications alone. The continuous-infusion anesthesia system is discontinued on postoperative day 3. Oral narcotics, a muscle relaxant, and a nonsteroidal anti-inflammatory agent are routinely prescribed upon hospital discharge and for at least several weeks after surgery.
- Patients with venous TOS are maintained on intravenous dextran for 48 hours and then switched to heparin or warfarin and clopidogrel. Anticoagulation and antiplatelet therapy are both discontinued 12 weeks after the operation, along with outpatient ligation of the AV fistula and follow-up venography.
- Patients are usually discharged from the hospital 4 to 6 days after the operation. The closed suction drain is removed as an outpatient procedure 7 to 10 days after surgery, when the daily output of serous fluid has decreased to less than 50 mL.

- Physical therapy is resumed the day after surgery and continued upon hospital discharge. Patients are advised to avoid excessive reaching overhead or heavy lifting with the affected upper extremity and are cautioned against activities that can result in muscle strain, spasm, and significant pain in the trapezius and other neck muscles.
- A gradual return to use of the upper extremity is encouraged, with the majority of patients permitted a cautious return to light-duty work activities by 4 to 6 weeks after the operation. Work restrictions are recommended to prevent heavy activity during the early stages of return to work, particularly to avoid excessive use of the upper extremity by lifting or repetitive activities that may contribute to postoperative complaints.
- Physical therapy is continued for as long as necessary to allow the patient to return to an optimal level of function, and patients are seen at least every 3 months in the first year to assess long-term results.

Postoperative Complications

- **Residual neurologic symptoms.** Symptoms of numbness and tingling in the hand or fingers are common early after thoracic outlet decompression, arising as a result of previous neurologic damage, intraoperative mobilization of the brachial plexus, and postoperative inflammation and perineural wound healing. The use of continuous local anesthetic infusions for pain control may also result in sensory neurologic symptoms. More pronounced neurologic dysfunction including motor deficiencies are rarely observed, particularly arm weakness and loss of handgrip strength but may represent temporary brachial plexus neuropraxia or pain-limited restrictions in mobility. Spontaneous resolution of such symptoms usually occurs within several days to weeks but may persist for several months. Patients with longstanding neurogenic TOS can often display residual symptoms of pain, dysesthesias, numbness, weakness, and other complaints that may not be eliminated by thoracic outlet decompression. Although these symptoms may be tolerable and are expected to gradually improve, the surgeon must provide continuing support and reassurance during the prolonged period of recovery and rehabilitation.
- **Pleural Effusion.** Mild to moderate pleural fluid collections are often observed on the side of surgery after supraclavicular decompression, consisting of serosanguineous fluid that can be expected to spontaneously resorb within several days to weeks. Although well tolerated by most patients, some may experience shortness of breath with exertion until the fluid has resolved. In such individuals chest radiographs are useful to distinguish the presence of a pleural effusion from the effects of diaphragmatic elevation because of phrenic nerve dysfunction.
- **Bleeding.** Postoperative bleeding is uncommon but can result in wound hematomas or when substantial may lead to a hemothorax. Early anticoagulation after operations for venous TOS can elevate the risk of bleeding complications. Although often self-limited, reexploration of the supraclavicular wound allows the operative site to be directly inspected and any specific site of bleeding to be controlled. Evacuation of hemothorax can usually be achieved through this approach as well, avoiding the need for chest tube placement.
- **Lymph leak.** If there is persistent or increasing drain output of lymphatic fluid of more than 250 mL/day, particularly when chylous in appearance and on the left side, a clear liquid diet is maintained, along with administration of octreotide to reduce the volume of lymph flow, and removal of the closed-suction drain is deferred until the leak has subsided. Early supraclavicular reexploration is recommended for persistent high-volume lymph leaks (>500 mL/day for >5 days) or those resulting in chylothorax.
- **Phrenic nerve dysfunction.** Elevation of the ipsilateral diaphragm on postoperative chest radiographs indicates the presence of phrenic nerve dysfunction,

which may be associated with shortness of breath on exertion or supine reclining, as well as lower lateral chest discomfort. Most individuals compensate satisfactorily with the contralateral diaphragm and intercostal muscles, and many become asymptomatic within a short period, but patients with severe underlying pulmonary disease may be at risk for significant disability. Postoperative phrenic nerve dysfunction is usually a temporary finding because of intraoperative mobilization of the nerve or postoperative infusion of local anesthetic, but on occasion phrenic neuropraxia can persist for several weeks; in rare situations, phrenic neuropraxia may be prolonged up to 9 to 10 months before signs of reinnervation appear. Most patients should be managed expectantly.

- **Long thoracic nerve dysfunction.** Postoperative dysfunction of the long thoracic nerve is occasionally observed after thoracic outlet decompression, resulting in a winged scapula defect because of weakness of the serratus anterior muscle. Scapular dysfunction because of this defect is readily detectable by physical examination, and it may interfere with shoulder girdle mechanics and physical therapy, thereby prolonging full recovery from operation. Although there is no specific treatment, long thoracic neuropraxia is usually self-limited and recovery can be expected within several months.

REFERENCES

1. Coote H: Exostosis of the left transverse process of the seventh cervical vertebra, surrounded by blood vessels and nerves; successful removal, *Lancet* 1:360-361, 1861.
2. Halsted WS: An experimental study of circumscribed dilatation of an artery immediately distal to a partially occluding band, and its bearing on the dilatation of the subclavian artery observed in certain cases of cervical rib, *J Exp Med* 24:271-286, 1916.
3. Murphy JB: Cervical rib excision: Collective review on surgery of cervical rib, *Clin John B Murphy* 5:227-240, 1916.
4. Adson AW, Coffey JR: Cervical rib: A method of anterior approach for relief of symptoms by division of the scalenus anticus, *Ann Surg* 85:839-857, 1927.
5. Ochsner A, Gage M, DeBakey M: Scalenus anticus (Naffziger) syndrome, *Am J Surg* 28:696-699, 1935.
6. Adson AW: Surgical treatment for symptoms produced by cervical ribs and the scalenus anticus muscle, *Surg Gynecol Obstet* 85:687-700, 1947.
7. Roos DB: Transaxillary approach for first rib resection to relieve thoracic outlet syndrome, *Ann Surg* 163:354-358, 1966.
8. Roos DB: Congenital anomalies associated with thoracic outlet syndrome, *Am J Surg* 132:771-778, 1976.
9. Machleder HI, Moll F, Verity MA: The anterior scalene muscle in thoracic outlet compression syndrome: Histochemical and morphometric studies, *Arch Surg* 121:1141-1144, 1986.
10. Sanders RJ, Jackson CG, Banchero N, et al: Scalene muscle abnormalities in traumatic thoracic outlet syndrome, *Am J Surg* 159:231-236, 1990.
11. Dale A: Thoracic outlet compression syndrome: Critique in 1982, *Arch Surg* 117:1437-1145, 1982.
12. Sanders RJ, Monsour JW, Gerber FG, et al: Scalenectomy versus first rib resection for treatment of the thoracic outlet syndrome, *Surgery* 85:109-121, 1979.
13. Qvarfordt PG, Ehrenfeld WK, Stoney RJ: Supraclavicular radical scalenectomy and transaxillary first rib resection for the thoracic outlet syndrome. A combined approach, *Am J Surg* 148:111-116, 1984.
14. Sanders RJ, Raymer S: The supraclavicular approach to scalenectomy and first rib resection: Description of technique, *J Vasc Surg* 2:751-756, 1985.
15. Reilly LM, Stoney RJ: Supraclavicular approach for thoracic outlet decompression, *J Vasc Surg* 8:329-334, 1988.
16. Sanders RJ: *Thoracic outlet syndrome: A common sequelae of neck injuries*, Philadelphia, 1991, J. B. Lippincott Company.
17. Hempel GK, Shutze WP, Anderson JF, et al: 770 consecutive supraclavicular first rib resections for thoracic outlet syndrome, *Ann Vasc Surg* 10:456-463, 1996.
18. Emery VB, Rastogi R, Driskill MR, et al: Diagnosis of neurogenic thoracic outlet syndrome. In Eskandari MK, Morasch MD, Pearce WH, Yao JST, editors: *Vascular surgery: Therapeutic strategies*, Shelton, Conn. 2010, People's Medical Publishing House, pp 129-148.
19. Melby SJ, Vedantham S, Narra VR, et al: Comprehensive surgical management of the competitive athlete with effort thrombosis of the subclavian vein (Paget-Schroetter syndrome), *J Vasc Surg* 47:809-820, 2008.

20. Sanders RJ, Pearce WH: The treatment of thoracic outlet syndrome: A comparison of different operations, *J Vasc Surg* 10:626-634, 1989.
21. Cheng SW, Reilly LM, Nelken NA, et al: Neurogenic thoracic outlet decompression: Rationale for sparing the first rib, *Cardiovasc Surg* 3:617-623, 1995.
22. Youmans CRJ, Smiley RH: Thoracic outlet syndrome with negative Adson's and hyperabduction maneuvers, *Vasc Surg* 14:318-329, 1980.
23. Sanders RJ, Hammond SL: Management of cervical ribs and anomalous first ribs causing neurogenic thoracic outlet syndrome, *J Vasc Surg* 36:51-56, 2002.
24. Sanders RJ: Pectoralis minor syndrome. In Eskandari MK, Morasch MD, Pearce WH, Yao JST, editors: *Vascular surgery: Therapeutic strategies*, Shelton, Conn. 2010, People's Medical Publishing House, pp 149-160.
25. Sanders RJ, Hammond SL, Rao NM: Observations on the use of seprafilm on the brachial plexus in 249 operations for neurogenic thoracic outlet syndrome, *Hand* 2:179-183, 2007.

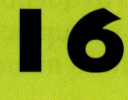

16 Transaxillary Rib Resection for Thoracic Outlet Syndrome

GEORGE J. ARNAOUTAKIS • JULIE ANN FREISCHLAG • THOMAS REIFSNYDER

Historical Background

The first anatomic descriptions of the thoracic outlet can be traced to 150 AD when Galen identified the presence of a cervical rib in human dissections. However, it was not until 1742 that Hunauld established the association between a cervical rib and upper extremity symptoms. In 1821 Cooper characterized the constellation of neurovascular symptoms involving the thoracic outlet. Ochsner called this the scalene santicus syndrome in 1936 and described the presence of muscle abnormalities secondary to repetitive trauma.[1] Peet and associates[2] first applied the term thoracic outlet syndrome (TOS) in 1956, which is applied to primary arterial, venous, and neurogenic pathologies.

In 1861 Coote[3] described the first operation to treat thoracic outlet pathology in a patient diagnosed as having an "exostosis" of the seventh cervical vertebra. Coote resected a portion of the transverse process, and the patient's symptoms improved. In 1910 Murphy[4] published the initial report describing first rib resection for the treatment of neurogenic TOS. Adson and Coffey[5] subsequently performed an anterior scalenectomy in 1927 but without concomitant rib resection. Because of high recurrence rates, Claggett resurrected the notion of first rib resection for treatment of TOS in 1962, adopting a posterior approach.[1] Because this was a morbid operation, Roos[6] introduced the transaxillary approach to first rib resection and scalenectomy in 1966. Other techniques have emerged in the ensuing decades, including supraclavicular scalenectomy with or without first rib resection, a combined supraclavicular and infraclavicular approach, and combinations thereof. More recently, thoracoscopic rib resection has been reported. This chapter focuses on transaxillary first rib resection and partial scalenectomy for TOS.

Indications

Patients with a diagnosis of TOS who are appropriate surgical candidates should undergo surgical decompression of the thoracic outlet. TOS is subdivided into three discrete entities: neurogenic, venous, and arterial. The optimal approach should be individualized depending on the patient's symptoms and anatomy and the surgeon's experience. The transaxillary approach is preferred by many surgeons because of its relative ease, low risk profile, and documented improvement in patients' quality of life.[7,8] This approach effectively decompresses the thoracic outlet and is generally reserved for patients with neurogenic or venous TOS. If vessel reconstruction is anticipated, a different approach should be used because the transaxillary approach limits proximal arterial exposure.

Careful history and physical examination enable classification of TOS. The neurogenic form accounts for the majority of cases in modern series (>95%).[9] Symptoms of neurogenic TOS, which is more prevalent in women, include paresthesia, pain, clavicle. From the surgeon's point of view the thoracic outlet can be visualized as an anatomic triangle: the two sides are the anterior and middle scalene muscles, with the first rib serving as the base of the triangle (Fig. 16-1, *inset* and Video 16-1). The artery and vein are appropriately colored in the figure. The scalene muscles, which originate from the lower cervical spine, may hypertrophy with repetitive neck motion or minor trauma. This hypertrophy is thought to contribute to compression of thoracic outlet structures, particularly in neurogenic TOS.

The subclavian artery and the five nerve roots (C5 to T1) to the brachial plexus are located within the thoracic outlet. The artery courses anterior to the brachial plexus nerve roots and exits the mediastinum in its course over the first rib behind the posterior border of the anterior scalene muscle. The cervical spine nerve roots join to form the initial trunks of the brachial plexus within the thoracic outlet and are located posterior to the subclavian artery. Subsequent merging and branching of these trunks into divisions, cords, and terminal nerves of the brachial plexus occurs outside the thoracic outlet. Other significant nerves within the thoracic outlet are the phrenic and long thoracic nerves. The phrenic nerve receives fibers from C3 to C5 and courses in a descending oblique direction from the lateral to the medial edge of the middle portion of the anterior scalene muscle. The phrenic nerve approaches the mediastinum posterior to the subclavian vein. The long thoracic nerve, composed of nerve fibers from C5 to C7, passes through the center of the middle scalene muscle and heads toward the chest wall to innervate the serratus anterior muscle.

The subclavian vein technically does not course through the thoracic outlet. It passes over the first rib anterior to the anterior scalene muscle. However, the middle segment of the vein remains susceptible to compression between the anteromedial first rib, the clavicle, and the subclavius muscle (see Fig. 16-1). Hypertrophy of the subclavius muscle and tendon may occur in athletes and is often implicated in venous TOS.

Several anatomic anomalies are relevant to the surgeon, as they predispose patients to the development of TOS. The most common is a cervical rib, and a preoperative chest radiograph is adequate for its detection. When present, cervical ribs appear as extensions of the transverse process of C7. Cervical ribs may be complete or partial, with the anterior end attaching to the first rib or floating freely. In addition, the anterior end may be fibrous and not calcified and thus not completely visualized on chest radiograph. By rigidly confining the thoracic outlet, cervical ribs render the neurovascular structures more prone to compression. Although cervical ribs are present in the general population with an incidence of 0.5% to 1%, they are found in 5% to 10% of all TOS patients.[13] A prominent C7 transverse process or bifid first rib is also associated with TOS.

AVOIDING INJURY TO THE BRACHIAL PLEXUS

The brachial plexus is rarely injured during a transaxillary first rib resection for TOS. However, because of the morbidity of neurologic injury, the surgeon should be vigilant on a few points. When a Machleder retractor is used to position the arm during the procedure, the arm should not be positioned in greater than 90 degrees of abduction (Fig. 16-2). The Machleder retractor should be adjusted periodically (every 20-25 minutes) to relieve tension on the brachial plexus. If an assistant is holding the arm, intermittent rest periods for the assistant also releases tension on the brachial plexus. Because the operative field is narrowly confined, the assistant holding retractor has an impaired view. Thus the operating surgeon must constantly monitor the placement of the retractor. In addition, the brachial plexus is vulnerable to injury when dividing the rib or when using the rongeur to smooth the posterior rib stump. A good rule when using the bone cutters or rongeur is to check positioning at least twice before cutting once. Positioning a Roos retractor in front of the brachial plexus and gently displacing the nerve bundle posteriorly offers protection when using the rongeur.

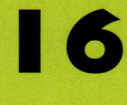

16 Transaxillary Rib Resection for Thoracic Outlet Syndrome

GEORGE J. ARNAOUTAKIS • JULIE ANN FREISCHLAG • THOMAS REIFSNYDER

Historical Background

The first anatomic descriptions of the thoracic outlet can be traced to 150 AD when Galen identified the presence of a cervical rib in human dissections. However, it was not until 1742 that Hunauld established the association between a cervical rib and upper extremity symptoms. In 1821 Cooper characterized the constellation of neurovascular symptoms involving the thoracic outlet. Ochsner called this the scalene santicus syndrome in 1936 and described the presence of muscle abnormalities secondary to repetitive trauma.[1] Peet and associates[2] first applied the term thoracic outlet syndrome (TOS) in 1956, which is applied to primary arterial, venous, and neurogenic pathologies.

In 1861 Coote[3] described the first operation to treat thoracic outlet pathology in a patient diagnosed as having an "exostosis" of the seventh cervical vertebra. Coote resected a portion of the transverse process, and the patient's symptoms improved. In 1910 Murphy[4] published the initial report describing first rib resection for the treatment of neurogenic TOS. Adson and Coffey[5] subsequently performed an anterior scalenectomy in 1927 but without concomitant rib resection. Because of high recurrence rates, Claggett resurrected the notion of first rib resection for treatment of TOS in 1962, adopting a posterior approach.[1] Because this was a morbid operation, Roos[6] introduced the transaxillary approach to first rib resection and scalenectomy in 1966. Other techniques have emerged in the ensuing decades, including supraclavicular scalenectomy with or without first rib resection, a combined supraclavicular and infraclavicular approach, and combinations thereof. More recently, thoracoscopic rib resection has been reported. This chapter focuses on transaxillary first rib resection and partial scalenectomy for TOS.

Indications

Patients with a diagnosis of TOS who are appropriate surgical candidates should undergo surgical decompression of the thoracic outlet. TOS is subdivided into three discrete entities: neurogenic, venous, and arterial. The optimal approach should be individualized depending on the patient's symptoms and anatomy and the surgeon's experience. The transaxillary approach is preferred by many surgeons because of its relative ease, low risk profile, and documented improvement in patients' quality of life.[7,8] This approach effectively decompresses the thoracic outlet and is generally reserved for patients with neurogenic or venous TOS. If vessel reconstruction is anticipated, a different approach should be used because the transaxillary approach limits proximal arterial exposure.

Careful history and physical examination enable classification of TOS. The neurogenic form accounts for the majority of cases in modern series (>95%).[9] Symptoms of neurogenic TOS, which is more prevalent in women, include paresthesia, pain, and impaired strength in the affected shoulder, arm, or hand, along with occipital headaches and neck discomfort. There is commonly an antecedent history of hyperextension neck injury or repetitive neck trauma. Patients frequently present with tenderness on palpation of the shoulder, mastoid region, or supraclavicular fossa or over the anterior scalene muscle. Three physical examination maneuvers support the diagnosis of neurogenic TOS:

- Rotation of the neck and tilting of the head to the opposite side to elicit pain in the affected arm.
- The upper limb tension test in which the patient first abducts both arms to 90 degrees with the elbows in a locked position, dorsiflexes the wrists, and finally tilts the head to the side. Each subsequent step imparts greater traction on the brachial plexus, with the first two positions causing discomfort on the ipsilateral side and the head tilt position causing pain on the contralateral side.
- The elevated arm stress test during which the patient raises both arms directly above the head and repeatedly opens and closes the fists. Characteristic upper extremity symptoms arise within 60 seconds in patients with neurogenic TOS.

A cold hand with discoloration may be present in neurogenic TOS. Vasospastic in nature, it should not be confused with the presentation of digital or forearm microemboli found in arterial TOS. A careful vascular physical examination should confirm the presence of normal circulation.

Patients with venous TOS typically present with acute onset of dull aching pain of the upper extremity, associated with arm edema and cyanosis. Paresthesias may be present but are because of hand swelling rather than thoracic outlet nerve involvement. A history of strenuous and repetitive work or athletics involving the affected extremity is common, and most patients are young. This specific condition is known as Paget-Schroetter syndrome or effort vein thrombosis, because the entrapped subclavian vein has progressed to thrombosis. Some patients present less acutely with nonthrombotic subclavian vein occlusion or stenosis manifested by intermittent swelling with activity. Regardless, the etiology of venous TOS is mechanical and treatment is ultimately aimed at eliminating not only the venous obstruction but also the muscular bands that have entrapped and damaged the vein.

Arterial TOS typically manifests in one of three ways: asymptomatic, arm claudication, or critical ischemia of the hand. The majority of these patients have a cervical rib that may or may not be fused to the first rib, which most commonly is posterior to the subclavian artery. The etiology is chronic repetitive injury to the subclavian artery as it exits the thoracic outlet. This injury may cause subclavian artery stenosis but more commonly leads to ectasia or a true aneurysm. In asymptomatic patients a pulsatile mass or supraclavicular bruit can be detected on physical examination. Arm claudication is caused by areas of stenosis, which may be fixed, because of longstanding injury, or dynamic and occur with the arm abducted or extended only. Critical ischemia is because of emboli of fibrin-enriched platelet aggregates that originate from an ulcerated mural thrombus in the aneurysmal segment. The aneurysm is typically small, may be subtle on imaging studies, and may be prone to embolize related to its position rather than its size.

Preoperative Preparation

- Preoperative physical therapy should be attempted for at least 8 weeks in patients with a diagnosis of neurogenic TOS. The aims of therapy are to improve posture and achieve greater range of motion. Patients with persistent symptoms of neurogenic TOS despite 8 weeks of physical therapy merit surgical intervention. At least 60% of patients improve with physical therapy and lifestyle alterations.
- A radiographically guided anterior scalene block with local anesthetic (lidocaine) injection may provide a few hours of symptomatic relief. Patients with suspected neurogenic TOS often present with a constellation of physical complaints, not

all of which are directly attributable to the disorder. A scalene block not only helps confirm the diagnosis but also simulates the expected postoperative result. This provides the patient and the surgeon with reassurance that surgical intervention will be beneficial and demonstrates which symptoms can be reliably expected to improve. As an alternative to surgical therapy patients can then opt for a onabotulinum toxin A (Botox, Allergan, Irvine, Calif.) injection. The Botox takes an average of 2 weeks to work and can be repeated once. This may provide symptomatic relief for 2 to 3 months, allowing participation in physical therapy. However, not all TOS patients respond to Botox. After two injections, the anterior scalene muscle becomes fibrotic and scarred and no longer responds as well to the Botox. This practice is especially helpful in patients who have had cervical spine fusions or shoulder operations, because they can strengthen the muscles of their neck and back, which may alleviate the TOS symptoms.

- Plain-film chest radiograph is recommended for all patients undergoing surgical intervention for TOS to rule out supernumerary cervical ribs.
- In young patients (<40 years of age) with a classic presentation of neurogenic TOS, there is no need for extensive preoperative testing. Older patients and those with a history of neck trauma should undergo magnetic resonance imaging to rule out cervical disc pathology.
- Nerve conduction studies are typically normal in neurogenic TOS but may be useful in ruling out nerve compression such as carpal tunnel or cubital compression syndrome.
- Duplex ultrasonography is the initial diagnostic modality to confirm pathology in patients with arterial TOS. Although useful to confirm axillosubclavian vein thrombosis in patients with suspected venous TOS, it is frequently unnecessary. Patients presenting acutely with classic signs and symptoms of venous TOS should undergo prompt venography for both diagnosis and therapeutic intervention. Patients with venous TOS should ultimately undergo imaging of the contralateral extremity with and without abduction, because the rate of bilateral venous compression ranges from 3% to 21%.[10]
- Therapeutic systemic anticoagulation with warfarin is initiated preoperatively only in patients with evidence of chronic venous TOS. Before surgery these patients are bridged from warfarin therapy to subcutaneous low-molecular-weight heparin.
- Prophylactic antibiotics are administered perioperatively. A first-generation cephalosporin is preferred. In patients with penicillin allergy, clindamycin or vancomycin is used.

Pitfalls and Danger Points

- **Incorrect diagnosis.** A successful operation hinges on an accurate preoperative diagnosis. A thorough history and physical examination and an anterior scalene block help to identify the correct neurogenic patients for an operation.
- **Brachial plexus injury.** Proper positioning and careful retraction help prevent excessive traction and injury to the brachial plexus.
- **Misidentification of the first rib.** Proper identification of the first rib requires careful attention on the part of the surgeon, because its anatomic position is more cephalad than is frequently expected.
- **Incomplete first rib resection.** Incomplete first rib resection has been associated with greater rates of recurrent TOS.[11,12]

Operative Strategy

SURGICAL ANATOMY OF THE THORACIC OUTLET

The thoracic outlet is a narrowly defined anatomic region consisting of the space between the neck and the shoulder above the thoracic cavity and beneath the clavicle. From the surgeon's point of view the thoracic outlet can be visualized as an anatomic triangle: the two sides are the anterior and middle scalene muscles, with the first rib serving as the base of the triangle (Fig. 16-1, *inset* and Video 16-1). The artery and vein are appropriately colored in the figure. The scalene muscles, which originate from the lower cervical spine, may hypertrophy with repetitive neck motion or minor trauma. This hypertrophy is thought to contribute to compression of thoracic outlet structures, particularly in neurogenic TOS.

The subclavian artery and the five nerve roots (C5 to T1) to the brachial plexus are located within the thoracic outlet. The artery courses anterior to the brachial plexus nerve roots and exits the mediastinum in its course over the first rib behind the posterior border of the anterior scalene muscle. The cervical spine nerve roots join to form the initial trunks of the brachial plexus within the thoracic outlet and are located posterior to the subclavian artery. Subsequent merging and branching of these trunks into divisions, cords, and terminal nerves of the brachial plexus occurs outside the thoracic outlet. Other significant nerves within the thoracic outlet are the phrenic and long thoracic nerves. The phrenic nerve receives fibers from C3 to C5 and courses in a descending oblique direction from the lateral to the medial edge of the middle portion of the anterior scalene muscle. The phrenic nerve approaches the mediastinum posterior to the subclavian vein. The long thoracic nerve, composed of nerve fibers from C5 to C7, passes through the center of the middle scalene muscle and heads toward the chest wall to innervate the serratus anterior muscle.

The subclavian vein technically does not course through the thoracic outlet. It passes over the first rib anterior to the anterior scalene muscle. However, the middle segment of the vein remains susceptible to compression between the anteromedial first rib, the clavicle, and the subclavius muscle (see Fig. 16-1). Hypertrophy of the subclavius muscle and tendon may occur in athletes and is often implicated in venous TOS.

Several anatomic anomalies are relevant to the surgeon, as they predispose patients to the development of TOS. The most common is a cervical rib, and a preoperative chest radiograph is adequate for its detection. When present, cervical ribs appear as extensions of the transverse process of C7. Cervical ribs may be complete or partial, with the anterior end attaching to the first rib or floating freely. In addition, the anterior end may be fibrous and not calcified and thus not completely visualized on chest radiograph. By rigidly confining the thoracic outlet, cervical ribs render the neurovascular structures more prone to compression. Although cervical ribs are present in the general population with an incidence of 0.5% to 1%, they are found in 5% to 10% of all TOS patients.[13] A prominent C7 transverse process or bifid first rib is also associated with TOS.

AVOIDING INJURY TO THE BRACHIAL PLEXUS

The brachial plexus is rarely injured during a transaxillary first rib resection for TOS. However, because of the morbidity of neurologic injury, the surgeon should be vigilant on a few points. When a Machleder retractor is used to position the arm during the procedure, the arm should not be positioned in greater than 90 degrees of abduction (Fig. 16-2). The Machleder retractor should be adjusted periodically (every 20-25 minutes) to relieve tension on the brachial plexus. If an assistant is holding the arm, intermittent rest periods for the assistant also releases tension on the brachial plexus. Because the operative field is narrowly confined, the assistant holding retractor has an impaired view. Thus the operating surgeon must constantly monitor the placement of the retractor. In addition, the brachial plexus is vulnerable to injury when dividing the rib or when using the rongeur to smooth the posterior rib stump. A good rule when using the bone cutters or rongeur is to check positioning at least twice before cutting once. Positioning a Roos retractor in front of the brachial plexus and gently displacing the nerve bundle posteriorly offers protection when using the rongeur.

TRANSAXILLARY RIB RESECTION FOR THORACIC OUTLET SYNDROME | 197

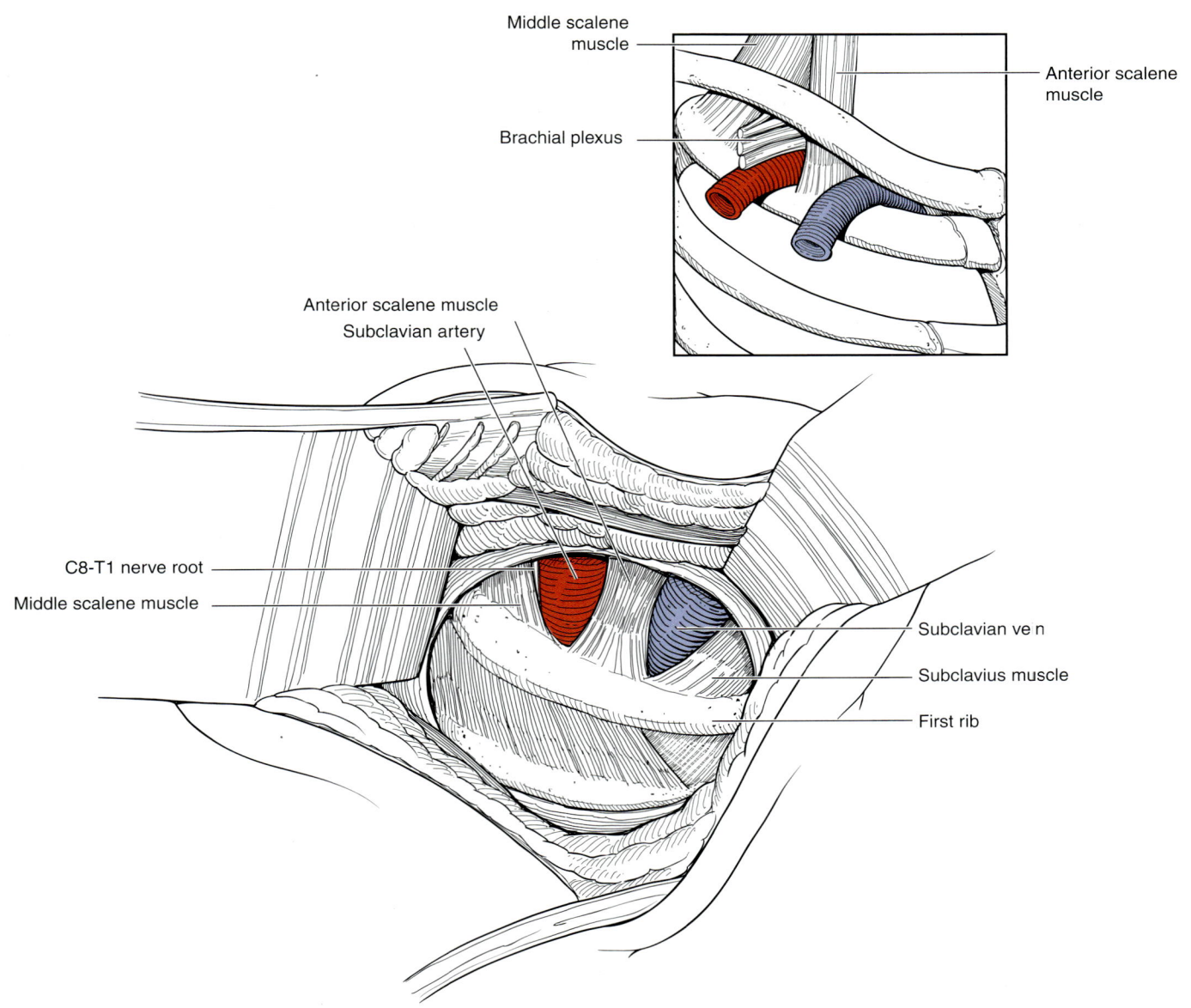

Figure 16-1. Thoracic outlet anatomy from the surgeon's perspective as viewed through the operative field in a transaxillary approach. *Inset,* Normal anatomic relationships of important thoracic outlet structures.

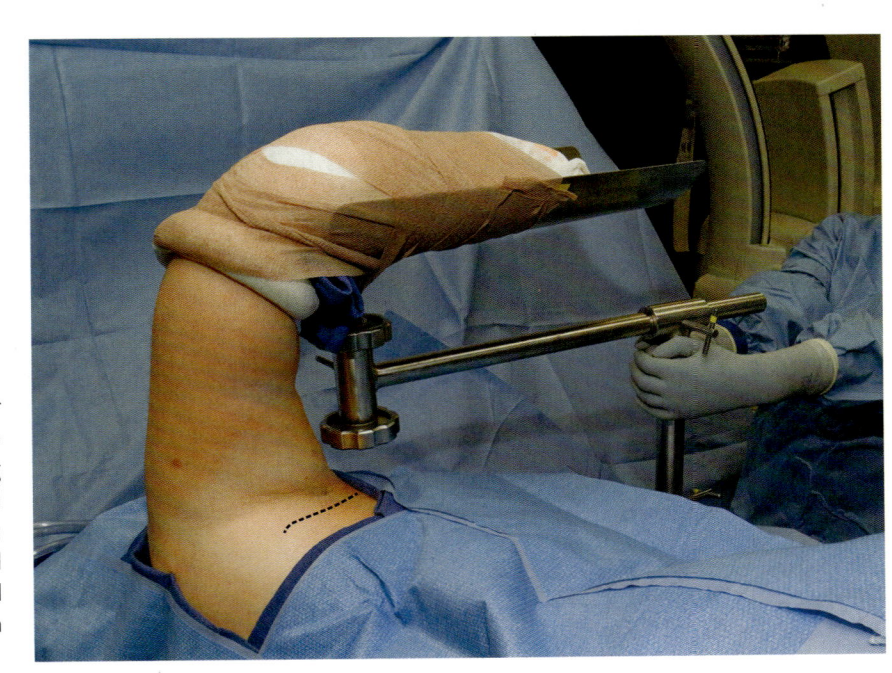

Figure 16-2. Proper patient positioning for right transaxillary first rib resection and use of the Machleder arm support with generous padding to prevent compression nerve injury. A padded axillary roll is placed under the dependent (left) axilla, and the patient is stabilized in the left lateral decubitus with the aid of a beanbag. The dashed line indicates the preferred location of the skin incision.

Operative Technique

INCISION

Induction of general anesthesia is performed, and if paralysis is required for endotracheal intubation, a short-acting neuromuscular blockade should be used to allow safer dissection near the brachial plexus. The patient is then moved to the lateral decubitus position using a beanbag to facilitate positioning. Care should be taken to pad the dependent axilla and support the head. The sterile field incorporates the arm, axilla, and shoulder. An adjustable Machleder arm support is affixed to the operating table, with the vertical support bar attached to the operating table at the level of the patient's chin. Generous padding around the patient's arm before placement in the arm holder protects the median and ulnar nerves from compression as they cross the elbow joint. After securing the arm in the retractor, the surgeon identifies the anterior border of the latissimus dorsi muscle and the posterior surface of the pectoralis major muscle. A transverse skin line incision should be made in the inferior axillary hairline extending between these two muscle borders.

EXPOSURE

Electrocautery is used to divide the subcutaneous tissue until thin areolar tissue superficial to the chest wall is encountered. A self-retaining cerebellar or Weitlaner retractor is then inserted into the wound. Upon encountering the chest wall—and if in the correct anatomic plane—gentle blunt dissection with the surgeon's fingers or a pair of Kittner or peanut dissectors easily separates the soft tissues from the chest wall. This dissection is cephalad, and the second rib rapidly comes into view. The intercostobrachial nerve is located in the second intercostal space. Although frequently difficult to avoid, care should be taken not to impart excess traction, because injury results in numbness or dysesthesia of the medial aspect of the proximal arm. Raising the Machleder arm support at this point allows for optimal access to the first rib and thoracic outlet. The aid of fiberoptic lighted Deaver retractors facilitates visualization during this portion of the dissection. Alternatively, the surgeon should wear a headlight. The first rib is identified near its insertion at the sternoclavicular joint and is generally encountered higher than anticipated. A Kittner or peanut dissector is then used to gently sweep away the loose fibrous tissue overlying the brachial plexus, subclavian artery and vein, and scalene muscles. There is occasionally a small branch of the subclavian artery that must be ligated and divided in order to fully expose the operative field.

The next step is to fully expose the rib. Depending on the patient's anatomy, it generally is easiest to first clear off the intercostal muscles laterally. A Cobb periosteal elevator works best, but any type of long elevator may be used (Fig. 16-3). The dissection proceeds in the anterior and posterior directions until all intercostal muscle attachments are divided from the rib. The elevator can then be used to elevate the first rib, thus separating the rib from the underlying parietal pleura. This mobilization should continue from behind the brachial plexus in the posterior direction to beyond the subclavian vein in the anterior direction. Attention is then directed to the superior border of the first rib, where the periosteal elevator is used to bluntly divide the scalene medius fibers at their attachment to the rib. The long thoracic nerve courses along the lateral edge of the scalene medius muscle but is generally not visualized. Sharp dissection is avoided during division of the scalene medius in order to protect the nerve. Closely adhering to the surface of the rib during blunt dissection is another measure to avoid injury to the long thoracic nerve.

The anterior scalene muscle should now be clearly identified as it arises from the medial superior aspect of the first rib (Fig. 16-4). A right-angled clamp is passed behind the anterior scalene muscle near its insertion on the scalene tubercle. Gently lifting the anterior scalene with the right-angled clamp protects the subclavian

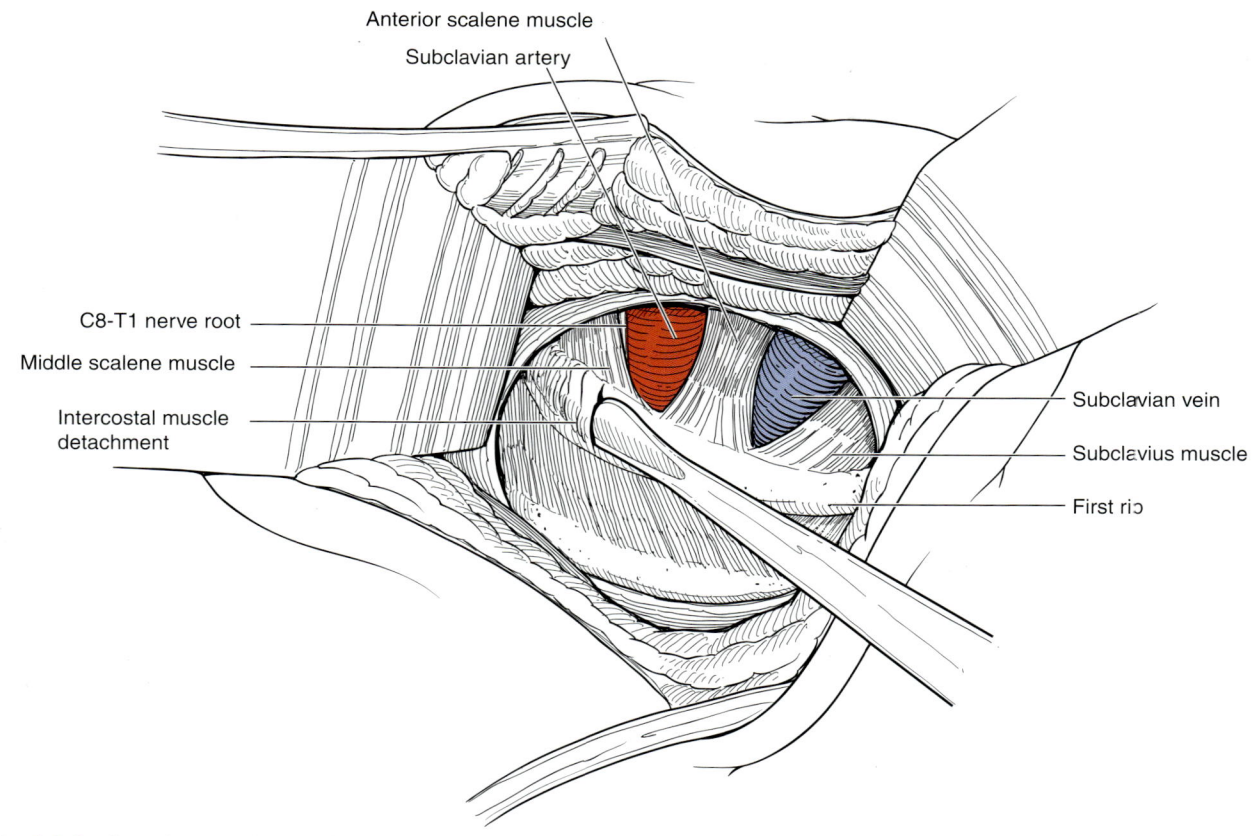

Figure 16-3. A periosteal elevator is used to dissect along the superior surface of the first rib in order to divide intercostal muscle attachments.

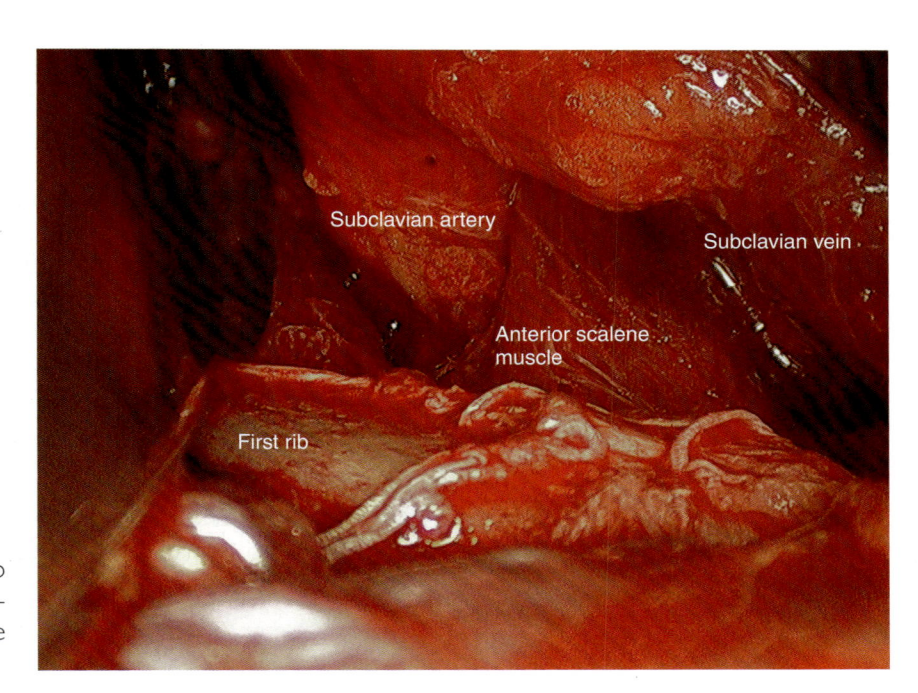

Figure 16-4. Gross anatomy from a close-up perspective, demonstrating the important relationships among the first rib, anterior scalene muscle, and subclavian vessels.

artery as it courses posterior to the muscle (Fig. 16-5). It is important to free several centimeters of the muscle before dividing it with Metzenbaum scissors. This maneuver facilitates resection of a portion of the anterior scalene muscle, which has been shown to reduce recurrence rates when compared with division at its insertion point on the rib.[14,15] Lastly, the subclavius muscle appears as a crescent-shaped ligamentous attachment to the first rib adjacent to the subclavian vein. Carefully, so as not to injure the subclavian vein, the subclavius muscle is sharply divided with scissors.

200 UPPER EXTREMITY VASCULAR DISEASE

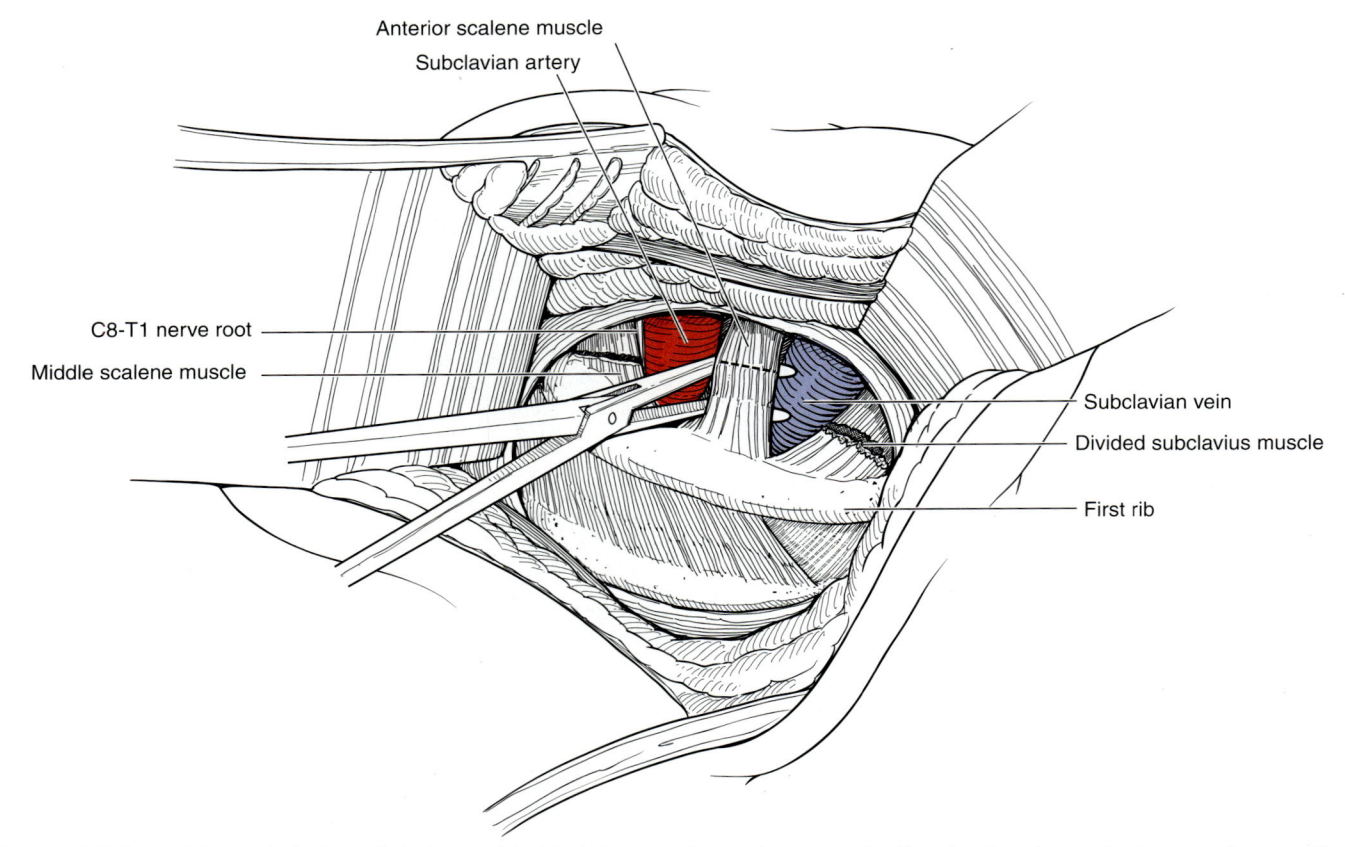

Figure 16-5. A right-angled clamp is insinuated behind the anterior scalene muscle. Gentle elevation pulls the muscle away from the underlying subclavian artery, thereby protecting the artery before dividing the muscle with scissors. The subclavius muscle is a crescent-shaped ligamentous attachment to the first rib adjacent to the subclavian vein. The subclavius muscle is sharply divided with scissors, taking care not to injure the subclavian vein.

RIB RESECTION

With the rib mobilized, a bone cutter is used to divide the first rib. Generally it is divided anteriorly and then posteriorly; however the patient's body habitus may make the reverse order easier (Fig. 16-6). In its anterior extent the rib is divided adjacent to the subclavian vein, and in the posterior direction it is divided just anterior to the brachial plexus; this ensures that the nerve roots are not inadvertently injured. The rib is then removed. A bone rongeur is used to remove the residual rib and to smooth the cut ends until there is no residual nerve impingement. A Roos retractor or similar instrument may be used to protect the nerves during use of the rongeur (Fig. 16-7).

It is important to ensure that no residual fibers from the anterior scalene muscle cross beneath the subclavian artery and insert onto the thickened surface at the apex of the pleura, known as Sibson's fascia. Any such fibers should be identified and divided.

CLOSURE

The surgical field is next inspected for bleeding. Temporarily packing the wound reliably controls minor bleeding. The wound is then reinspected, and hemostasis is completed with judicious use of electrocautery. The wound is then filled with saline. Several positive pressure ventilations are administered with saline left in the wound to assess for an air leak indicative of a postoperative pneumothorax. A small-caliber (12 Fr) chest tube is warranted in this situation. If the irrigation drains into the pleural space but there is no air leak, the pleura has been breached but a chest tube may not be necessary. In this situation a 12- or 14-Fr red rubber catheter is placed into the bed of the first rib and attached to gentle suction. The Machleder arm holder is lowered to facilitate a tension-free closure.

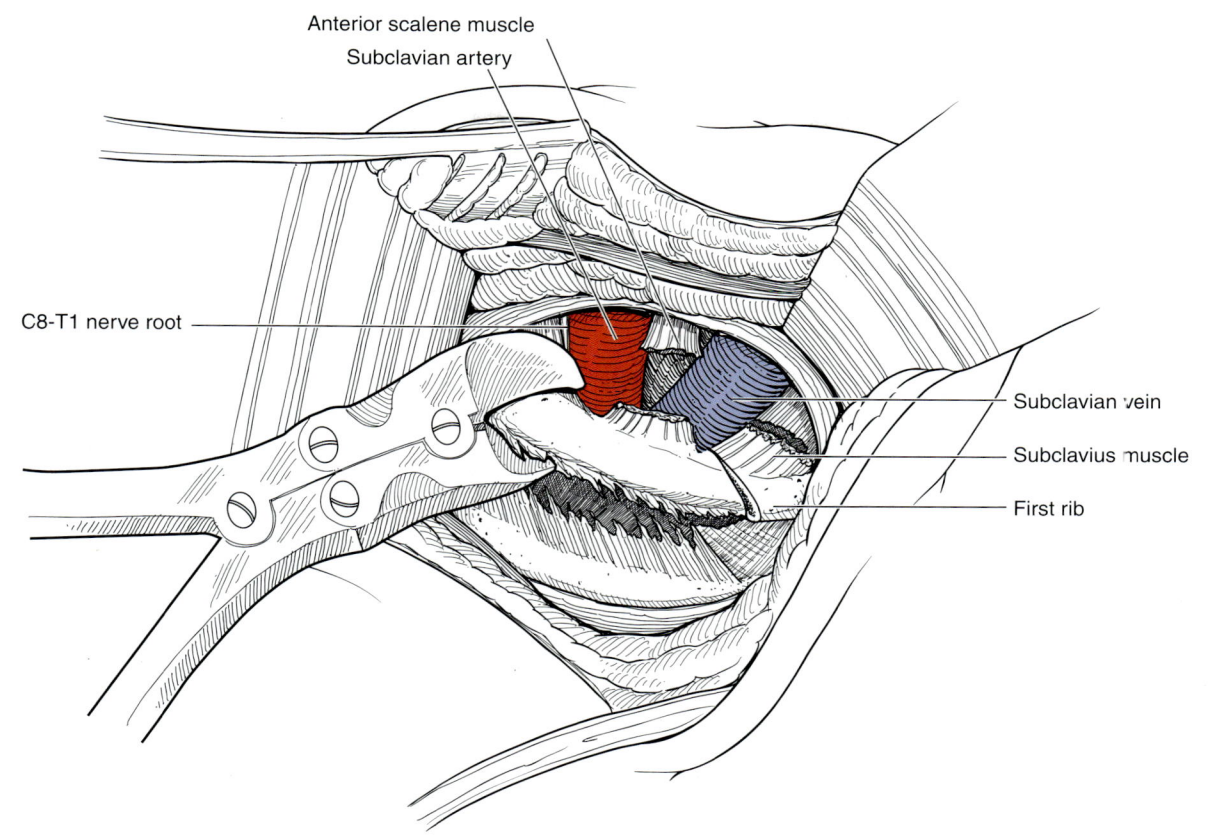

TRANSAXILLARY RIB RESECTION FOR THORACIC OUTLET SYNDROME

Figure 16-6. A bone cutter is used to divide the first rib in its anterior and posterior directions. Once removed, the rongeur is used to achieve smooth rib edges.

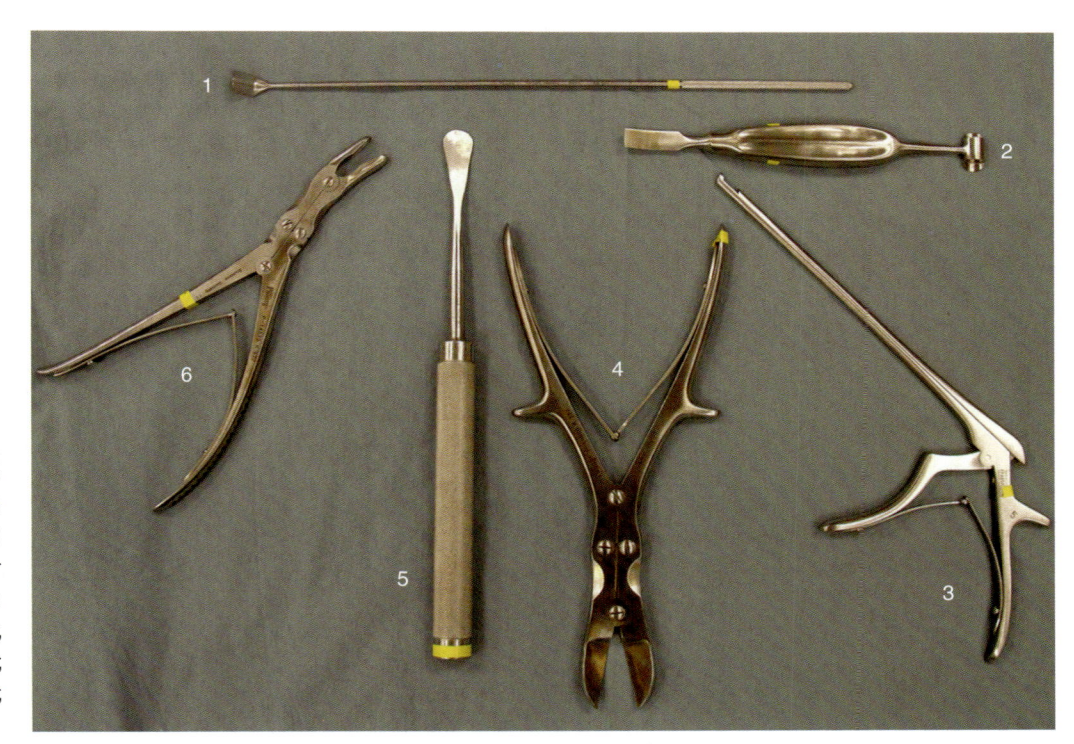

Figure 16-7. From the top of the image clockwise, the instruments depicted are (1) Roos retractor, (2) Alexander periosteotome, (3) Kerrison punch upbiting instrument, (4) double-action bone cutter, (5) Cobb periosteal elevator, and (6) rongeur.

The subcutaneous fascia is then closed around the tube on suction but is not tied. The anesthesia team then provides a sustained valsalva, and the fascial suture is tied as the suction tube is rapidly removed. This maneuver generally avoids a clinically significant postoperative pneumothorax. Closure is performed with an absorbable 2-0 suture in the fascia and a 4-0 subcuticular skin closure.

Postoperative Care

- A radiographic examination of the chest is performed in the recovery room. A small, clinically asymptomatic pneumothorax may be observed with a follow-up chest radiograph the next morning.
- Patients are discharged from the hospital on postoperative day 1 if adequate oral analgesia has been achieved.
- Activity is restricted by the amount of postoperative pain. Occasionally, a sling is required for patient comfort, but it is preferable to have the arm as mobile as tolerated.
- Physical therapy should be prescribed after 2 weeks in all patients undergoing transaxillary first rib resection, regardless of the cause, to restore range of motion and strength. For those with neurogenic TOS, 8 to 12 weeks of physical therapy may be required. If symptoms recur, more physical therapy may help. If symptoms recur after a year, Botox injections into the surrounding muscles that are in spasm may be helpful to facilitate participation in physical therapy.
- In patients with venous TOS, postoperative care varies depending on preoperative presentation. In patients who present with acute thrombosis, the most widespread practice is to attempt preoperative thrombolytic therapy and convert the patients to therapeutic anticoagulation with warfarin. An interval first rib resection and partial scalenectomy is then performed in approximately 4 weeks. Some evidence from patients treated at our institution suggests that there is no difference between patients treated preoperatively with thrombolytic therapy and patients treated with anticoagulation alone. At the time of first rib resection, patients are bridged from warfarin to low-molecular-weight heparin. After the procedure, to decrease the risk of bleeding complications, anticoagulation is withheld until 3 days after surgery. There is no universally accepted protocol on the postoperative management of patients with venous TOS. Patients with venous TOS typically undergo a follow-up venogram 2 weeks postoperatively with venous angioplasty if necessary. Patients are maintained on oral anticoagulation for 3 months, and if they remain asymptomatic, anticoagulation may be safely discontinued.[16,17]
- Patients with arterial TOS who have undergone a vascular reconstruction, as well as decompression, warrant antiplatelet therapy with aspirin regardless of the conduit type used (vein or prosthetic).

Postoperative Complications

- **Vascular injury.** A national query identified injury to the subclavian vessels as the most common complication after transaxillary rib resection for neurogenic TOS, occurring in 1% to 2% of cases.[18] Patients experiencing a vascular injury have greater lengths of stay, as well as increased hospital charges.[7] It is difficult to obtain proximal control of these vessels from the transaxillary approach; therefore the surgeon should exercise extreme caution when dissecting near these vessels.
- **Nerve injury.** Major nerve injury has been traditionally regarded as the most common complication after surgery for TOS. However, large contemporary series disprove this belief, with rates of brachial plexus injury for patients undergoing transaxillary first rib resection approaching 0%.[7,18] Temporary or permanent numbness of the upper medial arm because of excessive traction or division of the intercostobrachial nerve occurs in up to 10%. Frequently these symptoms improve over time.
- **Pneumothorax.** The complication of pneumothorax occurs in 2% to 10% of patients.[18] Accordingly, an upright chest radiograph is routinely performed in the recovery room. Radiographically detected pneumothoraces only require a chest tube if symptomatic or enlarging. Adhering closely to the inferior surface

of the first rib during blunt dissection helps protect against postoperative pneumothorax.
- **Recurrence.** Symptoms of TOS recur in 10% to 20% of patients.[12,15] Two intraoperative factors are known to reduce recurrence rates: (1) resecting a significant portion (2-3 cm) of the anterior scalene muscle, as opposed to simply dividing it at its insertion point, and (2) ensuring that the posterior edge of the first rib is resected sufficiently to leave as short a rib stump as technically feasible. Patients with spontaneous recurrence, compared with those who are reinjured, have worse outcomes when reoperation is performed. Most recurrences develop beyond 3 months but within 18 months of the initial operation,[18] and this finding reinforces the need to follow patients with neurogenic TOS for at least 2 years in order to ensure a successful operation.

REFERENCES

1. Atasoy E: History of thoracic outlet syndrome, *Hand Clin* 20(1):15-16, V, 2004.
2. Peet RM, Henriksen JD, Anderson TP, et al: Thoracic-outlet syndrome: Evaluation of a therapeutic exercise program, *Proc Staff Meet Mayo Clin* 31:281-287, 1956.
3. Coote H: Exostosis of the left transverse process of the seventh cervical vertebra, surrounded by blood vessels and nerves. Successful removal, *Lancet* 1:360-361, 1861.
4. Murphy T: Brachial neuritis caused by pressure of first rib, *Aus Med J* 15:582-585, 1910.
5. Adson AW, Coffey JR: Cervical rib: a method of anterior approach for relief of symptoms by division of the scalenus anticus, *Ann Surg* 85:839-857, 1927.
6. Roos DB: Transaxillary approach for first rib resection to relieve thoracic outlet syndrome, *Ann Surg* 163:354-358, 1966.
7. Chang DC, Lidor AO, Matsen SL, et al: Reported in-hospital complications following rib resections for neurogenic thoracic outlet syndrome, *Ann Vasc Surg* 21:564-570, 2007.
8. Chang DC, Rotellini-Coltvet LA, Mukherjee D, et al: Surgical intervention for thoracic outlet syndrome improves patient's quality of life, *J Vasc Surg* 49:630-635, 2009.
9. Sanders RJ, Hammond SL, Rao NM: Diagnosis of thoracic outlet syndrome, *J Vasc Surg* 46:601-604, 2007.
10. Burihan E, de Figueiredo LF, Francisco Junior J, et al: Upper-extremity deep venous thrombosis: Analysis of 52 cases, *Cardiovasc Surg* 1:19-22, 1993.
11. Geven LI, Smit AJ, Ebels T: Vascular thoracic outlet syndrome. Longer posterior rib stump causes poor outcome, *Eur J Cardiothorac Surg* 30:232-236, 2006.
12. Mingoli A, Feldhaus RJ, Farina C, et al: Long-term outcome after transaxillary approach for thoracic outlet syndrome, *Surgery* 118:840-844, 1995.
13. Urschel HC Jr: Anatomy of the thoracic outlet, *Thorac Surg Clin* 17:511-520, 2007.
14. Ambrad-Chalela E, Thomas GI, Johansen KH: Recurrent neurogenic thoracic outlet syndrome, *Am J Surg* 187:505-510, 2004.
15. Sanders RJ, Haug CE, Pearce WH: Recurrent thoracic outlet syndrome, *J Vasc Surg* 12:390-400, 1990.
16. de Leon RA, Chang DC, Hassoun HT, et al: Multiple treatment algorithms for successful outcomes in venous thoracic outlet syndrome, *Surgery* 145:500-507, 2009.
17. Fugate MW, Rotellini-Coltvet L, Freischlag JA: Current management of thoracic outlet syndrome, *Curr Treat Options Cardiovasc Med* 11:176-183, 2009.
18. Altobelli GG, Kudo T, Haas BT, et al: Thoracic outlet syndrome: Pattern of clinical success after operative decompression, *J Vasc Surg* 42:122-128, 2005.

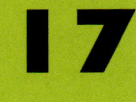

17 Endovascular Therapy for Subclavian-Axillary Vein Thrombosis

KARL A. ILLIG • ADAM J. DOYLE

Historical Background

Subclavian-axillary vein thrombosis, also referred to as Paget-Schroetter syndrome or "effort thrombosis," refers to primary thrombosis of the subclavian vein at the costoclavicular junction. Primary subclavian-axillary vein thrombosis is relatively rare, with a yearly incidence in the United States of 3000 to 6000 cases. A recent analysis suggests that less than 1000 first rib resections are performed for venous thoracic outlet syndrome yearly.[1] This is a disorder of the anterior part of the thoracic outlet region, where the subclavian vein passes through the intersection of the clavicle and first rib (Fig. 17-1), often seen in young, healthy patients who participate in vigorous activity that involves raising the arm above the head.[2]

Paget was the first to describe "gouty phlebitis" of the upper extremity in 1875, which was a spontaneous thrombosis of the subclavian vein.[3] von Schroetter postulated in 1884 that this entity resulted from a direct stretch injury to the vein caused by muscular strain.[4] Hughes termed the condition Paget-von Schroetter syndrome in 1949.[5]

Leaving this condition untreated results in residual upper extremity venous obstruction in up to 78% of cases and persistent symptoms and permanent disability in 41% to 91% and 39% to 68% of cases, respectively.[2] Anticoagulation alone results in "excellent or good" long-term results in only 10 of 35 (29%) patients.[6] Although significant differences exist, most recommend thrombolysis, followed by thoracic outlet decompression, most often by first rib resection. Decompression was initially thought best performed after an interval of a few months, but many now advocate immediate surgery to reduce the risk of rethrombosis. Secondary venous thrombosis is typically associated with a central catheter, with recommended treatment including anticoagulation and catheter removal.

Preoperative Preparation

- True effort thrombosis almost always produces acute symptoms, and the patient usually presents to the clinic or emergency department with a swollen, blue, painful arm. Clinical clues include a history of vigorous activity, often with the affected arm overhead, and even if the onset of swelling is acute, a history of intermittent swelling, discoloration associated with activity, or both is common. Patients may have prominent chest wall or shoulder collaterals.
- Duplex imaging should be performed to confirm the diagnosis.
- If duplex is negative or equivocal, computed tomography or magnetic resonance venography can be considered. The patient with a duplex ultrasound venous thrombosis should be anticoagulated, with intravenous access established in the contralateral extremity.

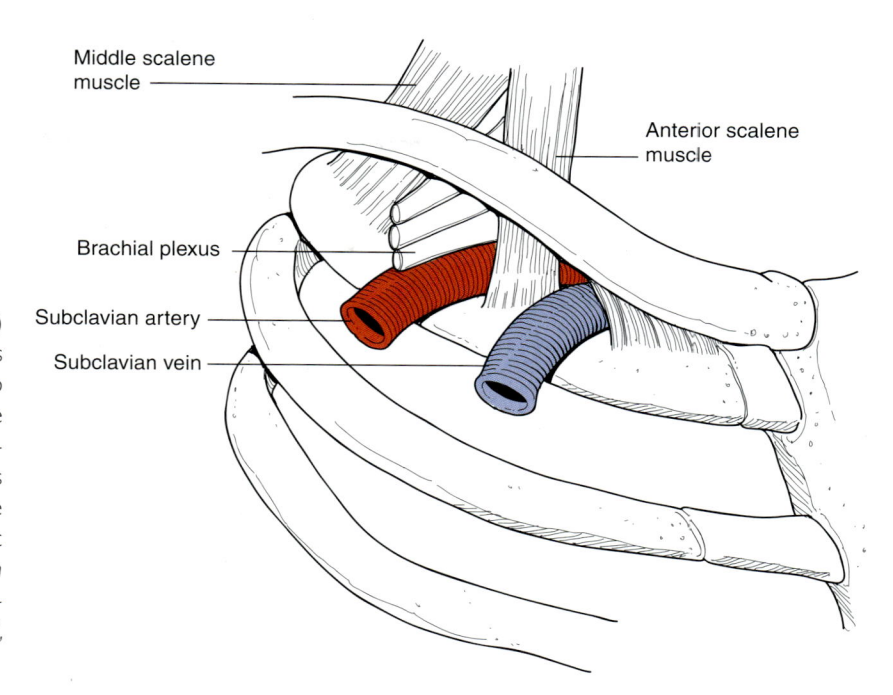

Figure 17-1. Anatomy of the venous (anterior) portion of the thoracic outlet. The vein passes through the junction of the clavicle and first rib anteriorly and is potentially compressed by the costoclavicular ligament anteriorly and the subclavius muscle and tendon superiorly. The venous thoracic outlet is anterior to the anterior scalene muscle; thus neurogenic and venous thoracic outlet syndromes are two different entities. *(From Illig KA, Doyle AJ: A comprehensive review of Paget-Schroetter syndrome. J Vasc Surg 51:1538-1547, 2010.)*

- Success of catheter-directed thrombolytic therapy rapidly decreases from onset of symptoms to intervention. Therefore, although not an emergency, treatment should be initiated within hours to a day or so after diagnosis unless contraindications exist. Although algorithms differ, pharmacologic or pharmacomechanical thrombolysis followed by transaxillary first rib resection during the same admission is an accepted approach. If thrombolysis is planned, pregnancy testing should be performed and renal function should be assessed.

Pitfalls and Danger Points

- Pulmonary embolism
- Vessel perforation
- Bleeding risk after thoracic outlet decompression is increased if surgery is performed within hours to days after thrombolysis.
- Venous occlusion while awaiting thoracic outlet decompression may occur in 10% to 33% of patients if surgery is delayed for months, but is uncommon (5%) if surgery is performed within several days of thrombolysis.

Endovascular Strategy

ANGIOGRAPHIC ANATOMY AND COLLATERALS

- The true deep system consists of the paired forearm veins that unite to form the paired brachial veins, surrounding the brachial artery in the antecubital fossa (Fig. 17-2). These vessels are the anatomic analogue of the tibial and popliteal veins in the leg. At the midupper arm or axilla, this system is usually joined by the basilic vein; at the lower border of the teres minor, this becomes the axillary vein; and at the lateral border of the first rib, it becomes the subclavian vein. The deep brachial vein joins the axillary vein in the axilla.
- The superficial system consists of the cephalic vein, which communicates with the deep system at the antecubital fossa and then joins the subclavian vein at the deltopectoral groove, and the basilic vein, which, as noted earlier, joins the deep system in the midupper arm or axilla after penetrating the superficial fascia and axillary sheath.

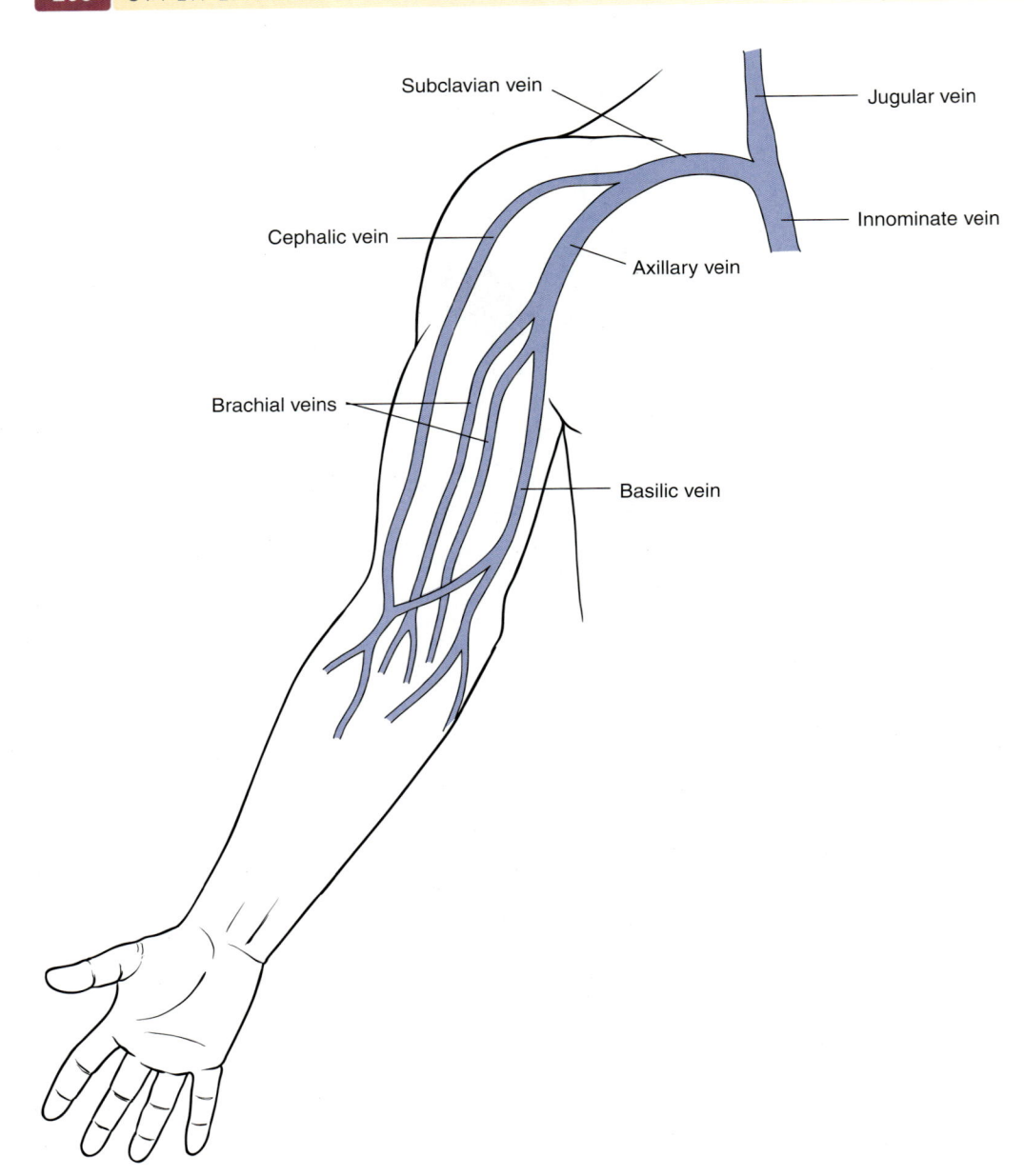

Figure 17-2. Anatomy of the veins of the arm. The basilic veins in the antecubital fossa and brachial vein just medial to it both provide access to the axillary-subclavian vein complex, whereas the cephalic vein does not enter the deep system until the deltopectoral groove is reached.

- Two main collateral pathways exist, collectively described as "first rib bypass collaterals,"[7] which become prominent in patients with subclavian-axillary vein thrombosis. The more prominent tend to occur cephalad to the costoclavicular junction and connect branches of the cephalic vein to the external and internal jugular veins, whereas the second pathway consists of branches of the deep brachial veins that connect to veins caudal to the junction, typically branches of the pectoral veins and intercostals (Fig. 17-3).
- The presence or absence of these collaterals on venography is a critically important marker for residual obstruction or successful thrombolysis, respectively.

TIMING

- **Thrombolysis—initiation.** Catheter-directed thrombolysis is most effective if performed as soon after thrombosis as possible. The success rate nears 100% if initiated within a few days of symptom onset but drops significantly if initiated after 7 to 14 days. In three series, no patient with symptoms persisting for longer than 7, 8, and 10 days, respectively, had successful lysis.[8-10] The success rate in patients at the University of Rochester with symptoms of less than 14 days' duration has been 84% over the past decade.[11]

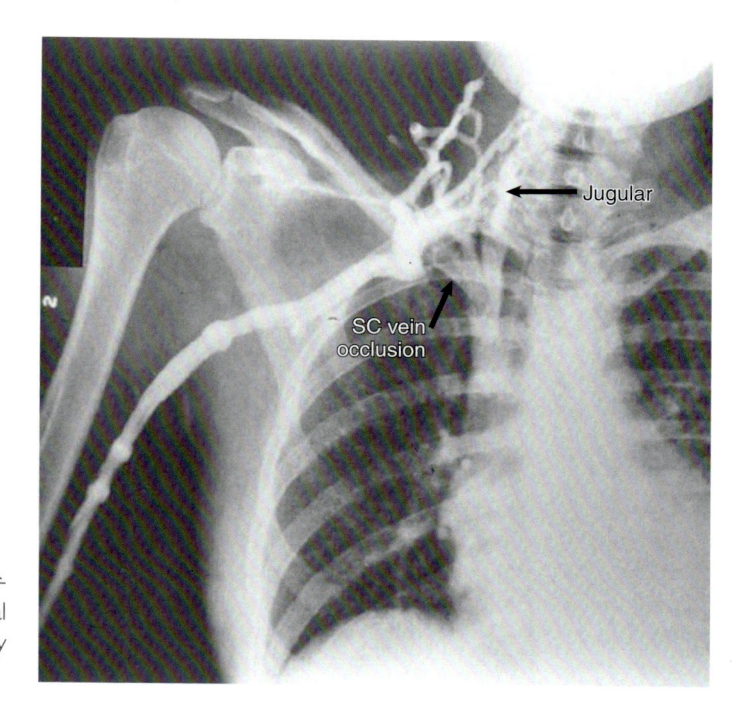

Figure 17-3. Venogram illustrating the "first rib bypass collaterals" connecting branches of the subclavian vein with the external jugular and jugular veins (arrow 1), pathognomic of hemodynamically significant venous occlusion (arrow 2) at this level.

- **Thrombolysis—duration.** Thrombolysis should be continued for approximately 48 hours before concluding that no further clot lysis can be achieved. Recent reports have demonstrated that pharmacomechanical lysis may be highly beneficial using the AngioJet (Medrad Interventional/Possis; Minneapolis, Minn.), EkoSonic (EKOS, Bothell, Wash.), or Trellis (Bacchus Vascular, Santa Clara, Calif.) systems with recanalization of the occluded vein within minutes to hours. If residual thrombus remains, a trial of standard catheter-based lytic infusion can be continued.
- **Decompression.** After clot dissolution, the thoracic outlet must be decompressed to relieve compression at the costoclavicular junction, although the timing of the second procedure has been the subject of debate. It was originally recommended that thoracic outlet decompression be delayed 3 months to allow the vessel to heal and to lessen the risk of surgical complications.[12] However, it was later recognized that rethrombosis occurs in up to one third of patients so treated. Most now recommend that decompression follow thrombolysis as soon as possible—ideally during the same admission. This may result in a somewhat higher complication rate but better long-term success; modern series following this algorithm show long-term symptom-free status in 95% to 100% of patients.[6,13]
- **Angioplasty and stenting before bony decompression.** After thrombolysis a significant number of patients are shown to have intrinsic venous defects, and essentially all have extrinsic compression at the costoclavicular junction. Angioplasty and even stenting of these patients is tempting, but the costoclavicular junction is unyielding, and angioplasty before decompression will commonly fail.[14] It has been suggested that angioplasty prior to decompression may worsen venous patency by further damaging the vein wall.[15] Stenting of the vein may also be complicated by stent fracture in some, deformation in nearly all, and rethrombosis rates as high as 40%.[14] Stents complicate subsequent repair and therefore should be avoided.
- **Angioplasty and stenting after bony decompression.** It is tempting to perform angioplasty, stenting, or both when residual defects are seen after thoracic outlet decompression. In one recent study stent patency was 64% at 3.5 years in 14 patients who were stented after decompression, compared with 100% at 4 years in 9 patients undergoing angioplasty alone.[16] Although this

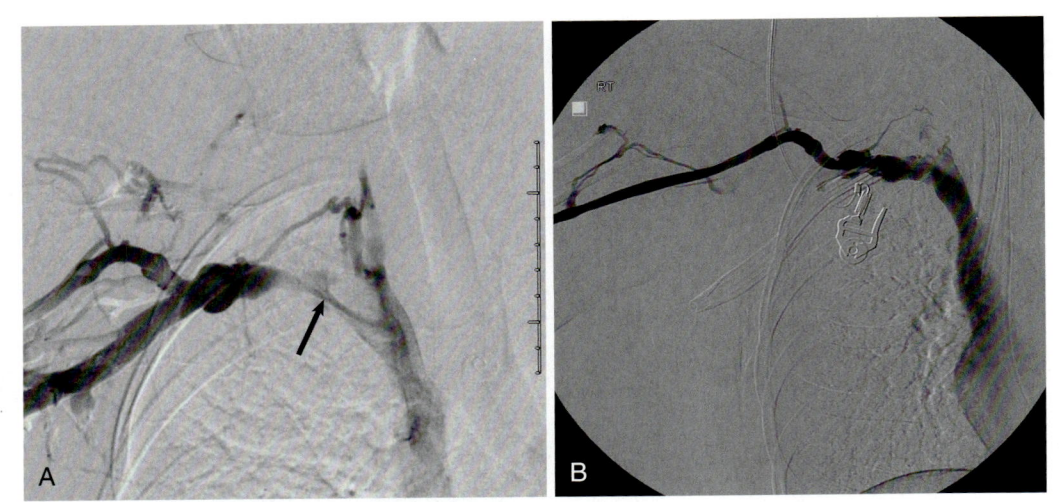

Figure 17-4. Venography illustrating the benefit of aggressive external surgical venolysis during first rib excision. **A,** Venography after thrombolysis but before decompression showing significant residual lesion *(arrow)* and prominent collaterals. **B,** Venogram after first rib excision and 360-degree circumferential venolysis to the level of the innominate vein without endoluminal intervention. The venous collaterals, evident before surgical venolysis, have disappeared.

may simply represent selection of more extensive residual lesions, some evidence suggests that postdecompression balloon angioplasty and observation alone for residual defects yield good long-term results. Anecdotal experience suggests that many "intrinsic" defects result from residual external scarring and that external venolysis can eliminate the need for endoluminal intervention in at least some cases (Fig. 17-4). Molina advocates aggressive direct venous reconstruction at the time of thoracic outlet decompression, which eliminates the need for angioplasty and stenting.[13,17] Many clinicians simply leave such lesions alone, citing the very high, long-term symptom-free status in almost all cases.

Endovascular Technique

An algorithm for decision making related to endoluminal intervention for axillary-subclavian vein thrombosis is presented in Figure 17-5.

ACCESS

The entire arm should be circumferentially prepped into the operative field to maximize sterility and surgical options. It is critically important to achieve access into the deep venous system—in order of preference, the basilic vein medial to the antecubital fossa, the brachial-axillary veins in the midupper arm, or the brachial veins surrounding the brachial artery in the antecubital fossa, which is less convenient for the patient. The cephalic or antecubital veins should not be used, because entry to the deep system is high in the arm at the deltopectoral groove. Therefore the axillary, brachial, and basilic veins may not be visualized or accessible. Even if pathology is central to the deltopectoral groove, access to central veins is difficult and there is a high rate of cephalic vein obliteration. The more central brachial-axillary veins within the axillary sheath are also a poor choice, because of the increased risk of axillary sheath hematoma. Access to all vessels is best performed using ultrasound guidance.

SHEATH PLACEMENT

After placement of a guidewire, a conventional sheath is placed. Because of the high likelihood of requiring intervention and the benign nature of venous access, a 6-Fr short, conventional sheath can be placed because manipulation is relatively straightforward.

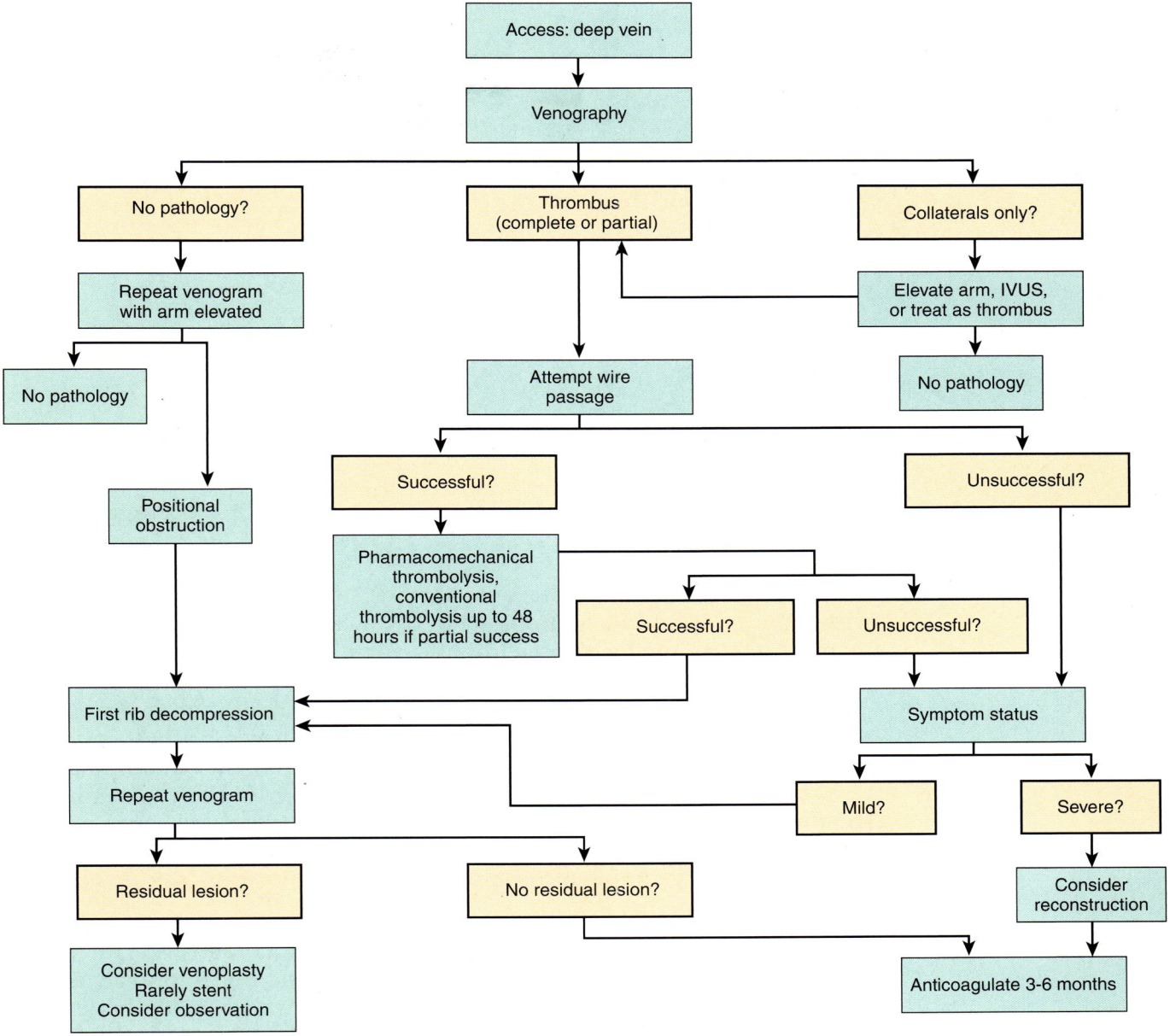

Figure 17-5. Algorithm for treatment of axillary-subclavian vein thrombosis. Beige colored boxes indicate critical decision points. *IVUS*, Intravascular ultrasound.

THROMBOLYSIS

The procedure begins with full diagnostic venography. Hand injection in aliquots of 20 cc of 50% contrast provides excellent visualization, although use of a power injector allows reduced radiation exposure to the surgeon. The entire arm central to the sheath should be imaged as the brachial vein is often partially or fully thrombosed, but attention should be focused on the costoclavicular junction. If complete thrombosis is present, a flow void with or without meniscus is typically seen (Fig. 17-6), and the arm drains via prominent collaterals. Even if the lesion does not appear critical, the presence of collaterals documents its hemodynamic significance. If inflow is brisk and collaterals are not observed, the test should be repeated with the arm abducted greater than 90 degrees. If stenosis, occlusion, or new collaterals are seen, venous compression at the costoclavicular junction is confirmed, although thrombolysis is not needed. Finally, if the situation is unclear, intravascular ultrasound can be used, although its sensitivity and specificity has not been well defined in this situation.

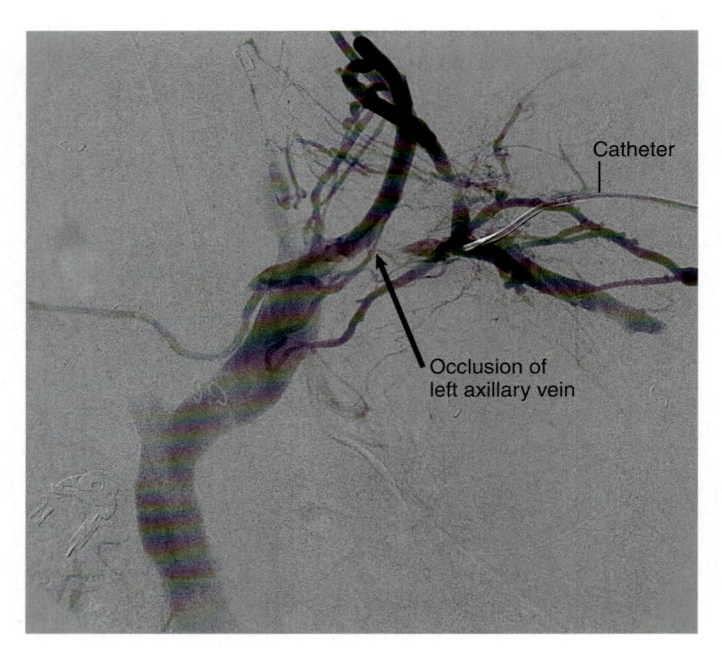

Figure 17-6. Venographic appearance of complete occlusion of the left axillary vein *(upward arrow)*. A catheter is in the left cephalic vein *(vertical line)*. Extensive first rib bypass collaterals are present, connecting primarily to the innominate vein.

As with any thrombolytic procedure, the first step is crossing the lesion with a wire. It is almost always appropriate to use a combination of an angled "vertebral" catheter along with a hydrophilic wire; if support is not adequate, the working sheath can be exchanged for a long sheath placed near the lesion. As with any attempt to cross a vascular occlusion, skill and experience are required to recognize extravascular wire passage. If needed, a puff of contrast through a catheter can distinguish an intraluminal from an extraluminal position. Extravascular wire passage in this circumstance is relatively benign and should be treated by withdrawing the wire and catheter to a confirmed intravascular location with another attempt through a different plane. The exception occurs in the treatment of lesions in the superior vena cava, where fatal tamponade can occur.

The observation that successful wire passage is a predictor of successful thrombolysis in occluded arterial segments does not seem to hold true in primary axillary-subclavian vein thrombosis. Wire passage is almost always possible, but in many patients the vein cannot be successfully opened. This may be due to the greater incidence of intrinsic fibrotic damage to the vein itself. Available options, including conventional pharmacologic thrombolysis or pharmacomechanical thrombolysis, are described as follows:

- **Conventional pharmacologic thrombolysis** is performed using conventional techniques. Venography is used to delineate the length of the thrombosed segment, and an infusion catheter is selected with an infusion length sufficient to treat the entire lesion. Frequently such lesions are shorter than the shortest available catheter; in this situation the excess length should be positioned peripheral to the occlusion. Although many pharmacologic options exist, a commonly used protocol includes tissue plasminogen activator (tPA) at a rate of 1 mg/hr through the infusion catheter, with heparin concomitantly infused through the sheath at a rate of 500 units/hr. Laboratory values do not need to be routinely monitored in this situation, and the patient may be admitted to a conventional floor bed. Ideally venography should be repeated at 8- to 12-hour intervals, but the very short segment being treated, low-pressure venous access, and young age of the majority of these patients makes reevaluation the next day safe. Should residual thrombus be noted, thrombolysis should be continued for up to 48 hours before concluding that maximum benefit has been achieved.

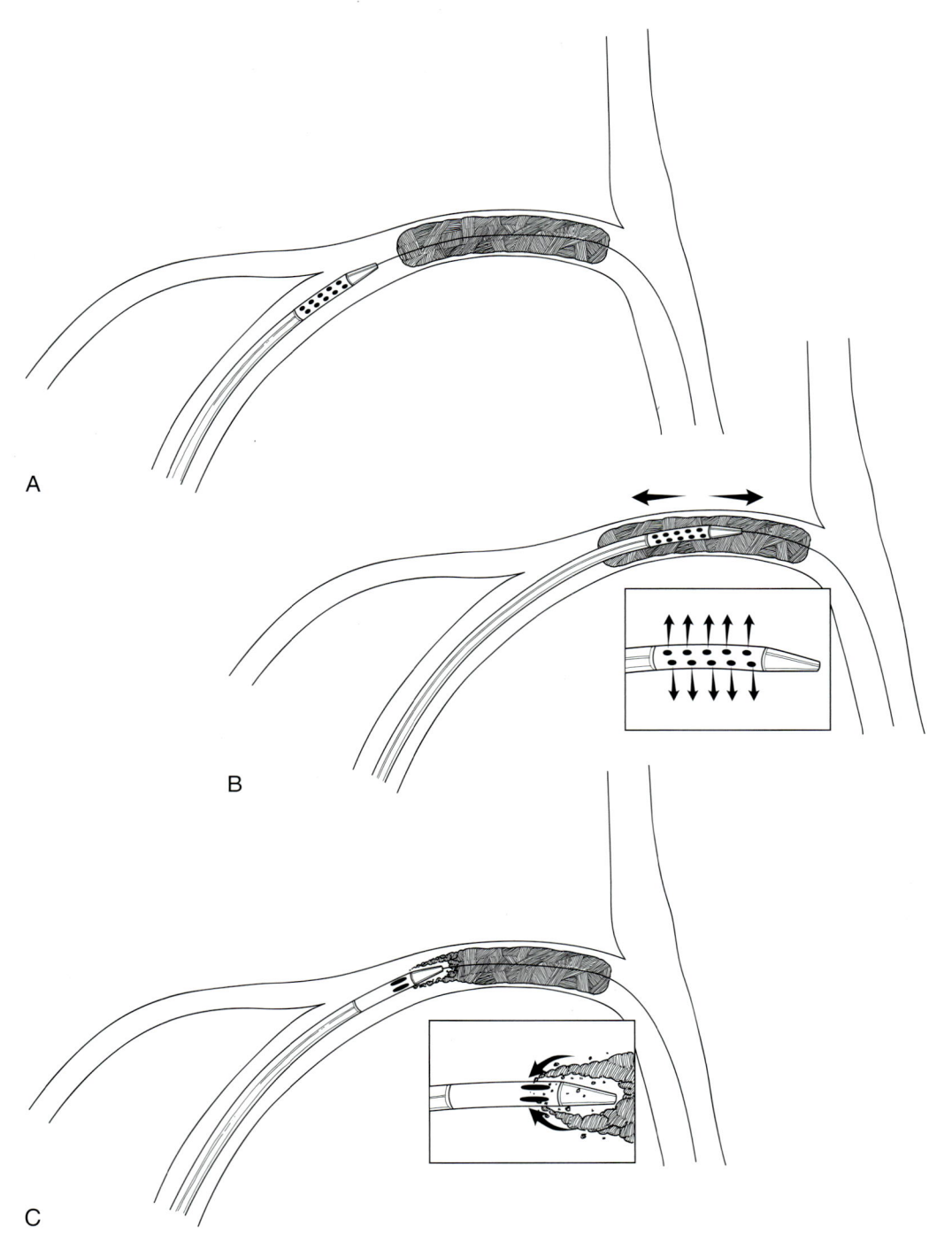

Figure 17-7. Process of pharmacomechanical thrombolysis using the AngioJet rheolytic thrombectomy device. **A,** The lesion is crossed with a wire. **B,** Using power pulse mode, the thrombus is laced with 10 mg of tPA. **C,** After a 20- to 30-minute dwell time for the thrombolytic agent, the tPA-laced thrombus is aspirated using a conventional AngioJet technique. Treatment of residual defects is individualized, but no further intervention should be considered until bony decompression has been performed.

- **Pharmacomechanical thrombolysis** is an excellent option and can be carried out with the AngioJet device, using the "power pulse spray" mode (Fig. 17-7). After wire passage a solution of 20 mg of tPA in 250 cc of saline solution is readied. Under fluoroscopic guidance, 10 mg of tPA is infused under pressure over 5 minutes to thoroughly impregnate the thrombus, followed by a 20- to 30-minute dwell time. Conventional AngioJet aspiration is then performed with saline followed by repeat imaging. If partial success is seen, aspiration is repeated. Once the vein is fully opened or further aspiration will be of little added benefit, the procedure is halted. If the vein is completely open, the sheath can be left in place for subsequent imaging at the time of thoracic outlet decompression, whereas if residual defects are seen, thrombolysis should be continued overnight followed by repeat imaging. If residual defects are thought to be extrinsic or fibrotic, continued thrombolysis is unlikely to be beneficial.

- The EkoSonic catheter, which uses endoluminal ultrasound to improve clot dissolution, or the Trellis device, which actively breaks up thrombus by means of a rotating wire, may also be used. Although the Trellis system is, in principle, suitable for long vessels without branches, the very short location of thrombus in this situation makes it less applicable, and descriptions of its use for axillary-subclavian vein thrombosis have not been reported.

ANGIOPLASTY AND STENTING

Angioplasty of residual lesions will not be of benefit unless the costoclavicular junction is decompressed and may, in fact, be unnecessary after decompression. Angioplasty should be reserved for significant residual lesions after first rib resection; therefore, if surgery is performed soon after thrombolysis, the sheath should be left in place for repeat imaging during surgery. Stenting before decompression may be harmful and should rarely be needed even after decompression.

Some controversy exists regarding management of the vein that remains completely occluded after complete, aggressive endovascular intervention. Some recommend first rib resection because a significant number of such patients spontaneously recanalize[18] and the majority become symptom free. Forcible dilation and stenting may lead to eventual stent fracture and rethrombosis.

COMPLETION STUDIES

If a residual defect is observed, the sheath may be left in place for venography immediately after first rib resection with the need to perform angioplasty individualized.

Postoperative Care

- A **chest radiograph** is obtained in the recovery room and on the first postoperative day to exclude a pneumothorax. Radiographic examination also confirms removal of the correct rib and may be performed in the operating room if there is any question. After thrombolysis the risk of bleeding is significant, and close attention paid to both physical examination and findings on the chest radiograph.
- **Anticoagulation.** Heparin is administered intravenously at 500 units/hr beginning 6 hours after surgery, with transition to full anticoagulation by 12 to 18 hours. Warfarin is administered on the evening of the first postoperative day and in young, healthy adults an oral dose of 10 mg on each of the first two days after surgery is an appropriate loading dose. Discharge is almost always possible before the international normalized ratio is between 2.0 and 3.0, and in this situation the patient may be bridged with self-injected, subcutaneous low-molecular-weight heparin. Anticoagulation is continued for 3 to 6 months.
- **Analgesia.** The patient is placed on a patient-controlled anesthesia pump immediately after surgery, and on the first postoperative day oral narcotic analgesia is begun.
- **Drains.** If a drain is left, it can be removed by the first postoperative day assuming there is no significant bleeding, the drainage is not chylous, and no pneumothorax is seen.
- **Physical therapy.** Active range of motion maneuvers should begin on the first postoperative day, with active rehabilitation begun in 3 to 4 weeks.
- **Postoperative imaging.** The patient is seen 3 to 4 weeks after surgery for examination and duplex ultrasound imaging. The patient is reassessed at 6 months

and if the vessel is patent, warfarin is discontinued, and the patient reevaluated at 1 year and yearly thereafter. If the vessel remains occluded, warfarin can be continued with follow-up every 6 months, if there are no contraindications to its use. Coumdain should be discontinued if recanalization has not occurred by 2 years.

Complications

- **Access site complications.** Local access complications are quite minor, because the venous system alone is involved. Inadvertent arterial puncture can cause axillary sheath hematoma or distal ischemia or emboli, but this can be minimized by the use of ultrasound-guided access techniques and access via the relatively peripheral basilic vein.
- **Local bleeding.** Local bleeding is common but relatively minor and can be managed by pressure, reinforcing the dressing, or occasionally placing a purse string suture around the catheter.
- **Systemic bleeding.** Systemic bleeding is rare. Routine monitoring of fibrin degradation products is not necessary, and most patients can be monitored on a surgical floor.
- **Pulmonary embolism.** Clinically relevant pulmonary embolism is exceedingly rare during venous thrombolysis, but subclinical embolism is probably frequent.[11]
- **Morbidity.** A recent review showed that complications after first rib resection occurred in up to 5.6% of patients.[1] Bleeding complications after subsequent thoracic outlet decompression are significantly increased if surgery is performed within hours to days after thrombolysis. These can manifest as a wound hematoma or hemothorax if communication with the pleural space has occurred.

REFERENCES

1. Lee JT, Jordan SE, Illig KA: Clinical incidence and prevalence: Basic data on the current scope of the problem. In Illeg KA, Thompson RW, Frieschlag JA, et al, editors: *Thoracic outlet syndrome*, London, 2013, Springer-Verlag.
2. Illig KA, Doyle AJ: A comprehensive review of Paget-Schroetter syndrome, *J Vasc Surg* 51:1538–1547, 2010.
3. Paget J: *Clinical lectures and essays*, London, 1875, Longmans, Green & Co.
4. von Schroetter L: Erkrankungen der gefasse. In Nothnagel CWH, et al, editors: *Handbuch der pathologie und therapie*, Wein, 1884, Holder.
5. Hughes ES: Venous obstruction in upper extremity, *Brit J Surg* 36:155-163, 1948.
6. Urschel HC Jr, Razzuk MA: Paget-Schroetter syndrome: What is the best management? *Ann Thorac Surg* 69:1663-1668, 2000.
7. Adams JT, McEvoy RK, DeWeese JA: Primary deep venous thrombosis of the upper extremity, *Arch Surg* 91:29-42, 1965.
8. Zimmerman R, Morl H, Harenberg J, et al: Urokinase therapy of subclavian-axillary vein thrombosis, *Klin Wochenschr* 59:851-856, 1981.
9. Wilson JJ, Zahn CA, Newman H: Fibrinolytic therapy for idiopathic subclavian-axillary vein thrombosis, *Am J Surg* 159:208-211, 1990.
10. Adelman MA, Stone DH, Riles TS, et al: A multidisciplinary approach to the treatment of Paget-Schroetter syndrome, *Ann Vasc Surg* 11:149-154, 1997.
11. Doyle AJ, Wolford HY, Davies MG, et al: Management of effort thrombosis of the subclavian vein: Today's treatment, *Ann Vasc Surg* 21:723-729, 2007.
12. Machleder HI: Evaluation of a new treatment strategy for Paget-Schroetter syndrome: Spontaneous thrombosis of the axillary-subclavian vein, *J Vasc Surg* 17:305-317, 1993.
13. Molina JE, Hunter DW, Dietz CA: Paget-Schroetter syndrome treated with thrombolytics and immediate surgery, *J Vasc Surg* 45:328-334, 2007.
14. Meier GH, Pollak JS, Rosenblatt M, et al: Initial experience with venous stents in external axillary-subclavian vein thrombosis, *J Vasc Surg* 24:974-983, 1996.
15. Lee MC, Grassi CJ, Belkin M, et al: Early operative intervention after thrombolytic therapy for primary subclavian vein thrombosis: An effective treatment approach, *J Vasc Surg* 27:1101-1108, 1998.

16. Kreienberg PB, Chang BB, Darling RC 3rd, et al: Long-term results in patients treated with thrombolysis, thoracic inlet decompression, and subclavian vein stenting for Paget-Schroetter syndrome, *J Vasc Surg* 33:s100-s105, 2001.
17. Molina JE: Treatment of chronic obstruction of the axillary, subclavian, and innominate veins, *Int J Angiol* 8:87-90, 1990.
18. deLeon R, Chang DC, Busse C, et al: First rib resection and scalenectomy for chronically occluded subclavian veins: What does it really do? *Ann Vasc Surg* 22:395-401, 2008.

Section 5

THE THORACIC AORTA

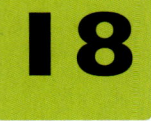

18 Direct Surgical Repair of Aneurysms of the Thoracic and Thoracoabdominal Aorta

HAZIM J. SAFI • ANTHONY L. ESTRERA

Historical Background

The first surgeon to repair a thoracoabdominal aortic aneurysm (TAAA) was Etheredge[1] in 1955 in a patient with a Type IV TAAA using a homograft. In 1956 DeBakey and associates[2] reported the surgical treatment of four patients with TAAA by resection and homograft replacement. A Dacron graft was used as a shunt between the descending thoracic aorta and infrarenal abdominal aorta. Sequentially, the celiac axis, superior mesenteric artery, and both renal arteries were revascularized, limiting ischemic time for the liver, stomach, bowels, and kidneys to 10 to 15 minutes. Subsequent reports utilized Dacron grafts instead of homografts for primary reconstruction of the aorta with Dacron side arms to each visceral vessel, as the primary approach for repair from the 1950s to the late 1970s.

In 1965 Crawford[3] ushered in the modern era of TAAA and descending thoracic aortic aneurysm (DTAA) repair. Three principles of repair were formulated: (1) the inclusion technique, as originally described by Matas, Javid, and Creech,[3,4] in which the aneurysm wall is not excised, thus avoiding damage to surrounding structures; (2) the reattachment of the renal arteries, superior mesenteric artery, and the celiac axis into the larger graft, by either creating an orifice in the body of the graft or beveling the anastomosis, as described by Carrel[5]; and (3) reattachment of the intercostal arteries to prevent paraplegia, as initially described by Spencer[6-8] in a canine model. From the 1970s until the 1990s, the "clamp and sew" technique was the primary surgical approach for treatment.

Beginning in the 1960s, multiple approaches to prevent paraplegia were introduced. As an early adjunct, cerebrospinal fluid drainage (CSFD) was described by Miyamoto and colleagues[9] in 1960, as well as by Blaisdell and Cooley[10] in 1962. Although the benefit of reduced cerebrospinal fluid (CSF) pressure during TAAA repair was demonstrated in a canine model, CSFD did not gain clinical popularity until the 1980s. The use of perfusion catheters from the descending aorta to both renal arteries, the celiac axis, and the superior mesenteric artery was first described by Korompai and Hayward in 1975.[11]

Although Hollier and co-workers[12] confirmed the benefits of CSFD, Crawford and associates[13] initially reported that CSFD did not improve outcomes. Despite this early controversy, subsequent studies have demonstrated the benefit of CSFD during TAAA repair.[14]

The use of distal aortic perfusion (DAP) or partial bypass was first reported in 1956 by DeBakey and associates[15] and later by Connolly and colleagues[16] to reduce distal ischemia and cardiac afterload. The benefit of DAP was confirmed in multiple studies conducted in the 1980s and 1990s.[17]

Preoperative Preparation

- **Cardiac evaluation.** Echocardiography is obtained to determine ventricular function and the presence of valvular abnormalities. Normal ventricular function is a predictor of good outcome after TAAA repair. Severe valvular dysfunction should be treated before aortic repair if repair is not urgent. Cardiac evaluation should include a physical examination and determination of exercise tolerance. If coronary artery disease is identified, then the extent and location of disease and associated symptoms determine the order of repair. Drug-eluting stents should be avoided as TAAA repair mandates discontinuation of clopidogrel. If required, coronary artery bypass grafting should be performed at least 6 weeks before repair.
- **Pulmonary function.** Pulmonary function tests and arterial blood gases are obtained as a routine. Patients with severe chronic obstructive pulmonary disease, as suggested by a forced expiratory volume in 1 second (FEV1) of less than 0.8 L/min, should be evaluated by a pulmonologist and receive bronchodilators as well as pulmonary rehabilitation before repair.
- **Nutritional and gastrointestinal status.** Large aneurysms may cause "aortic dysphagia" as a result of intrinsic compression of the lower esophagus leading to a nutritionally depleted state that may benefit from preoperative enteral alimentation.
- **Renal function.** Preoperative renal function is a strong predictor of postoperative mortality after TAAA repair,[18] and glomerular filtration rate (GFR) is more sensitive than serum creatinine in predicting postoperative outcome.[18] Patients with renal dysfunction may benefit from admission before surgery for intravenous hydration. Advanced, irreversible renal failure constitutes a relative contraindication to surgery.

Operative Strategy

A classification for thoracoabdominal aortic aneurysm describes five anatomic types: Type I extends from the left subclavian artery to just above the renal arteries; Type II from the left subclavian to the aortic bifurcation; Type III from the sixth intercostal space to the aortic bifurcation; Type IV from the twelfth intercostal space to the aortic bifurcation; and Type V from the sixth intercostal space to just above the renal arteries (Fig. 18-1). This classification has been used in the prediction of complications, especially the risk of spinal cord ischemia, which is highest for Type II TAAA.

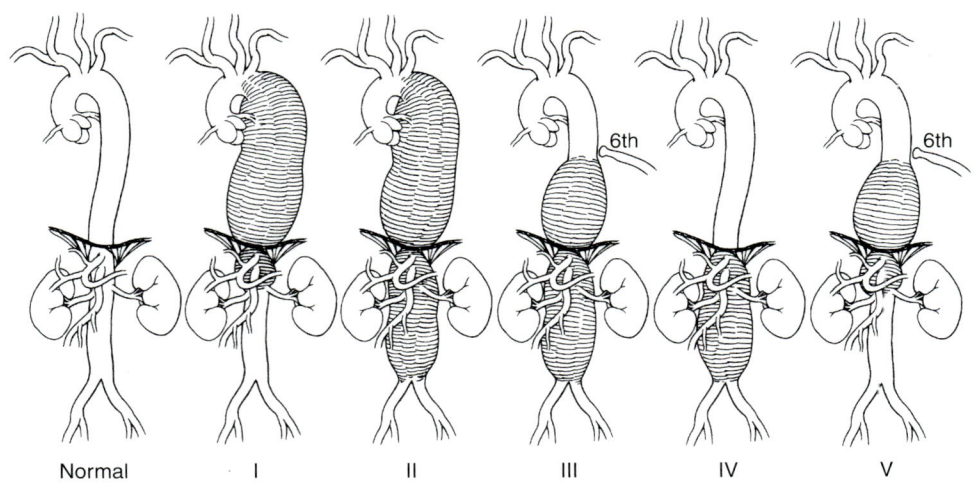

Figure 18-1. Modified Crawford anatomic classification of TAAAs. *(From Rutherford RB: Vascular surgery, ed 6. Philadelphia, 2005, Saunders, p 1491, Fig. 103-2.)*

A separate classification scheme has been devised for those aneurysms confined to the descending thoracic aorta. Type A extends distal to the left subclavian artery to the sixth intercostal space; Type B arises between the sixth and twelfth intercostal spaces, above the diaphragm; and Type C extends distal to the left subclavian artery to the twelfth intercostal space.

AVOIDING SPINAL CORD ISCHEMIA

Spinal cord protection may be achieved through distal aortic perfusion by cannulating both the left atrium or the left lower pulmonary vein and the femoral artery or distal aorta, either directly or through use of a Dacron graft, as a sleeve for the cannula, sutured end to side to the left common femoral artery. In addition, CSFD should be employed to maintain the CSF pressure less than 10 mm Hg, both intraoperatively and extending 3 days postoperatively. Although disputed by some,[19-21] patent intercostal arteries in the T8-T12 distribution should be reattached at the time of surgery.[22] Somatosensory-evoked potentials (SSEPs) and motor-evoked potentials (MEPs)[23] may be helpful in pursuing a selective approach to intercostal revascularization.

AVOIDING VISCERAL ISCHEMIA

Avoiding visceral ischemia relies on sequential aortic clamping, DAP with retrograde perfusion, and direct visceral and renal artery perfusion using balloon perfusion catheters. DAP with sequential aortic clamping allows for retrograde flow to the abdominal aorta, avoiding ischemia to the visceral and renal arteries. Visceral and renal artery perfusion with balloon-tip catheters requires a centrifugal pump with two perfusion heads to allow infusion of blood to the celiac axis and superior mesenteric artery, and cold crystalloid into the renal arteries, maintaining renal temperature below 68°F (20°C).

COAGULOPATHY

Patients should be evaluated for history of bleeding and easy bruising. Although aspirin discontinuation is not mandatory, clopidogrel and warfarin should be discontinued. Intraoperatively, meticulous attention to hemostasis is mandatory and reduces coagulopathy. In cases of persistent coagulopathy, vacuum-assisted closure of the abdomen may be instituted. Infusion of platelet-rich plasma after repair may also be considered.

AVOIDING EMBOLIZATION

Transesophageal echocardiography and computed tomography (CT) or magnetic resonance imaging (MRI) may be used to determine the degree of atheromatous plaque in the proximal descending thoracic aorta. If atheromatous disease is severe, profound hypothermic circulatory arrest and reconstruction without clamping may be considered.

AVOIDING DIAPHRAGMATIC PARALYSIS

Radial division of the diaphragm to the aorta has traditionally provided good exposure but rendered most of the diaphragm paralyzed, adversely affecting respiratory function. As an alternative, partial division of the anterior muscular portion of the diaphragm can be performed, avoiding injury to the phrenic nerve, followed by division of the crus of the diaphragm to create an aortic hiatus for the graft (Fig. 18-2). This approach has reduced the incidence of diaphragmatic paralysis and has aided expeditious extubation.[24]

AVOIDING INJURIES TO THE VAGUS NERVE

The vagus nerve enters the chest cavity, lies in front of the transverse aortic arch near the left subclavian artery and the recurrent laryngeal nerve, and then runs parallel to the descending thoracic aorta, as well as the esophagus. With dissection initiated at the level of the hilum of the lung and progressing cephalad, the vagus nerve is

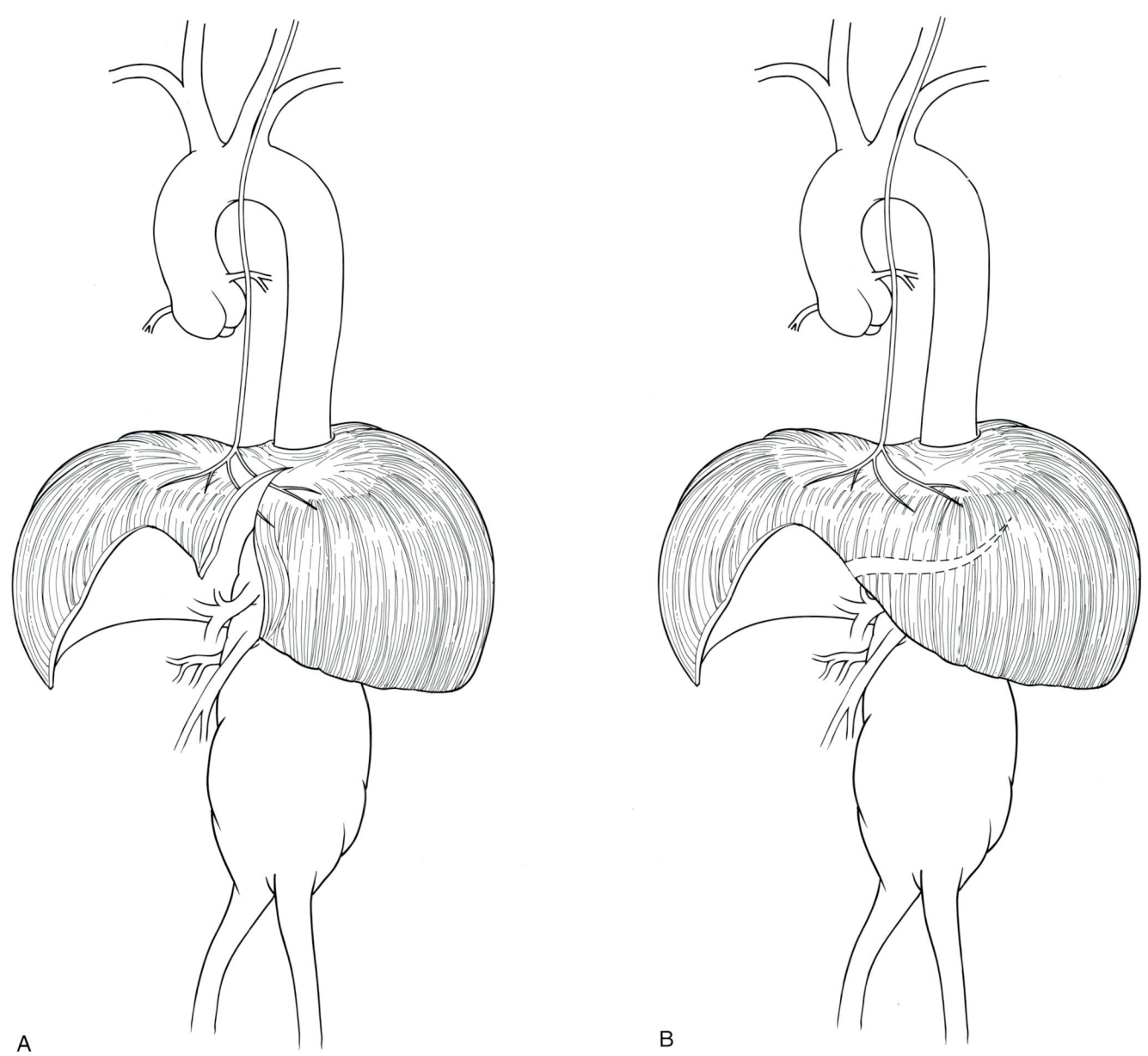

DIRECT SURGICAL REPAIR OF ANEURYSMS OF THE THORACIC AND THORACOABDOMINAL AORTA

Figure 18-2. A, Radial division of the diaphragm provides excellent exposure but may adversely affect postoperative pulmonary function. **B,** Partial lateral division of the diaphragm combined with opening of the aortic hiatus (*not shown*) and sparing of the phrenic nerve has been associated with enhanced postoperative recovery of diaphragmatic and pulmonary function.

dissected away from the descending thoracic aorta until the concave portion of the transverse arch is reached, and the atretic ductus arteriosus is divided where the recurrent laryngeal nerve curves around the transverse arch and ascends to the neck.

AVOIDING INJURIES TO THE ESOPHAGUS

The esophagus is located directly behind the thoracic aorta. When performing the proximal anastomosis in patients with DTAA and TAAA, the aorta is circumferentially divided and lifted off the esophagus to prevent an inadvertent esophagograft fistula (Fig. 18-3).

SOMATOSENSORY- AND MOTOR-EVOKED POTENTIAL MONITORING

Neuromonitoring is led by a neurologist or neurophysiologist, in conjunction with anesthesia. SSEPs are recorded bilaterally at three levels. A baseline SSEP tracing is obtained before the start of the operation. All subsequent tracings are compared with baseline. An abnormal response is defined as a 10% change in latency or 50% change in amplitude. The evaluation of three channels allows one to distinguish spinal cord injury from peripheral nerve ischemia or cerebral injury.[25]

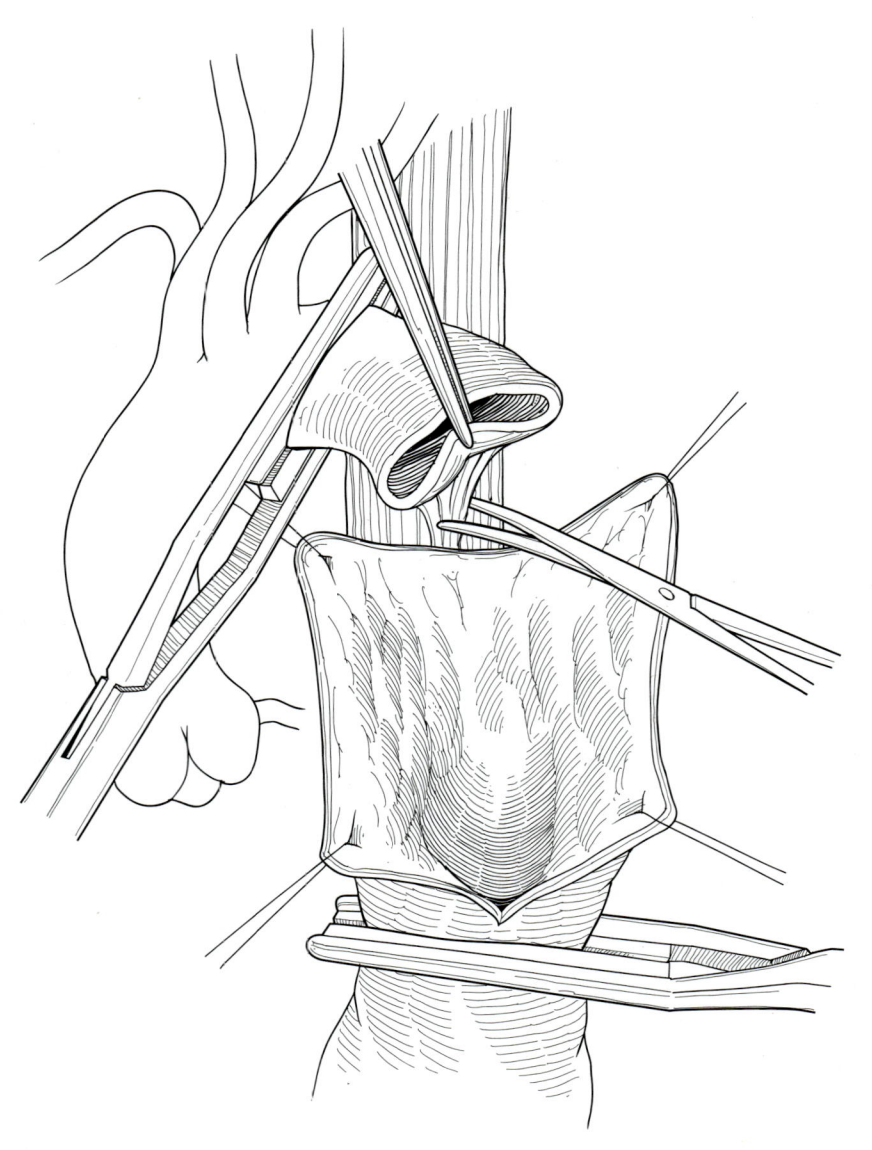

Figure 18-3. During the proximal anastomosis in the presence of a DTAA and TAAA, the thoracic aorta is circumferentially divided and elevated off the esophagus to prevent esophagograft fistula.

For MEP monitoring, electrodes are placed at C3 and C4 and myogenic responses are recorded bilaterally with electrodes placed in the abductor digiti minimi, tibialis anterior, and abductor hallucis muscles. Compound muscle action potentials are checked throughout the operation as present or absent.[25]

INTRAOPERATIVE CORRECTIVE MEASURES

If there are signs of potential spinal cord dysfunction based on an abnormal SSEP or MEP finding, a series of corrective measures may be instituted, including increasing the mean blood pressure to at least 80 mm Hg and distal aortic pressure to at least 60 mm Hg. CSF pressure may be reduced by gravity drainage and hemoglobin increased by transfusion. Furthermore, additional patent intercostal arteries should be reimplanted, especially those between T4 to T7 and L1, as necessary.

Operative Considerations

POSITIONING

The patient should be positioned with the shoulder blades at a right angle to the edge of the operating table, stabilized by a bean bag, with both axillas well padded. The hips are tilted 60 degrees so that both femoral arteries are accessible. The left knee should be flexed and a pillow placed between both lower extremities (Fig. 18-4). The patient is secured to the table with the bean bag vacuumed into a supportive shape. Tape can be used where feasible but should not compromise exposure. The table should then

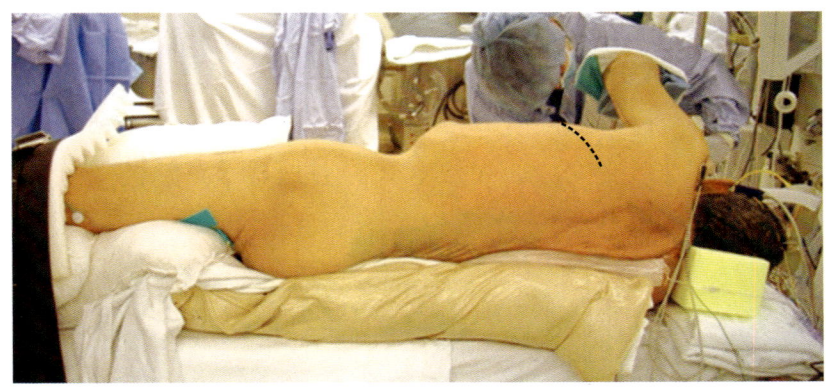

Figure 18-4. The patient should be positioned on a bean bag with shoulders at right angles to the edge of the operating table and hips tilted at 60-degree angles. Both axillas and legs are well padded and the electrocautery grounded by placing the Bovie pad on the posterior thigh. The superior portion of the skin incision and the selected thoracic interspace to enter the thoracic cavity is dictated by the proximal extent of the aneurysm. The thoracic interspaces are defined by counting up from the tip of the twelfth rib. The proximal portion of the incision is made in the eighth intercostal space (top of the ninth rib) for a Type IV TAAA, the sixth intercostal space (top of the seventh rib) for a Type III/V TAAA, and the fifth intercostal space (top of the sixth rib) for a Type I/II TAAA, where the fourth or fifth rib can be shingled or divided posteriorly, if more proximal exposure is required in the thoracic cavity.

be flexed and the kidney rest elevated at the flexion point, just above the dependent iliac crest, for greater lateral flexion and to improve access to the retroperitoneal space.

INCISION

An incision, which extends from just medial to the tip of the scapula to the costal cartilage along the sixth rib, can be applied to Type A DTAAs, as well as Type I or II TAAAs. For most thoracoabdominal aneurysms, the incision begins, as described previously, at or below the level of the scapula depending upon the proximal extent, which is then carried down along the anterolateral margin of the abdominal wall, lateral to the rectus sheath, to the level of the umbilicus or pubis as dictated by the distal extent of the aneurysm. This incision may be used for Type III, IV, and V TAAAs. The superior portion of the skin incision and the selected thoracic interspace to enter the thoracic cavity is dictated by the proximal extent of the aneurysm. The thoracic interspaces are defined by counting up from the tip of the twelfth rib. The proximal portion of the incision is made in the eighth intercostal space (top of the ninth rib) for a Type IV TAAA, the sixth intercostal space (top of the seventh rib) for a Type III/V TAAA, and the fifth intercostal space (top of the sixth rib) for a Type I/II TAAA, where the fourth or fifth rib can be shingled or divided posteriorly, if more proximal exposure is required in the thoracic cavity.

RETROPERITONEAL OR TRANSPERITONEAL THORACOABDOMINAL EXPOSURE

The left kidney and the viscera are mobilized medially, exposing the aorta from the aortic hiatus to the iliac bifurcation. The retroperitoneal approach is preferred because it prevents the viscera, and especially the small bowel, from obscuring the operative field, facilitates closure, and decreases water and heat loss.

DISTAL AORTIC PERFUSION

The left inferior pulmonary vein is used for aortic outflow. On exposure of the left inferior pulmonary vein, the pericardium is incised and the pericardial cavity entered. A pledgeted 3-0 polypropylene pursestring suture is placed in the left inferior pulmonary vein, followed by a transverse incision. The vein is dilated, and the cannula is inserted into the left atrium and connected to the centrifugal pump and inline heat exchanger (Fig. 18-5). Although the femoral artery can be directly cannulated, it may be preferable to suture an 8-mm graft onto the femoral artery, as a sleeve for the cannula, to prevent warm ischemia to the left leg. As an alternative to avoid accessing the femoral artery, the distal aortic anastomosis can be performed initially using a premanufactured,

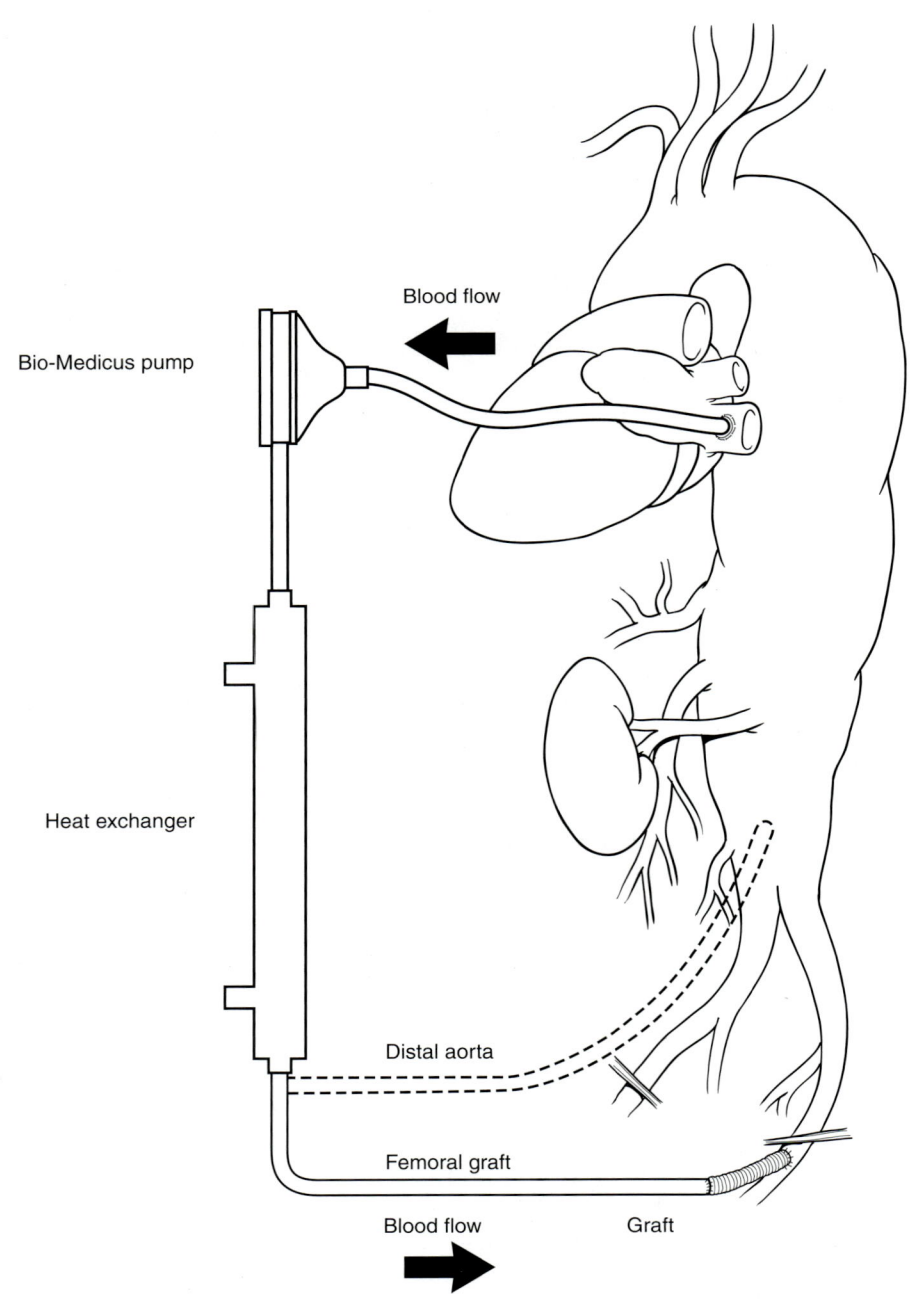

Figure 18-5. Distal aortic perfusion is established with an outflow cannula inserted into the left inferior pulmonary vein and inflow cannula inserted into the left common femoral artery or distal abdominal or thoracic aorta.

single-arm branched aortic graft.[26] The single arm is then connected to the inflow portion of the distal perfusion circuit.

An advantage of using a left atrial to left femoral bypass using a centrifugal or Bio-Medicus pump is the ability to maintain proximal pressure above 100 mm Hg and distal pressure above 60 mm Hg. In addition, the presence of an inline heat exchanger allows the patient to be effectively warmed during the later stages of the procedure.

SELECTION OF A SITE FOR PROXIMAL CONTROL

The proximal clamp is placed either proximal or distal to the left subclavian artery for Type I or II thoracoabdominal aortic aneurysms, as well as for Type A thoracic aneurysms, depending on the presence of atheromatous debris (Fig. 18-6).

SELECTION OF A SITE FOR DISTAL CONTROL

Sequential clamping of the distal aorta is preferred to reduce the distal ischemic period, and is often feasible because of turns and buckles in the descending thoracic aorta.

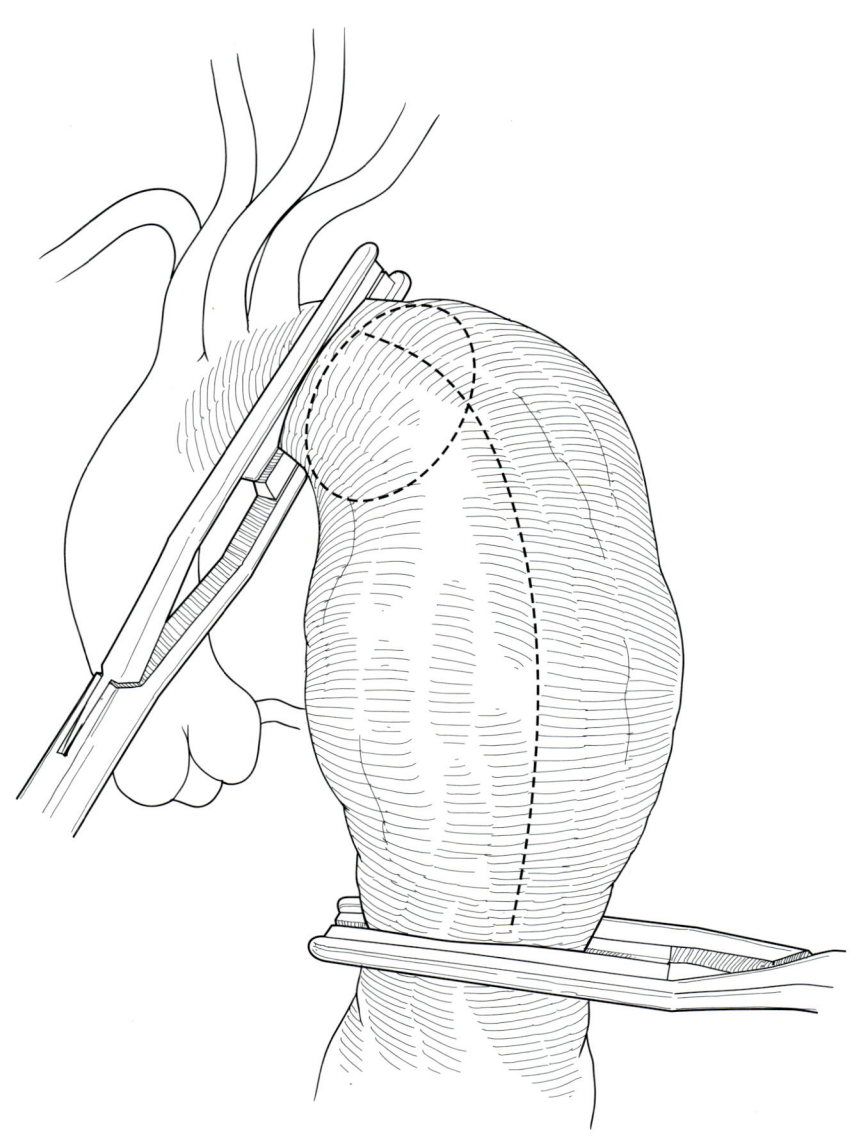

Figure 18-6. The proximal aortic clamp is placed just proximal or distal to the left subclavian artery, depending on the presence of atheromatous debris and the extent of the thoracic or thoracoabdominal aortic aneurysm.

USE OF BALLOON CATHETERS FOR VASCULAR CONTROL

Balloon catheters are not used for proximal or distal aortic control, but balloon-tip 3-Fr Fogarty catheters can be used to occlude the intercostal arteries, especially T8 to T12 (Fig. 18-7). A perfusing balloon-tip catheter can be used in celiac axis, superior mesenteric artery, and both renal arteries (Fig. 18-8).

CONSIDERATIONS IN THE PRESENCE OF CHRONIC DISSECTION

In chronic type A or chronic type B dissection, there is a partition or flap between the false and the true lumen that has to be excised. The distal anastomosis is typically created in a fenestrated fashion without attempting to incorporate the flap or septum into the anastomosis, since it is difficult to discern the true from false lumen.

Operative Technique for Repair of a Descending Thoracic Aortic Aneurysm

INCISION (MODIFIED THORACOABDOMINAL INCISION)

The incision begins at the inferior tip of the scapular, moving along the curve of the sixth rib to the costal cartilage. The fifth intercostal space is entered after the left lung is deflated. A wedge is cut in the costal cartilage to facilitate reapproximation.

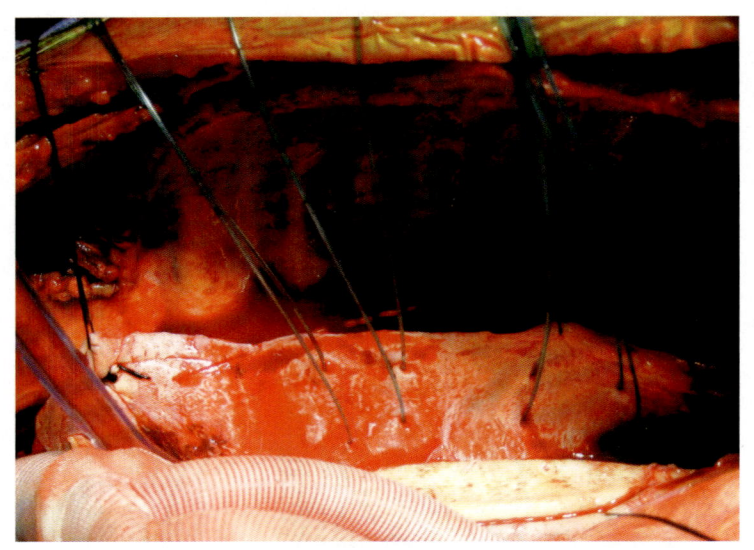

Figure 18-7. Small-caliber balloon catheters are used to temporarily occlude intercostal arteries before reattachment.

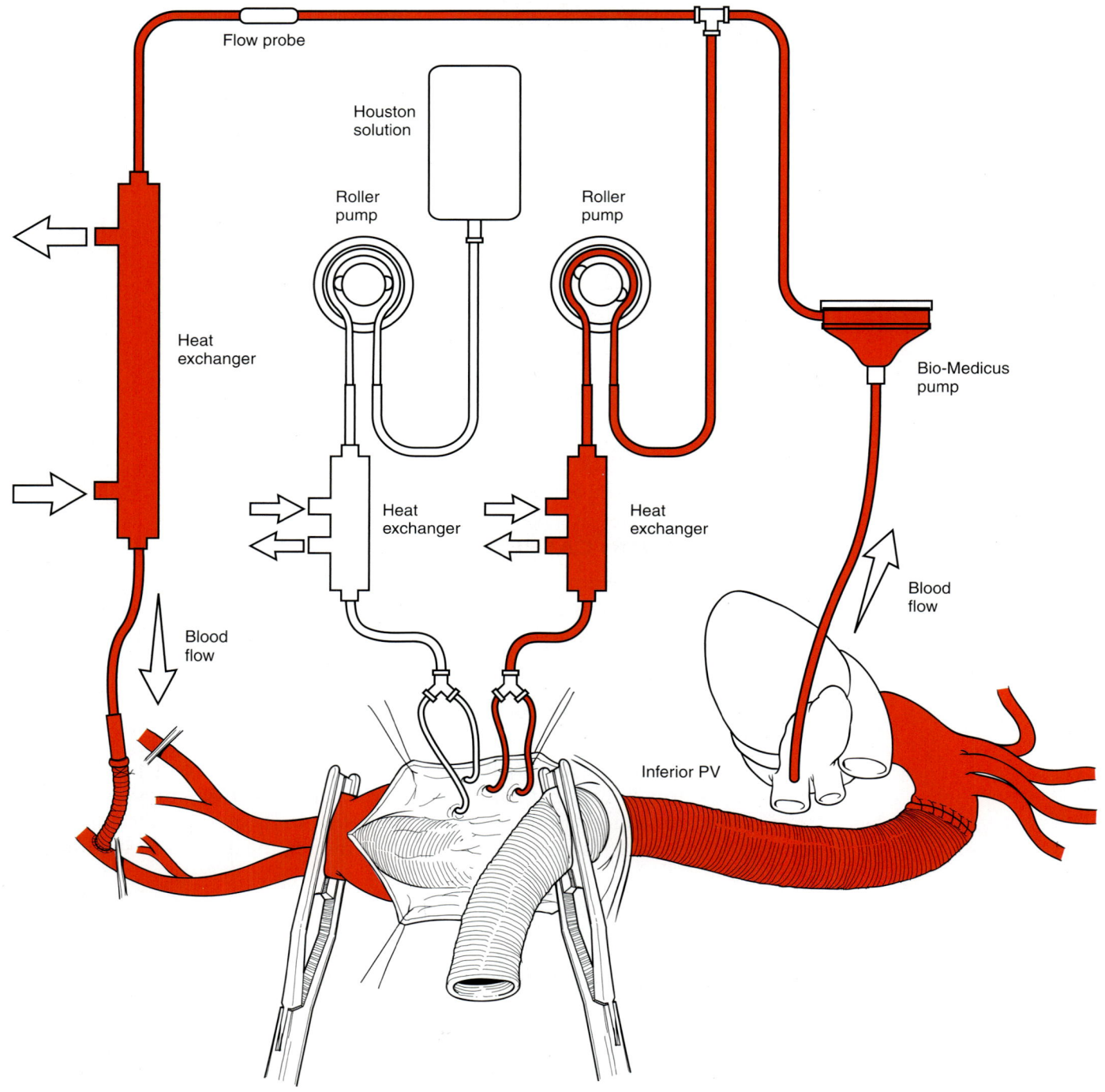

Figure 18-8. Balloon perfusion catheters are placed in the celiac, superior mesenteric, and renal arteries. Separate perfusion circuits are used for both the renal arteries (cold crystalloid) and the visceral vessels (tepid blood at 32°-34° C). *PV,* Pulmonary vein.

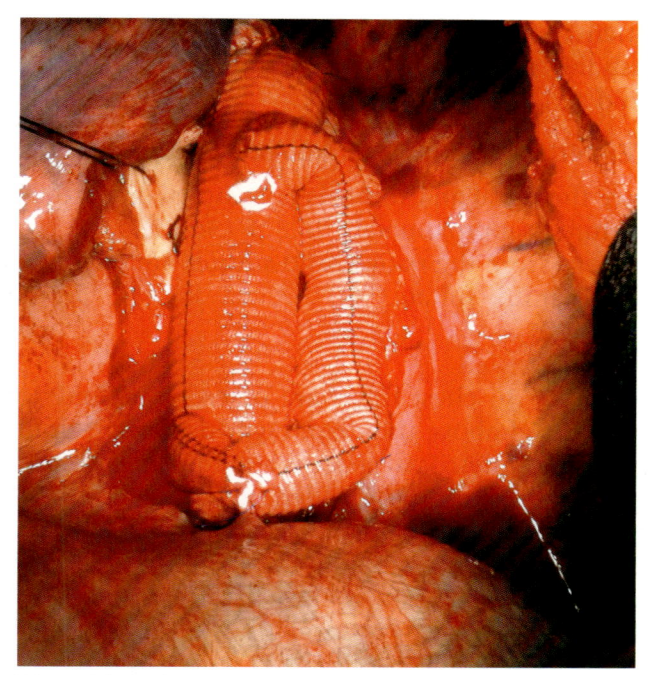

Figure 18-9. Loop Dacron graft (12 or 14 mm) is used to create a side-to-side anastomosis to revascularize patent intercostal arteries T8-T12.

PROXIMAL ANASTOMOSIS

In performing the proximal anastomosis, suture choice depends on the quality of the aorta. Most frequently, 3-0 polypropylene is sufficient. In cases of acute dissection in younger patients with traumatic injury, 4-0 polypropylene is preferred. In patients with thick or calcified aorta, running 2-0 polypropylene is used. Beginning with the posterior anastomosis, the posterior wall is selectively reinforced using pledgeted suture of 3-0 or 4-0 polypropylene or a felt strip. Once that is completed, the anterior anastomosis is continued. This anastomosis is checked for hemostasis by releasing the clamp occluding the graft. Any bleeding portions of the anastomosis are reinforced using interrupted pledgeted sutures.

REIMPLANTATION OF INTERCOSTAL ARTERIES

The order of reattachment of the intercostal arteries depends on neurologic monitoring at the time of aortic clamping. If changes in MEPs and SSEPs are observed early during the clamp period, the important patent intercostal arteries (T8-T12) are reattached immediately side to side using a separate graft as a "loop graft" (Fig. 18-9 and Video 18-1) in younger patients, in those with connective tissue disorders such as Marfan syndrome, or as an island patch in older patients. If changes in neuromonitoring are not observed, patent intercostal arteries are temporarily occluded using 3-Fr Fogarty balloon-tip catheters and the rest of the procedure completed. If changes in neuromonitoring are not observed, then patent intercostal arteries are oversewn. In Marfan syndrome, as in other genetically associated thoracic aneurysms, guided reimplantation of the intercostal arteries is performed. Prior approaches described reimplantation of intercostal vessels with a Carrel patch or by direct bypasses, but reattachment using a 14- to 16-mm Dacron tube loop graft is now preferred. Specifically, patent intercostal arteries are reattached as a side-to-side anastomosis to the body of the smaller Dacron graft, and then each end is anastomosed to the main body of the aortic graft. This approach reduces the risk of graft thrombosis as compared with direct end-to-end anastomosis from a side arm graft.

DISTAL ANASTOMOSIS

Prior to the completion of the distal anastomosis, the distal clamp is released to fill the graft with blood and evacuate the graft of all air and debris by placing the patient in the head-down position. The proximal clamp is then slowly released to flush the graft in a prograde manner. Coordination with anesthesia is required to avoid sudden hypotension.

WEANING FROM DISTAL AORTIC PERFUSION

Once the distal anastomosis is completed and the patient's nasopharyngeal temperature is approximately 96.8°F (36°C), DAP is discontinued. All cannulae are removed from the patient and sutures are secured. Heparinization is reversed using protamine sulfate.

CLOSURE

Three No. 36 chest tubes are placed; one anteriorly, one posteriorly, and one right angled above the diaphragm to prevent fluid accumulation in the phrenic sulcus. The intercostal space is closed using interrupted No. 2 braided absorbable sutures. The lung is expanded, and the pericostal sutures are secured. A No. 1 absorbable monofilament suture (polydioxanone) is used to close the muscular fascia, first reapproximating the serratus anterior muscle and then the latissimus dorsi muscle. The skin is closed subcuticularly with skin staples or sutures. The patient is placed in the supine position, and if there are no complications, the double lumen tube is exchanged for a single lumen tube.

Operative Technique for Repair of a Type I Thoracoabdominal Aortic Aneurysm

Repair of a Type I TAAA is similar to DTAA repair, except the incision is carried 2 to 5 cm below the costal margin. This allows adequate exposure for reflection of the diaphragm inferiorly, exposing the celiac axis and superior mesenteric artery. If greater caudal exposure is required, then the diaphragm is partially and circumferentially split along its anterior margin. The retroperitoneal space is entered, and the abdominal contents are reflected medially.

The aorta is opened, thrombus removed, and the lower intercostal arteries are identified. If there is substantial bleeding from intercostal arteries (i.e., T8-T12), 2- or 3-Fr balloon-tip catheters may be used for control. Revascularization of the intercostal vessels is dictated by MEP and SSEP, as described previously, with surgical options, including use of a loop graft, as outlined earlier in this chapter. The abdominal aorta containing the orifices of the celiac axis and superior mesenteric artery is examined to determine whether a clamp can be placed infrarenally. If a Dacron graft is attached to the left common femoral artery, flow from the left heart assist device is to the left lower extremity. The celiac and superior mesenteric arteries are identified, and if the extent of the aneurysm requires extension of the aortotomy, the orifices of the left and right renal arteries may be visible. The graft is bevelled and sutured to the abdominal aorta. The distal clamp is released, and hemostasis assessed. The proximal clamp is released, restoring pulsatile flow to the celiac axis, superior mesenteric artery, and both renal arteries. The patient is rewarmed to a nasopharyngeal temperature of 36°C.

Operative Technique for Repair of a Type II Thoracoabdominal Aortic Aneurysm

INCISION

Repair of a Type II TAAA requires exposure from the left subclavian to the aortic bifurcation. The incision extends along the top of the sixth rib from the level of the scapula across the costal margin and inferiorly along the lateral margin of the abdominal wall to below the umbilicus. In thinner patients, this allows access to the iliac vessels. Access to the external iliac arteries may require extension of the incision to the pubis. The crus of the diaphragm is divided to create an aortic hiatus.

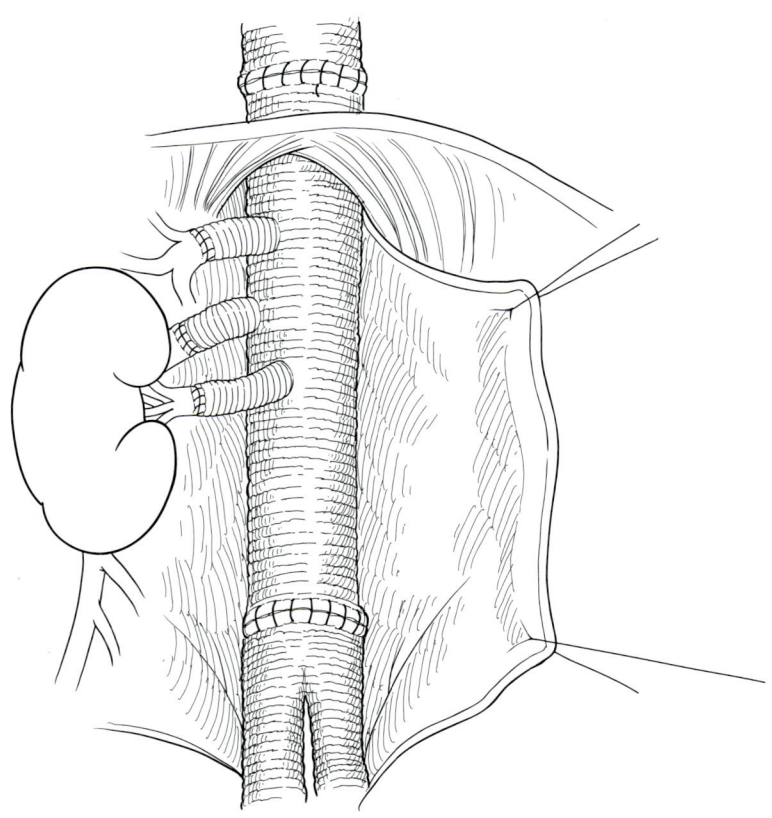

DIRECT SURGICAL REPAIR OF ANEURYSMS OF THE THORACIC AND THORACOABDOMINAL AORTA

Figure 18-10. Reattachment of the celiac, superior mesenteric, and left renal artery using a premanufactured side branched thoracoabdominal aortic graft (STAG).

Management of the proximal part of the reconstruction and intercostal vessels is as described earlier.

REIMPLANTATION OF VISCERAL VESSELS

Once the proximal anastomosis is performed, the visceral aorta is opened after the infrarenal aorta is clamped. When the infrarenal abdominal aorta is too large for clamping, the visceral aorta is opened and the celiac and superior mesenteric arteries are perfused with a perfusing catheter with tepid blood (32°-34°C). The left and right renal arteries are perfused with cold crystalloid solution. The kidney temperature is maintained below 20°C. If a clamp cannot be placed onto the abdominal aorta, then DAP is halted and a premanufactured Dacron graft with a side branch is sutured to the aortic bifurcation using 3-0 or 2-0 polypropylene sutures (Fig. 18-10). The clamp is applied to the graft and flow is restored to the pelvic circulation via the side-arm graft. Alternatively, placing clamps on the common iliac arteries also allows continuous pelvic perfusion.

The ostia of the visceral and renal vessels are examined and cleaned of atheromatous debris. If the ostia are close (i.e., >2 cm apart), then a single island patch can be created or reattached. If a vessel, most frequently the left renal artery, is separated from the other vessels, then a separate interposition bypass graft is performed using a 10-mm Dacron tube graft. In cases of Marfan syndrome or other connective tissue disorders, in patients younger than 60 years, or with ostial separation of greater than 3 cm, a premanufactured side-branched thoracoabdominal aortic graft (STAG) is used, with separate bypasses to each of the vessels (see Fig. 18-10).[26] This is performed consecutively, starting with the celiac and superior mesenteric arteries and ending with the left renal artery. Creating buttons for each ostium facilitates suturing using running 4-0 polypropylene.

In the presence of a chronic aortic dissection, the septum between the false and the true lumen is excised, and patent intercostal arteries are identified and revascularized.

CLOSURE

Closure of the chest is similar to DTAA and Type I TAAA closure. The diaphragm is reapproximated using a running monofilament No. 1 permanent suture. The abdomen is closed in layers, using a running monofilament No. 1 permanent suture for both fascial layers of the oblique musculature.

Operative Technique for Repair of a Type III Thoracoabdominal Aortic Aneurysm

The incision for a Type III TAAA is similar to that for a Type V thoracoabdominal aneurysm, which may be approached through the fifth intercostal space on top of the sixth rib. In this region, circumferential division of the descending thoracic aorta is not required because the thoracic aorta is not adjacent to the esophagus. The visceral and renal vessels are addressed as with Type II TAAA.

Operative Technique for Repair of a Type IV Thoracoabdominal Aortic Aneurysm

INCISION

In approaching repair of a Type IV TAAA, the chest is opened in the seventh intercostal space on top of the eighth rib to provide access to the distal descending thoracic aorta.

EXPOSURE OF THE AORTA

The aorta is prepared for clamping at the level of the diaphragm. The remainder of the procedure is similar to a Type II TAAA.

RECONSTRUCTION

In a Type IV TAAA, the option exists to initially revascularize the celiac, superior mesenteric artery, and left renal artery, in a sequential fashion using a multi-side arm graft, which originates from the normal descending thoracic aorta. Typically, a 14 × 6 mm bifurcated graft is used on which two additional side arms are attached. After the celiac, superior mesenteric, and left renal arteries are revascularized, the distal thoracic aorta and iliac arteries are clamped, the aneurysm is opened, and the fourth side arm is used to revascularize the right renal artery. The aorta is then reconstructed with an interposition graft. Given the sequential nature of visceral vessel reattachment, DAP is not typically required.

Postoperative Care

- All patients are cared for in an intensive care unit.
- Blood pressure is maintained at a mean arterial pressure above 80 mm Hg by judicious use of blood and blood component therapy.
- Hemoglobin should be maintained above 10 g/dL.
- CSF pressure is monitored and maintained below 10 mm Hg. Close attention is paid to the character of the flow of the CSF drain. If the fluid is not clear or is bloody, then a neurologic examination is performed and a CT scan of the head is obtained. If there is no evidence of bleeding, CSF drainage is continued or a new catheter inserted in a different site. If the catheter is kinked or dislodged, it is replaced urgently, even if noted in the middle of the night.[27]

Complications

- **Mortality.** Early mortality for open repair of TAAA remains between 10% and 14% and is independently related to calculated GFR.[18] With normal renal function, GFR of more than 90 mL/min/1.73 m^2, mortality from TAAA repair is 5%.

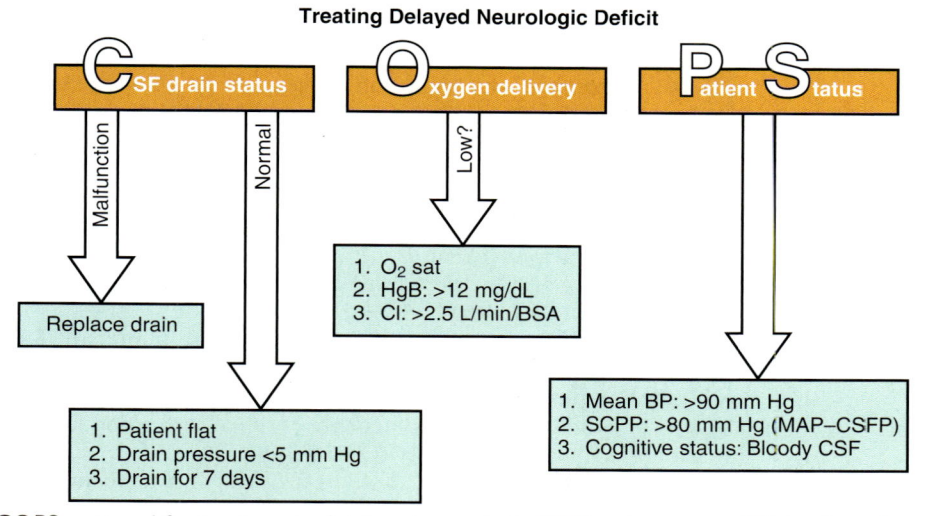

Figure 18-11. The COPS protocol for treatment of delayed paraplegia. *BP,* Blood pressure; *BSA,* body surface area; *CI,* cardiac index; *CSFP,* cerebrospinal fluid pressure; *HgB,* hemoglobin; *MAP,* mean arterial pressure; O_2 *sat,* oxygen saturation; *SCPP,* spinal cord perfusion pressure.

- **Paraplegia.** Much improvement in the prevention of paraplegia has occurred over the past 2 decades. Use of DAP and CSFD, in combination with moderate hypothermia, has reduced the overall paraplegia rate after DTAA and Type I TAAA from 15% to less than 1% and after Type II TAAA from 33% to less than 4%.[28] Although it remains difficult to unequivocally prove the benefit of intercostal reattachment, indirect evidence with improvement of MEP and SSEP responses suggests cord perfusion is improved with potential benefit. This contrasts with those who argue against this adjunct based on the collateral network concept of spinal cord circulation.[29]

- **Delayed paraplegia.** Delayed paraplegia or paraparesis occurring after a period of normal motor function remains a devastating complication. Although rare, poor CSFD and low blood pressure are predictive of delayed paraplegia.[30] The peak incidence is in the second postoperative day and the CSF drain status, oxygen delivery, and patient status (COPS) protocol should be instituted (Figure 18-11). The patient is placed flat, and if the spinal catheter is still in place, then drained freely for 7 days.[27] The hemoglobin level is kept above 10 g/dL, and cardiac output is kept at an optimal level (cardiac index 2.5 L/min/m^2). In more than 75% of cases, strength may be regained.[31] MRI or CT imaging should be used to exclude epidural hematoma.

- **Renal failure.** Risk factors for renal dysfunction include extent of aneurysm, involvement of the left renal artery, use of visceral perfusion, and preoperative renal dysfunction. Renal dysfunction occurs in as many as 35% of cases and is most common in Type II TAAA. Fortunately, the renal dysfunction encountered is temporary and most patients recover, with only 3% requiring permanent dialysis.[32] Myoglobinuria that occurs from warm ischemia to the leg with direct femoral artery occlusion for arterial cannulation may contribute to renal dysfunction after TAAA.[33] Therefore a sutured graft to the femoral artery may be used to prevent lower leg ischemia during cannulation.[34]

- **Gastrointestinal complications.** The incidence of gastrointestinal (GI) complications is approximately 7%.[35] The mortality rate associated with GI complications is 39.5%. Risk factors for the occurrence of GI complications are visceral involvement of the aortic repair and low preoperative GFR.

- **Pulmonary complications.** Pulmonary complications may occur in as many as 20% of patients undergoing TAAA repair. Risk factors for prolonged ventilation (>72 hours) include increasing age, current smoking, total cross-clamp time, units of packed red blood cells transfused, and division of the diaphragm.[24]

REFERENCES

1. Etheredge S, Yee J, Smith J, et al: Successful resection of a large aneurysm of the upper abdominal aorta and replacement with homograft, *Surgery* 138:1071-1081, 1955.
2. DeBakey ME, Creech O Jr, Morris GC: Aneurysm of the thoracoabdominal aorta involving the celiac, mesenteric and renal arteries. Report of four cases treated by resection and homograft replacement, *Ann Surg* 179:763-772, 1956.
3. Crawford ES: Thoraco-abdominal and abdominal aortic aneurysms involving renal, superior mesenteric, celiac arteries, *Ann Surg* 179:763-772, 1974.
4. Crawford ES, Crawford JL, Safi HJ, et al: Thoracoabdominal aortic aneurysms: Preoperative and intraoperative factors determining immediate and long-term results of operations in 605 patients, *J Vasc Surg* 3:389-404, 1986.
5. Lawrie GM: Profiles in cardiology. The scientific contributions of Alexis Carrel, *Clin Cardiol* 10:428-430, 1987.
6. Laschinger JC, Cunningham JN Jr, Nathan IM, et al: Experimental and clinical assessment of the adequacy of partial bypass in maintenance of spinal cord blood flow during operations on the thoracic aorta, *Ann Thorac Surg* 36:417-426, 1983.
7. Cunningham JN Jr, Laschinger JC, Merkin HA, et al: Measurement of spinal cord ischemia during operations upon the thoracic aorta: Initial clinical experience, *Ann Surg* 196:285-296, 1982.
8. Grossi EA, Krieger KH, Cunningham JN Jr, et al: Venoarterial bypass: A technique for spinal cord protection, *J Thorac Cardiovasc Surg* 89:228-234, 1985.
9. Miyamoto K, Veno A, Wada T, et al: A new and simple method of preventing spinal cord damage following temporary occlusion of the thoracic aorta by withdrawing cerebrospinal fluid, *J Cardiovasc Surg* 16:188-197, 1960.
10. Blaisdell FW, Cooley DA: The mechanism of paraplegia after temporary thoracic aortic occlusion and its relationship to spinal fluid pressure, *Surgery* 51:351-355, 1962.
11. Korompai FL, Hayward RH: Preservation of visceral perfusion during resection of thoraco-abdominal aneurysm, *Cardiovasc Dis* 2:349-351, 1975.
12. Hollier LH, Symmonds JB, Pairolero PC, et al: Thoracoabdominal aortic aneurysm repair. Analysis of postoperative morbidity, *Arch Surg* 123:871-875, 1988.
13. Crawford ES, Svensson LG, Hess KR, et al: A prospective randomized study of cerebrospinal fluid drainage to prevent paraplegia after high-risk surgery on the thoracoabdominal aorta, *J Vasc Surg* 13:36-45, 1991.
14. Coselli JS, Lemaire SA, Koksoy C, et al: Cerebrospinal fluid drainage reduces paraplegia after thoracoabdominal aortic aneurysm repair: Results of a randomized clinical trial, *J Vasc Surg* 35:631-639, 2002.
15. DeBakey ME, Creech O Jr, Morris GC Jr: Aneurysm of the thoracoabdominal aorta involving the celiac, mesenteric and renal arteries. Report of four cases treated by resection and homograft replacement, *Ann Surg* 179:763-772, 1956.
16. Connolly JE, Wakabayashi A, German JC, et al: Clinical experience with pulsatile left heart bypass without anticoagulation for thoracic aneurysms, *J Thorac Cardiovasc Surg* 62:568-576, 1971.
17. Coselli JS, LeMaire SA: Left heart bypass reduces paraplegia rates after thoracoabdominal aortic aneurysm repair, *Aneurysms Thorac Surg* 67:1931-1934, 1999.
18. Huynh TT, van Eps RG, Miller CC III, et al: Glomerular filtration rate is superior to serum creatinine for prediction of mortality after thoracoabdominal aortic surgery, *J Vasc Surg* 42:206-212, 2005.
19. Safi H, Miller CI, Carr C, et al: The importance of intercostal artery reattachment during thoracoabdominal aortic aneurysm repair, *J Vasc Surg* 27:58-68, 1998.
20. Etz CD, Halstead JC, Spielvogel D, et al: Thoracic and thoracoabdominal aneurysm repair: Is reimplantation of spinal cord arteries a waste of time? *Ann Thorac Surg* 82:1670-1677, 2006.
21. Estrera AL, Sheinbaum R, Miller CC III, Harrison R, Safi HJ: Neuromonitor-guided repair of thoracoabdominal aortic aneurysms, *J Thorac Cardiovasc Surg* 140:S131-S135, 2010.
22. Safi H, Miller CI, Carr C, et al: The importance of intercostal artery reattachment during thoracoabdominal aortic aneurysm repair, *J Vasc Surg* 27:58-68, 1998.
23. Estrera AL, Sheinbaum R, Miller CC III, et al: Neuromonitor-guided repair of thoracoabdominal aortic aneurysms, *J Thorac Cardiov Surg* 140:S131-S135, 2010.
24. Engle J, Safi HJ, Miller CC III, et al: The impact of diaphragm management on prolonged ventilator support after thoracoabdominal aortic repair, *J Vasc Surg* 29:150-156, 1999.
25. Keyhani K, Miller CC III, Estrera AL, et al: Analysis of motor and somatosensory evoked potentials during thoracic and thoracoabdominal aortic aneurysm repair, *J Vasc Surg* 49:36-41, 2009.
26. De Rango P, Estrera AL, Miller CC III, et al: Operative outcomes using a side-branched thoracoabdominal aortic graft (STAG) for thoraco-abdominal aortic repair, *Eur J Vasc Endovasc* 41:41-47, 2011.
27. Estrera AL, Sheinbaum R, Miller CC, et al: Cerebrospinal fluid drainage during thoracic aortic repair: Safety and current management, *Ann Thorac Surg* 88:9-15, 2009.

28. Safi HJ, Miller CC III, Huynh TT, et al: Distal aortic perfusion and cerebrospinal fluid drainage for thoracoabdominal and descending thoracic aortic repair: Ten years of organ protection, *Ann Surg* 238:372-380, 2003.
29. Etz CD, Luehr M, Kari FA, et al: Paraplegia after extensive thoracic and thoracoabdominal aortic aneurysm repair: Does critical spinal cord ischemia occur postoperatively? *J Thorac Cardiov Surg* 135:324-330, 2008.
30. Azizzadeh A, Huynh TT, Miller CC III, et al: Postoperative risk factors for delayed neurologic deficit after thoracic and thoracoabdominal aortic aneurysm repair: A case-control study, *J Vasc Surg* 37:750-754, 2003.
31. Estrera AL, Miller CC III, Huynh TT, et al: Preoperative and operative predictors of delayed neurologic deficit following repair of thoracoabdominal aortic aneurysm, *J Thorac Cardiov Surg* 126:1288-1294, 2003.
32. Safi HJ, Estrera AL, Azizzadeh A, et al: Progress and future challenges in thoracoabdominal aortic aneurysm management, *World J Surg* 32:355-360, 2008.
33. Miller CC III, Villa MA, Sutton J, et al: Serum myoglobin and renal morbidity and mortality following thoracic and thoraco-abdominal aortic repair: Does rhabdomyolysis play a role? *Eur J Vasc Endovasc Surg* 37:388-394, 2009.
34. Miller CC III, Grimm JC, Estrera AL, et al: Postoperative renal function preservation with nonischemic femoral arterial cannulation for thoracoabdominal aortic repair, *J Vasc Surg* 51:38-42, 2010.
35. Achouh PE, Madsen K, Miller CC III, et al: Gastrointestinal complications after descending thoracic and thoracoabdominal aortic repairs: A 14-year experience, *J Vasc Surg* 44:442-446, 2006.

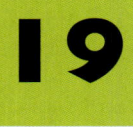

19 Endovascular Repair of the Aortic Arch and Thoracoabdominal Aorta

TIMOTHY A.M. CHUTER

Historical Background

The first multibranched stent grafts,[1,2] like the first bifurcated stent grafts, were of unibody design, whereby the entire stent graft was inserted whole and deployed using a system of catheters. Downstream access to the branches made the arch version slightly simpler than the thoracoabdominal version, but both showed a high degree of irreducible complexity that has limited application to a small group of highly skilled users in Japan.[3]

Modular multibranched stent grafts, combining a primary stent graft with one or more covered stents, vary mainly in the type of intercomponent connection. The first modular systems for thoracoabdominal aortic aneurysm (TAAA)[3] and aortic arch aneurysm (ArAA)[4] repair used longitudinally oriented cuffs, like the attachments sites on a typical bifurcated modular stent graft. The first modular system for ArAA repair was simply an upside-down bifurcated stent graft, with one long leg extending back along the line of insertion into the innominate artery and the other opening into the aorta as an attachment site for a descending thoracic aortic extension.[4]

The first hybrid operations for TAAA[5] and ArAA[6] were reported more than a decade ago, and these techniques have probably been used more widely than other methods of endovascular repair. The snorkel technique was first described as a way to treat juxtarenal aneurysm.[7] The expanded use of this technique for ArAA and TAAA is a relatively recent phenomenon.[8-11]

Indications

The most common indication for endovascular repair is the presence of a large asymptomatic aortic aneurysm. Although data on the natural history of TAAA and ArAA are not as robust as those for abdominal aortic aneurysm, it is clear that the risk of rupture depends mainly on aneurysm size; in addition, female sex, a positive family history, symptoms related to the aneurysm, and the presence of chronic obstructive pulmonary disease have been demonstrated to increase rupture risk in natural history studies. At the University of California at San Francisco (UCSF) procedures of this type are generally performed under research protocols, which require a minimum aneurysm diameter of 60 mm. Factors that increase the diameter threshold include serious comorbid conditions that raise the risks of surgery or shorten life expectancy, thereby reducing the benefit of freedom from rupture. Factors that reduce the diameter threshold include female gender, pseudoaneurysm, saccular aneurysm, and symptoms or signs of imminent rupture.

The long-term effects of aortic dissection include false lumen dilatation and aneurysm formation, yet dissection remains an uncommon indication for endovascular repair of the aortic arch[12] and thoracoabdominal aorta for the following reasons: the true lumen is often narrow, and origins of the aortic branches may be separated by the septum between the true and the false lumens, especially within the dissected thoracoabdominal aorta. These factors do not usually impede hybrid repairs, which use bypass grafts to circumvent complex luminal anatomy. Often patients with aneurysms of chronic dissection etiology are younger, afflicted with syndromic conditions, or both such that open repair remains the mainstay of treatment.

Patient Selection

Patient selection depends on an assessment of the relative risks of observation, open surgical repair, and various endovascular alternatives. The lack of good long-term data on outcome relegates endovascular repair to a subsidiary role in the management of ArAA and TAAA. Endovascular repair offers a last resort for patients whose large aneurysms preclude observation and whose poor physical condition precludes open surgery. Most candidates for endovascular repair of ArAA or TAAA have already undergone a full assessment of their fitness for operation, including tests of cardiac, pulmonary, and renal function. These patients usually present with well-documented indications for treatment in the form of aneurysm diameter measurements. The feasibility of endovascular repair depends on general anatomic factors, such as the state of the implantation sites, the proximity of aortic branches, the diameter of the iliac arteries, and the presence of mural thrombus. Other site- and device-specific anatomic factors relate to the potential pitfalls of a particular technique. For example, transcarotid insertion of an ascending aortic bifurcated stent graft requires a large right carotid artery, and the multibranched repair of a TAAA requires a luminal diameter of at least 20 mm at the level of the visceral arteries.

Preoperative Preparation

- **Cardiopulmonary function.** Cardiac risk stratification for TEVAR procedures in general is neither evidence-nor consensus guidelines-based; applying the same paradigm used in open repair appears illogical. Recent placement of a coronary stent, especially a drug-eluting stent, requires antiplatelet therapy such as clopidogrel to be maintained throughout the perioperative period. The risk of intraoperative hemorrhage is lower for a completely endovascular technique, but a hybrid repair may be contraindicated.
- **Preoperative imaging.** Preoperative imaging provides the anatomic data needed for patient selection, operative planning, and stent-graft sizing. Moreover, preoperative imaging is necessary to identify areas of stenosis or branching that might limit access to the aorta and its branches. In general, the more complicated the stent graft, the greater the need for precise anatomic data. This is particularly true of fenestrated stent grafts, because the distribution of fenestrations has to match the distribution of aortic branches. Modular branched stent grafts are more forgiving. Imaging techniques include computed tomography (CT), magnetic resonance imaging or magnetic resonance angiography, catheter angiography, and intravascular ultrasound (IVUS).
  - **Contrast-enhanced spiral CT imaging.** High-resolution three-dimensional (3D) data sets yield orthogonal reconstructions for diameter measurements, multiplanar reconstructions for length measurements, and 3D representations such as shaded surface displays for assessments of angulation, profile, and relative position. Generic 3D reconstructions seldom provide the necessary level of anatomic detail. Image processing software such as that provided by TeraRecon (iNtuition) and OsiriX (OsiriX MD) allow the operator to make measurements and identify potential pitfalls by processing raw digital imaging and communications in medical files. Alternatively, services such as

M2S can provide preprocessed data in an accessible form, together with the software for analysis and display.

- **Magnetic resonance imaging.** Magnetic resonance imaging yields a volumetric data set suitable for 3D analysis but lacks spatial resolution. The quality of magnetic resonance angiography is enhanced by the intravenous administration of gadolinium. However, rare, but serious side effects of gadolinium have almost eliminated its role in patients with poor renal function.
- **Angiography.** Catheter angiography is reserved for the evaluation and possible preoperative treatment of specific CT findings, such as renal artery or celiac stenosis.
- **IVUS.** Although IVUS is a potentially useful intraoperative adjunct in the presence of aortic dissection, it has no preoperative role. IVUS can provide accurate measurements of implantation site diameter, but so can CT angiography. IVUS-derived length measurements are unreliable.
- **Hybrid surgical and endovascular repairs.** The physiologic stress of a hybrid repair may be reduced by staging the open surgical and endovascular procedures or by performing interventions to avoid the need for surgical intervention.
- **Preoperative intervention of a branch artery stenosis.** The goal of preoperative intervention is to create a wide, metal lined, radiopaque arterial orifice that lies flush to the surface of the artery.

Endovascular Strategy

ANATOMIC CONSIDERATIONS

ArAAs and TAAAs are more difficult to treat than aneurysms of the descending thoracic and infrarenal abdominal aorta. The surgeon cannot simply exclude an aneurysm from the circulation when its branches supply organs such as the brain or the abdominal viscera, which cannot tolerate ischemia.

Although four basic methods of branch preservation are used in all cases involving endovascular repair of ArAA, TAAA, and common iliac aneurysm, each branched segment has specific anatomic features, which affect the choice of one endovascular technique over another. The aortic arch is wide, curved, close to the aortic valve, and far from the femoral arteries. Its branches are accessible in the root of the neck. The thoracoabdominal aorta is narrower, straighter, farther from the aortic valve, and closer to the femoral arteries. Its branches stay within the abdomen. The common iliac artery has only two branches: one remains within the pelvis, whereas the other passes over the rim of the pelvis into the groin.

BASIC TECHNIQUES FOR BRANCH ARTERY PRESERVATION

Hybrid repair[5,6,13,14] involves surgical bypass from a remote artery to each branch of the aneurysmal segment. The "debranched" aneurysm can then be treated using standard endovascular techniques. Alternatively, if the aneurysm involves only part of the branched aortic segment, the bypass may originate from one of the branches and terminate on another. The most common example of this approach is a left carotid-subclavian bypass before TEVAR repair (see Chapter 20), which is a modest "surgical component" to the hybrid procedure. At the other end of the spectrum would be a four-vessel renal or visceral debranching procedure to permit endovascular graft repair of a thoracoabdominal aorta. Debranching is a major surgical procedure.

The following types of stent grafts are used:

- A fenestrated stent graft[7,15,16] has strategically located holes in its wall (see Chapter 27). The goal of using a fenestrated stent graft is to perfuse vital arterial branches without perfusing the aneurysm (type III endoleak).

- A branched stent graft[1-4,12,17,18] has small side branches, each of which conveys blood from the lumen of the stent graft to the lumen of the corresponding arterial branch. A fenestrated stent graft can be converted into a branched stent graft by substituting a covered stent for the usual uncovered bridging stent.
- A snorkel, or chimney, stent[8-11] runs alongside the stent graft from the nondilated aorta into a branch artery. The aortic stent graft seldom conforms perfectly to the outer surface of the stent, leaving channels through which blood can flow past the target artery into the aneurysm (type I endoleak). Multiple snorkels create multiple channels and multiple opportunities for endoleak.

CHOICE OF TECHNIQUE

There are too few published data regarding the results of endovascular ArAA and TAAA repair to support definite statements about the relative merits of hybrid repair, fenestrated stent grafts, branched stent grafts, and snorkels. Nevertheless, the following generalizations are probably valid: The surgical portion of a hybrid repair is familiar and well tested, and the endovascular portion is relatively simple and predictable. Snorkels and fenestrations both rely upon the creation of a hemostatic seal between the wall of the stent graft and the wall of the aorta. They tend to leak when the branches originate from a dilated segment of the aorta. In the creation of a branch, the intercomponent connection between the margin of a fenestration and a balloon-expanded covered stent is less secure, less hemostatic, and less forgiving than the connection between the lumen of a cuff and a self-expanding covered stent. The axially oriented branches of a cuffed stent graft are able to vary in length and orientation to accommodate variations in branch distribution. As a result, off-the-shelf cuffed stent grafts can be combined with other stent grafts and covered stents for multibranched endovascular repair of a symptomatic TAAA.

Device characteristics are often less important in the choice of technique than the availability of high-level endovascular skills and complex endovascular technology. The stent grafts used for hybrid and snorkel techniques are simple and widely available. Thousands of fenestrated stent grafts have been implanted by hundreds of surgeons. The technique may be complicated, but it is at least familiar. Simple fenestrations can be converted to branches with nothing more than the substitution of a covered stent for an uncovered stent. Few centers worldwide have used more than a dozen cuffed branched stent grafts. Unfamiliarity with the necessary techniques is one barrier to more widespread use; high cost is another. The multibranched stent graft is assembled from many components, each of which is sold separately. Fenestrated and cuffed stent grafts are now commercially available throughout the world with several notable exceptions, including the United States and Japan.

Modular Branched Repair of Aneurysms of the Aortic Arch

The following description focuses on modular multibranched techniques of ArAA repair because both snorkel technique and hybrid repair use standard endovascular devices and standard techniques, all of which are adequately described in other chapters. Only modular multibranched stent grafts have the potential to replace open surgery as the mainstay of treatment. Hybrid repair involves too much surgery, and snorkels and fenestrations involve too great a risk of endoleak. Small fenestrations require precise alignment, which is difficult to achieve in the curves of the aortic arch. Stent-graft misalignment can occlude cerebral flow, causing a stroke. Large fenestrations and scallops require less precise placement with a lower risk of stroke, but are more likely to be associated with an increased risk of endoleak. Unibody multibranched stent grafts are too complicated for widespread use.

Modular, multibranched stent grafts fall into two groups, transcervical and transfemoral, based on the route of insertion. Both require the tip of the delivery system to cross the aortic valve. The transcervical route is shorter and straighter. The delivery system does not have to navigate the aortic arch, and stent-graft orientation is easier to control. The basic form of transcervical stent graft, with only one supraaortic branch, requires little aortic instrumentation once the stent graft is in place, because blood flows to the innominate artery through a limb of the primary (bifurcated) stent graft. However, insertion of a large-caliber delivery system often requires access to the innominate artery. The necessary exposure negates some advantages of endovascular repair.

The transfemoral route is long and curved, and the delivery system tends to enter the aortic arch in one orientation and exit in another. In addition, the large-caliber delivery system with a short soft tip tracks poorly around the tight bends of the aneurysmal aortic arch. These barriers to transfemoral delivery require low-profile stents and fabrics, kink-resistant sheaths, precurved sheaths, and twist-prevention mechanisms, all of which have taken years to develop. Extensive in vitro testing and short-term results of early clinical experience suggest that transfemoral grafts have great promise.

MODULAR TRANSCERVICAL BIFURCATED STENT GRAFT

Device Design

The bifurcated stent graft (Fig. 19-1) is an upside-down version of the type of long- and short-leg devices used to treat abdominal aortic aneurysm. The long, thin leg trails back along the route of insertion into one of the supraaortic trunks, usually the innominate artery (Fig. 19-2, A). Carotid-carotid and carotid-subclavian bypass grafts distribute blood to the left carotid and left subclavian arteries (Fig. 19-2, B). The short, wide leg opens into the aorta to form an attachment site for an extension to the descending thoracic aorta.

The delivery system is a short (30-40 cm), wide (22-24 Fr) version of the TX2 delivery system (Cook Medical, Bloomington, Ind.). Trigger wires attach the trunk of the stent graft and the long limb to the central portion of the delivery system.

Implantation Procedure

A bifurcated stent graft is inserted into the aortic arch as follows:

1. A pacing catheter is inserted into the right ventricle through a femoral or subclavian vein. Ideally, capture rates in excess of 200 beats per minute allow the heart to be paced to standstill. Alternatively, the pacing catheter provides a means of restoring cardiac rhythm after adenosine-induced arrest. Either way, the catheter's performance should be tested at the time of insertion.

2. The patient is placed in the supine position on a radiolucent operating table. A left brachial access site is included in the surgical field and covered before tucking the arms at the patient's sides to improve supraclavicular exposure of the supraaortic trunks. A draped table to the right of the patient's neck serves as an angiographic runway.

3. Left carotid-subclavian bypass and carotid-carotid bypass are performed in the standard fashion. The wounds can be left open or closed loosely with a few staples. Definitive closure is performed at the end of the operation.

4. If the right carotid artery is too small to admit the primary delivery system, a conduit to the distal innominate artery is needed. Transcervical exposure of the innominate artery is sometimes difficult. A little traction on the carotid and subclavian arteries helps. Access is not through the end of the conduit but through a puncture site on the side of the conduit.

5. Heparin (100 units per kilogram of body weight) is given intravenously and supplemented throughout the rest of the operation to keep the activated clotting time (ACT) above 300 seconds.

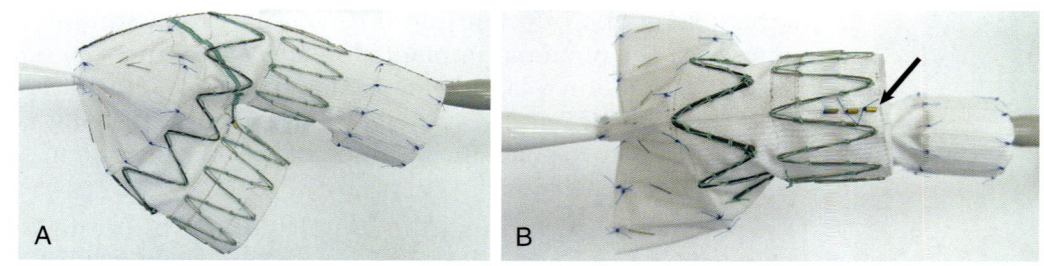

Figure 19-1. A, The transcervical version of the arch stent graft showing where the delivery system attaches to the trunk and long limb of the stent graft, leaving the short limb free to open inside the ascending aorta. **B,** A lateral view of the transcervical arch stent graft showing markers *(arrow)* on the short limb of the stent graft.

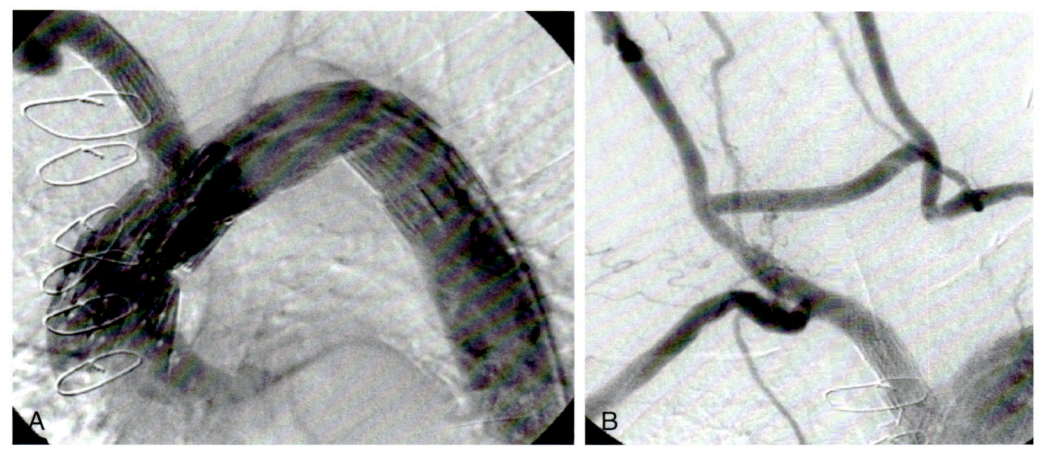

Figure 19-2. A, Completion angiography showing a bifurcated stent graft within the aortic arch. **B,** Completion angiography of the surgically modified brachiocephalic circulation showing multiple bypass grafts connecting the innominate artery with the rest of the brachiocephalic circulation.

6. One pigtail catheter is inserted through a sheath in the surgically exposed common femoral artery, advanced up to the proximal ascending aorta, connected to the contrast injector, and flushed carefully. Another pigtail catheter is advanced through the right carotid (or the innominate conduit) and spun through the aortic valve into the left ventricle, where it is exchanged for a double-curved Lunderquist (Cook Medical) wire. The intersection of the pigtail catheter and the Lunderquist wire marks the proximal margin of the innominate artery.

7. The primary delivery system is inspected under fluoroscopy before insertion to check the orientation of the stent graft and identify all markers. The delivery system is inserted over the Lunderquist wire into the left ventricle. Only one radiopaque marker matters, the one at the distal end of the short leg of the bifurcated stent graft. This should be proximal to the innominate orifice and oriented toward the lesser curvature of the aortic arch. At this point in the procedure blood flows through the carotid-carotid bypass from left to right.

8. Angiograms are performed through the femoral pigtail to confirm the position of the innominate artery.

9. During a brief period of adenosine-induced asystole (or pacer-induced ventricular standstill), the stent graft is deployed by withdrawing the sheath to the innominate bifurcation (Fig. 19-3, *A*), the proximal attachment is released by removing the trigger wire, and the tip of the delivery system is removed from the ventricle by loosening the pin vise and withdrawing the central cannula.

10. The pigtail catheter is carefully removed from the perigraft space and replaced with a selective catheter, which is directed into the distal end of the short limb

of the stent graft. Correct positioning is confirmed by spinning the catheter at the level of the proximal implantation site, where there is too little space to permit free rotation of a catheter tip that happens to lie outside the lumen of the stent graft. The selective catheter is then removed, leaving a double-curved Lunderquist wire to guide the insertion of the delivery system of a descending thoracic aortic extension.

11. Flow is established through the long leg of the bifurcated stent graft, up the repaired right carotid artery, and through the carotid-carotid bypass before implanting the second (descending thoracic aortic) stent graft. As soon as the second stent graft opens, it directs all flow from the short leg of the bifurcated stent graft into the descending thoracic aorta, whereupon prograde flow into the proximal left carotid and left subclavian arteries ceases.

12. The descending thoracic stent graft is deployed in the usual way. Barbs and a 1.5-stent-length overlap ensure a secure hemostatic intercomponent connection.

13. The repair is completed by occluding the left common carotid and subclavian arteries to prevent retrograde leakage (type II endoleak) into the aneurysm. The common carotid is divided and oversewn or plugged with an occluder

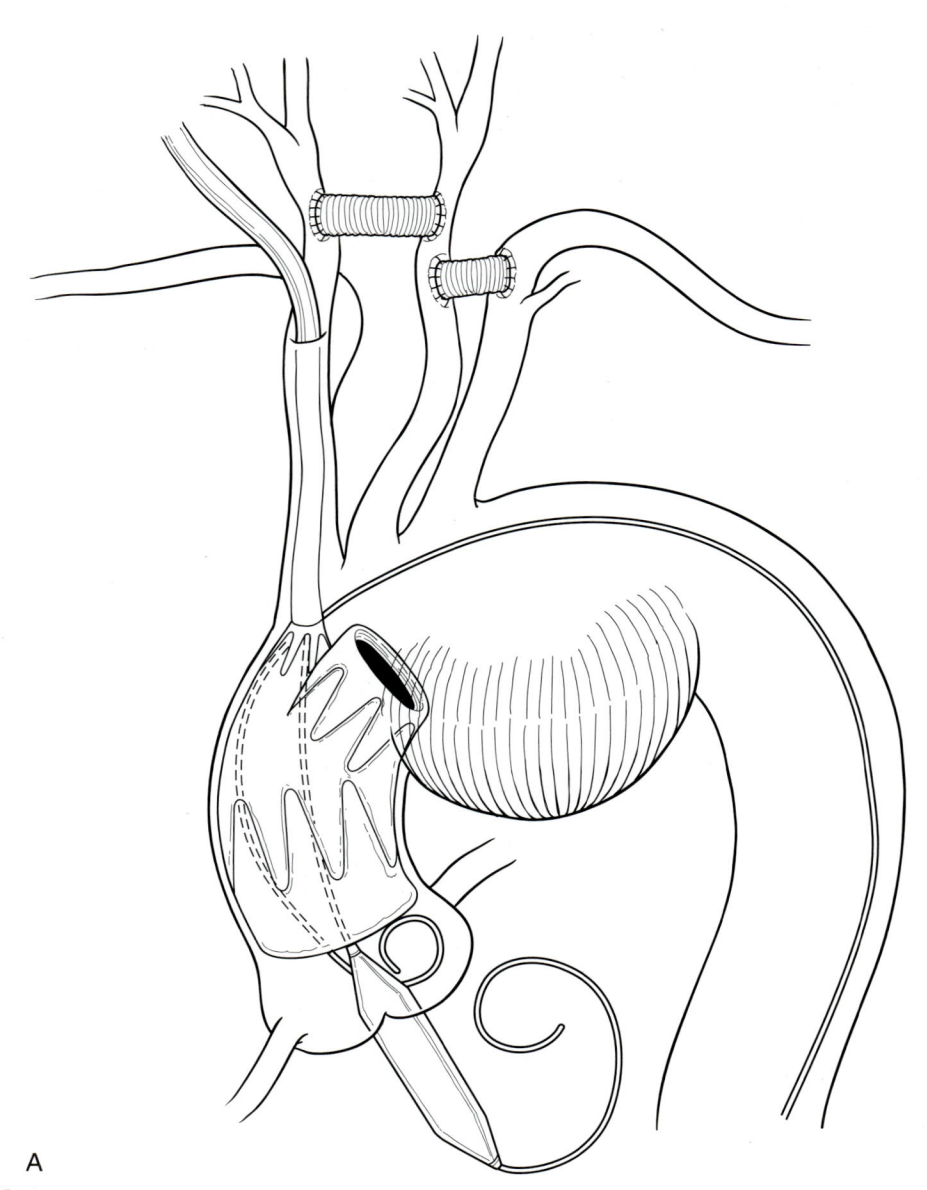

Figure 19-3. A, Insertion of a bifurcated stent graft through the right carotid artery into the ascending thoracic aorta.

device. The subclavian artery is plugged with an Amplatzer II (AGA Medical, Plymouth, Minn.) proximal to the internal mammary and vertebral origins (see Fig. 19-3, *B*).

Pitfalls and Danger Points

- **Stroke.** Stroke may be caused by embolism of atheromatous debris from the ascending aorta and arch, embolism of air, or occlusion of flow through one or more supraaortic trunks. In theory the simplicity of a bifurcated ascending aortic stent graft minimizes the risk of stroke by limiting the extent of proximal aortic instrumentation. Carotid-carotid and carotid-subclavian bypass substitutes for additional stent-graft branches. Both stent-graft delivery systems are flushed under saline until long after the last bubbles emerge from the end of the sheath. The left carotid and left subclavian arteries provide an alternate source of flow to both sides of the brain, whereas the right-sided arteries are occupied by the primary stent-graft delivery system.
- **Left ventricular perforation.** There is no remedy for left ventricular perforation. A stiff Lunderquist wire provides some protection by directing the tip of the delivery system along a curved path around the wall of the ventricle. A Meier wire is not a suitable substitute. When pushed, the Meier wire tends to fold at the point of transition from stiff to floppy with a functionally stiff end that, likewise, can perforate the ventricle.

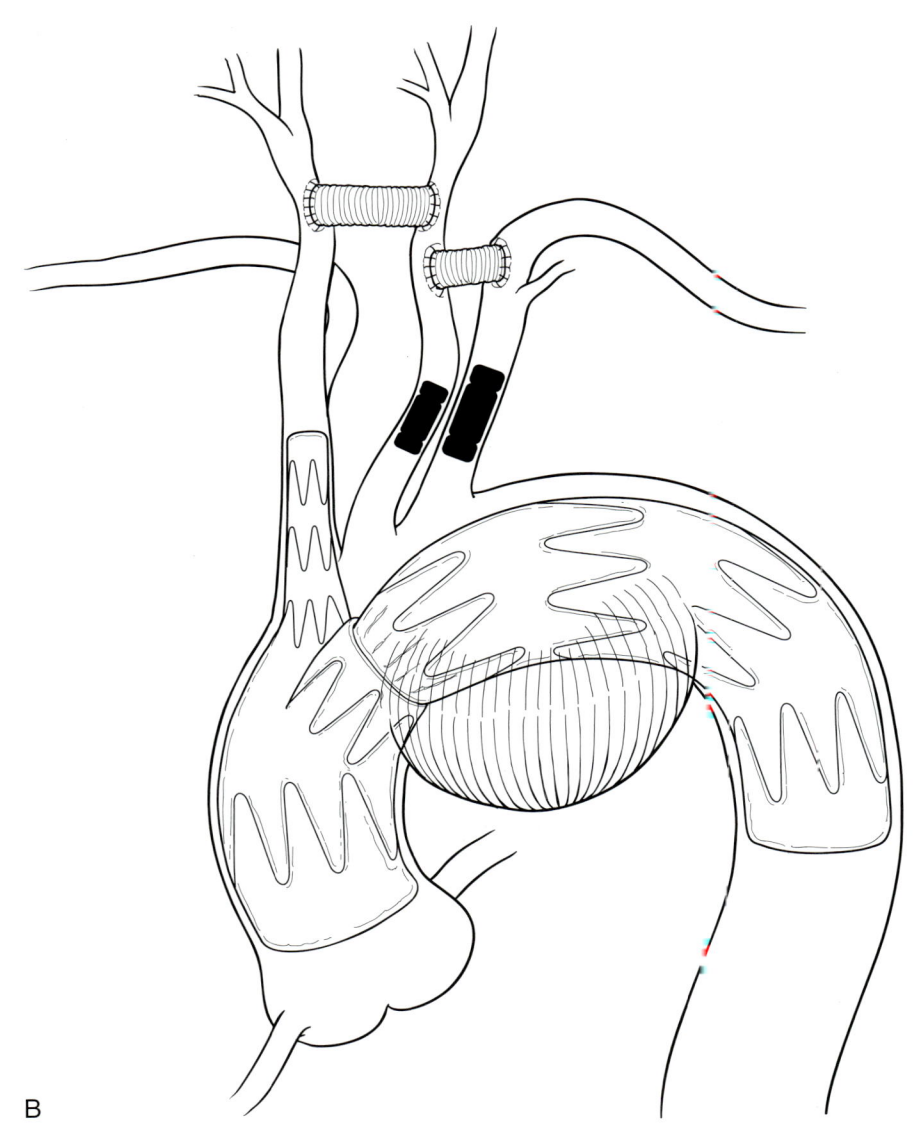

B

Figure 19-3, cont'd **B,** The completed repair.

- **Device displacement.** The tip of the second delivery system (the descending thoracic extension) can catch on the distal margin of the first (bifurcated) stent graft, pushing it upstream. In theory upstream migration of the proximal end could result in coronary occlusion. In practice this is unlikely. It is almost impossible to move one end of the Gianturco stent exoskeleton by pushing on the other. The stent graft collapses but does not move. However, there is a real risk that the collapsing trunk of the bifurcated stent graft will pull its long limb out of the innominate artery. The resulting gap is easy to bridge with a stent-graft extension as long as the right-sided guidewire remains in place. Stent-graft migration can be prevented by applying traction to the distal end of the bifurcated stent graft via its still-attached delivery system during introduction of the delivery system for the second stent graft. Alternatively, the risk of snagging is much reduced if the second delivery system has a long, tapered tip.

MODULAR TRANSFEMORAL MULTIBRANCHED STENT GRAFT

Device Design

The transfemoral multibranched stent graft (Fig. 19-4, A) used for ArAA repair resembles the multibranched stent graft used for TAAA repair. Both are self-expanding combinations of polyester fabric and Z stent, have barbs, and have a tapered trunk bearing multiple short branches (cuffs), which serve as attachment sites for extensions to the visceral arteries. The main difference is in the direction of branch insertion: the branches of an arch stent graft are inserted through access sites in the supraaortic trunks or their downstream branches, whereas the branches of a thoracoabdominal aortic stent graft are inserted through a remote access site. Consequently, the cuffs of the arch stent graft are designed to facilitate catheterization from the perigraft space to the lumen, whereas the cuffs of the thoracoabdominal stent graft are designed to facilitate catheterization from the lumen of the stent graft to the perigraft space.

The multibranched ArAA stent graft has two funnel-shaped cuffs (see Fig. 19-4, B), measuring 12 and 8 mm in diameter (see Fig. 19-4, C), on the outer curvature of the stent graft. Radiopaque markers indicate the proximal and distal ends of each cuff.

The ArAA delivery system is based upon the TX2 delivery system, but instead of one trigger wire there are four wires, each controlling a separate aspect of stent-graft deployment. A fixed curve in the proximal 15 cm of the delivery system (see Fig. 19-4, D) helps ensure proper orientation of the stent graft within the aortic arch.

Implantation Procedure

The transfemoral insertion of a multibranched stent graft has many elements in common with the transcervical insertion of the bifurcated stent graft described earlier: proper orientation is critical, the tip of the delivery system enters the left ventricle, and the primary stent graft is deployed during a short period of adenosine-induced asystole or rapid ventricular pacing.

Two fundamental differences, the route of insertion and the number of branches, affect all other details of stent-graft implantation. The transfemoral version has branches to both sides of the brachiocephalic circulation. A large proximal branch goes to the innominate artery, and a smaller distal branch goes to the left carotid artery or left subclavian artery, depending on individual anatomy and the position of the stent graft at the time of deployment. Carotid-carotid bypass is therefore unnecessary. Large-caliber transcervical access is unnecessary because the primary stent graft is delivered through the femoral artery. Only the branches are inserted through the neck.

ENDOVASCULAR REPAIR OF THE AORTIC ARCH AND THORACOABDOMINAL AORTA

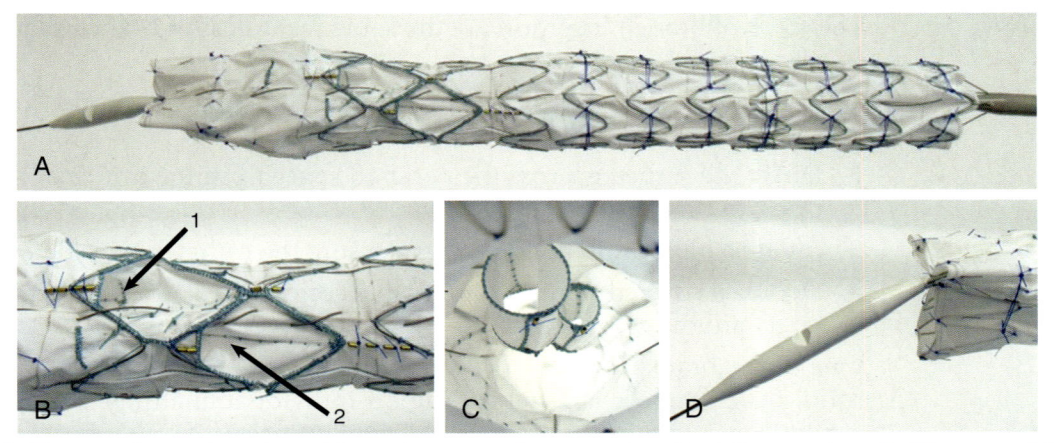

Figure 19-4. A, The transfemoral version of the arch stent graft mounted on its delivery system. **B,** Close-up of the outer aspect of the superior surface showing the external orifices of the proximal *(arrow 1)* and distal *(arrow 2)* cuffs. **C,** Close-up of the inner aspect of the superior surface through the proximal end of the stent graft showing the proximal and distal cuffs. **D,** The proximal end of the stent graft showing the orientation notch in the tip of the delivery catheter and the inherent curve of the delivery catheter.

1. The patient is placed in the supine position on a radiolucent operating table. Both arms, both groins, and both sides of the neck are included in the surgical field. After carotid-subclavian bypass, both arms are extended on arm boards to facilitate transbrachial access.
2. Left carotid-subclavian bypass is performed in the standard fashion. The wounds are usually left open or closed loosely with a few staples. Definitive closure is performed at the end of the operation.
3. Heparin (100 units per kilogram of body weight) is given intravenously and supplemented throughout the rest of the operation to keep the ACT above 300 seconds.
4. One pigtail catheter is inserted through a sheath in the surgically exposed right brachial artery, advanced into the proximal ascending aorta, connected to the contrast injector, and flushed carefully.
5. Another pigtail catheter is advanced through a surgically exposed femoral artery into the ascending thoracic aorta and spun through the aortic valve into the left ventricle, where it is exchanged for a double-curved Lunderquist wire. The pigtail catheter and the Lunderquist wire usually cross at the proximal margin of the innominate artery.
6. The primary delivery system is inspected under fluoroscopy to check the orientation of the stent graft and identify all markers.
7. The delivery system is inserted over the Lunderquist wire into the left ventricle.
8. Angiograms are performed through the femoral pigtail to confirm the position of the innominate artery, the sinotubular ridge just distal to the sinuses of Valsalva at the junction with the tubular segment of the ascending aorta, and the left coronary artery. The proximal or caudal end of the stent graft should be just distal to the left carotid artery, and the cuff markers should be just proximal to the corresponding arterial orifices.
9. During a brief period of adenosine-induced asystole (or pacer-induced ventricular standstill), the sheath is withdrawn. The stent graft is deployed by removing all but one of the trigger wires. Partial removal of the last trigger wire releases the tip of the delivery system, which can then be removed from the ventricle by loosening the pin vise and withdrawing the central cannula. It is sometimes helpful to maintain attachment between the distal or cephalad end of the first (cuff-bearing) stent graft and its delivery system to prevent displacement of the first aortic stent graft during insertion of the second stent graft.

The steps of branch insertion are the same regardless of branch diameter and cuff location:

1. Introduce a catheter through a branch (brachial or carotid) of the targeted supraaortic trunk (Fig. 19-5, *A*).
2. Direct the catheter across the perigraft space from the orifice of the supraaortic trunk to the corresponding cuff.
3. Inflate a balloon in the cuff to make sure the catheter is in the intended cuff.
4. Deploy a covered stent or stent graft to bridge the gap between the cuff and the target artery.

One of the branches goes to the innominate artery. The other goes to the left carotid, or left subclavian, depending on individual anatomy. A bovine trunk, for example, is an indication for a subclavian branch.

In some cases the distal end of the cuff-bearing stent graft is long enough, and wide enough, to reach the distal implantation in the descending thoracic aorta. If not, a second thoracic aortic stent graft is required (see Fig. 19-5, *B*).

Whichever supraaortic trunk is not occupied by a branch of the stent grafts has to be occluded to prevent a large type II endoleak. The proximal carotid can be transected anywhere below the carotid-subclavian bypass, because this segment of the artery has no important proximal branches. The subclavian artery is easier to occlude using an Amplatzer II plug because the site of occlusion has to be below

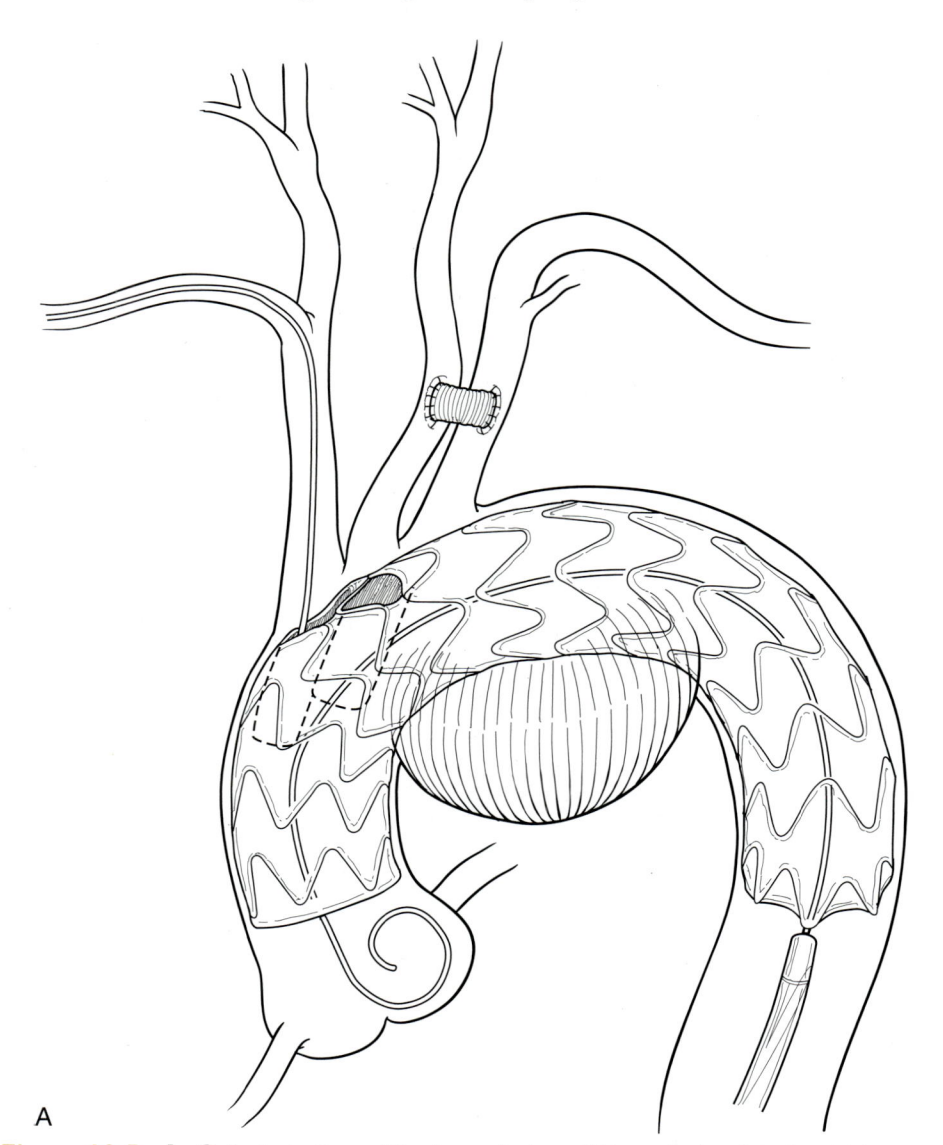

Figure 19-5. A, Catheterization of the innominate cuff through the right brachial artery.

the internal mammary and vertebral branches, and this segment of the subclavian artery may be outside the exposed surgical field.

Pitfalls and Danger Points

- Left ventricular perforation
- Stroke
- Device displacement
- **Impaired perigraft flow.** The primary cuff-bearing component of the multi-branched stent graft extends all the way through the arch. The only sure way for blood to reach the supraaortic trunks is through the cuffs into the perigraft space. If the stent graft bows upward and outward against the superior surface of the arch and eliminates the perigraft space, not only might the outer surface of the graft occlude the orifices of the supraaortic trunks, but the inner surface of the aorta might occlude the cuffs, cutting off the only route of blood flow to the brain. Signs of inadequate supraaortic flow include reduced brachial and carotid pulses; failure to observe a perigraft space on flush angiography, through a transbrachial catheter, of the aortic arch; and failure to note the supraaortic trunks on flush angiography of the stent-graft lumen. The remedy is to reestablish the perigraft space by pushing the graft away from the vault of aortic arch using a sheath, balloon, or snare.

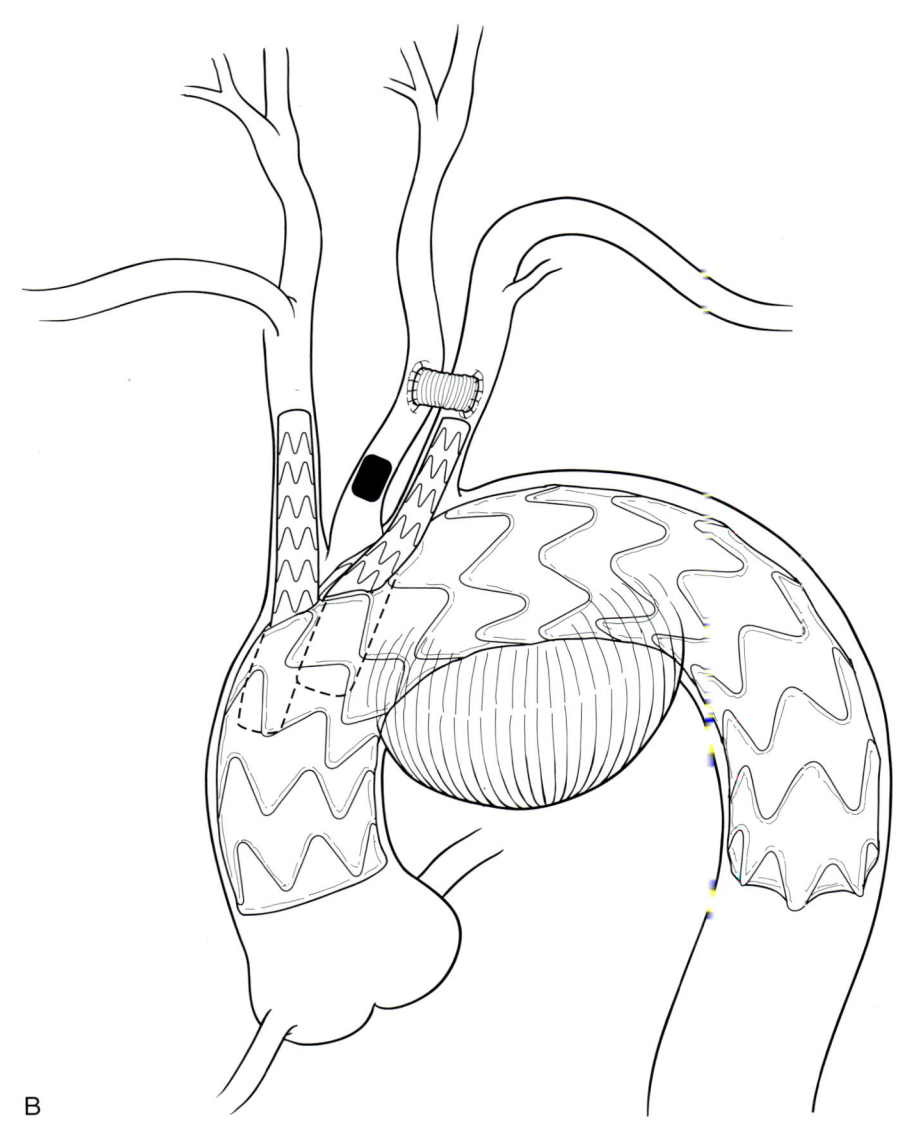

Figure 19-5, cont'd B, All cuffs of the stent graft are connected to branches of the aorta and an occlusion device is deployed in the left common carotid artery.

- **Device malorientation.** The stent graft has to be deployed in the correct orientation and the correct position to permit catheterization of the cuffs and branch insertion. Because all supraaortic trunks tend to point toward the aortic valve, the cuffs are never likely to be too far upstream. However if they are downstream of the target orifices, catheterization may be impossible. The curved delivery system generally ensures proper orientation of the stent graft. If the notched tip of the delivery system is not in the same plane as the supraaortic trunks by the time the stent graft reaches the intended level, the delivery system has to be withdrawn, rotated, and inserted again. Attempts to rotate the delivery system within the aortic arch are generally futile and likely to cause embolism. The chances of successful branch insertion are increased by the multitude of potential combinations, matching three supraaortic trunks with two cuffs. The most proximal cuff is intended for the innominate branch, but the other cuff can provide attachment for a branch to either of the left-sided supraaortic trunks. It is also conceivable that a single branch could provide inflow to all supraaortic trunks through a series of bypass grafts in the root of the neck, as it does with the transcervical, bifurcated stent graft.

Endovascular Repair of Thoracoabdominal Aortic Aneurysms

At UCSF a completely endovascular method of TAAA repair is used based on a cuff-bearing, multibranched modular stent graft. Most TAAAs can be treated using off-the-shelf stent grafts of standard design.

MODULAR TRANSFEMORAL MULTIBRANCHED STENT GRAFT

Device Design

The standard central (branched) stent graft has a tapered trunk and four caudally oriented cuffs: two for the renal arteries, one for the celiac artery, and one for the superior mesenteric artery (Fig. 19-6). The graft fabric extends to the proximal end of the barbed proximal stent.

The central component is designed for use with a variety of proximal and distal extensions. Some are specifically made for this purpose (Fig. 19-7); others are taken from the TX2 and Zenith inventory (Cook Medical). The choice of extension is dictated by the extent of disease and the pattern of prior repair. Because assembly of the composite modular stent graft starts proximally (upstream) and ends distally (downstream), the proximal end of each successive stent graft has to be as wide as or wider than the distal end of the one that preceded it.

The barbs secure the intercomponent connection. The potential for barb-generated injury to the fabric of the stent graft is mitigated by the overlap between two stent grafts with two layers of fabric.

The branched stent-graft delivery system (20- to 22-Fr inner diameter) has trigger wires for proximal attachment, stent-graft expansion, and distal attachment. There is no top cap as in the standard Zenith abdominal aortic stent-graft.

Implantation Procedure

The implantation of a multibranched thoracoabdominal stent graft proceeds as follows:

1. The left arm is extended on an arm board. The right arm is tucked. Both groins and the medial aspect of the left arm are prepped and draped. An additional preparation table extends from the left hand as a runway for transbrachial catheters, sheaths, and wires.

ENDOVASCULAR REPAIR OF THE AORTIC ARCH AND THORACOABDOMINAL AORTA 245

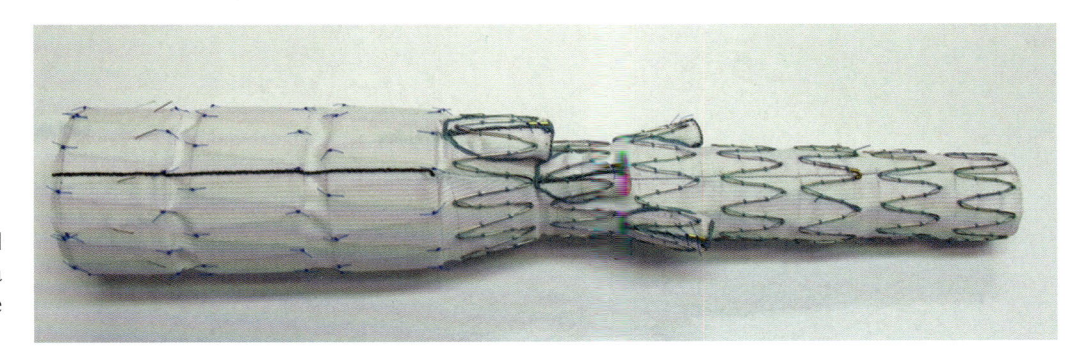

Figure 19-6. The standard TAAA stent graft showing a taper from 34 to 18 mm in the region of the cuffs.

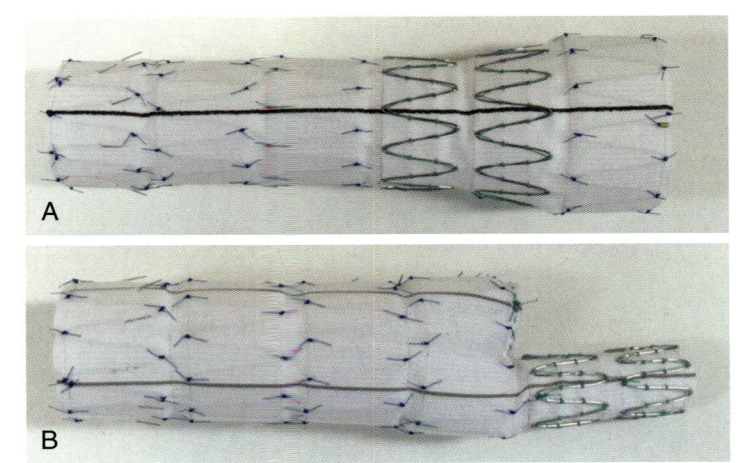

Figure 19-7. A, The tubular distal extension for cases with a long aortic implantation site from prior open surgical repair of an abdominal aortic aneurysm. **B,** The bifurcated distal extension for cases with no aortic implantation site. Note the inversion of the contralateral limb attachment site.

2. One set of viewing screens is positioned to the left of the patient's left hip. Another viewing screen is positioned above the left arm.
3. The common femoral arteries and the proximal left brachial artery are exposed surgically.
4. In cases with a previously created iliofemoral bypass graft (conduit), the route of access depends on the location of the distal anastomosis. If the anastomosis is on the distal external iliac artery, the femoral artery is exposed and punctured in the usual way and the first guidewire is directed anteriorly into the bypass. If the distal anastomosis is to the distal common femoral artery, surgical exposure is limited to isolation of the graft at the inguinal ligament.
5. Before arterial puncture heparin is given intravenously at 100 units per kilogram of body weight. It is then supplemented to keep the ACT above 300 seconds.
6. Fluoroscopy examination of the delivery system confirms orientation and allows marker identification.
7. The aortic stent-graft delivery system is inserted over a stiff (Lunderquist) guidewire through one femoral artery (or conduit). The other femoral artery is provides access for the selective catheterization of one of the visceral arteries.
8. The branched stent graft is deployed by reference to the position of the visceral catheter (Fig. 19-8, *A*). The primary goal is to place the corresponding cuff 15 to 20 mm above the corresponding arterial orifice. The decision as to which artery to catheterize is based on an assessment of which cuff is likely to end up closest to its arterial orifice. Ideally, the cuff-to-artery distance would be the same for all four branches, but this is seldom the case because the cuffs and arteries are frequently distributed differently. A secondary goal is to avoid aortic flush angiography and minimize contrast load. Selective visceral angiograms require only 5 to 8 mL of half-strength contrast.

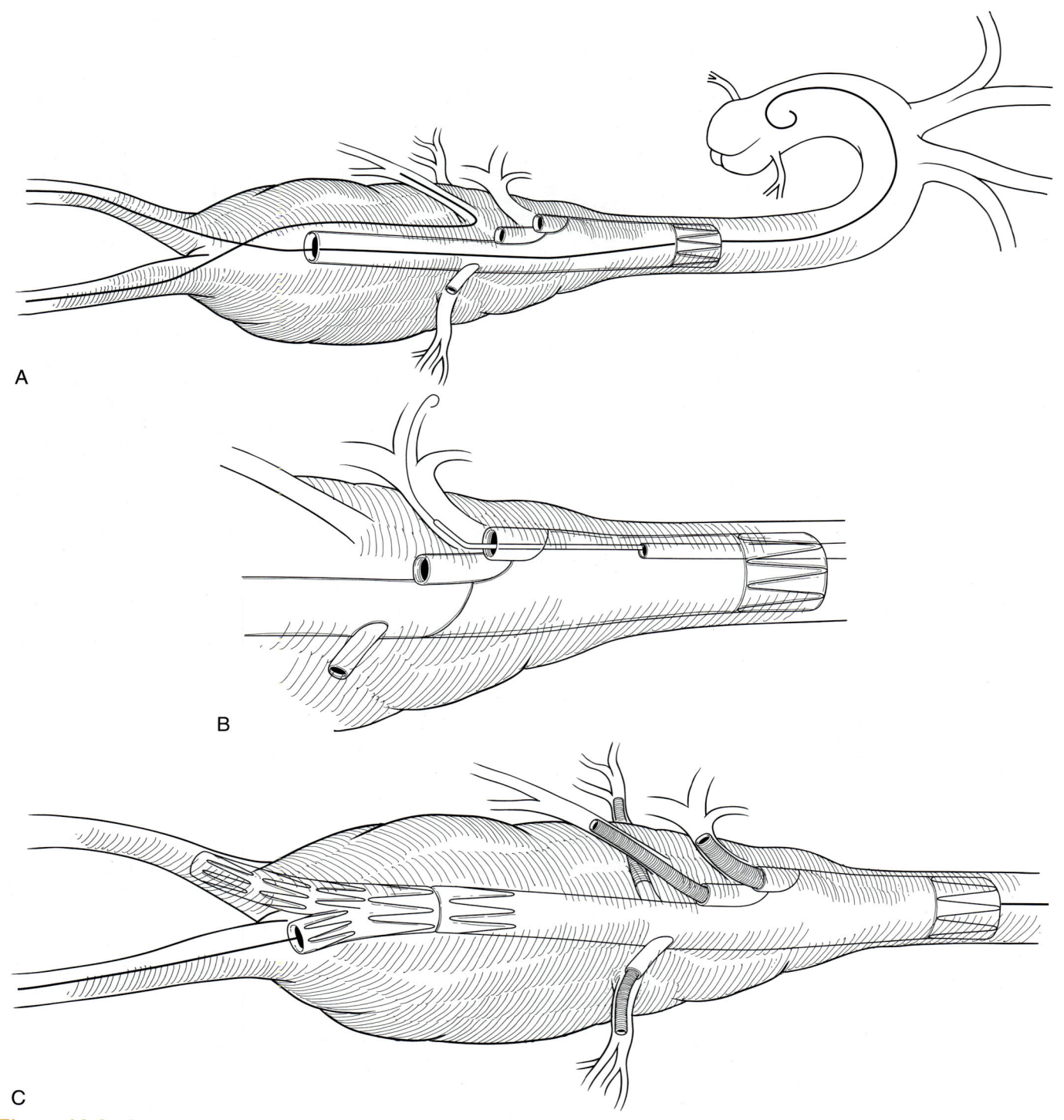

Figure 19-8. **A,** The multibranched thoracoabdominal stent graft is deployed by reference to the position of a catheter in the superior mesenteric artery. **B,** Transbrachial catheterization of the celiac artery. **C,** Covered stents are inserted through the caudally oriented cuffs into all four branches of the thoracoabdominal aorta.

9. Sheath withdrawal is followed by the removal of all three trigger wires. Cuffed branched stent grafts benefit little from constraining wires, or indwelling catheters, because the trunk is tapered and the cuffs are relatively easy to catheterize.

10. Once all aortic (and aortoiliac) stent grafts are in place, their delivery systems are removed and the primary access artery is repaired to restore lower extremity blood flow. The contralateral access sheath is smaller and less likely to obstruct flow. Its removal is generally postponed until the end of the

operation. In the meantime this sole remaining femoral sheath serves as the exit site for a small (0.014-inch) left brachial-femoral guidewire.

The left brachial sheath (usually a 10- to 12-Fr Flexor sheath; Cook Medical) and brachial-femoral guidewire are inserted as follows:

1. Once the main stent graft is in place, withdraw the catheter from the visceral artery and redirect it into the lumen of the main stent graft (usually through a cuff but sometimes through the contralateral iliac limb attachment site).
2. Advance the catheter to the arch.
3. Replace the catheter with a 5-Fr sheath.
4. Insert a three-loop snare through the sheath.
5. Insert a long vertebral catheter and floppy wire through the left subclavian artery into the waiting snare. Pull the wire out through the contralateral femoral access sheath.
6. Exchange the short left brachial sheath for a 40- to 45-cm, 10- to 12-Fr Flexor sheath. Apply traction to both ends of the brachial-femoral wire. Advance the Flexor sheath through the arch, taking care to ensure that its dilator does not push back.
7. Reinsert the long (125 cm) vertebral catheter over the brachial-femoral guidewire.
8. Replace the original 0.035-inch brachial-femoral guidewire with another of even greater length (260-300 cm) and smaller diameter (0.014 inch).
9. Apply tension to both ends of the brachial femoral guidewire using two small hemostatic clamps: one at the orifice of the femoral sheath and the other attached through elastic rubber loops to a fold in the arm drapes.
10. Puncture the margin of the left brachial Flexor sheath and introduce a guidewire.

The remainder of the procedure involves the insertion of a series of covered stents that connect each cuff with a visceral artery and constitute the branches of the stent graft. The dimensions of the covered stent vary, but insertion always has the following steps:

1. Pass a catheter over the 0.035-inch guidewire, through the small accessory left brachial sheath, and down the longer Flexor sheath into the lumen of the stent graft. An additional sheath at the puncture site in the margin of the primary left brachial sheath may help with hemostasis, especially during catheter and delivery system exchanges.
2. Direct the catheter out through one of the cuffs, across the perigraft space, and into the corresponding target artery (Fig. 19-8, B).
3. Confirm the catheter position angiographically using a small volume (5-8 mL) of half-strength contrast.
4. Replace the catheter with a self-expanding Fluency (Bard Medical, Covington, Ga.) covered stent (Fig. 19-8, C, and Fig. 19-9), maintaining access using a stiff guidewire.
5. Provide additional support to the lumen of the covered stent and additional stability to its position by implanting another, slightly longer, uncovered stent.

Take the following steps to preserve spinal perfusion:

1. Drain 20 mL of cerebrospinal fluid immediately before inserting the last branch of the stent graft. Drain another 10 mL/hr for the remainder of the operation.
2. Infuse intravenous fluid, blood, or pressors to maintain a systolic pressure of at least 120 mm Hg for the remainder of the operation.
3. Assess lower extremity neurologic function at the end of the operation. The presence of a deficit is an indication for additional cerebrospinal fluid drainage and more aggressive blood pressure support.

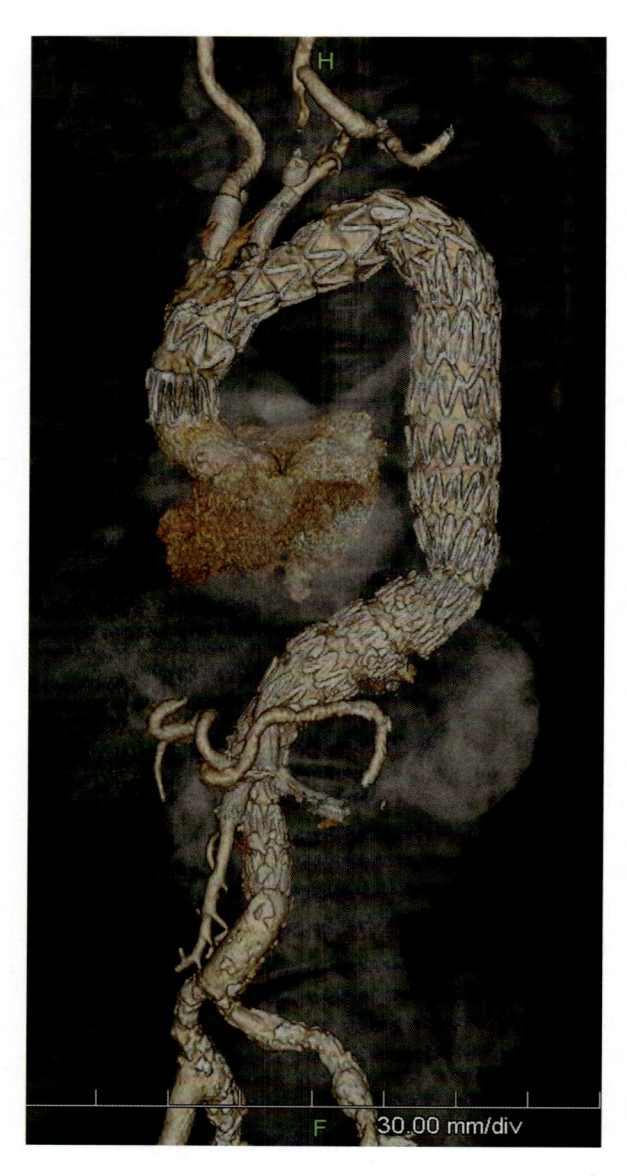

Figure 19-9. A surface-rendered CT angiography after endovascular repair of arch and thoracoabdominal aortic aneurysms.

Pitfalls and Danger Points

- **Embolism.** The presence of shaggy mural thrombus is a relative contraindication to repair. The procedure is designed to minimize the risk of embolic stroke. Transbrachial interventions are performed through the left arm and left subclavian artery, not the right arm and innominate artery. Transbrachial interventions are performed through a long sheath with its tip inside the stent graft.

- **Spinal ischemia.** In the UCSF experience, as many as 20% of patients develop lower extremity neurologic changes because of ischemia of the spinal cord or lumbosacral plexus, but few (5%) have permanent deficits. Early identification, prompt cerebrospinal fluid drainage, and avoidance of hypotension are most important. Vigilance for delayed-onset neurologic deficits is imperative.

- **Device misalignment.** In theory, inaccurate stent-graft design or insertion could result in cuff misalignment and failed branch insertion. In practice, moderate degrees of misalignment are surprisingly well tolerated. The situation is only irretrievable when a caudally oriented cuff lies caudal to the corresponding visceral artery orifice.

- **Impaired perigraft flow.** In areas of aortic luminal narrowing, the lack of a perigraft space may impair visceral perfusion and complicate branch placement. However, this is rarely a problem, except in cases of aortic dissection with true lumen compression. The narrow 18-mm diameter trunk of the stent graft helps ensure a perigraft space. Inflation of an angioplasty balloon can also help open the perigraft space and allow a catheter to pass. Branch compression has not been a problem in these cases, perhaps because of the additional luminal support provided to the branch by most self-expanding stents.

- **Difficult access to a target visceral vessel.** The path from the left brachial artery to the lumen of a visceral artery is long and tortuous. When the tip of a catheter, sheath, or stent delivery system encounters resistance in the form of an acute angle or irregular plaque, there is a tendency for the sheath to loop into the ascending aorta and the tip of the guidewire to push back. The support provided by a stiff guidewire (Rosen or Amplatz, Cook Medical), a kink-resistant brachial sheath, and tension on a brachial-femoral guidewire all help prevent looping. A zigzag bend on a guidewire helps move the tip of the delivery system away from the offending cuff or plaque. A 6-Fr Shuttle Select sheath mounted on a 6.5-Fr JB-1 catheter (Cook Medical) may pass where the blunt-ended Fluency delivery system will not. If so, lining the path from the cuff to the target artery with a Wallstent eliminates most impediments to Fluency insertion. The result is a Fluency-and-Wallstent sandwich, which is expensive but stable.

- **Access in a short, acutely angulated renal artery.** It can be difficult to gain a stable guidewire position in a short, acutely angulated renal artery without risking injury to the tiny downstream branches. The safest option is a Rosen guidewire with a short floppy segment and a 1.5-mm J tip. The orientation of the imaging system is important. The renal orifice is often seen best in the contralateral obliquity, but the rest of the renal artery is seen best in the ipsilateral obliquity.

REFERENCES

1. Saito N, Kimura T, Odashiro K, Toma M, et al: Feasibility of the Inoue single-branched stent-graft implantation for thoracic aortic aneurysm or dissection involving the left subclavian artery: Short-to-medium-term results in 17 patients, *J Vasc Surg* 41:206-212, 2005.
2. Inoue K, Iwase T, Sato M, et al: Transluminal endovascular branched graft placement for a pseudoaneurysm: Reconstruction of the descending thoracic aorta including the celiac axis, *J Thorac Cardiov Surg* 114:859-861, 1997.
3. Chuter TAM, Gordon RL, Reilly LM, et al: An endovascular system for thoracoabdominal aortic aneurysm repair, *J Endovasc Ther* 8:25-33, 2001.
4. Chuter TA, Schneider DB, Reilly LM, et al: Modular branched stent graft for endovascular repair of aortic arch aneurysm and dissection, *J Vasc Surg* 38:859-863, 2003.
5. Quinones-Baldrich W, Jimenez JC, DeRubertis B, et al: Combined endovascular and surgical approach (CESA) to thoracoabdominal aortic pathology: A 10-year experience, *J Vasc Surg* 49:1125-1134, 2009.
6. Criado FJ, Clard NS, Barnatan MF: Stent graft repair in the aortic arch and descending thoracic aorta: A 4-year experience, *J Vasc Surg* 36:1121-1128, 2002.
7. Greenberg RK: Aortic aneurysm, thoracoabdominal aneurysm, juxtarenal aneurysm, fenestrated endografts, branched endografts and endovascular aneurysm repair, *Ann NY Acad Sci* 1085:187-196, 2006.
8. Hiramoto JS, Schneider DB, Reilly LM, et al: A double-barrel stent-graft for endovascular repair of the aortic arch, *J Endovasc Ther* 13:72-76, 2006.
9. Criado FJ: Chimney grafts and bare stents: Aortic branch preservation revisited, *J Endovasc Ther* 14:823-824, 2007.
10. Ohrlander T, Sonesson B, Ivancev K, et al: The chimney graft: A technique for preserving or rescuing aortic branch vessels in stent-graft sealing zones, *J Endovasc Ther* 15:427-432, 2008.
11. Sugiura K, Sonesson B, Akesson M, et al: The applicability of chimney grafts in the aortic arch, *J Cardiovasc Surg* 50:475-481, 2009.
12. Verhoeven EL: Endovascular reconstruction of aortic arch by modified bifurcated stent graft for Stanford type A dissection, *Asian J Surg* 30:296-297, 2007.
13. Bergeron P, Mangialardi N, Costa P, et al: Great vessel management for endovascular exclusion of aortic arch aneurysms and dissections, *Eur J Vasc Endovasc Surg* 32:38-45, 2006.

14. Muehling BM, Bischoff G, Schelzig H, et al: Hybrid procedures for complex thoracoabdominal aortic aneurysms: Early results and secondary interventions, *Vasc Endovascular Surg* 44:110-115, 2010.
15. Anderson JL, Berce M, Hartley DE: Endoluminal aortic grafting with renal and superior mesenteric artery incorporation by graft fenestration, *J Endovasc Ther* 8:3-15, 2001.
16. Sonesson B, Resch T, Allers M, et al: Endovascular total aortic arch replacement by in situ stent graft fenestration technique, *J Vasc Surg* 49:1589-1591, 2009.
17. Imai M, Kimura T, Toma M, et al: Inoue stent-graft implantation for thoracoabdominal aortic aneurysm involving the visceral arteries, *Eur J Vasc Endovasc Surg* 35:462-465, 2008.
18. Chuter TA, Rapp JH, Hiramoto JS, et al: Endovascular treatment of thoracoabdominal aortic aneurysms, *J Vasc Surg* 47:6-16, 2008.

20 Endovascular Treatment of Thoracic Aneurysms

VENKATESH G. RAMAIAH • ALEXANDER KULIK

Historical Background

Aneurysms of the descending thoracic aorta (DTA) affect an estimated 3 to 4 per 100,000 adults. The surgical treatment of DTA aneurysms began in the 1950s through pioneering work by DeBakey, Cooley, and others.[1] Over the years, a number of advances have been made in the surgical techniques and perioperative care of patients with DTA aneurysms. Cerebrospinal fluid (CSF) drainage is now routinely applied, and there has been a shift away from the clamp-and-sew approach to the routine use of left-heart bypass, total cardiopulmonary bypass, or hypothermic circulatory arrest.[2-4] This progress has enabled patients to undergo surgical resection with improved outcomes and morbidity. Nevertheless, many patients with DTA aneurysms are denied open surgical repair because of older age and multiple comorbidities. The concept of using an endovascular stent graft in patients with thoracic aortic disease emerged out of the desire to avoid the hazards of open surgery in this high-risk population.

Initially introduced by Parodi and colleagues[5] for the treatment of abdominal aortic aneurysms (AAAs), endovascular stent-graft technology has been applied for DTA aneurysms for nearly 2 decades.[6] Led by favorable outcomes with stent-graft repair of abdominal aneurysms, the group at Stanford University first applied stent-graft technology for the treatment of DTA aneurysms in the early 1990s. Thirteen high-risk nonoperable patients with DTA aneurysms were treated with custom-designed stent grafts, each constructed with self-expanding Gianturco Z stents (Cook Medical, Bloomington, Ind.) placed with Dacron (DuPont, Wilmington, Del.) grafts. Deployed through peripheral vascular access, the grafts enabled the exclusion and depressurization of the aneurysmal sac without the need for thoracotomy and aortic cross-clamping. Placement of these stents was successful in all patients, with thrombosis of the aneurysm surrounding the stent occurring in 12 of the 13 patients.[6] With favorable early results, the study was then extended to the treatment of 103 additional patients with DTA aneurysms, many of whom were deemed unsuitable for conventional open surgical repair. Highly satisfactory results were achieved.[7]

The first-generation "homemade" devices were limited because of the inflexible delivery system, making it difficult to navigate a tortuous aorta or to achieve secure fixation across an angled aortic arch. Years of experience with the endovascular repair of DTA aneurysms and AAAs have led to refinements in stent-graft technology and the commercial production of stent grafts. The Gore thoracic aortic graft (TAG) thoracic endoprosthesis (W.L. Gore and Associates, Newark, Del.) became the first thoracic stent graft to be approved by the U.S. Food and Drug Administration (FDA) for the treatment of DTA aneurysms in 2005. Approval subsequently followed for the Talent system (Medtronic Vascular, Santa Rosa, Calif.) and the TX2 Zenith system (Cook Medical). These grafts are manufactured with polytetrafluoroethylene (PTFE) or polyester for the graft material and nitinol or stainless steel for the stent material. Available DTA stent grafts feature less stiff and lower-profile delivery systems (20- to 28-Fr access), less porous graft material, greater flexibility, and a wider variety of available sizes.

Endovascular approaches have emerged as less invasive treatment options for patients with DTA aneurysms. They are well tolerated, even in elderly patients, and are associated with both shorter stays in the intensive care unit and decreased blood transfusion requirements. Perioperative mortality and paraplegia risk compare favorably with open surgical repair rates.

Indications

An aneurysm of the DTA is defined as a localized or diffuse dilatation, with a diameter at least 50% greater than the adjacent normal-sized aorta. In an average-height older man with a normal distal aortic arch diameter of 2.8 cm, dilatation of the proximal DTA of 5.6 cm or greater is defined as aneurysmal.[4] The most common risk factors for aneurysmal degeneration of the aorta include smoking, chronic obstructive pulmonary disease, hypertension, atherosclerosis, bicuspid aortic valve, and genetic disorders.

In an asymptomatic patient with a DTA aneurysm, the risk of rupture or dissection increases to more than 40% per year when the aorta grows larger than 7 cm in diameter.[8] Therefore intervention of an asymptomatic DTA aneurysm before it reaches 6 cm preempts most ruptures and dissections.[4] For asymptomatic patients who are in excellent health and anatomically suitable for endovascular repair, DTA aneurysms 5.5 cm or larger in diameter and eccentric saccular aneurysms greater than 2 cm in width are potential candidates for repair.[9] In contrast to asymptomatic aneurysms, aneurysms associated with symptoms should be treated regardless of size, if there are no contraindications, because symptoms are believed to be indications of impending rupture. As a result of compression or erosion into surrounding structures, DTA aneurysms may lead to back pain, abdominal pain, hoarseness, dysphagia, dyspnea, hemoptysis, or hematemesis. Spinal cord compression or thrombosis of spinal arteries may result in paraparesis or paraplegia. Embolization of atheromatous debris could lead to distal ischemia involving the viscera, kidneys, or lower extremities. Acute rupture leads to cardiovascular collapse.

Available thoracic aortic stent grafts are only approved by the FDA for the treatment of DTA aneurysms. However, they are commonly applied "off label" for the management of other thoracic aortic pathology, including penetrating atherosclerotic ulcer (PAU), intramural hematoma (IMH), aortic dissection, and traumatic aortic transection. A PAU represents rupture of an atherosclerotic plaque, with penetration into the internal elastic lamina of the aorta. Although slow growing, PAU may lead to saccular aneurysm formation, severe pain, and aortic rupture.[10] An IMH is thought to result from the spontaneous rupture of the aortic vasa vasorum, with hemorrhage into the aortic media. IMH may be associated with pain and can lead to an intimal tear and aortic dissection. Enlarging or symptomatic PAU and IMH represent appropriate indications for DTA stent-graft repair. The endovascular management of aortic dissection and traumatic aortic disruption are discussed in other chapters of this book.

Preoperative Preparation

- **Cardiac evaluation.** A noninvasive myocardial stress test should be performed, such as exercise treadmill testing, dobutamine stress echo cardiography, or a persantine thallium study. Coronary angiography may be warranted if significant coronary artery disease is identified.
- **Carotid artery duplex imaging** should be obtained.
- **Imaging the vascular anatomy.** Computed tomography (CT) angiography with the possibility of three-dimensional (3D) reconstruction provides excellent

visualization of the aorta, including aneurysm diameter, thrombus characteristics, branch vessel anatomy, and extent of calcification. Magnetic resonance imaging (MRI) is also capable of providing angiographic images and 3D reconstruction. Although it avoids ionizing radiation, MRI cannot be used in emergency circumstances or for patients with implanted pacemakers. Thin-slice CT angiography of the thorax, abdomen, and pelvis with distal arterial runoff and 3D reconstruction of the aorta should be obtained (Fig. 20-1).

- **Assessment of aortic landing zones.** Appropriate length and diameter of the aorta are required proximal and distal to the aneurysm for DTA stent-graft repair (Fig. 20-2). The landing zones should be long enough to allow safe deployment between the aneurysm and the brachiocephalic arteries proximally and the celiac artery distally. In general, proximal and distal landing zones must be 2 cm in length and free of thrombus and calcification to achieve adequate seal and prevent endoleak. Available devices are 22 to 46 mm in diameter, and because stent grafts are oversized by 10% to 20%, landing zone diameters must be larger than 19 mm and smaller than 43 mm in diameter.
- **Assessment of iliofemoral vascular access.** Size, tortuosity, and calcification of the iliofemoral vasculature must be examined preoperatively to determine the need for an iliac artery conduit.

Pitfalls and Danger Points

- **Avoiding stroke.** The risk of stroke after DTA stent-graft repair was noted to be as high as 8% in early reports and was thought to be related to the manipulation of catheters and sheaths in and around the aortic arch and its branches.[6] Older stent-graft delivery systems required the handling of large, stiff sheaths and dilators. Newer deployment systems only require a guidewire to pass through the arch and therefore are associated with less manipulation, with recent reports documenting a stroke risk of 3% to 4%.[11-18] Coverage of the left subclavian artery may increase the risk of posterior circulation strokes, particularly if the right vertebral artery is absent or stenotic. However, the majority of strokes are atheroembolic. Therefore arch wire and catheter manipulations should be kept to a minimum.

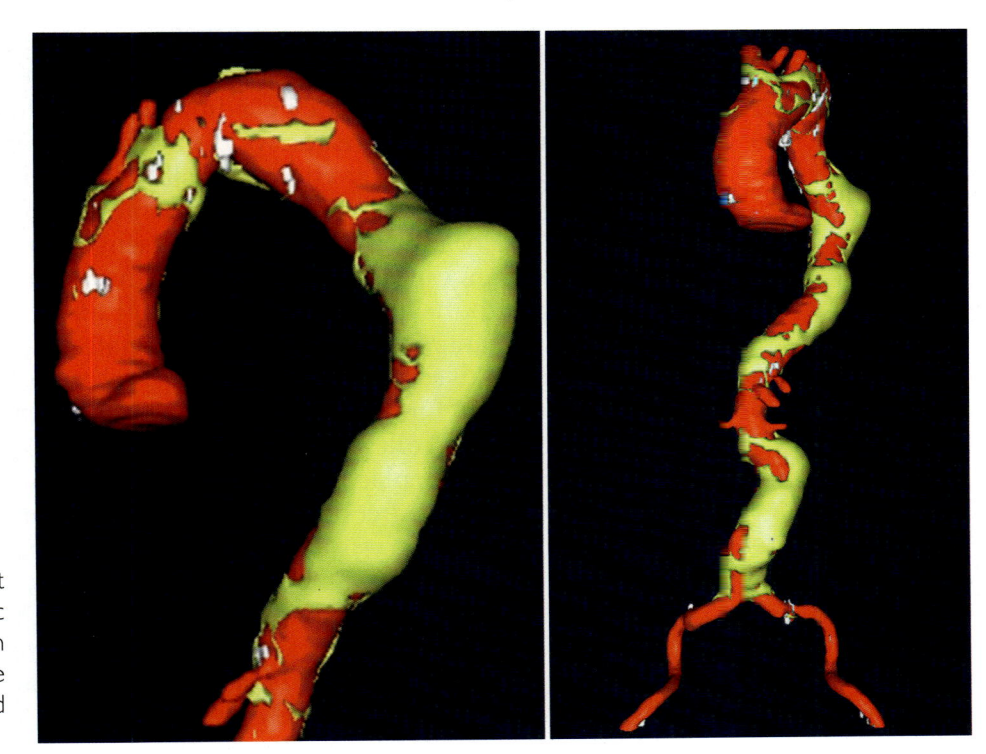

Figure 20-1. Reconstructed chest CT scan demonstrating a thoracic aortic aneurysm measuring 6 cm in diameter with iliac vessels of adequate size and with minimal tortuosity and calcium.

THE THORACIC AORTA

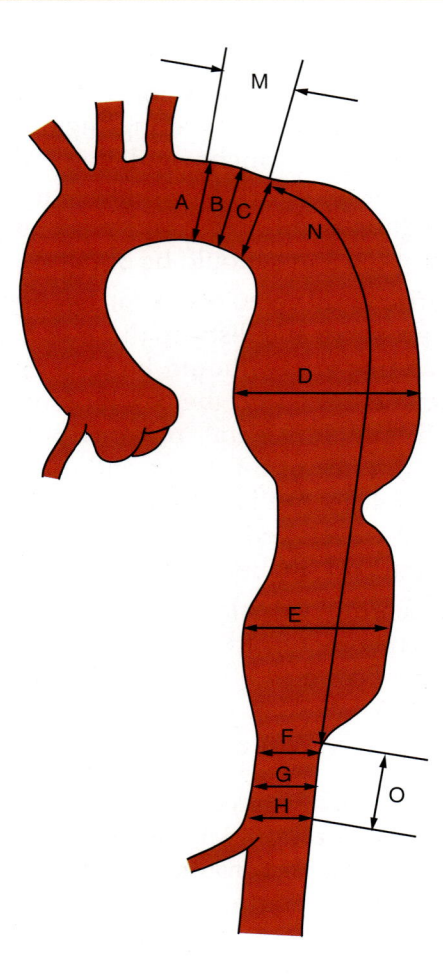

Figure 20-2. The anatomic suitability for endovascular repair is assessed using a standardized preoperative worksheet. Representative anatomic measures for treatment planning are presented. A, Proximal implantation site (30-mm diameter). B, 1 cm proximal to the implantation site. C, 2 cm from implantation site (32-mm diameter). D, Aneurysm diameter (60 mm). E, Secondary aneurysm (not applicable). F, 2 cm distal to the implantation site. G, 1 cm from the distal implantation site (29-mm diameter). H, Distal implantation site (28-mm diameter). M, Aneurysm length (5 cm). N, Distal neck (3 cm from aneurysm to celiac axis). O, Total treatment length (9 cm).

- **Avoiding paraplegia.** Spinal cord ischemic injury has been reported at a rate of 2% to 4% after DTA stent-graft repair.[11-18] The risk of paraplegia or paraparesis is greatest if collateral blood supply to the spinal cord has been compromised during previous aortic intervention, such as through an open or endovascular abdominal aortic aneurysm repair or by the presence of unilateral or bilateral occlusion of the internal iliac artery. Likewise, the risk of paraplegia increases if extensive thoracic aortic coverage or coverage of left subclavian artery is planned for the current DTA intervention. Because large patent intercostal arteries cannot be reimplanted during stent-graft repair, care should be taken to avoid excessive distal coverage of the DTA, and the patency of as many intercostal arteries as possible should be maintained. The left subclavian artery supplies the superior portion of the anterior spinal artery via the vertebral artery and may therefore represent an important collateral source of spinal perfusion, especially in patients with prior abdominal aortic aneurysm repair. Some reports have suggested coverage of the left subclavian artery increases the risk of paraplegia during DTA stent-graft repair and have recommended routine preoperative revascularization with carotid-subclavian bypass, but others have found this not to be the case.[14,15] If concerns are raised about compromised spinal cord collateral perfusion, or if long aortic coverage is required, a CSF drain may be placed immediately before surgery. The drain is left in position for 48 hours. After the procedure, the patient's blood pressure is raised to 140- to 160-mm Hg systolic to encourage collateral blood flow to the spinal cord. If delayed neurologic injury arises after surgery, elevating systemic blood pressure and instituting CSF drainage can occasionally reverse neurologic deficits. For patients with concomitant abdominal aortic aneurysm and DTA aneurysm, the repair is staged and the larger aneurysm treated first, with the assumption that collateral circulation to the spinal cord will develop during the interval period.

- **Avoiding arm ischemia.** A significant proportion of DTA aneurysms lie close to the left subclavian artery. Therefore stent-graft coverage across the subclavian origin is sometimes necessary to ensure adequate fixation of the device at the proximal landing zone and to exclude the aneurysm. Preemptive revascularization of the left subclavian artery before covering its origin is required in the setting of a dominant left vertebral artery, previous coronary artery bypass graft surgery with a patent left internal mammary artery graft, and functioning arteriovenous fistula in the left upper extremity. In the absence of these absolute indications, controversy exists regarding whether routine preoperative revascularization of the left subclavian artery is required. Some centers have reported complications associated with coverage of the left subclavian artery, such as left arm claudication or vertebrobasilar insufficiency, and advocate revascularization of the left subclavian artery before DTA stent-graft repair. The authors have observed that only 2% of patients develop postoperative left upper extremity ischemia, and thus advocate an expectant approach.[14,19] Subclavian artery revascularization can be performed expediently for the treatment of left upper extremity ischemia. To identify patients who require a left carotid-subclavian bypass, preprocedural carotid and vertebral duplex ultrasound imaging and CT angiography can be used to evaluate the patency, size, and location of the vertebral arteries; to rule out an aortic arch origin of the left vertebral artery; and to document an intact circle of Willis.

- **Avoiding proximal type I endoleaks.** A proximal type I endoleak is the most common type of endoleak seen after DTA stent-graft repair and represents a lack of apposition between the graft and the aortic wall, leading to active arterial flow within the aneurysmal sac. A type I endoleak is more common in the thoracic aorta than in the abdominal aorta because of the short and frequently angled attachment zone in the aortic arch. Achieving proximal anchorage of at least 2 cm is necessary to avoid a proximal type I endoleak. Although type I endoleaks occasionally seal spontaneously, the failure of sealing usually results in persistent sac pressurization, leaving the patient at risk of future aneurysmal rupture. Therefore identification and management of a proximal type I endoleak at the time of the initial stent-graft repair is critical.[20] Proximal type I endoleaks can be visualized with aortography after stent-graft deployment. A proximal type I endoleak can often be corrected with angioplasty using a large-diameter, compliant balloon. Balloon angioplasty helps ensure that the stent graft is fully expanded and improves contact with the aortic wall. Should the endoleak persist despite angioplasty, consideration should be given to placement of a stent-graft extension to lengthen the seal zone. This may require coverage of the left subclavian artery and stent-graft deployment at the origin of the left common carotid artery to increase the length of the proximal landing zone. Alternatively, aortic arch debranching techniques with carotid-carotid bypass can be considered to further lengthen the proximal landing zone (Figs. 20-3 and 20-4). In certain circumstances a proximal type I endoleak can be treated with the deployment of a balloon-mounted bare metal stent to the proximal portion of the stent graft to enhance apposition of the stent graft to the aortic wall.

- **Avoiding distal type I endoleak.** A distal landing zone of at least 2 cm is required to avoid a distal type I endoleak at the time of DTA stent-graft repair. Should a distal type I endoleak be identified after stent-graft deployment, balloon angioplasty may be applied as an initial step to ensure that the stent graft is fully expanded distally and to improve graft contact with the aortic wall. A persistent distal type I endoleak may necessitate the distal deployment of a stent-graft extension or a balloon-mounted bare metal stent to lengthen the seal zone or improve graft contact with the aortic wall. If the endoleak persists and the distal landing zone extends to the origin of the celiac artery, either visceral debranching of the celiac artery can be performed via laparotomy or the celiac artery can be embolized and covered with a distal graft extension (Figs. 20-5 and 20-6). This latter approach, without celiac artery revascularization, increases the risk of visceral ischemia.

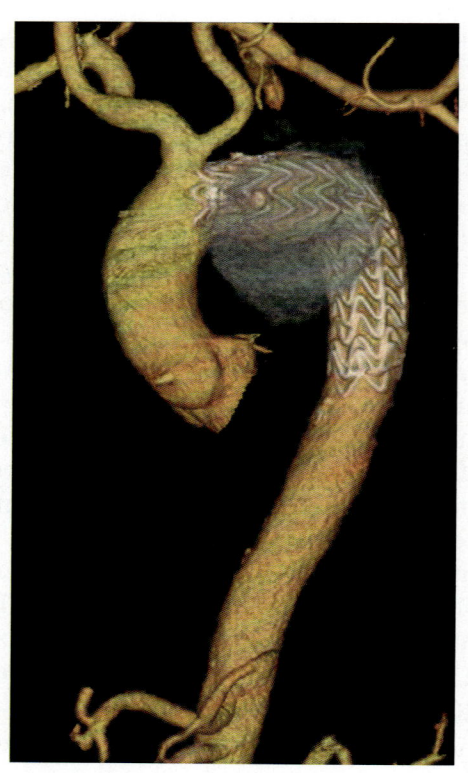

Figure 20-3. CT scan demonstrating carotid-subclavian bypass with placement of a thoracic endograft just distal to the common origin of the innominate artery and left carotid artery.

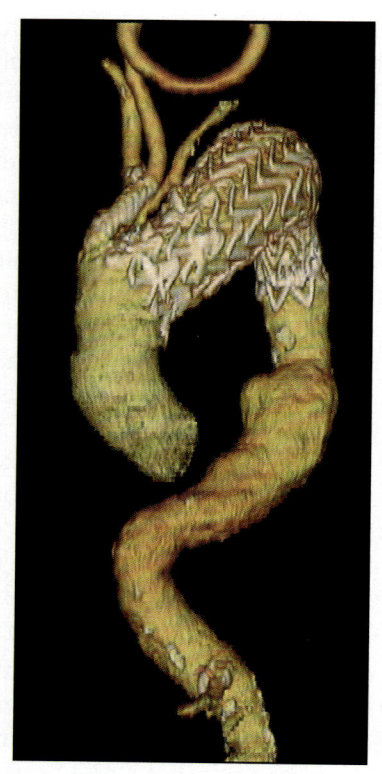

Figure 20-4. CT scan showing a carotid-carotid bypass and the satisfactory position of the endograft.

- **Avoiding proximal type II endoleaks.** Retrograde filling of the excluded aorta from a patent subclavian artery may predispose patients to type II endoleaks.19 These endoleaks can be treated at a delayed interval should they persist.
- **Avoiding visceral ischemia.** Purposeful coverage of the celiac artery during DTA stent-graft repair should be avoided to reduce the risk of visceral complications. If the distal sealing zone proximal to the celiac artery is of insufficient length and sacrificing the celiac artery is anticipated, angiographic evaluation should

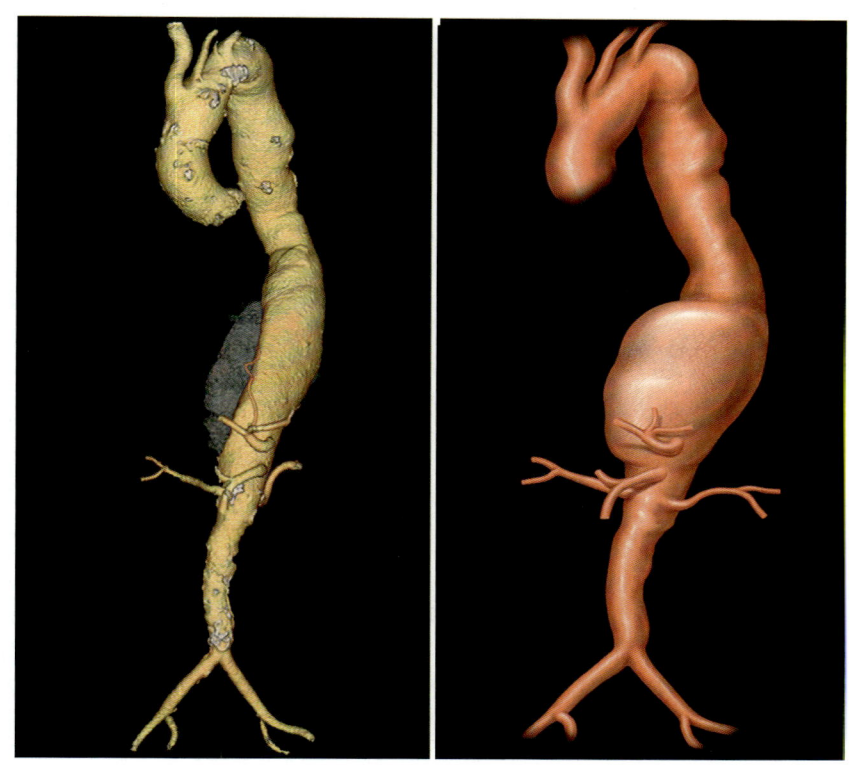

Figure 20-5. CT scan of a thoracoabdominal aneurysm before repair.

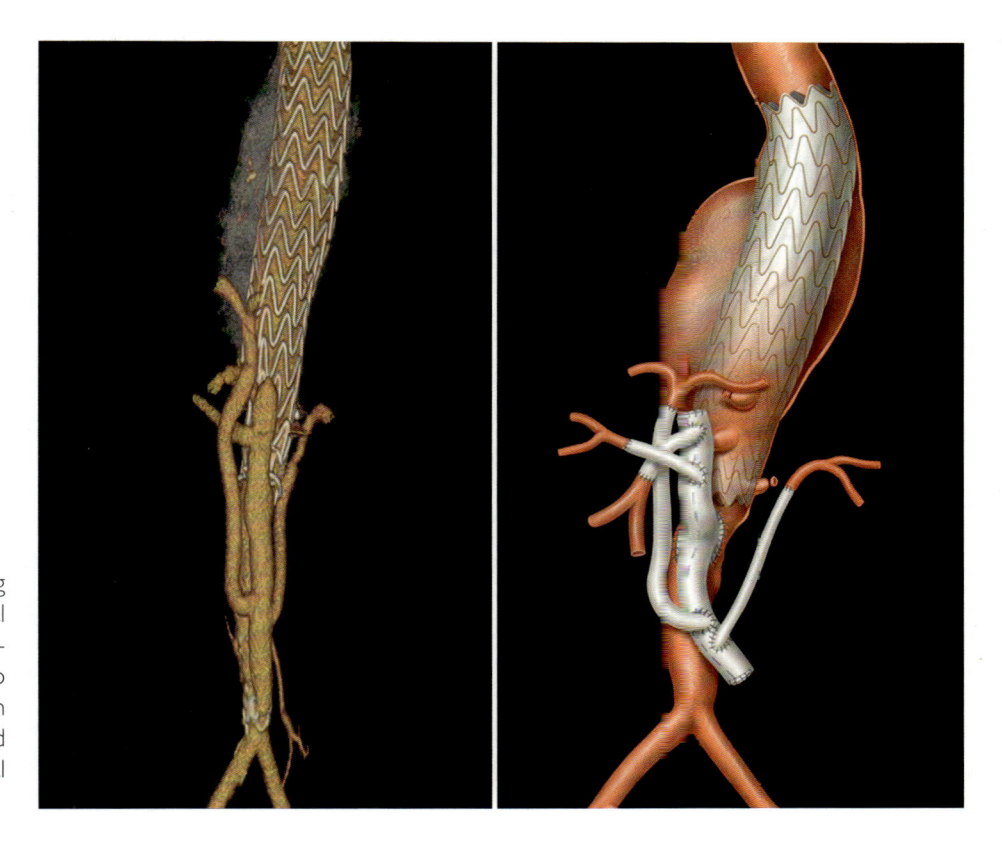

Figure 20-6. CT scan illustrating hybrid repair of a thoracoabdominal aneurysm using a thoracic endovascular graft and operative bypass grafts to the celiac, superior mesenteric, and both renal arteries arising from a bifurcated graft anastomosed to the infrarenal aorta.

first be performed to assess the collateral circulation between the celiac artery and the superior mesenteric artery. Temporary balloon occlusion of the celiac artery and selective angiography of the superior mesenteric artery determine whether sufficient collateral supply is supplied by the superior mesenteric artery via the gastroduodenal artery. Coil embolization of the celiac artery can then be performed, allowing a distal stent-graft extension to be deployed up to the origin of the superior mesenteric artery. Experience with coverage of the celiac artery to extend the distal landing zone remains limited.

Endovascular Strategy

ACCESS VESSEL TORTUOSITY AND SIZE

Adequate vascular access is critical for DTA stent-graft deployment, and preoperative imaging must include an assessment of the iliofemoral vasculature. Current DTA stent-graft devices require a large-caliber delivery system that ranges from 20 to 24 Fr (0.7-0.8 cm) in outer diameter. Therefore the presence of small, tortuous, or calcified iliac vessels may prove to be hazardous in advancing the sheaths necessary for stent-graft deployment, and such patients are at increased risk of iliac artery rupture. Tortuous iliac vessels force the relatively stiff delivery catheter to assume a variety of angles as it negotiates the curves, increasing friction and decreasing the "pushability" of the device at each of these bends (Fig. 20-7). Excessive force can lead to iliac artery injury. Fortunately, iliac artery tortuosity can be overcome with the use of superstiff guidewires such as the Amplatz SuperStiff or Meier guidewire (Boston Scientific, Natick, Mass.) or Lunderquist wires (Cook Medical). These wires straighten the iliac system and enable improved tracking of the device into position.

Serial dilatation with Coons dilators (Cook Medical) may be attempted for patients with small iliofemoral vessels or to treat mild to moderate atherosclerotic lesions. Focal iliac stenosis can also be treated by balloon angioplasty to enable the introduction of the delivery devices, followed by the deployment of balloon-expandable stents at the conclusion of the procedure (Fig. 20-8). However, the safest and most commonly used technique in the face of calcified or small iliofemoral vessels is to obtain retroperitoneal exposure of the common iliac artery and construct an iliofemoral conduit using a 10-mm Dacron graft (Figs. 20-9 and 20-10). The stent graft may be delivered through the conduit after the proximal anastomosis is performed to the common iliac artery, and the conduit is either tunneled under the inguinal ligament or brought out through a lower abdominal wall stab incision to traverse an acutely angulated graft-host vessel anastomosis. After deployment of the graft, if needed, the conduit can be grafted to the common femoral artery to complete an iliofemoral bypass. The rate of retroperitoneal conduit use was 15% in the Gore TAG phase II trial and up to 22% in reported series.[21]

Alternative techniques available to manage suboptimal femoral artery access include direct cannulation of the iliac artery after retroperitoneal exposure. Two purse strings of 4-0 polypropylene sutures may be used to secure hemostasis after the removal of the sheath. Deployment of a Gore TAG device without a sheath (the bareback technique) can be used in the setting of small or diseased iliofemoral vessels. This technique is not recommended in the instructions of use (W.L. Gore) and exposes the iliac artery to potential graft-induced trauma. An endoluminal conduit may also be considered for delivery of a stent graft through a small calcified iliac vessel that may otherwise require a retroperitoneal conduit. A covered stent 8 to 10 mm in diameter, such as a Viabahn (W.L. Gore), iCast (Atrium Medical, Lebanon, N.H.), or Fluency (Bard Medical, Covington, Ga.) graft, is deployed via a femoral sheath into the common iliac artery covering the origin of the internal iliac artery (Fig. 20-11). An oversized noncompliant balloon is used to dilate the iliac artery and crack the calcified plaque from within the endoconduit. The aortic endograft is then placed through the conduit into the aorta. The major risk of this technique is the potential for dislodging the endograft with use of large delivery systems.

After stent-graft deployment, it is prudent to keep a guidewire in the aorta upon removal of the delivery sheath. Should iliac artery injury be suspected during insertion of the delivery system, blood products and an aortic occlusion balloon should be available in the operating room (Fig. 20-12). A retrograde iliac angiogram can be performed on removal of a delivery sheath to assess for an iliac artery injury, and if rupture exists, an occlusive balloon can be advanced and inflated. A covered stent can be used to cover the area of extravasation, or the injured vessel can be exposed and repaired primarily.

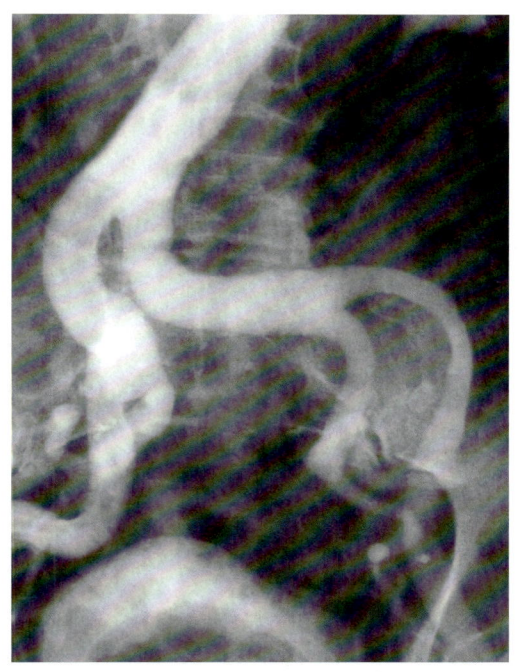

Figure 20-7. Illustration of tortuous iliac vessels. Iliac artery tortuosity is often overcome with the use of superstiff guidewires to straighten the iliac system and enable improved tracking of the endovascular graft.

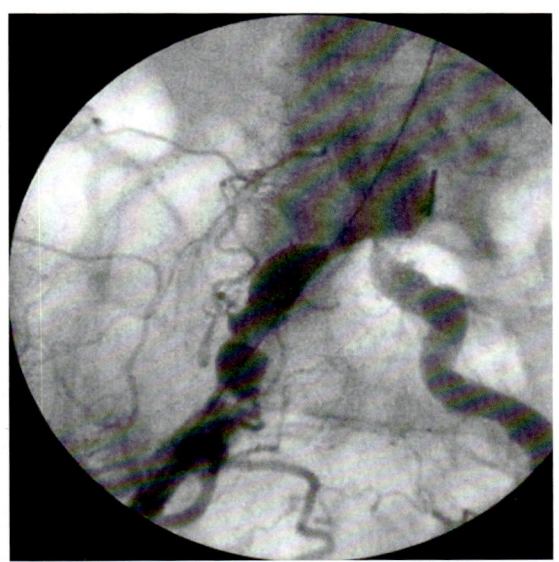

Figure 20-8. Retrograde iliac angiogram demonstrating tortuous iliac arteries with areas of stenosis. A focal iliac stenosis can be treated by balloon angioplasty to enable the introduction of the delivery devices, followed by the deployment of balloon-expandable stents at the conclusion of the procedure.

AORTIC ARCH

Accurate placement of a stent graft in a curved or tortuous aortic arch can be challenging. A small amount of distal migration during deployment of the stent graft can result in inadequate proximal fixation and necessitate the placement of a proximal cuff to achieve seal. Deployment of a stent graft across a severe arch angulation may result in "bird beaking" of the endograft and a proximal type I endoleak. Device collapse is the most serious complication. If necessary, the landing zone may be extended proximally by aortic arch debranching through placement of a left carotid-subclavian bypass, a carotid-carotid bypass, or both. During graft deployment in the aortic arch, it is critical to lower the blood pressure and cardiac output to ensure accurate deployment and prevent migration. This can be achieved with the administration of vasodilators, adenosine, rapid ventricular pacing, or a sustained Valsalva maneuver.

260 THE THORACIC AORTA

Common Iliac artery

Common femoral artery

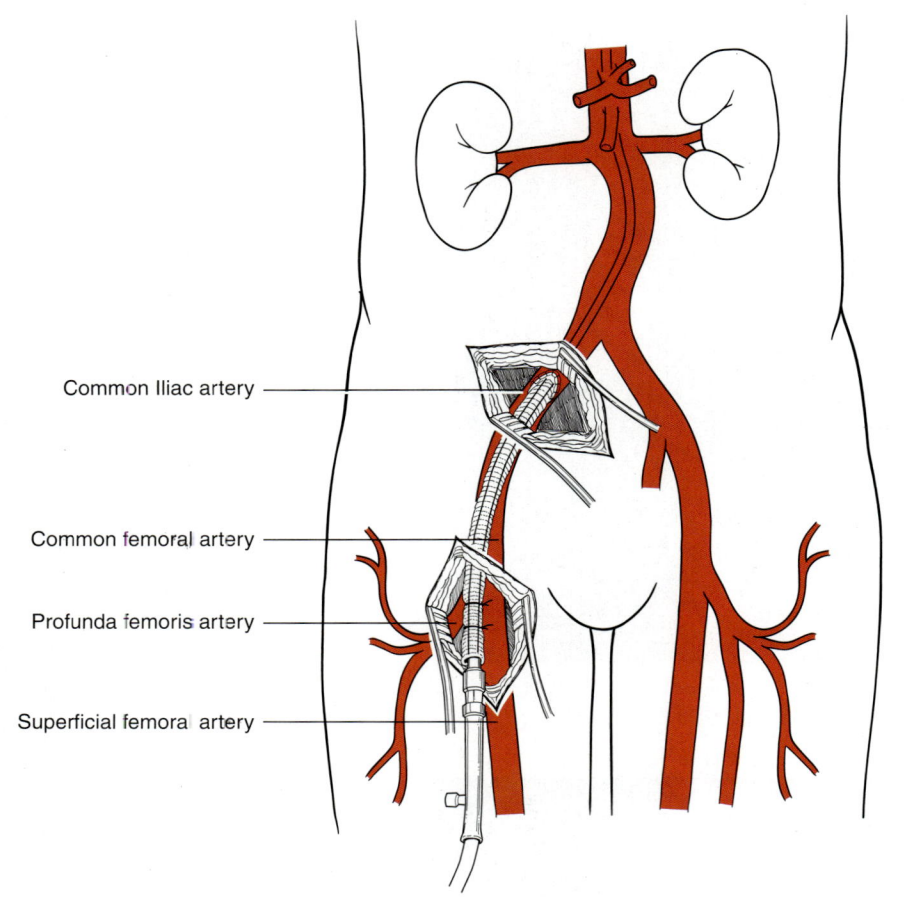

Profunda femoris artery

Superficial femoral artery

Figure 20-9. A right retroperitoneal incision with a 10-mm conduit sewn to the right common iliac artery and connected to a device delivery sheath for deployment of endoluminal graft to the thoracic aorta.

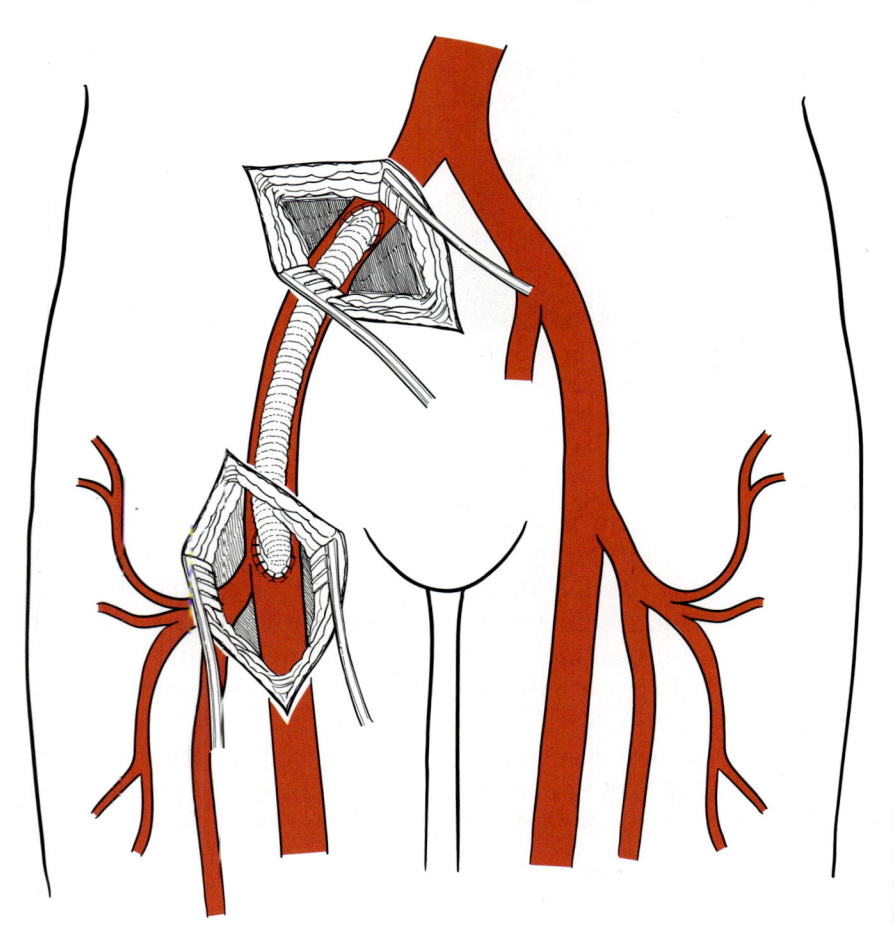

Figure 20-10. A retroperitoneal iliac conduit sewn as an end-to-side bypass graft to the right common femoral artery to create an iliofemoral bypass graft.

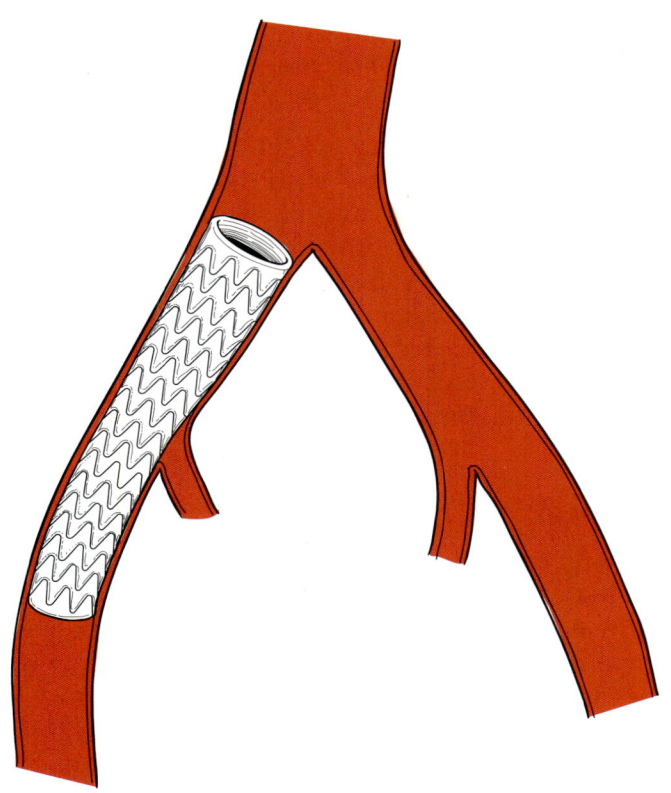

Figure 20-11. Endoconduit is placed in the right common and external iliac arteries using a Viabahn endograft to facilitate dilation of a vessel that may be prone to rupture for subsequent passage of a thoracic endograft.

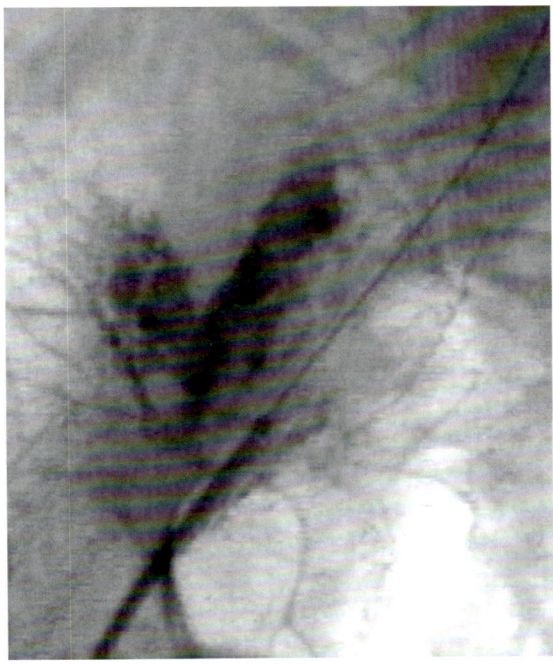

Figure 20-12. A retrograde iliac angiogram demonstrating extravasation of contrast indicative of an iliac artery rupture after removal of a device sheath.

AORTIC TORTUOSITY

Tortuosity of the aorta can often be overcome with the use of superstiff guidewires, such as the Lunderquist wire. This leads to straightening of the iliofemoral system, as well as the thoracoabdominal aorta and the aortic arch, improving the pushability of stent-graft delivery system. Care must be exercised during placement of the wire's tip to avoid iatrogenic injury to the aorta or supraaortic branches, which could lead to aortic rupture or stroke. A curved Lunderquist wire can be used that features a flexible distal tip to minimize the risk of trauma to the aortic arch and aortic valve.

An alternative technique available to manage severe aortic tortuosity is the use of brachiofemoral access wires that can help straighten the most angulated of vessels. This technique, also known as "body floss," involves right brachial artery catheterization, advancement of a 260-cm guidewire and catheter into the descending aorta, and subsequent retrieval of the guidewire from the common femoral artery using a snare or through an arteriotomy (Fig. 20-13). The technique requires that a protective guiding catheter be placed over the brachial artery wire to protect the left subclavian artery from injury. As the delivery sheath is passed into the aorta, firm tension is placed on both ends of the wire to straighten the aorta.

LANDING ZONES

The proximal and distal landing zones must be at least 2 cm long to achieve adequate exclusion of the DTA aneurysm. Insufficient proximal or distal landing zones may necessitate extraanatomic bypass to provide additional fixation length. Minimal tapering of the aortic diameter over the length of the landing zone is also suggested (<15%), and the least amounts of tortuosity and angulation are desirable to ensure adequate exclusion. Additional factors to consider in the evaluation of the landing zones include the presence of thrombus and calcification. Circumferential thrombus and extensive calcification at a landing zone may not allow adequate seal, resulting in endoleaks. Information regarding the characteristics of the landing zones, such as their length and diameter and the presence of thrombus, may be obtained with preoperative imaging. Intraoperative evaluation of the aortic landing zones can also be performed with intravascular ultrasound (IVUS).

Selection and Sizing of an Endovascular Graft

PREOPERATIVE IMAGING

The imaging evaluation of a patient with a DTA is critical for endovascular stent-graft repair. Inaccurate sizing of the diameter or the length of the graft can result in failure to exclude the aneurysm, device migration, device collapse, or inadvertent exclusion of aortic branches. Preoperative imaging with a contrast-enhanced CT scan of the chest, abdomen, and pelvis is usually sufficient for sizing of the aorta for stent-graft repair. However, accurate aortic diameters may be difficult to measure when the aorta transverses through the thoracic cavity, yielding oblique cross sections. The 3D reconstruction of CT scan images provides true orthogonal (short axis) aortic cross-sectional images for the determination of aortic diameters at proximal and distal landing zones (TeraRecon, San Mateo, Calif.; M2S, West Lebanon, N.H.). If a preoperative CT scan is unavailable or CT images are of limited quality, IVUS and contrast angiography may be performed during the DTA stent-graft procedure.

Compared with the diameter of the landing zones, the stent-graft devices are upsized by 10% to 20% to achieve adequate exclusion. Downsizing may result in inadequate exclusion, predisposing the patient to stent-graft migration or endoleak. However, oversizing greater than 20% may be associated with stent-graft collapse or aortic dissection. Available devices enable the safe treatment of aortic diameters between 19 and 43 mm. Stent grafts are generally deployed in a proximal-to-distal sequence. However, if the proximal landing zone is larger than the distal landing zone or precise deployment is required at the level of the celiac artery, it may be advantageous to deploy the stent grafts in a distal-to-proximal sequence.

INTRAOPERATIVE IMAGING

The primary modality of intraoperative imaging for DTA stent-graft repair is fluoroscopy, using either a portable or fixed C arm. IVUS is used routinely to supplement fluoroscopic imaging. IVUS enables measurement of the aortic diameter at the proximal and distal landing zones and the length of the aorta requiring coverage; identification of the aortic branches, such as the left subclavian artery and celiac artery; and identification of calcium or thrombus at the landing zones. IVUS also enables surgeons to limit the intravenous contrast load in patients with compromised renal function (Fig. 20-14).

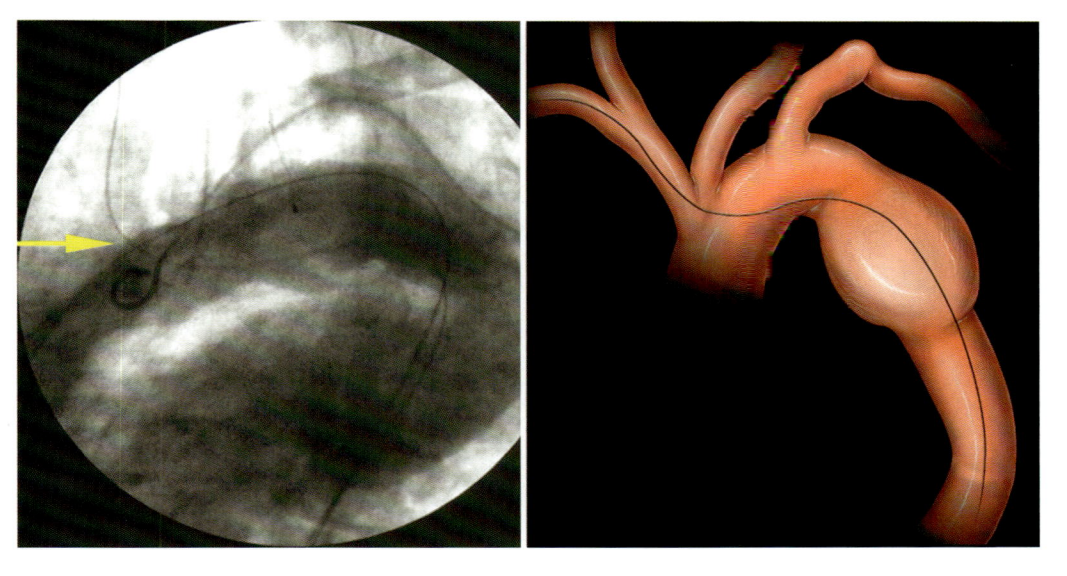

Figure 20-13. Angiogram demonstrating an extremely angulated arch with a large thoracic aortic aneurysm and a brachiofemoral wire *(yellow arrow)* in place.

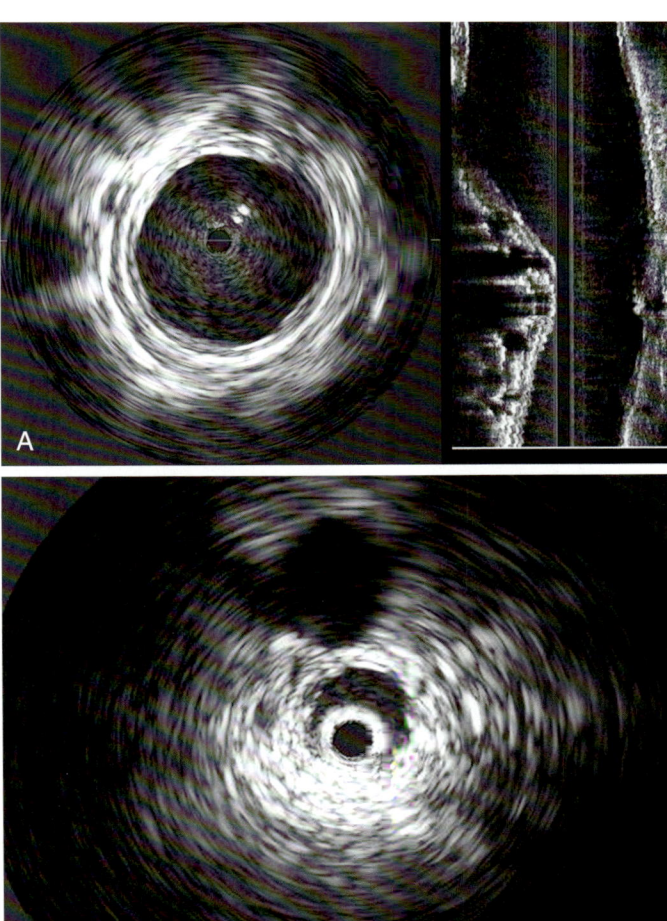

Figure 20-14. A, Intravascular ultrasound (IVUS) demonstrating the distal neck of a thoracic aortic aneurysm with no demonstrable thrombus. **B,** IVUS demonstrating a common iliac artery measuring 8.5 mm without thrombus and with mild calcification.

For optimal angiographic imaging of the aortic arch, the C arm is placed in a left anterior oblique position of 45 to 50 degrees. For imaging of the celiac artery, however, the C arm is placed in a full lateral position. Before deployment, the stent graft is positioned and a diagnostic arteriogram is obtained to confirm the location of the aneurysm and the landing zones. Digital subtraction angiography may be useful to enhance visualization of the aorta and remove background images, including bony structures. Road mapping may also facilitate stent-graft positioning by providing an aortogram image superimposed onto the live image. This enables visualization of the left subclavian and celiac arteries and accurate graft position during deployment (Fig. 20-15).

Endovascular Technique for Repair of a DTA Aneurysm

The femoral artery usually provides adequate vascular access for the deployment of a DTA stent graft. The right common femoral artery is exposed through a small, oblique incision at the level of the inguinal ligament. Proximal and distal control is obtained with umbilical tapes and tourniquets. The right femoral artery is directly punctured with an 18-Ga needle, and a 0.035-inch soft-tip, flexible, angled guidewire is introduced in a retrograde fashion using the Seldinger technique. The wire is positioned into the aortic arch under fluoroscopic guidance. The right femoral artery is cannulated with a 9-Fr sheath. Percutaneous access of the left common femoral artery is performed with an 18-Ga needle, a flexible guidewire, and a 5-Fr sheath using fluoroscopy. Heparin is administered (70 units per kilogram of body weight) to achieve an activated clotted time greater than 200 seconds.

A 5-Fr pigtail catheter is advanced through the left groin sheath into the aortic arch under fluoroscopy. The fluoroscopic C arm is then positioned in a left anterior oblique angle at 45 to 50 degrees, and a thoracic arch aortogram is performed via the 5-Fr pigtail catheter to visualize the orifices of the arch vessels and the DTA aneurysm. Subsequently, IVUS is performed using an 8.2-Fr probe (Volcano Corp., Rancho Cordova, Calif.) through the right-groin 9-Fr sheath to evaluate the size of aneurysm, the presence of thrombus and calcium, the proximal neck diameter and length, and the distal neck diameter and length. An 260-cm Lunderquist Extra Stiff wire is then exchanged through the IVUS catheter and positioned in the ascending aorta.

Next, the right 9-Fr sheath is exchanged for the DTA stent-graft device in the case of current devices from Medtronic Vascular and Cook Medical or for an introducer sheath when using the device produced by W.L. Gore. Once the endograft is in place, but before deployment, an arteriogram is obtained to confirm the location of the aneurysm and position of the endograft in relation to the landing zones. This is facilitated by road mapping for precise deployment. Before stent-graft deployment, systemic blood pressure is reduced to less than 100 mm Hg to minimize device migration. The stent graft is then deployed, and the pigtail is withdrawn over a wire from behind the deployed graft and repositioned within the aortic lumen for the next aortogram.

Should a second stent graft be necessary, it is exchanged with the first device over the Lunderquist guidewire. A minimum overlap of 5 cm is necessary to avoid a type III or junctional endoleak. The landing zones, as well as the junction between endografts, should be ballooned to achieve optimal apposition of the stent grafts and prevent endoleak. Under fluoroscopic guidance, ballooning is performed in a proximal-to-distal sequence. A compliant balloon is used, and aggressive ballooning avoided to minimize the risk of aortic dissection or stent fracture.

A completion angiogram is performed to confirm satisfactory exclusion of the DTA aneurysm and absence of endoleak. The delivery system is then withdrawn from the femoral artery. If a vascular injury is suspected, the Lunderquist guidewire should be left in place. A sheath may then be repositioned in the femoral artery, and a retrograde iliac angiogram can be obtained. Should an arterial injury be identified, proximal control can be achieved with the inflation of an occlusive balloon. If no injury suspected or identified, all wires and sheaths are removed and the right common femoral artery is closed in a transverse fashion with restoration of flow after appropriate prograde and retrograde flushing. The sheath puncture site in the left femoral artery can be managed with direct pressure or through use of a vascular closure device.

DEPLOYMENT OF A GORE TAG ENDOGRAFT

The TAG stent graft is an expanded PTFE tube reinforced with an external nickel-titanium (nitinol) self-expanding stent along the entire surface of the graft. A circumferential PTFE sealing cuff is located on the external surface of the graft at the base of each flared, scalloped end to enhance sealing and eliminate endoleaks. At the base of the flares are two radiopaque gold bands, which serve as guides during implantation and follow-up. The original TAG device graft material was constructed from two PTFE layers with two longitudinal wires. Because of frequent wire fracture, the graft was subsequently redesigned with removal of the wires and the strength and porosity of the graft were modified by adding a third PTFE layer. The TAG graft is available in 26- to 40-mm diameters and in 10-, 15-, and 20-cm lengths. Depending on the device size, an introducer sheath (size 20, 22, or 24 Fr) is required (Fig. 20-16). The stent graft is constrained within a PTFE sleeve.

A deployment knob is located at the control end of the delivery catheter and has a deployment line that runs the entire length of the catheter, connecting it to the sleeve. Turning and then pulling the deployment knob removes the deployment

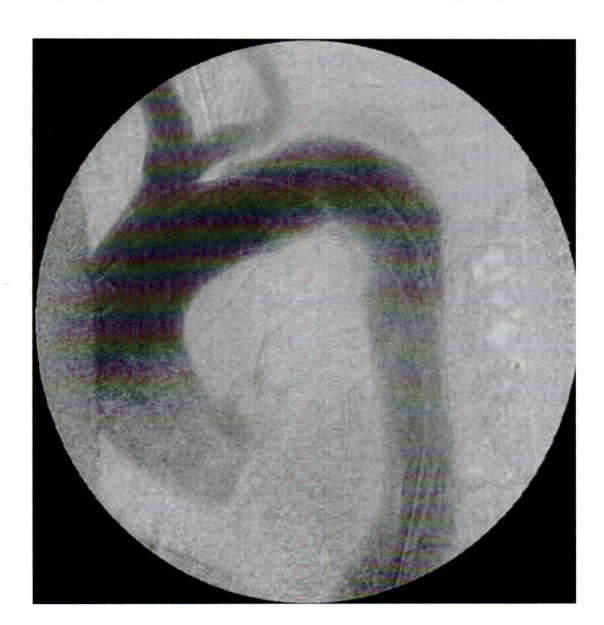

Figure 20-15. An arch angiogram demonstrating a bovine arch with placement of a thoracic endograft across the origin of the left subclavian artery.

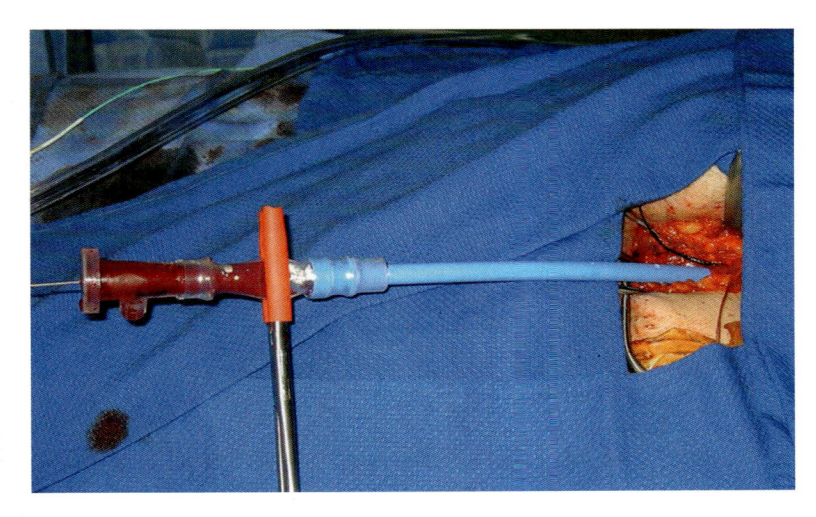

Figure 20-16. A 22-Fr delivery sheath (W.L. Gore) introduced through the femoral artery for deployment of an endoluminal graft.

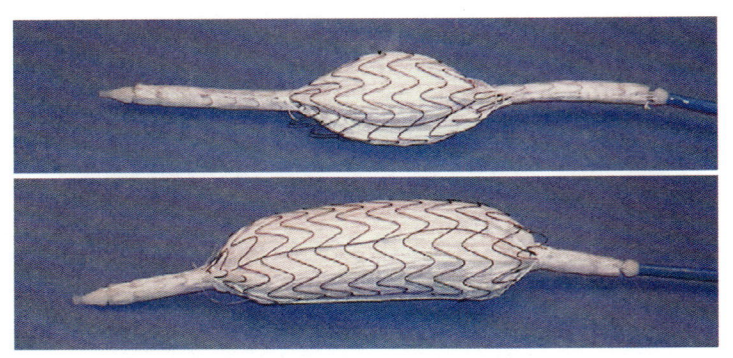

Figure 20-17. A partially deployed TAG device (W.L. Gore).

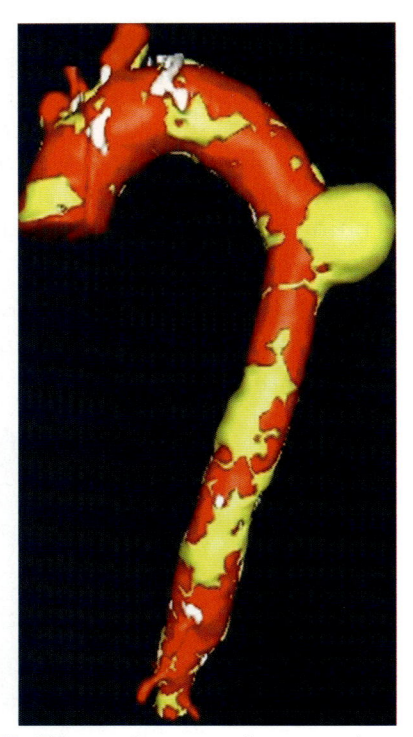

Figure 20-18. A 3D CT scan demonstrating a saccular aneurysm of the DTA.

line from the stent graft, thereby deploying it. The self-expanding deployment mechanism allows the graft to expand centrally and then propagate in both antegrade and retrograde directions simultaneously (Fig. 20-17). Rapid intraluminal expansion of the device minimizes the displacing forces related to high arterial blood flow. When multiple stent grafts of differing diameters are deployed, an overlap of at least 3 cm is recommended. If the deployed devices are of the same diameter, a 5-cm overlap is recommended. Intraluminal profiling and device expansion are performed with a trilobed balloon (W.L. Gore), which permits continuous blood flow during inflation (Figs. 20-18 through 20-20).

DEPLOYMENT OF A ZENITH ENDOGRAFT

The Zenith stent graft is a one-piece (TX1) or two-piece (TX2) modular endovascular graft system. The device is composed of Dacron fabric sewn to self-expanding, stainless steel Z stents. The Z stents are sutured on the external surface of the graft except at the distal and proximal graft margins, where they are attached to the inner surface. Gold radiopaque markers are stationed near the edge of the graft material to enhance visualization of graft ends. Proximal caudally oriented barbs and distal cranially oriented barbs are designed to prevent graft migration.

The TX1 system is intended for use in relatively short DTA aneurysms that are less than 12 cm in length. This device can be up to 202 mm in length. The TX2 system, in which the proximal and distal fixation systems are on separate components, is

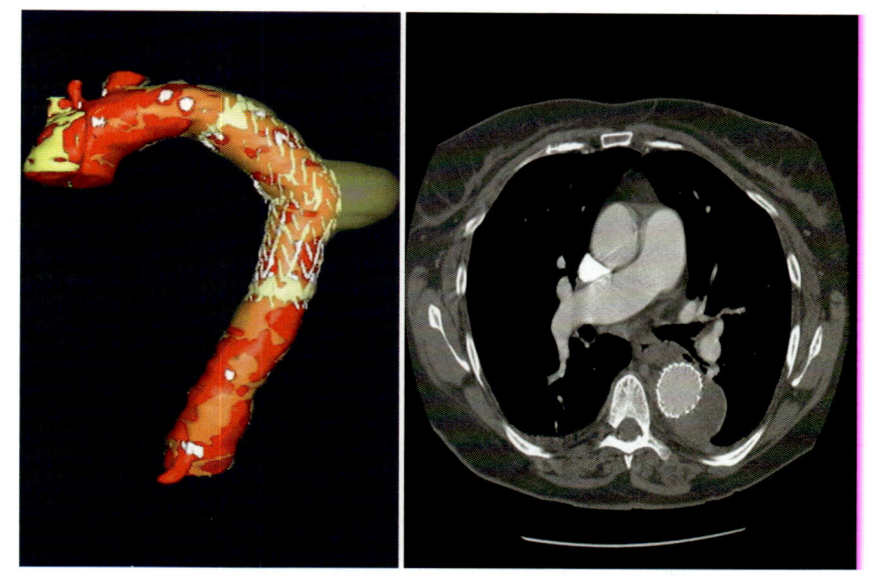

Figure 20-19. Successful exclusion of the descending thoracic aneurysm.

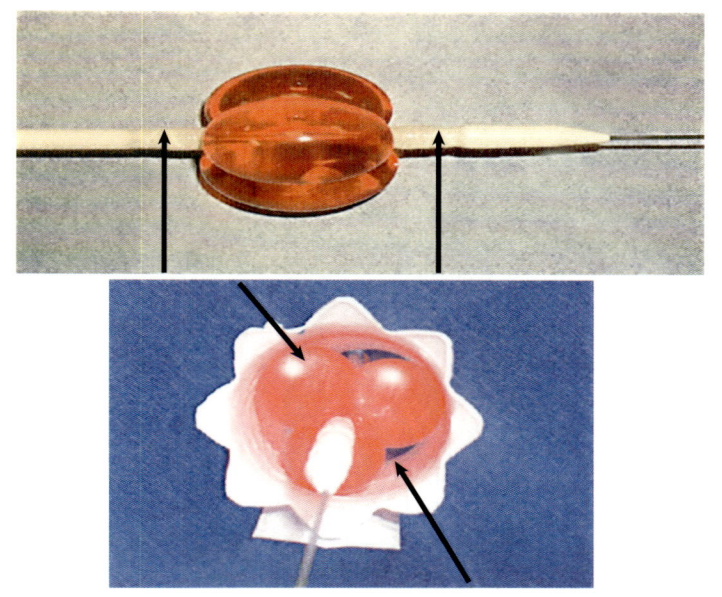

Figure 20-20. A trilobed balloon used for profiling the TAG stent graft (W.L. Gore)

intended to be used for DTA aneurysms longer than 12 cm (Figs. 20-21 through 20-23). The first component (TX2P) is sized from the proximal sealing segment to the distal end of the aneurysm, whereas the distal component (TX2D) is sized from the proximal portion of the aneurysm to the distal seal. TX2D features an optional uncovered distal stent for supplemental fixation. The TX2 components range in length from 120 to 207 mm. The graft diameters range from 22 to 42 mm, and the graft profiles range from 18 to 22 Fr.

The Zenith endograft is introduced through a preloaded sheath with a hydrophilic coating. The devices are attached to the delivery system using trigger wires. The device is deployed by manually retracting the outer sheath of the delivery system while holding the stent graft in position. When positioning is certain, trigger wires are removed to allow release of the metal barbs for secure fixation to the aortic wall. Balloon fixation is usually not required. If two components are used, TX2D is seated within TX2P using a minimum overlap of two stents.

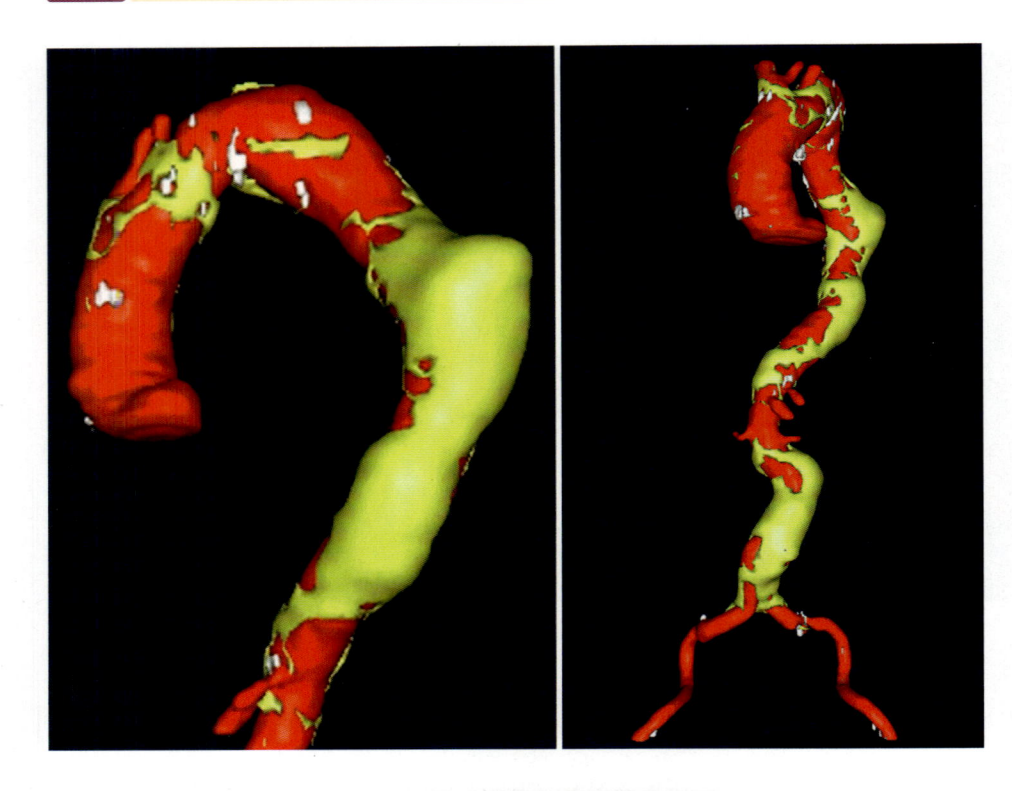

Figure 20-21. A 3D CT scan demonstrating a 6-cm thoracic aortic aneurysm with iliac vessels of adequate size, minimal tortuosity, and calcium.

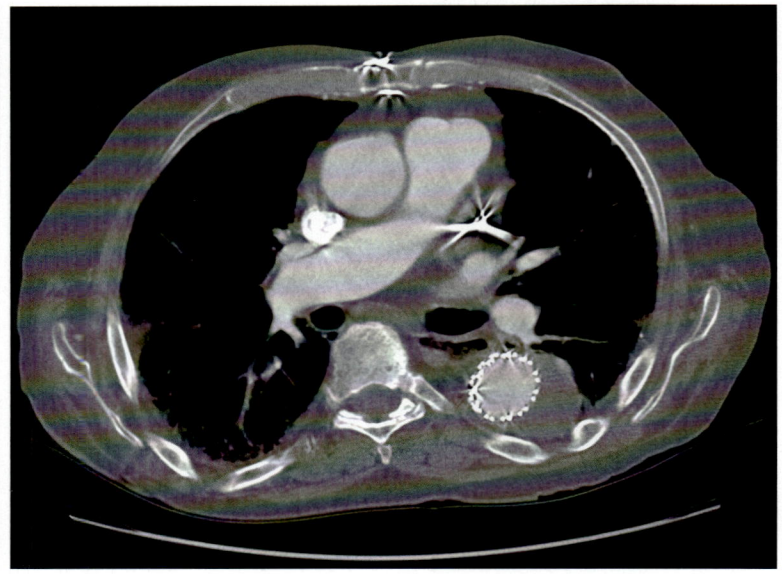

Figure 20-22. Postoperative transverse CT image demonstrating exclusion of a thoracic aneurysm without a detectable endoleak using a TX2 graft (Cook Inc.).

DEPLOYMENT OF A MEDTRONIC VASCULAR ENDOGRAFT

The Talent thoracic stent-graft system (Medtronic Vascular) is composed of a polyester (Dacron) graft sewn to self-expanding nitinol rings interconnected by a longitudinal wire (Fig. 20-24). Radiopaque "figure of 8" markers are sewn to the graft material to aid in visualization during fluoroscopy. The Talent device is a modular system consisting of grafts 22 to 46 mm in diameter and 112 to 116 mm in length. Four graft configurations are available, including proximal and distal main components and proximal and distal extension grafts. The proximal main and distal extension grafts are designed with uncovered bare springs to allow placement of these devices across the left subclavian artery proximally or the celiac artery distally. Each graft is preloaded onto an inner catheter and compressed in a 20- to 25-Fr PTFE sheath. The Talent device is deployed by pulling back an outer catheter via a gearing, ratchetlike mechanism, allowing the device to self-expand and contour to the aorta (Figs. 20-25 through 20-27). A Reliant balloon (Medtronic Vascular) may be used to ensure proper apposition of the graft to the aorta after deployment.

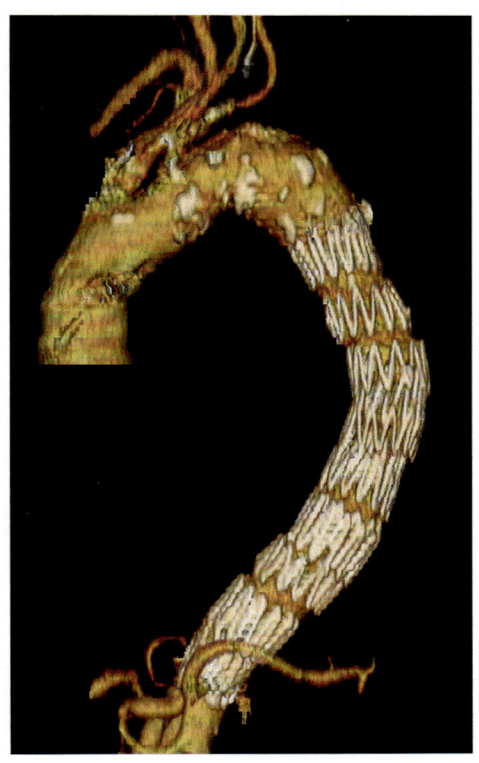

Figure 20-23. Postoperative 3D CT image illustrating treatment of a descending thoracic aneurysm with a TX2 graft (Cook Inc.).

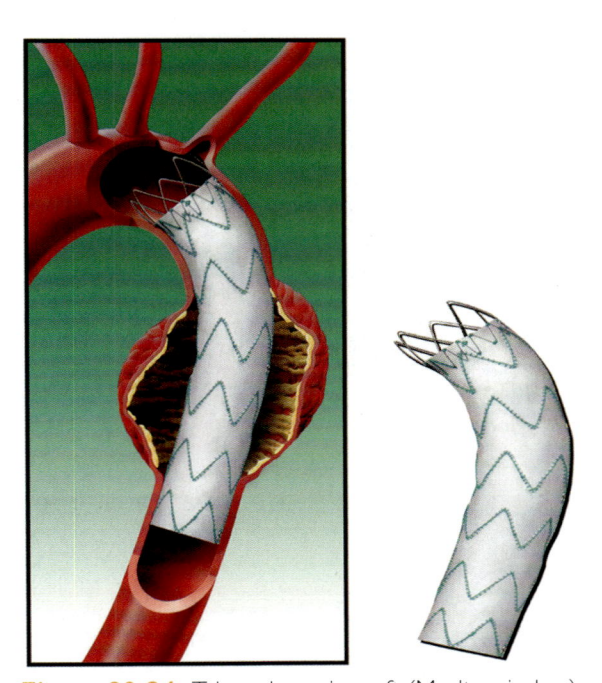

Figure 20-24. Talent thoracic graft (Medtronic, Inc.).

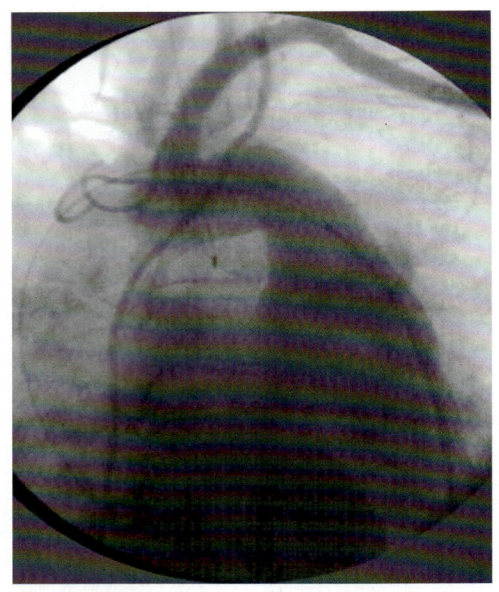

Figure 20-25. Thoracic aortogram demonstrating a descending thoracic aortic aneurysm measuring 9 cm in its maximum diameter.

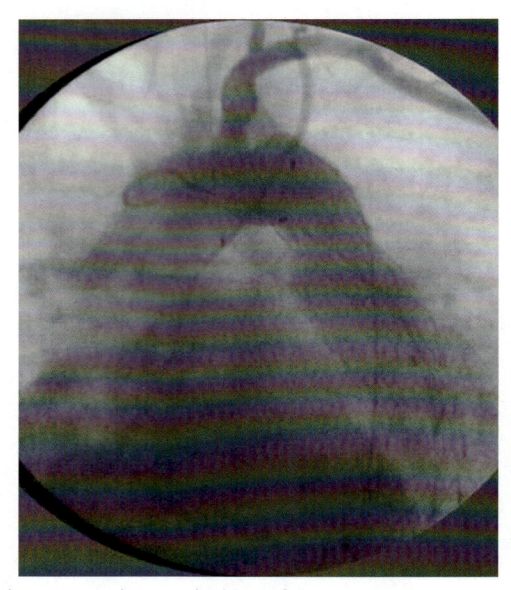

Figure 20-26. Completion angiogram demonstrating exclusion of thoracic aortic aneurysm using a Talent endograft (Medtronic, Inc.).

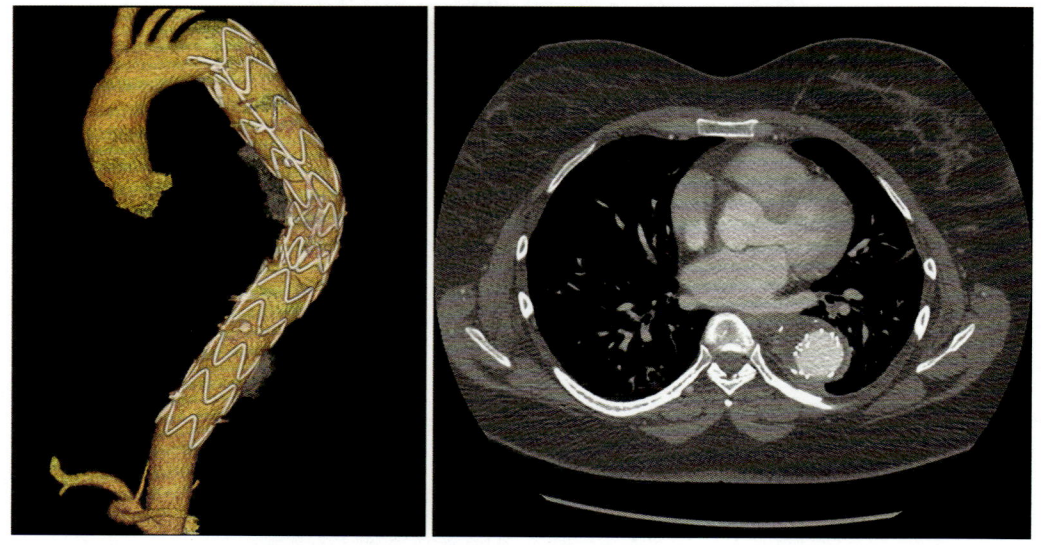

Figure 20-27. CT scan demonstrating exclusion of a thoracic aneurysm without visualized endoleak.

The Valiant thoracic stent-graft system (Medtronic Vascular) has incorporated a number of modifications of the Talent system in an effort to improve deployment accuracy, device flexibility, and technical ease of use. The long connecting bar of the Talent device has been removed, columnar support been optimized through stent spacing, and eight bare peak wires are present, compared with the five bare peak wires found in the Talent stent graft, to reduce force and stress at each point of contact. The Valiant device is available in closed web, straight, and tapered lengths ranging from 100 to 227 mm, and its proximal neck diameters range from 24 to 46 mm with a 2-mm increment. A distal bare spring device is available to avoid covering the celiac artery. Controlled ratcheted deployment is achieved using the Xcelerant delivery system.

Postoperative Care

- **Intensive care unit monitoring.** Patients are monitored in an intensive care unit for 48 hours. Hemodynamic parameters, pulse oximetry, and telemetry are monitored continuously, and standard resuscitation protocols are implemented.
- **Neurologic assessment.** Patients are allowed to emerge from anesthesia expeditiously for early neurologic assessment
- **Spinal cord perfusion.** To optimize collateral spinal cord perfusion, systolic blood pressure is maintained between 140 and 160 mm Hg for the first 48 hours after stent-graft repair. If spinal cord injury is suspected and CSF drainage has not yet been performed, rescue maneuvers include the institution of spinal drainage with maintenance of CSF pressure below 10 mm Hg for 3 days postoperatively, elevation of systemic pressure, volume expansion, and administration of steroid therapy.
- **Postoperative imaging.** Contrast-enhanced CT angiography of the chest, abdomen, and pelvis are obtained on the first or second postoperative day in patients with normal renal function to assess for endoleak and graft positioning.
- **Discharge planning.** Patients are typically discharged on the second or third postoperative day and seen within 2 to 3 weeks to evaluate the incision site.
- **Postoperative surveillance.** Follow-up contrast-enhanced CT scans are obtained at 3, 6, and 12 months and yearly thereafter. Serial CT angiography is the most widely used imaging modality for endoleak detection, although magnetic resonance angiography may also be useful for device surveillance. Published series have noted secondary interventions are required in 6% to 12% of patients after DTA stent-graft repair.[11-18,22]

Complications

- **Mortality, stroke, and paraplegia rates.** Results using the first-generation devices from Stanford University confirmed the feasibility of DTA stent-graft repair, with a reported operative mortality rate of 9%, stroke rate of 7%, and paraplegia rate of 3%.[6,7] Risk factors for death included older age, previous stroke, and designation as a nonoperative candidate. In patients with PAU, the stent-graft operative mortality rate was up to 12%, reflecting a higher-risk population.[10] At the Arizona Heart Institute, rates of operative mortality, stroke, and spinal cord injury after DTA stent-graft repair in 289 patients treated between 2000 and 2006 were 4.8%, 3.8%, and 4.2%, respectively.[14] Early data from the Gore TAG trial suggested that DTA stent-graft repair reduced the perioperative risk compared with open techniques. However, a recent metaanalysis noted similar rate of complications between endovascular and open repair when stratified to anatomic classification of thoracic aneurysm. Gleason and Benjamin[3] compared DTA outcomes from the 5 largest series of open surgical repair (1716 cases) with pooled data from the 17 largest series of endovascular stent-graft repair (1342 cases). Outcomes were nearly identical for open surgery compared with stent-graft repair (operative mortality of 4.8% vs. 6.3% for open vs. stent, $p = 0.51$; paraplegia in 2.9% vs. 1.4% for open vs. stent, $p = 0.11$; stroke in 3.2% vs. 2.4% for open vs. stent, $p = 0.52$).[3]

- **Peripheral vascular complications.** The incidence embolism, thrombosis, and vascular trauma may be as high as 14%.[21]
- **Aortic dissection.** Acute aortic dissection may occur with the use of oversized endografts and aggressive balloon dilatation.
- **Stent-graft migration or fracture.** These can occur with all endografts, and highlights the need for continued surveillance.
- **Endoleak.** At the Arizona Heart Institute, endoleaks were noted in 38 patients (15.3%) in a series of 249 DTA stent-graft patients, including 15 distal type I endoleaks, 13 proximal type I endoleaks, 8 type II endoleaks, and 2 type III endoleaks.[20] Twelve patients (4.8%) required reintervention using an additional stent graft and 4 patients (1.6%) required open conversion. Most type II endoleaks recognized on the initial postoperative CT scan resolve spontaneously. Type II endoleaks that persist can be treated with coil embolization or, if related to retrograde flow from the left subclavian artery, by deployment of a vascular plug via the ipsilateral brachial artery.[19]

REFERENCES

1. DeBakey ME, Cooley DA: Successful resection of aneurysm of thoracic aorta and replacement by graft, *J Am Med Assoc* 152:673-676, 1953.
2. Kulik A, Castner CF, Kouchoukos NT: Replacement of the descending thoracic aorta: Contemporary outcomes using hypothermic circulatory arrest, *J Thorac Cardiovasc Surg* 139:249-255, 2010.
3. Gleason TG, Benjamin LC: Conventional open repair of descending thoracic aortic aneurysms, *Perspect Vasc Surg Endovasc Ther* 19:110-121, 2007.
4. Svensson LG, Kouchoukos NT, Miller DC, et al: Expert consensus document on the treatment of descending thoracic aortic disease using endovascular stent-grafts, *Ann Thorac Surg* 85(Suppl 1):S1-41, 2008.
5. Parodi JC, Palmaz JC, Barone HD: Transfemoral intraluminal graft implantation for abdominal aortic aneurysms, *Ann Vasc Surg* 5:491-499, 1991.
6. Dake MD, Miller DC, Semba CP, et al: Transluminal placement of endovascular stent-grafts for the treatment of descending thoracic aortic aneurysms, *N Engl J Med* 331:1729-1734, 1994.
7. Demers P, Miller DC, Mitchell RS, et al: Midterm results of endovascular repair of descending thoracic aortic aneurysms with first-generation stent grafts, *J Thorac Cardiov Surg* 127:664-673, 2004.
8. Coady MA, Rizzo JA, Hammond GL, et al: Surgical intervention criteria for thoracic aortic aneurysms: A study of growth rates and complications, *Ann Thorac Surg* 67:1922-1926, 1999.
9. Diethrich EB, Ramaiah VG, Kpodonu J, Rodriguez-Lopez JA: Endovascular and hybrid management of the thoracic aorta: A case-based approach, *Hoboken: Blackwell Publishing Ltd*, 2008.
10. Demers P, Miller DC, Mitchell RS, et al: Stent-graft repair of penetrating atherosclerotic ulcers in the descending thoracic aorta: Mid-term results, *Ann Thorac Surg* 77:81-86, 2004.
11. Fattori R, Nienaber CA, Rousseau H, et al: Results of endovascular repair of the thoracic aorta with the Talent Thoracic stent graft: The Talent Thoracic Retrospective Registry, *J Thorac Cardiov Surg* 132:332-339, 2006.
12. Patel HJ, Williams DM, Upchurch GR Jr, et al: Long-term results from a 12-year experience with endovascular therapy for thoracic aortic disease, *Ann Thorac Surg* 82:2147-2153, 2006.
13. Stone DH, Brewster DC, Kwolek CJ, et al: Stent-graft versus open-surgical repair of the thoracic aorta: Mid-term results, *J Vasc Surg* 44:1188-1197, 2006.
14. Wheatley GH III, Gurbuz AT, Rodriguez-Lopez JA, et al: Midterm outcome in 158 consecutive Gore TAG thoracic endoprostheses: Single center experience, *Ann Thorac Surg* 81:1570-1577, 2006.
15. Buth J, Harris PL, Hobo R, et al: Neurologic complications associated with endovascular repair of thoracic aortic pathology: Incidence and risk factors. A study from the European Collaborators on Stent/Graft Techniques for Aortic Aneurysm Repair (EUROSTAR) registry, *J Vasc Surg* 46:1103-1110, 2007.
16. Brown KE, Eskandari MK, Matsumura JS, et al: Short and midterm results with minimally invasive endovascular repair of acute and chronic thoracic aortic pathology, *J Vasc Surg* 47:714-722, 2008.

17. Greenberg RK, Lu Q, Roselli EE, et al: Contemporary analysis of descending thoracic and thoracoabdominal aneurysm repair: A comparison of endovascular and open techniques, *Circulation* 118:808-817, 2008.
18. Hughes GC, Daneshmand MA, Swaminathan M, et al: "Real world" thoracic endografting: Results with the Gore TAG device 2 years after U.S. FDA approval, *Ann Thorac Surg* 86:1530-1537, 2008.
19. Peterson MD, Wheatley GH III, Kpodonu J, et al: Treatment of type II endoleaks associated with left subclavian artery coverage during thoracic aortic stent grafting, *J Thorac Cardiov Surg* 136:1193-1199, 2008.
20. Preventza O, Wheatley GH III, Ramaiah VG, et al: Management of endoleaks associated with endovascular treatment of descending thoracic aortic diseases, *J Vasc Surg* 48:69-73, Jul 2008.
21. Bavaria JE, Appoo JJ, Makaroun MS, et al: Endovascular stent grafting versus open surgical repair of descending thoracic aortic aneurysms in low-risk patients: A multicenter comparative trial, *J Thorac Cardiov Surg* 133:369-377, 2007.
22. Makaroun MS, Dillavou ED, Wheatley GH, et al: Five-year results of endovascular treatment with the Gore TAG device compared with open repair of thoracic aortic aneurysms, *J Vasc Surg* 47:912-918, 2008.

21 Endovascular Treatment of Aortic Dissection

KARTHIKESHWAR KASIRAJAN

Historical Background

Acute dissection of the thoracic aorta was first described by Nichools (1699-1778) in referring to the autopsy findings of King George II. Traditionally, acute uncomplicated type B dissection has been managed medically with an effective medical regimen directed toward lowering blood pressure and dP/dt first introduced by Palmer and Wheat in 1967.[1] The 30-day mortality for acute uncomplicated type B dissection decreased from 40% in the 1960s to less than 10% at present. However, between 20% and 30% of patients remain at risk for developing a delayed aneurysm, with catastrophic aortic rupture in approximately 18% of patients. Dialetto and associates[2] reported that 28.5% of uncomplicated type B dissections managed medically progress to aneurysmal dilatation at a mean of 18.1 ± 16.9 months. Risk factors for aneurysmal degeneration were patency of the false lumen and distal aortic diameter of 40 to 45 mm or larger.

The first attempt at surgical repair was reported in 1935 by Gurin and colleagues,[3] who created a distal reentry point in the iliac artery to decompress the false lumen. Similar to early attempts to contain abdominal aortic aneurysms by cellophane wrapping, this technique was attempted by Abbott in 1949.[4] In 1955 DeBakey and co-workers[5] introduced a revolutionary surgical treatment that involved excision of the intimal tear, obliteration of the false lumen, and either direct reanastomosis or insertion of a prosthetic graft. Nevertheless, open surgery for symptomatic type B thoracic aortic dissection carries a mortality rate of 20% to 80%, especially in the presence of bowel ischemia. This motivated the development of less invasive techniques, such as fenestration and endovascular stent-graft therapy. The first series that described thoracic endovascular aortic repair (TEVAR) for treatment of type B aortic dissection was reported by Dake and associates in 1999.[6]

Indications

Medical management of uncomplicated type B thoracic aortic dissection remains the current standard of care, although the role of endovascular grafting for such patients is an active area of clinical investigation.[7-9] Indications for intervention include symptomatic type B dissection that manifests with aortic rupture or end-organ ischemia to the limbs or the gut (Box 21-1). Endovascular intervention, when feasible, is preferred over open surgical repair for symptomatic disease due to its lower risk of mortality and morbidity.[10-11] However, an extraanatomic axillofemoral or femoral-femoral bypass remains an option for the treatment of isolated lower extremity ischemia in the presence of type B thoracic aortic dissection. Persistent chest pain, despite adequate blood pressure management, has been considered an indication for intervention. However, wide variation exists in the definition of persistent pain from 48 hours to 14 days. TEVAR should be used in patients with syndromic connective tissue disorders only when other options are not practical. In contrast to type B dissections, all type A dissections are managed by immediate referral for direct surgical repair.

| Box 21-1 | INDICATIONS FOR THORACIC STENT-GRAFT PLACEMENT |

- Rupture
- Limb ischemia
- Visceral ischemia
- Acute false lumen enlargement
- Penetrating ulcer
- Aortic diameter >4 cm at site of thoracic dissection
- Refractory hypertension with back pain
- Persistent back pain despite adequate blood pressure control
- Partial false lumen thrombosis

Preoperative Preparation

- **Intensive care unit monitoring.** Suspicion of acute aortic dissection should involve immediate admission to the intensive care unit with blood pressure control and diagnostic evaluation.
- **Considerations in the differential diagnosis.** Other causes for chest and back pain need to be excluded, such as acute myocardial infarction (electrocardiogram or cardiac enzymes) and pulmonary embolism (chest computed tomography [CT] angiogram).
- **Pain and blood pressure control.** Immediate pain and blood pressure control can be achieved with morphine sulfate and intravenous beta-blockers (labetalol, metoprolol, or esmolol). Refractory hypertension requires vasodilating drugs (sodium nitroprusside) or angiotensin-converting enzyme inhibitors. Medical therapy should remain the first line of treatment in patients with uncomplicated acute type B dissection. Abdominal pain in the presence of type B dissection carries the diagnosis of bowel ischemia until proven otherwise.
- **Preoperative hydration.** The risk of renal dissection, presence of hypotension, and use of contrast for preoperative and intraoperative imaging can result in acute renal failure. Special attention to adequate hydration is mandatory.
- **Imaging.** A transesophageal echo can confirm the diagnosis of aortic dissection and discern between types A and B dissections.[12] Nonetheless, a multidetector CT scan provides the best assessment of the thoracic aorta, with 64-slice multidetector technology capable of providing a CT angiogram from neck to groin in about 1 minute. CT imaging confirms the diagnosis, differentiates between type A and type B dissection, and identifies branch vessel involvement and possible contained rupture.

Pitfalls and Danger Points

- **Visceral ischemia.** Abdominal pain in the presence of type B dissection carries the diagnosis of bowel ischemia until proven otherwise. Patients need an initial CT diagnosis, followed by stent-graft exclusion of the entry point in the thoracic aorta, and may require exploratory laparotomy. If gut hypoperfusion persists despite proximal stent-graft exclusion and true lumen enlargement, stenting of the visceral vessel into the true lumen is recommended (Fig. 21-1). Visceral bypass may be required when extensive dissection into the branch vessel has occurred. In the presence of dead bowel, resection and a second look laparotomy is the preferred approach.
- **Differentiating between the true and the false lumen of the thoracic aorta.** Deployment of the stent graft in the true lumen with exclusion of the entry tear is axiomatic in TEVAR of dissection. The operator should

276 THE THORACIC AORTA

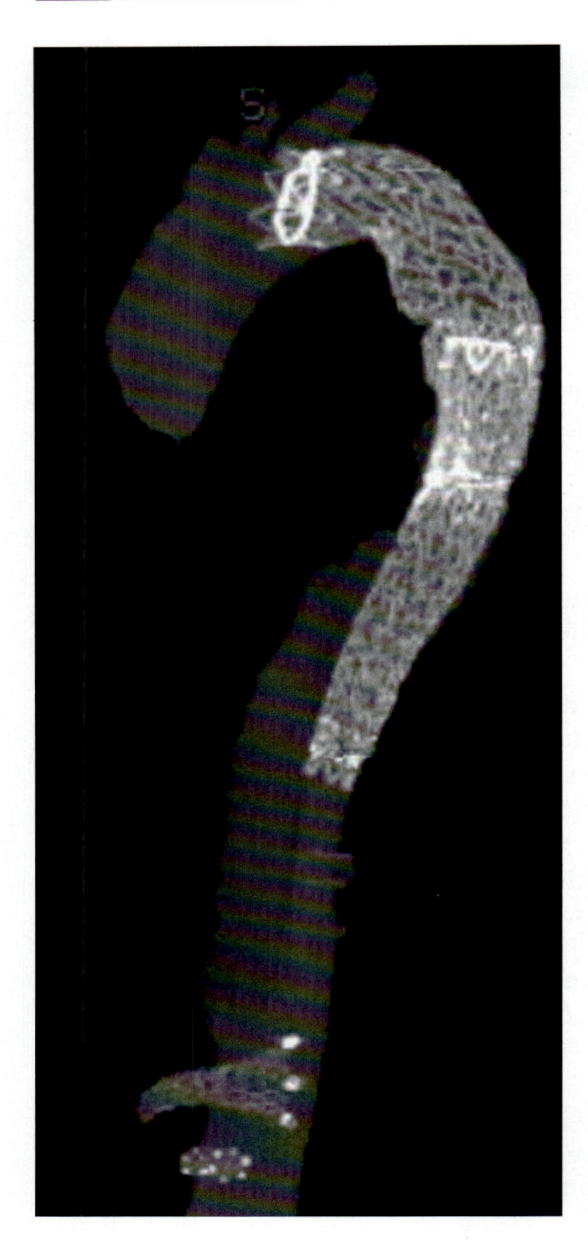

Figure 21-1. Proximal thoracic stent-graft exclusion of the entry tear with additional stents placed into the superior mesenteric artery and celiac axis for intestinal ischemia. Note the location of the visceral stents, extending across the false lumen into the true lumen.

understand the relative orientations of true and false lumen as depicted on the CT angiogram and verify this orientation intraoperatively with intravascular ultrasound (IVUS). The true lumen is typically smaller than the false lumen and darker in contrast (Fig. 21-2). During initial guidewire manipulation, if the wire is located in the false lumen, it typically does not easily follow the arch to the ascending aorta but instead curls just distal to the left subclavian artery. However, the absence of this sign should not be used as a confirmation of true lumen catheterization. Reliable guidewire positioning in the true lumen includes careful assessment of the CT angiogram to select the appropriate access vessel, intraoperative verification by IVUS imaging, and right brachial access if retrograde transfemoral passage does not reliably afford true lumen wire position. On the arch angiogram, contrast first fills the true lumen and typically fills the false lumen a few seconds later (Fig. 21-3). It is vital to confirm that the guidewire is located in the true lumen from the femoral artery to the arch, and IVUS is the most reliable predictor of the guidewire's course. Inability to adequately differentiate true from false lumen can result in a variety of complications, including rupture, creation of large reentry tears, development of type A dissection, and acute true lumen occlusion (Fig. 21-4).

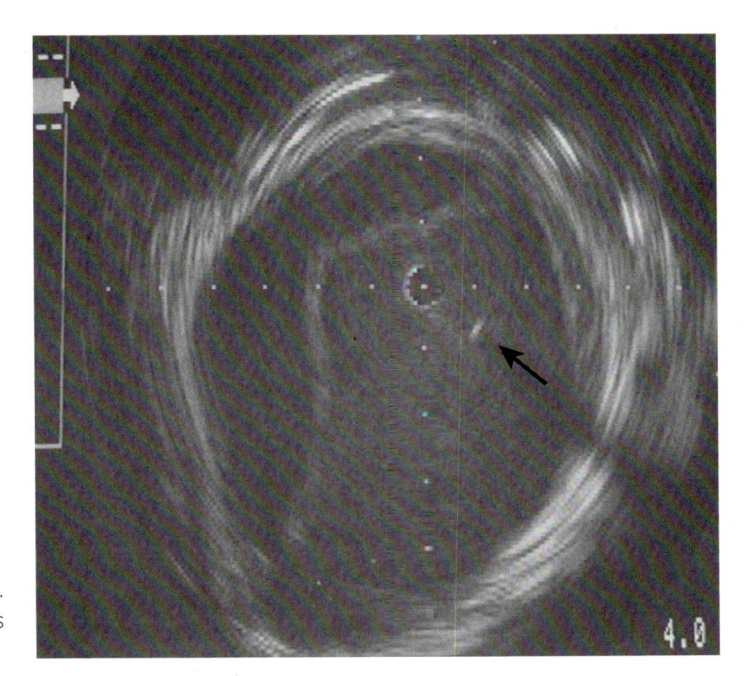

ENDOVASCULAR TREATMENT OF AORTIC DISSECTION   277

Figure 21-2. IVUS catheter located in the false lumen *(arrow)*. Typically, the false lumen is the larger of the two lumens and is lighter in tone.

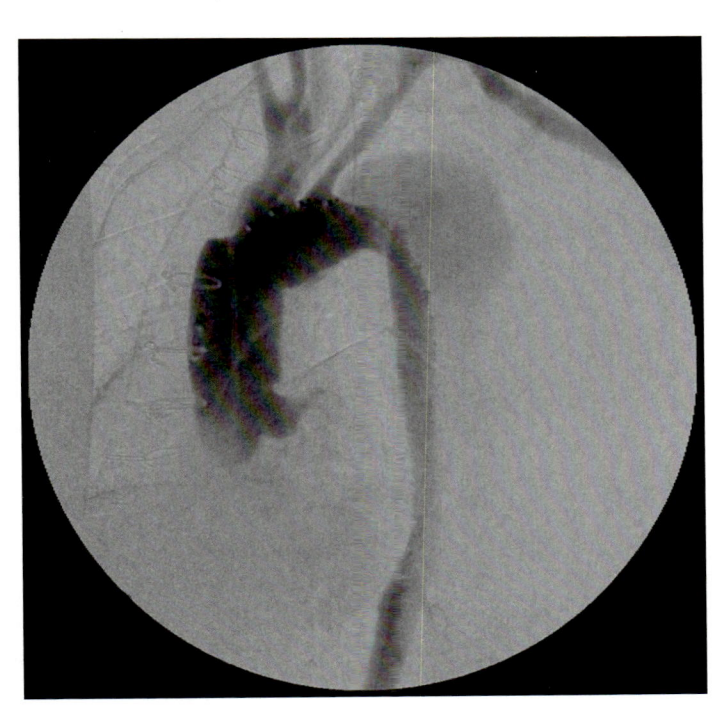

Figure 21-3. Diagnostic angiogram demonstrating rapid early filling of the relatively compressed true lumen, with delayed blush seen in the false lumen.

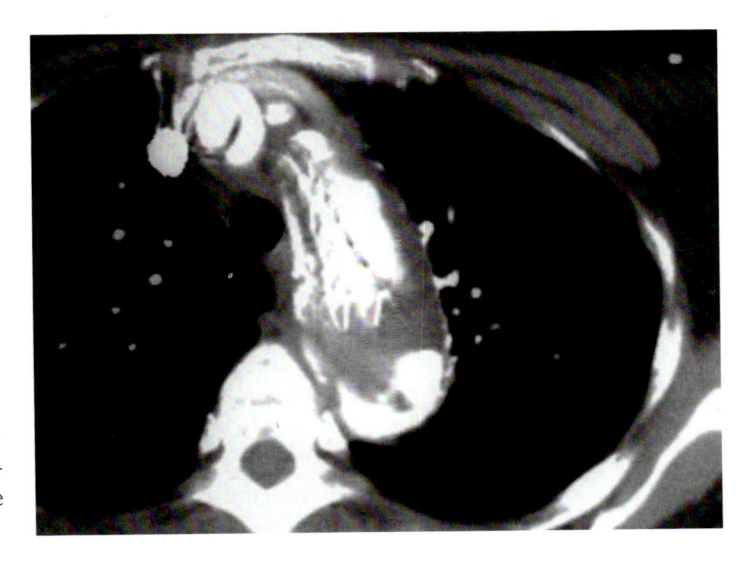

Figure 21-4. Acute true lumen compression with inadvertent stent-graft deployment in the false lumen and acute type A conversion.

- **Arterial access.** Large-diameter devices require large access sheaths. The most frequently encountered complication in thoracic stent-graft trials has involved iliofemoral access-related complications. Vascular trauma or thrombosis of the iliac vessels was noted in 14% of patients in the W.L. Gore-sponsored TEVAR multicenter trial. Femoral access complications most commonly are encountered when using a 24-Fr sheath in patients with borderline iliac diameters. Smaller iliac diameters, combined with calcification and tortuosity, further increase the risk of iliac dissection or rupture. Preoperative planning should involve CT imaging to the level of the common femoral artery. Both contrast and noncontrast CT scans need to be evaluated to assess the smallest iliac diameter and extent of calcification. Tortuosity is best evaluated with a three-dimensional reconstruction or conventional angiogram. As a rule, if a conduit is thought to be necessary, it is almost always necessary. It is also important to watch the sheath move into the aorta at all times using fluoroscopy. The sheath is ideally introduced over a stiff Lunderquist or Meier wire. Most iliac artery injuries are commonly noticed during sheath withdrawal. Hence, if excessive force is required to introduce a sheath, despite the sheath moving forward, an iliac tear may be encountered during sheath withdrawal. If the sheath is not easily withdrawn, it may be advisable to plan for an iliac artery exposure with the sheath in place or to have a contralateral femoral sheath (12 Fr) and an aortic Reliant or Coda occlusion balloon readily available for emergency control of the aorta. It is also important not to lose wire access, because iliac artery injuries may be temporarily tamponaded by reintroducing the sheath and dilator until a definitive repair is undertaken.
- **Iliac artery pseudoaneurysm.** During sheath withdrawal an intimal flap may be noted adherent to the sheath. After the closure of the femoral arteriotomy, a completion pelvic angiogram may identify an iliac artery pseudoaneurysm that may result in delayed rupture. If two or more devices are required, an introducer sheath is advisable to prevent trauma to the iliac or femoral artery during each subsequent introduction.
- **Vascular tortuosity.** The descending thoracic aorta can have acute angles that may prevent the device from easily tracking across the curvatures. Various maneuvers may help overcome this problem. First, use of a stiffer Lunderquist wire placed proximally in the aortic root may provide more support. If this does not help, the use of a stiff "buddy wire" from the contralateral femoral access may help straighten the descending thoracic aorta. Lastly, the use of a brachio-femoral wire ("body floss" technique) may prevent buckling of the wire in the descending thoracic aorta. Because most patients with an acute type B dissection have minimal atherosclerotic arch disease, the risk of arch embolization may be lower than in patients with thoracic aneurysms. Right brachial artery access via a percutaneous sheath allows easy cannulation of the true lumen, especially in patients with difficult true lumen catheterization via the femoral route. Significantly, this technique frequently allows the device to track across a tortuous descending thoracic aorta by preventing the wire from buckling.
- **Avoiding the generation of a de novo type A dissection.** Routine ballooning of endografts in patients with dissection may not be advisable, especially in the proximal location, because this carries the risk of producing a cerebrovascular accident or type A conversion (Fig. 21-5). Ballooning should be reserved for treatment of an endoleak or inadequate graft expansion. Mean blood pressure below 70 mm Hg also helps prevent proximal extension of the dissection flap during the endograft procedure, as well as reduce the risk of distal graft migration.

Endovascular Strategy

PREOPERATIVE IMAGING

CT angiography is the initial imaging modality of choice. Magnetic resonance angiography is valuable in patients with severe iodinated contrast allergy, renal

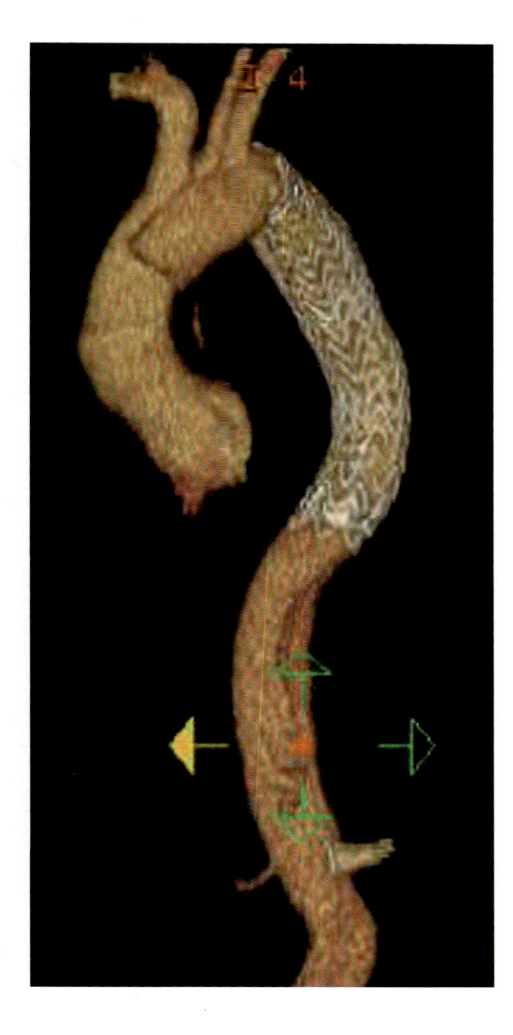

Figure 21-5. Proximal extension of the dissection into the arch as a complication of balloon dilatation of the proximal seal zone.

failure, or pregnancy. Magnetic resonance angiography has less spatial resolution than CT angiography. In addition, magnetic resonance angiography is sensitive to the presence of metal, with surgical clips and stents producing significant image artifacts. Patients with pacemakers, defibrillators, and certain cardiac valves cannot undergo a magnetic resonance angiography. CT imaging is generally preferred for evaluation of branch vessels and obtaining measurements for stent-graft placement. Echocardiography is often limited to the unstable patient or unreliable CT or magnetic resonance imaging because of excessive patient movement. Intraoperative transesophageal echocardiography can help exclude type A dissection after stent-graft placement.

DIFFERENTIATING BETWEEN TYPE A AND TYPE B DISSECTIONS

Type A dissection remains treatable solely by open surgery, and it is rare that type A dissection manifests with an isolated entry point in the descending aorta. Stent grafts inserted in the descending thoracic aorta for type A dissection can often be fatal because of abrupt closure of the exit point, resulting in rapid pressurization of the false lumen in the ascending aorta with attendant aortic valve insufficiency and aortic rupture into the pericardial space.

DEFINING THE EXTENT OF TREATMENT

The extent of coverage depends on the indication. Generally, coverage of the entry tear promotes false lumen thrombosis and aortic remodeling (Fig. 21-6). Most tears occur a few centimeters distal to the left subclavian artery. This portion of the thoracic aorta is usually highly angulated, because it represents the transition from the arch to the descending thoracic aorta, and it is best to avoid landing stent grafts in this angle. The stent graft is preferably landed just distal

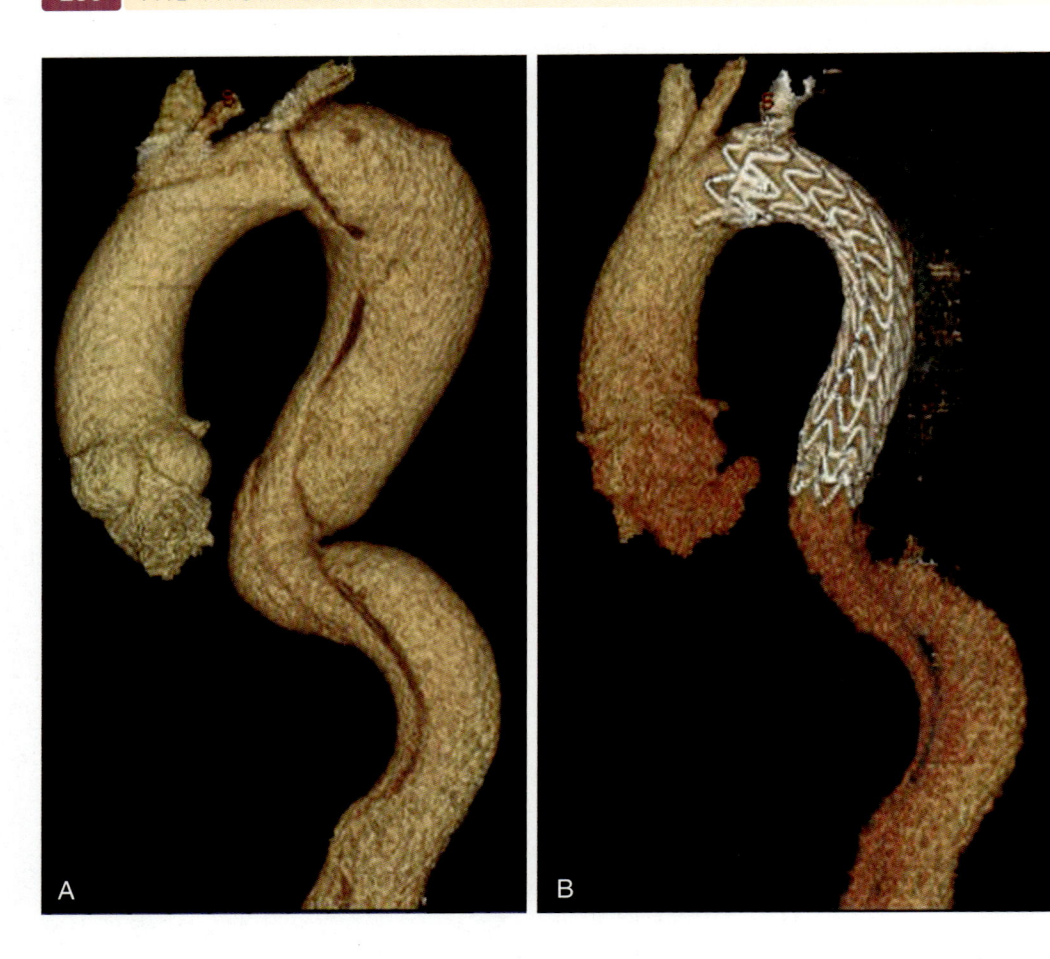

Figure 21-6. A, Typical CT scan appearance of an acute type B dissection with the entry point just distal to the left subclavian artery. **B,** Stent-graft elimination of the entry point typically causes false lumen thrombosis across the stented segment, despite distal reentry points.

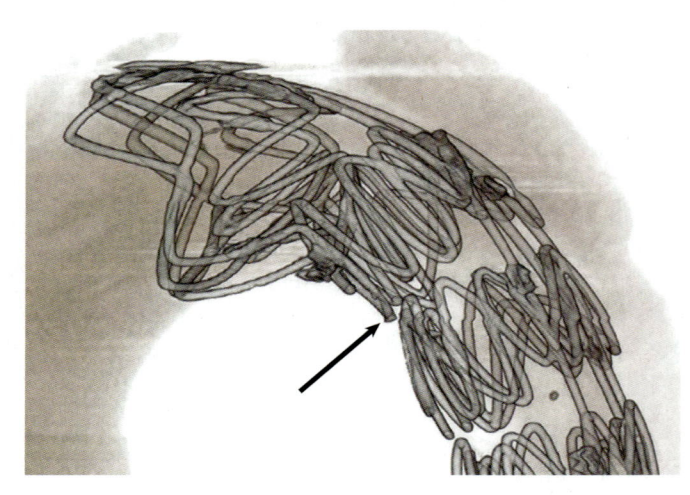

Figure 21-7. Proximal wire flip noted *(arrow)* along the inner curve of the aorta because of improper selection of the proximal landing zone.

to the origin of the left common carotid artery. This allows the proximal portion of the stent graft to have circumferential wall opposition. Landing the stent graft distal to this location may result in inadequate inner curve opposition that may result in stent-graft compression or collapse, acute type A conversion, or anchor wire flips (Fig. 21-7). The portion of the aorta just distal to the left common carotid artery and proximal to the distal end of the left subclavian artery provides the most stable landing zone. This requires a carotid-subclavian bypass in certain patient subsets (Box 21-2). Thoracic stent grafts 15 cm in length are often adequate, and it is best to use a stent graft that is less than 20 cm in length. The only exception to this rule is free rupture, where coverage is advisable from a point distal to the left common carotid artery to the celiac axis. This posture relates to the fact that the extent of coverage in patients with aortic dissection has been correlated with an increased incidence of paraplegia because of the presence of multiple open intercostal vessels.

Box 21-2	ARCH VESSEL RELOCATION TO EXTEND THE PROXIMAL THORACIC ENDOVASCULAR AORTIC REPAIR LANDING ZONE

Total

Ascending aorta to innominate and left common carotid arteries

Partial

Carotid-subclavian bypass
Carotid-carotid bypass
Carotid-axillary bypass

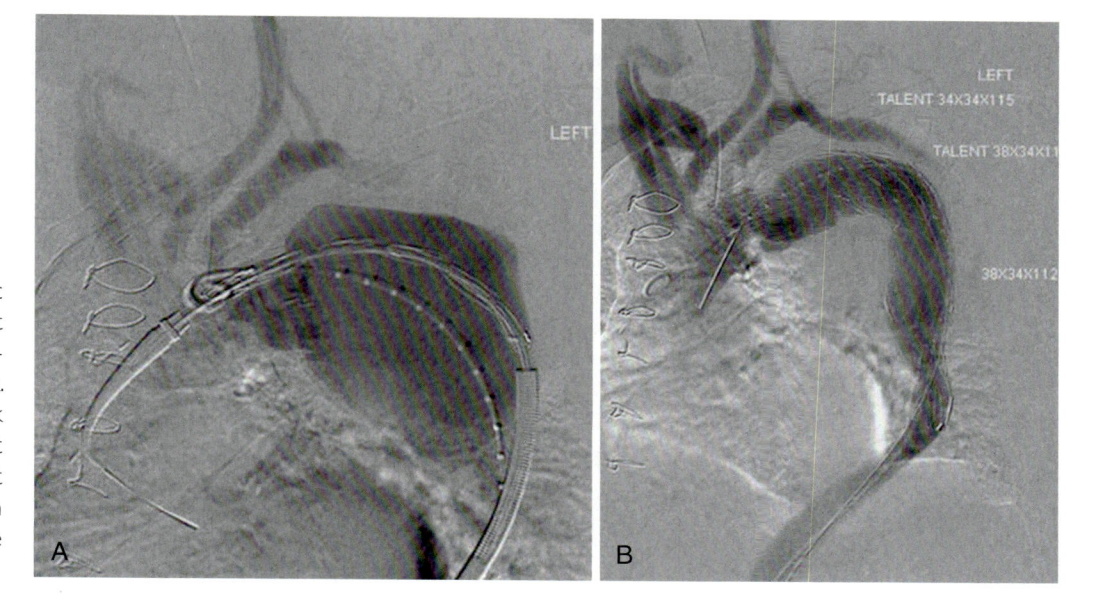

Figure 21-8. A, Diagnostic angiogram with thoracic stent graft in place before deployment in the elephant trunk. Note metal clips used to mark the distal end of the elephant trunk. **B,** Thoracic stent-graft exclusion of the false lumen with a proximal landing zone in the elephant trunk.

THORACIC ENDOVASCULAR AORTIC REPAIR AFTER ELEPHANT TRUNK REPAIR

Thoracic stent grafts are well suited for the second stage of the elephant trunk procedure. After an arch replacement, the distal end of the graft that is left free floating in the proximal portion of the descending aorta can be used as the proximal landing zone (Fig. 21-8, A). This requires a few important steps during the initial operative intervention for arch replacement. The elephant trunk needs to be at least 6 cm long at the time of the open procedure, because these grafts have a tendency to foreshorten after implantation. Radiopaque markers placed at the distal end of the elephant trunk make cannulation and stent-graft placement easier. During the stent-graft procedure, difficulty may be encountered in cannulating the elephant trunk from the femoral approach, because the graft floats freely within the descending thoracic aorta. A transbrachial wire quickly solves this problem, preferably using a right brachial artery access, which allows easier C arm mobility and straight cannulation of the elephant trunk. This wire can be tracked to the exposed femoral artery or snared via a separate femoral snare and then used to deliver the stent graft. Endograft coverage should include at least 2 cm of the Dacron graft and extend 15 to 20 cm distally (Fig. 21-8).

FENESTRATION OR ENDOGRAFT REPAIR

Fenestration was one of the first percutaneous options described for the treatment of patients with malperfusion syndromes. This technique has largely been abandoned in favor of thoracic stent-graft therapy and selective branch vessel stenting. Fenestration, if performed, is done close to the target organ that is compromised. For example, a thoracic aortic fenestration is often ineffective in relieving limb ischemia. Fenestration for limb ischemia needs to be performed close to the aortic bifurcation. Fenestration is rarely required to relieve end-organ ischemia and should be avoided if possible. Extensive areas of fenestration in the thoracic aorta and the visceral segment often result in rapid false lumen enlargement during follow-up. In patients with prior fenestration and false lumen aneurysm, few endovascular options are available, leading to a complex open procedure.

AVOIDING STROKE

Stroke continues to be one of the major adverse events after proximal thoracic stent-graft procedures. Unlike paraplegia after TEVAR, the vast majority of strokes are irreversible, making them debilitating events. Hence, identifying patients at high risk for a stroke is important. Dissection patients are unique in that left subclavian coverage is often required. This results in an acute interruption in the blood flow to the left vertebral artery unless a carotid-subclavian bypass has been performed. Current data do not support the routine use of carotid-subclavian bypass in all patients, requiring sacrifice of the left subclavian artery. However, attention needs to be paid to certain critical anatomic variations of the vertebral arteries that can result in a devastating stroke unless recognized. These include (1) dominant left vertebral artery, (2) left vertebral artery ending in the posterior inferior cerebellar artery (PICA) and not the basilar artery (sacrificing this vessel can result in a left vertebrobasilar stroke), (3) right vertebral artery terminating in the PICA (sacrificing the left vertebral artery can result in an extensive brainstem infarct), and (4) innominate or right subclavian occlusion or stenosis. A computed tomography, magnetic resonance, or intraoperative angiogram demonstrating the cervical and intracranial portions of both vertebral arteries is mandatory before covering the left subclavian artery. If any of the preceding variants is noted, a left carotid-to-subclavian revascularization can prevent a devastating stroke. Fortunately, carotid-subclavian bypass procedures are required in less than 10% of patients for the previously mentioned indications.

In addition, patients with extensive atherosclerosis of the arch should have limited arch manipulation with wires, catheters, and the stent graft. In such patients, bare spring devices that allow transcarotid fixation should not be used. Balloon dilatation of the proximal portion of the stent graft also has the potential for releasing debris to the brain and should be avoided in patients with dissection and in those with extensive plaque burden in the arch.

AVOIDING PARAPLEGIA

Unlike with degenerative aneurysm, the extent of TEVAR coverage in patients with dissection can predict the risk of paraplegia. Degenerative aneurysms typically have extensive intraluminal thrombus, resulting in occlusion of intercostals to a varied degree. This preocclusive state of intercostal vessels minimizes the risk of paraplegia in most patients with degenerative aneurysms. Unlike a degenerative aneurysm, most intercostal vessels are open in patients with dissection. Hence, long-segment coverage can often result in paraparesis or paraplegia. With the exception of rupture, stent-graft coverage is limited to 15 or 20 cm. Only proximal entry point coverage is required in most patients. In the acute phase this can result in total aortic remodeling despite the presence of reentry points in most patients.[13-15] Routine cerebrospinal fluid drainage is not required, given the low risk of paraplegia (<2%) with short-segment entry point coverage. Motor- and sensory-evoked potentials are not routinely performed, because the predictive value has not been well established. In addition, TEVAR for dissections may be conducted under local anesthesia unless a left subclavian artery revascularization is required, preventing the use of motor- or sensory-evoked potentials.

AVOIDING RUPTURE

TEVAR for rupture requires extensive coverage from the left common carotid artery to the celiac axis to prevent flow to the false lumen from reentry points. An abdominal aortogram in these patients often indicates an iliac artery reentry that

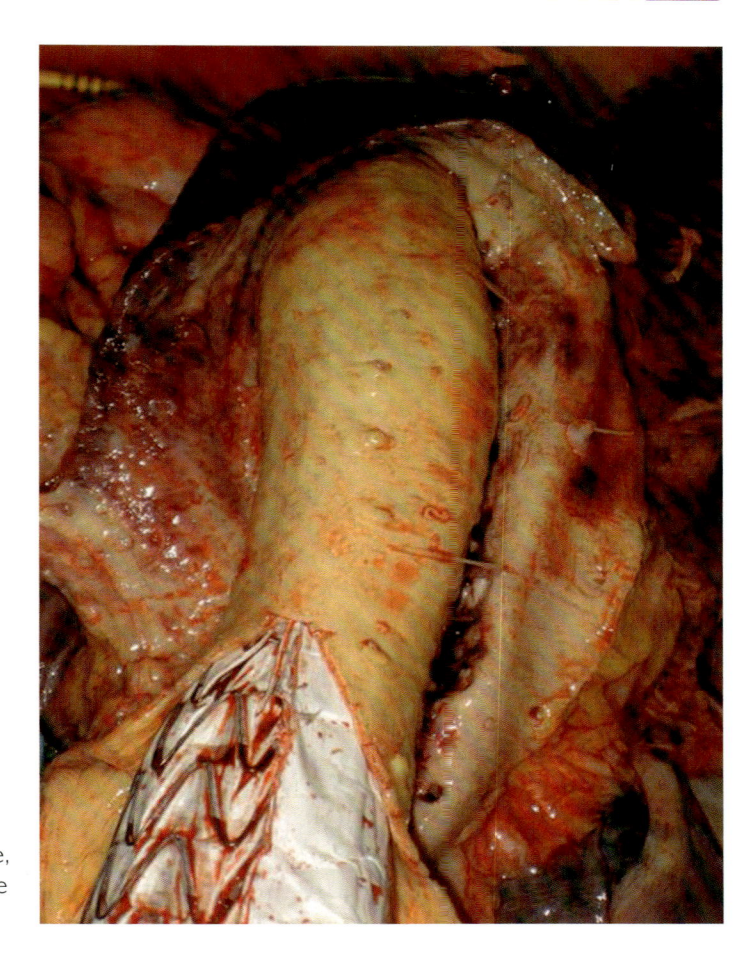

Figure 21-9. Aggressive balloon dilatation resulting in rupture, evident in the splitting of the septum between true and false lumen.

may also require placement of a covered stent. Because of the risk of paraplegia, routine cerebrospinal fluid drains are placed after TEVAR and correction of coagulopathy.

Iatrogenic rupture can also occur with improper wire and sheath manipulation. It is common for the initial wire to be located in the false lumen. IVUS helps confirm the position of the wire in the true lumen. As mentioned earlier, the true lumen on IVUS is typically the smaller of the two channels and is often darker in contrast because of laminar flow patterns. Excessive manipulation in the false lumen or inadvertent sheath or endograft insertion in the false lumen can result in rupture because of the fragile nature of the false lumen. The leading point of all inserted devices always needs to be fluoroscopically visualized during manipulation and advancement to avoid perforation or rupture. Aggressive balloon dilatation should also be avoided to prevent rupture at the distal end of the stent graft (Fig. 21-9).

AVOIDING VISCERAL ISCHEMIA

Visceral ischemia can involve the celiac artery, superior mesenteric artery, or renal arteries. Any patient with complaints of abdominal pain should be considered to have bowel blood flow compromise to the intestines. The arterial flow pattern can be easily determined by preoperative CT angiography or magnetic resonance angiography. In patients with abdominal pain, the proximal entry point is covered with a stent graft, and then the target artery is stented back to the true lumen (see Fig. 21-1). This is followed by an exploratory laparotomy if radiographic or clinical signs of mesenteric is-chemia are evident. Dead bowel needs to be resected, with the patient brought back for a second look in 24 hours. Dead bowel on exploration carries a mortality rate in excess of 60%.

Renal ischemia typically manifests as uncontrolled hypertension or as a renal infarct as seen on CT or magnetic resonance imaging. Unlike an atherosclerotic renal artery stenosis, the renal compromise in a patient with dissection typically is a dynamic flow restriction. The false lumen compresses the true lumen leading into the kidney, resulting in elimination of flow during the diastolic phase. Stenting the renal artery across the false lumen to prevent this dynamic compression can help alleviate this problem. Typically, the renal artery is cannulated from the true lumen across the false lumen to the level of the nondissected renal artery. Large self-expanding (8×30-mm nitinol) stents are then placed extending from the distal renal artery, across the false lumen, and into the true lumen. Balloon-expandable stents should be avoided.

Hybrid Procedures

Refer to Box 21-2 for the various types of arch debranching procedures.

TOTAL AORTIC ARCH DEBRANCHING

The technique of total debranching involves proximal relocation of all vessels from the aortic arch with the exception of the left subclavian artery. The left subclavian artery in most patients is occluded proximally with coils or an occlusion plug at the time of stent-graft repair to prevent a retrograde type II endoleak. This converts the distal ascending aorta and the arch to a proximal landing zone for the thoracic stent graft. The technique involves a median sternotomy and isolation of the proximal ascending aorta or a prior ascending aortic graft, followed by exposure of the innominate artery and the left common carotid artery. The brachiocephalic vein may be ligated for ease of exposure, and significant postoperative arm swelling is unusual. A 12-mm Dacron graft is anastomosed to the right lateral wall of the proximal ascending aorta using a side-biting clamp. Even those patients with ejection fractions of less than 20% have been able to tolerate a side-biting clamp with little cardiac stress. The graft is typically taken off the lateral wall to avoid compression during closure of the median sternotomy. The distal end is then anastomosed to the innominate artery in an end-to-end manner. Usually an 8-mm side limb is sewn to the 12-mm Dacron before the innominate bypass is performed, which is then anastomosed to the left common carotid artery in an end-to-end fashion (Fig. 21-10, A). The proximal stumps of the innominate and the left common carotid arteries are then ligated.

The entire arch and the distal ascending aorta are then used as the proximal landing zone (see Fig. 21-10, B). The transfemoral route is preferred for thoracic stent-graft placement. In patients with a severely angled aortic arch, both arch debranching and stent-graft placement are done in a single setting, which allows the stent graft to be manipulated across the arch using manual compression during device tracking. A temporary side limb can also be sewn to the graft off the ascending aorta for antegrade graft deployment. This is especially useful in patients with an acute aortic arch angulation.

CAROTID-CAROTID AND CAROTID-SUBCLAVIAN BYPASS

Extraanatomic bypasses allow the proximal end of the stent graft to cover the origins of the left common carotid artery and the left subclavian artery, landing the endograft just distal to the innominate artery. Indications for revascularization of the left subclavian artery are given in Box 21-3.

The ability to avoid an intracavitary procedure allows for a quicker recovery with minimal morbidity. The technique of carotid-carotid bypass is quite similar to the exposure for a carotid endarterectomy but is performed at a more proximal location in the common carotid artery. The common carotid artery is located on both sides of the neck. The surgeon should take care to remain close to the artery to avoid any cranial nerve injury. A subcutaneous tunnel can be used for an 8-mm ringed expanded polytetrafluoroethylene graft, unless the patient is very thin. In this case, a retropharyngeal tunnel can be used, taking care to stay just anterior to

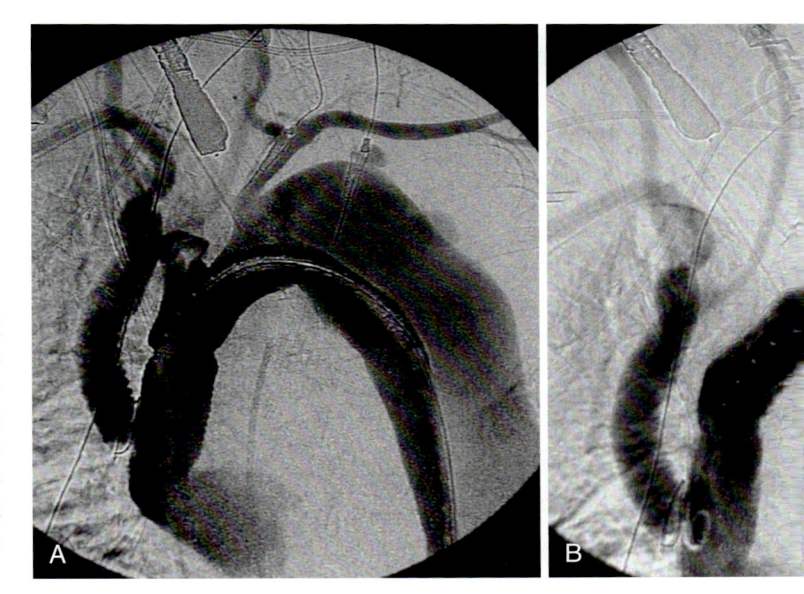

Figure 21-10. A, Typical ascending aortic debranching with grafts to the innominate and left common carotid arteries. **B,** Completion angiogram after endograft placement demonstrating flow to cerebral circulation via the ascending aortic grafts and flow elimination in the false lumen.

Box 21-3	INDICATIONS FOR LEFT CAROTID-SUBCLAVIAN BYPASS

- Left internal mammary artery for coronary artery bypass
- Dominant left vertebral artery
- Right subclavian artery or innominate artery stenosis
- Aberrant origin of left vertebral artery off the arch
- Left brachial artery occlusion
- Aberrant right subclavian artery origin to the left of the left subclavian artery
- Total arch and abdominal visceral vessel debranching
- Left or right vertebral artery terminating in the PICA
- Presence of an arteriovenous fistula or graft in the left arm for dialysis

the prevertebral fascia (Fig. 21-11). If simultaneous carotid-carotid and carotid-subclavian bypasses are required, one option is to perform a right common carotid to left subclavian bypass, followed by transection and reimplantation of the left common carotid artery onto the graft (Fig. 21-12). This allows for fewer anastomoses and ease of tunneling. In certain patients it may be difficult to surgically ligate the left subclavian artery proximal to the vertebral artery. In this instance, the subclavian artery can be occluded using a vascular plug at the time of stent-graft placement.

Endovascular Technique

TECHNIQUE FOR AORTIC FENESTRATION

Although rarely required with the advent of TEVAR, a variety of techniques may be used for fenestrating the septum to equalize pressure across the true and the false lumen and treat end-organ ischemia.[16] This may involve simple balloon dilatation, stent placement, or slicing across the septum with a guidewire. The technically challenging portion of the procedure involves wire access across the septum at the site of the flow compromise. Typically, femoral access is obtained in both common femoral arteries and an attempt is made to manipulate the wire across the septum. If this is not possible with a variety of preshaped catheters, the needle provided with the Outback catheter (Cordis Corp., Bridgewater, N.J.), Pioneer catheter (Medtronic Vascular, Santa Rosa, Calif.), or the transjugular intrahepatic portosystemic shunt kit can be used. To prevent the needle tip from inadvertently perforating the normal aortic wall, a balloon is inflated in the true lumen and the needle tip (advanced via the false lumen) is used to indent and subsequently

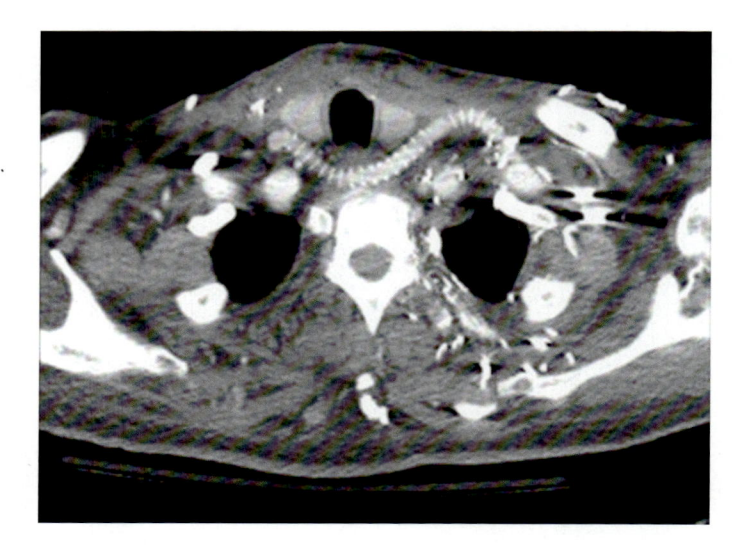

Figure 21-11. Prevertebral location of a left-to-right carotid-carotid bypass.

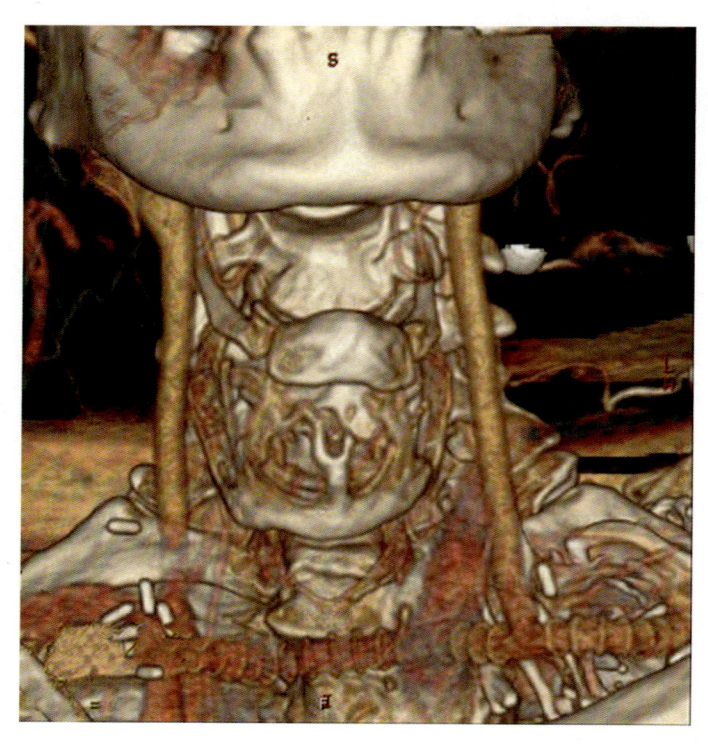

Figure 21-12. Right-to-left carotid-subclavian bypass, with reimplant of the left common carotid artery on to the bypass.

puncture the balloon, thereby gaining access from the false lumen to the true lumen. The needle is then substituted for a wire, and a 16-mm or larger balloon can be used to create a large fenestration. If the fenestration tends to collapse, a large Wallstent or nitinol stent can be inserted across the fenestration. An IVUS can also be used, along with fluoroscopic imaging, to puncture across the septum, especially with the aid of the Pioneer catheter. The other technique involves snaring the wire across the septum to have through-and-through wire access. In this situation one wire is exiting the common femoral artery from the true lumen and the other wire is exiting the contralateral femoral artery via the false lumen. A sawing motion and gentle downward traction result in a linear tear in the septum, causing the fenestration. Because most fenestrations are done to equalize the pressure in both lumens, a pressure recording in both the false and the true lumen may confirm the adequacy of the size of the fenestration.

TECHNIQUE FOR ENDOGRAFT PLACEMENT

Preoperative attention is directed at access vessel sizing and thoracic stent-graft sizing with information obtained from the CT angiography or magnetic resonance angiography. The endograft size is based on the normal nondissected thoracic aorta

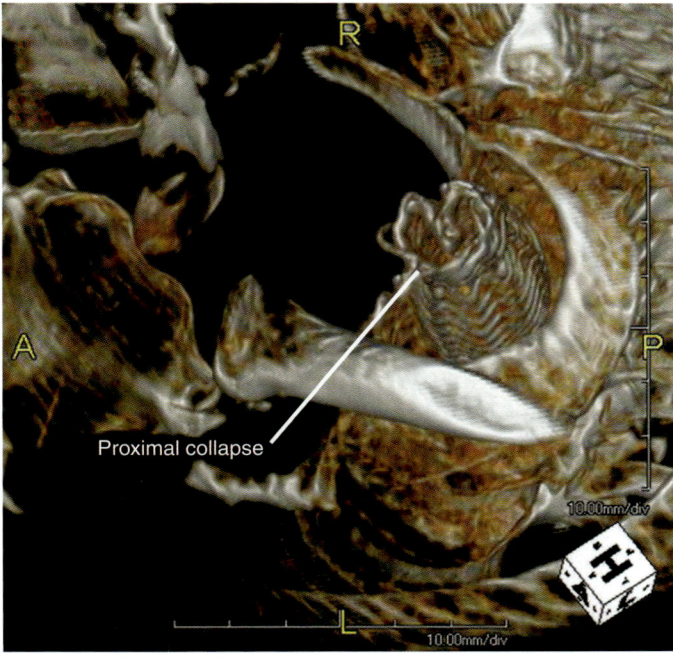

Figure 21-13. Thoracic stent-graft infolding because of inadequate expansion.

between the left common carotid artery and the left subclavian artery. Attention need not be paid to the small size of the true lumen in the dissected portion, because it rapidly enlarges with adequate coverage of the entry point. Oversizing is kept to a minimum (10%), and a typical length of 15 cm is often adequate. Guidewire location in the true lumen is confirmed by IVUS before stent-graft insertion. Typically, the graft is deployed just to the left of the left common carotid artery. Completion angiogram confirms adequate entry point seal. Balloon dilation is avoided unless graft compression or inadequate expansion is noted (Fig. 21-13). Aggressive balloon dilation can result in rupture, or type A conversion. IVUS is performed before completion to confirm adequate graft expansion, no proximal flap extension, and adequate true lumen expansion distal to the stented segment. In patients with acute type B dissection, the immediate completion IVUS can be quite dramatic with rapid false lumen reapproximation.

Postoperative Care

- **Hemodynamic monitoring.** All patients are best managed in an intensive care unit setting. Mean blood pressure should be maintained at or below 70 mm Hg to prevent graft collapse or conversion to type A aortic dissection. Pressures may need to be maintained higher in patients with paraplegia or stroke.
- **Neurologic monitoring.** Patients should be constantly evaluated for any change in peripheral and central neurologic status.
- **Spinal cord perfusion.** Cerebrospinal pressure should be maintained below 10 mm Hg by use of a lumbar drain for 3 days postoperatively.
- **Postoperative surveillance.** In patients with normal renal function, contrast-enhanced CT angiography of the chest, abdomen, and pelvis should be obtained before discharge to assess flow in the false lumen and graft positioning. Follow-up contrast-enhanced CT scans are obtained at 3, 6, and 12 months and yearly thereafter.

Complications

- **Delayed paraplegia.** Although paraplegia may develop days after initial TEVAR, often in association with malfunction of a lumbar drain, an alternate cause may be endograft collapse that leads to low distal perfusion pressure.

- **Late stroke.** Conversion to an acute type A dissection or device collapse may cause a stroke.
- **Visceral ischemia.** Unexplained lactic acidosis or abdominal pain in awake patients suggests visceral ischemia, which should prompt further imaging studies.
- **Renal dysfunction.** Decreased urine output may be due to contrast nephropathy or compromised renal blood flow. Temporary dialysis may be required.
- **Acute lung injury.** The etiology is unclear, but some researchers have speculated that acute lung injury may be secondary to acute bronchial artery occlusion. Prolonged ventilatory support and tracheostomy may be required in some patients.
- **Endograft collapse.** A significant pressure difference between the upper and the lower extremity suggests device collapse, which can be confirmed by a bedside chest radiograph or a CT scan. In intubated patients this condition may manifest as sudden onset of severe hypertension. Treatment involves relining the graft, balloon dilatation, or use of large balloon-expandable stents.
- **Persistent flow in the false lumen.** Given the presence of multiple potential entry and reentry points that may be challenging to visualize, it remains difficult to predict those patients at risk for persistent false lumen flow. Such patients require continued surveillance for aneurysmal degeneration of the false lumen.

REFERENCES

1. Palmer RF, Wheat MW Jr: Treatment of dissecting aneurysms of the aorta, *Ann Thorac Surg* 4:38-52, 1967.
2. Dialetto G, Covino FE, Scognamiglio G, et al: Treatment of type B aortic dissection: Endoluminal repair or conventional medical therapy? *Eur J Cardiothorac Surg* 27:826-830, 2005.
3. Gurin D, Bulmer JW, Derby R: Dissecting aneurysms of the aorta: Diagnosis and operative relief of arterial obstruction due to this cause, *N Y State J Med* 35:1200, 1935.
4. Abbott OA: Clinical experiences with application of polythene cellophane upon aneurysms of thoracic vessels, *J Thorac Surg* 18:435, 1949.
5. DeBakey ME, Cooley DA, Creech O Jr: Surgical considerations of dissecting aneurysm of the aorta, *Ann Surg* 142:586-610, 1955.
6. Dake MD, Kato N, Mitchell RS, et al: Endovascular stent-graft placement for the treatment of acute aortic dissection, *N Engl J Med* 340:1546-1552, 1999.
7. Parsa CJ, Schroder JN, Daneshmand MA, et al: Midterm results for endovascular repair of complicated acute and chronic type B aortic dissection, *Ann Thorac Surg* 89:97-102, 2010.
8. Khoynezhad A, Gupta PK, Donayre CE, et al: Current status of endovascular management of complicated acute type B aortic dissection, *Future Cardiology* 5:581-588, 2009.
9. Nienaber CA, Rousseau H, Eggebrecht H, et al: Randomized comparison of strategies for type B aortic dissection: The Investigation of Stent Grafts in Aortic Dissection (INSTEAD) trial, *Circulation* 120:2519-2528, 2009.
10. Sachs T, Pomposelli F, Hagberg R, et al: Open and endovascular repair of type B aortic dissection in the Nationwide Inpatient Sample, *J Vasc Surg* 52:860-866, 2010.
11. Cambria RP, Crawford RS, Cho JS, et al: A multicenter clinical trial of endovascular stent graft repair of acute catastrophes of the descending thoracic aorta, *J Vasc Surg* 50:1255-1264, 2009.
12. Evangelista A, Avegliano G, Aguilar R, et al: Impact of contrast-enhanced echocardiography on the diagnostic algorithm of acute aortic dissection, *Eur Heart J* 31:472-479, 2010.
13. Conrad MF, Crawford RS, Kwolek CJ, et al: Aortic remodeling after endovascular repair of acute complicated type B aortic dissection, *J Vasc Surg* 50:510-517, 2009.
14. Khoynezhad A, Donayre CE, Omari BO, et al: Midterm results of endovascular treatment of complicated acute type B aortic dissection, *J Thorac Cardiov Surg* 138:625-631, 2009.
15. Kische S, Ehrlich MP, Nienaber CA, et al: Endovascular treatment of acute and chronic aortic dissection: Midterm results from the Talent Thoracic Retrospective Registry, *J Thorac Cardiov Surg* 138:115-124, 2009.
16. Slonim SM, Miller DC, Mitchell RS, et al: Percutaneous balloon fenestration and stenting for life-threatening ischemic complications in patients with acute aortic dissection, *J Thorac Cardiov Surg* 117:1118-1127, 1999.

22 Endovascular Treatment of Traumatic Thoracic Aortic Disruption

MARK A. FARBER • MARC A. CAMACHO

Historical Background

Traumatic aortic injury is the result of a high-velocity or deceleration injury to the wall of the aorta, which most commonly occurs at the level of the ligamentum arteriosum, proximal to the third intercostal artery. Of those patients who reach the hospital, the lesion is most often a noncircumferential injury limited to the intima and media. It may range from subintimal hemorrhage, with or without an intimal tear, to complete transection. If all three layers are involved, rapid exsanguination occurs. However, if the adventitial layer is intact, tamponade from peri-aortic tissue with resultant pseudoaneurysm formation allows patients to reach nearby medical facilities. Traumatic aortic injury is an unstable condition that can cause rapid patient deterioration anytime after injury.

The principle of early diagnosis and treatment was first established by Parmley and associates in 1958,[1] who reviewed 275 cases of traumatic aortic rupture. Of the 38 (13.8%) patients who reached the hospital alive, 3 patients died within 1 hour and 23 (61%) died of rupture within 1 week of admission. Subsequent studies have demonstrated that as many as 70% of patients survive with surgical treatment.[2] Through the advancement of minimally invasive techniques, most traumatic aortic injuries are now repaired using an endovascular approach.[3,4]

Indications

Delayed repair of thoracic aortic injury may be considered in select, stable patients where the injury is more than 4 hours old, such as high-risk elderly patients with major comorbidities or those with associated head injury, pulmonary injury, and coagulopathy. An anatomic injury grading scheme (grades I-IV) has been developed to identify those patients with a grade I or II injury who may be appropriate for a more conservative approach (Fig. 22-1).[5] Unfortunately, it is not possible to differentiate those intimal injuries that display a more stable course from those that will progress to rupture. Approximately 10% of stable patients will rupture before repair. Thus patients should be considered for emergent repair in the presence of hemodynamic instability, an enlarging mediastinal hematoma, or worsening pleural effusion.

Preoperative Preparation

- Patients with suspected thoracic aortic injury should be transferred to a level I trauma center for treatment of their associated traumatic injuries, as well as for respiratory and cardiovascular stabilization.
- Computed tomography (CT) angiography has a sensitivity of nearly 100% for diagnosing traumatic aortic transection.[6] Although the diagnosis of aortic

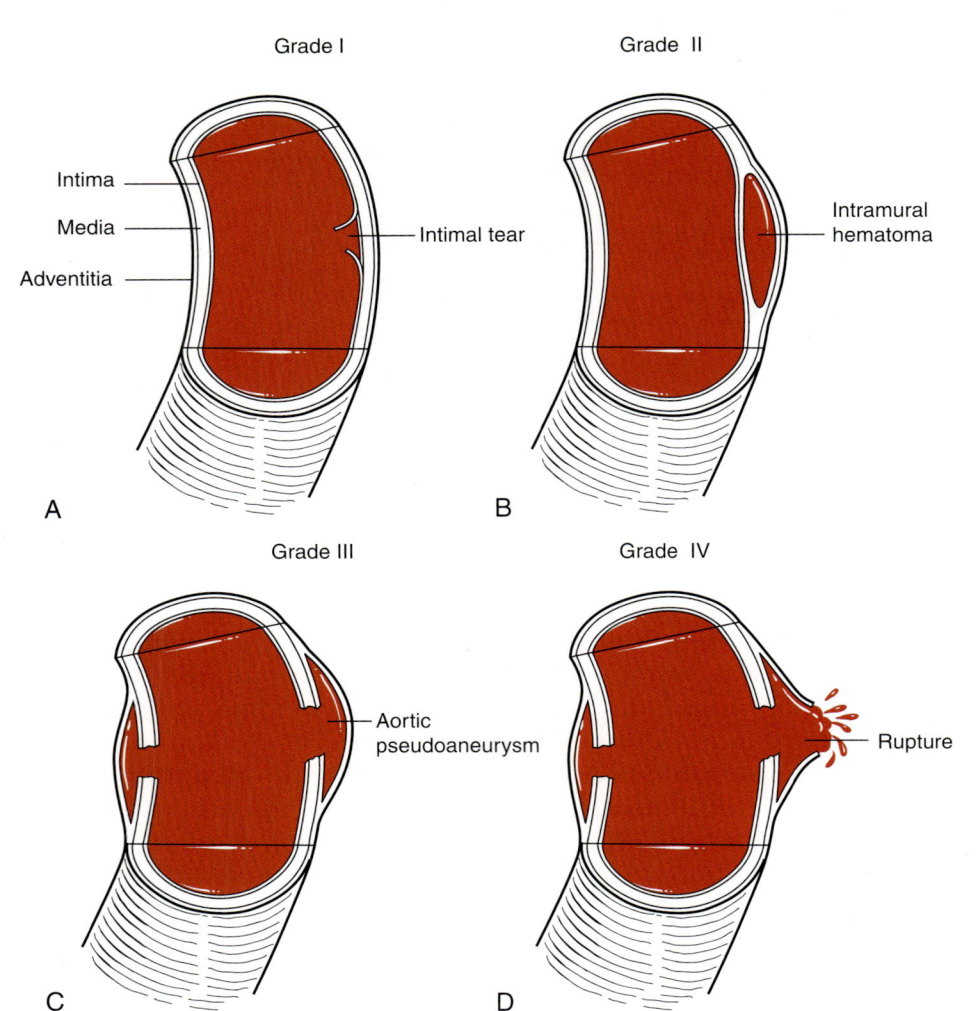

Figure 22-1. Grading scheme of traumatic aortic injury of the thoracic aorta. **A,** Grade I: Intimal tear; **B,** Grade II: Intramural hematoma, **C,** Grade III: Aortic pseudoaneurysm, **D,** Grade IV: Rupture. (From Azizzadeh A, Keyhani K, Miller C, et al: Blunt traumatic aortic injury: Initial experience with endovascular repair. J Vasc Surg 49:1403-1408, 2009.)

injury can be made by transesophageal echocardiography, it is not as sensitive as CT angiography.

- Signs of aortic disruption on chest radiography may include a widened mediastinum, a rightward shift of the trachea, blurring of the aortic knob, opacification of the juncture between the aorta and the pulmonary trunk, and a left-sided hemothorax (Table 22-1).[7-9]
- In the presence of suspected aortic injury, strict blood pressure control is mandatory with beta-blockade and afterload reduction to reduce aortic wall stress.
- If the patient is unstable, with evidence of possible aortic disruption on chest radiograph, transfer to the operating room is recommended for angiography and repair if an aortic injury is confirmed.
- Three-dimensional CT imaging facilitates preoperative planning, including endograft selection and assessment of access vessel tortuosity and caliber. Because endovascular repair often requires coverage of the left subclavian artery, knowledge of the vertebral anatomy and prior history of coronary artery bypass grafting with a left internal mammary artery graft is critical. Concomitant pelvic fracture is a relative contraindication to use of the iliac vessels for access.
- Head CT imaging can exclude occult brain injuries where anticoagulation should be avoided.

Endovascular Strategy

SIZING OF AN ENDOVASCULAR GRAFT

Knowledge of each device's performance with respect to oversizing and flexibility is critical to avoiding device collapse or failure to exclude the site of aortic injury.

TABLE 22-1 Frequency of Abnormal Radiographic Signs in Patients With Suspected Traumatic Aortic Injury of the Thoracic Aorta

Sign	Suspected Thoracic Aortic Injury on Chest Radiograph* (%)	Angiographic Confirmation of Injury (%)
Mediastinum > 8 cm	76	27
Indistinct descending aortic arch contour	76	5
Indistinct aortic contour	12	85
Trachea displaced to the right	61	78
Nasogastric tube or esophagus displaced to the right	67	87
Left main stem bronchus displaced inferiorly	53	84
Pleural apical cap	37	68
Fracture of rib 1 or 2	17	70

From Kadir S: Arteriography of the thoracic aorta. In Kadir S, editor: *Diagnostic angiography*, Philadelphia, 1986, Saunders, pp 124-171.
*Given that chest radiographic examination may fail to identify a traumatic thoracic injury in as many as 11% of patients, CT angiography is recommended in any patient with a suspected injury. Data from Matsumura JS, Cambria RP, Dake MD, et al: International controlled clinical trial of thoracic endovascular aneurysm repair with the Zenith TX2 endovascular graft: 1-year results. *J Vasc Surg* 47:247, 2008.

In the instance of traumatic injury, the aortic diameter may be reduced because of hypovolemia and may lead to an underestimation of the true aortic diameter. Critical measurements include the orthogonal diameter of the aorta 2 cm proximal to the cephalad extent of the injury, as well as the diameter of the aorta 8 to 10 cm distal to the proximal sealing region. The proximal extent typically involves the subclavian artery and almost never involves the left common carotid artery.

EXTENT OF REPAIR

Critical attention should be paid to the degree of curvature of the aorta in the proximal sealing region, because this may affect both device performance and device selection. Apposition to the inner curvature is paramount to avoid device malfunction. Most repairs can be accomplished with a 10-cm-long device. In rare circumstances, aortic injury can extend a variable distance down the aorta, necessitating a longer length of coverage.

Endovascular Technique

The ipsilateral groin is typically accessed either percutaneously or using an open exposure with the patient in the supine position. Secondary access may be obtained from either the left brachial artery or the contralateral femoral artery using the Seldinger technique. Heparin is recommended unless contraindicated by the presence of a brain injury. In these circumstances, repair can be undertaken without need for anticoagulation by avoiding vessel loop occlusion of the profunda and superficial femoral arteries. In some instances iliac or aortic exposure may be necessary if the delivery catheters are too large for femoral arterial insertion. In young individuals without evidence of atherosclerosis, vessel elasticity will often allow the passage of standard endovascular devices despite smaller vessel size.

Once access is obtained, angiographic identification of the lesion is performed to accurately identify its location. The orthogonal angle of the image intensifier with respect to the site of injury can be determined by inspection of preoperative CT images and is typically greater than 45 degrees of left anterior oblique. When CT imaging has not been undertaken, intravascular ultrasound (IVUS) can be used as an adjuvant to angiography to locate the precise proximal and distal extent of the aortic injury. Final selection of device diameter may be determined from IVUS imaging, because hypovolemic patients may have a under distended aorta on initial CT imaging.

Device selection should be based on proximal and distal aortic diameters and lesion length. Available devices can treat aortic luminal diameters ranging from 16 to 42 mm, with treatment lengths ranging from 10 to 20 cm. The device should be deployed along the inner curvature of the aorta, because the radius of curvature

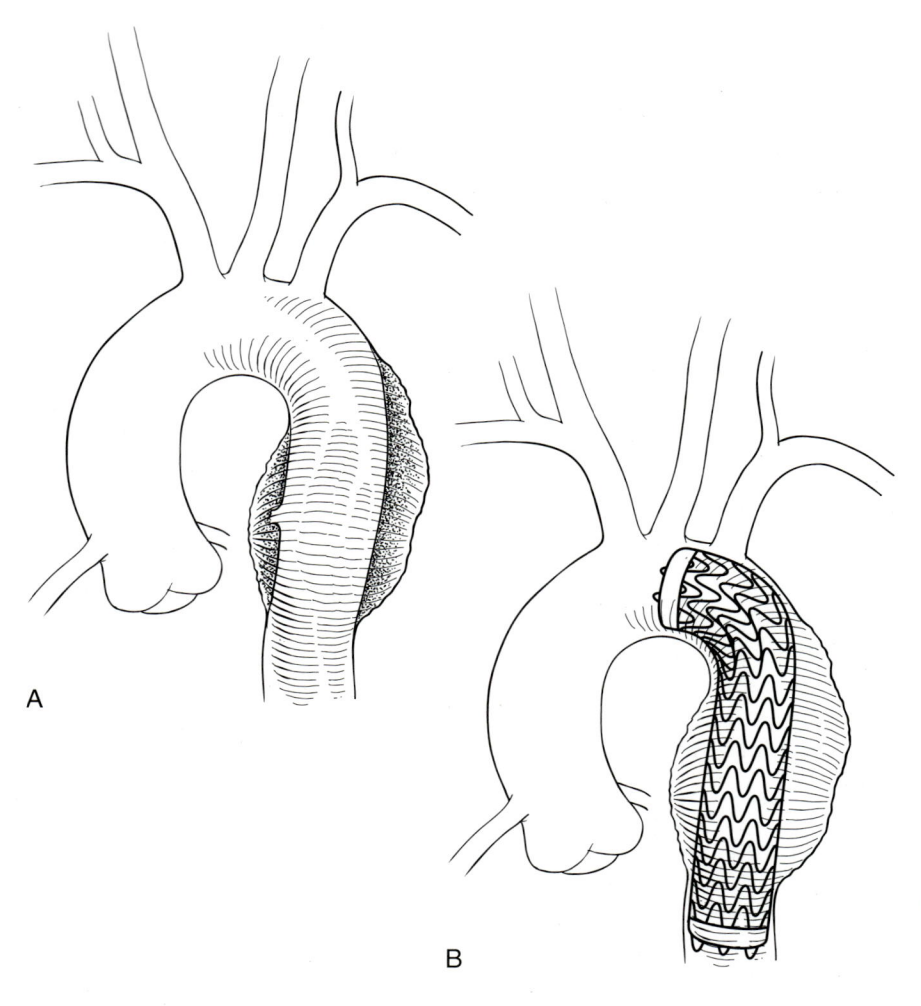

Figure 22-2. Thoracic aortic injury (**A**) before and (**B**) after endovascular repair. The endograft covers the left subclavian artery.

is often smaller in older patients with degenerative aortic pathology and can result in inappropriate positioning of the device. If subclavian artery coverage is required, preoperative imaging helps determine whether carotid-subclavian transposition or bypass is required or, in select cases, if a branched or fenestrated device should be used.

Device deployment in hyperdynamic individuals may require temporarily induced cardiac arrest with adenosine for more accurate device placement. Once the device is deployed, evaluation of lesion exclusion and device apposition to the aortic wall can be conducted with IVUS or angiography. If malapposition or endoleak exists, balloon molding with a compliant or semicompliant balloon may be required. However, overaggressive ballooning can exacerbate aortic injury and should be avoided.

At the conclusion of the procedure, an angiogram is obtained after replacing the delivery sheath with a 6- to 8-Fr sheath, while maintaining wire access, in order to exclude access artery dissection or rupture (Figs. 22-2 and 22-3).

Postoperative Care

- Once the aortic injury has been excluded by endovascular repair, systolic blood pressure may be increased as desired for optimal treatment of associated traumatic brain injury.
- Since extensive thoracic aortic coverage is rarely needed, the risk of paraplegia is low. If postoperative paraplegia or paraparesis is present, traumatic or ischemic injury should be evaluated. If an ischemic etiology is likely, lumbar drain placement should be considered and mean arterial pressure maintained above 90 mm Hg.

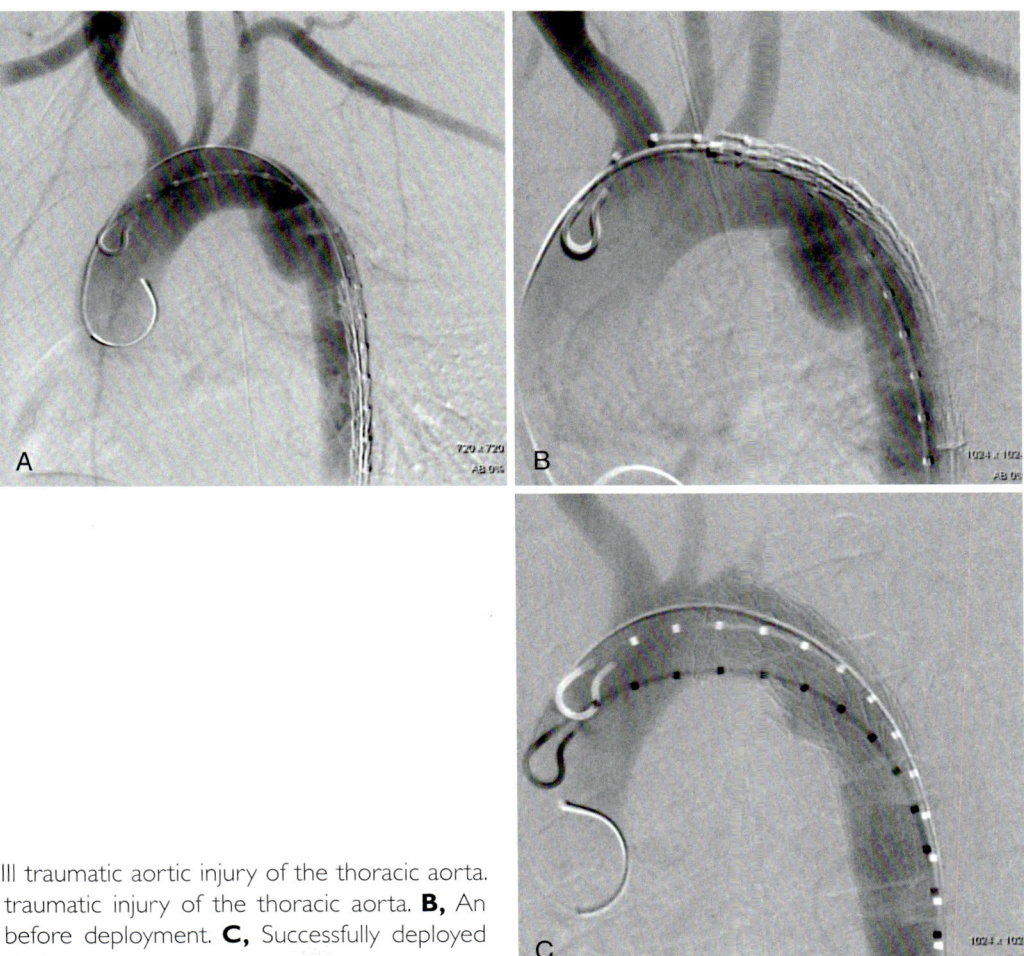

Figure 22-3. Repair of a grade III traumatic aortic injury of the thoracic aorta. **A,** An aortogram demonstrates traumatic injury of the thoracic aorta. **B,** An endovascular stent is positioned before deployment. **C,** Successfully deployed stent covering the injury and left subclavian artery.

- Device surveillance should be conducted in the first 24 to 48 hours with either CT imaging or conventional chest radiographs in four views (anteroposterior, lateral, right anterior oblique, and left anterior oblique) Careful inspection of these radiographs should be conducted to identify device collapse, position, stent fracture, or migration.
- Follow-up surveillance consists of a chest radiograph and chest CT angiogram at 1, 6, and 12 months and yearly thereafter to monitor integrity of the repair, as well as to exclude device collapse, stent fracture, or migration Once lesion exclusion has been confirmed at 12 months, follow-up imaging with a noncontrast CT is appropriate, with additional imaging conducted as needed.

Complications

- **Mortality and morbidity.** Mortality and morbidity rates after thoracic endovascular aortic repair (TEVAR) varies with aortic pathology but are as high as 12% and 19% in series limited to the treatment of traumatic aortic injury. This, of course, is considerably higher than elective TEVAR treatment of degenerative thoracic aneurysm.[10-15]
- **Stroke.** Stroke may result from thromboembolic events related to catheter manipulations in the presence of atherosclerotic arch disease or ischemic complications from coverage of critical branch vessels. Posterior strokes can occur with coverage of the left subclavian artery in the presence of a dominant left vertebral anatomy.
- **Spinal cord ischemia.** Paraplegia is rare after TEVAR for traumatic aortic injury, due to the limited length of required aortic coverage.
- **Access complications.** Avoidance of iliac artery injury requires careful preoperative planning and device selection.

- **Arm ischemia.** Severe upper extremity ischemia is rare, but if present can be managed with elective carotid-subclavian bypass or transposition.
- **Device collapse.** Device collapse has a reported incidence of 0.8% due to graft oversizing, small aortic lumen, or lack of aortic arch conformability.[13] Simple angioplasty of the collapsed device is generally unsuccessful and placement of additional devices or stents is most often required.
- **Device migration.** Caudal device migration of more than 10 mm can occur in up to 1% to 3% of patients over a 6- to 12-month period after TEVAR, but is even less frequent after traumatic aortic injury because of higher surface area contact of the device and aortic wall.[10-13]

REFERENCES

1. Parmley LF, Mattingly TW, Manion WC: Nonpenetrating traumatic injury of the aorta, *Circulation* 17:1086-1101, 1958.
2. Kirsh MM, Behrendt DM, Orringer MB, et al: The treatment of acute traumatic rupture of the aorta: A 10-year experience, *Ann Surg* 184:308-316, 1976.
3. Demetriades D, Velmahos GC, Scalea TM, et al: Operative repair or endovascular stent graft in blunt traumatic thoracic aortic injuries: Results of an American Association for the Surgery of Trauma multicenter study, *J Trauma* 64:561, 2008.
4. Xenos ES, Abedi NN, Davenport DL, et al: Meta-analysis of endovascular vs open repair for traumatic descending thoracic aortic rupture, *J Vasc Surg* 48:1343, 2008.
5. Azizzadeh A, Keyhani K, Miller C, et al: Blunt traumatic aortic injury: Initial experience with endovascular repair, *J Vasc Surg* 49:1403-1408, 2009.
6. Sammer M, Wang E, Blackmore CC, et al: Indeterminate CT angiography in blunt thoracic trauma: Is CT angiography enough? *AJR Am J Roentgenol* 189:603-608, Sep 2007.
7. Kadir S: *Diagnostic angiography*, Philadelphia, 1986, Saunders, 124–171.
8. Ekeh AP, Peterson W, Woods RJ, et al: Is chest x-ray an adequate screening tool for the diagnosis of blunt thoracic injury? *J Trauma* 65:1088-1092, Nov 2008.
9. Matsumura JS, Cambria RP, Dake MD, et al: International controlled clinical trial of thoracic endovascular aneurysm repair with the Zenith TX2 endovascular graft: 1-year results, *J Vasc Surg* 47:247, 2008.
10. Bavaria JE, Appoo JJ, Makaroun MS, et al: Endovascular stent grafting versus open surgical repair of descending thoracic aortic aneurysms in low-risk patients: A multicenter comparative trial, *J Thorac Cardiov Surg* 133:369, 2007.
11. Stone DH, Brewster DC, Kwolek CJ, et al: Stent-graft versus open-surgical repair of the thoracic aorta: Mid-term results, *J Vasc Surg* 44:1188, 2006.
12. Makaroun MS, Dillavou ED, Wheatley GH, et al: Five-year results of endovascular treatment with the Gore TAG device compared with open repair of thoracic aortic aneurysms, *J Vasc Surg* 47:912, 2008.
13. Demetriades D, Velmahos GC, Scalea TM, et al: Diagnosis and treatment of blunt thoracic aortic injuries: Changing perspectives, *J Trauma* 64:1415-1419, 2008.
14. Neschis DG, Moainie S, Flinn WR, et al: Endograft repair of traumatic aortic injury: A technique in evolution: A single institution's experience, *Ann Surg* 250:377-382, 2009.
15. Mohan IV, Hitos K, White GH, et al: Improved outcomes with endovascular stent grafts for thoracic aortic transections, *Eur J Vasc Endovasc Surg* 36:152-157, 2008.

Section 6

THE ABDOMINAL AORTA AND ILIAC ARTERIES

23 Direct Surgical Repair of Aneurysms of the Infrarenal Abdominal Aorta and Iliac Arteries

ANDRES SCHANZER • MICHAEL BELKIN

Historical Background

Abdominal aortic aneurysms were first described by the sixteenth-century anatomist Vesalius.[1] Before the advent of modern surgical techniques, numerous management methods focusing on aneurysm ligation, induced thrombosis, or wrapping were attempted, all with little success. It was not until 1951, when Dubost and associates[2] performed the first successful abdominal aortic aneurysm repair using an aortic homograft, that the management of abdominal aortic aneurysms entered the modern era. That achievement prolonged the patient's life by 8 years and stood in stark contrast to the dismal results associated with prior methods of treatment. The next major advance occurred in 1953, when Blakemore and Voorhees first used a prosthetic graft to repair an aortic aneurysm.[3] Despite these early advances, operative mortality rates were approximately 20%.[4] Subsequent improvements in anesthetic management and operative technique reduced mortality rates to between 4% and 9% by the 1970s.[5] Chief among these advances was the adoption of the graft inclusion technique, as advocated by Creech.[6] Refinements in preoperative cardiac evaluation and optimization, in addition to intraoperative cardiac and fluid management, have contributed to further reductions in perioperative mortality to less than 5%.[7,8]

Preoperative Preparation

- Transabdominal ultrasonography is an excellent screening tool for determining the maximum diameter of an abdominal aortic aneurysm. Once the decision is made to proceed with repair, computed tomography (CT) angiography is essential for operative planning. Arteriography is seldom used in contemporary practice. However, in patients with extensive aortoiliac occlusive disease or a significant renal artery stenosis, catheter interventions may reduce the extent of open abdominal aortic aneurysm repair.
- Evaluation of cardiac risk is based on clinical history, electrocardiogram (ECG), and noninvasive testing in select patients deemed to be at high risk.
- An abdominal aortic aneurysm is an indicator of increased cardiovascular risk,[9] and both perioperative statin[10] and antiplatelet[11] therapy are beneficial. Beta-blockade has also been thought to provide benefits, although recent publications have questioned this understanding.[12]
- Prophylactic antibiotics, an intraoperative nasogastric tube, arterial blood pressure monitoring, a central venous catheter, a Foley catheter, large-bore intravenous access, and an epidural catheter are standard tenets in open aortic surgery.

Pitfalls and Danger Points

- **Proximal and distal aortic control.** A plan for the positioning of the aortic clamp and the extent of resection should be defined before operative intervention. The plan should be based on the surgical anatomy as determined by CT imaging.
- **Venous injuries.** To avoid injury to the renal vein, wide mobilization by ligation of renal vein branches is preferred, or if needed, the renal vein is divided close to the inferior vena cava with dependence on adrenal, gonadal, and renal lumbar vein branches for venous drainage. To minimize the risk of iliac vein or cava injury, dissection of the aorta and iliac arteries should be limited to non-circumferential, anterior, lateral, and medial exposure.
- **Impaired distal perfusion.**
  - **Distal embolization.** Manual retraction of the aneurysm sac during dissection of the aortic neck may be required but should be as gentle as possible with appropriate use of a lap pad. In addition, distal iliac clamps should be placed before the proximal aortic clamp.
  - **Iliac artery clamp injury.** To avoid an obstructing plaque, the iliac artery should be carefully palpated and assessed and the clamp should be positioned in a noncalcified portion of the vessel or angled so that the posterior plaque is compressed against the anterior wall rather than crushed.
- **Retrograde ejaculation or impotence.** To avoid retrograde ejaculation or impotence, the autonomic sympathetic fibers along the left side of the aortic bifurcation, inferior mesenteric artery, and left common iliac artery should be preserved, along with internal iliac artery flow.
- **Intestinal injury.** Preventing duodenal injury requires careful dissection of the third portion of duodenum off the proximal portion of aneurysm while avoiding thermal injury.
- **Ureteral injury.** The ureters are at risk for injury where they cross anterior to the distal common iliac arteries.
- **Bowel ischemia.** Maintenance of flow to at least one internal iliac artery is essential. Reimplantation of the inferior mesenteric artery should be considered if backbleeding is sluggish despite restoration pelvic flow, mesenteric Doppler signals are weak, and the sigmoid colon is dusky.
- **Retraction injury.** Self-retaining retractor traction injury is a risk for nerves or other structures, such as the spleen and superior mesenteric artery.

Operative Strategy

TRANSPERITONEAL EXPOSURE

The major benefit of the transabdominal technique relates to the broad abdominal exposure that this approach provides (Box 23-1). Careful intraoperative examination of the abdomen may reveal a concomitant pathology, including malignancy (4%-12%), cholelithiasis (4%-19%), or diverticulitis.[13] Direct evaluation of the left colon for evidence of ischemia is particularly important in patients with compromised hypogastric or collateral perfusion, such as those who have had a prior colectomy. Another advantage of the transabdominal approach is the ease of exposure and repair of aneurysms extending into the right iliac artery. Although seldom necessary, exposure of the right femoral vessels for thrombectomy or distal anastomosis is also straightforward. Similarly, exposure of the right renal artery for bypass or endarterectomy, as well as subsequent evaluation of blood flow, is best performed via the transabdominal approach. Familiarity with transabdominal exposure for most surgeons results in an easy, expeditious repair.

The disadvantages of the transabdominal approach relate primarily to aneurysm morphology and prior surgical history (Box 23-1). Although juxtarenal aneurysms

> **Box 23-1 TRANSABDOMINAL APPROACH TO ANEURYSM REPAIR**
>
> *Advantages*
> 1. Familiar anatomy to most surgeons
> 2. Broad abdominal exposure and complete abdominal exploration
> 3. Ease of exposure of right femoral, iliac, and renal arteries
>
> *Disadvantages*
> 1. Surgery in "hostile" abdomen: multiple previous operations
> 2. Abdominal wall stomas
> 3. Difficult aortic anatomy: suprarenal aneurysm, recurrent aneurysm, inflammatory aneurysm, and horseshoe kidney

> **Box 23-2 RETROPERITONEAL APPROACH TO ANEURYSM REPAIR**
>
> *Advantages*
> 1. Improved exposure to the suprarenal aorta and visceral segment
> 2. Improved exposure of complex aortic aneurysms: suprarenal aneurysm, recurrent aneurysm, inflammatory aneurysm, and horseshoe kidney
> 3. Avoidance of hostile abdomen and abdominal wall ostomies
> 4. Balance of literature suggesting fewer gastrointestinal complications: ileus or small bowel obstruction
>
> *Disadvantages*
> 1. Limited familiarity of many surgeons with anatomy
> 2. Limited visualization of abdominal contents
> 3. Difficult or limited exposure of right femoral, iliac, and renal arteries
> 4. Increased incisional pain and long-term wound problems

can be exposed and repaired via a transabdominal approach, true suprarenal aneurysms are difficult to address via this approach and generally require complex modifications, such as a medial visceral rotation. Similarly, in patients with an inflammatory aneurysm or a proximal anastomotic pseudoaneurysm, proximal control may be difficult to achieve via the transabdominal technique. Patients with an aneurysm in the presence of a horseshoe kidney also are difficult to repair via the transabdominal approach. In addition, patients with multiple past abdominal operations often have severe adhesions, which may complicate and prolong the surgical exposure or increase risk of an inadvertent enterotomy with an attendant risk of graft infection. Bowel or urinary stomas also complicate exposure and repair via the transabdominal approach.

RETROPERITONEAL EXPOSURE

The retroperitoneal approach greatly facilitates exposure of the suprarenal aorta, left renal artery, and proximal mesenteric vessels (Box 23-2). Other advantages of the retroperitoneal approach arise when anterior exposure of the aneurysm is complicated by concurrent pathology, such as abdominal adhesions, stomas, and horseshoe kidney, or in the presence of an inflammatory aneurysm or anastomotic pseudoaneurysm.

A number of disadvantages for the retroperitoneal approach have been noted (Box 23-2). Although the abdominal cavity can be entered if intraabdominal pathology is suspected, abdominal contents are generally not inspected. Exposure of the right iliac and femoral vessels is cumbersome and may require a counter incision for sufficient iliac artery exposure. Transaortic right renal endarterectomy

DIRECT SURGICAL REPAIR OF ANEURYSMS OF THE INFRARENAL ABDOMINAL AORTA AND ILIAC ARTERIES

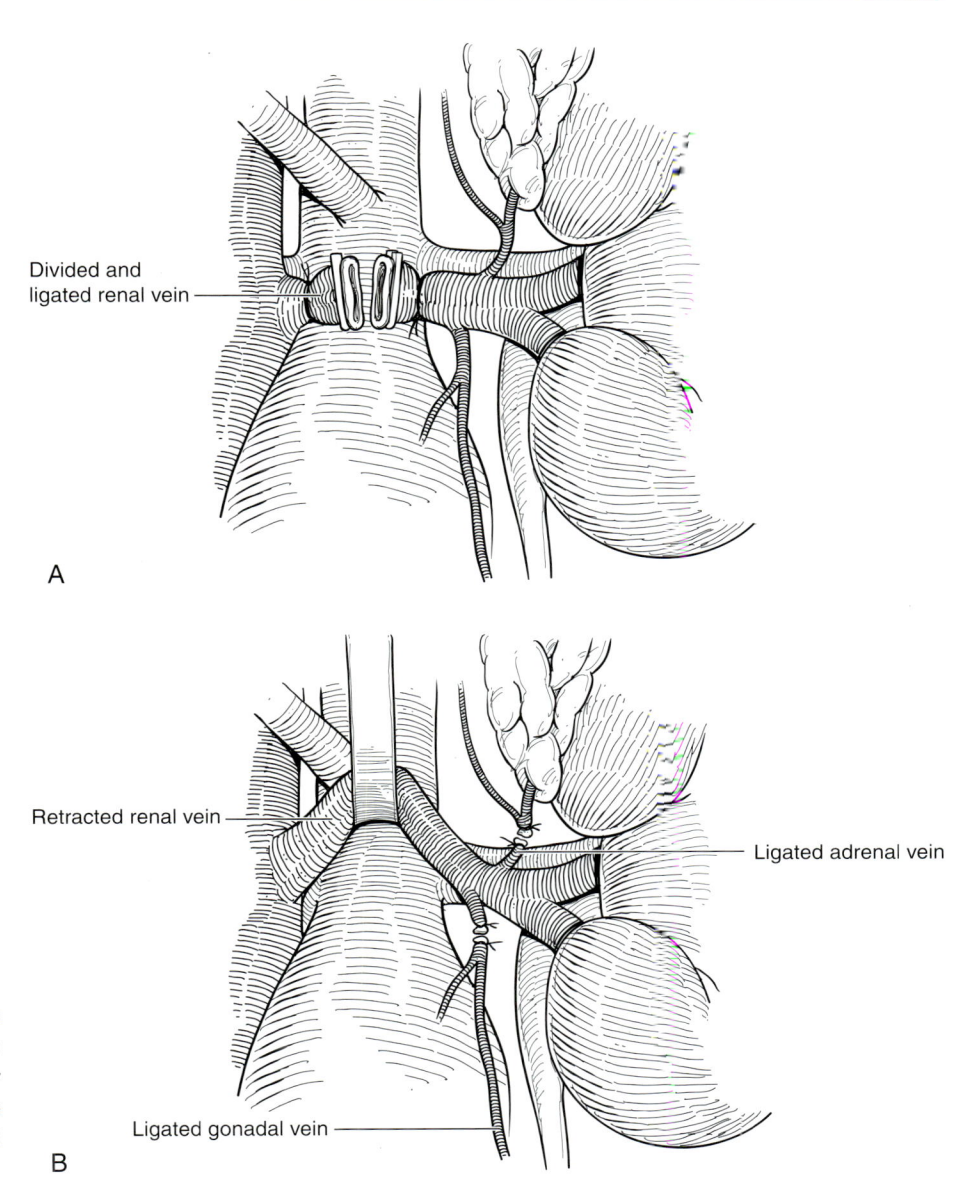

Figure 23-1. For improved exposure of the aortic neck, the left renal vein can either be (**A**) divided or (**B**) extensively mobilized, with ligation and division of the adrenal vein superiorly and the gonadal vein inferiorly.

is possible via left retroperitoneal exposure; however, subsequent evaluation of renal blood flow for the detection and repair of related technical problems is difficult. Direct surgery on the right renal artery is not possible via a left flank exposure. The retroperitoneal incision may be more painful beyond the perioperative period than are the midline incisions of the transabdominal approach, and the former incision is frequently complicated by a permanent protrusion around the incision. This usually represents weakness of the abdominal wall musculature because of denervation rather than frank herniation.

DIVISION OF THE RENAL VEIN

Renal vein division is not necessary in most cases, especially with complete circumferential dissection of the renal vein and with ligation and division of the adrenal, gonadal, and renal lumbar branches that facilitate retraction of the renal vein (Fig. 23-1). In the case of a reoperative field or suprarenal aneurysm, where the dissection is more challenging, division of the renal vein with an endoscopic vascular stapler can be helpful technique and is well tolerated.[14]

ASSESSMENT OF THE QUALITY OF THE INFRARENAL AORTIC NECK

Based on the high quality of contemporary CT imaging, aortic neck quality, including calcification, thrombus, and aneurysmal degeneration, can be anticipated preoperatively and the most appropriate location for clamp placement can be determined. Intraoperative digital palpation helps locate the most suitable position for clamp placement to minimize the risk of plaque perforation of the aortic neck, but it cannot discern aortic mural debris as a source of embolization.

SITE SELECTION FOR DISTAL EXPOSURE AND CONTROL

A tube graft configuration with the distal anastomosis sewn directly into the aortic bifurcation is the preferred repair method if the common iliac arteries are not aneurysmal, with approximately 60% of infrarenal AAAs amenable to tube graft repair. As a guideline, if the common iliac arteries are greater than 2 cm in diameter, a bifurcated graft is required, but it may be modified according to the age and fitness of the particular patient. Late reoperation for iliac aneurysm disease is rarely required. If severe iliac artery occlusive disease is present, an aortobifemoral configuration is used to ensure adequate lower extremity arterial perfusion. Alternatively, preemptive endovascular treatment followed by open tube grafting may be an option in select patients.

BALLOON CATHETERS FOR VASCULAR CONTROL

In the setting of severe calcification, balloon occlusion catheters may be less traumatic, safer, and more effective in providing vascular control compared with other catheters. Fogarty catheters with balloon diameters between 5 and 7 mm work well in most iliac arteries. Large compliant balloons are used rarely for proximal aortic control.

ASSESSMENT OF THE ADEQUACY OF COLONIC PERFUSION

Visual inspection of the colon at the conclusion of aneurysm repair is generally adequate to assess colonic viability. Patients with internal iliac artery occlusion, previous colonic surgery, and a large inferior mesenteric artery that has not been reimplanted are at greater risk for bowel ischemia. Assessment of Doppler signals at the colonic antimesenteric border or use of a Wood's lamp with fluorescein to evaluate intestinal perfusion may be helpful in high-risk patients. If colonic perfusion appears marginal, the inferior mesenteric artery should be reimplanted and a second-look operation is prudent.

RUPTURED ANEURYSM

The retroperitoneal hematoma of a ruptured aneurysm often dissects out the proximal aortic neck, but care must be taken to avoid injury to the left renal vein, which is often suspended and not easily visualized in the hematoma. Initial control of the supraceliac aorta may be necessary in some situations. Exposure is obtained by incising the gastrohepatic ligament, entering the lesser sac, and retracting the stomach and esophagus to the patient's left while retracting the liver and diaphragm superiorly. It is useful to have a nasogastric tube in place to assist in identifying the esophagus so as to avoid injury to this structure during the dissection. The crura of the diaphragm is incised, digital dissection is used to expose each side of the supraceliac aorta, and a cross-clamp placed over the surgeon's fingers to the level of the vertebral body.

INFLAMMATORY ANEURYSM

In the setting of an inflammatory aneurysm, the anatomic plane between the duodenum and the aorta becomes obscured by inflammation and fibrosis, thereby increasing the risk of a duodenal injury during dissection. Similarly, this process can involve the vena cava, left renal vein, and ureters. Because both the retroperitoneal approach and endovascular repair do not require mobilization of these structures, these approaches are preferred. In some cases the diagnosis of an inflammatory aneurysm is made at the time of transabdominal aortic aneurysm repair by the presence of a white fibrotic reaction over the anterior surface of the aneurysm that extends to the level of the aortic neck. To avoid injury to the duodenum, it may be necessary to dissect the duodenum sharply off the aneurysm by superficially incising the aneurysm wall with a No. 15 blade beneath the duodenum.

HORSESHOE KIDNEY

A horseshoe kidney poses a technical challenge because of limited access to the aorta and the presence of multiple renal arteries arising from the aorta and iliac arteries.[15] If approached transabdominally, the renal isthmus should not be divided unless it is extremely atrophic. The graft should be tunneled beneath the kidney, and arteries that are sufficiently large to supply distinct areas of renal parenchyma should be reimplanted. There may also be duplicated ureters lying more anteriorly than encountered in normal anatomy. A retroperitoneal approach avoids these challenges and is the recommended approach.

TRANSPLANTED KIDNEY

The inflow for a transplanted kidney is generally based on either the common or the external iliac artery. Continuous retrograde perfusion to the transplanted kidney can be achieved by the creation of a temporary, nontunneled, axillofemoral artery bypass, which is removed at the conclusion of the operation.

VENOUS ANOMALIES

A retroaortic left renal vein, circumaortic anterior and posterior renal vein, and left-sided or duplicated inferior vena cava are the most common venous anomalies that can be found during abdominal aortic aneurysm repair.[15] Renal vein anomalies usually do not hinder aortic exposure. A left-sided vena cava usually crosses anteriorly to the right side at the level of the renal veins and may need to be mobilized to facilitate aortic exposure. A retroaortic left renal vein, which is present in 4% of the population, typically crosses to the inferior vena cava obliquely and more caudally than the typical anterior renal vein. Accordingly, circumferential dissection of the aortic neck can occur cephalad to the retroaortic vein. However, vigilance is paramount to avoid intraoperative injury.

AORTOCAVAL FISTULA

If an aortic aneurysm has eroded into the vena cava, surgical treatment consists of conventional aneurysm repair with suture ligation of the fistula from within the aneurysm. Sponge stick compression of the vena cava, above and below the fistula and from within the aneurysm sac, ensures venous control and minimizes the risk of pulmonary embolization of air or mural thrombus.

Operative Technique for Repair of an Infrarenal Aortic Aneurysm

INCISION

The abdomen is opened and explored through a midline incision. The length of the incision is dictated by the extent of the aneurysm and the planned repair. The incision for a tube graft is extended from the xiphoid to the midway point between the umbilicus and the pubis. The incision for a bifurcated graft is extended to above the pubis.

EXPOSURE OF THE ABDOMINAL AORTA

The transverse colon and omentum are displaced superiorly. The small bowel is then either packed into the right upper quadrant of the abdomen or eviscerated into moist towels. Exposure of the operative field is facilitated by a mechanical self-retaining retractor system fixed to the operating table. The peritoneum is incised with scissors along the inferior border of the third and fourth portions of the duodenum, and the duodenum is retracted laterally to the patient's right. The peritoneum and areolar tissue overlying the aorta are opened longitudinally with the scissors or cautery, exposing the anterior surface of the aneurysm.

The peritoneal incision over the aorta is carried superiorly to the level of the left renal vein and inferiorly to below the aortic bifurcation. The aorta, just above the aneurysm and below the left renal vein, is freed from its surrounding tissues by a combination of sharp and gentle blunt dissection anteriorly and laterally (Fig. 23-2). No attempt is made to dissect behind the aorta, and the neck of the aneurysm is not encircled with tape. The dissection along the lateral walls of the aorta is continued far enough posteriorly that the neck of the aneurysm can be compressed easily by an occluding clamp, which is applied at this level. Juxtarenal and pararenal aneurysms may require division of the left renal vein (see Fig. 23-1). Dissection of the lateral walls of the aneurysm is limited to facilitate retractor placement, which assists in opening up the operative field and providing exposure during the dissection of the more proximal aortic neck. Mobilization of the aneurysm wall from the inferior vena cava is unnecessary, but visualization of the anterior surface of the vena cava is common.

EXPOSURE OF THE ILIAC ARTERIES

The anterior and lateral walls of both common iliac arteries are exposed by sharp dissection without separating these vessels from the common iliac veins posteriorly.

PROXIMAL AND DISTAL CONTROL

Intravenous heparin is administered at 80 units per kilogram of body weight (4000-6000 units in an average adult). Large, straight Fogarty vascular clamps are applied after systemic anticoagulation to both common iliac arteries, and a Fogarty or DeBakey reversed angle aortic clamp is applied to the aortic neck. Clamps may be angled in the presence of a calcified plaque so as to avoid plaque rupture or inadvertent perforation of the vessel wall by the plaque.

AORTIC INCISION

The superficial, adventitial layer of the aneurysm is incised longitudinally with electrocautery to minimize bleeding from the aortic wall (Fig. 23-3). The aneurysm is then opened with Mayo scissors. Each end of the aneurysm is incised laterally to increase exposure to the aneurysm cavity. All mural thrombus and loose atherosclerotic debris are evacuated from the lumen of the aneurysm. Inadvertent impaction of thrombus or atherosclerotic debris into the origins of the iliac arteries should be avoided.

Bleeding lumbar arteries are oversewn with figure-eight sutures of 3-0 polypropylene. The origin of the inferior mesenteric artery is sutured if backbleeding is present and if prior control was not obtained with a tape and collar or vessel loop.

PROXIMAL ANASTOMOSIS

In the absence of iliac aneurysms, a tube graft of collagen-impregnated knitted Dacron can be performed. The posterior wall of the aorta is not divided, although circumferential division of the proximal aortic cuff is a matter of surgeon preference. A double-armed running 3-0 polypropylene suture is used for the anastomoses. Strength can be added to the posterior suture line of the anastomosis by taking generous bites that incorporate both the normal aortic neck and aneurysm wall. In the presence of calcified plaque, a limited endarterectomy of the sewing ring may be necessary. The suture is carried around each side of the neck of the aneurysm and tied anteriorly. The proximal anastomosis is then tested for leaks by clamping the tube graft and releasing the aortic clamp briefly. Alternatively, the graft can be filled with saline using a bulb syringe to assess the anastomosis. Leaks, which may occur around the 3- and 9-o'clock positions, are repaired with figure-eight sutures or pledgeted horizontal mattress 3-0 polypropylene sutures. The aortic clamp is then placed on the graft just distal to the proximal anastomosis, a lap pad placed over the suture line, and a fixed retractor used to gently compress the lap pad.

DISTAL ANASTOMOSIS

After evacuating all blood from the graft with a sucker, the graft is distracted and cut to appropriate length to avoid redundancy or excessive tension for anastomosis to the aortic bifurcation using a double-armed, continuous running 3-0 polypropylene

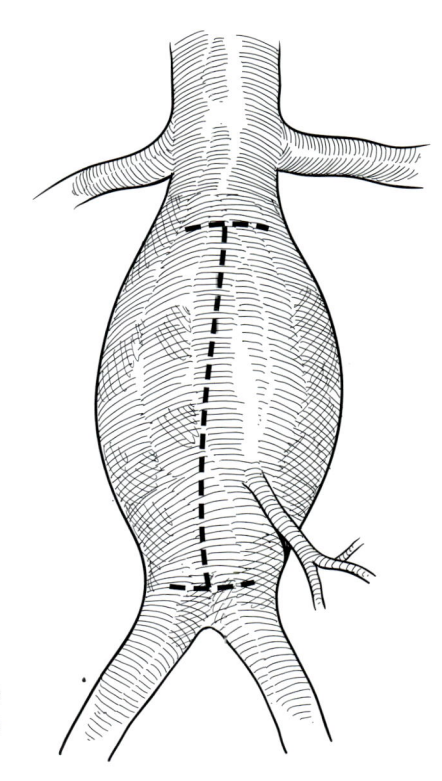

DIRECT SURGICAL REPAIR OF ANEURYSMS OF THE INFRARENAL ABDOMINAL AORTA AND ILIAC ARTERIES

Figure 23-2. The aorta is exposed via a transperitoneal approach by reflecting the large intestine superiorly, reflecting the small intestine and duodenum to the right, and incising the retroperitoneum longitudinally.

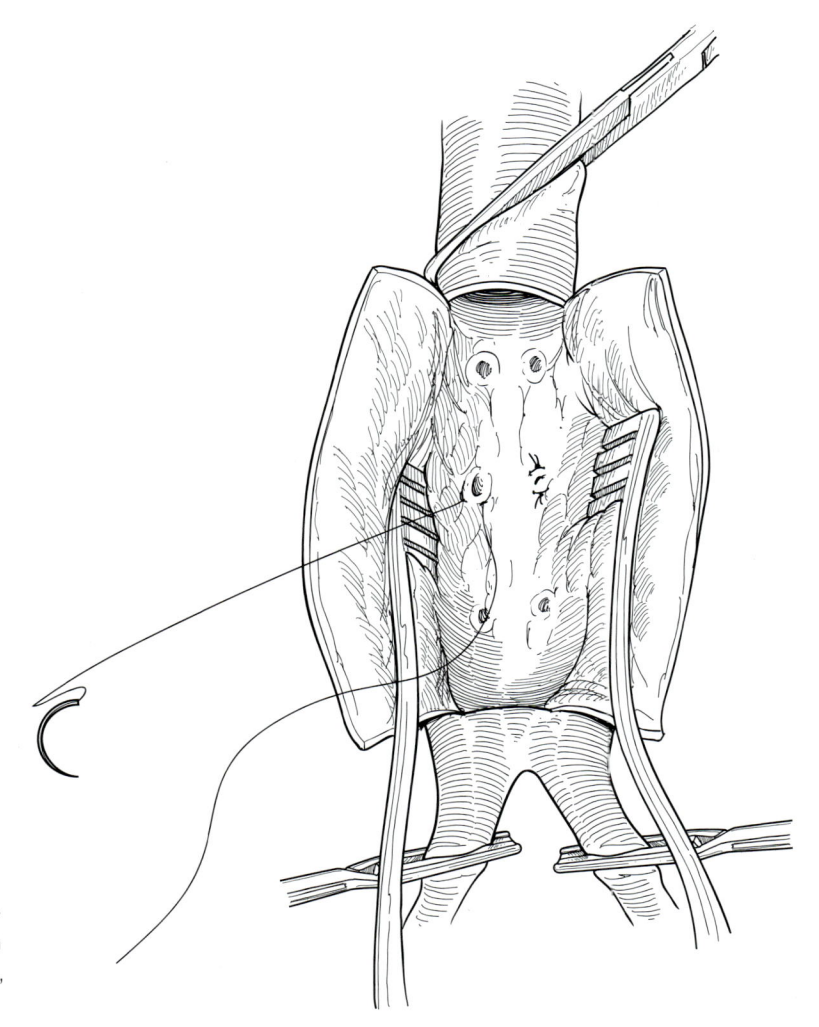

Figure 23-3. Vascular clamps are placed to provide inflow and outflow control. The aneurysm is then opened longitudinally, the mural thrombus is extracted, and the lumbar arteries are oversewn.

suture. In cases of calcification of the aortic bifurcation, judicious endarterectomy may be required to facilitate suturing.

Prograde flushing of the graft and retrograde flushing of the iliac arteries are conducted before the suture line is completed and tied anteriorly. One iliac clamp is released, and the anastomosis is inspected for leaks, which are repaired as necessary (Fig. 23-4). The proximal aortic clamp is then gradually released while blood pressure is monitored. The second iliac clamp is released once hemodynamic stability is ensured. The iliac arteries are inspected for adequate pulsation, and the presence of good femoral pulses is determined by palpation. The absence of a femoral pulse indicates either iliac thrombosis or flow-limiting plaque, which should be addressed immediately. Intraoperative evaluation of lower extremity circulation is mandatory and typically assessed by the presence of pedal Doppler signals.

REIMPLANTATION OF AN INFERIOR MESENTERIC OR ACCESSORY RENAL ARTERY

To reimplant either an inferior mesenteric artery or an accessory renal artery, a side-biting Satinsky clamp is placed on the aortic graft. The branch vessel is then sewn directly to the aortic graft in an end-to-side configuration using a single running 5-0 polypropylene suture, which is facilitated by using the aortic tissue surrounding the origin of the vessel as a Carrel patch.

GRAFT COVERAGE

Residual bleeding in the aneurysm wall is sutured, ligated, or electrocoagulated, and the aneurysm wall is closed over the prosthesis with a running 3-0 polypropylene suture. This is helpful both for hemostasis and for exclusion of the prosthetic graft from the duodenum and other viscera. The posterior peritoneum and periaortic lymphatic tissue are then approximated over the aorta by a running absorbable suture to provide another layer between the prosthesis and the posterior wall of the duodenum.

CLOSURE

Protamine sulfate is used selectively for heparin reversal depending on the duration of aneurysm repair and the appearance of the operative field. The abdomen is then closed with a continuous No. 1 polydioxanone suture to the rectus fascia and staples to the skin.

Operative Technique for Repair of an Iliac Aneurysm

If common iliac aneurysms are present, an operative procedure is followed similar to that used for repair of an infrarenal aortic aneurysm. However, clamps are applied to the external iliac arteries, taking care to avoid injury to the ureters, which usually cross the common iliac arteries distally. Although the distal right iliac system can be easily exposed by extending the posterior peritoneal incision, the left external iliac artery is best approached through a separate incision lateral to the sigmoid colon. Depending on the size of the common iliac artery aneurysm, it may not be possible to clamp the internal iliac artery directly, and balloon occlusion may be required. The iliac aneurysms are opened longitudinally in a staged manner with a lateral T extension at each end. The iliac limbs of a bifurcated graft are sutured to the common iliac arteries from within the iliac aneurysm (Fig. 23-5). Limited endarterectomy to remove dense calcium may be necessary. If it is necessary to anastomose the limb to the external iliac artery, the internal iliac artery orifice can be oversewn from within the aneurysm sac. If restoration of flow to the internal iliac artery is required, the distal end of a side limb graft can be first sewn to the orifice of internal iliac artery and the proximal end of the limb, then sewn in an end-to-side manner to the main iliac graft limb.

In the case of a large left iliac aneurysm, it may be more convenient to exclude the aneurysm by oversewing the orifice of the nonaneurysmal common iliac

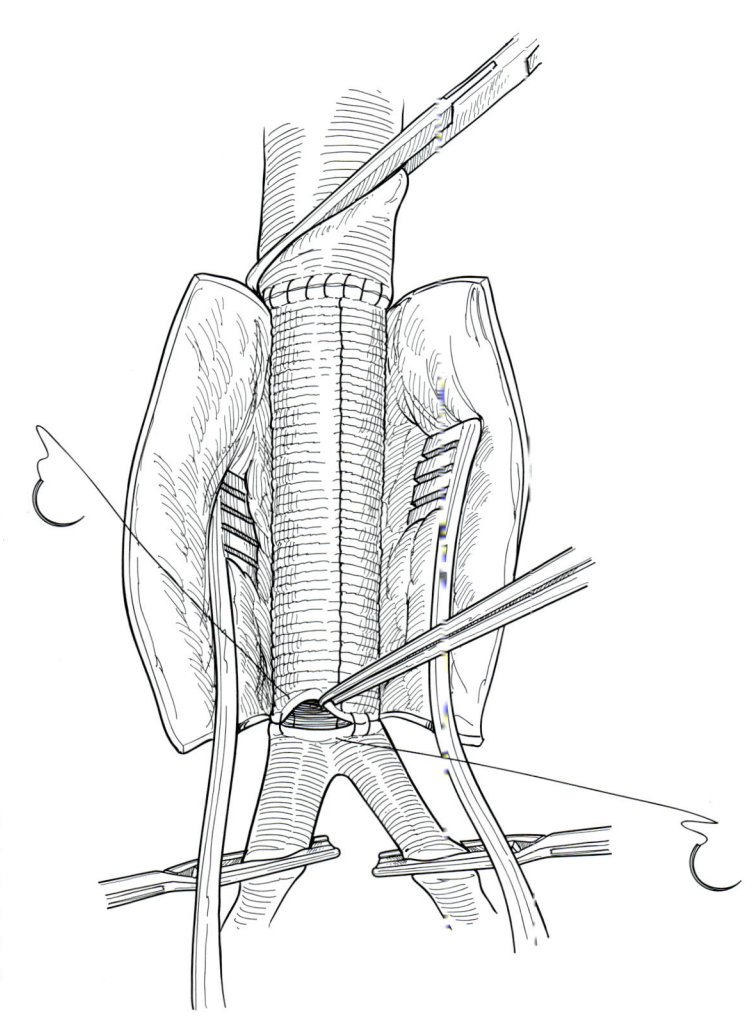

Figure 23-4. The proximal and distal anastomoses are completed with 3-0 polypropylene suture, with special attention given to obtaining large bites of the posterior wall. When necessary, limited endarterectomy of proximal, distal, or both sewing rings is performed to obtain adequate tissue for suture placement. If suture line bleeding occurs, horizontal mattress sutures with pledgets are placed.

artery. The left limb of the graft is then anastomosed end to side to the external iliac artery inferior to the sigmoid mesentery or, if necessary, to the femoral artery.

Operative Technique for Retroperitoneal Exposure

The patient is placed on an air-evacuating beanbag in a right lateral decubitus position with the shoulders elevated approximately 60 degrees and the legs and pelvis positioned relatively flat (Fig. 23-6). An oblique flank incision is made from the tip of the eleventh rib extending toward the lateral edge of the rectus at the level of the umbilicus. A more cephalad incision in the ninth interspace, as a thoracoabdominal incision, is performed for suprarenal aneurysms across the costal margin. This is supplemented with limited lateral division of the diaphragm. The underlying musculature is divided, leaving the posterior rectus sheath and the adherent peritoneum beneath intact. The retroperitoneal space is entered laterally at the level of the costal margin, and all abdominal contents are gently retracted medially by bluntly sweeping the peritoneal membrane off of the anterior and lateral aspects of the abdominal wall. As the peritoneal membrane is dissected off of the posterior rectus sheath, the sheath can be incised to improve the medial exposure. If a tear in the peritoneal membrane is created, this can be approximated with 3-0 polyglactin 910 (Vicryl) suture.

For infrarenal aortic aneurysm repair, we generally prefer to leave the left kidney in situ by developing a plane anterior to Gerota fascia. Alternatively, the kidney can be elevated and moved anteromedially with the rest of the abdominal contents. This is preferred for juxtarenal and suprarenal lesions, where suprarenal cross-clamp application is intended. Once the retroperitoneal plane has

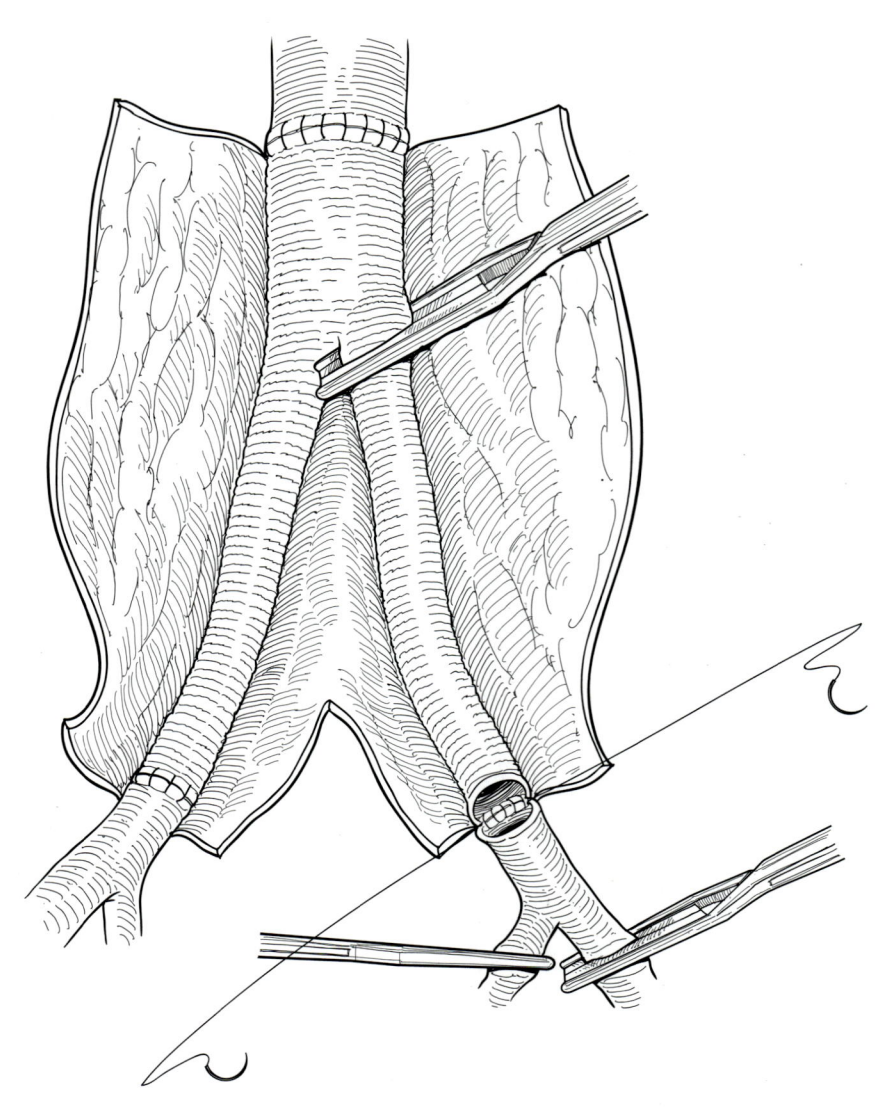

Figure 23-5. When the aortic aneurysm involves the iliac arteries, a bifurcation graft extending to the iliac bifurcation is required. Distal control is obtained either by clamping the distal common iliac arteries or by placing separate clamps on the external and internal iliac arteries. Exposure of the left iliac bifurcation usually requires mobilization of the sigmoid colon mecially.

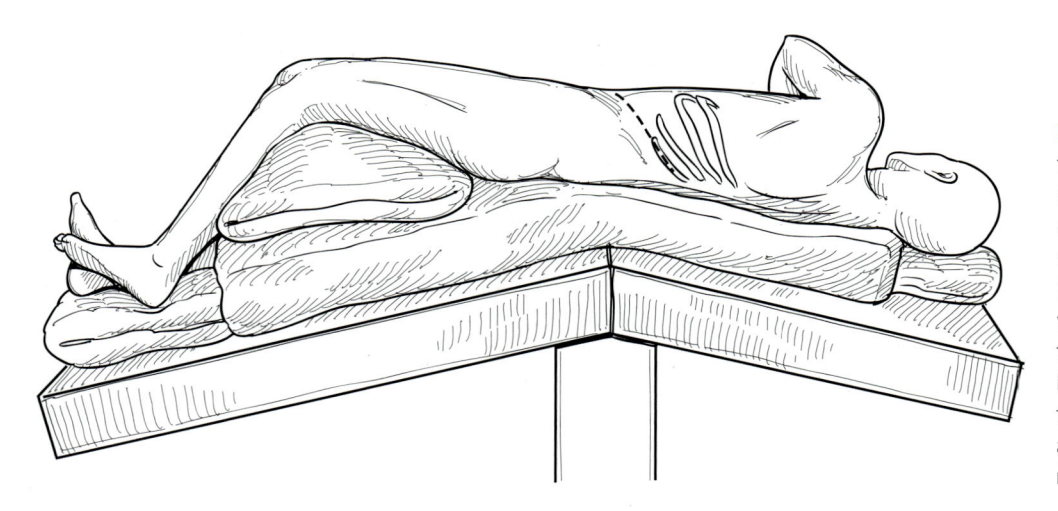

Figure 23-6. The patient is positioned on a beanbag in a modified right decubitus position with the chest at 60 degrees and the pelvis nearly flat. The operating table bed is flexed and the kidney rest elevated to open the space between the costal margin and the pelvic brim. The incision begins at the tip of the eleventh or twelfth rib and extends obliquely toward the midline.

been developed, the entire abdominal aorta and left iliac system can be easily visualized.

Aneurysm repair involves essentially the same steps as those described for a transabdominal approach. Access to the right common iliac artery can be achieved by dividing the inferior mesenteric artery, which facilitates sweeping of the peritoneal structures off the aneurysm and aortic bifurcation.

Postoperative Care

- If appropriate, the patient is extubated in the operating room. Dosing of the epidural catheter plays a significant role in the success of early intubation by providing adequate pain control for proper pulmonary mechanics.
- Patients are monitored with an arterial line, central line, Foley catheter, and nasogastric tube in the intensive care unit for a minimum of 24 hours. Vasoactive agents are used to avoid hypertension or hypotension, with volume infusion used as needed.
- Patients are usually prescribed bed rest on the day of operation and encouraged to ambulate the next day. Until patients are ambulating regularly, they are given subcutaneous heparin for deep venous thrombosis prophylaxis.
- Perioperative antibiotics consisting of a cephalosporin or, in the case of a penicillin allergy, vancomycin are administered for 24 hours after the operation.
- Epidural catheters are used for pain control in the perioperative period. If there is a contraindication to epidural catheter placement, a patient-controlled analgesia device is used.
- Aspirin and statin therapy for atherosclerotic risk reduction are prescribed for all patients being discharged. Where appropriate, antihypertensive therapy is also instituted.
- Patients are seen postoperatively at 1 month and then evaluated with a noncontrast CT scan at 1 year and 5 years.

Complications

- **Cardiac complications.** Most cardiac ischemic events occur within 72 hours of surgery. Intensive care monitoring during this period, with a focus on ensuring adequate oxygen delivery to the heart, is recommended for patients with high cardiac risk. A postoperative ECG should be routine for all patients undergoing abdominal aortic aneurysm repair.
- **Hemorrhage.** Bleeding from either an arterial suture line or a venous injury is usually recognized intraoperatively and is less likely to manifest postoperatively. More commonly, diffuse bleeding after substantial intraoperative blood loss results from a combination of hypothermia and exhausted coagulation factors and platelets. Aggressive rewarming, accompanied by factor replacement, is the treatment of choice.
- **Colon ischemia.** Sigmoid colon blood flow can be jeopardized by disruption of blood flow to the inferior mesenteric artery or the internal iliac arteries by either vessel ligation or atheromatous embolization. This condition occurs more frequently after repair of a ruptured aneurysm than after an elective repair. Recognition of colon ischemia is often difficult, so it is important to maintain a high index of clinical suspicion. Bloody stools, diarrhea, abdominal distention, acidemia, or unexplained fever, leukocytosis, and oliguria should prompt urgent flexible sigmoidoscopy. Isolated mucosal injury often resolves with fluid resuscitation and bowel rest, whereas full-thickness necrosis necessitates bowel resection.
- **Renal failure.** The most common cause of renal dysfunction after aneurysm repair relates to embolization of atheromatous debris into the renal arteries. Gentle manipulation of the aortic neck and careful cross-clamp placement can help minimize this risk. When the pararenal volume of atheromatous debris or thrombus is substantial, occlusion of the renal arteries before aortic clamping with vessel loops or tapes and collars may be prudent with release of occlusion tapes after aortic clamp placement. Although renal protective benefits are controversial, furosemide to maintain high urine volume and mannitol to serve as

an oxygen radical scavenger have been advocated by some groups. Direct renal artery instillation of a cold renal preservation solution has been used to limit ischemic renal injury in the circumstance of suprarenal cross-clamp application.

- **Impaired distal perfusion.** Lower extremity ischemia may occur secondary to either iliac plaque disruption or embolization of debris. Plaque disruption results in the loss of a femoral pulse, and treatment options include aorta to femoral artery bypass, femoral-femoral bypass, and retrograde stent placement. Embolization is generally less amenable to definitive treatment, but in the case of a large embolus, surgical retrieval may be possible. More frequently, emboli are small and result in patchy areas of dusky skin or in digital ischemia with trash foot or trash buttocks syndrome in the severest cases.
- **Impaired sexual function.** Impotence or retrograde ejaculation may result from autonomic sympathetic nerve injury or decreased arterial inflow to the internal iliac arteries.

REFERENCES

1. Friedman SG: *A history of vascular surgery*, ed 2, Malden, Mass., 2005, Blackwell Publishing.
2. Dubost C, Allary M, Oeconomos N: Resection of an aneurysm of the abdominal aorta: Re-establishment of the continuity by a preserved human arterial graft, with result after five months, *Arch Surg* 64:405-408, 1952.
3. Blakemore AH, Voorhees AB Jr: The use of tubes constructed from vinyon N cloth in bridging arterial defects: Experimental and clinical, *Ann Surg* 140:324-334, 1954.
4. DeBakey ME, Crawford ES, Cooley DA, et al: Aneurysm of abdominal aorta analysis of results of graft replacement therapy one to eleven years after operation, *Ann Surg* 160:622-639, 1964.
5. Hicks GL, Eastland MW, DeWeese JA, et al: Survival improvement following aortic aneurysm resection, *Ann Surg* 181:863-869, 1975.
6. Creech O Jr: Endo-aneurysmorrhaphy and treatment of aortic aneurysm, *Ann Surg* 164:935-946, 1966.
7. Brady AR, Fowkes FG, Greenhalgh RM: Risk factors for postoperative death following elective surgical repair of abdominal aortic aneurysm: Results from the UK Small Aneurysm Trial, *Br J Surg* 87:742-749, 2000.
8. Lederle FA, Wilson SE, Johnson GR, et al: Immediate repair compared with surveillance of small abdominal aortic aneurysms, *N Engl J Med* 346:1437-1444, 2002.
9. Young JR, Hertzer NR, Beven EG, et al: Coronary artery disease in patients with aortic aneurysm: A classification of 302 coronary angiograms and results of surgical management, *Ann Vasc Surg* 1:36-42, 1986.
10. Schouten O, Boersma E, Hoeks SE, et al: Fluvastatin and perioperative events in patients undergoing vascular surgery, *N Engl J Med* 361:980-989, 2009.
11. Antiplatelet Trialists Collaboration: Collaborative overview of randomised trials of antiplatelet therapy I: Prevention of death, myocardial infarction, and stroke by prolonged antiplatelet therapy in various categories of patients, *BMJ* 308:81-106, 1994.
12. Devereaux PJ, Yang H, Yusuf S, et al: Effects of extended-release metoprolol succinate in patients undergoing non-cardiac surgery (POISE trial): A randomised controlled trial, *Lancet* 371: 1839-1847, 2008.
13. Weinstein ES, Langsfeld M, DeFrang R: Current management of coexistent intra-abdominal pathology in patients with abdominal aortic aneurysms, *Semin Vasc Surg* 8:135-143, 1995.
14. Samson RH, Lepore MR Jr, Showalter DP, et al: Long-term safety of left renal vein division and ligation to expedite complex abdominal aortic surgery, *J Vasc Surg* 50:500-504, 2009.
15. Starr DS, Foster WJ, Morris GC Jr: Resection of abdominal aortic aneurysm in the presence of horseshoe kidney, *Surgery* 89:387-389, 1981.
16. Baldridge ED Jr, Canos AJ: Venous anomalies encountered in aortoiliac surgery, *Arch Surg* 122:1184-1188, 1987.

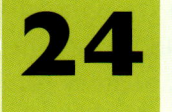

24 Direct Surgical Repair of Juxtarenal and Suprarenal Aneurysms of the Abdominal Aorta

JAMES H. BLACK III

Historical Background

The surgical management of abdominal aortic aneurysms was first pursued by direct aortic ligation as reported by Matas[1] in 1923. Likewise, beginning in 1906, Halsted and Reid[2] at the Johns Hopkins Hospital attempted to treat suprarenal aortic aneurysms in five patients by the placement of partially occlusive metal bands. Subsequent strategies included the induction of partial or complete thrombosis of aortic aneuryms by translumbar placement of intraluminal wires to increase wall thickness and reduce the risk of rupture.[3] In 1949 Nissen wrapped Albert Einstein's aortic aneurysm with cellophane, borrowing upon a technique described by Rea.[4] Einstein eventually succumbed to rupture 6 years later.[5] Complete resection of an abdominal aortic aneurysm and graft replacement was reported in 1951 by Dubost and colleagues,[6] but this technique was often complicated by major bleeding from adherent nearby major venous structures. The modern technique of endoaneurysmorrhaphy with intraluminal graft placement was popularized by Creech[7] in the 1960s and is the current approach for most aortic aneurysms, including juxtarenal abdominal aortic aneurysms (jAAAs) and suprarenal abdominal aortic aneurysms (sAAAs). The application of a left retroperitoneal approach to address extensive aneurysms of the abdominal aorta is credited to Williams.[8]

Indications

The surgical repair of asymptomatic jAAAs and sAAAs carries a greater incidence of postoperative complications than the surgical repair of infrarenal aortic aneurysms.[9] As a consequence, a 6-cm diameter is considered the threshold for repair of asymptomatic aneurysms. A slightly lower threshold (5.5 cm) may be considered for women, given a presumed increased risk for rupture.[10] Symptomatic jAAAs and sAAAs should be repaired urgently.

Preoperative Preparation

- Beta-blocker should be initiated before surgery with a target heart rate of less than 70 beats per minute.[11]
- Aspirin and statin therapy may reduce perioperative cardiovascular risk and should be maintained throughout the recovery period.[12]
- Thienopyridines should be halted 7 to 10 days before surgery because of risk of excessive bleeding, but should be resumed in the postoperative period if used as part of a dual antiplatelet regimen for patients who have received a drug-eluting coronary stent.[12]

- Double lumen endotracheal intubation is not necessary for left lung isolation for jAAA and sAAA repairs.
- Intraoperative arterial line monitoring of blood pressure is recommended.
- Intravenous access with large bore central lines should be established for rapid infusion, and pulmonary artery catheterization is mandatory for patients with cardiac dysfunction.
- Intraoperative autotransfusion devices are preferred to return collected red blood cells from the aneurysmal sac and bleeding lumbar vessels.
- Systemic normothermia should be maintained.
- Perioperative prophylactic antibiotics should be given for 24 hours with intraoperative redosing for every 1500 mL blood loss.

Pitfalls and Danger Points

- Intraoperative hemorrhage from a proximal anastomosis constructed to inhospitable aortic tissue or an iatrogenic venous injury to an unrecognized retroaortic left renal vein
- Precipitous hemodynamic changes during aortic clamping and reperfusion leading to myocardial injury and renal dysfunction
- Visceral ischemia from embolization during dissection and clamping of the proximal aorta or due to unrecognized stenosis of the visceral vessels
- Colonic ischemia from interruption of the inferior mesenteric artery or collateral blood supply from the pelvis

Operative Strategy

RETROPERITONEAL OR TRANSPERITONEAL EXPOSURE

For a jAAA, a retroperitoneal or transperitoneal approach may be used. Randomized trials have not demonstrated major differences in outcomes for either approach. In general, a transperitoneal approach affords rapid access to the abdomen and ease of bilateral iliac exposure when large iliac aneurysms are present, but upper abdominal organs limits access to the visceral segment of the abdominal aorta. The left renal vein may be divided to facilitate suprarenal aortic clamping during a transperitoneal approach, but left renal dysfunction may ensue. The left retroperitoneal approach facilitates exposure of the upper abdominal aorta for cross clamping at or above the superior mesenteric artery or celiac axis—a strong advantage in a sAAA—but limits access to the right iliac artery and may require intraluminal right iliac control (Box 24-1).

SELECTION OF SITE FOR PROXIMAL AORTIC CONTROL

Preoperative computed tomography (CT) imaging is mandatory to determine the level of proximal aortic control. Features that suggest an appropriate clamp site include lack of significant calcification or mural thrombus, along with a normal aortic diameter. A jAAA implies the aneurysm extends to the lowest

---

Box 24-1 | RELATIVE INDICATIONS FOR RETROPERITONEAL EXPOSURE

- "Hostile" abdomen secondary to multiple prior transperitoneal operations or presence of a stoma
- Inflammatory aortic aneurysm
- Horseshoe kidney
- Need for suprarenal endarterectomy

renal artery, necessitating aortic clamping above the renal arteries so that an anastomosis can be performed across the lower border of the renal arteries. In practice, a clamp may be placed across the jAAA neck if not overly burdened by atheroma, mural thrombus, or calcification to allow the surgeon to open the jAAA, evacuate the blood and mural thrombus, control lumbar vessels, with subsequent placement of the clamp above the renal arteries when performing the anastomosis. If feasible, such a strategy significantly reduces the period of renal ischemia.

For a sAAA, the aneurysm extends to involve varying portions of the renal artery origins and/or the visceral vessels. The segment of aorta between the celiac and the superior mesenteric artery may be more normal in caliber, but the presence of orificial disease near the superior mesenteric artery may preclude clamping in this area. If this visceral segment of the abdominal aorta is heavily diseased, the proximal clamp should be applied above the celiac axis to avoid embolization of debris into the visceral vessels. The supraceliac segment of aorta is also more easily exposed that the region between the superior mesenteric artery and celiac axis.

Operative Technique

CONTROL OF THE SUPRARENAL AORTA

The suprarenal aorta can be approached from either a transperitoneal or retroperitoneal exposure. In the transperitoneal exposure, the duodenum is mobilized to the right with the root of the mesentery. The retroperitoneal tissues along the lower border of the pancreas are opened, and the inferior mesenteric vein should be divided from its confluence onto the splenic vein to allow a static retraction device to reflect the pancreas cephalad. The left renal vein is appreciated coursing across the aorta and overlying the renal artery origins. By sacrificing the lumbar and gonadal branches to the left renal vein seen just left of the aorta, the left renal vein can be retracted to expose the suprarenal aorta for clamp application.

CONTROL OF THE SUPRACELIAC AORTA

In the retroperitoneal exposure of the jAAA or sAAA, the left-sided abdominal structures are reflected medially. The left retroperitoneal space is developed cephalad, and the spleen is displaced medially until the left crural fibers of the diaphragm are appreciated. The suprarenal aorta is covered by the left crural diaphragmatic muscle and a layer of thick fascia, which is continuous with the pleura. Both layers can be divided with electrocautery after a clamp or index finger is insinuated beneath these layers to develop a surgical plane along the left side of the aorta. Short, direct arteriolar perforators to the crus are rarely encountered during this maneuver, but if encountered, direct suture repair of the aortic wall with pledgeted 4-0 polypropylene sutures placed in horizontal-mattress fashion may be required. Sharp dissection is used to dissect the retroperitoneal tissues from the region surrounding the origins of the visceral vessel to allow secure clamping, and reduce bleeding as well as embolization during proximal aortic clamping. The anterior and posterior tissues just above the celiac axis are easily mobilized to allow proximal aortic control.

RETROPERITONEAL EXPOSURE

Incision for a Juxtarenal Abdominal Aortic Aneurysm

The tenth interspace is selected as the site of incision for most patients with a jAAA (Fig. 24-1). The incision is carried posteriorly along the superior border of the eleventh rib for 4 to 6 inches. In some patients, a limited incision in the diaphragm is required to separate the tenth and eleventh ribs, but this may be repaired primarily during closure and a left pleural tube is not required. The

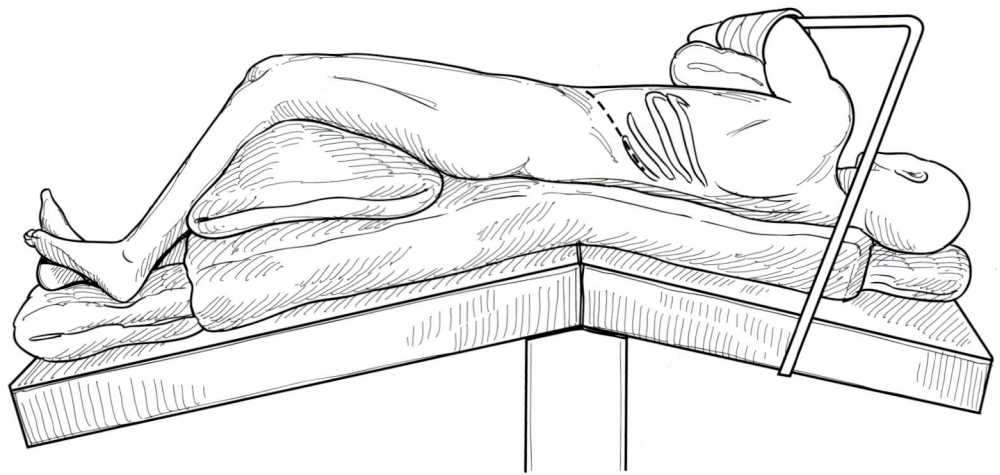

Figure 24-1. Patient positioning and incision for a retroperitoneal approach to the abdominal aorta. The patient is turned on the right side with the shoulders nearly vertical and the hips rotated as horizontal as possible. The operative table is flexed with the patient's flank positioned on the table break. A kidney rest fixed to the table may also be used to further elevate and flatten the region of the torso between the lower costal margin and iliac crest. The left flank and both groins may be prepped into the field, but right groin exposure may be limited. The patient position is stabilized by the use of a bean bag. Although the depicted incision courses onto the tip of the twelfth rib, it can and should be varied to the interspace above depending on the proximal extent of the aortic aneurysm and the patient's body habitus. For example, an incision in the tenth interspace, over the eleventh rib, is required for optimal exposure of most juxtarenal aortic aneurysms.

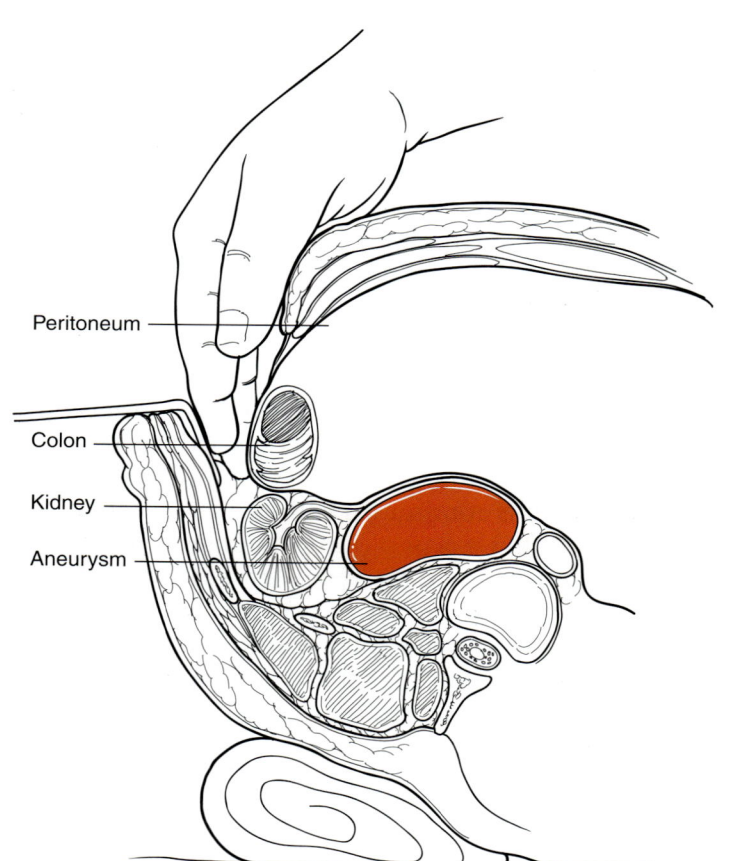

Figure 24-2. Developing the appropriate retroperitoneal plane in performing a left-sided medial visceral rotation. Typically the left kidney is elevated out of its bed, but there are circumstances (e.g., retroaortic left renal vein) in which the plane is developed anterior to the kidney, which is left in situ.

retroperitoneal plane is entered at the tip of the eleventh rib (Fig. 24-2) and the peritoneal sac bluntly swept from the undersurface of the anterior abdominal wall. The anterior abdominal incision should be kept parallel to the course of the rib to avoid crossing the intercostals nerve bundles as they merge onto the abdominal wall, thus reducing the risk of denervating the flank muscle with resultant muscle bulging. The anterior portion of the incision is carried forward to the lateral border of the rectus, which may curve caudally to the umbilicus or below, in the case of iliac artery involvement.

Incision for a Suprarenal Abdominal Aortic Aneurysm

The ninth or tenth interspace is the choice of incision for most patients with a sAAA (see Fig. 24-1). The incision is carried posterior along the rib for 4 to 6 inches. The ninth and tenth ribs are fused on the costal margin anteriorly, and the bridge of cartilage must be divided with electrocautery or bone-cutting scissors after dissection of the anterior abdominal muscular attachments. Typically, the superior epigastric artery must be ligated under the divided costal margin. With the costal margin divided, the retroperitoneum and diaphragm are evident. The diaphragm is opened for 4 to 6 inches to facilitate blunt retroperitoneal mobilization of the left-sided abdominal viscera. The peritoneal sac is bluntly mobilized from the under surface of the anterior abdominal wall muscles. The incision is carried anteriorly and parallel to the course of the tenth rib and then curves downward, lateral to the left rectus muscle, beyond the level of the umbilicus.

REPAIR OF A JUXTARENAL AORTIC ANEURYSM WITH ILIAC ARTERY INVOLVEMENT

Incision

With the patient in a supine position, a midline incision is made from the xiphoid to the pubis. The peritoneum is entered, and after inspection of the abdominal contents, the transverse mesocolon is reflected onto the lower chest and wrapped with a warm towel to prevent desiccation. The small bowel is kept intracavitary and packed to the right abdomen with a wet towel, whereas the duodenum is mobilized at the root of the mesentery from the retroperitoneum as it lies on the jAAA. A static retraction device is fixed to the table. Wide retraction blades are placed against the small bowel and mesocolon, and shallow blades are placed to steady the left abdominal wall and the bilateral lower quadrants.

Exposure of the Abdominal Aorta

The fibrofatty retroperitoneal tissue is opened in the midline to expose the jAAA. With electrocautery dissection, the retroperitoneum is mobilized from the anterior aorta and the inferior mesenteric artery is identified and dissected. If the inferior mesenteric artery is patent, it may need to be reimplanted into the aortic graft depending upon the adequacy of colonic perfusion. The tissues overlying the common iliac arteries are opened and suitable sites selected for distal control.

Exposure of the Iliac Arteries

For patients with aneurysmal involvement of both common iliac arteries, individual control of iliac bifurcation vessels facilitates construction of the distal anastomosis. The dissection plane should adhere to the vessel wall during exposure of the iliac artery bifurcation to reduce the risk of ureteral injury. The exposure of the internal iliac vessels may be obscured by the presence of a large common iliac artery aneurysm, and intraluminal control of the internal iliac after opening the aneurysm may be the only option for control. If the internal iliac artery can be visualized, it should be mobilized along its lateral walls, but not circumferentially, to avoid iatrogenic iliac vein injury. Once the iliac bifurcations are dissected free of the surrounding structures, lower quadrant shallow retraction devices are replaced with deeper retractors to "hook and hold" the ureters and colonic structures lateral to the region for distal anastomosis.

Division of the Renal Vein

In the transperitoneal approach for a jAAA, mobilization of the renal vein is key to securing a suitable suprarenal cross-clamp. If the neck of the aneurysm is tortuous, consideration should be given to early division of the left renal vein, with preservation of the left gonadal and adrenal veins for left renal drainage. In many patients, simple downward traction on the aneurysm may straighten the neck and facilitate dissection of the left renal vein with gentle blunt dissection. If such a maneuver appears to facilitate visualization of the suprarenal neck, then renal vein division is likely not needed. Ligation of the left lumbar and gonadal veins on the lower edge of the left renal vein will allow its cephalad mobilization. Once mobilized, a narrow and deep static retraction blade is placed under the left renal vein. The vein is retracted cephalad to expose the suprarenal aorta to the origin of the superior mesenteric artery.

Proximal and Distal Control

Before clamp application, the patient should be anticoagulated with intravenous heparin (100 IU/kg). The right renal artery and superior mesenteric artery may occasionally originate so close to each other to render clamping below the superior mesenteric artery yet above both renal arteries impossible. If the aortic neck intervening between the right and the often lower left renal artery is normal, a cross-clamp can be applied at that site for proximal control, with only left renal ischemia induced by clamping. If the aorta in the pararenal region is not hospitable for secure control, supraceliac control of the aorta should be obtained (Box 24-2). Although backbleeding will occur from the celiac artery and the superior mesenteric artery, this can be controlled with a compliant intraluminal endovascular aortic balloon inserted coaxially through the surgical graft.

When feasible, distal control of the iliac vessels is performed initially, followed by clamping of the superior mesenteric artery to reduce the risk of visceral embolization upon proximal aortic clamping. Thereafter, surgeon and anesthesia communication are key to ensure appropriate control of blood pressure before applying suprarenal or supraceliac clamps so that the proximal aortic pressure does not rise unexpectedly with a detrimental increase in cardiac afterload.

Aortic Incision

The incision of the jAAA should follow the center line with blunt evacuation of mural thrombus. The autotransfusion device should be used to salvage blood from the aneurysmal sac and lumbar vessels. In the presence of an underlying chronic aortic dissection, lumbar artery blood loss can be substantial and nonautologous transfusion should be anticipated. The center line aortotomy should avoid the aortic tissue in the immediate vicinity of the inferior mesenteric artery, leaving an aortic cuff in case later reimplantation is required (see Chapter 23). If back bleeding from the

---

Box 24-2 STEPS FOR TRANSPERITONEAL CONTROL OF THE SUPRACELIAC AORTA

1. The triangular ligament of the left lobe of the liver is incised and liver reflected medially and cephalad.
2. The stomach and gastroesophageal junction should be retracted toward the left lower quadrant. The presence of a nasogastric tube is palpated to avoid injuring the esophagus.
3. The diaphragm is incised vertically and anterior to the upper abdominal aorta.
4. Blunt finger mobilization can free surrounding pleural and mediastinal tissues and define the lateral boundaries of the supraceliac aorta and the spine lying posterior.
5. The supraceliac aorta is clamped with a long, straight clamp while the index and middle fingers of the surgeon's other hand are kept in place to guide the jaws of the clamp to the appropriate position.

inferior mesenteric artery is noted, control can easily be achieved with a vessel loop or cotton tape and small rubber collar.

Proximal Anastomosis

With hemostasis of the aneurysmal sac achieved, the junction between the aneurysmal aortic wall and the smooth intimal surface of the aortic neck define a sewing ring of aorta suitable for the proximal anastomosis. If such tissues are not observed at, or just below, the renal vessels, then the anastomosis can be carried out above the renal vessels, with separate jump grafts to each renal artery. Such a situation can be anticipated by a preoperative CT scan, and a surgical graft preconstructed with appropriate "side arm" grafts available before proximal clamping.

The proximal anastomosis should be performed with a 3-0 polypropylene suture with felt reinforcement using either interrupted or running suture lines, dictated by surgeon preference. Preoperative CT imaging or intraoperative plastic aortic neck sizers, which are included along with most vascular grafts, can help guide selection of an appropriate diameter graft. Typically a graft is selected that is 2 mm less than the outer wall neck diameter by either method. In a jAAA, it is not advisable to formally divide the aortic neck, which may injure posterior retroaortic veins. Therefore a standard endoaneurysmorrhaphy technique with Creech bites along the posterior row is advised.

If direct reconstructions of the renal vessels are required, then the side-arm grafts can be anastomosed end-to-side to the midportion of either renal artery. The proximal renal vessels are ligated to prevent bleeding at the original orifice. Alternatively, the side-arm grafts can be anastomosed to the renal artery origins, but the physical space to do so may be limited if the pararenal aorta is nearly normal in diameter.

Distal Anastomosis With Side Graft to External Iliac Artery

When the aneurysm involves the common iliac artery, the distal anastomosis can assume several configurations. If the origins of the internal and external iliac arteries are of normal caliber and in close proximity, an end-to-end anastomosis can be performed to the distal common iliac artery. In very large iliac aneurysms the origins of these vessels can be a distance apart, and a single end-to-end anastomosis to both is not possible. In this case, it is often best to take the limb of the bifurcated Dacron graft and first perform an end-to-end anastomosis to the internal iliac artery using a parachute or standard technique. With the length of the internal iliac limb slightly redundant, the end of the external iliac artery can be anastomosed either to the side of the internal iliac graft limb or to a separate side graft.

Graft Coverage

Once reperfusion of the aortic branches and lower extremities is confirmed by continuous wave Doppler, protamine should be administered for reversal of the systemic anticoagulation. The interior of the aneurysmal sac should be reinspected for latent bleeding from lumbar arteries after pelvic and lower extremity reperfusion. The aneurysm sac is approximated over the repair to isolate the repair from the abdominal contents. The midline retroperitoneal tissues are also closed to isolate the repair from the duodenum.

REPAIR OF A SUPRARENAL AORTIC ANEURYSM

Incision

The patient is turned on the right side with the shoulders nearly vertical and the hips rotated as horizontal as possible. The operative table is flexed with the patient's flank positioned on the table break. The left flank and both groins may be prepped into the field, but right groin exposure may be limited in the obese patient. For sAAAs (Video 24-1), the incision to gain access into the left retroperitoneal space is performed through the ninth interspace and carried onto the anterior abdominal wall to the lateral border of the rectus and then curved caudally to the umbilicus or below (see Fig. 24-1). A static retraction device is used to hold the peritoneal sac medially. A shallow body wall retractor placed against the tenth rib and a right angle retractor held in parallel to the left iliac vessels in the left lower quadrant usually suffices for the lateral and inferior exposure. On the superior and medial portions of the wound, a deep right angle retractor can be used to displace the ninth rib cephalad and a wide fan-type retractor positioned against the peritoneal sac. Separate, deep, narrow blades can be used to visualize the visceral vessels and the right iliac artery. If not a critical vessel, division of the inferior mesenteric artery can facilitate displacement of the peritoneal contents to the patient's right for improved access to the right iliac artery.

Exposure of the Abdominal Aorta

Once the abdominal structures and ureter are reflected from the left retroperitoneum (see Fig. 24-2), the pulse of the left renal artery is identified. In most patients the left renolumbar vein orients the dissection toward the left renal artery, which is now dissected back to its aortic origin. Proceeding cephalad, the median arcuate ligament and curs is opened; it is often easiest to identify the celiac axis and work down the aorta sharply to the superior mesenteric artery, which is usually surround by fibrous tissues and a nerve plexus. In addition, when the sAAA neck is tortuous, the origin of the superior mesenteric artery may appear nearly behind the course of the left renal artery. In such cases, circumferential dissection of retroperitoneal tissue from around the left renal artery opens a space to identify its origin (Fig. 24-3). The left retroperitoneal tissue is divided with electrocautery or between ties over the abdominal aorta.

Exposure of the Iliac Arteries

The left common iliac artery is exposed for subsequent clamping. The left retroperitoneal approach renders the left iliac artery in plain view, but the ureter should be bluntly reflected under the retractor to avoid injury. In thinner patients, the retroperitoneum can be mobilized to the right side of the aorta to identify the origin of the right common iliac artery for clamping. If necessary, the right iliac artery can be identified and controlled intraluminally.

Proximal and Distal Control

Unfractionated heparin (100 IU/kg) is administered intravenously. Clamps are applied distally to proximally, with separate atraumatic vascular clamps placed on the superior mesenteric artery and the celiac axis. Vasodilators should be titrated to accommodate the increase in afterload with aortic clamping. Once the blood pressure is stable, the supraceliac aorta is cross-clamped.

Aortic Incision

The aortotomy is opened longitudinally, with care taken to position the aortotomy close to the level of the anterior portion vertebral bodies so that arterial incision runs posterior to the left renal artery orifice (Fig. 24-4) up to the level of the normal proximal aorta. Cold renal artery perfusion may decrease the risk of renal ischemic injury,[13] but should be balanced against adverse effects of systemic hypothermia. The left renal artery is excised and cold saline is flushed before performing the proximal anastomosis.

Proximal Aortic Anastomosis

In a typical sAAA, the aorta may be suitable for anastomosis near the origins of the right renal artery extending upward to the superior mesenteric artery. However, the aorta posteriorly overlying the spine may not be suitable for the construction of an anastomosis. Although the back wall of the aorta is not divided, the proximal aspect of the longitudinal aortic incision should be "T'd" and extended posteriorly to the spine to reveal the bevel of the native aorta to be anastomosed.

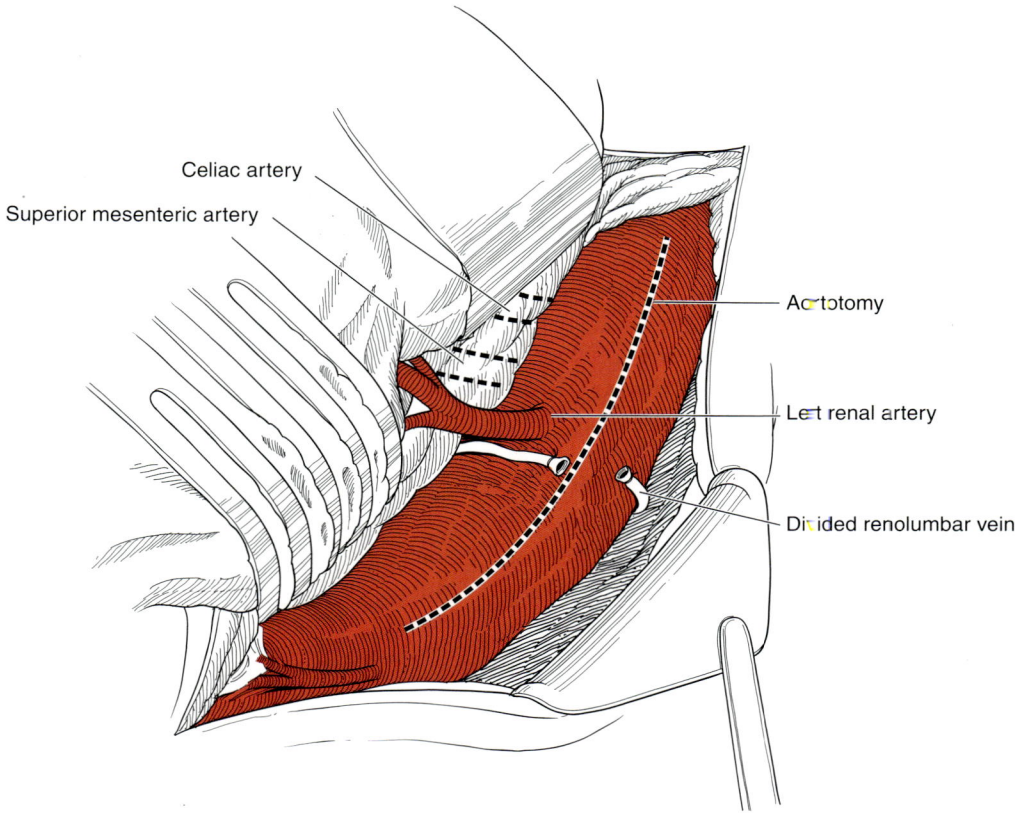

DIRECT SURGICAL REPAIR OF JUXTARENAL AND SUPRARENAL ANEURYSMS OF THE ABDOMINAL AORTA | 317

Figure 24-3. Orientation of an aortotomy posterior to a left renal artery origin. The left renolumbar vein is divided.

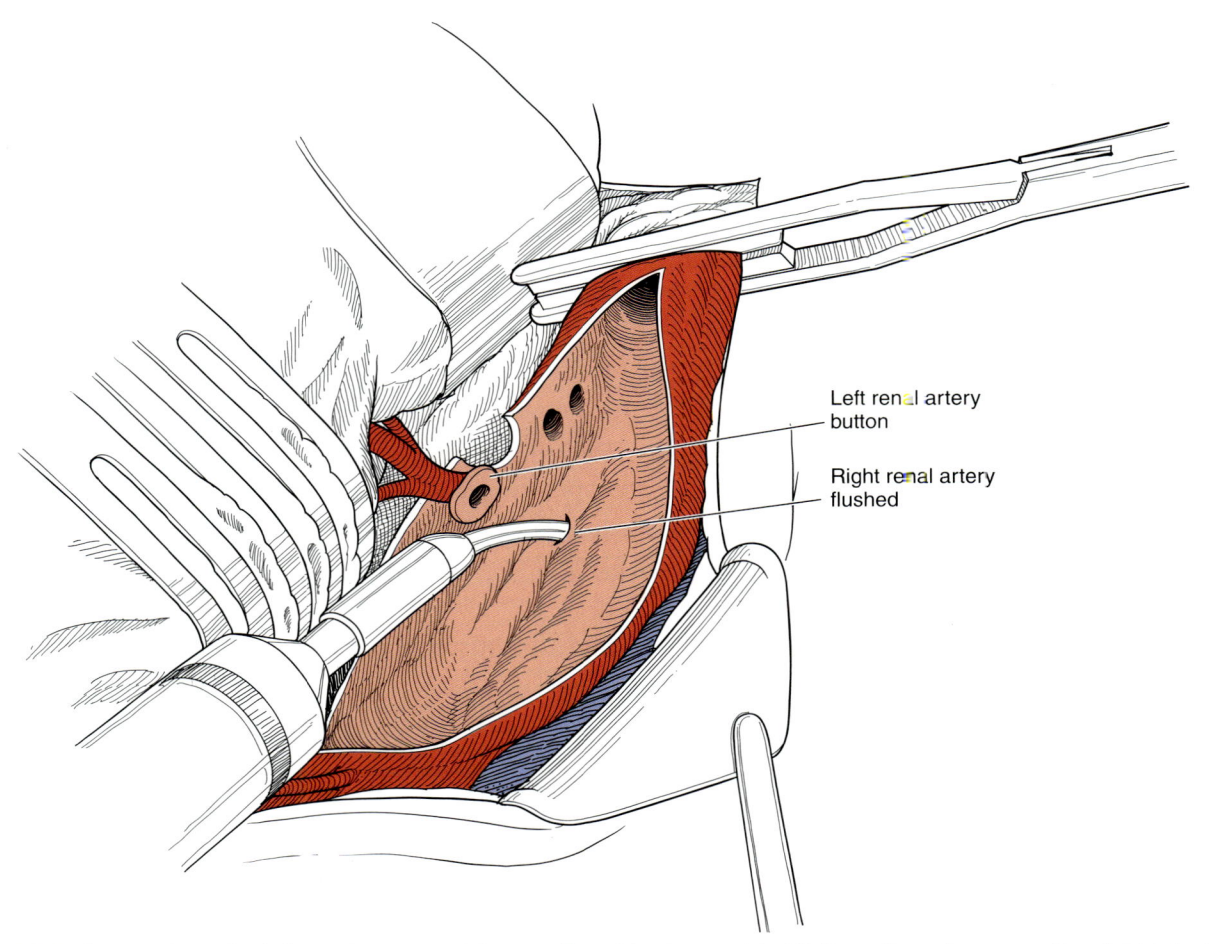

Figure 24-4. Amputation of a left renal artery origin as a Carrel button and instillation of renal preservation fluid into the right kidney. The left renal artery can be reimplanted as such a Carrel button onto the aortic graft or preferably can be reconstructed with a side-arm graft.

Consequently, the graft is cut at a 45-degree angle to accommodate the origins of the right renal artery, superior mesenteric arteric artery, and if needed, the celiac artery off the native aorta. An endoaneurysmorrhaphy technique is used for the posterior suture line of the anastomosis, which travels posteriorly and cephalad with each stitch. If the quality of the aorta is poor, then felt strip reinforcement can be used along the posterior row and anterior row by passing the stitch through the strip after the needle exits the aortic tissue. The left renal artery can be reimplanted as a Carrel patch or reconstructed with a side-arm graft previously placed on the main aortic graft. The advantage of the latter is to allow a space to clamp the aortic graft so that visceral and right renal artery perfusion can be restored before revascularization of the left kidney (Fig. 24-5). In this figure, the extent of the reconstruction could legitimately be classified an extent IV thoracoabdominal aneurysm (i.e., the graft itself is carried cephalad to the celiac axis origin).

Distal Aortic Anastomosis

The distal aortic anastomosis can be performed to the aortic bifurcation, the origins of the iliac arteries, or the iliac artery bifurcation, as required. If feasible, performing the distal anastomosis at the aortic bifurcation to expedite the operation is preferred. Addressing small or moderate aneurysmal disease of the iliac arteries can be deferred as the need to intervene for later iliac aneurysms after prior aortic aneurysm repair is low.[14]

Closure

With reperfusion of the visceral and renal vessels as well as both lower extremities, protamine should be administered. The aneurysm sac is approximated over the surgical repair using 0 silk sutures, with attention paid to avoiding kinking the left renal artery reconstruction as the kidney assumes its usual location in the left retroperitoneum. Closed or open suction tubes are tunneled from the paraaortic area and out the anterior abdominal wall to evacuate postoperative blood. The hiatus of the diaphragm is reapproximated with 0 silk sutures as is the diaphragm near the costal margin. A left pleural tube is not required but is sometimes desirable in patients with borderline pulmonary status to drain any effusion that develops during the first few days after surgery.

The anterior abdominal wall is closed in a single layer with running or interrupted sutures. The divided costal margin is reapproximated with No. 2 absorbable suture, and the chest wall muscles are approximated with a No. 2 absorbable suture.

Postoperative Care

- Extubation should be deferred until the patient is normothermic. Extubation is often considered on postoperative days 1 or 2.
- Hemodynamic monitoring and serial hemoglobin checks are advisable.
- Preoperative beta-blocker therapy, aspirin, and statin medications should be reinitiated.
- Prophylactic antibiotics are administered for the first 24 hours postoperatively.

Postoperative Complications

- **Mortality.** Postoperative mortality after surgical repair of a jAAA is 1% to 3% in most centers,[15] with mortality after repair of a sAAA ranging between 3% and 10%.[16,17]
- **Renal function.** Postoperative deterioration in renal function is not uncommon (10%-20%) among patients who require suprarenal aortic cross-clamp application, but a requirement for dialysis is rare (<1%) in patients with normal preoperative renal function.[17]

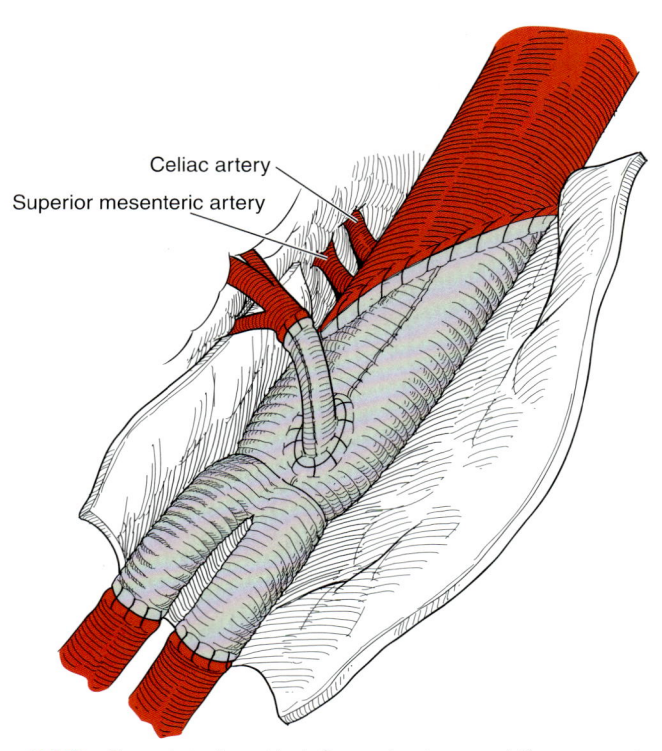

Figure 24-5. Completed aortic, left renal artery, and iliac reconstruction.

- **Cardiac morbidity.** Cardiac complications are becoming less frequent with improvements in perioperative anesthesia, beta-blocker administration, intensive care unit monitoring, and preoperative screening for underlying cardiac disease.
- **Gastrointestinal morbidity.** Gastrointestinal complications may manifest insidiously in sedated patients. The extent to which technical factors, such as time to pelvic reperfusion and inferior mesenteric artery reimplantation contribute to the risk of colonic ischemia is not well defined.

REFERENCES

1. Matas R: Ligation of the abdominal aorta: Report of the ultimate result, one year, five months, and nine days after the ligation of the abdominal aorta for aneurysm of the bifurcation, *Ann Surg* 81:457, 1925.
2. Reid MR: Aneurysms in the Johns Hopkins Hospital, *Arch Surg* 12:1-21, 1926.
3. Power DA: The palliative treatment of aneurysms by "wiring" with Colt's apparatus, *Br J Surg* 9:27, 1921.
4. Rea CE: The surgical treatment of aneurysm of the abdominal aorta, *Minn Med* 31:153, 1948.
5. Cohen JR, Graver LM: The ruptured abdominal aortic aneurysm of Albert Einstein, *Surg Obstet Gynecol* 170:455, 1990.
6. Dubost C, Allary M, Oeconomos N: Resection of an aneurysm of the abdominal aorta: Reestablishment of the continuity by a preserved arterial graft, with result after five months, *Arch Surg* 64:405, 1952.
7. Creech O: Endo-aneurysmorrhaphy and treatment of aortic aneurysm, *Ann Surg* 164:935, 1966.
8. Williams GM, Schlossberg L: *Atlas of aortic surgery*, Baltimore, 1997, Williams and Wilkins, pp 77-90.
9. Chaikof EL, Brewster DC, Dalman RL, et al: The care of patients with an abdominal aortic aneurysm: The Society for Vascular Surgery Guidelines, *J Vasc Surg* 50:1S-48S, 2009.
10. Brown LC, Powell JT: For UK Small Aneurysm Trial participants: Risk factors for aneurysm rupture in patients kept under ultrasound surveillance, *Ann Surg* 230:289-296, 1999.
11. Feringa HH, Bax JJ, Boersma E, et al: High-dose beta blockers and tight heart rate control reduce myocardial ischemia and troponin T release in vascular surgery patients, *Circ* 114:I344-I349, 2006.
12. ACC/AHA 2007 Guidelines on Perioperative Cardiovascular Evaluation and Care for Noncardiac Surgery: Executive Summary, *Circ* 116:1971-1996, 2007.
13. LeMaire SA, Jones MM, Conklin LD, et al: Randomized comparison of cold blood and cold crystalloid renal perfusion for renal protection during thoracoabdominal aortic aneurysm repair, *J Vasc Surg* 49:11-19, 2009.

14. Conrad MF, Crawford RS, Pedraza JD, et al: Long term durability of open abdominal aortic aneurysm repair, *J Vasc Surg* 46:669-675, 2007.
15. Knott AW, Kalra A, Duncan AA, et al: Open repair of Juxtarenal aortic aneurysms remains a safe option in the era of fenestrated endografts, *J Vasc Surg* 47:695-701, 2008.
16. Jean-Claude JM, Reilly LM, Stoney RJ, et al: Pararenal aortic aneurysms: The future of open aortic repair, *J Vasc Surg* 29:902-912, 1999.
17. Chong T, Nguyen L, Owens CD, et al: Suprarenal aortic cross clamp position: A reappraisal of its effects on outcomes for open abdominal aortic aneurysm repair, *J Vasc Surg* 49:873-880, 2009.

25 Endovascular Treatment of Aneurysms of the Infrarenal Aorta

ATUL S. RAO • MICHEL S. MAKAROUN

Historical Background

Volodos and colleagues[1] performed the first stent graft repair of an aortic pathology in 1987 in Kharkov, Union of Soviet Socialist Republics, but Parodi, Palmaz, and Barone[2] are credited with pioneering and popularizing the technique in the early 1990s. Scott and Chuter[3] were the first to repace the early single tube structure with a bifurcated device, extending the ability to exclude more complex aortoiliac aneuryms. Numerous innovations have been subsequently introduced to improve fixation, correct early failure modes, and extend these devices to effectively treat more challenging aneurysmal anatomy. Three large, randomized prospective trials confirmed an early advantage to endovascular aneurysm repair (EVAR) in both mortality and morbidity when compared with open surgical repair.[4-6] The survival benefit of EVAR is largely limited to the first 2 years after the procedure; associated comorbidities are the main cause of late deaths.[7,8]

Current endovascular devices intended for EVAR come in a variety of configurations. Although most devices consist of modular components that are assembled in situ to improve ease of device delivery, some endografts are composed of a single or unibody construction. Bifurcated devices are used in most patients, but tapered aortomonoiliac devices, which would necessitate an associated femoral-femoral bypass for lower extremity revascularization, also are available for challenging iliac and distal aortic anatomy. Both passive and active infrarenal or suprarenal fixation systems are also available to improve attachment of the device to the aortic wall.

Preoperative Preparation

- **Physical examination.** Most asymptomatic aneurysms are discovered incidentally on imaging studies, and 75% of aneurysms greater than 5 cm are palpable on physical examination.[9]
- **Ultrasound screening.** Ultrasound identifies aneurysms in 3% to 10% of patients in targeted screening studies.[10,11] A screening ultrasound should be considered for male adults older than 65 years with a smoking history or family history of aortic aneurysm.[12]
- **Ultrasound surveillance.** Small aneurysms between 3.5 and 4.4 cm in diameter can be followed with an annual ultrasound examination. Aneurysms between 4.5 and 5.4 cm in greatest dimension should be evaluated with an ultrasound examination every 6 months. Aneurysms 5.5 cm or larger should be evaluated by contrast-enhanced computed tomography (CT) imaging for possible repair.[13] Note that measurements in the minor axis provide a closer estimate of centerline measurements, and these are usually smaller than the greatest diameter measurements.
- **Preoperative imaging.** Three-dimensional (3D) CT imaging with fine (0.6 to 2.5 mm) cuts is required for preoperative measurements and graft selection.

Workstation image processing with curved linear reformats facilitates accurate diameter, angle, and centerline length measurements. The infrarenal neck length is measured from the lowest renal artery to the start of the aneurysm, and diameters at several locations should be obtained to assess the extent of tapering within the neck. The diameter of the common iliac arteries should be measured at several points before the iliac bifurcation, with special focus on the intended landing zone. The distance from the aortic bifurcation to the iliac bifurcation should be recorded on both sides.

- **Preoperative risk assessment.** Preoperative risk assessment should be performed, with particular attention given to renal function. Patients with marginal renal function may be prehydrated, and sodium bicarbonate, *N*-acetylcysteine, and isosmolar contrast agents may be considered.
- **Preoperative vascular examination.** A comprehensive pulse examination should be performed and documented before the procedure.
- **Management of anticoagulation and antiplatelet agents.** Cessation of chronic anticoagulation is necessary before EVAR, but antiplatelet agents can be continued unless epidural anesthesia is planned.
- **Anesthesia.** EVAR can be performed under general, epidural, or local anesthesia with sedation. If the patient is awake, sedation should be minimized to allow breath-holding during abdominal digital subtraction. Intraoperative arterial monitoring is advisable, but central venous monitoring can be used selectively.
- **Prophylaxis of infection and deep venous thrombosis.** Perioperative antibiotics and subcutaneous heparin are administered.

Pitfalls and Danger Points

- **Device selection.** Appropriate preoperation sizing is critical to the success of EVAR. Undersized grafts lead to endoleaks and graft migration. Significantly oversized grafts can lead to aortic injury or infolding (Fig. 25-1).
- **Arterial injury.** Calcified and narrow femoral and iliac arteries are at risk for injury at the time of the introduction and removal of the device delivery system. Wire access should be maintained until the end of the procedure to allow endovascular rescue in the event of an injury. Depending upon the deployment system, an iliac conduit may be necessary when the iliac artery is deemed too small to facilitate passage of sheaths. Oversized noncompliant balloons should be avoided in the aortic neck and the iliac arteries, and balloon inflation should be confined within the fabric of the endograft.
- **Unintended coverage of arterial branches.** Precise angiographic imaging is mandatory throughout the procedure. The C arm should be oriented orthogonal to the branch vessel of interest to avoid parallax. For example, cranial angulation should be used to image the aortic neck, and caudal angulation should be used when imaging the iliac arteries. Right or left oblique projections should be used to visualize the ostia of the renal arteries and the iliac artery bifurcation.
- **Embolization and thrombosis.** Device and wire manipulation should be kept to a minimum to limit the risk of embolization. Postdeployment imaging should ensure that limbs are not kinked to avoid subsequent limb thrombosis.
- **Endoleak.** Types I and III endoleaks at the aortic and iliac attachments sites and graft component junctions, respectively, are associated with a persistent risk of aortic rupture. A neck that has an angulation greater than 60 degrees, is less than 15 mm in length, or is lined with substantial thrombus and calcification is associated with an increased risk of a type IA endoleak. An aortic extension piece or a balloon-expandable Palmaz stent may be needed to treat a proximal type IA endoleak. Junctional type III leaks are avoided by ensuring that optimal component overlap is achieved.

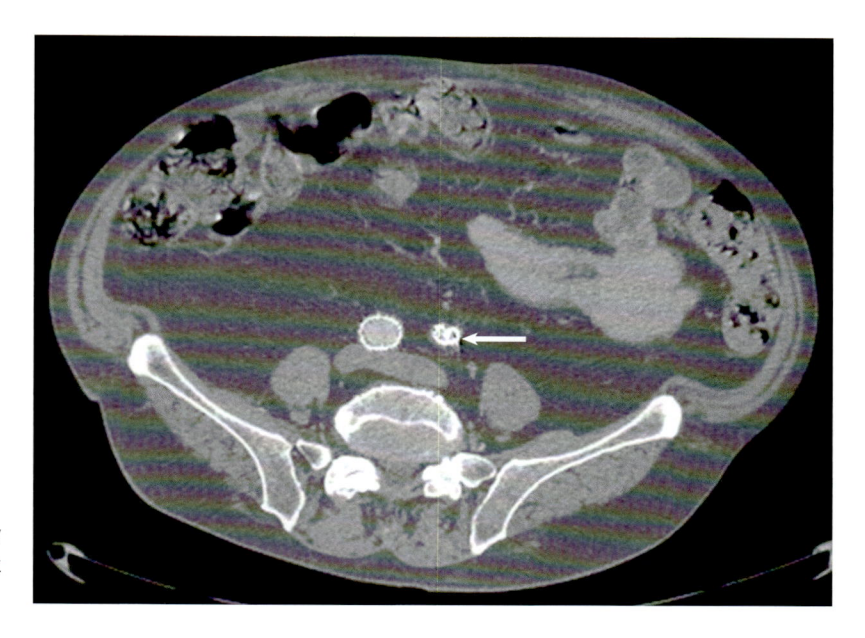

Figure 25-1. CT scan after EVAR. The arrow denotes an infolded left iliac limb as a result of graft oversizing.

Endovascular Strategy

GRAFT SIZING OR SELECTION

Endograft diameters at seal zones are typically oversized by 10% to 20%.[14,15] Endograft length should be selected to extend from the most caudal renal artery to the iliac bifurcations, with best estimates obtained from line of flow measurements. It is important to anticipate the potential need for alternative or additional sizes, including proximal and distal extensions. For bifurcated, modular grafts with single docking limbs, such as Excluder (W.L. Gore and Associates, Newark, Del.), the ipsilateral side of deployment should be chosen to assure the appropriate graft length and iliac diameter. Additional flexibility exists when using a bifurcated device with bilateral iliac docking limbs, such as in the Zenith device (Cook Medical, Bloomington, Ind.). In the case of severe unilateral, external iliac artery occlusive disease, an aortouniiliac graft, with planned occlusion of the common iliac artery on the contralateral side and femoral-femoral bypass, is an alternative option.

PERCUTANEOUS DEPLOYMENT

Percutaneous EVAR can be performed in more than 90% patients, with a success rate exceeding 95%, shorter operative times, and fewer wound complications compared with open surgical repair. However, access vessel diameters less than 5 mm are at greater risk for percutaneous failure. Maintaining wire access while assessing hemostasis allows reintroduction of the sheath after EVAR in case femoral artery exposure is required. The most widely used approach uses the preclose technique with suture-mediated closure devices (Prostar XL or Perclose ProGlide, Abbott Vascular, Redwood City, Calif.). Contraindications to percutaneous closure include circumferential or anterior wall calcification of the common femoral artery, stenosis or small-caliber femoral artery, and high femoral bifurcation.

ADJUNCTIVE ILIAC ANGIOPLASTY

A stenotic external or common iliac artery may prevent introduction of a large endograft sheath, which can be pretreated by balloon angioplasty at the time of EVAR. Although the presence of a dissection in the external iliac artery requires stent placement after the completion of endograft deployment, if noted within the common iliac artery, stenting is not necessary because it will be covered by the endograft iliac limb. Stent deployment for iliac occlusive disease before endograft introduction should be avoided.

ILIAC ARTERY CONDUIT

Small-caliber external iliac arteries, severe calcification, and occlusive disease or excessive tortuosity may impede device delivery. As an alternative, an iliac artery conduit provides direct access to the common iliac artery. Iliac conduits can be performed either 1) via open surgical anastomosis of a prosthetic graft to more proximal healthy iliac artery, or 2) via endoluminal placement of covered stent graft or iliac limb followed by balloon angioplasty. Planned conduits have a lower complication rate than emergency conduits performed after a failed attempt to introduce an endograft.[16]

Endovascular Technique

ARTERIAL ACCESS

Open Femoral Artery Exposure

A short oblique incision parallel to the inguinal ligament is made 1 to 2 cm above the inguinal crease on both sides. Dissection to the femoral sheath is performed with ligation of lymphatics and venous branches. The common femoral artery is dissected for a short segment distal to the inguinal ligament and controlled with vessel loops. In the presence of significant occlusive disease, the distal external iliac artery is exposed, because it may provide a less calcified point of access. An anterior wall puncture needle is inserted into a disease-free portion of the artery, and a 0.035-inch J wire is advanced into the proximal aorta. A short 6- to 8-Fr femoral sheath is placed over the wire into the common femoral artery. In tortuous iliac arteries or large aneurysm sacs, an angled 5-Fr catheter, such as a Kumpe (KMP; Cook Medical) or Berenstein catheter (Infiniti Medical, Menlo Park, Calif.) may help direct the wire into the proximal aorta. On the ipsilateral side, the wire is replaced with an exchange-length, stiff Amplatz or Lunderquist wire. A pigtail angiographic catheter with multiple 1-cm marks is introduced from the contralateral side and placed into the aorta, and heparin is administered.

Percutaneous Access

Many practitioners do not routinely use ultrasound in the course of gaining percutaneous access. However, for those who advocate this approach, the ultrasound probe is used to identify the common femoral artery and the femoral bifurcation. The best location for common femoral artery puncture is determined by the extent of calcification on the anterior wall and plaque both anteriorly and posteriorly. A small stab incision is made in the skin inferior to the expected arterial puncture site. Blunt dissection with a hemostat is then carried down through the subcutaneous tissue to the anterior wall of the common femoral artery under ultrasound scan guidance. A micropuncture needle is inserted into the common femoral artery under direct visualization with the ultrasound probe. Fluoroscopy is used to confirm puncture over the femoral head.

A microsheath and a 0.035-inch wire are inserted into the common femoral artery, followed by a 7-Fr dilator. After dilation of the artery and subcutaneous tissue, a 6-Fr Perclose ProGlide device is inserted over the wire into the common femoral artery. Because the wire exits the side of the device, it is removed as soon as the ProGlide device approaches the incision to avoid arterial injury. Pulsatile blood flow from the marker lumen confirms proper positioning of the device within the common femoral artery. The ProGlide device is then fired and the wire is replaced before the device is withdrawn from the common femoral artery. The sutures are not tied down, because they are secured to the sterile drapes with a Kelly clamp. A second ProGlide device is inserted into the same artery over the wire, confirmation of intraarterial placement is obtained, the wire is removed, the device is fired, the wire is then replaced, and the sutures are secured with a Crile clamp to distinguish the second knot from the first. A 7-Fr, 25-cm sheath is then inserted into the common femoral artery.

The preceding steps are repeated on the contralateral groin, leaving two sets of untied ProGlide sutures in each groin. Two devices are deployed at 11:59 and 12:01, with the goal of slightly offsetting the devices without puncturing the sidewall of the common femoral artery to avoid narrowing the vessel or failure to puncture the vessel wall. The patient is then heparinized. If there is hemorrhage around the 7-Fr sheath, a 12-Fr sheath is inserted over an Amplatz or Lunderquist wire. Serial dilations are used with Coons dilators before placement of the large sheath and device.

Iliac Artery Conduit

An oblique lower abdominal wall incision is made between the umbilicus and the inguinal ligament. The abdominal wall muscle layers are divided until the preperitoneal fat is encountered. The peritoneum is swept medially and superiorly, exposing the iliac arteries, which are controlled at the bifurcation. An end-to-side anastomosis is fashioned using a 10-mm Dacron graft at the junction of the common and external iliac arteries. This location allows deployment into the distal common iliac artery and patching of the origin of the external, normally the most diseased portion. In thin patients the Dacron graft may be brought out directly through the retroperitoneal incision, whereas in larger patients it can be brought through a separate distal stab incision in the abdominal wall. The conduit is clamped distally, and the device sheath can then be placed through a puncture or small incision in the anterior surface of the graft. After EVAR, the conduit is either divided and oversewn near the iliac anastomosis or tunneled under the inguinal ligament and anastomosed to the common femoral artery as an iliofemoral bypass graft.

Endovascular Conduit

Alternatively, one can use a covered stent graft or iliac limb in the iliac system as an endovascular conduit.[17,18] To accomplish this, once wire access across the iliac is obtained, a covered stent graft or iliac limb is deployed in the region of stenosis. This is then balloon angioplastied to profile. Larger sheaths now can be passed into the aorta through the iliacs.

ANGIOGRAPHY

An initial aortoiliac angiogram is obtained using a marker pigtail catheter, which is placed at the level of the renal arteries using a Power injection run of 15 mL/sec for a total of 15 mL (Fig. 25-2), although in smaller aortas a rate of 10mL/sec

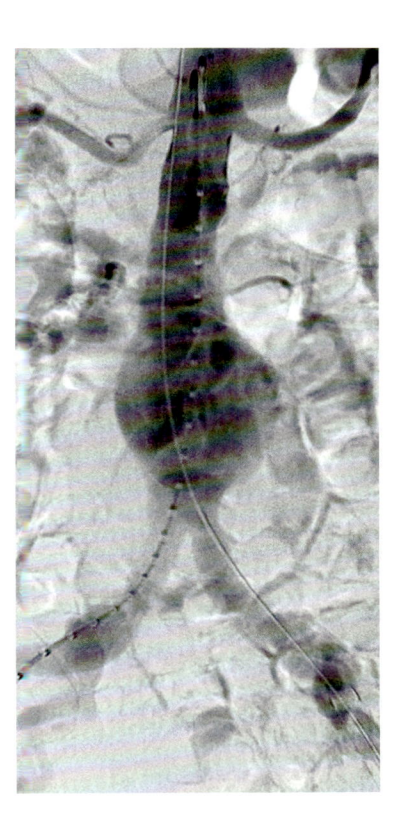

Figure 25-2. Initial angiogram. Note the pigtail catheter placed at the level of the renal arteries.

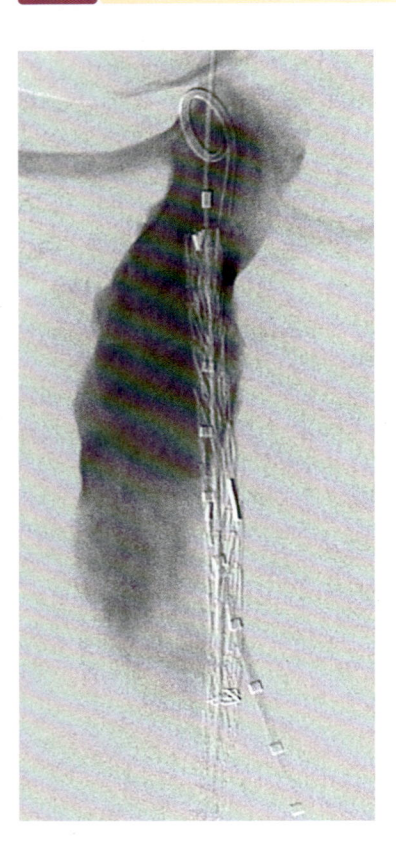

Figure 25-3. Angiogram obtained before deployment of the main body of the graft. A magnified image is recommended to allow precise placement of the graft relative to the renal artery ostia. The C arm has been angulated cranially to minimize parallax.

may be more appropriate. Larger volumes may be needed in the presence large aneurysm sacs or in patients with low cardiac output. The number and location of main and accessory renal arteries are identified, and the patency of the internal iliac arteries is assessed. The length of device is confirmed.

Magnified angiography to guide proximal device deployment is performed after the main body is advanced from the ipsilateral side (Fig. 25-3). Based on preoperative CT imaging, an oblique projection may be used to best visualize the origin of the most caudal renal artery, along with cranial angulation and appropriate magnification. Power injection runs of 15 mL/sec for a total volume of 5 to 7 mL confirm positioning of the device with respect to the most caudal renal artery.

Angiography for contralateral limb length selection and deployment is performed after cannulation of the contralateral gate (Fig. 25-4). The C arm is oriented caudally and in an LAO orientation for the right iliac artery or in a right anterior oblique orientation for the left iliac artery. A marker pigtail is placed over a stiff wire within the iliac vessel, and a retrograde injection is performed through the sheath to ascertain the location of the origin of the internal iliac artery.

A broad, nonmagnified image of the aorta to the iliac bifurcation is obtained after device deployment using a Power injection run of 15 mL/sec for a total volume of 15 mL (Fig. 25-5). Digital subtraction with a breath hold and image acquisition for a prolonged period is necessary to identify endoleaks. All devices have several radiopaque markers at the proximal end of the fabric. Aligning them with cranial angulation of the image intensifier provides the best projection for accurate evaluation of the proximal extent of the endograft in relation to the renal arteries. The catheter may be repositioned proximally, distally, or within the endograft to differentiate among endoleak types.

GRAFT DEPLOYMENT AND CANNULATION OF THE CONTRALATERAL GATE

The main device is advanced to the desired location from the planned side (Fig. 25-6). It is oriented under fluoroscopy before insertion and during deployment.

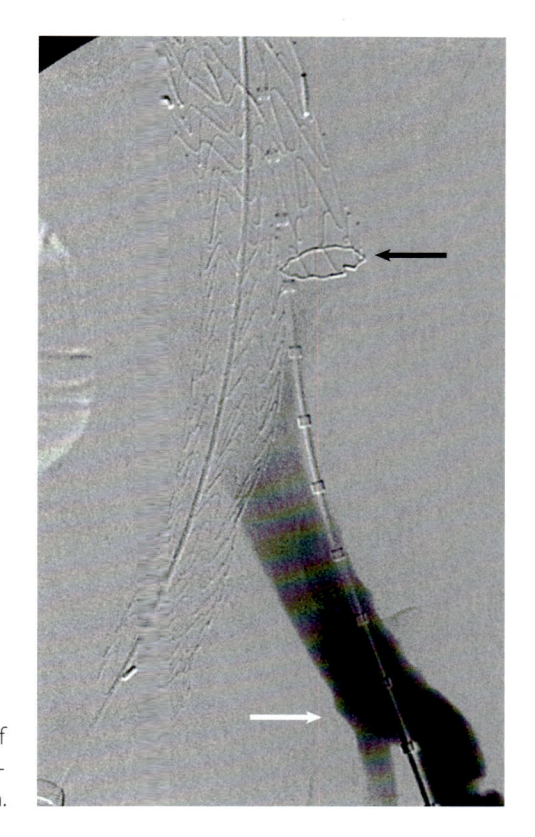

Figure 25-4. Measurement of contralateral limb length. Retrograde injection of contrast from the sheath into the left iliac artery. The *black arrow* denotes the contralateral gate of the bifurcated graft. The *white arrow* denotes the iliac artery bifurcation.

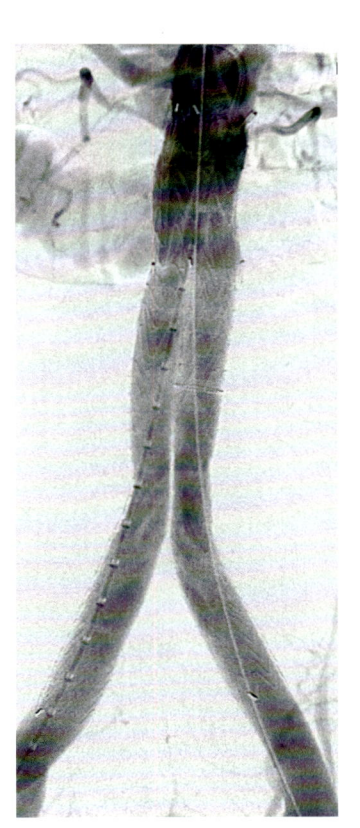

Figure 25-5. Completion angiogram. Broad, nonmagnified image obtained with power injection of 15 mL/sec of 15 mL of contrast. Image acquisition is prolonged to allow visualization of endoleaks.

All devices have radiopaque markers that are unique to the device to facilitate orientation, proper positioning, and various steps of deployment. Markers indicate the proximal extent of the fabric, the origin and orientation of the gate, and the distal end of the device. Although it is important to properly orient the gate to permit cannulation of the contralateral limb, crossing the limbs may be necessary to assist in cannulation and avoid kinking of the endograft in the distal aorta,

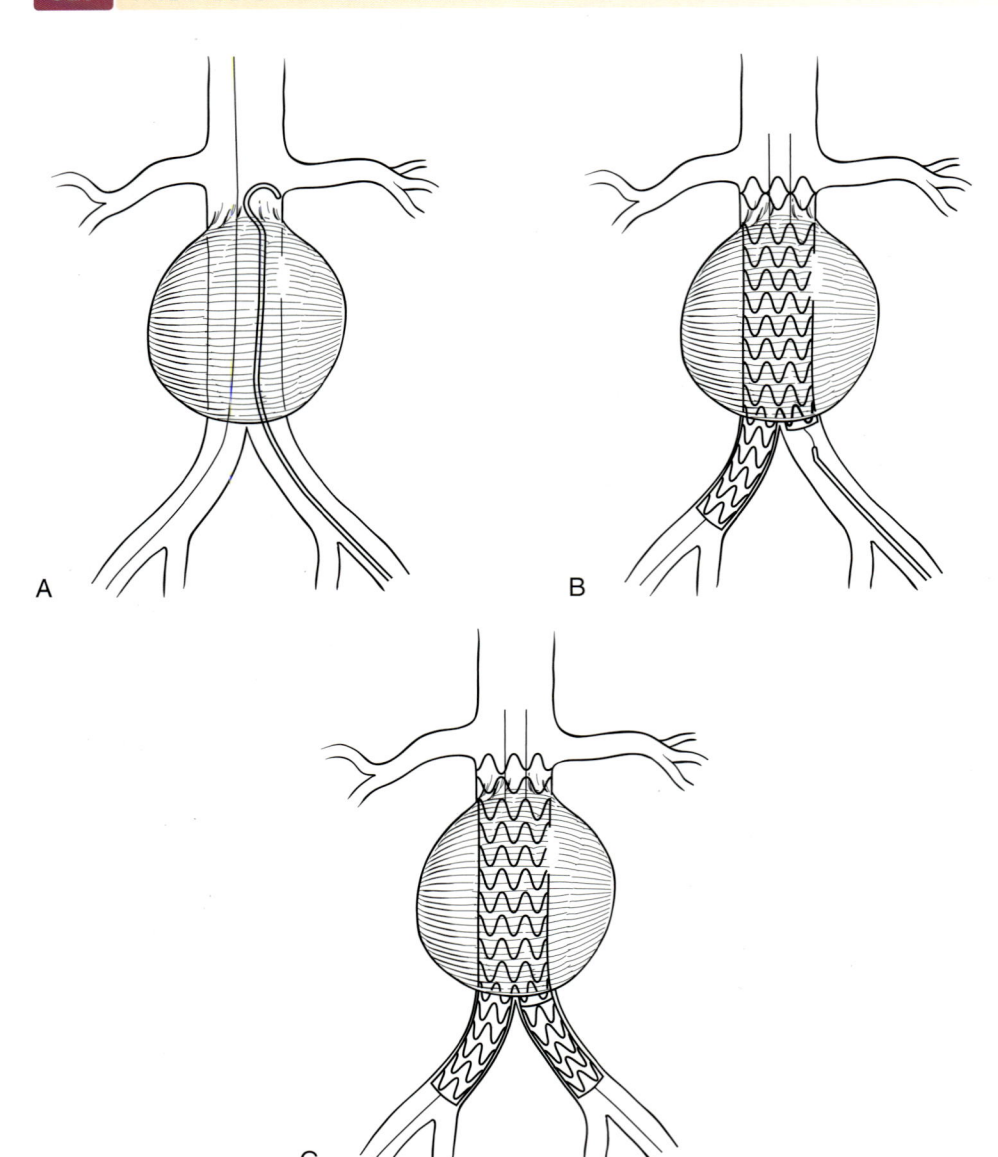

Figure 25-6. Overview of graft deployment. **A,** Positioning of the main body of the endograft in proximity to renal arteries, with a pigtail catheter at the level of the renal arteries via the contralateral iliac artery. **B,** Deployment of the main body and opening of the contralateral gate. The pigtail catheter is moved down into aneurysm sac before deployment. Then the pigtail catheter is exchanged for an angled multipurpose catheter, and the contralateral gate is cannulated. **C,** After cannulation of the contralateral gate and exchange for a stiff wire, the contralateral limb of the graft is deployed, and ballooning of the proximal and distal seal zones and graft overlap junctions is performed.

especially when the origin of the common iliac artery is significantly angulated from the aorta or there is a limited distance to the hypogastric artery (Fig. 25-7).

To cannulate the contralateral gate, a stiff, angled hydrophilic wire is placed through the marker pigtail in the contralateral limb side, and the marker pigtail is replaced with an angled multipurpose (KMP) catheter. A torquing device on the Glidewire (Terumo Medical Corp., Somerset, N.J.) is helpful in negotiating the gate, but a variety of strategies can be used to assist in cannulating the contralateral gate. To better visualize the gate, the C arm can be repositioned to obtain different oblique views and a number of shaped catheters can be used to better negotiate angulated entry to the gate. If the aneurysm sac where the gate resides is large, an 8-Fr guiding catheter can be used to introduce a third catheter angle. If repeated attempts at cannulation have failed, a soft Glidewire can be advanced over the graft bifurcation from the ipsilateral side using a directional catheter, such as a Sos Omni or VS1 catheter, to be snared after passing through the contralateral gate. Alternatively, a wire can be advanced through the body of the graft to the contralateral gate from a left brachial artery approach. Once the contralateral gate is cannulated, the wire should be exchanged for a pigtail catheter that is rotated within the neck of the aneurysm to ensure the catheter is within the main body and has not traversed outside the graft. A stiff wire is then placed through the gate to allow the introduction of the contralateral limb.

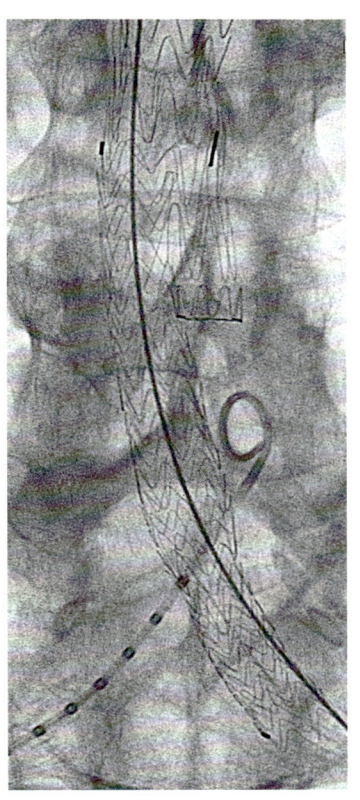

Figure 25-7. Intentional crossing of limbs of the graft to facilitate cannulation of the contralateral gate.

ENDOGRAFT DEPLOYMENT

Excluder Endograft

The Excluder C3 device (W.L. Gore) requires the use of an 18-Fr, 30-cm-long sheath for deployment in most cases. The ipsilateral sheath should preferably be advanced into the aorta but can be left in the iliac artery during a difficult device introduction. A contralateral 12-Fr sheath is required for 12- and 14-mm iliac limbs, whereas an 18-Fr sheath is recommended for larger limbs and should be advanced through the contralateral gate. The sheath should be withdrawn to expose the device before deployment. Lower profile devices that require smaller sheath sizes have been recently introduced.

Rapid deployment of the Excluder device is achieved by releasing a constraining sleeve around the endograft. The Excluder C3 delivery system offers the advantage of a repositionable main trunk. When using this device, the outer deployment knob is released to deploy the main trunk and ipsilateral limb. The ipsilateral limb remains constrained, however. The proximal trunk of the C3 can be reconstrained to allow repositioning of the device until the inner knob is released, thereby freeing the constraint and fixing the main trunk. Finally, after cannulation of the contralateral gate, the innermost knob is released, thereby deploying the remainder of the ipsilateral limb. The 3-cm overlap zone between the body and the contralateral limb should be ballooned with a 14-mm × 4-cm balloon. The short delivery mechanism only requires 180-cm-long stiff wire and 65-cm-long catheters. Sheaths can be left in place after device delivery and can be used for wire, catheter, and balloon exchanges or for deployment of additional components.

Endurant Endograft

The Endurant device, the next generation of endograft from Medtronic (Medtronic Vascular, Santa Rosa, Calif.), is packaged within hydrophilic sheaths and is delivered directly over a stiff 0.035-inch guidewire. It is approved for the treatment of aortic aneurysms with proximal infrarenal necks as short as 10 mm in length. Deployment involves a very accurate, slow retraction of the sheath to expose the device using a handle rotation mechanism. The Endurant device, like its predecessor the Talent graft but unlike the prior generation AneuRx (both also FDA approved), has a suprarenal uncovered stent but also has anchor pins for active fixation. In addition, the suprarenal stent of the Endurant remains constrained until it is released at the desired position. After device delivery is complete, the sheath must be replaced with a standard introducer sheath that has a hemostatic valve for introduction of balloons, catheters, or other limbs.

Zenith Endograft

The Zenith device (Cook Medical) consists of a main body and bilateral limb extensions, is packaged within a hydrophilic sheath, and is delivered over a 0.035-inch wire. The delivery mechanism requires 260-cm-long wires and 100-cm-long pigtail catheters. The main body is opened gradually by manually retracting the sheath to expose the endograft. The proximal attachment is a suprarenal stent with hooks that remains constrained by a cap until the desired position in the neck is achieved. Release of the proximal stent fixes the main body in position. The ipsilateral limb remains constrained, whereas the contralateral gate is cannulated, a retrograde angiogram is obtained, and the contralateral limb length is confirmed and deployed. The ipsilateral leg is then deployed, and the proximal cap is retrieved. The dilator and graft carrier are removed, but the sheath, which has a hemostatic valve, remains in place. The ipsilateral limb is then extended to the iliac bifurcation. Cook now has released more flexible, nitinol-based iliac limbs to minimize kinking. Because the sheath is quite long, retrograde injections require a large volume of contrast to simply fill the sheath.

PowerLink and AFX Endograft

The PowerLink and AFX (Endologix, Irvine, Calif.) are unibody grafts that are packaged within their own sheaths. The AFX device is housed in a 17-Fr sheath, while the PowerLink uses a 19-Fr sheath. Deployment begins by capturing a wire attached to the contralateral leg of the device transfemorally. A double lumen catheter facilitates this procedure, and the device is advanced above the bifurcation and exposed. It is retracted to the aortic bifurcation before full deployment, and a proximal extension is added to complete the procedure.

Ovation Prime Endograft

The Ovation Prime (TriVascular, Santa Rosa, Calif.) is a three piece, modular bifurcated graft with an uncovered suprarenal stent and active anchor fixation. Its sealing zone is comprised of two polymer-filled rings that enhance sealing in irregular necks, including reverse tapers. It is delivered via a low-profile 14-Fr sheath, which makes it a valuable option in treating aneurysms in patients with small iliac arteries. Once the main body is deployed, a polymer is used to fill sealing rings in the main trunk. Once the polymer has hardened, the contralateral gate is cannulated and extended with an iliac limb, followed by similar extension on the ipsilateral side.

Aorfix Endograft

The Aorfix (Lombard Medical Technologies, Oxfordshire, UK) is a two-piece modular device with a fish mouth--shaped proximal end with hooks for active fixation. It is packaged within its own sheath, with 22-Fr ipsilateral and 20-Fr contralateral sheath sizes. Cannulation of contralateral gate and limb extension follows deployment of main body and ipsilateral limb. It is approved for highly angulated proximal necks, up to 90-degree angulations.

Aortouniiliac Graft

In the case of severely tortuous, calcific, or occlusive unilateral iliac artery disease that precludes safe passage of bifurcated grafts, an aortouniiliac graft can be used (Figs. 25-8 and 25-9). Deployment is simple because there is no need to cannulate a contralateral gate. The contralateral common iliac should be occluded, if patent,

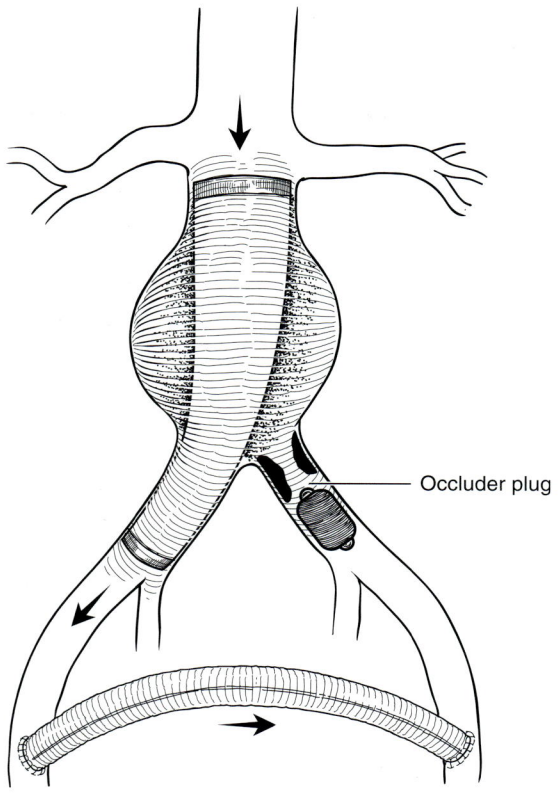

Figure 25-8. Aortouniiliac configuration, with a contralateral iliac occluder device and femoral-femoral crossover bypass.

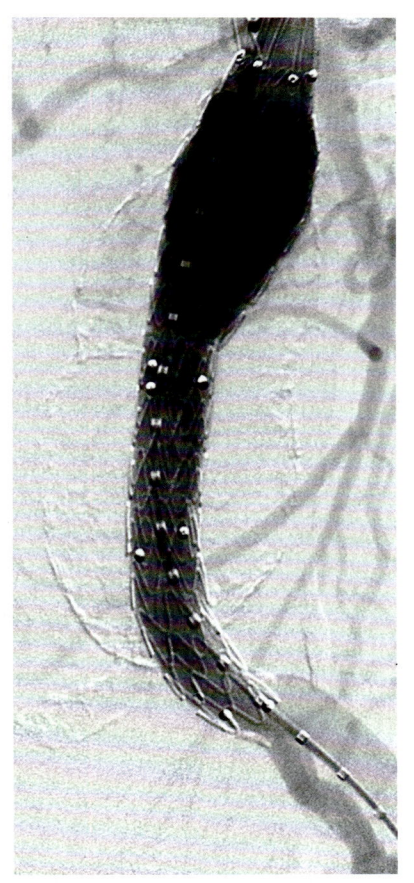

Figure 25-9. Angiogram after deployment of an aortouniiliac device.

which can be achieved by a variety of endovascular occluders. A femoral-femoral bypass may be needed to perfuse the contralateral lower extremity.

MANAGEMENT OF INTRAOPERATIVE COMPLICATIONS

Rupture of the Aorta or Iliac Vessels

Patients with heavily calcified or small-caliber vessels are at risk for this potentially catastrophic outcome. Many such events can be successfully managed via endovascular techniques.[19] The key to endovascular repair is maintaining wire access until the completion of all graft-related procedures. A high index of suspicion is needed, because injury may not always be immediately obvious. Balloon occlusion above the suspected point of rupture provides control, and an aortic occlusion balloon, such as an Equalizer, Reliant, or Coda balloon, can be placed in the supraceliac aorta if the site of rupture is unclear. If the endograft has not yet been deployed, it may be possible to deploy the prosthesis by maintaining aortic balloon occlusion, alternating the side of the occlusion balloon while deploying each module of the graft.[20] If the endograft has been deployed, aortic or iliac extensions are used to exclude the ruptured segment. Open conversion is required if the source of bleeding is unclear or endovascular repair is not feasible. Aortic balloon occlusion should be maintained during conversion until a cross-clamp can be placed.

Arterial Dissection

Predisposing factors for dissection, which most commonly occurs in the iliac or femoral arteries, includes heavily calcified or atheroma-laden arteries and severe tortuosity.[21] Many of these injuries can go unnoticed at the time of graft deployment and may lead to subsequent limb occlusion.[22] Most dissections that are flow limiting can be treated with bare metal stents or with an iliac limb extender.

Distal Embolization

Atherosclerotic debris can result in distal embolization. In addition, inadequate heparinization can lead to thrombosis, especially in the presence of severe, preexistent lower extremity occlusive disease. A discrepant pulse examination at the completion of the procedure should be evaluated with angiography, and thrombectomy should be performed as needed. Limited distal embolization of small plaque fragments may result in postoperative pain and discoloration of toes and should be managed expectantly.

Limb Occlusion

Failure to recognize poor flow or kinking of limbs contributes to late limb thrombosis. Predisposing risk factors include unsupported fabric grafts,[23] graft kinking or infolding, stenosis, small graft diameter, and extension to external iliac artery.[24,25] Completion angiography should be performed after removing all stiff wires, which may mask the presence of a kinked limb.

Renal Artery Occlusion

Deployment of an endograft close to a renal artery may lead to orificial stenosis or occlusion. In the absence of proximal hooks or barbs, inflation of a low-pressure balloon near the bifurcation of the endograft or use of a transfemoral wire with gentle downward traction may expose the renal orifice in some cases. If the orifice is only partially occluded, wire access can be attempted via the femoral or brachial artery and a balloon-expandable stent can be deployed. If bilateral occlusion has occurred, open conversion or renal artery bypass may be necessary.

Bleeding

Percutaneous suture delivery allows for less invasive device delivery. However, failure of these sutures can result in brisk bleeding that necessitates emergent femoral artery open exposure. Maintaining wire access allows for advancement of the sheath to control bleeding during open exposure. If the sheath cannot be

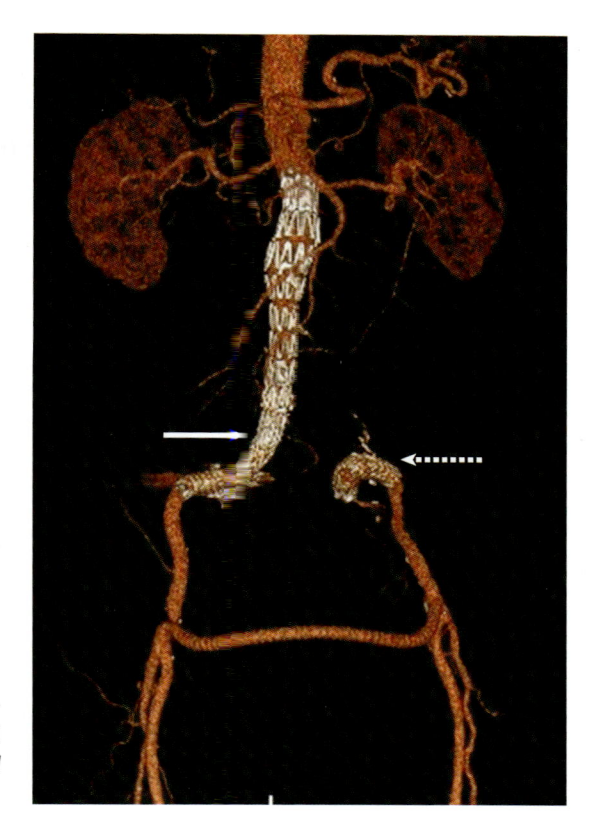

Figure 25-10. 3D reconstruction of a CT angiogram performed after placement of an aortouniiliac device *(thick arrow)*, and right to left femoral-femoral bypass with left external to internal iliac artery endovascular bypass *(dashed arrow)*.

advanced because of partial suture closure of the artery, manual pressure and maintenance of wire access can facilitate the exposure of the artery.

ADJUNCTIVE TECHNIQUES IN ENDOVASCULAR ANEURYSM REPAIR

Hypogastric Artery Occlusion

Concomitant common iliac artery aneurysmal disease may preclude obtaining an adequate distal seal unless the graft is extended into the external iliac artery. Hypogastric artery occlusion is necessary to avoid type II endoleak but may not be needed if the internal iliac artery is diseased at its origin or arises from a nondilated segment of the distal common iliac artery to be covered with the endograft. Although some prefer to use coil embolization of the hypogastric artery several weeks before definitive endograft placement, embolization may be performed at the time of endografting. Access to the internal iliac artery can be from the ipsilateral or the contralateral femoral artery based on the angulation and tortuosity of the aortoiliac segment. A sheath or guiding catheter should be placed at the origin of the internal iliac artery to protect from unwanted deployment of occlusion devices. An Amplatzer occlusive plug (St. Jude Medical, St. Paul, Minn.) can provide occlusion of the proximal internal iliac artery in one step. Otherwise, multiple appropriately sized coils should be deployed in the first portion of the hypogastric artery rather than in the distal branches to minimize risk of buttock claudication.[26]

External Iliac to Internal Iliac Artery Bypass

To avoid bilateral internal iliac artery occlusion, a bypass to the internal iliac artery can be considered. An end-to-end anastomosis to the internal iliac is performed, and the graft is anastomosed to the distal external iliac or femoral artery in an end-to-side manner. An alternative approach is to deploy an aortouniiliac device followed by an endovascular external to internal iliac artery bypass (Fig. 25-10). The recent development of an endoprosthesis with internal iliac branches may further limit the need for hypogastric artery occlusion in the future.

Postoperative Care

- Patients are observed in the postanesthesia care unit for 1 to 2 hours with continuous hemodynamic monitoring and frequent assessment of lower extremity peripheral pulses and neurologic function.
- Patients are discharged on the first postoperative day provided that they are ambulating, voiding, and tolerating a diet and that pain is well controlled with oral medication.
- Outpatient assessment and CT imaging are initially performed at 1 month. If an endoleak or other abnormality is noted on the 1-month scan, follow-up imaging is obtained at 6 months. Otherwise, CT imaging need not be obtained until 12 months, and if a stable or shrinking aneurysm is observed without endoleak, annual follow-up is conducted with duplex imaging, and a CT scan is obtained at 5 years.

Postoperative Complications

- **Cardiac.** Routine postoperative electrocardiogram or cardiac isoenzymes are not recommended but may be appropriate in select cases based on preoperative risk assessment.
- **Renal.** Patients are hydrated for several hours after the procedure, and serum creatinine is measured on the first postoperative day.
- **Access site complications.** The groins are visually inspected in the recovery area and periodically on the floor.
- **Buttock claudication.** Unilateral internal iliac artery occlusion leads to buttock claudication in about one third of patients, and pelvic ischemia may occur with acute bilateral hypogastric artery occlusion.

REFERENCES

1. Volodos NL, Karpovich IP, Troyan VI, et al: Clinical experience in the use of self-fixing synthetic prosthesis for remote endoprosthetics of the thoracic and abdominal aorta and iliac arteries through the femoral artery and as intraoperative endoprosthesis for aorta reconstruction, *Vasa Suppl* 33:93-95, 1991.
2. Parodi JC, Palmaz JC, Barone HD: Transfemoral intraluminal graft implantation for abdominal aortic aneurysms, *Ann Vasc Surg* 5:491-499, 1991.
3. Scott RA, Chuter TA: Clinical endovascular placement of bifurcated graft in abdominal aortic aneurysm without laparotomy, *Lancet* 343:413, 1994.
4. Prinssen M, Verhoeven E, Buth J, et al: A randomized trial comparing conventional and endovascular repair of abdominal aortic aneurysms, *N Engl J Med* 351:1607-1618, 2004.
5. Endovascular Aneurysm Repair Trial participants: Comparison of endovascular aneurysm repair with open repair in patients with abdominal aortic aneurysm (EVAR trial 1), 30-day operative mortality results: Randomized controlled trial, *Lancet* 364:843-848, 2004.
6. Lederle FA, Freischlag JA, Kyriakides TC, et al: Outcomes following endovascular vs open repair of abdominal aortic aneurysm: A randomized trial, *JAMA* 302:1535-1542, 2009.
7. Blankensteijn JD, de Jong S, Prinssen M, et al: Two-year outcomes after conventional or endovascular repair of abdominal aortic aneurysms, *N Engl J Med* 352:2398-2405, 2005.
8. Endovascular Aneurysm Repair Trial participants: Endovascular aneurysm repair versus open repair in patients with abdominal aortic aneurysm (EVAR trial 1): Randomized controlled trial, *Lancet* 365:2179-2186, 2005.
9. Lederle FA, Simel DL: The rational clinical examination: Does this patient have abdominal aortic aneurysm? *JAMA* 281:77-82, 1999.
10. Webster MW, Ferrell RE, St Jean PL, et al: Ultrasound screening of first-degree relatives of patients with an abdominal aortic aneurysm, *J Vasc Surg* 13:9-13, 1991.
11. Lederle FA, Johnson GR, Wilson SE, et al: The aneurysm detection and management screening program: Validation cohorts and final results, *Arch Intern Med* 160:1425-1430, 2000.
12. U.S. Preventive Services Task Force: Screening for abdominal aortic aneurysm: Recommendation statement, *Ann Intern Med* 142:198-202, 2005.
13. Chaikof EL, Brewster DC, Dalman RL, et al: SVS practice guidelines for the care of patients with an abdominal aortic aneurysm: Executive summary, *J Vasc Surg* 50:880-896, 2009.
14. Prehn JV, Schlosser F, Muhs BE, et al: Oversizing of aortic stent grafts for abdominal aneurysm repair: A systematic review of the benefits and risks, *Eur J Vasc Endovasc Surg* 38:42-53, 2009.

15. Sternbergh WC, Money SR, Greenberg RK, et al: Influence of endograft oversizing on device migration, endoleak, aneurysm shrinkage, and aortic neck dilation: Results from the Zenith multicenter trial, *J Vasc Surg* 39:20-26, 2004.
16. Abu-Ghaida AM, Clair DG, Greenberg RK, et al: Broadening the applicability of endovascular aneurysm repair: The use of iliac conduits, *J Vasc Surg* 36:111-117, 2002.
17. Hinchliffe RJ, Ivancev K, Sonesson B, et al: "Paving and cracking": An endovascular technique to facilitate the introduction of aortic stent-grafts through stenosed iliac arteries, *J Endovasc Ther* 14:630-633, 2007.
18. Peterson BG, Matsumura JS: Internal endoconduit: An innovative technique to address unfavorable iliac artery anatomy encountered during thoracic endovascular aortic repair, *J Vasc Surg* 47:441-445, 2008.
19. Fernandez JD, Craig JM, Garrett E, et al: Endovascular management of iliac rupture during endovascular aneurysm repair, *J Vasc Surg* 50:1293-1300, 2009.
20. Malina M, Veith F, Ivancev K, et al: Balloon occlusion of the aorta during endovascular repair of ruptured abdominal aortic aneurysm, *J Endovasc Ther* 12:556-559, 2005.
21. Tillich M, Bell RE, Paik DS, et al: Iliac arterial injuries after endovascular repair of abdominal aortic aneurysms: Correlation with iliac curvature and diameter, *Radiology* 219:129-136, 2001.
22. Hingorani AP, Ascher E, Marks N, et al: Iatrogenic injuries of the common femoral artery (CFA) and external iliac artery (EIA) during endograft placement: An underdiagnosed entity, *J Vasc Surg* 50:505-509, 2009.
23. Baum RA, Shetty SK, Carpenter JP, et al: Limb kinking in supported and unsupported abdominal aortic stent-grafts, *J Vasc Interv Radiol* 11:1165-1171, 2000.
24. Carroccio A, Faries PL, Morrissey NJ, et al: Predicting iliac limb occlusions after bifurcated aortic stent grafting: Anatomic and device-related causes, *J Vasc Surg* 36:679-684, 2002.
25. Cochennec F, Becquemin JP, Desgranges P, et al: Limb graft occlusion following EVAR: Clinical pattern, outcomes, and predictive factors of occurrence, *Eur J Vasc Endovasc Surg* 34:59-65, 2007.
26. Lin PH, Chen AY, Vij A: Hypogastric artery preservation during endovascular aortic aneurysm repair: Is it important? *Semin Vasc Surg* 22:193-200, 2009.

26 Special Problems in the Endovascular Treatment of the Infrarenal Aorta

W. CHARLES STERNBERGH III

Historical Background

Aortic endograft technology has evolved significantly since the initial U.S. commercial release in late 1999. Second- and third-generation endografts have come to market, providing improvements in fixation, sizing, versatility, tractability, and delivery profile. These device improvements have made it possible to treat challenging anatomy that would not have been feasible in the early days of endovascular aneurysm repair (EVAR). However, anatomic limitations continue to persist despite the improvements that have been incorporated among currently available endografts. Thus the ability to safely "push" the anatomic envelope is predicated on the ability of the experienced operator to make wise decisions with regards to patient and device selection.

Preoperative Preparation

- Detailed examination of computed tomography (CT) angiography imaging is critical to evaluate concerns regarding the aortic neck, iliac access, or maintenance of hypogastric perfusion.
- All measurements related to selection of the size of the endograft should be made by the operator.
- The presence of anatomic constraints should anticipate the potential need for adjunctive techniques.
- A stock of ancillary devices (stents, wires, catheters, and sheaths) that could be required should be available.

Pitfalls and Danger Points

- Persistent type IA endoleak may occur from poor patient selection, inaccurate endograft placement, or both.
- Iliac perforation and hemorrhage can occur from overly aggressive attempts at treating challenging iliac anatomy.
- Iliac limb occlusion from kinking, external compression, or excessive oversizing may be observed, particularly if endografts extend into the external iliac arteries.
- Colonic ischemia can result from atheroemboli or simultaneous bilateral hypogastric occlusion.

Endovascular Strategy for Unfavorable Anatomy

ACCESS VESSELS

Severe iliac occlusive disease, calcification, and tortuosity can combine to make access for EVAR difficult. Although these challenges can frequently be overcome with adjunctive techniques when only a single anatomic problem is present, the combination of multiple anatomic access issues may make EVAR difficult or impossible to perform. Commercially available endografts are 14 to 20 Fr and thus require a minimum 5- to 7-mm iliac diameter for passage. Although focal areas of iliac occlusive disease can be readily treated to gain access to the aorta, a diffusely diseased iliac artery can be more problematic. Use of longer angioplasty balloons or hydrophilic Coons dilators (over a stiff wire) can sometimes be helpful in these situations. The placement of uncovered stents in the iliac vessel should be avoided before EVAR. Finally, a surgically placed iliofemoral conduit can be considered if the patient is anatomically suitable. Placement of the proximal iliac artery anastomosis typically is performed at the iliac bifurcation, allowing deployment of the ipsilateral endograft limb in the common iliac artery.

An alternate method of obtaining access in a patient with extensive iliac occlusive disease is to create an "internal endoconduit" by placing a covered stent in the external iliac vessel, which is then aggressively angioplastied to the required diameter. The covered stent protects against extensive dissection, free rupture of the native vessel caused by the aggressive angioplasty, or both. There must be a sufficient proximal and distal seal zone for the covered stent for this approach to be safe. Although these techniques have been anecdotally reported with successful outcomes,[1,2] larger series are needed to establish the safety of this approach.

Significant iliac tortuosity can often be straightened with use of a very stiff guidewire, such as the Lunderquist or Amplatz (Cook Medical, Bloomington, Ind.) guidewires. Severe circumferential calcification in association with tortuosity must be approached cautiously, because even the stiffest guidewire may not straighten the vessel. Rarely, a second "buddy wire" may be helpful in this situation. Superstiff wires should be exchanged for a soft J wire before completion arteriography. Otherwise, an apparent high-grade stenosis may be seen in the external iliac artery that is caused by the vessel "accordioning" on the wire. These pseudolesions disappear with replacement of the stiff wire for a more flexible wire and thus do not require intervention.

"Through and through" access or brachial-femoral access was commonly used in the early period of EVAR to manage tortuous and challenging access vessel anatomy. It is rarely needed today given the development of smaller hydrophilic delivery systems.

AORTIC NECK

Aortic necks that are less than 15 mm in length, highly angulated (>60 degrees), and conical are considered suboptimal for EVAR using current commercial devices. Aortic necks with multiple adverse anatomic features have a substantially higher risk of poor immediate and long-term outcome.

AORTIC BIFURCATION

Proximal limb diameters range from 12 to 16 mm, so placing two limbs in a small terminal aorta with an aortic bifurcation diameter of less than 20 mm can significantly constrict the limbs of a bifurcated endograft. After placement of the limbs, bilateral "kissing" angioplasty with noncompliant balloons usually ameliorates this issue. If there is significant residual stenosis, the placement of kissing balloon-expandable stents should be considered.

ENDOGRAFT SELECTION

Bifurcated endografts such as Endurant (Medtronic, Minneapolis), Excluder (Gore, Flagstaff, Ariz.), Ovation (Trivascular, Santa Rosa, Calif.), Powerlink (Endologix, Irvine, Calif.), or Zenith (Cook Medical) are used in more than 95% of EVARs. An aortouniiliac configuration may be preferable in the presence of a small calcific terminal aorta, severe unilateral iliac occlusive disease, treatment of a displaced shortbodied endograft, or when there is a need to preserve hypogastric flow using a retrograde approach.

Type I Endoleak Treatment

Initial treatment of a type IA endoleak should be guided by the position of the endograft to the lowest renal artery. If this distance is less than 3 mm, the seal zone should be angioplastied with a compliant molding balloon such as Coda (Cook Medical) or Reliant (Medtronic). If the distance is more than 5 mm, placement of an aortic cuff should be considered to increase the seal zone. Compliant balloon angioplasty of the aortic neck should be performed after cuff placement. It is essential that proper fluoroscopic gantry position is used to accurately assess the distance between the endograft and the renal arteries before these adjunctive treatments are employed. Frequently, significant cranial tilt and left or right obliquity are required to achieve a perpendicular axis to the aortic neck and lowest renal artery. The gantry position should be adjusted until the radiopaque markers on the proximal edge of the stent graft are in alignment.

GIANT PALMAZ STENT PLACEMENT

If a type IA endoleak persists despite these maneuvers, placement of a giant Palmaz (Cordis Corp., Bridgewater, N.J.) stent is indicated[3] (Fig. 26-1). Placement of this stent provides greater radial strength in the seal zone and eliminates the type I endoleak in most cases. A 3010, 4010, or 5010 Palmaz stent is hand-mounted on an appropriately sized valvuloplasty balloon (Z-Med, B. Braun Interventional Systems, Bethlehem, Pa.) in a slightly asymmetric manner, such that the more proximal (cranial) extent of the balloon inflates first. Choose a balloon size to match the diameter of the aortic neck. The choice of stent length depends on the diameter of the neck and the length of the main body of the endograft. The stent foreshortens significantly as it is expanded. Although the Palmaz 5010 is 5 cm in length at 10 mm of expansion, it shortens to about 33.8 cm at 28 mm.[3] We typically use a Palmaz 5010 length for a long-body device such as Zenith. If this technique is used with a short-body bifurcated device (Endurant, Excluder, Ovation), a shorter stent (Palmaz 4010 or 3010) and balloon may be required so as not to intrude on the iliac flow divider distally.

The existing main body delivery sheath, or comparably sized sheath, is advanced beyond the intended deployment zone. The Palmaz stent is then carefully delivered through the sheath to the intended deployment area. Continuous fluoroscopic observation of the stent during this maneuver is prudent, confirming that its position relative to the balloon does not change. To prevent the stent from "watermelon seeding" with cranial displacement during balloon inflation, the distal two thirds of the stent is constrained in the delivery sheath while the initial balloon deployment is performed (Fig. 26-2, *A*). Because the stent in slightly asymmetrically mounted, stent displacement should not occur. After the proximal portion of the stent is expanded, the sheath in carefully retracted and the remainder of the stent is deployed (Fig. 26-2, *B*). Finally, a compliant molding balloon is used to expand the stent to the aortic neck (Fig. 26-2, *C*). This final step is critical when a conical neck is being treated.

Embolization of the Internal Iliac Artery

When a common iliac aneurysm is present, endograft repair must extend to the external iliac artery. Decision making is focused on the excluded hypogastric artery. The most frequently used approach is embolization of the proximal hypogastric artery to eliminate the possibility of a type II endoleak. Such embolization can be performed with standard coils or occlusion plugs (Amplatzer II). In most anatomic circumstances this is most easily performed antegrade from the contralateral femoral artery. If the angle between the hypogastric artery and the external iliac artery is less acute than typical, an ipsilateral retrograde approach can be used. In either case, the key is to provide a stable delivery platform for the coils or plugs. It is always important to ensure that the catheter position is stable before

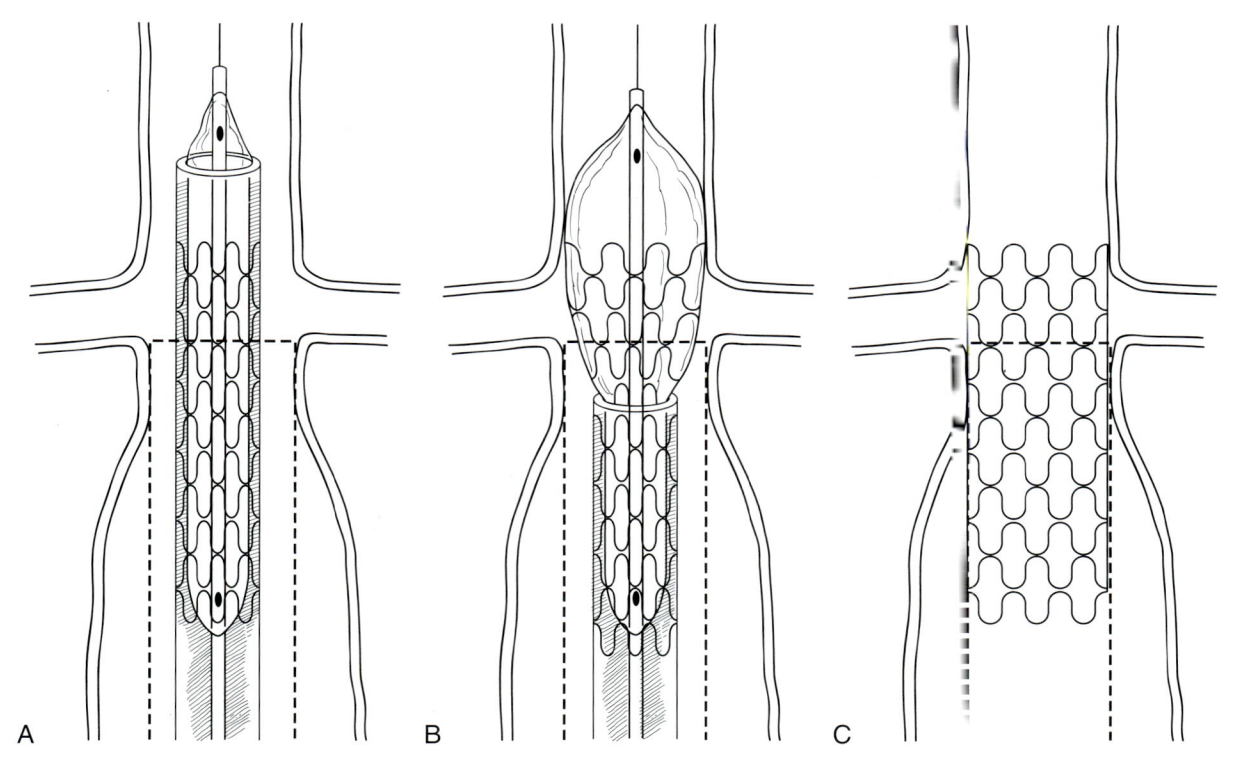

SPECIAL PROBLEMS IN THE ENDOVASCULAR TREATMENT OF THE INFRARENAL AORTA

Figure 26-1. Diagram sequence of the modified deployment technique of a giant Palmaz stent in the perirenal aorta for repair of a type IA endoleak. The dotted line represents the previously placed endograft for EVAR. Details of the endograft have been omitted from this illustration for clarity of imaging of the giant Palmaz stent device. **A,** The stent (Palmaz 3010, 4010, or 5010) is hand-crimped off-center on a valvuloplasty balloon. The balloon-mounted stent is then positioned at the intended area of deployment through the sheath under fluoroscopic guidance. **B,** The sheath is partially retracted and the balloon is inflated, deploying the proximal (cranial) portion of the stent. The off-center mounting of the stent ensures that it will not inadvertently be displaced superiorly or otherwise "watermelon seed" cranially, whereas the sheath prevents caudal displacement. **C,** Fully deployed stent. (*From Kim JM, Tonnessen BH, Noll ER Jr, et al: A technique for increased accuracy in the placement of giant Palmaz stents for treatment of type I endoleaks following EVAR. J Vasc Surg 48:755-757, 2008.*)

Figure 26-2. A, Initial deployment of the giant Palmaz stent. The cranial portion of the stent is expanded while the distal half is still constrained in the delivery sheath. **B,** The delivery sheath is withdrawn and the valvuloplasty balloon is completely inflated to expand the caudal portion of the Palmaz stent. **C,** A compliant molding balloon (Coda or Reliant) is used to flare the stent distally in this patient with a conical aortic neck.

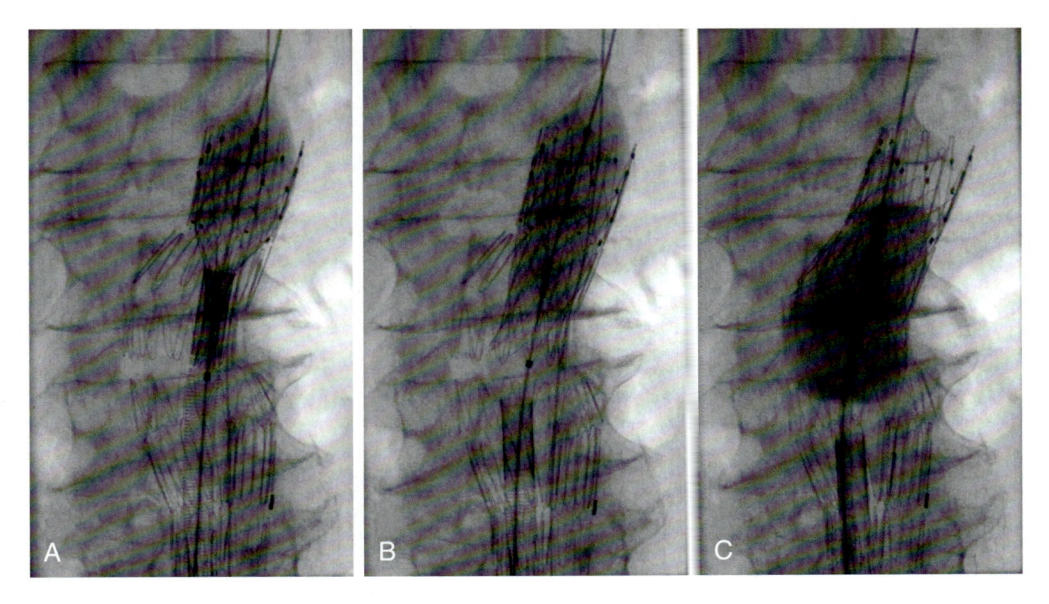

introducing coils. This can be confirmed by advancing a straight delivery wire (Newton wire guides, Cook Medical) 1 to 2 cm past the catheter tip. If the catheter starts to "back out" with this maneuver, the delivery platform is not sufficiently stable. Introduction of coils in this situation may lead to malpositioned coils that may embolize into the femoral artery.

Ideally, hypogastric arterial embolization is performed in the proximal aspect of the vessel, preserving the distal branches.[4] This approach preserves distal collateral flow and lessens the incidence of buttock claudication. If bilateral hypogastric embolization is planned, a staged approach is recommended.

Preservation of Flow to the Internal Iliac Artery

Preservation of flow to the hypogastric artery can be achieved by several methods. The most intuitive method to preserve flow to the hypogastric artery is the use of a branched endograft specifically designed for this purpose. Although not yet commercially available in the United States, such devices are undergoing clinical trials and are in use in other parts of the world.

EXTERNAL ILIAC TO INTERNAL ILIAC ENDOGRAFT

A second endovascular option to preserve hypogastric artery flow is placement of a covered stent from the hypogastric artery into the ipsilateral external iliac artery.[5] Combined with a contralateral aortouniiliac endograft and a femoral-femoral bypass, this provides retrograde arterial flow to the hypogastric artery from the external iliac artery. The usually tight angle between the hypogastric artery and the external iliac artery makes this innovative option realistic only in highly selected cases. To perform this procedure, a guidewire is placed retrograde from the common femoral artery to a distal branch of the ipsilateral hypogastric artery. This needs to be a stiff wire that supports passage of an appropriately sized, low-profile, self-expanding, covered stent such as the Viabahn (Gore) or Fluency (Bard Peripheral Vascular, Tempe, Ariz.). Tracking the stent into this position is difficult if there is a normal tight angle between the vessels. If the diameter of the hypogastric artery is significantly less than the external iliac artery, two covered stents may be required for accurate sizing. Covered stents such as the Viabahn do not conform well with excessive oversizing; significant eccentric infolding may occur that greatly increases the risk of thrombosis or endoleak. This problem may be reduced somewhat with the Fluency graft. Once the covered stent is in place, an open femoral-femoral bypass is performed that provides retrograde flow to the hypogastric artery and antegrade flow to the extremity (Fig. 26-3).

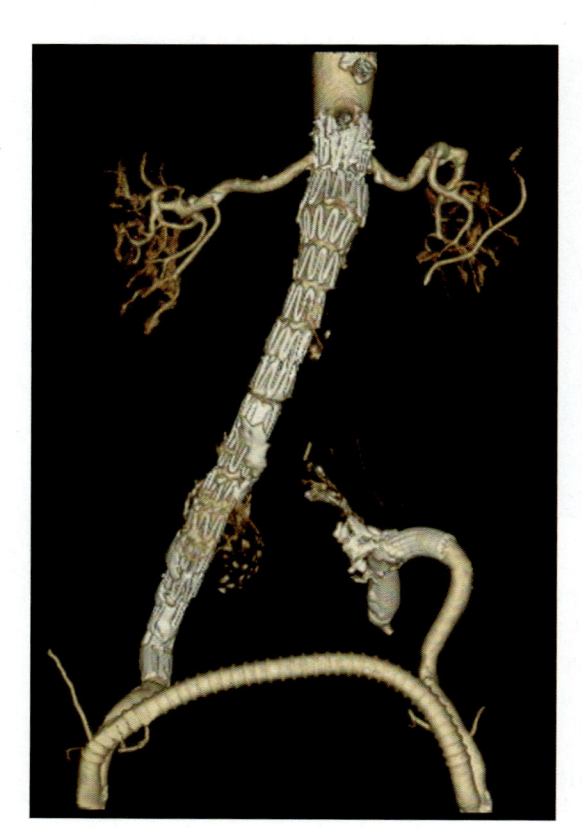

Figure 26-3. Three-dimensional CT angiogram demonstrating a patient treated with an aortouniiliac endograft, right to left femoral-femoral bypass with 8-mm polytetrafluoroethylene bypass graft, and preservation of left hypogastric artery flow by placement of a covered stent from the left hypogastric artery to the left external iliac artery. The femoral-femoral bypass provides retrograde flow to the hypogastric artery and prograde flow to the left limb.

Deployment of an Aortouniiliac Endograft

Although bifurcated endografts are used in more than 95% of EVARs, an aortouniiliac endograft with a femoral-femoral bypass is a valuable option in selected cases. These circumstances include severe unilateral iliac occlusive disease, a very narrow terminal aorta (<15 mm) that cannot otherwise accommodate two iliac limbs, or secondary treatment for migration of a short-body endograft. Both Medtronic and Cook now offer a aorto-uni-iliac endograft. These devices have a suprarenal stent with active fixation, identical to the bifurcated devices and consist of a two-piece system with an extender iliac limb allowing treatment of a variety of lengths and distal diameters.

Deployment of the proximal device is identical to that of a bifurcated endograft. The distal limb is then deployed with a minimum of 3-cm overlap proximally, extending distally to the terminal common iliac artery. The contralateral iliac artery is then occluded if it is not already chronically occluded. This is performed using a retrograde femoral approach with either a specifically designed Zenith component "plug" or through the use of a large vessel occlusion device (Amplatzer II). Placement of the occlusion device in the common iliac artery allows retrograde perfusion of the ipsilateral hypogastric artery, decreasing the incidence of buttock claudication. If the hypogastric artery is chronically occluded, then open ligation of the terminal external iliac artery achieves the same result. This can be performed through the existing femoral incision with minimal mobilization of the inguinal ligament. The ligature should be placed proximal to patent medial or lateral circumflex vessels to allow continued perfusion via the femoral-femoral bypass as these vessels are important sources of collateral flow to the pelvis. A standard femoral-femoral bypass is performed with an 8-mm synthetic conduit.

Type II Endoleak Treatment

Type II endoleaks are frequently seen on initial completion arteriograms after placement of the aortic endograft. Because most of these are lumbar endoleaks and inferior mesenteric arterial endoleaks, which resolve spontaneously, there is rarely a role for treatment in the acute setting. Treatment of a persistent type II endoleak is indicated if more than 5 mm in aneurysm sac growth is noted on follow-up imaging. Before treatment of a presumed type II endoleak, it is important to ensure that the endoleak is not a type I or type III endoleak.

Treatment options for type II endoleaks include transarterial selective coil embolization, translumbar glue or coil embolization of the aneurysm sac and feeding vessels, or by laparoscopic or open operative clipping of the offending branch vessel.[7-10] Translumbar embolization has emerged for many as the preferred therapy, because it is minimally invasive, often with durable results. With the patient prone, the aneurysm sac is punctured via a translumbar approach. Accessing the specific area of endoleak in the sac provides the best results. Injection of contrast should confirm filling of one or more collateral vessels. Biologically compatible glue is then slowly injected, with the goal of proximally occluding the feeding vessels, as well as the nidus of the endoleak. A fairly rapidly setting polymer is highly desirable. Embolization of the lumbar or inferior mesenteric arterial vessels carries some risk of spinal cord or left colon ischemia, respectively. Coils may also be delivered via a translumbar approach with less risk of end-organ ischemia but may be more difficult to deliver into the feeding vessels.

Transarterial coil embolization is usually successful in the near term, but may be associated with a fairly high recurrence rate.[8] Other collateral pathways frequently open over time, and the type II endoleak returns. More durable results with transarterial coiling may be achieved if the aneurysm sac can be accessed though the feeding vessel, allowing embolization at the nidus of the endoleak. Persistently patent lumbar arteries are typically fed from a distal branch of the ipsilateral hypogastric artery. Selective catheterization (3-Fr Tracker catheter) of this feeding distal vessel allows placement of small occluding coils. A patent inferior mesenteric artery can be accessed via the arc of Riolan from the superior mesenteric artery arcade. A microcatheter is advanced to the proximal inferior mesenteric artery and coils are placed. To maximize collateral flow to the colon, it is ideal to place the coils proximal to the first branches of the inferior mesenteric artery.

Postoperative Care

- **Follow-up imaging.** A CT scan is typically obtained 4 weeks after the intervention to access for endoleak. Long-term surveillance can be performed with yearly duplex ultrasound in patients without early endoleak.[11] However, patients with marginal aortic necks and those needing secondary procedures for endoleak should undergo more frequent surveillance with periodic CT imaging.

REFERENCES

1. Peterson BG, Matsumura JS: Internal endoconduit: An innovative technique to address unfavorable iliac artery anatomy encountered during thoracic endovascular aortic repair, *J Vasc Surg* 47:441-445, 2008.
2. Hinchliffe RJ, Ivancev K, Sonesson B, et al: "Paving and cracking": An endovascular technique to facilitate the introduction of aortic stent-grafts through stenosed iliac arteries, *J Endovasc Ther* 14:630-633, 2007.
3. Kim JM, Tonnessen BH, Noll ER Jr, et al: A technique for increased accuracy in the placement of giant Palmaz stents for treatment of type I endoleaks following EVAR, *J Vasc Surg* 48:755-757, 2008.
4. Kritpracha B, Pigott JP, Price CI, et al: Distal internal iliac artery Embolization: A procedure to avoid, *J Vasc Surg* 37:943-948, 2003.
5. Bergamini TM, Rachel ES, Kinney EV, et al: External iliac artery-to-internal iliac artery endograft: A novel approach to preserve pelvic inflow in aortoiliac stent grafting, *J Vasc Surg* 35:120-124, 2002.
6. Thomas BG, Sanchez LA, Geraghty PJ, et al: A comparative analysis of the outcomes of aortic cuffs and converters for endovascular graft migration, *J Vasc Surg* 51:1373-1380, 2010.
7. Kasirajan K, Matteson B, Marek JM, et al: Technique and results of transfemoral superselective coil embolization of type II lumbar endoleak, *J Vasc Surg* 38:61-66, 2003.
8. Stavropoulos SW, Park J, Fairman R, et al: Type 2 endoleak embolization comparison: Translumbar embolization versus modified transarterial embolization, *J Vasc Interv Radiol* 20:1299-1302, 2009.
9. Nevala T, Biancari F, Manninen H, et al: Type II endoleak after endovascular repair of abdominal aortic aneurysm: Effectiveness of embolization, *Cariovasc Inter Rad* 33:278-284, 2010.
10. Richardson WS, Sternbergh WC III, Money SR: Minimally invasive treatment of type II endoleaks from patent inferior mesenteric artery following endovascular abdominal aortic aneurysm repair, *J Laparoendosc Adv Surg Techniques* 13:355-358, 2003.
11. Sternbergh WC III, Greenberg RK, Chuter TAM, et al: Redefining post-operative surveillance after EVAR: Recommendations based on 5 year follow-up in the U.S. Zenith multi-center trial, *J Vasc Surg* 48:278-285, 2008.

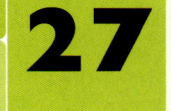

27 Endovascular Treatment of Aneurysms of the Juxtarenal and Pararenal Aorta

RONALD M. FAIRMAN • GRACE J. WANG

Historical Background

Juxtarenal aneurysms refer to abdominal aortic aneurysms with an infrarenal neck less than or equal to 1 cm in length, and pararenal aneurysms refer to abdominal aortic aneurysms that involve one or both orifices of the renal arteries. Browne and associates[1] first described the design of a fenestrated graft in 1999 in which holes were placed within an endograft for deployment of uncovered balloon-expandable stents from the aortic graft into the renal arteries. The principle of fenestrated technology was extended above the infrarenal segment by Anderson[2] in 2005 to treat aneurysms involving the visceral arteries. The first report of branched endograft used for the treatment of a thoracoabdominal aneurysm was reported in 2001 by Chuter and colleagues.[3] Branched and fenestrated grafts offer a complete endovascular solution. Fenestrated grafts are now commercially available in the United States. As an alternative to fenestrated and branched endografts, Greenberg and associates[4] were the first to describe a "snorkel" or "chimney graft" technique in 2003, with placement of a stent into the renal artery alongside the endograft to treat a juxtarenal aortic aneurysm. Others have extended this technique to treat pararenal aneurysms during endovascular aneurysm repair (EVAR).[5] Hybrid, or combined open and endovascular, approaches are another option for treatment of complex aortic aneurysms involving visceral vessels and were first reported in 1999 by Quinones-Baldrich and co-workers.[6]

Preoperative Preparation

- A detailed analysis is required of axial images and three-dimensional reconstructed images of the aorta using TeraRecon (San Mateo, Calif.) or M2S (West Lebanon, N.H.) devices. The radial orientation of visceral vessels is often related to in terms of the hands of a clock.
- The diameter of each vessel and the distance of each vessel origin from the edge of the graft, as well as from each other, are recorded. The endograft is manufactured accordingly.
- Preoperative hydration should be considered for patients with compromised renal function.
- Spinal catheter drainage is recommended if coverage of a long segment of thoracic aorta is planned in addition to treatment of the visceral segment of the aorta.
- Perioperative antibiotics and subcutaneous heparin for prophylaxis of deep venous thrombosis are routinely administered.

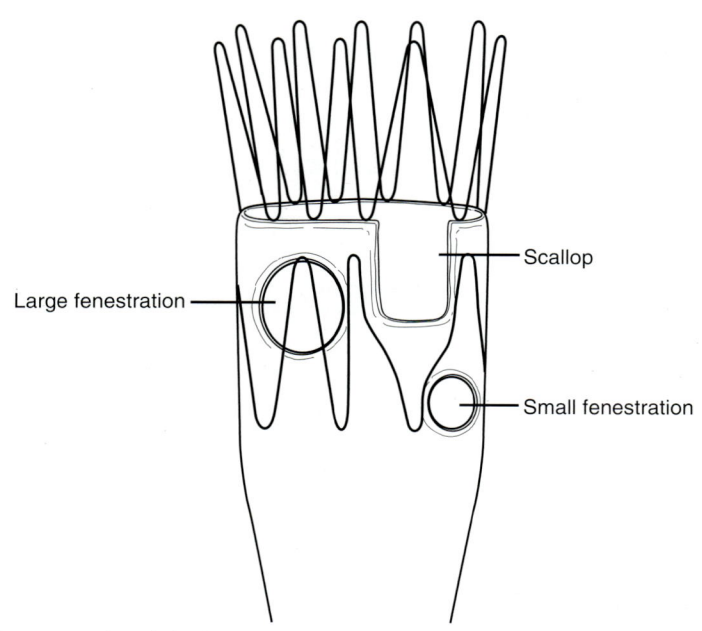

Figure 27-1. A fenestrated graft is depicted with a scallop, a small fenestration, and a large fenestration.

Endovascular Strategy

Endovascular repair of the visceral segment of the aorta uses stent-graft exclusion of the aneurysm with preservation of flow to important branch vessels (Videos 27-1 through 27-12). Flow to the renal, celiac, and superior mesenteric arteries is preserved with transarterial access. When the branch vessel arises from where the stent graft is attached, a simple hole, or fenestration in the stent graft, is sufficient. When the branch vessel arises from an aneurysmal portion of the aorta, however, flow between the stent-graft component and the branch vessel must be achieved with a branched graft to traverse the distance between the stent and the origin of the vessel.[7]

FENESTRATED GRAFTS

Current fenestrated stent grafts are manufactured by Cook Medical (Bloomington, Ind.). The graft is composed of woven polyester and the stent component is of stainless steel. Radiopaque markers on the front and back of the graft provide reference points for orientation. Fenestrations are categorized into three types: scallops, small fenestrations, and large fenestrations (Fig. 27-1). Scallops are open to the free margin of the graft, small fenestrations occupy the spaces between stent struts, and large fenestrations are crossed by stent struts. The fenestrations are sized and positioned on the stent graft according to the relative positions of the origins of the branch vessels. Because of device constraints, with small fenestrations located between stents, the stent graft cannot be a perfect replica of aortic anatomy. Tortuosity in the path from the femoral artery to the aorta can dramatically shift the geometric relationships between the origins of the branch vessels and their corresponding fenestrations. The more fenestrations in a stent graft, the fewer degrees of freedom allowable with respect to slight adjustments in orientation during deployment. There is some flexibility in the system because of stent-graft oversizing, where the orifice of the fenestration can be forced into the proper position with a guiding catheter. The use of a bridging stent allows patency when this alignment is strained.[7-9]

BRANCHED GRAFTS

Unlike fenestrated grafts, branched stent grafts allow a zone of overlap between the main stent graft and the covered stent within the branch vessel, preventing component separation and endoleak. The orientation of the branch component is parallel to the axis of the primary stent graft and aorta, and in most cases, the

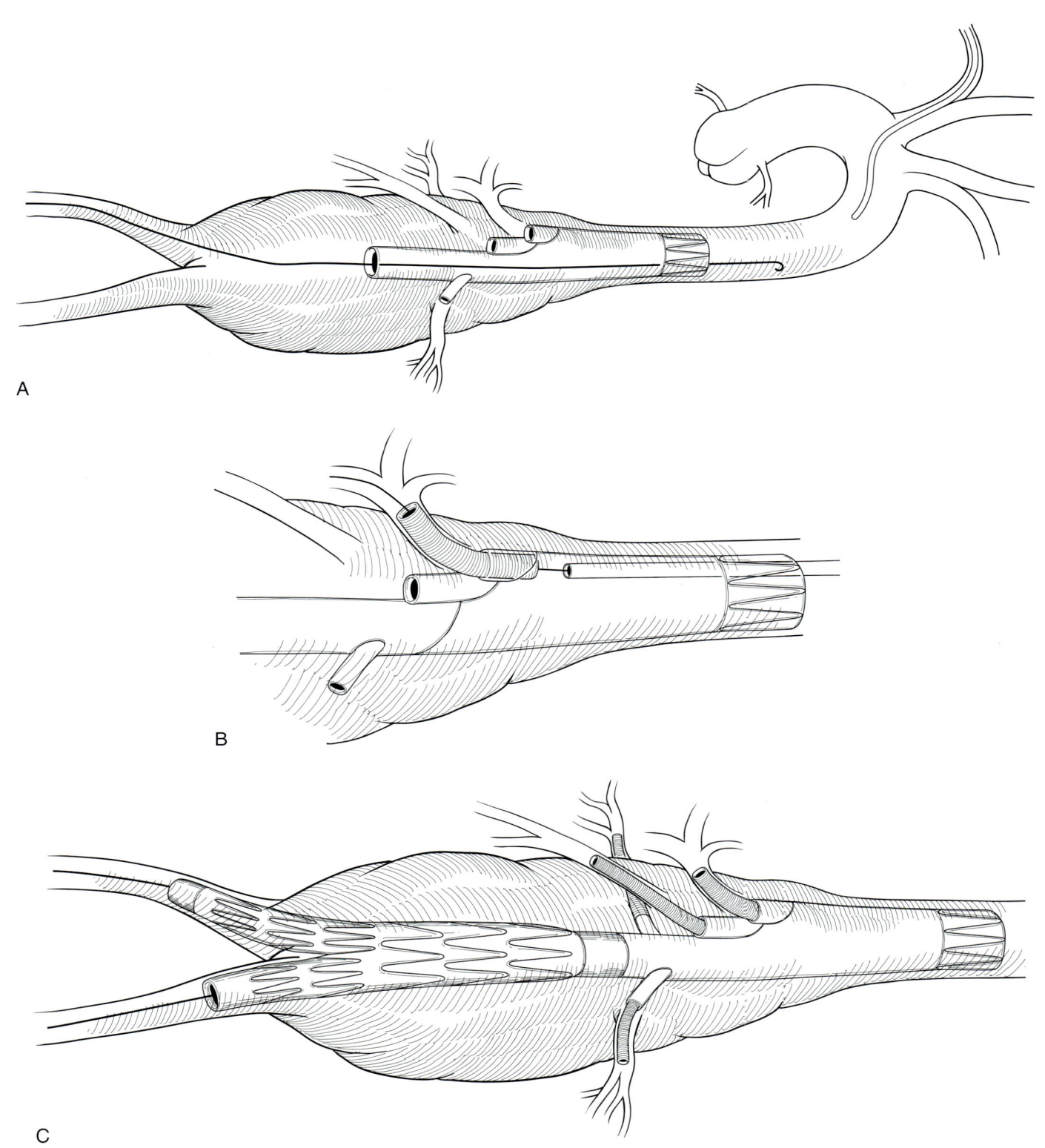

Figure 27-2. A, A branched graft is positioned cranial to the visceral segment, with caudally oriented branches of the stent graft. **B,** The visceral extension is deployed into the target vessel, as well as the branch component of the branched stent graft. **C,** The branched graft is shown with all four visceral extensions in their target arteries, as well as the infrarenal component.

inner orifice of the branch is cranial to the origin of the target vessel. The relatively indirect route allows more flexibility in cannulation of the branch vessels compared with the fenestrated approach and is the preferred approach when targeting a greater number of branch vessels. Generally, the target vessels are caudally oriented; thus the branches of the stent graft are typically caudally oriented and more easily cannulated through the brachial approach (Fig. 27-2, A). Occasionally, the renal arteries are cranially oriented, dictating a different branch takeoff from the main graft, and are more easily cannulated compared with the femoral approach.

Endovascular Technique

FENESTRATED GRAFT IMPLANTATION

Fenestrated grafts consist of a fenestrated main body component, a bifurcated component, and bridging stents. Bilateral common femoral arteries are exposed, and the patient is systemically heparinized. The delivery system of the fenestrated stent graft is inserted, and an aortogram is performed. The stent graft is then positioned and oriented to match each fenestration with the appropriate target vessel. The sheath is withdrawn, and then the stent graft is deployed and repositioned as appropriate.

Wire and catheter traversal through the fenestration into the target vessel is achieved, followed by transgraft bridging sheath insertion into the target vessel. The constraining trigger wire on the upper attachment system is then removed, the delivery system is withdrawn, and the bridging stent is deployed and ballooned to create a flared end. The infrarenal bifurcated stent graft is then inserted and deployed.

BRANCHED GRAFT IMPLANTATION

There are three major components of the branched stent-graft system: a thoracoabdominal component with multiple branches for each visceral artery, an infrarenal aortic component consisting of a main aortic trunk and two iliac limbs, and small stent grafts used to extend each branch of the thoracoabdominal component into the visceral branches of the aorta. After bilateral femoral artery exposure and systemic heparinization, the thoracoabdominal stent-graft delivery system is inserted over a stiff wire and an angiographic catheter is inserted through the contralateral side. An aortogram is performed to locate the celiac artery, and the thoracoabdominal stent graft is positioned with the distal end 1 to 2 cm above the celiac artery orifice. The sheath is withdrawn, and a confirmatory arteriogram is performed before removal of safety wires, releasing both ends of the stent graft. The delivery system is removed. Attention is then directed toward cannulating the graft branches.

Because most branches are caudally oriented, most cannulations are performed from the brachial or axillary artery. Cranial-oriented branches may be cannulated from the femoral approach. Brachial access is achieved with a short 7-Fr sheath. The descending thoracic aorta is catheterized, and a stiff guidewire is inserted. The short sheath is exchanged for a long 10-Fr Flexor sheath. Using a combination of a smaller sheath or guiding catheter and an angled catheter, branches of the stent graft are cannulated, followed by access into the corresponding visceral artery. The guidewire is exchanged for a long Rosen wire, and a sheath or guiding catheter is advanced at least 2 cm into the visceral artery. The catheter is exchanged for the delivery system of the visceral extension. The visceral extension is deployed with 15-mm overlap into the visceral artery, as well as the branch of the stent graft (Fig. 27-2, B). These steps are repeated for all involved visceral arteries.

The infrarenal component is then deployed into the thoracoabdominal component, followed by deployment of the iliac limbs (Fig. 27-2, C). A completion arteriogram is performed; all sheaths, wires, and catheters are removed; and the brachial artery repaired. If cannulation of the branches proves difficult and time consuming, this portion of the procedure may be delayed for hours or days, given that visceral perfusion is maintained through the perigraft space.

SNORKEL OR CHIMNEY GRAFT TECHNIQUE

In some patients the stent graft partially covers the renal artery orifice and adjunctive renal artery stenting is required.[10] In the "encroachment" technique the

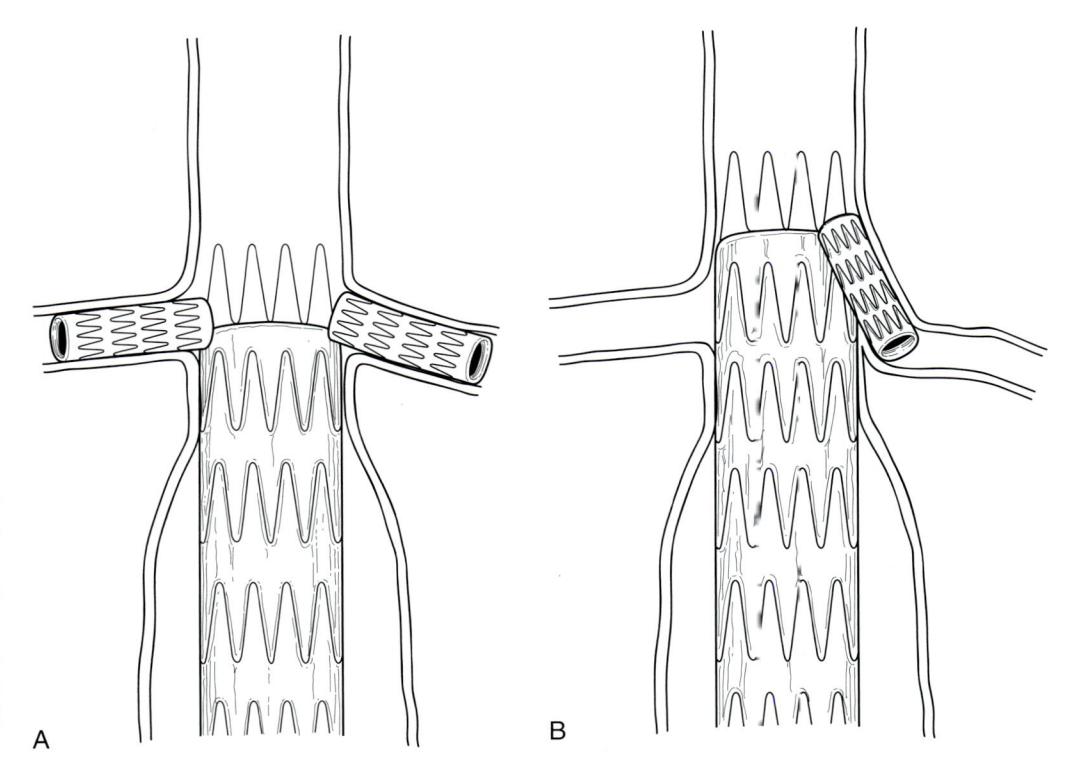

ENDOVASCULAR TREATMENT OF ANEURYSMS OF THE JUXTARENAL AND PARARENAL AORTA

Figure 27-3. A, The encroachment technique allows preservation of renal blood flow with a stent deployed transaxially. **B,** The snorkel technique allows preservation of renal blood flow with a renal artery stent deployed parallel to the stent graft.

superior margin of the stent graft is pushed inferiorly by the renal stent. In the snorkel technique a covered stent is deployed parallel to the main stent graft, protruding proximally, like a chimney, to preserve flow to the branch vessel covered by the graft. The snorkel technique provides an alternative to fenestrated stent grafts in urgent cases or to reestablish flow to a branch vessel unintentionally compromised during EVAR (Fig. 27-3). Transbrachial access is critical for the snorkel maneuver.

HYBRID SURGICAL AND ENDOVASCULAR APPROACHES

Hybrid procedures have included renal revascularization by splenorenal or hepatorenal bypass, when celiac artery coverage is not intended, or use of the iliac artery for revascularization of the renal, superior mesenteric, and hepatic arteries (Fig. 27-4).[11,12] These procedures debranch a segment of aorta, allowing stent-graft coverage of visceral vessels. The renal arteries often arise from the aorta at different levels. Thus, the surgeon may plan to cover the lowest renal, with use of a splenorenal or hepatorenal artery bypass for the other. As more visceral vessels are targeted for revascularization, however, morbidity and mortality increase.[12,13] The Viabahn open revascularization technique has been described as a simple rapid alternative to the creation of standard sutured anastomoses by placement of a self-expanding stent graft into renal or visceral arteries, using a Seldinger technique, after surgical identification of the origin of the arteries.[14] The end of the stent outside of the artery is then sutured to the main graft.

Postoperative Care

- Patients are observed in the intensive care unit overnight, with continuous hemodynamic monitoring and frequent assessment of peripheral pulses, renal function, and neurologic function.
- Augmentation of blood pressure using pressors to improve spinal cord blood flow may be needed to minimize the risk of spinal cord ischemia.
- Postoperative assessment, including computed tomography and ultrasound imaging, plain radiographs, and measurement of renal function, is performed at 1, 6, and 12 months and annually thereafter.

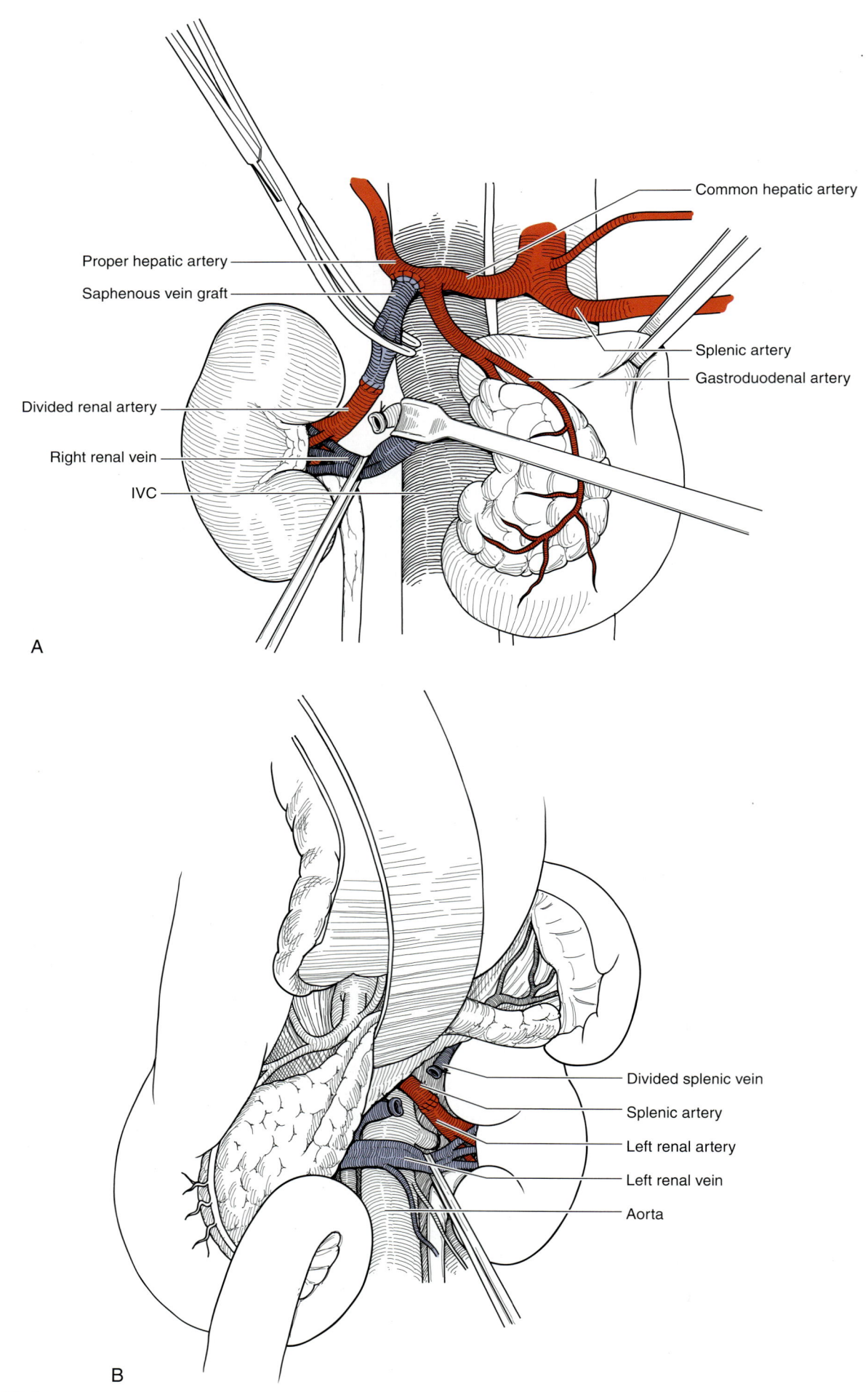

Figure 27-4. Hepatorenal (**A**) and splenorenal (**B**) bypass used in association with a hybrid endovascular repair. *IVC,* Inferior vena cava.

Postoperative Complications

- **Endoleak.** At the completion of a fenestrated EVAR, proximal and distal type I endoleaks have been reported in 6% of patients, and type II endoleaks have been reported in 7% of patients. Type II endoleaks also have been noted in approximately 20% of patients at 1- and 2-year follow-ups.[15-18]
- **Visceral vessel stenosis.** At the completion of a fenestrated EVAR, target vessel occlusion has been noted in 3% of patients. Renal artery stenosis or occlusion has been observed in up to 10% of patients at late follow-up.[17,18] In a recent systematic review of 629 patients with follow-ups between 15 and 25 months, pooled estimates for branch vessel patency, renal impairment, and secondary interventions were 93.2%, 22.2%, and 17.8%, respectively.[19]
- **Spinal cord ischemia**
- **Component separation**

REFERENCES

1. Browne TF, Hartley D, Purchas S, et al: A fenestrated covered suprarenal aortic stent, *Eur J Vasc Endovasc Surg* 18:445-449, 1999.
2. Anderson JL, Adam DJ, Berce M, et al: Repair of thoracoabdominal aortic aneurysms with fenestrated and branched endovascular stent grafts, *J Vasc Surg* 42:600-607, 2005.
3. Chuter TA, Gordon RL, Reilly LM, et al: Multi-branched stent-graft for type III thoracoabdominal aortic aneurysm, *J Vasc Interv Radiol* 12:391-392, 2001.
4. Greenberg RK, Clair D, Srivastava S, et al: Should patients with challenging anatomy be offered endovascular aneurysm repair? *J Vasc Surg* 38:990-996, 2003.
5. Ohrlander T, Sonesson B, Ivancev K, et al: The chimney graft: A technique for preserving or rescuing aortic branch vessels in stent-graft sealing zones, *J Endovasc Ther* 15:427-432, 2008.
6. Quinones-Baldrich WJ, Panetta TF, Vescera CL, et al: Repair of type IV thoracoabdominal aneurysm with a combined endovascular and surgical approach, *J Vasc Surg* 30:555-560, 1999.
7. Chuter TA: Fenestrated and branched stent-grafts for thoracoabdominal, pararenal and juxtarenal aortic aneurysm repair, *Semin Vasc Surg* 20:90-96, 2007.
8. Greenberg RK: Aortic aneurysm, thoracoabdominal aneurysm, juxtarenal aneurysm, fenestrated endografts, branched endografts, and endovascular aneurysm repair, *Ann N Y Acad Sci* 1085:187-196, 2006.
9. Verhoeven EL, Muhs BE, Zeebregts CJ, et al: Fenestrated and branched stent-grafting after previous surgery provides a good alternative to open redo surgery, *Eur J Vasc Endovasc Surg* 33:84-90, 2007.
10. Hiramoto JS, Chang CK, Reilly LM, et al: Outcome of renal stenting for renal artery coverage during endovascular aortic aneurysm repair, *J Vasc Surg* 49:1100-1106, 2009.
11. Fulton JJ, Farber MA, Marston WA, et al: Endovascular stent-graft repair of pararenal and type IV thoracoabdominal aortic aneurysms with adjunctive visceral reconstruction, *J Vasc Surg* 41:191-198, 2005.
12. Patel R, Conrad MF, Paruchuri V, et al: Thoracoabdominal aneurysm repair: Hybrid versus open repair, *J Vasc Surg* 50:15-22, 2009.
13. Chiesa R, Tshomba Y, Melissano G, et al: Hybrid approach to thoracoabdominal aortic aneurysms in patients with prior aortic surgery, *J Vasc Surg* 45:1128-1135, 2007.
14. Donas KP, Lachat M, Rancic Z, et al: Early and midterm outcome of a novel technique to simplify the hybrid procedures in the treatment of thoracoabdominal and pararenal aortic aneurysms, *J Vasc Surg* 50:1280-1284, 2009.
15. O'Neill S, Greenberg RK, Haddad F, et al: A prospective analysis of fenestrated endovascular grafting: Intermediate-term outcomes, *Eur J Vasc Endovasc Surg* 32:115-123, 2006.
16. Bicknell CD, Cheshire NJ, Riga CV, et al: Treatment of complex aneurysmal disease with fenestrated and branched stent grafts, *Eur J Vasc Endovasc Surg* 37:175-181, 2009.
17. Greenberg RK, Sternbergh WC III, Makaroun M, et al: Intermediate results of a United States multicenter trial of fenestrated endograft repair for juxtarenal abdominal aortic aneurysms, *J Vasc Surg* 50:730-737, 2009.
18. GLOBALSTAR Registry: Early results of fenestrated endovascular repair of juxtarenal aortic aneurysms in the United Kingdom, *Circulation* 125:2707-2715, 2012.
19. Linsen MAM, Jongkind V, Nio D, et al: Pararenal aortic aneurysm repair using fenestrated endografts, *J Vasc Surg* 56:238-246, 2012.

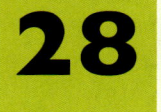

28 Direct Surgical Repair of Aortoiliac Occlusive Disease

ROBERT S. CRAWFORD • DAVID C. BREWSTER

Historical Background

The distal aorta and iliac segments are among the most common sites of chronic atherosclerotic disease. This disease is usually segmental, generally produces a constellation of characteristic symptoms, and is amenable to durable surgical reconstruction. Direct surgical correction of aortoiliac occlusive disease (AIOD) has developed rapidly since the 1940s and 1950s. Although AIOD commonly coexists with disease below the inguinal ligament, correction of inflow disease alone can often provide effective symptomatic relief[1] and is of paramount importance if durable results of further distal arterial revascularization are to be expected.

Indications

Accurate assessment of disease severity is performed on the basis of the history and physical examination and a combination of imaging and physiologic testing. A history of intermittent claudication, diminished sexual potency, and absent femoral pulses accurately describes the triad of Leriche syndrome. Some patients with AIOD present with proximal claudication symptoms in the thigh, hip, and buttock distribution, whereas others with significant inflow disease may complain principally of calf claudication. Disabling symptoms of intermittent claudication that significantly impair a patient's occupation or desired lifestyle can be considered appropriate indications for intervention. Ischemic rest pain and tissue necrosis are unequivocal indications for revascularization.

On physical examination, audible bruits over the lower abdomen or groins, elevation pallor, rubor of dependency, and shiny atrophic skin are all characteristic findings. Areas of ischemic ulceration, necrosis, or gangrene are often observed in advanced stages of the disease. Some patients may present with distal microemboli secondary to thromboembolism, the so-called blue toe syndrome.

With regard to conservative management, complete cessation of smoking, weight reduction, treatment of hypertension and diabetes, antiplatelet therapy, and aggressive serum lipid lowering are all desirable. A regular exercise program may enhance ambulatory function by improving muscle metabolic function. Finally, pharmacologic agents, such as cilostazol (Pletal), may provide benefit in a limited number of patients based on previous trials; however, this is rarely successful in patients with severe disease.

Preoperative Preparation

- Pulmonary, renal, or coagulation function abnormalities should be addressed. Corrective action, such as a brief period of chest physiotherapy and bronchodilator medication and correction of a prerenal cause of renal impairment, should be pursued.
- Evaluation of the carotid circulation should be performed.

DIRECT SURGICAL REPAIR OF AORTOILIAC OCCLUSIVE DISEASE

- Preoperative coronary evaluation is necessary and the most important modifiable risk factor in patients undergoing vascular operations. Open aortic reconstruction qualifies as a high-risk procedure compared with, for example, percutaneous endovascular revascularization. Preoperative thallium imaging has been used to identify high-risk patients for perioperative myocardial infarction[2]; however, most such tests suffer from a poor predictive value, and it is best to manage all vascular patients as potentially having coronary disease.
- Segmental limb Doppler pressure measurements and pulse volume recordings are useful for diagnostic confirmation, establishing an objective baseline and localizing the disease process. They also provide useful quantification to establish whether a lesion has the potential to heal without revascularization. The addition of pre- and post- exercise ankle-brachial indices adds diagnostic sensitivity to noninvasive studies.
- Angiography has long been considered the gold standard for delineating the location, extent, and severity of AIOD, but advances in imaging have allowed computed tomography angiography and magnetic resonance angiography to often obviate the need for catheter-based angiography. In select patients, measurements of femoral artery pressures may be of considerable value. In assessing the hemodynamic significance of AIOD, a resting peak systolic pressure difference of more than 5 mm Hg, or a fall of more than 15% when reactive hyperemia is induced pharmacologically by intraarterial administration of 30 mg of papaverine or by inflation of an occluding thigh cuff for 3 to 5 minutes, implies hemodynamically significant inflow disease.
- Assessment of infrainguinal runoff is indicated because the status of the distal vessels has a considerable influence in the outcome of the proximal procedure. It also helps plan for adjunctive future distal bypass procedures.
- Appropriate antibiotic prophylaxis (cefazolin) should be administered before the operation and through the perioperative period.
- A radial artery cannula is routine in many units. Selective placement of a Swan-Ganz pulmonary artery catheter is reserved for select patients such as those with significant cardiac disease, likely requiring suprarenal clamps, or at risk of having significant hemodynamic disturbances.
- A combination of epidural and general anesthesia is used, which limits postoperative pain medication administration.

Operative Strategy

A simple classification by disease pattern (type I-III) can affect symptom presentation, affect progression of the disease, and help determine the appropriate operative strategy (Fig. 28-1). Type I lesions are confined to the distal abdominal aorta and common iliac arteries. This least common pattern of disease usually occurs in younger patients presenting with symptoms of claudication in the hips and buttock region. At least half of these patients are women, usually heavy smokers with a characteristic pattern called hypoplastic aortic syndrome. Type II patients (about 25% of cases) present with disease that is confined to the abdomen. Type III patients (about 65%) have disease that extends above and below the inguinal ligament, are typically older, are more greatly affected by diabetes and hypertension, and manifest symptoms of more advanced ischemia.

END-TO-END VERSUS END-TO-SIDE PROXIMAL ANASTOMOSIS

An end-to-end aortic anastomosis is preferred for most patients for several reasons. All flow is through the graft, which avoids competitive flow and an increased risk of graft limb thrombosis. An end-to-end anastomosis provides a superior hemodynamic configuration with less perianastomotic turbulence and less recurrent atheroma or anastomotic aneurysms. It is less likely to cause distal atheromatous

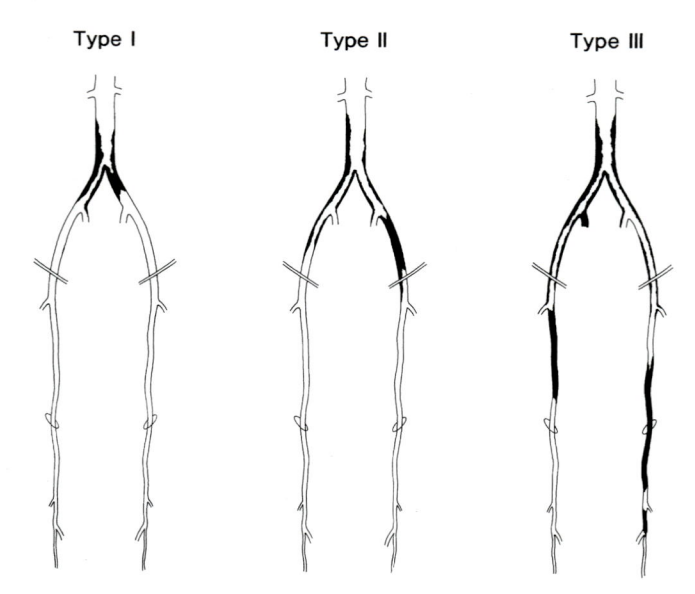

Figure 28-1. Patterns of aortoiliac occlusive disease. In type I localized disease is confined to the distal abdominal aorta and common iliac arteries. In type II more widespread intraabdominal disease is present. In type III the pattern denotes multilevel disease with associated infrainguinal occlusive lesions, which may require concomitant treatment. *(From Brewster CD: Direct reconstruction for aortoiliac occlusive disease. In Cronenwett JL, Johnston KW, editors: Rutherford's vascular surgery, ed 6, Philadelphia, 2005, Saunders, p 1106, Fig. 79-1.)*

embolization and is easier to cover with retroperitoneal tissue, with less chance of graft-enteric fistula.

An end-to-side anastomosis is preferred for certain anatomic configurations, such as for patients with a sizable accessory renal artery arising from the infrarenal abdominal aorta, patients with a patent inferior mesenteric artery that needs to be maintained, and patients in whom most disease is located in the external iliac arteries. In this instance, retrograde flow to the hypogastric arteries to maintain pelvic circulation may be limited, which can lead to impotence, colonic ischemia, or even lumbosacral spinal or cauda equina syndrome.

PROCEDURE SELECTION

The optimal method of revascularization represents a controversial area in the management of aortoiliac disease.[3,4] Surgical risk, extent of disease, personal bias, and previous surgical training may all play parts in decision making. Anatomic or direct reconstructive procedures, extraanatomic bypasses, and catheter-based methods each plays a role.

For low-risk, young patients with extensive disease and mild comorbid conditions, aortobifemoral grafting is the preferred choice and remains the gold standard. Angioplasty, femoral-femoral bypass, or unilateral iliofemoral grafting may be considered for patients with limited disease. Aortoiliac endarterectomy may be used for a small number of patients with distal aortic disease, confined to the distal aorta and common iliac arteries, although stenting has largely replaced this open surgical method in contemporary practice. For high-risk patients with bilateral iliac disease or heavy retroperitoneal scarring or contamination, an axillobifemoral bypass can be considered even though it may have lower long-term patency.

Aortoiliac Endarterectomy

Appropriate for patients with type I disease, aortoiliac endarterectomy is only infrequently performed today. Its advantages include the lack of prosthetic material, no infective potential, and continuity of antegrade inflow to the hypogastrics. Contraindications include evidence of aneurysmal change, total occlusion of the aorta to the level of the renal arteries, and extension of the disease into the external iliac and distal vessels. Although percutaneous transluminal angioplasty (PTA) and stents have replaced endarterectomy as first-line therapy for localized aortoiliac disease for many patients in current practice, endarterectomy remains

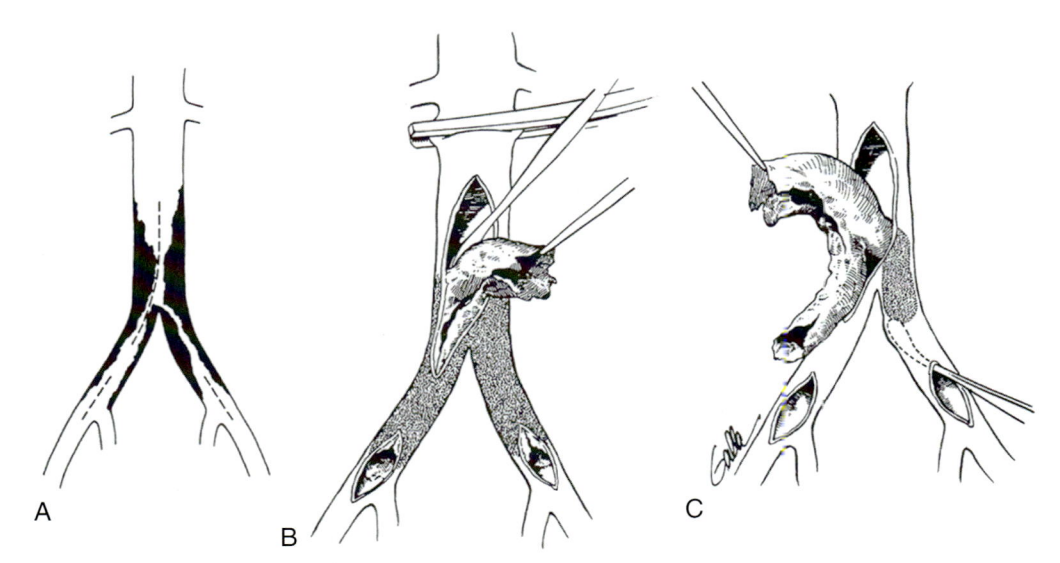

Figure 28-2. Steps in aortoiliac endarterectomy. **A,** Occlusive disease is limited to the distal aorta and common iliac arteries. Location of typical arteriotomies is indicated by dotted lines. **B,** The endarterectomy plane is achieved, and atheromatous disease is removed from the level of the proximal aortic clamp to the bifurcation. **C,** A satisfactory endpoint is attained at the iliac bifurcation, and endarterectomy is carried proximally. Tacking sutures may be necessary to secure an adequate endpoint. **D,** Operative specimen removed by endarterectomy. *(From Brewster CD: Direct reconstruction for aortoiliac occlusive disease. In Cronenwett JL, Johnston KW, editors: Rutherford's vascular surgery, ed 6. Philadelphia, 2005, Saunders, p 1114, Fig. 79-5.)*

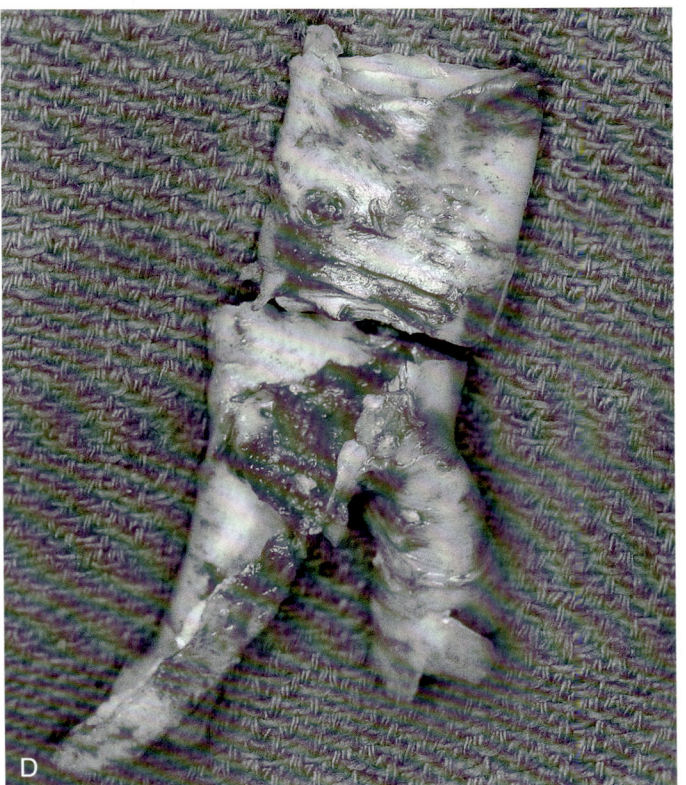

a viable option for select patients and cases (Fig. 28-2). From a technical standpoint, the atherosclerotic disease should terminate at the iliac bifurcation to obtain satisfactory results and achieve a good endpoint no farther than 1 to 2 cm into the external iliac arteries. Bilateral longitudinal arteriotomies, one extending from the distal aorta into one common iliac artery and the other confined to the common iliac artery, are performed. The proper endarterectomy plane, to the level of the external elastic lamina, should be obtained. Patch closure, either with vein or prosthetic, can be used. Tacking sutures may also be used to secure the distal endpoint.

Graft Selection

Both Dacron and polytetrafluoroethylene (PTFE) grafts are used in current practice. Dacron grafts are preferred by many surgeons because of flexibility and easy handling, although they have been known to dilate by 10% to 20% when exposed

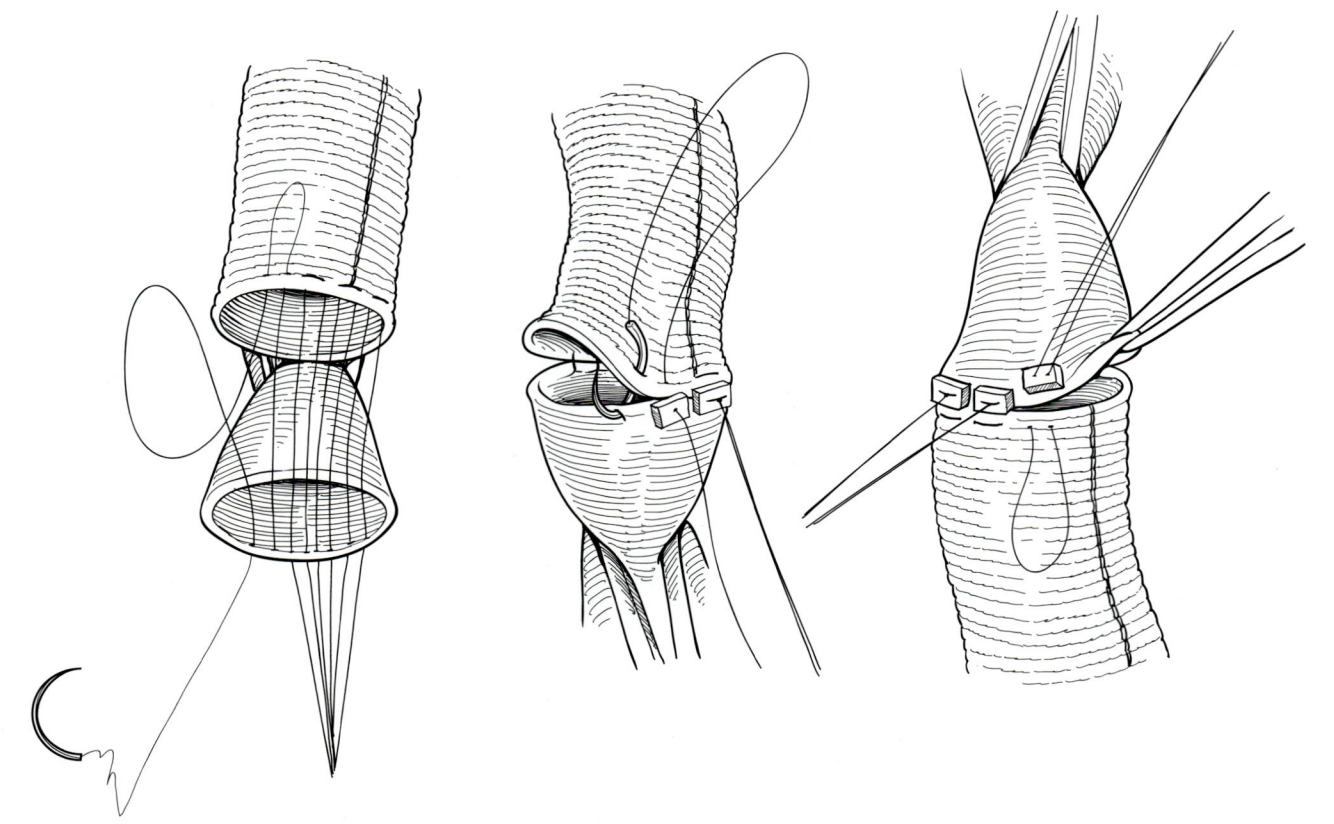

Figure 28-3. Technique of interrupted pledgeted sutures for proximal aortic anastomosis. This is preferred with a fragile or endarterectomized aortic cuff.

to arterial pressure.[5] Proper sizing of the graft, more than graft type, prevents the development of sluggish flow and later potential fragmentation and dislodgement of laminar clot, which often builds up in oversized grafts. A graft that is 16 × 8 or 14 × 7 mm for female patients is a frequently used size.

Totally Occluded, Calcified, and Small Aortas

Surgical management of patients with a totally occluded aorta hinges upon extension of the occlusion into the juxtarenal segment. Occlusion that is limited to the distal aorta, usually up to a patent inferior mesenteric artery or lumbar branch, is managed in the usual way with placement of an aortic graft. With extension of thrombus into the juxtarenal segment, however, the operative approach requires control of the aorta above the renal arteries and protection of the renal arteries with bulldog clamps to avoid migration of thrombus into the renal arteries. After removal of the occluding thrombus in the juxtarenal aorta, relocation of the clamp to an infrarenal position is typically possible. Graft implantation is then carried out in the usual fashion.

A second problem may arise with dense calcification of the aorta. The anastomosis can usually be accomplished in these circumstances by constructing it close to the renal arteries, where the aorta may be more normal, or by endarterectomizing the proximal aortic cuff to the level of the proximal clamp. In this case interrupted pledgeted sutures are recommended for the anastomosis (Fig. 28-3).

A third special circumstance arises with the management of the small aorta. Arbitrary definitions have been made about what constitutes a small aorta; a hypoplastic aortic syndrome has also been defined. Some advocate endarterectomy for this group of patients. If a bypass is needed, an end-to-side anastomosis is preferred. Smaller grafts are also in order, and some data suggest that PTFE should be the preferred conduit for these cases.[6] Most importantly, stringent technical detail must be exercised because of the small aortic diameter.

ADJUNCTIVE OR ALTERNATIVE PROCEDURES

Associated Renal or Visceral Lesions

No general recommendations are appropriate for simultaneous correction of renal arterial disease; instead, each case must be considered individually, because concomitant revascularization may increase morbidity and mortality.[7] The same type of caution must be exercised when dealing with concomitant visceral arterial disease. Care should be taken to preserve a patent large inferior mesenteric artery when significant disease exists in both the celiac and the superior mesenteric arteries.

Simultaneous Distal Lower Extremity Bypass Grafting

The decision to perform simultaneous distal grafting is one that requires sound clinical judgment. Reasons may include a more complete correction of distal ischemia and avoidance of the complications implicit in reoperative groin surgery. Experience has shown a technically sound inflow procedure is usually sufficient if there is reasonable evidence of severe aortoiliac disease, as documented by preoperative imaging, absent femoral pulses, or both. This, in combination with an intraoperative finding of a profunda femoris artery of adequate size and length, usually predicts a good clinical response[1] to inflow operation alone. However, if the proximal disease is only a modest component of the ischemic problem, simultaneous distal revascularization may be appropriate, particularly if severe tissue loss, the need for amputations in the foot, or both are present.[8]

Thoracic Aorta to Femoral Artery Bypass

Cases in which the abdominal aorta may be difficult to access because of previous abdominal operations, sepsis, radiation therapy, or occlusion at the juxtarenal level may suggest the use of the thoracic aorta as the inflow segment in low-risk patients. Rarely the ascending and more typically the lower descending aorta may be used with potentially more durability than axillofemoral reconstructions.

Operative Technique for Aortobifemoral Bypass

INCISION

The infrarenal abdominal aorta may be exposed by a variety of approaches. A long midline incision provides the best exposure and is preferred. A retroperitoneal approach may also be used (shoulders and torso rotated 45 degrees to the right, with the hips and extremities maintained as horizontal as possible to facilitate femoral artery exposure). The incision is made obliquely in the left flank, starting at the tip of the twelfth rib toward the midline below the umbilicus. This incision is good for patients with right-sided stomas and previous abdominal surgery, including aortic surgery. The retroperitoneal approach may reduce ileus and postoperative cardiopulmonary stress.

EXPOSURE OF THE ABDOMINAL AORTA

After the incision is made from xiphoid to pubis, the abdominal organs are explored for other pathologies. The abdominal aorta is then exposed using a standard infrarenal approach. The transverse colon and greater omentum are retracted cephalad and secured with a wet towel. We prefer to have the entire small bowel eviscerated, covered with a lap pad, and the descending and sigmoid portions of the colon retracted laterally and caudally. Next the parietal peritoneum between the duodenum and the inferior mesenteric vein is incised along the long axis of the aorta. The inferior mesenteric vein may need to be divided for optimal exposure of the proximal aorta. Care is taken to preserve the autonomic nerve fibers on the anterolateral aspect of the aorta down to the left common iliac artery; these are involved in male sexual function. The fourth portion of the duodenum is mobilized, and the dissection is carried to expose the left renal vein as it crosses anterior to the aorta. Distally, the aorta is exposed past the origin of the inferior mesenteric artery. This allows construction of the proximal anastomosis and of the graft limb tunnels.

EXPOSURE OF THE FEMORAL ARTERIES

Bilateral oblique groin incisions are preferred because they are easy to close and provide technical flexibility. The incision is carried partially above the anatomic position of the inguinal ligament to ensure adequate exposure. Lymphatic tissue is divided between clamps to minimize the occurrence of lymphatic leaks. The caudal border of the inguinal ligament is divided to ensure enough space for tunneling of the graft. When performing this, care must be taken to ligate the superficial circumflex vein that courses on top of the distal external iliac artery to avoid injury and bleeding during the creation of the tunnel (Fig. 28-4). The common, superficial, and profunda femoral arteries should be dissected out and controlled. Sizable branches of the femoral arteries should be controlled with loops and preserved if possible.

EXPOSURE OF THE DISTAL PROFUNDA

Profundaplasty may need to be performed at the same time as aorto bifemoral grafting, as suggested by preprocedural imaging. To perform this adequately, at least 2 to 3 cm of the profunda must be exposed. This may require separate control of an early bifurcating profunda and ligation of a nearly constant femoral vein branch, which courses anterior to the profunda in its early course.

TUNNEL CONSTRUCTION

After completion of the dissection, tunnels are made by gentle blunt dissection, with the index fingers, simultaneously from the groins and the aortic bifurcation. Care must be made to construct the tunnel underneath the ureters and thus avoid possible hydronephrosis. Long Penrose drains, 16 Fr red rubber catheters, or umbilical tapes can be passed through the tunnels to facilitate later passage of the graft limbs (see Fig. 28-4).

AORTIC DIVISION AND CLOSURE OF THE DISTAL AORTA

The patient is systemically heparinized, and the aorta is clamped just caudal to the left renal vein and either caudal or cephalad to the inferior mesenteric artery. The aorta is the transected. Patent lumbar branches are ligated. The transected distal aortic end is oversewn with 3-0 vascular suture. Pledgeted sutures may be used for closure in a calcified distal aorta after a limited local endarterectomy of calcific plaque.

Proximal Graft Anastomosis

END-TO-END AORTIC ANASTOMOSIS

The graft is cut 3 to 4 cm from its bifurcation to construct a prosthesis with a short body or stem. This configuration facilitates retroperitoneal closure over the graft and allows separation of the anastomosis from the duodenum. It also diminishes the takeoff angle of the limb, which prevents kinking and potential graft limb thrombosis. The standard anastomosis is constructed using a 3-0 running polypropylene suture run from both the posterior and the anterior midline clockwise and counterclockwise, and it is tied in the lateral aspect of the aorta. Thromboendarterectomy of the proximal aortic cuff up to the proximal clamp can be performed in cases of significant disease at the site of the intended proximal graft anastomosis. In this event, an interrupted, pledgeted suture technique is recommended because of the thinness and possible fragility of the remaining adventitia of the endarterectomized aortic wall (Fig 28-5, and see Fig. 28-3).

END-TO-SIDE AORTIC ANASTOMOSIS

Totally occluding an aortic segment with proximal and distal aortic clamps is preferred in lieu of using a side-biting clamp. The anastomosis is placed as cephalad

DIRECT SURGICAL REPAIR OF AORTOILIAC OCCLUSIVE DISEASE 357

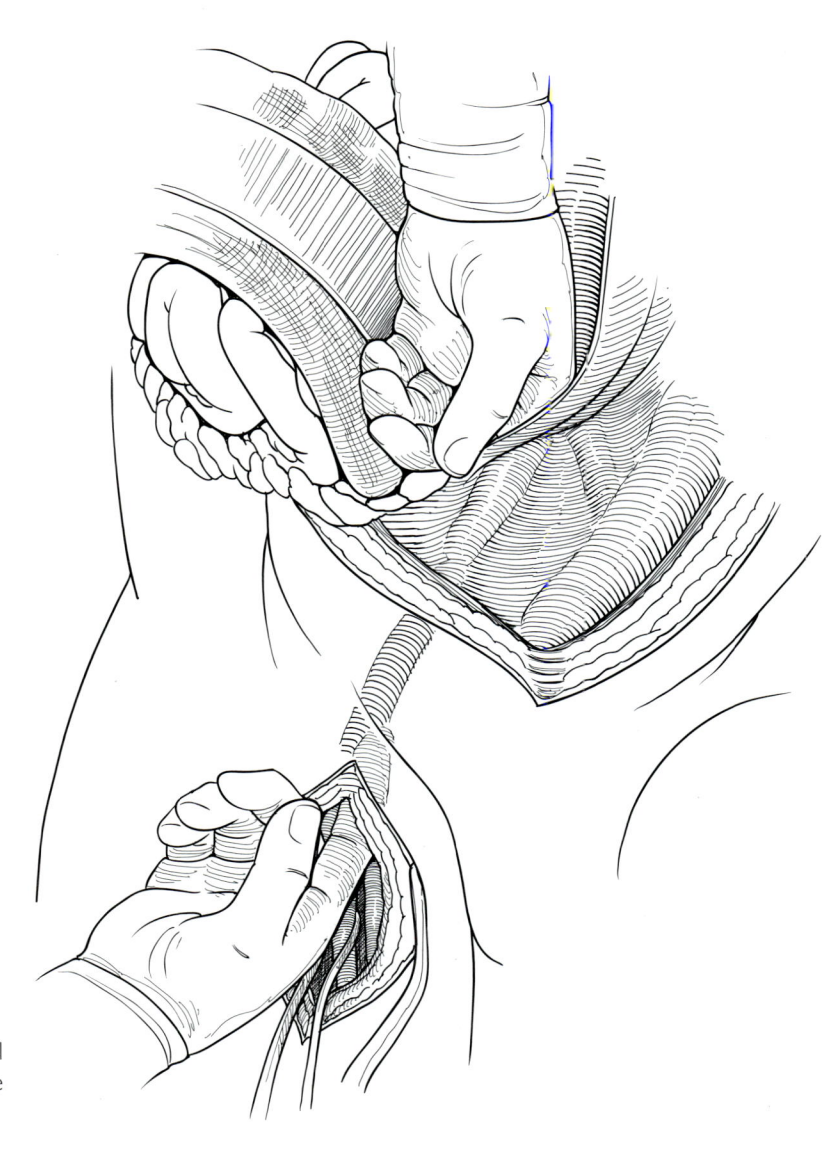

Figure 28-4. Creation of the retroperitoneal tunnel to the femoral artery. Care must be taken to place the graft limb underneath the ureter.

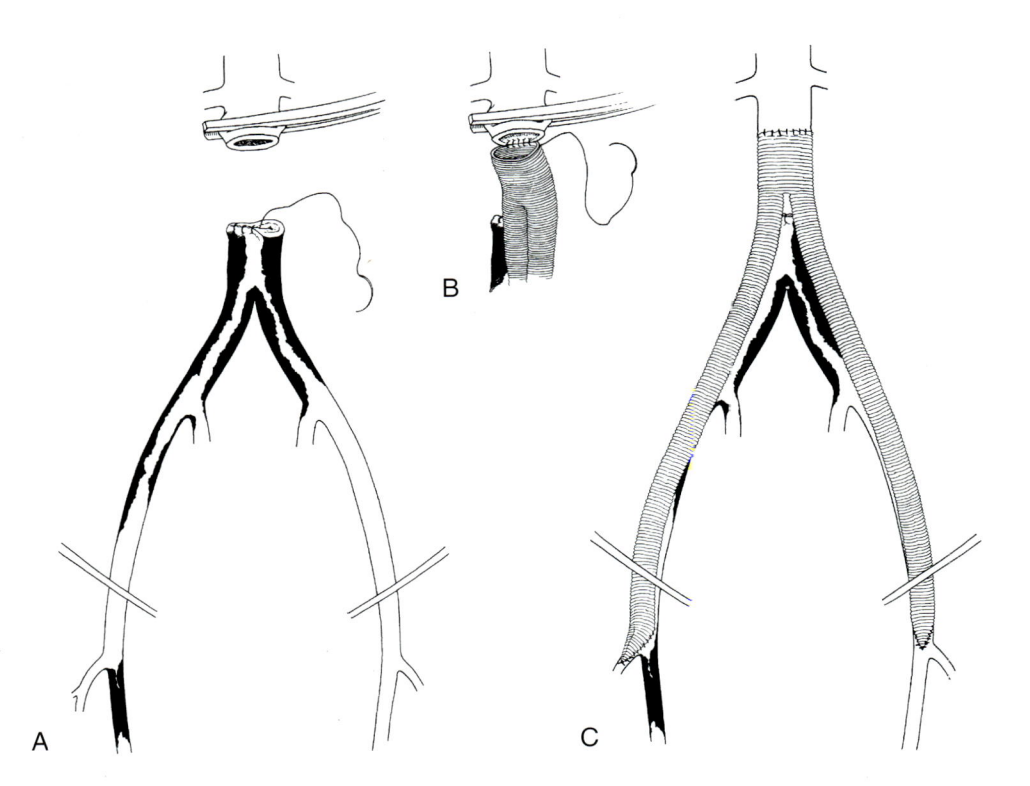

Figure 28-5. Aortofemoral graft. **A,** A segment of diseased aorta is resected, and the distal aortic stump is oversewn. **B,** End-to-end proximal anastomosis. **C,** Completed reconstruction. *(From Brewster CD: Direct reconstruction for aortoiliac occlusive disease. In Cronenwett JL, Johnston KW, editors: Rutherford's vascular surgery, ed 6. Philadelphia, 2005, Saunders, p 1115, Fig. 79-6.)*

as possible by cutting the graft with a bevel of approximately 60 degrees (anterior to posterior) that extends close to the aortic bifurcation. The edges of the aortic arteriotomy may be trimmed to produce a more elliptical opening for the anastomosis. The anastomosis is then performed with two 3-0 sutures, which are placed one at the toe and one at the heel and tied to each other at the lateral aspect of the aorta. Appropriate backbleeding is performed to prevent debris from embolizing to the distal circulation (Fig. 28-6).

FEMORAL ANASTOMOSIS

Graft limbs are then passed down into the femoral region with the aid of the previously placed Penrose drains and a large DeBakey aortic clamp. Care is taken to avoid twisting the graft limbs. The femoral anastomosis must ensure good flow to the profunda femoris arteries (Fig. 28-7). Because of this, the profunda arteries should be evaluated by both preoperative imaging and intraoperatively by passage of 3.5- to 4.0-mm dilators at the time of anastomosis to ensure that no significant stenotic lesion are present. A standard end-to-side anastomosis to the common femoral artery is performed with 5-0 vascular suture using either a toe-and-heel mattress technique or a parachute technique. In the case of significant profunda disease at the origin, the femoral arteriotomy should be carried down into the profunda and across the stenosis, and in most circumstances, profundaplasty can be performed concomitantly. Under these circumstances, three to five interrupted mattress sutures are recommended for placement at the toe of the anastomosis. A common femoral artery endarterectomy can also be performed before the anastomosis if significant disease is found. If needed, tacking sutures can be placed at the endarterectomy endpoint to prevent subsequent intimal flap formation. In either case, sutures must be passed outside to inside on the graft and inside to outside on the artery. This prevents plaque from being lifted from the vessel wall and acting as an obstructing flap that can potentially obstruct flow. Establishment of adequate graft flow to the profunda femoris artery in patients with significant disease or occlusion of the superficial femoral artery is of utmost importance for patency. After alerting the anesthesia team in advance, and performing the appropriate flushing maneuvers (vigorous limb flushing and backbleeding of the native arterial system), the anastomosis is completed and vascular clamps are removed. Performance of a perfect femoral anastomosis is perhaps the most important predictor of late graft patency. In difficult cases of extensive redo groin surgery, if appropriate tissue is not available to cover the anastomosis, or both, closure may be assisted by rotating a Sartorius flap onto the site of the anastomosis at the end of the procedure. Experience shows this is infrequently necessary.

ILIOFEMORAL BYPASS

With advances in catheter-based methods of revascularization, including angioplasty and stenting, unilateral iliac disease requiring open (direct) surgical reconstruction is less frequent. When endovascular approaches are not possible, unilateral iliofemoral grafting, femoral-femoral bypass, or localized iliac endarterectomy represent options with demonstrated efficacy and durability. Methods of unilateral reconstruction can also be combined with simultaneous local endarterectomy procedures, profundaplasty, or with distal bypasses or distal endovascular interventions.[9,10]

Complications

EARLY COMPLICATIONS

- **Bleeding.** Meticulous attention to hemostasis throughout, providing appropriate postoperative blood pressure control and avoidance of venous injury, are all important. Aside from this, correct management of intraoperative anticoagulation, prevention of postoperative coagulopathy, and prompt administration of blood products as guided by laboratory values are essential.

DIRECT SURGICAL REPAIR OF AORTOILIAC OCCLUSIVE DISEASE | 359

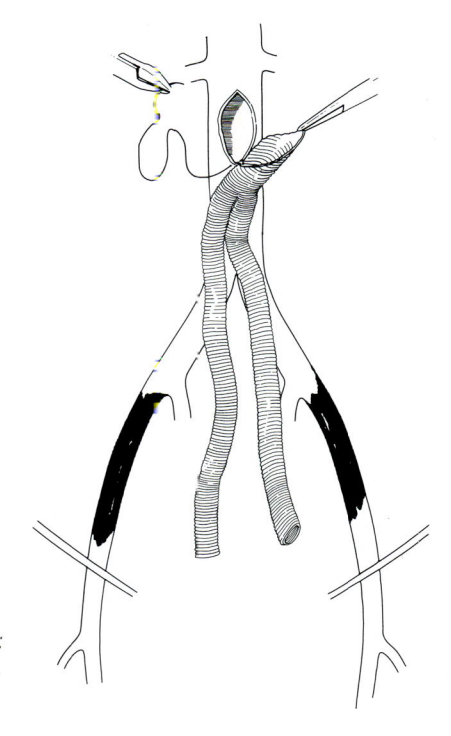

Figure 28-6. Technique of end-to-side proximal aortic anastomosis. (From Brewster CD: Direct reconstruction for aortoiliac occlusive disease. In Cronenwett JL, Johnston KW, editors: Rutherford's vascular surgery, ed 6. Philadelphia, 2005, Saunders, p 1116, Fig. 79-7.)

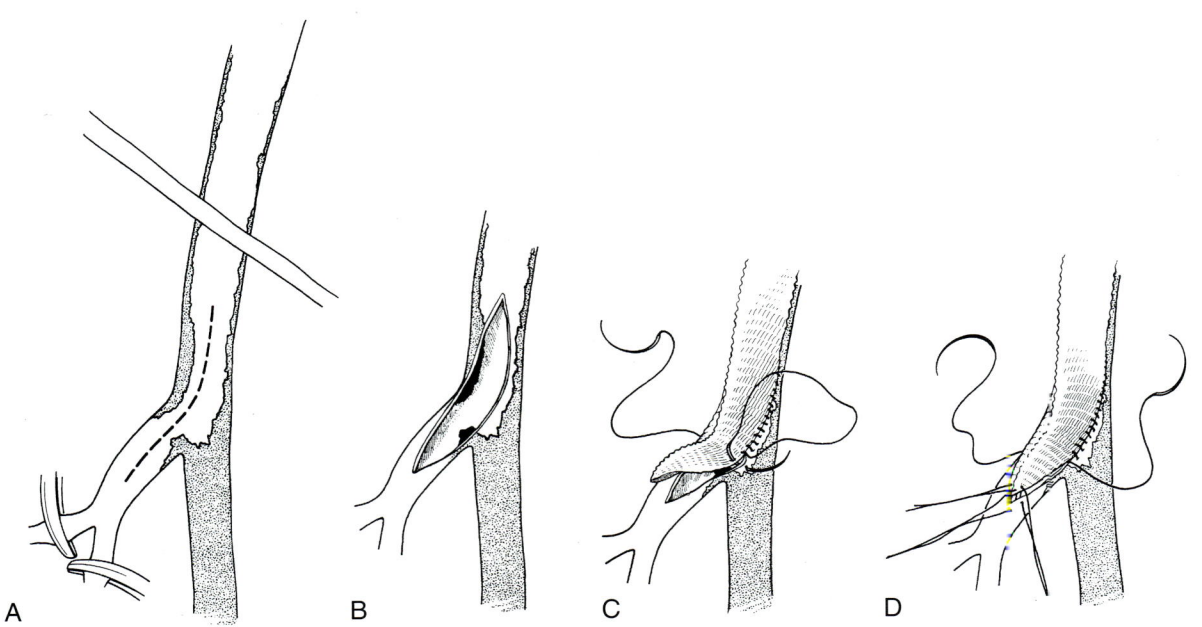

Figure 28-7. Femoral anastomosis in a patient with multilevel disease. **A,** With associated femoropopliteal occlusive disease, disease at the orifice of the profunda femoris artery may limit graft limb runoff and subsequent patency. **B,** The common femoral artery arteriotomy is extended into the proximal profunda femoris artery, distal to the orificial stenosis. **C,** The heel of the long, beveled graft hood is anastomosed to the common femoral artery. **D,** The femoral anastomosis is completed with the tip of the graft extended down the profunda femoris artery, thus achieving a patch profundaplasty. Three to five interrupted sutures are first placed at the tip and are not tied down, facilitating visualization and accurate placement without constriction. These distal sutures can then be run up the sides of the arteriotomy with closure at the midpoint of the medial and lateral walls of the arteriotomy. (From Brewster CD: Direct reconstruction for aortoiliac occlusive disease. In Cronenwett JL, Johnston KW, editors: Rutherford's vascular surgery, ed 6. Philadelphia, 2005, Saunders, p 1117, Fig. 79-8.)

- **Acute limb ischemia.** Acute limb ischemia occurs in up to 3% of patients in the early postoperative period after aortofemoral grafting.[11] Kinking or twisting of the graft limb, poor or inadequate runoff, inadvertent dislodgement of debris from proximal vessels, embolization of the clot from insufficient anticoagulation during clamping, and inadequate termination of endarterectomy, causing distal flap formation, are all recognized causes of graft failure. Recognition of an early problem can be difficult, because perfusion in the distal extremities often requires 4 to 6 hours after the procedure to improve. Thromboembolectomy of the graft limbs can be performed via groin incisions, with simultaneous correction of a technical problem if present. More distal occlusions in the tibial vessels may require a popliteal incision for correction, bailout distal bypass, or both.

- **Renal failure.** More commonly encountered in elective aortic surgery for aneurysm and especially in emergent cases, renal failure is an uncommon complication in reconstructions done for occlusive disease.[12] Avoidance of intraoperative (declamping) and postoperative hypotension, adequate volume replacement, management of postreperfusion myoglobinuria, and avoidance of nephrotoxic drugs are all important in preventing renal failure. More worrisome, renal failure resulting from embolism of atheromatous debris during clamping of a diseased juxtarenal segment must be avoided. Clamping a less diseased supraceliac segment or separate control of the renal arteries during aortic cross-clamping can avoid potentially irreversible renal injury.

- **Ureteral injury.** A related issue is the protection of the ureters during these procedures, especially in circumstances of reoperative surgery, wherein placement of ureteral stents may be advisable. Attention to anatomic relationships is of great importance to avoid injury. Hydronephrosis may be seen during the postoperative period, where it is usually of no clinical significance but sometimes can be a sign of late complications, such as infection or extrinsic obstruction.[13]

- **Intestinal ischemia.** Given its mortality rate (50%-75%) and incidence (2%),[14] intestinal ischemia represents a significant complication in surgery for AIOD. Two anatomic distributions deserve emphasis. The first is the more commonly encountered left colon ischemia. The second, more diffuse small and large bowel ischemia is uncommon but frequently lethal. Prolonged or vigorous retraction of the root of the mesentery can compromise superior mesenteric artery flow, which should be evaluated at the completion of the procedure. Diarrhea, sepsis, abdominal distention, and unexplained metabolic acidosis should raise clinical suspicion in the early postoperative period. Evaluation of preoperative imaging is of vital importance, because certain anatomic situations increase the risk of intestinal ischemia. The first is the status of the hypogastric arteries. Reconstruction must ensure flow to at least one hypogastric, directly or retrograde, from the femoral arteries. A second, perhaps most important, modifiable factor in the development of intestinal ischemia is the reimplantation of a large patent inferior mesenteric artery. Reimplantation is particularly advisable in cases where a large inferior mesenteric artery is identified in a patient with significant occlusive disease of the superior mesenteric artery.

- **Retrograde ejaculation and impotence.** Impaired sexual function may occur as a result of injury to the autonomic sympathetic nerve fibers along the left side of the aortic bifurcation, inferior mesenteric artery, and left common iliac artery. This is particularly troubling in young patients, and care should be taken to preserve those fibers. Patients should be counseled about these risks prior to the procedure.

LATE COMPLICATIONS AND LONG-TERM RESULTS

- **Mortality and morbidity.** Significant reduction in perioperative morbidity and mortality rates have been obtained with advances in anesthetic and intensive care management. Patients with localized AIOD, as opposed to those with multilevel disease and associated coronary and visceral occlusive disease, tend to have improved perioperative mortality, as well as long-term mortality.

- **Graft patency.** Graft patency of 85% to 90% at 5 years and 70% to 75% at 10 years has been documented in many reports. Graft occlusion is the most common late complication, and the most common scenario is occlusion of one limb in the setting of progressive profunda femoris occlusive disease, because most patients already have chronic superficial femoral artery occlusions.[15] Failure at the proximal anastomosis is usually a technical problem related to not placing the graft close enough to the renal arteries. This occurs with greater frequency in those patients who continue to smoke. Thromboembolectomy with the use of a graft thrombectomy catheter to clean out an occluded limb, along with correction of any outflow problem, is an adequate way to deal with graft occlusion. Extension of a graft to the femoral level via the retroperitoneal approach can be used for a failed aortoiliac graft. Finally, femoral-femoral grafts can be used when the occlusion is more chronic.

REFERENCES

1. Brewster DC, Perler BA, Robison JG, et al: Aortofemoral graft for multilevel occlusive disease. Predictors of success and need for distal bypass, *Arch Surg* 117:1593-1600, 1982.
2. Brewster DC, Okada RD, Strauss HW, et al: Selection of patients for preoperative coronary angiography: Use of dipyridamole-stress–thallium myocardial imaging, *J Vasc Surg* 2:504-510, 1985.
3. Brewster DC: Direct reconstruction for aortoiliac occlusive disease. In Cronenwett JL, Johnston KW, editors: *Rutherford's vascular surgery*, ed 6, Philadelphia, 2005, Saunders.
4. Brewster DC: Current controversies in the management of aortoiliac occlusive disease, *J Vasc Surg* 25:365-379, 1997.
5. Nunn DB, Carter MM, Donohue MT, et al: Postoperative dilation of knitted Dacron aortic bifurcation graft, *J Vasc Surg* 12:291-297, 1990.
6. Burke PM Jr, Herrmann JB, Cutler BS: Optimal grafting methods for the small abdominal aorta, *J Cardiovasc Surg (Torino)* 28:420-426, 1987.
7. Tarazi RY, Hertzer NR, Beven EG, et al: Simultaneous aortic reconstruction and renal revascularization: Risk factors and late results in eighty-nine patients, *J Vasc Surg* 5:707-714, 1987.
8. Dalman RL, Taylor LM Jr, Moneta GL, et al: Simultaneous operative repair of multilevel lower extremity occlusive disease, *J Vasc Surg* 13:211-219, 1991. discussion 9-21.
9. Brewster DC, Cambria RP, Darling RC, et al: Long-term results of combined iliac balloon angioplasty and distal surgical revascularization, *Ann Surg* 210:324-330, 1989. discussion 31.
10. Faries PL, Brophy D, LoGerfo FW, et al: Combined iliac angioplasty and infrainguinal revascularization surgery are effective in diabetic patients with multilevel arterial disease, *Ann Vasc Surg* 15:67-72, 2001.
11. Brewster DC: Reoperation for aortofemoral graft limb occlusion. In Veith F, editor: *Critical problems in vascular surgery*, St. Louis, 1989, Quality Medical Publishing, pp 341-351.
12. Diehl JT, Cali RF, Hertzer NR, et al: Complications of abdominal aortic reconstruction. An analysis of perioperative risk factors in 557 patients, *Ann Surg* 197:-9-56, 1983.
13. Wright DJ, Ernst CB, Evans JR, et al: Ureteral complications and aortoiliac reconstruction, *J Vasc Surg* 11:29-35, 1990. discussion 35-37.
14. Brewster DC, Franklin DP, Cambria RP, et al: Intestinal ischemia complicating abdominal aortic surgery, *Surgery* 109:447-454, 1991.
15. Nevelsteen A, Suy R: Graft occlusion following aortofemoral Dacron bypass, *Ann Vasc Surg* 5:32-37, 1991.

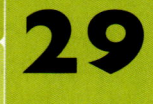

29 Extraanatomic Repair of Aortoiliac Occlusive Disease

JOSEPH R. SCHNEIDER

Historical Background

Extraanatomic procedures were developed as alternatives to direct aortofemoral bypass for patients deemed to be at high risk for direct aortic surgery or for those presenting with a "hostile" abdomen, an infection of the native aortoiliac arterial system, or prior prosthetic replacement of the aortoiliac system. The first extraanatomic procedure to be described for treatment of aortoiliac occlusive disease was the femoral-femoral bypass, which was first reported by Freeman in 1952.[1] In 1962 Vetto[2] provided the first comprehensive description of a significant number of cases with an analysis of clinical outcomes. Axillofemoral bypass was first reported by Blaisdell[3] and Louw[4] in 1963, and by 1968 growing experience supported this option as a safe alternative to direct aortic reconstruction.[5] The feasability of thoracofemoral bypass was first reported in 1961,[6] but it was not until the 1980s and 1990s that retrospective reviews reported long-term outcomes for patients treated with this approach.[7-10] Balloon thromboembolectomy was introduced by Fogarty and colleagues in 1963,[11] with reports of its utility for treatment of aortoiliac embolism appearing soon thereafter.[12,13]

Preoperative Preparation

- **Prophylactic antibiotics.** Extraanatomic bypass is nearly always performed with prosthetic material, either expanded polytetrafluoroethylene (ePTFE) or polyester. Infection of these grafts is associated with a high risk of loss of life or limb. Thus preexisting infection should be treated to the extent possible before placing the grafts, and antibiotics administered to reduce the risk of secondary graft infection.

- **Risk assessment.** Cardiac, pulmonary, and renal function should be assessed and optimized.

- **Emergent or urgent intervention.** Arterial embolectomy is implicitly an urgent or emergent procedure in most cases, so preoperative care is usually limited to volume resuscitation, transfusion, and other measures to optimize organ function. Mortality related to arterial embolectomy remains high,[14] due to advanced age and associated comorbidities, particularly cardiac disease.

Pitfalls and Danger Points

- **Injury to the axillary and subclavian arteries, veins, and brachial plexus.** The axillosubclavian artery is characteristically less robust than the femoral artery, and injury from dissection, clamp placement, or sutures tearing through the artery is more likely. Injury could conceivably require transection of the clavicle, sternotomy, or thoracotomy to facilitate repair. The axillary artery and vein and brachial plexus may also be injured during tunneling of the axillofemoral graft.

- **Disruption of the axillary artery anastomosis.** The axillary artery anastomosis should be placed as medial (adjacent to the clavicle) as possible and to allow some redundancy in the axillary end of the axillofemoral graft. This will minimize the risk of "axillary pullout," or disruption of the axillary anastomosis with arm abduction.[15] The axillofemoral graft should also be placed in the midaxillary line to reduce the risk of kinking during torso flexion.

- **Bladder or bowel injury.** Bladder or bowel injury is possible when tunneling a femoral-femoral graft if the graft is placed in the retrofascial space or if the patient has a suprapubic hernia, particularly if there has been previous surgery in this area.

- **Iatrogenic injury during embolectomy.** Embolectomy leads to arterial perforation, rupture, and dissection. The catheter should not be "forced" when advancing it, (i.e., if the catheter meets with resistance it should be withdrawn a significant distance and then readvanced and rotated somewhat to try to "give a different look" to the catheter tip). The surgeon must learn to get tactile information from both hands, (i.e., a sense of resistance when advancing the catheter and drag on the catheter when withdrawing with the balloon inflated), and a sense of the resistance to inflation using the syringe. Pulling back on an overinflated balloon can do irreparable damage in the short term and produces significant vasospasm, particularly in the infrapopliteal arteries.

Femoral-Femoral Bypass

INCISION AND EXPOSURE

Femoral-femoral bypass depends on the ability of one "donor" iliac artery to supply enough blood flow to perfuse both the donor and the "recipient" legs (Fig. 29-1). Oblique, groin-crease incisions may be used, but longitudinal groin incisions centered over the femoral arteries and beginning approximately at the inguinal ligament provide the most flexibility and are preferred by most surgeons. Incision length depends on patient habitus. Anastomoses to the common femoral artery may extend onto the deep or superficial femoral artery and may occasionally be made directly to the deep or superficial femoral arteries. This decision is most often made after exposure, inspection, and palpation of the femoral arteries, but it is also predicted by complete preoperative imaging. The extent of dissection to control femoral arteries and the use of vascular clamps, silicone elastomer (Silastic) vessel loops, or occasionally balloon catheters are dictated by the site of anastomosis, surgeon preference, and whether there has been previous surgical exposure of the femoral arteries.

Figure 29-1. Typical configuration for femoral-femoral bypass with bilateral longitudinal groin incisions, a suprapubic subcutaneous tunnel, and a generally continuous arc to avoid kinking of the graft. Longitudinal skin incisions are generally the most versatile for this operation. *(From Schneider JR: Extra-anatomic bypass. In Cronenwett JL, Johnston KW, editors: Rutherford's vascular surgery, ed 7. Philadelphia, 2010, Saunders, pp 1633-1652.)*

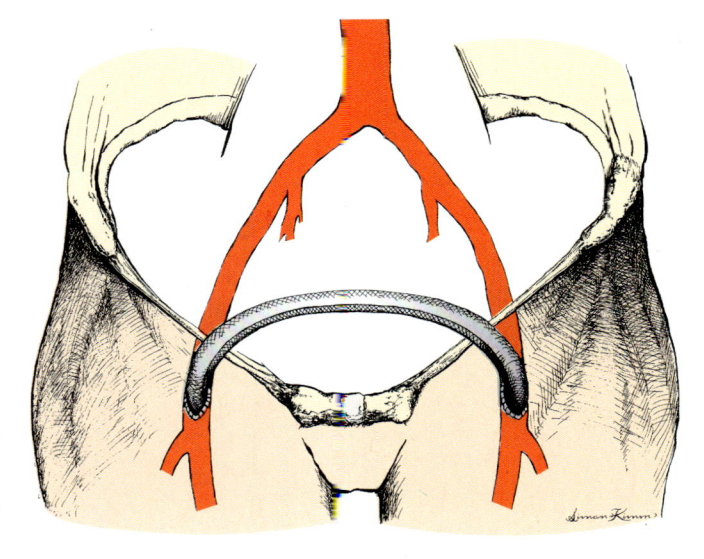

TUNNELING OF THE BYPASS GRAFT

Most femoral-femoral grafts are placed in the immediately prefascial subcutaneous position. The tunnel should begin in line with the planned arteriotomy to be used for anastomosis and should be made in a continuous arc, avoiding abrupt right-angle turns to reduce the risk of graft kinking and subsequent thrombosis. The tunnel can be made bluntly with index fingers from both sides, with fingers meeting in the midline. A large clamp, such as a curved DeBakey aortic clamp, or uterine packing forceps may be used to complete the tunnel, but the surgeon must be careful not to perforate the fascia or a hollow viscus in an unsuspected hernia. The same clamp may be used to pull the graft from one side to the other, taking care that the graft does not twist during passage. Some surgeons prefer larger-diameter grafts, but there is no evidence that grafts larger than 6 mm in diameter perform better hemodynamically or that patency is improved with larger-diameter grafts.[16] A 6-mm-diameter, externally supported ePTFE graft is an acceptable choice, but there is also no evidence that external support or the use of ePTFE as opposed to polyester is associated with better outcomes.[17]

ANASTOMOSIS

Systemic heparin or another suitable anticoagulant is administered, and in most cases a longitudinally oriented or slightly oblique arteriotomy is created in a convenient place for anastomosis. Making the anastomosis on a more distal portion of the femoral system, such as the deep or superficial femoral artery, may be dictated by local anatomy and may reduce the tendency of the graft to kink in the sagittal plane in patients with protuberant abdomens. As with most end-to-side anastomoses, arteriotomies are made about three times as long as the graft diameter. The graft ends are spatulated by placing a curved hemostat on the graft and then using a scalpel to cut the ePTFE graft along the inside of the hemostat curve. An end-to-side graft to artery anastomosis is then created using running 5-0 or 6-0 polypropylene or CV-5 or CV-6 polytetrafluoroethylene (PTFE) suture. The donor-side anastomosis is usually performed first, although either side may be completed first and the anastomoses may be performed simultaneously if there are two surgeons. For at least one anastomosis, preferably the recipient side, the suture is not tied to complete the anastomosis until the clamps and vessel loops have been briefly released to fill the graft with blood and to allow expulsion of air and thrombus or other debris.

CLOSURE

A sterile, handheld continuous wave Doppler probe is used to interrogate outflow on both donor and recipient sides and to ensure that flow is qualitatively better on the recipient side, as evident by a higher Doppler frequency shift, with the graft open than with the graft clamped. Anticoagulant may then be reversed, the wounds may be closed with running subcutaneous absorbable suture, and the skin may be closed with staples in most cases.

Axillofemoral Bypass

SELECTION OF A DONOR ARTERY

The versatility of the axillofemoral bypass depends on the ability of one axillosubclavian artery to supply enough blood flow to adequately perfuse both the donor arm and one (axillounifemoral bypass) or more often both (axillobifemoral bypass) legs. Either axillary artery may be a donor artery, but the donor vessel is almost always the ipsilateral axillary artery in the case of axillounifemoral bypass (Fig. 29-2). However, if there is any suggestion of a stenosis in the proposed donor side, as evident by a weak brachial or radial pulse, or presence of a lower blood pressure than in the contralateral arm, then preoperative angiography is warranted.

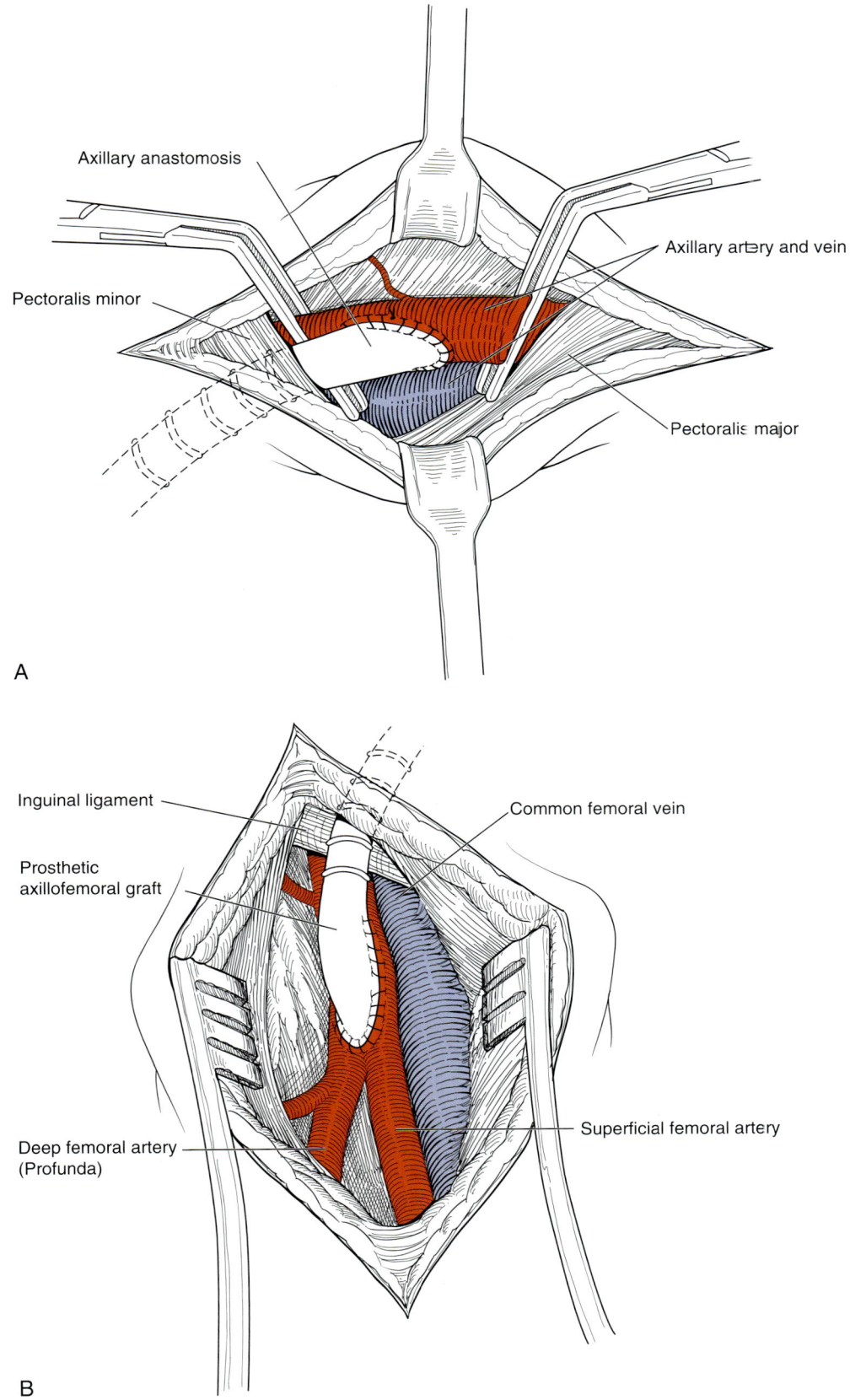

Figure 29-2. Configuration of an axillobifemoral bypass based on the right axillary artery. **A,** The donor axillary artery is exposed using a transverse incision inferior to the clavicle and the artery is controlled from the clavicle medially to the pectoralis minor muscle laterally. **B,** The graft is tunneled posterior to the pectoralis minor muscle and then subcutaneously in the midaxillary line.

Continued

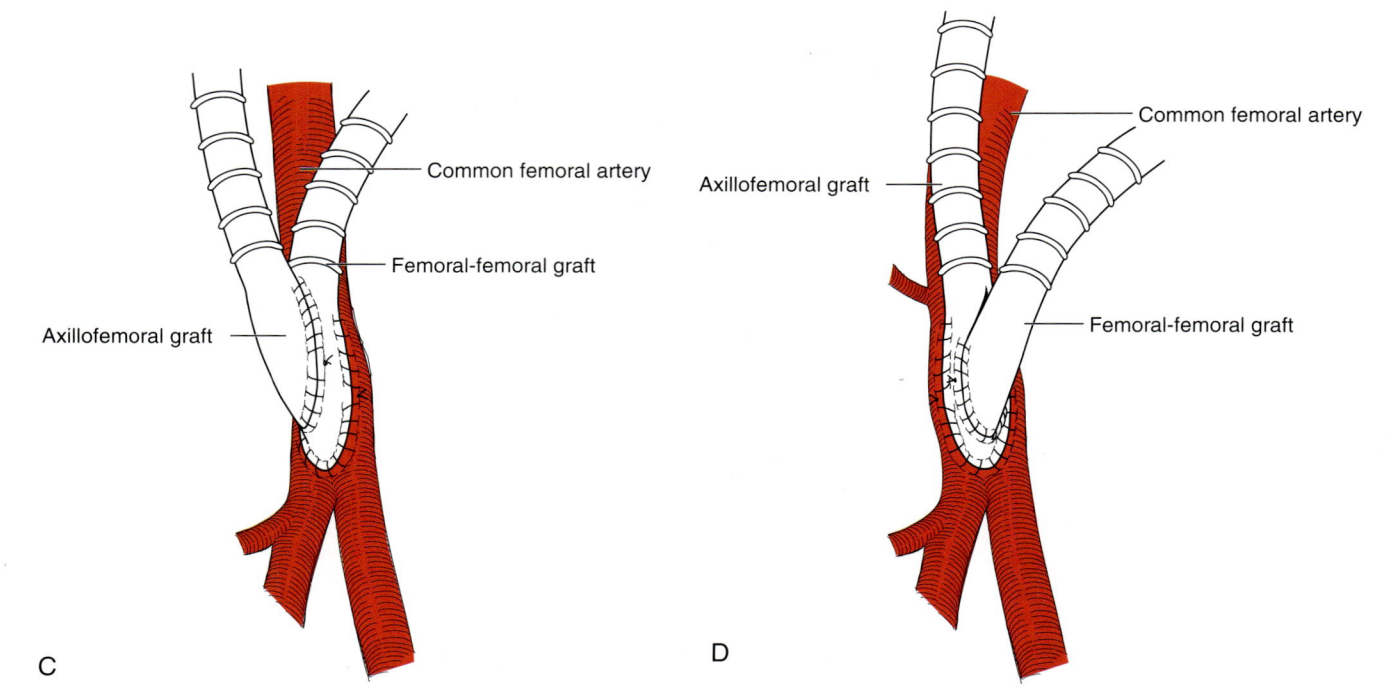

Figure 29-2, cont'd. C, A femoral-femoral graft is first placed, followed by the anastomosis of the distal axillofemoral graft limb to the ipsilateral hood of the femoral-femoral graft. **D,** The distal axillofemoral graft limb is anastomosed to the femoral artery followed by the anastomosis of the ipsilateral side of a femoral-femoral graft to the hood of the axillofemoral graft.

INCISION AND EXPOSURE

The operation is performed with the patient supine but with elevation of the flank ipsilateral to the donor artery using a soft roll or gel pad. In most cases the procedure is performed under general anesthesia. Wide prepping and draping are essential to allow exposure of the ipsilateral clavicle, lower neck, anterior chest and sternum, flank, abdomen, and both groins. The ipsilateral arm is abducted to 90 degrees and may be prepped into the field with the hand and lower arm placed in a stockinette. Groin incisions are made as described earlier. The first portion of the axillary artery, between the clavicle and the pectoralis minor muscle, is exposed using a transverse incision about 5 cm in length that is placed a few centimeters inferior to the midportion of the clavicle. The deep fascia is incised parallel to the incision, and the pectoralis major muscle fibers are split, exposing the fat containing the axillary artery and vein and their branches. The artery is dissected free of the surrounding tissues, and small branches are ligated as necessary from the clavicle medially to the medial edge of the pectoralis minor muscle. At least one large venous branch crossing the artery is almost always encountered, ligated, and divided to allow exposure of the artery. Division of the pectoralis minor insertion may improve exposure.

TUNNELING THE BYPASS GRAFT

A subcutaneous tunnel is created between the axillary artery and the ipsilateral groin incision. The tunnel is brought posterior to the pectoralis minor muscle. These tunnels are most conveniently made with a tubular tunneler. Early descriptions included placement of an intermediate incision at the midpoint of the tunnel, but this is not necessary with a 65-cm-long Gore tunneler (W.L. Gore and Associates, Newark, Del.). The graft is passed through the tubular tunneler, taking care not to allow it to twist during passage. An externally supported 8-mm ePTFE graft can be used. The use of larger grafts may predispose the patient to thrombosis. There is no evidence that external support or a specific graft material is associated with superior results.[17]

AXILLARY ANASTOMOSIS

The patient is systemically anticoagulated with heparin or another suitable anticoagulant, the axillary artery is controlled with clamps, and a 1.5- to 2-cm longitudinal arteriotomy is created in the axillary artery. Since the axillary artery is easily kinked when elevated into the wound following clamp placement, care should be taken not to puncture the back wall during the performance of the arteriotomy. Alternatively, the thoracoacromial branch can be divided near its take off from the axillary artery and used as an entry point for Potts scissors. The axillary end of the graft is spatulated using a hemostat, and an end-to-side graft to axillary artery anastomosis is created using running 5-0 or 6-0 polypropylene or CV-5 or CV-6 PTFE suture. In addition to medial placement of the axillary anastomosis, some redundancy of the graft in the axilla reduces the risk of axillary pullout because of excess traction upon abduction of the arm.[15]

FEMORAL ANASTOMOSIS

If the graft is placed in the axillounifemoral configuration, then the distal anastomosis is made to the femoral arterial system. In the case of an axillobifemoral configuration, two common approaches have been described for the distal anastomoses. The preferred approach is to first place the femoral-femoral graft, create an oval graftotomy in the ipsilateral anastomotic "hood" of the femoral-femoral graft, and then anastomose the spatulated femoral end of the axillofemoral graft to the femoral-femoral graftotomy (Fig. 29-2, C). An alternative approach is to first place an axillounifemoral graft, create an oval graftotomy on the femoral anastomotic hood of the axillounifemoral graft, and then perform the ipsilateral anastomosis of the femoral-femoral graft to this graftotomy (Fig. 29-2, D). A number of other approaches have been described for revascularization of target femoral arteries.[17] Grafts are also available with manufactured femoral-femoral "side arm" components. Prior to completing the distal anastomoses, the grafts are flushed to allow expulsion of air, thrombus, or other debris.

CLOSURE

A sterile, handheld Doppler probe is used to interrogate outflow, ensuring augmented flow with the graft open than when clamped. It is important to assess flow in the donor arm distal to the axillary anastomosis by checking the radial pulse after completing all anastomoses. Poor flow in the donor-side hand implies a technical defect, thrombosis, or occult flow-limiting lesion, which must be addressed immediately to assure adequate flow in the donor arm. A running subcutaneous absorbable suture is used to close the subcutaneous tissue and the skin closed with staples or suture.

Thoracofemoral Bypass

INCISION AND EXPOSURE

Technique for thoracofemoral bypass is not standardized and different approaches have been described.[17] Figure 29-3 provides a general illustration of the placement of a descending aorta to femoral artery graft. The operation is performed with the left chest elevated 45 degrees, and the pelvis is maintained as close to horizontal as possible to facilitate femoral artery exposure. The bypass is based on the descending thoracic aorta, which is exposed through a left thoracotomy, usually in the seventh, eighth, or ninth interspace. A double lumen endotracheal tube is required to allow deflation of the left lung during exposure and anastomosis to the descending aorta. If a patent femoral-femoral graft is present, then only the left groin need be exposed. If bypass is required to both legs, then exposure of both groins is necessary.

TUNNELING OF THE BYPASS GRAFT

Blind tunneling of the graft from the chest to the left groin without an abdominal counterincision has been described, although, others have recommended use of

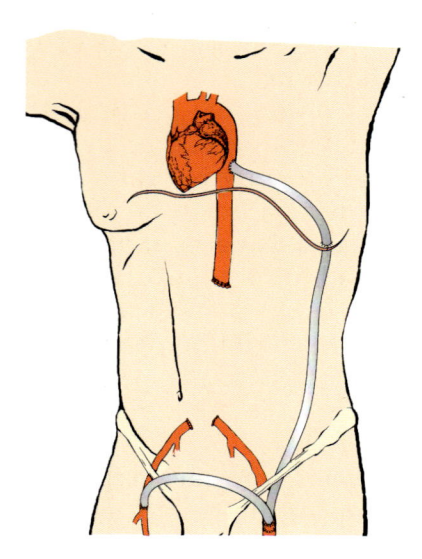

Figure 29-3. A thoracofemoral bypass is performed with the left chest elevated 45 degrees with the descending aorta approached through a left thoracotomy. *(From Schneider JR: Extra-anatomic bypass. In Cronenwett JL, Johnston KW, editors:* Rutherford's vascular surgery, *ed 7. Philadelphia, 2010, Saunders, pp 1633-1652.)*

a left flank retroperitoneal exposure as a counterincision. The former is preferred when tunneling a single graft from the chest to the left groin, but the latter approach facilitates passage of a limb in the abdominal retrofascial space to the right groin. If an abdominal counterincision is not used, an olive-tipped or tubular tunneling device is passed from the left groin exposure into the retroperitoneal space, keeping the tunnel lateral to the iliac arteries, and then over the anterior surface of the psoas major muscle posterior to the left kidney, tail of pancreas, and spleen until the tip of the tunneler can be palpated through the posteromedial left hemidiaphragm. The diaphragm is incised over the tip of the tunneler, and the tunneler is advanced into the left chest. Care must be taken to prevent the graft from twisting during passage. When a left flank retroperitoneal counterincision is used, the diaphragm is opened and the graft brought through the diaphragmatic defect under direct vision and advanced to the left groin. The retrofascial preperitoneal tunnel to the right groin should be created before anticoagulation with a combination of blunt finger dissection and the use of a DeBakey aortic clamp or ring forceps. The graft may be placed in the tunnel before performing the aortic anastomosis, but some surgeons prefer to pass the graft through the tunnel after completion of the aortic anastomosis, believing that the pressurized graft is less likely to twist during passage. A 14 × 7 or 16 × 8 mm bifurcated polyester graft is recommended when bypassing to both legs. These grafts may not be long enough to reach the right femoral artery, and the redundant part of the left limb should be salvaged and sewn to the right limb to provide sufficient length. A 10-mm polyester or ePTFE graft is appropriate when the bypass is to be brought only to the left groin.

ANASTOMOSIS

The aorta is exposed by incising the mediastinal pleura over a suitable segment to allow the aortic anastomosis to be superior enough to the diaphragm to prevent acute angulation and kinking of the graft. This generally requires division of the inferior pulmonary ligament, taking care not to injure the inferior pulmonary vein. Anticoagulation is administered before clamping the aorta. Depending on the size and quality of the aorta, it may be possible to use a partial occlusion sidebiting clamp; the proximal anastomosis is generally easier with complete control and clamping both above and below the site of proposed anastomosis. A Cosgrove or similar articulated clamp is preferred to control the aorta superiorly and any suitable vascular clamp, placed in such a way that it will not impede the aortic anastomosis, is used inferiorly. A longitudinal aortotomy is made with a length appropriate for what is essentially a right-angle, side-to-end, aorta-to-graft anastomosis, performed with running 3-0 polypropylene suture. Distal anastomoses are performed conventionally to native femoral or iliac arteries or to preexisting grafts, as indicated. A Doppler probe is used to confirm that flow is enhanced in the outflow arteries. Anticoagulation is reversed, a single chest tube is placed, and all wounds are closed.

Aortoiliac Embolectomy

Acute lower extremity ischemia related to aortoiliac occlusion may be caused by saddle embolism, thrombosis of either preexistent aortoiliac occlusive disease, aortic aneurysm, or acute aortic dissection.[18] Whereas the source of embolism is nearly always cardiac, in contemporary practice the nature of the cardiac disease has shifted from rheumatic valve pathology to ischemic heart disease.[14] Furthermore, the range of possible percutaneous endovascular techniques for thrombus removal continues to expand.[19,20] Acute ischemia may result from causes other than embolism, and none of these is likely to be successfully treated with embolectomy. Some surgeons have argued that all patients with acute ischemia except those with atrial fibrillation should undergo imaging studies,[21] but this necessarily increases the ischemic time before reperfusion. The patient with atrial fibrillation, sudden onset profound ischemia of one leg with good contralateral pulses or of both legs with no premorbid history suggestive of chronic lower extremity ischemia, is best taken directly to surgery for attempted transfemoral aortoiliac embolectomy. The patient with sinus rhythm and a history suggestive of generalized atherosclerosis with less severe ischemia is better served with a preoperative or intraoperative conventional transarterial catheter-based or preoperative computed tomography angiogram to aid in planning an intervention. Unfortunately, the choice is not always clear, and the surgeon must balance the imperative to rapidly reperfuse the limb against the risk of proceeding without imaging only to find a problem more anatomically complex than simple embolism.

INCISION AND EXPOSURE

The importance of early heparin anticoagulation to prevent distal thrombus propagation in acute arterial occlusion was recognized many years ago.[13,22,23] Anticoagulation must be continued during and after the operation, but this is associated with a higher risk of surgical site hematoma. A radiolucent operating table deck is highly desirable in case angiography is required during surgery. A power injector for contrast, a portable C-arm fluoroscopy unit, and an inventory of guidewires, appropriate sheaths, and catheters are the minimum equipment necessary to perform aortic and pelvic angiography. As discussed previously, angiography may be performed before any attempted embolectomy or if the nature of the problem requires something more complex than embolectomy. Patients are draped with the lower abdomen and both groins prepped and the legs prepped circumferentially. A longitudinal groin incision is preferred, because it allows more flexibility with respect to control and reconstruction of the femoral arteries. Only the symptomatic side need be controlled if the process is unilateral, but if a "saddle" aortic bifurcation or bilateral iliac emboli are suspected, then both femoral arteries are exposed and controlled. If embolectomy is deemed appropriate, deep and superficial femoral branches are controlled with Silastic loops at points where the arteries are minimally diseased with an adequate region for arteriotomy. The common femoral artery is often more diseased, and it may be difficult to find a place where a Potts loop will control but not damage the artery. In these cases control is usually maintained with a Cooley or similar clamp oriented transversely or parallel to the predominantly posterior plaque. In the case of a saddle embolus, the contralateral femoral artery is clamped before creating an arteriotomy in the ipsilateral common femoral artery.[24,25]

FEMORAL ARTERIOTOMY AND EMBOLECTOMY

If the femoral arteries are minimally diseased, then a transverse arteriotomy is placed, extending half of the circumference of the artery in the distal common femoral artery at a point that allows visualization of the superficial and deep femoral artery origins inside the artery (Fig. 29-4, *A*). However, if the femoral artery

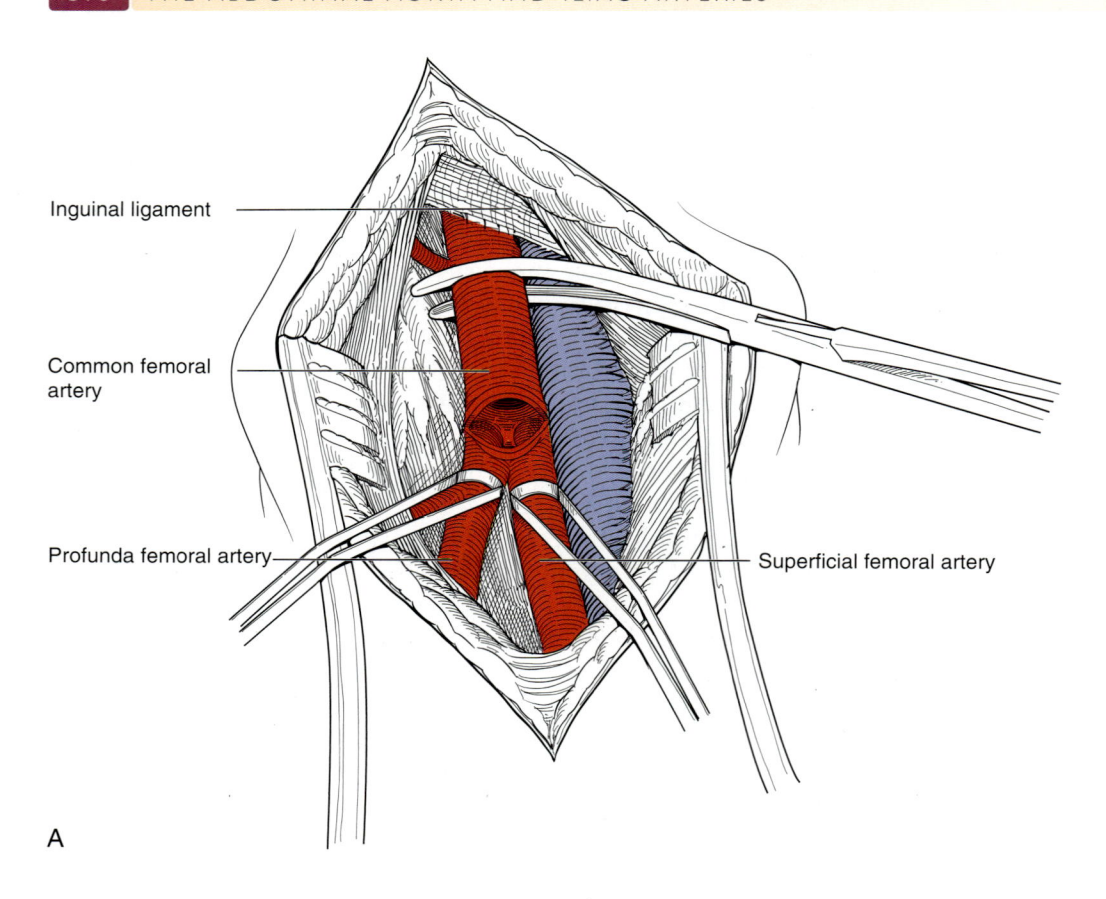

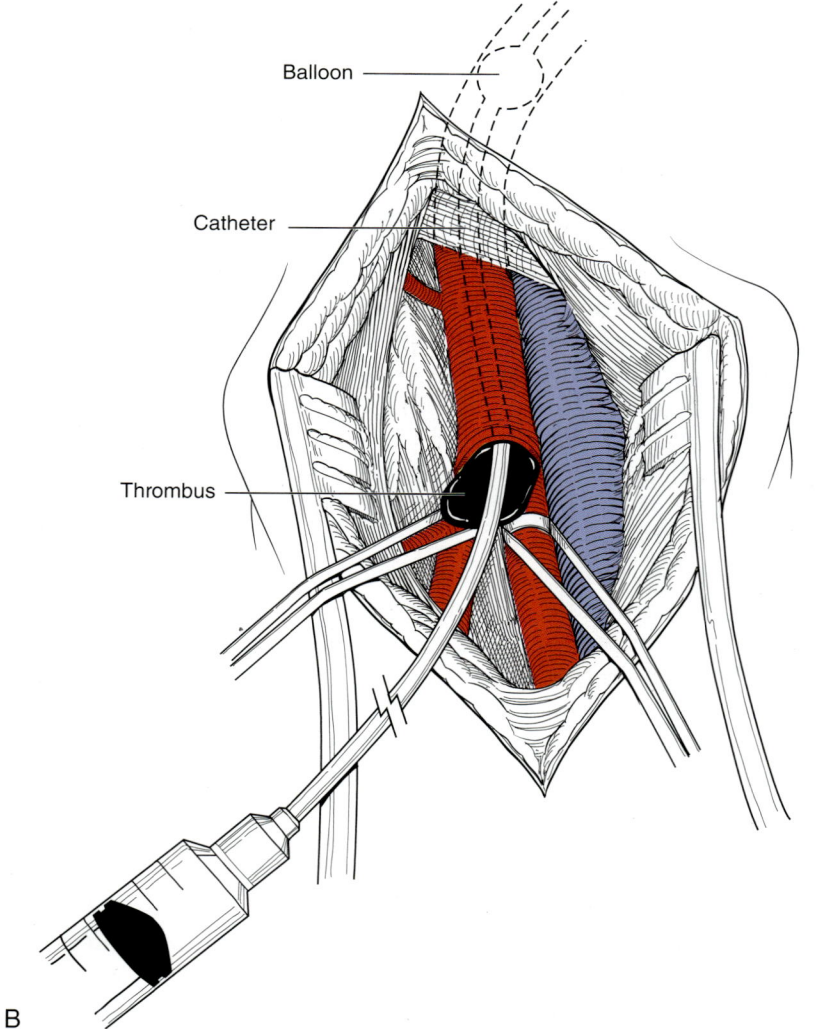

Figure 29-4. Transfemoral aortoiliac embolectomy. **A,** When possible, a transverse arteriotomy is created in the distal common femoral artery to allow visualization of the deep and superficial femoral artery orifices and is extended to about half of the circumference of the artery. A longitudinal arteriotomy may be appropriate when the artery is highly diseased, anticipating either patch closure or use of the arteriotomy as the inflow or outflow site for a bypass graft. **B,** The balloon is then inflated, withdrawing it slightly during inflation and feeling for both increased "drag" on the catheter and increased resistance to inflation, which indicate the balloon has reached the diameter of the vessel. Embolic material is expelled through the arteriotomy as the balloon catheter is withdrawn and is ideally followed by brisk bleeding.

is diseased, then it may be better to place a longitudinal arteriotomy, anticipating possible endarterectomy, patch closure, or bypass. A 5- or 6-Fr balloon embolectomy catheter is advanced proximally into the iliac arteries (see Fig. 29-4, B), with a clamp in place on the contralateral common femoral artery, if an aortic or saddle embolus is suspected. Embolectomy catheters are marked with bands in 10-cm increments. The balloon should not pass beyond 30 cm, because the catheter might inadvertently enter and damage a visceral artery. A single operator should control the balloon-inflating syringe while withdrawing the catheter so as to sense unusual resistance to withdrawal of the catheter.[25] Blood loss is often substantial but may be minimized most commonly by finger pressure on the femoral artery or with Potts Silastic loops. A change in resistance to withdrawal of the catheter associated with the need to deflate the balloon indicates a stenosis, which may need to be addressed if inflow is not adequate following embolectomy. The catheter may be passed multiple times until there is both brisk bleeding and no further return of embolic material. The artery may then be flushed with heparinized saline (10 units of heparin per milliliter saline) and clamped. The process is repeated on the contralateral side if necessary. After this, the procedure should be repeated on the original ipsilateral side in case balloon catheter use from the contralateral side has sent emboli into the ipsilateral side.

Appropriately sized 3- or 4-Fr balloon embolectomy catheters are then passed into the superficial and deep femoral arteries until there is no further return of embolic material. Passage of a catheter approximately 10 to 15 cm into the deep femoral artery is usually adequate. Whether performing an embolectomy of the deep femoral artery or infrageniculate vessel, care should be taken to avoid inadvertent arterial injury by overinflating the embolectomy balloon.

CLOSURE

If satisfied with forward and backbleeding, then the arteriotomies are closed with polypropylene or PTFE sutures and distal perfusion assessed by pulse examination and Doppler interrogation. If there are concerns about the adequacy of embolectomy, angiography is easily performed through a suitable cannula in the superficial femoral artery with hand injection of contrast material. Some balloon catheters are designed to allow passage over a guidewire. Indeed, in contemporary practice, "simple embolectomy" procedures often evolve into hybrid endovascular operations. This may facilitate passage of the balloon catheter "over the wire" after fluoroscopically directed subselection of vessels with a guidewire passed distally from the femoral arteriotomy. Transverse arteriotomies are closed primarily, but longitudinal arteriotomies are closed with a patch unless the artery is large.

CONSIDERATIONS FOR FASCIOTOMY

The need for adjunctive fasciotomies to treat compartment syndrome was recognized early in the embolectomy experience.[13] It is critical to include fasciotomy in the initial procedure if the anterior, lateral, or posterior compartments are palpably "firm" after reperfusion, measured compartment pressures are elevated, or there is a history of ischemia exceeding 6 hours. If fasciotomy is not performed, the patient must be frequently reexamined during the first 24 hours. Anticoagulation should be continued after cardiogenic emboli, because recurrence is common.

REFERENCES

1. Freeman NE, Leeds FH: Operations on large arteries: Application of recent advances, *California Medicine* 77:229-233, 1952.
2. Vetto RM: The treatment of unilateral iliac artery obstruction with a trans-abdominal, subcutaneous, femoro-femoral graft, *Surgery* 52:343-545, 1962.
3. Blaisdell FW, Hall AD: Axillary-femoral artery bypass for lower extremity ischemia, *Surgery* 54:563-568, 1963.

4. Louw JH: Splenic-to-femoral and axillary-to-femoral bypass grafts in diffuse atherosclerotic occlusive disease, *Lancet* 281:1401-1402, 1963.
5. Mannick JA, Nabseth DC: Axillofemoral bypass graft. A safe alternative to aortoiliac reconstruction, *New Engl J Med* 278:461-466, 1968.
6. Stevenson JK, Sauvage LR, Harkins HN: A bypass homograft from thoracic aorta to femoral arteries for occlusive vascular disease: Case report, *Ann Surgery* 27:632-637, 1961.
7. Feldhaus RJ, Sterpetti AV, Schultz RD, et al: Thoracic aorta-femoral artery bypass: Indications, technique, and late results, *Ann Thoracic Surg* 40:588-592, 1985.
8. McCarthy WJ, Rubin JR, Flinn WR, et al: Descending thoracic aorta-to-femoral artery bypass, *Arch Surg* 121:681-688, 1986.
9. Canepa CS, Schubart PJ, Taylor LM Jr, et al: Supraceliac aortofemoral bypass, *Surgery* 101: 323-328, 1987.
10. Kalman PG, Johnston KW, Walker PM: Descending thoracic aortofemoral bypass as an alternative for aortoiliac revascularization, *J Cardiovasc Surg* 32:443-446, 1991.
11. Fogarty TJ, Cranley JJ, Krause RJ, et al: A method for extraction of arterial emboli and thrombi, *Surgery, Gynecol Obstet* 116:241-244, 1963.
12. Cranley JJ, Krause RJ, Strasser ES, et al: Catheter technique for arterial embolectomy: A seven-year experience, *J Cardiovasc Surg* 11:44-51, 1970.
13. Fogarty TJ, Daily PO, Shumway NE, et al: Experience with balloon catheter technic for arterial embolectomy, *Am J Surg* 122:231-237, 1971.
14. Abbott WM, Maloney RD, McCabe CC, et al: Arterial embolism: A 44 year perspective, *Am J Surg* 143:460-464, 1982.
15. Taylor LM Jr, Park TC, Edwards JM, et al: Acute disruption of polytetrafluoroethylene grafts adjacent to axillary anastomoses: A complication of axillofemoral grafting, *J Vasc Surg* 20:520-526, 1994.
16. Schneider JR, Besso SR, Walsh DB, et al: Femorofemoral versus aortobifemoral bypass: Outcome and hemodynamic results, *J Vasc Surg* 19:43-55, 1994.
17. Schneider JR: Aortoiliac Disease: Extra-anatomic bypass. In Cronenwett JL, Johnston KW, editors: *Vascular surgery*, vol 2, ed 7, Philadelphia, 2010, Saunders, pp 1633.
18. Kornmesser TW, Trippel OH, Haid SP: Acute occlusion of the abdominal aorta. In Bergan JJ, Yao JST, editors: *Surgery of the aorta and its body branches*, New York, 1979, Grune & Stratton, p 329.
19. Sharafuddin MJ, Hicks ME: Current status of percutaneous mechanical thrombectomy. Part III. Present and future applications, *J Vasc Intervent Radiol* 9:209-224, 1998.
20. Sharafuddin MJ, Hicks ME: Current status of percutaneous mechanical thrombectomy. Part II. Devices and mechanisms of action, *J Vasc Intervent Radiol* 9:15-31, 1998.
21. Cambria RP, Abbott WM: Acute arterial thrombosis of the lower extremity. Its natural history contrasted with arterial embolism, *Arch Surg* 119:784-787, 1984.
22. Haimovici H, Escher DJ: Aortoiliac stenosis: diagnostic significance of vascular hemodynamics, *Arch Surg* 72:107-117, 1956.
23. Panetta T, Thompson JE, Talkington CM, et al: Arterial embolectomy: A 34-year experience with 400 cases, *Surg Clin North Am* 66:339-353, 1986.
24. Livesay JJ, Atkinson JB, Baker JD, et al: Late results of extra-anatomic bypass, *Arch Surg* 114: 1260-1267, 1979.
25. Fecteau SR, Darling RC III, Roddy SP: Arterial thromboembolism. In Rutherford RB, editor: *Vascular surgery*, vol 1, ed 6, Philadelphia, 2005, Saunders, pp 971.

30 Endovascular Treatment of Aortoiliac Occlusive Disease

RICHARD J. POWELL

Historical Background

In 1964 Dotter and Judkins[1] first reported percutaneous transluminal angioplasty as a technique for treating atherosclerotic stenoses and occlusions. Application of this method for the treatment of iliac occlusive disease was reported in 1974.[2] In February 1974 Grüntzig and Hopff[3] introduced the clinical use of a new balloon catheter, and in 1979 Grüntzig and Kumpe[4] reported a 2-year patency rate of 87% for treatment of iliac lesions with this technique. In 1985 Tegtmeyer and colleagues[5] first reported the two-balloon technique for angioplasty in the region of the aortic bifurcation, commonly called the "kissing balloon" technique. In 1987 Johnston and co-workers[6] prospectively analyzed the results of 984 iliac angioplasties alone and noted an initial success rate of 88%, with continued success at 5 years of 48%. In 1992 Palmaz and associates[7] reported the results of a multicenter trial of 486 patients with iliac artery disease treated with balloon-expandable stents. Initial success was achieved in 99% of patients, with continued success at 43 months of 68%. In 1995 long-term results for treatment of iliac lesions with self-expanding stents were reported.[8] In 2004 the outcomes of iliac stenting using two different self-expanding stents were compared in a multicenter prospective randomized trial, with similar 1-year primary patency of greater than 90%.[9] The role of primary iliac stenting or angioplasty with selective stenting was assessed in the Dutch Iliac Stent Trial Study,[10] a prospective randomized, multicenter study. Similar outcomes were reported for both groups, with approximately 80% of treated iliac artery segments remaining free of repeat revascularization procedures at 5 years.[11] In a recent systematic review of 19 nonrandomized cohort studies, 4-year primary patency for Trans-Atlantic Inter-Society Consensus (TASC II) classes C and D aortoiliac lesions ranged from 69% to 88%, with most clinicians reporting 4-year primary patency of between 75% and 80%.[12]

Indications

Endovascular treatment for aortoiliac occlusive disease is indicated for lifestyle-limiting claudication, nocturnal metatarsalgia, or ischemic ulceration. Less frequent indications include treatment of vasculogenic impotence and atheroembolization to the lower extremities. Aortoiliac lesions most suitable for endovascular therapy can be guided by the newly revised TASC II guidelines (Fig. 30-1 and Table 30-1).[13] Endovascular therapy is a first-line therapy for symptomatic patients with TASC II A and B lesions, whereas surgical therapy is usually considered for TASC II D lesions and for low-risk patients with TASC II C disease. Although less durable than open surgical options, endovascular therapy may be applicable for high-risk patients with advanced associated comorbidities, such as severe chronic obstructive pulmonary disease, unreconstructable coronary artery disease, and low cardiac ejection fraction with TASC II C and D level disease in the setting of critical limb ischemia.

374 THE ABDOMINAL AORTA AND ILIAC ARTERIES

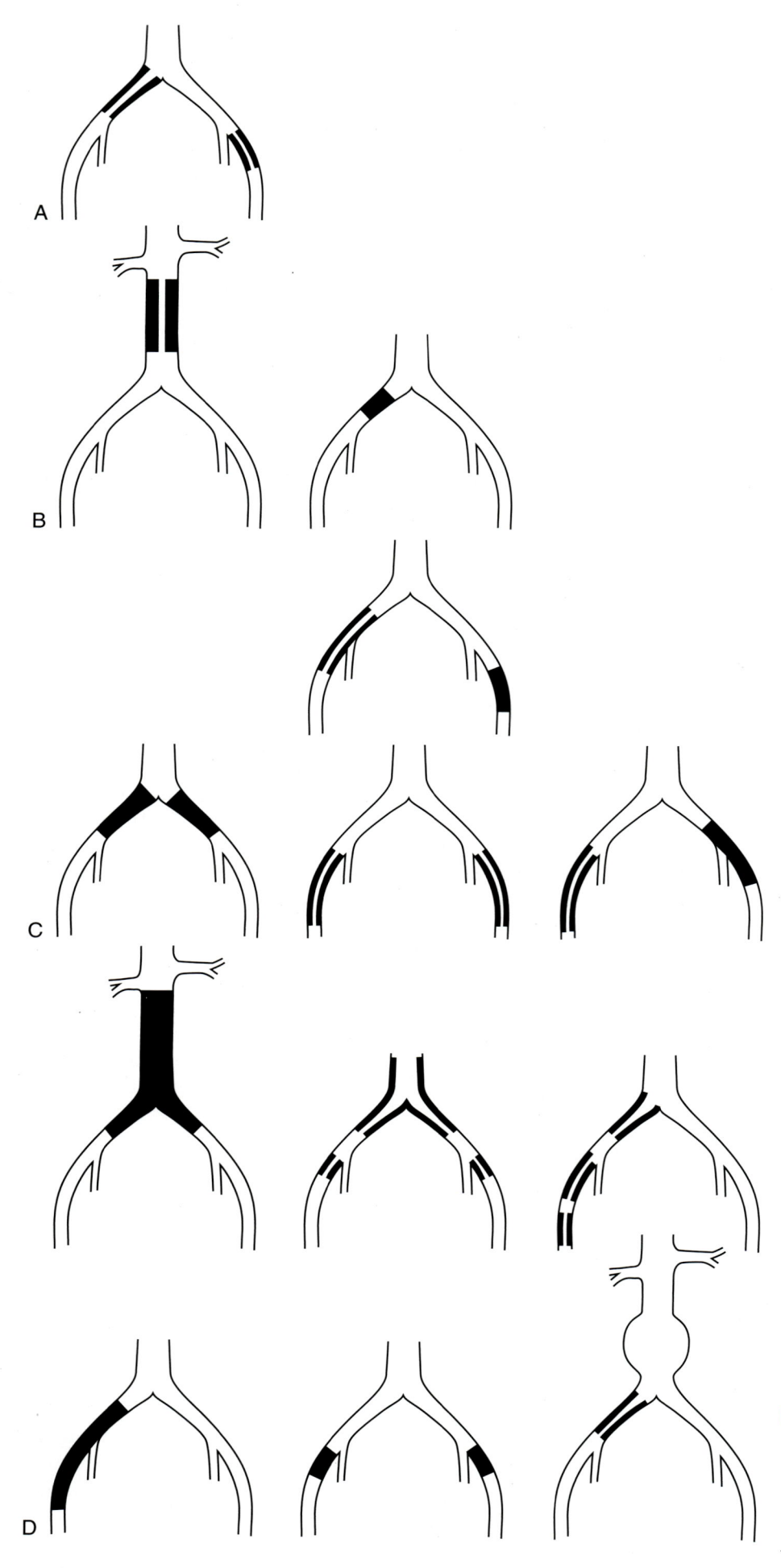

Figure 30-1. TASC II classification of aortoiliac lesions. See Table 30-1. (From Norgren L, Hiatt WR, Dormandy JA et al: Inter-Society Consensus for the management of peripheral arterial disease [TASC II]. J Vasc Surg 45:S5-S67, 2007, Fig. F1.)

TABLE 30-1 Trans-Atlantic Inter-Society Consensus Classification of Aortoiliac Lesions

Lesion Type	Guidelines
A	Unilateral or bilateral stenoses of the CIA Unilateral or bilateral single short (≤3 cm) stenosis of the EIA
B	Short (≤3 cm) stenosis of the infrarenal aorta Unilateral CIA occlusion Single or multiple stenoses totaling 3-10 cm and involving the EIA but not extending into the CFA Unilateral EIA occlusion not involving the origins of the internal iliac artery or the CFA
C	Bilateral CIA occlusions Bilateral EIA stenoses 3-10 cm long not extending into the CFA Unilateral EIA stenosis extending into the CFA Unilateral EIA occlusion that involves the origins of the internal iliac artery and/or the CFA Heavily calcified unilateral EIA occlusion with or without involvement of the origins of the internal iliac artery and/or the origins CFA
D	Infrarenal aortoiliac occlusion Diffuse disease involving the aorta and both iliac arteries and requiring treatment Diffuse multiple stenoses involving the unilateral CIA, EIA, and CFA Unilateral occlusions of both the CIA and the EIA Bilateral occlusions of the EIA Iliac stenoses in patients with abdominal aortic aneurysm requiring treatment and not amenable to endograft placement or with other lesions requiring open aortic or iliac surgery

From Norgren L, Hiatt WR, Dormandy JA, et al: Inter-Society Consensus for the management of peripheral arterial disease (TASC II). *J Vasc Surg* 45:S5-S67, 2007, Table F1.
CFA, Common femoral artery; *CIA*, common iliac artery; *EIA*, external iliac artery.

Preoperative Preparation

- The use of aspirin (81-325 mg/day) or clopidogrel (75 mg/day) during the preoperative and postoperative periods is an accepted adjunct to diminish perioperative complications.
- Patients should undergo noninvasive physiologic arterial studies such as ankle-brachial index and toe pressure measurements if indicated. Additional diagnostic studies are indicated to assess the location and extent of arterial occlusive disease, as well as the degree of calcification.
- The use of arteriography as a diagnostic tool is rarely indicated. Less invasive imaging modalities are available that can provide anatomic detail without exposing the patient to an invasive procedure.
- Duplex arterial mapping (DAM) of the aortoiliac segment and common femoral arteries can provide an adequate assessment of the location of hemodynamically significant lesions. This modality is especially useful in patients with renal insufficiency who are at risk from contrast-induced renal dysfunction. Drawbacks to DAM include only a semiquantitative assessment of the degree of iliac calcification, the inability to adequately image the iliac system in certain patients because of overlying bowel gas or body habitus, and the need for a significant time commitment and a highly trained vascular technologist.
- Magnetic resonance arteriography has developed to the point that it can provide reliable assessment of the aortoiliac arterial segment, though there continues to be institutional variability in the accuracy of this modality. The major drawback to magnetic resonance arteriography is that it does not provide an accurate assessment of the degree of calcification of the aortoiliac lesions. Gadolinium-enhanced magnetic resonance arteriography is contraindicated in patients with renal insufficiency.
- Computed tomography (CT) arteriography has been used with success to evaluate the aortoiliac segment before intervention. The major drawbacks to this imaging modality include exposure to ionizing radiation and the need for iodinated contrast, with the associated risk of contrast-induced renal dysfunction. In appropriate patients CT arteriography gives an accurate assessment of lesion location, lesion extent, and degree of calcification. Based on CT arteriography evaluation, the severity of aortoiliac and femoral disease can be classified according to TASC II guidelines.

- Use of preprocedural fluids and low-osmolar or isosmolar contrast agents decreases the risk for contrast-induced nephropathy, defined as an increase in serum creatinine greater than 25% or 0.5 mg/dL (44.2 µmol/L) within 3 days of intravascular contrast administration in the absence of an alternative cause. Although the effect may be small, preprocedural treatment with *N*-acetylcysteine (NAC) may reduce the risk for contrast-induced nephropathy. Because free radicals are postulated to mediate contrast-induced nephropathy, alkalinizing renal tubular fluid with bicarbonate has been shown to reduce injury. The use of NAC and bicarbonate may have an additive protective effect. Patients with a baseline serum creatinine of at least 1.5 mg/dL should receive an intravenous bolus of 3 mL/kg/hr (154 mEq/L sodium bicarbonate in dextrose and water) for 1 hour immediately before contrast injection.[14,15] Patients should receive the same fluid regimen at a rate of 1 mL/kg/hr during contrast exposure and for 6 hours after the procedure. NAC at 1200 mg taken orally twice daily the day before and the day of contrast administration is also recommended. Diuretics should be withheld on the day of contrast injection.

Pitfalls and Danger Points

- **Stent migration or embolization**
- **Subintimal dissection.** Intraarterial catheter placement should be confirmed after crossing an occlusion by aspiration of blood.
- **Iliac artery or aortic rupture**
- **Atheroembolization**
- **Iliac occlusion.** Plaque disruption or narrowing of the contralateral common iliac artery occurs during ipsilateral common iliac artery intervention.
- **Late restenosis.** Risk factors include TASC II C or D lesions and lesions in the external iliac artery.

Endovascular Strategy

Depending on the location and extent of the disease determined by preoperative imaging, an ipsilateral retrograde, contralateral, bilateral femoral, or brachial approach can be planned.

INITIAL INTRAOPERATIVE IMAGING

An arteriographic examination is performed at the time of intervention and includes oblique pelvic imaging of the iliac arteries to determine the location of internal iliac artery and common femoral artery bifurcation disease. A contralateral oblique projection opens the iliac artery bifurcations, whereas the ipsilateral oblique projection is most useful for the femoral artery bifurcations. Imaging of the infrainguinal runoff is a requisite before intervention in most patients to ensure that the etiology of distal occlusion is because of preexisting disease rather than embolization during the course of intervention.

ASSESSING HEMODYNAMIC SIGNIFICANCE

Pressure measurements across the lesion should be obtained in moderate stenoses by connecting the hub of the catheter and the side arm of the vascular sheath to the intraarterial pressure monitor. The catheter should be at least 1-Fr smaller than the sheath. Other options include the pullback method of withdrawing an end-hole catheter over a 0.014-inch guidewire across a lesion from proximal to distal or through use of a pressure wire. A peak-to-peak systolic pressure gradient at rest of 10 mm Hg or greater is indicative of a hemodynamically significant lesion. In the absence of a resting gradient due to a distal superficial femoral artery occlusion, hemodynamic significance can be determined by measuring the

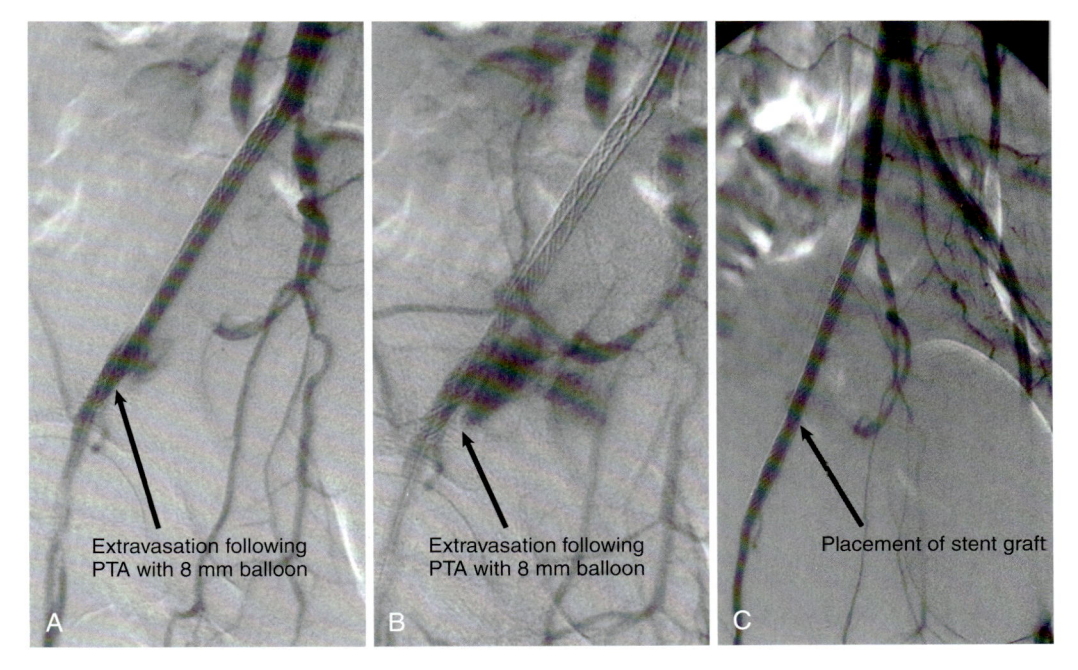

Figure 30-2. Ruptured external iliac artery treated with a stent graft. **A** and **B,** After placement of a bare metal stent and dilatation with an 8-mm balloon. **C,** Stent graft placed to achieve hemostasis. *PTA,* Percutaneous transluminal angioplasty.

A — Extravasation following PTA with 8 mm balloon
B — Extravasation following PTA with 8 mm balloon
C — Placement of stent graft

pressure gradient after intraarterial administration of nitroglycerin (100-200 mcg) to dilate distal runoff vessels in the affected extremity.

CONCOMITANT COMMON FEMORAL ARTERY DISEASE

The determination to proceed with a percutaneous endovascular therapy or an open femoral approach is based on the presence of significant common femoral artery disease. Patients with at least 30% to 50% stenosis of the common femoral artery on imaging studies are usually treated with a hybrid approach that entails open femoral endarterectomy and patch angioplasty and simultaneous aortoiliac stent or stent-graft placement. In patients with less severe common femoral artery disease, a percutaneous approach alone is appropriate.

CALCIFICATION

The presence of severe calcification has significant implications on operative or interventional planning. Circumferential calcification more than 1 mm thick is a relative contraindication to aortoiliac angioplasty and stenting. Consideration should be given to the use of stent grafts in patients who have extensive calcification of the aortoiliac segment and are poor candidates for open surgery, particularly of the external iliac artery segment in elderly females. Potential advantages of a stent graft are decreased risk of bleeding and the ability to more aggressively dilate the iliac segment (Fig. 30-2).[1] A larger arterial sheath may be required, although recent improvements in design have reduced the sheath profile necessary for these devices.

LESIONS ABOVE THE AORTIC BIFURCATION

Aortic angioplasty and stenting for lesions above the aortic bifurcation are frequently exophytic and calcified. Acceptance of an imperfect angiographic result is critical to avoiding aortic rupture. Primary stent placement to trap potential atheroembolic debris should be considered for exophytic lesions or for those patients who present with a recent history of atheroembolization. The use of a stent graft should also be considered because of the risk of rupture.

Endovascular Technique

ARTERIAL ACCESS

The procedure begins with placement of an arterial sheath to facilitate catheter exchanges. Common iliac artery disease is treated through an ipsilateral approach.

If the common iliac artery is occluded, contralateral flush catheter placement should be considered so that a complete diagnostic study before intervention is performed and the contralateral common iliac artery protected from injury during ipsilateral common iliac artery intervention. External iliac artery disease is generally approached from the contralateral side, which allows for extension of treatment into the proximal portion of the common femoral artery, if needed (Fig. 30-3).

CROSSING THE ILIAC ARTERY LESION

Retrograde Approach

The iliac artery lesion is crossed with the use of a catheter-guidewire combination. A floppy-tipped guidewire is used to cross the lesion first, followed by an angle tip catheter. In difficult cases hydrophilic guidewires may be used (Fig. 30-3, *B*). With the catheter across the lesion, aspiration of blood ensures the intraluminal position of the catheter tip.

Antegrade Approach

In many instances the guidewire may follow a subintimal path in retrograde attempts to recanalize an occluded iliac artery. Once this happens it may be difficult to redirect the guidewire into the lumen. In this instance, an antegrade approach from the contralateral common femoral artery is frequently successful, especially if the common iliac artery is not flush occluded. A hooked catheter is used to probe the occlusion. The lesion can then be crossed in most instances (5%-20% failure rate) with the use of a hydrophilic guidewire. As soon as the guidewire has crossed the lesion and lies within the ipsilateral external iliac artery lumen, it is snared from the ipsilateral common femoral artery. A short catheter is then inserted in a retrograde fashion over the wire end into the abdominal aorta proximal to the lesion. Intraarterial catheter placement is confirmed through aspiration of blood from the aortic catheter. The hydrophilic guidewire is then removed, and a working guidewire is inserted to facilitate the intervention.

COEXISTENT COMMON FEMORAL ARTERY DISEASE

With common femoral artery disease noted on preoperative imaging, an open femoral approach is prudent (Fig. 30-4). The common femoral artery is exposed from the circumflex femoral branches distally to the femoral bifurcation. The common femoral artery is punctured under direct vision, and the iliac lesion is crossed before endarterectomy. This technique allows no doubt in intraluminal wire placement distally at the endarterectomy site. When the guidewire cannot be passed retrograde, a percutaneous approach from the contralateral femoral artery, or the brachial artery, can be used to allow crossing of the iliac lesion. The guidewire can then be brought out through the femoral artery.

BRACHIAL ARTERY ACCESS

There is occasionally a flush occlusion of the occluded common iliac artery; therefore contralateral crossing of the lesion is generally unsuccessful. Crossing the lesion can be attempted from the brachial approach or retrograde ipsilateral approach. A left brachial artery approach decreases the risk of an aortic dissection and facilitates "pushability" of the wire and catheter. The presence of a left subclavian artery stenosis precludes this approach or otherwise requires pretreatment.

REENTRY CATHETERS

Recent development of reentry catheters has increased the ability to cross complete arterial occlusions from a retrograde ipsilateral approach. The hydrophilic guidewire in the subintimal space beyond the occlusion is exchanged for a 300-cm-long, 0.014-inch guidewire using a hydrophilic catheter. The catheter is then removed, and a reentry catheter is advanced into the level of the aortic

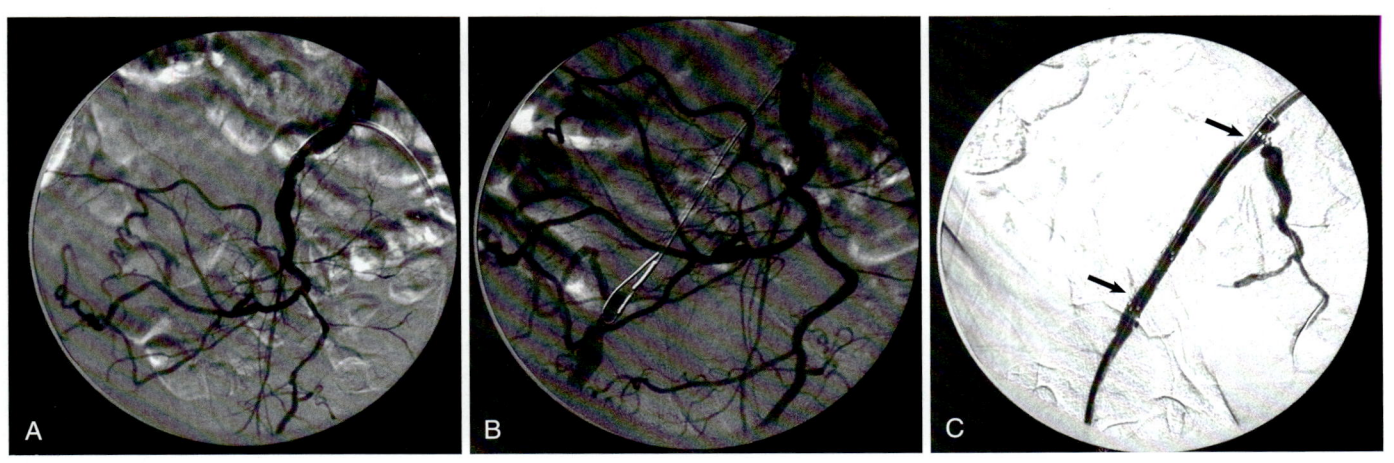

ENDOVASCULAR TREATMENT OF AORTOILIAC OCCLUSIVE DISEASE   379

Figure 30-3. A, External iliac artery occlusion being approached from the contralateral common femoral artery. **B,** Subintimal crossing of the complete occlusion with a reentry catheter. **C,** Contralateral placement of a bare metal stent *(arrows)* into the external iliac artery with extension to the proximal portion of the common femoral artery.

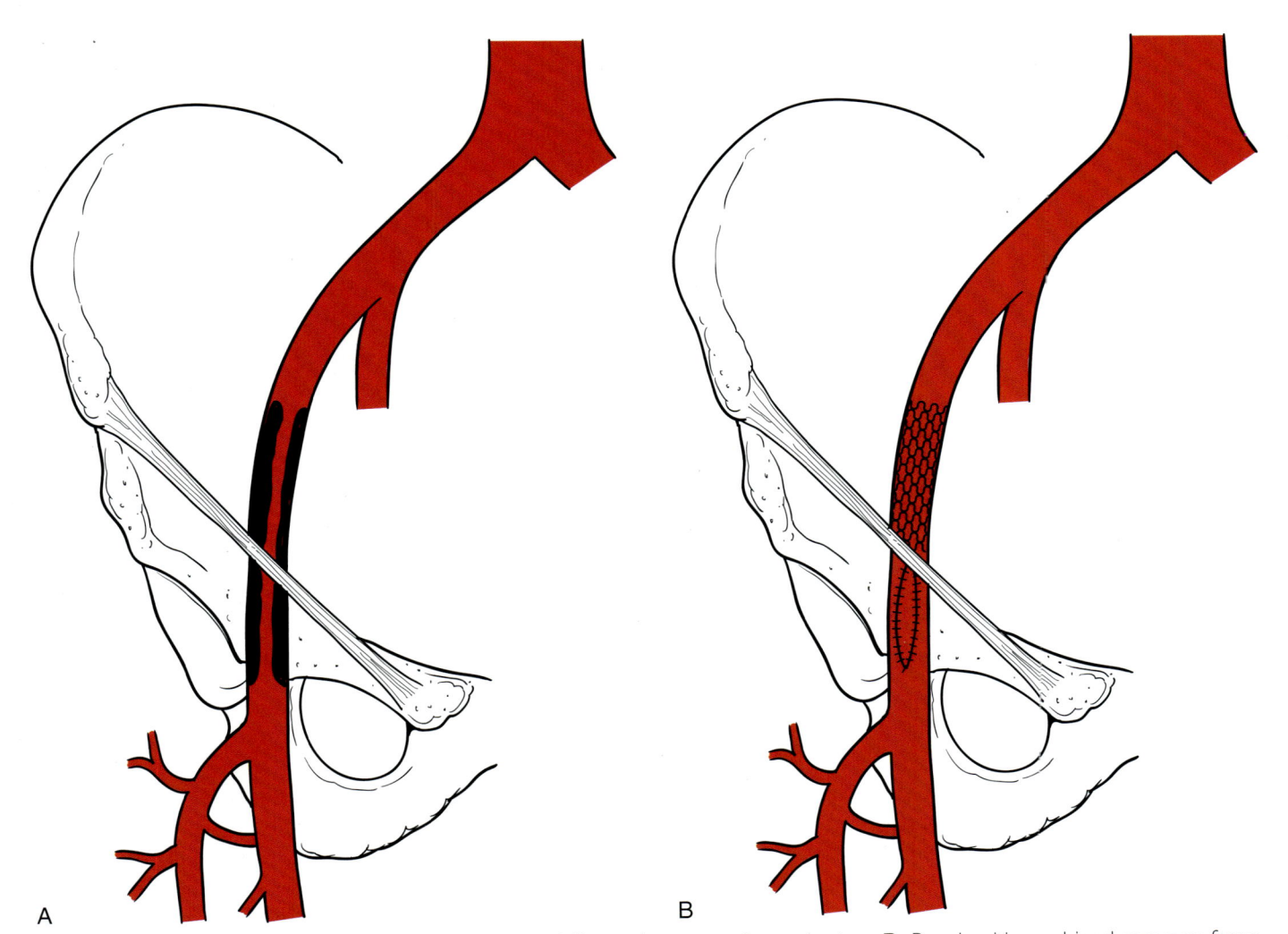

Figure 30-4. A, Severe occlusive disease of the external iliac and common femoral artery. **B,** Repair with combined common femoral endarterectomy and external iliac artery stenting. Either a bare metal or a covered stent may be used.

bifurcation under continuous fluoroscopy (Fig. 30-5, *A*). An angiogram is performed via a catheter advanced through a contralateral access sheath to confirm traversal of the occlusion and that the lateral exit port of the catheter is at the aortic bifurcation above the occlusion. The precise location and orientation of the lateral exit port is confirmed by aligning the fluoroscopic guiding markers or with intravascular ultrasound, depending on catheter type (see Fig. 30-5).

The nitinol needle is advanced through the lateral exit port under continuous fluoroscopy. Applying firm but guarded forward pressure while briskly deploying the cannula contributes to successful puncture. Free passage of the 0.014-inch guidewire indicates true lumen access, which is confirmed by contrast injection through the catheter. The catheter is then exchanged for a 4- or 5-Fr catheter. Frequently the subintimal tract requires balloon angioplasty before placement of the catheter or stent. A 3-mm-diameter angioplasty balloon is typically used to dilate the intimal puncture site to enable catheter passage and exchange for a 0.035-inch guidewire to facilitate stenting, which can be performed conventionally (Fig. 30-6).

AORTIC BIFURCATION DISEASE

Lesions at the aortic bifurcation are traditionally treated using a kissing balloon technique. However, simultaneous balloon dilatation at the origins of both common iliac arteries is often advocated, even in the presence of a unilateral lesion, to protect the contralateral common iliac artery from dissection or plaque dislodgement with subsequent embolization. Because calcified lesions at the aortic bifurcation are not amenable to balloon dilatation alone, "kissing stents" or the aortic reconstruction technique may be necessary (see Fig. 30-6, *C*). Although concerns have been raised that the proximal portion of the stents, which extend into the distal aorta (aortic advancement) may serve as a nidus for thrombus formation, low complication rates have been reported with this procedure. Smith and co-workers[16] challenged this long established practice. In a retrospective review of 175 patients with unilateral ostial iliac artery lesions treated with angioplasty or stenting without contralateral protection, only two patients developed mild stenosis of the contralateral unprotected common iliac artery.

CONCOMITANT FEMORAL ARTERY ENDARTERECTOMY

Wire access is left in place, proximal and distal control is obtained, and longitudinal arteriotomy is created, allowing standard subintimal endarterectomy. Patch angioplasty is then performed. Before completion of the patch angioplasty, the patch is punctured in the center with an 18-Ga needle, and the guidewire is brought out through the center of the patch. The patch angioplasty is then completed and flow is restored. Iliac stenting is subsequently performed such that the distal endpoint of the stent is just proximal to the endarterectomy and patch angioplasty (see Fig. 30-4).

SELECTION OF BALLOON AND STENT DIMENSIONS

Balloon and stent oversizing by 5% to 10% is recommended except for heavily calcified lesions that may rupture. The optimal vessel diameter is judged from the adjacent normal arterial segment or from the equivalent vessel on the contralateral side. Calibrated imaging systems facilitate diameter and length measurements, but a calibrated catheter can be inserted for vessel measurements. The length of the balloon or stent should cover the diseased area without damaging the normal vessel. If in doubt, it is wise to initially undersize when dilating a lesion. With self-expanding stent placement this rule does not apply, because an undersized stent cannot be exchanged for an optimal one. Balloon inflation should be gradual to avoid trauma to the adjacent normal vessel. The lesion is identified by the presence of a waist on the balloon, which disappears when the lesion is successfully dilated. Mild pain during dilation because of stretching of the adventitia is common; excessive and persistent pain may indicate arterial

ENDOVASCULAR TREATMENT OF AORTOILIAC OCCLUSIVE DISEASE

Figure 30-5. Reentry catheter. **A,** Outback catheter. The cannula *(large arrow)* is deployed with free passage of the guidewire into the true lumen of the aorta. Note the L configuration *(small arrow)*. **B,** Outback LTD catheter. The cannula *(large black arrow)* is deployed, and the 0.014-inch guidewire *(small black arrow)* is advanced through it. The nose cone *(large white arrow)* has the radiopaque "LT" orientation marker. The catheter shaft is indicated with the small white arrow.

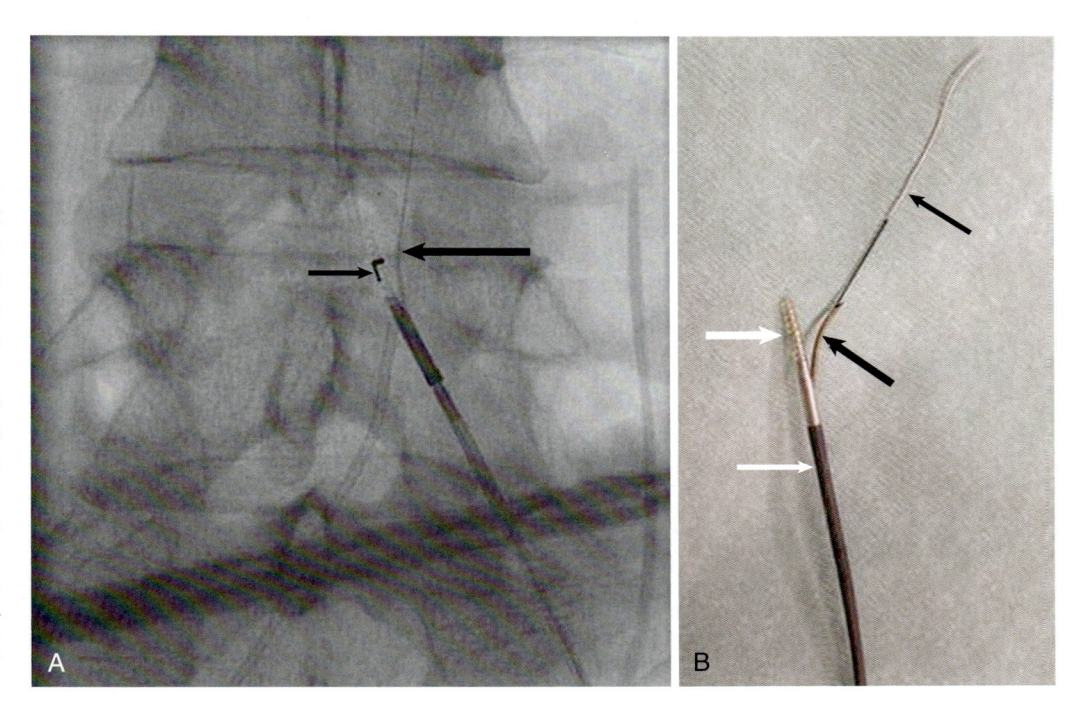

Figure 30-6. Results using a reentry catheter. **A,** Pelvic arteriogram showing complete occlusion of the left common and external iliac arteries. **B,** Glide catheter advancement into the aorta after reentry at the aortic bifurcation. **C,** Retrograde placement of a stent graft into the common iliac artery. Note the contralateral bare metal common iliac stent.

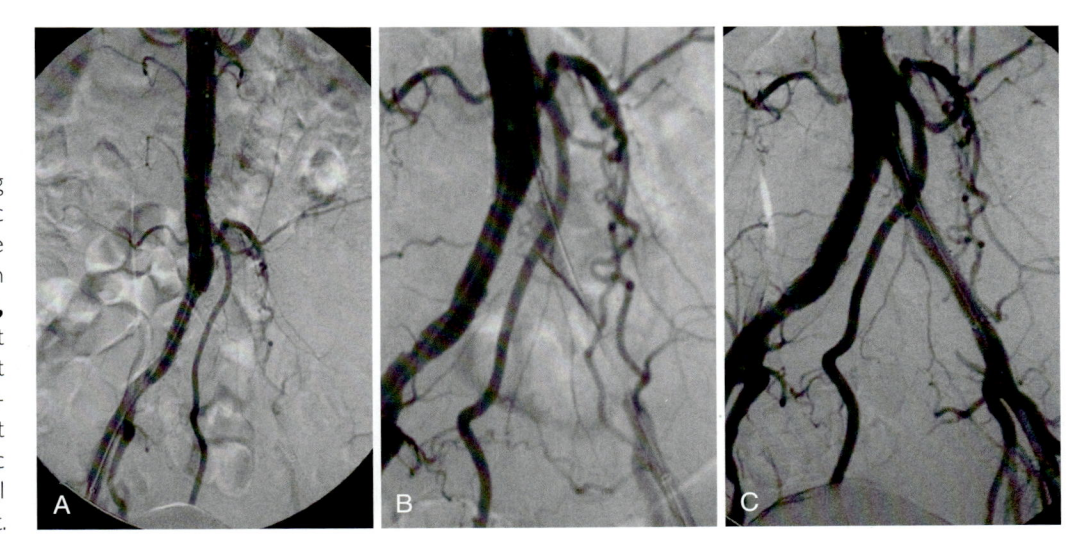

rupture (see Fig. 30-2, *A* and *B*). Technical success is judged by a residual stenosis of less than 20% and a systolic pressure gradient of less than 10 mm Hg.

The placement of a balloon-expandable stent requires the sheath to be advanced beyond the lesion, especially if primary stenting is performed of a severe stenosis to avoid dislocation of the stent. The balloon-mounted stent is positioned across the lesion using bone landmarks or road mapping. The sheath is then retracted, and the balloon is inflated to expand the stent. Self-expanding stents are mounted on a carrier device; constrained by an outer sheath. The introducer sheath does not need to cross the lesion. Stent deployment is achieved by holding the carrier device with one hand while retracting the outer sheath with the other. Selection of a stent for an iliac artery depends on the operator's familiarity with specific devices and the lesion's characteristics, including length and tortuosity. Eccentric, calcified short lesions typically occur at the aortic bifurcation and may be best treated with a balloon-expandable stent because of high precision of placement. If the path is tortuous or the stent is to be placed from the contralateral side, self-expanding stents are useful because of their flexibility. Stent grafts, either balloon expandable or self-expanding, are playing an increasingly important role and are especially useful in patients with calcified or small iliac segments with potential for arterial rupture.[17]

Postoperative Care

- **Antiplatelet therapy.** Antiplatelet therapy should be started preoperatively and continued after the endovascular procedure.
- **Clinical surveillance.** Interval history, examination of peripheral pulses, and measurement of ankle-brachial indices, should be performed in the immediate postoperative period, every 6 months for at least 2 years, and annually thereafter.

REFERENCES

1. Dotter CT, Judkins MP: Transluminal treatment of arteriosclerotic obstruction. Description of a new technique and a preliminary report of its application, *Circulation* 30:654-670, 1964.
2. Dotter CT, Rosch J, Anderson JM, et al: Transluminal iliac artery dilatation: Nonsurgical catheter treatment of atheromatous narrowing, *JAMA* 230:117-124, 1974.
3. Grüntzig A, Hopff H: Perkutane rekanalisation chronischer arterieller Verschlüsse mit einem neuen dilatationskatheter. Modifikation der Dotter-Technik, *Dtsch Med Wochenschr* 99:2502-2505, 1974.
4. Grüntzig A, Kumpe DA: Technique of percutaneous trans-luminal angioplasty with the Grüntzig balloon catheter, *Am J Roentgenol* 132:547-552, 1979.
5. Tegtmeyer CJ, Kellum CD, Kron IL, et al: Percutaneous transluminal angioplasty in the region of the aortic bifurcation. The two-balloon technique with results and long-term follow-up study, *Radiology* 157:661-665, 1985.
6. Johnston KW, Rae M, Hogg-Johnston SA, et al: 5-year results of a prospective study of percutaneous transluminal angioplasty, *Ann Surg* 206:403-413, 1987.
7. Palmaz JC, Laborde JC, Rivera FJ, et al: Stenting of the iliac arteries with the Palmaz stent: Experience from a multicenter trial, *Cardiovasc Intervent Radiol* 15:291-297, 1992.
8. Martin EC, Katzen BT, Benenati JF, et al: Multicenter trial of the Wallstent in the iliac and femoral arteries, *J Vasc Interv Radiol* 6:843-849, 1995.
9. Ponec D, Jaff MR, Swischuk J, et al: The Nitinol SMART stent vs Wallstent for suboptimal iliac artery angioplasty: CRISP-US Trial results, *J Vasc Interv Radiol* 15:911-918, 2004.
10. Tetteroo E, van der Graaf Y, Bosch JL, et al: Randomised comparison of primary stent placement versus primary angioplasty followed by selective stent placement in patients with iliac-artery occlusive disease. Dutch Iliac Stent Trial Study Group, *Lancet* 351:1153-1159, 1998.
11. Klein WM, van der Graaf Y, Seegers J, et al: Long-term cardiovascular morbidity, mortality, and reintervention after endovascular treatment in patients with iliac artery disease: The Dutch Iliac Stent Trial Study, *Radiology* 232:491-498, 2004.
12. Jongkind V, Akkersdijk GJM, Yeung KK, et al: A systematic review of endovascular treatment of extensive aortoiliac occlusive disease, *J Vasc Surg* 52:1376-1383, 2010.
13. Norgren L, Hiatt WR, Dormandy JA, et al: Inter-Society Consensus for the management of peripheral arterial disease (TASC II), *J Vasc Surg* 45:S5-S67, 2007.
14. Merten GJ, Burgess WP, Gray LV, et al: Prevention of contrast-induced nephropathy with sodium bicarbonate: A randomized controlled trial, *JAMA* 291:2328-2334, 2004.
15. Briguori C, Airoldi F, D'Andrea D, et al: Renal insufficiency following contrast media administration trial (REMEDIAL): A randomized comparison of 3 preventive strategies, *Circulation* 115:1211-1217, 2007.
16. Smith JC, Watkins GR, Taylor FC, et al: Angioplasty or stent placement in the proximal common iliac artery: Is protection of the contralateral side necessary? *J Vasc Interv Radiol* 12:1395-1398, 2001.
17. Rzucidlo EM, Powell RJ, Zwolak RM, et al: Early results of stent-grafting to treat diffuse aortoiliac occlusive disease, *J Vasc Surg* 37:1175-1180, 2003.

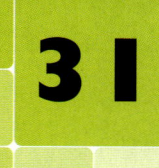

31 Special Problems in the Endovascular Treatment of Aortoiliac Occlusive Disease

DANIEL G. CLAIR • JESSICA M. TITUS

Historical Background

In recent years there has been a shift in the treatment of aortoiliac occlusive disease (AIOD) from open surgical treatment to endovascular interventions.[1] Endovascular treatment for Trans-Atlantic Inter-Society Consensus (TASC) class A lesions is considered standard.[2] Recommendations are not as clear for more complex disease, including TASC class B and C lesions, but even these are often treated with interventional therapy with excellent results.[3-6] As catheter-based interventions have advanced, the treatment spectrum has widened to include TASC class D lesions (Table 31-1). Although, a surgical approach continues to be recommended for patients with low operative risk for complex aortic and iliac TASC class D lesions, recent studies have revealed comparable technical success and durability when compared with open reconstruction.[6-8] A hybrid approach for treating occlusive disease that extends into the femoral arteries has further increased endovascular options for AIOD.[8-10]

Preoperative Care

- Preoperative physical examination should include a determination of ankle-brachial index; assessment of severity of comorbidities, including renal, cardiac, and functional limitations; and estimated life expectancy. Patients who cannot tolerate general anesthesia and have limited life expectancy, minimal functional performance, or a hostile abdomen may be better served with endovascular treatment.

- Preoperative imaging is performed to determine the extent of aortoiliac disease, with particular attention given to associated common femoral artery or infrainguinal disease. Computed tomography angiography is preferred over conventional angiography and magnetic resonance angiography because of its capacity to assess arterial calcification. In patients with renal insufficiency (estimated glomerular filtration rate of less than 45 mL/min/1.73 m^2), hydration is recommended before and after the imaging.

- Optimization of comorbidities should be undertaken as follows:
  - Patients with significant renal insufficiency should be admitted before intervention for hydration. Volume loading with sodium bicarbonate and N-acetylcysteine has been shown to reduce risk of renal failure.[11-13]
  - Smoking cessation reduces graft failure, risk of myocardial infarction, and progression of peripheral artery disease.[14,15]
  - Perioperative beta-blockade is recommended for patients with cardiac disease.[16]
  - Aspirin is recommended at a daily dosage of 162 to 325 mg, and clopidogrel (75 mg daily) has been found to reduce the risk of ischemic events.[17,13]

TABLE 31-1 Outcomes for Aortoiliac Stenting for TASC Class B, C, and D Lesions

Study	No. Patients (technical success rate, %)	Follow-up (yr)	Primary Patency (%)	Secondary Patency (%)	Limb Salvage (%)
Uher et al.[4]	73 (97)	3	69	81	NR
Henry et al.[5]	105 (88)	6	52	66	NR
Leville et al.[6]	92 (91)	3	76	90	97
Kashyap et al.[8]	86 (100)	3	74	95	98
Rzucidlo et al.[10]	34 (100)	1	70	88	100

NR, Not reported.

- Most endovascular procedures can be performed under local anesthesia and sedation. However, if a hybrid procedure is planned, regional or general anesthesia is recommended. Cardiac stress testing has been recommended for patients undergoing vascular surgery,[19,20] but recent evidence suggests a selective approach to testing may be appropriate based on the application of a cardiac risk index.[21,22]

Pitfalls and Danger Points

- **Rupture.** Increased risk in small, calcified vessels is often observed in female patients. The external iliac artery is most vulnerable. In high-risk situations an access sheath should be selected at the outset that allows delivery of a covered stent.
- **Dissection**
- **Embolization**
- **Thrombosis.** Activated clotting time (ACT) should be maintained between 250 and 300 seconds during interventions.
- **Access site bleeding**

Endovascular Strategy

The TASC classification of aortic and iliac artery occlusive disease provides a framework for considering endovascular options and outcomes (see Table 30-1). Endovascular treatment is preferred for TASC class A and B lesions. However, surgery should be considered for treatment of TASC class C and D disease in patients at low operative risk, with endovascular approaches reserved for high-risk patients or those with other factors, such as a hostile abdomen, that would complicate surgical repair.

UNFAVORABLE ANATOMIC FEATURES FOR INTERVENTIONS ON COMMON AND EXTERNAL ILIAC ARTERIES

Large irregular calcifications, especially close to the aortic or iliac bifurcation, increase concern for vessel rupture during stenting or dilation and may require a covered stent. Extension of disease into the common femoral artery precludes stenting in this region, and a hybrid procedure with femoral endarterectomy should be considered.

ADJUNCTIVE THROMBOLYSIS AND PERCUTANEOUS MECHANICAL THROMBECTOMY

Motarjeme and associates[23] found that a short course of thrombolysis may assist in crossing an aortoiliac occlusive lesion. However, most lesions can be crossed without the need for thrombolysis, and its routine use is not necessary. Thrombolysis may reduce the juxtarenal thrombus burden before stent placement as a means to decrease renal emboli. The role of percutaneous mechanical thrombectomy in subacute or chronic disease is not well defined, with an inherent risk of distal embolization.[24]

AVOIDING EMBOLIZATION, DISSECTION, AND RUPTURE

Minimizing wire and catheter manipulation across a lesion at high risk for embolization, such as those that are heavily calcified with an irregular plaque or ulceration, is prudent and should dictate early intraoperative anticoagulation. In heavily calcified vessels, a low-profile, predilation balloon should be considered followed by primary stenting. Aggressive balloon dilation after stent placement may reduce the risk of embolization, because the stent traps potential embolic debris.

It is often difficult to avoid dissection in a heavily calcified iliac artery. Intravascular ultrasound (IVUS) may be used before dilation to confirm vessel diameter and lesion length, and thus reduce the potential for vessel rupture by assuring appropriate device sizing. Self-expanding rather than balloon-expandable stents also allow for a more controlled dilation, with covered stents permitting dilation in vessels at risk for rupture. If there is concern that vessel dilation is inadequate, IVUS may be used to confirm that an appropriate vessel diameter has been achieved. Pain may be noted with iliac angioplasty, but severe pain may be a sign of rupture.

Endovascular Technique

AORTIC OCCLUSION

Sheath Placement

Antegrade recanalization is easier than retrograde traversal of a lesion, and access sites should be planned for the arm and both groins. Using a 4-Fr sheath, retrograde brachial artery access is obtained and the wire is manipulated through the descending thoracic and abdominal aorta to the point of occlusion. A flush aortogram is performed, including the abdomen and pelvis, with careful and extended imaging of the vessels beyond the occlusion to determine precisely where the vessel reconstitutes. A multi-purpose angled (MPA) catheter, such as one from Cook Medical (Bloomington, Ind.) or a straight catheter, such as a Quick-Cross (Spectranetics, Colorado Springs, Colo.), is then advanced to the level of the occlusion.

Crossing a Lesion

An angled Glidewire (Terumo Medical Corp., Somerset, N.J.) is manipulated through the occlusion "cap" using a drilling technique. This involves advancing the catheter to the level of the occlusion, with forward force maintained on the catheter to keep it in position, and then rapidly spinning the wire to "drill" through the occlusion, advancing the catheter as a pathway is created (Fig. 31-1). The most difficult part of the occlusion to traverse is the proximal cap, which is often hard to penetrate. Once access through the cap is achieved, the surgeon can more easily advance the wire. After passing the wire and advancing the catheter through the occlusion, an intraluminal position is confirmed by removing the wire and noting blood return through the catheter. Pressure measurement through the catheter or a contrast injection is performed to assure luminal reentry. When crossing the lesion and reentering the true lumen of the aorta proves challenging, a combination of antegrade and retrograde access can be used to achieve through-and-through arm to groin access.

Access in the ipsilateral groin is obtained, and the wire from above is snared to gain brachial-femoral access. A sheath and catheter can then be advanced from the groin through the occlusion to the level of the thoracic aorta. The brachial catheter is pulled back but left in place for later use. The aortic tract is dilated with a 4- to 5-mm balloon.

To achieve access through the contralateral iliac artery, the MPA catheter from the arm is advanced through the previously accessed aortic segment. The use of an angled catheter is helpful, because it allows the wire to be directed within the small aortic channel toward the intended iliac system. Once the catheter is in position and

386 THE ABDOMINAL AORTA AND ILIAC ARTERIES

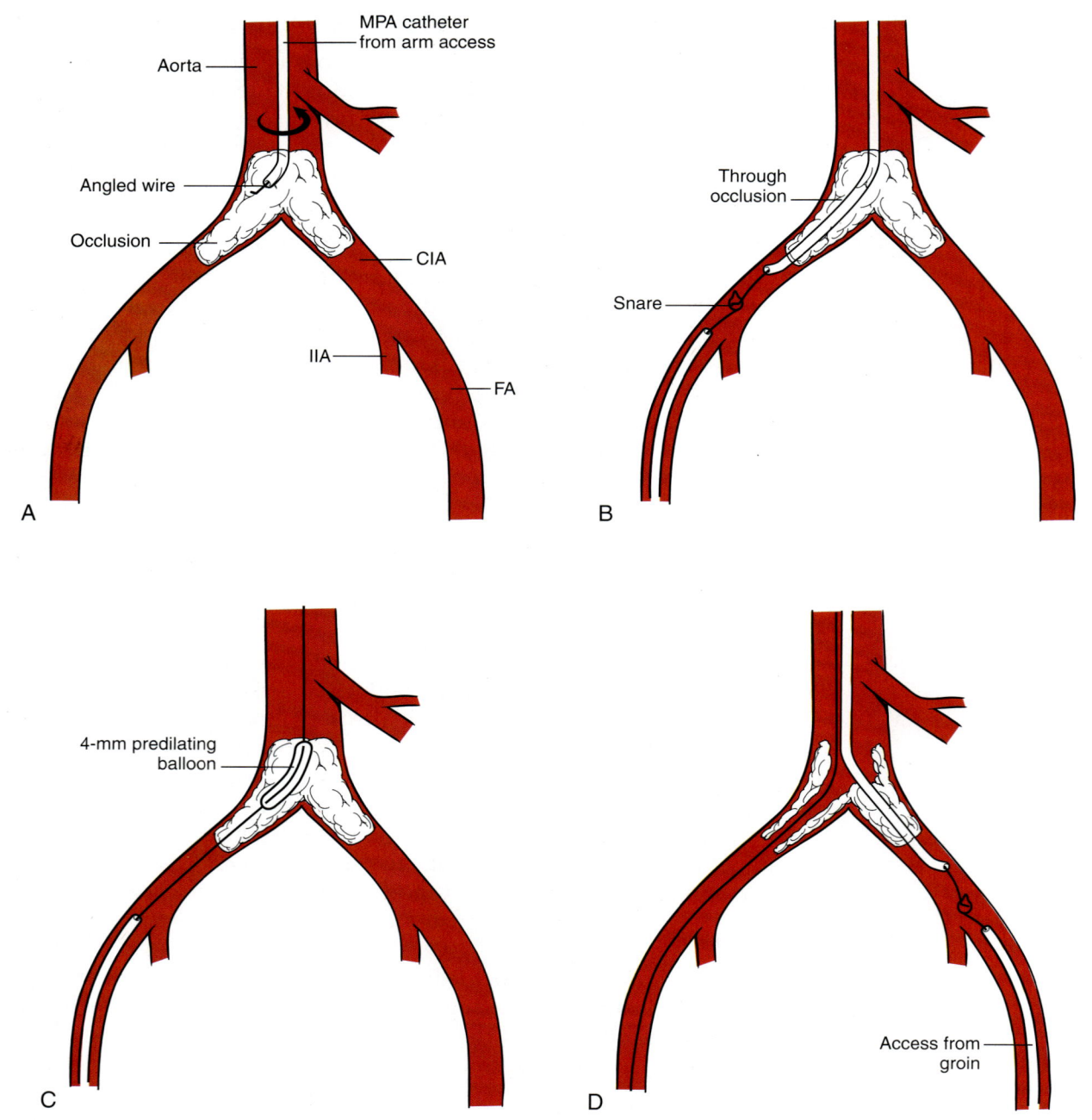

Figure 31-1. Technique for crossing an aortic occlusion. **A,** Wire from a brachial access point is used to cross the aortic occlusion in an antegrade fashion using the drill technique. **B,** Access is gained from the groin, and this wire is snared from below and brought through the occlusion. **C,** The tract is predilated using a 4-mm balloon. **D,** The brachial access is again used to cross through the occlusion to the contralateral groin, and the wire is similarly snared from below. *CIA,* Common iliac artery; *FA,* femoral artery; *IIA,* internal iliac artery.

aimed appropriately, recanalized antegrade access is achieved with the drilling technique, as used in the aorta. Lumen reentry is again confirmed. The wire from the arm is snared from the groin, and a sheath and catheter from the groin are advanced through the occlusion into the thoracic aorta. There is now access from each groin above the level of the occlusion. Dilation of the iliac artery should be performed with a low-profile 4- to 5-mm angioplasty balloon to assure access across the occlusion is maintained. The brachial catheter is removed, but the sheath is left in place in the aorta above the occlusion for imaging during intervention.

Angioplasty and Stenting

Routine stenting is recommended.[25,26] IVUS can assist in determining the diameter of the aorta and iliac arteries, and a calibrated catheter can be used to determine stent length. A self-expanding 12- to 14-mm stent is generally adequate through the aortic channel. The aortic stent should be placed within 1 cm of the bifurcation, delivered from either groin, and dilated to 8 to 10 mm. The wire from the opposite groin must be manipulated to regain access into the aortic stent. If difficulty exists, brachial access may be used for antegrade entry through the aortic stent, followed by snaring of the wire.

With access from both groins through the aortic stent, kissing iliac stents can be placed to recreate the bifurcation. Balloon-expandable stents are used in this position to facilitate precise and symmetric placement, with both stents placed about 5 mm into the aortic stent and dilated to adequate size.

COMMON ILIAC ARTERY OCCLUSION

Sheath Placement

Three methods of access can be used to treat iliac lesions: ipsilateral groin access with retrograde recanalization, contralateral groin access with use of a reverse-curved catheter for antegrade recanalization, and brachial access with antegrade recanalization. Any combination of these methods may be used or required for crossing a difficult lesion. An occlusion in the iliac system tends to have an increased plaque diameter proximally within the vessel, which makes true lumen reentry difficult when attempted in a retrograde fashion. Nonetheless, although retrograde recanalization may be difficult, an initial attempt is appropriate, because ipsilateral groin access is required to deliver a stent.

Crossing a Lesion

Either a drill technique or a subintimal technique may be used to recanalize the lesion. In the latter approach, a subintimal dissection plane is created using a slightly angled 4- to 5-Fr catheter with an angled hydrophilic guidewire (Fig. 31-2). Once the wire is advanced across the cap of the lesion and pushed forward, it naturally forms a J loop. The wire loop and catheter are continually advanced through the plane until a loss of resistance is felt. At this point the occlusion has been passed, and the native lumen should be reentered beyond the level of the occlusion. Confirmation that the catheter passed over this wire is within the true lumen is obtained by observing blood in the catheter and contrast injection that fills the true lumen.

In difficult long-segment lesions, the subintimal technique may be used from both proximal and distal access sites. Within the subintimal plane, the wire from either a proximal or a distal approach can be snared from the other access site. In some circumstances the manipulation of snare and wire within this plane proves challenging, and the wires may not reside in the same subintimal plane. In this situation dilation of the subintimal tract with a small-diameter, 4-mm balloon can be used to enlarge the subintimal space and in some instances to directly connect the channels in which the wires reside. After dilation, a second attempt at snaring the wire should prove successful. Use of a reentry device is another option.

Angioplasty and Stenting

In the case of occlusion, routine stenting should be performed.[26] Balloon-expandable stents should be used in the common iliac arteries, especially if the iliac orifice is involved. If the occlusion abuts within 5 mm or less of the aortic bifurcation, consideration should be given to placement of kissing iliac stents. If there is adequate distance from the bifurcation, a unilateral stent may be placed, but it may be necessary to protect the contralateral side using simultaneous balloon occlusion. This maneuver prevents embolization down the contralateral leg and limits narrowing of the contralateral orifice from associated displacement of the aortic bifurcation.

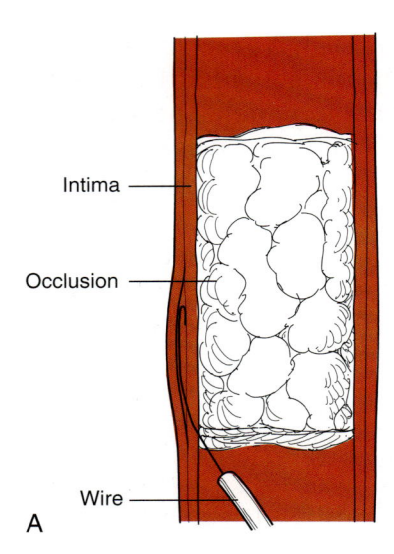

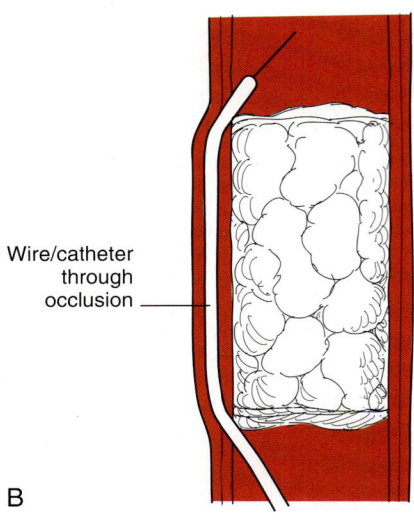

Figure 31-2. Subintimal technique for crossing an occlusion. **A,** Wire is passed into the subintimal plane. The characteristic J loop is formed. **B,** Once past the occlusion, the wire reenters the true lumen, forming a new channel to bypass the occlusion.

EXTERNAL ILIAC ARTERY OCCLUSION

Sheath Placement

Treatment of an external iliac artery occlusion is performed from either the contralateral groin or the arm, because stenting may be required close to the inguinal ligament. Access and closure from the ipsilateral groin are difficult given the proximity of the access site to the area of treatment.

If the occlusion extends into the common femoral artery, a hybrid procedure is recommended. This involves a limited groin incision with exposure of the common femoral, superficial femoral, and profunda femoris arteries. Either conventional endarterectomy with a saphenous vein patch or eversion endarterectomy may be performed. Eversion endarterectomy involves transecting the common femoral artery close to the bifurcation, which is then everted both proximally and distally to remove the plaque (Fig. 31-3). Transection close to the bifurcation is especially important when disease extends into the superficial femoral and profunda femoris arteries, because this provides access to both vessels during distal eversion. The common femoral artery is reapproximated by a running suture on the back wall and with interrupted sutures on the front wall.

Crossing a Lesion

A subintimal technique is favored in the external iliac artery, because the disease segment tends to be longer.

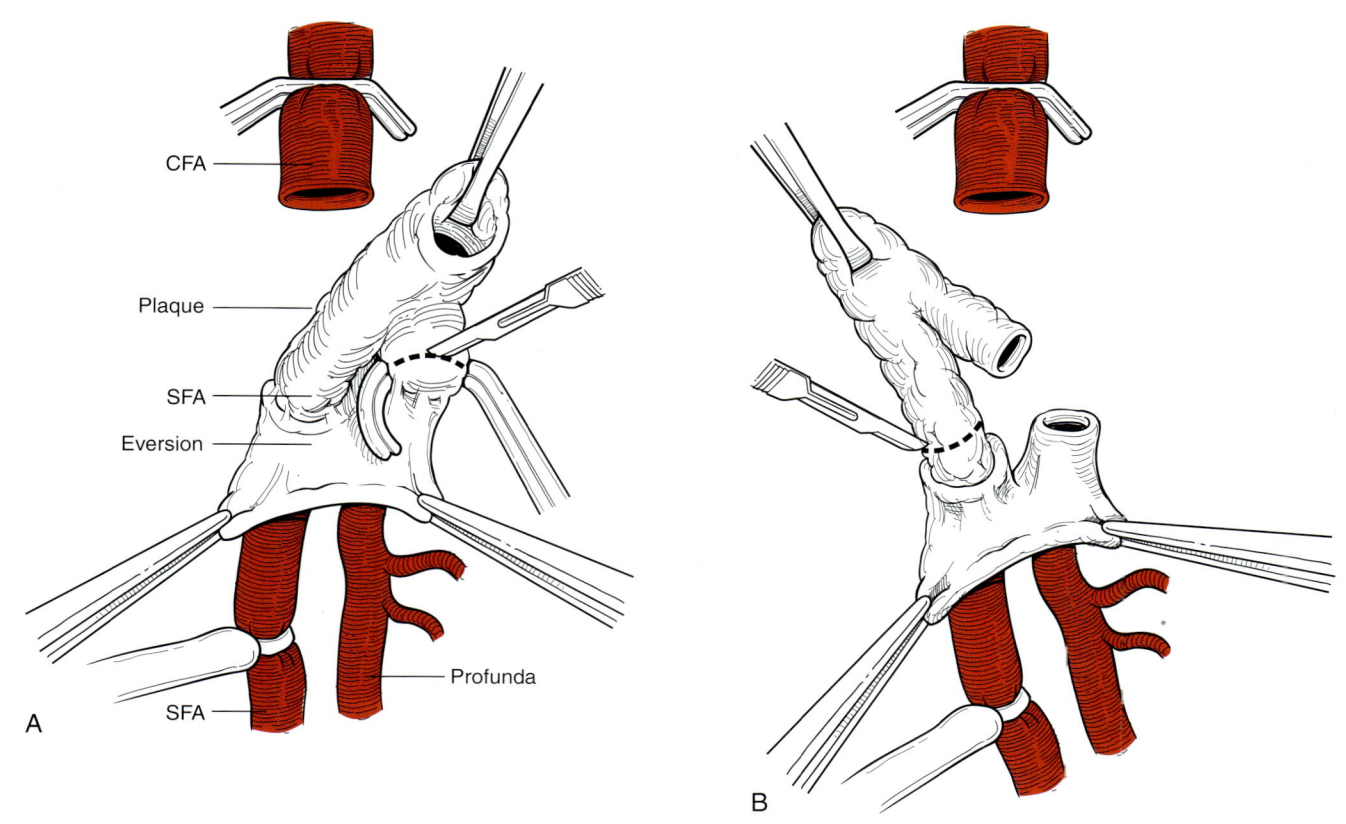

Figure 31-3. Eversion femoral endarterectomy technique. Arteriotomy is made close to the bifurcation to allow eversion of both the superficial femoral artery and the profunda femoris artery, if needed CFA, Common femoral artery; SFA, superficial femoral artery.

Angioplasty and Stenting

Routine stenting is recommended for treatment of an occlusion. Self-expanding stents are preferred, because the external iliac artery is subjected to flexion and extension with hip motion. The external iliac artery is more susceptible to rupture than the common iliac artery because of its small size and propensity for calcification.

Management of Arterial Dissection, Embolization, Occlusion, and Rupture

Arterial dissection can occur after angioplasty or overdilation of heavily calcified vessels. Dissection can be recognized by the presence of contrast on either side of the dissection flap. It may be treated by low-pressure, extended-duration balloon inflation as an attempt to "tack down" the dissection flap. However, stenting should be performed if the dissection is flow limiting.

If significant distal embolization or occlusion has occurred, it is important to ensure that the patient is adequately heparinized. Embolic debris may be retrieved using an aspiration catheter, mechanical thrombectomy device, or in some situations atherectomy with or without use of a thrombolytic agent. If these approaches fail, open embolectomy may be required.

Vessel rupture can be recognized in the awake patient by complaints of severe pain with subsequent hypotension. If significant pain is noted with dilation but vessel diameter is not optimal, slow, gradual dilation can be performed with frequent contrast injections around the shaft of the balloon to assess for rupture. If rupture occurs, the balloon can be inflated at the level of the rupture to occlude flow and a covered stent can be placed over the perforation. Dilation of the balloon above or below the site allows continued bleeding from the rupture. The sheath may often be inadequate for delivery of a covered stent and need to be replaced. If the patient requires balloon occlusion for hemodynamic stability, then access must be achieved from an alternate site and occlusion is performed above the area of the injury during sheath replacement. A covered stent can then be deployed, and the proximal occluding balloon can be deflated.

If the patient remains stable with balloon deflation, the larger sheath should be readied, along with the covered stent; the balloon should be deflated rapidly; and the sheath and balloon should be removed simultaneously. After upsizing of the sheath, balloon reinflation allows time to infuse volume and assess the tear and the extent of the artery that needs to be treated. Imaging can be performed around the shaft of the balloon, and the stent graft can be deployed after removal of the balloon. If the perforation is near the bifurcation or in the aorta, an aortic occlusion balloon should be delivered from the contralateral groin. Bilateral proximal iliac artery covered stents may be necessary. Rupture of the aorta or iliac arteries is rare if adequate imaging and appropriate device sizing have been performed.

Postoperative Care

- All patients are admitted postoperatively for overnight observation and assessment of renal function.
- Patients with renal insufficiency are continued on sodium bicarbonate and N-acetylcysteine.
- Clopidogrel should be continued for 4 to 6 weeks.[17]
- An office evaluation and noninvasive imaging, including duplex ultrasound and segmental lower extremity pressures, are performed in 4 to 6 weeks. If an aortic intervention was performed, CT angiography may also be considered.

Complications

- **Renal insufficiency.** The risk of renal failure may be higher when performing an intervention for a chronic infrarenal occlusion.[27]
- **Local wound complications.** Rates of pseudoaneurysm, bleeding, and thrombosis related to access site vary from 1% to 3%.[28] Complication risk may be higher with brachial access, warranting consideration of operative exposure rather than percutaneous puncture.[29]

REFERENCES

1. Upchurch GR, Dimick JB, Wainess RM, et al: Diffusion of new technology in health care: The case of aorto-iliac occlusive disease, *Surgery* 136:812-818, 2004.
2. Park KB, Do YS, Kim DI, et al: The TransAtlantic InterSociety Consensus (TASC) classification system in iliac arterial stent placement: Long-term patency and clinical limitations, *J Vasc Interv Radiol* 18:193-201, 2007.
3. Carnevale FC, De Blas M, Merino S, et al: Percutaneous endovascular treatment of chronic iliac artery occlusion, *Cardiovasc Inter Rad* 27:447-452, 2004.
4. Uher P, Nyman U, Lindh M, et al: Long-term results of stenting for chronic iliac artery occlusion, *J Endovasc Ther* 9:67-75, 2002.
5. Henry M, Amor M, Ethevenot G, et al: Percutaneous endoluminal treatment of iliac occlusions: Long-term follow-up in 105 patients, *J Endovasc Surg* 5:228-235, 1998.
6. Leville CD, Kashyap VS, Clair DG, et al: Endovascular management of iliac artery occlusions: Extending treatment to TransAtlantic Inter-Society Consensus class C and D patients, *J Vasc Surg* 43:32-39, 2006.
7. Sixt S, Alawied AK, Rastan A, et al: Acute and long-term outcome of endovascular therapy for aortoiliac occlusive lesions stratified according to the TASC classification: A single-center experience, *J Endovasc Ther* 15:408-416, 2008.
8. Kashyap VS, Pavkov ML, Bena JF, et al: The management of severe aortoiliac occlusive disease: Endovascular therapy rivals open reconstruction, *J Vasc Surg* 48:1451-1457, 2008. 1457 e1–e3.
9. Nishibe T, Kondo Y, Dardik A, et al: Hybrid surgical and endovascular therapy in multifocal peripheral TASC D lesions: Up to three-year follow-up, *J Cardiovasc Surg (Torino)* 50:493-499, 2009.
10. Rzucidlo EM, Powell RJ, Zwolak RM, et al: Early results of stent-grafting to treat diffuse aortoiliac occlusive disease, *J Vasc Surg* 37:1175-1180, 2003.
11. Merten GJ, Burgess WP, Gray LV, et al: Prevention of contrast-induced nephropathy with sodium bicarbonate: A randomized controlled trial, *JAMA* 291:2328-2334, 2004.

12. Kelly AM, Dwamena B, Cronin P, et al: Meta-analysis: Effectiveness of drugs for preventing contrast-induced nephropathy, *Ann Intern Med* 148:284-294, 2008.
13. Eisenberg RL, Bank WO, Hedgock MW: Renal failure after major angiography can be avoided with hydration, *AJR Am J Roentgenol* 136:859-861, 1981.
14. Tonstad S, Farsang C, Klaene G, et al: Bupropion SR for smoking cessation in smokers with cardiovascular disease: A multicentre, randomised study, *Eur Heart J* 24:946-955, 2003.
15. Faulkner KW, House AK, Castleden WM: The effect of cessation of smoking on the accumulative survival rates of patients with symptomatic peripheral vascular disease. *Med J Aust* 1:217-219, 1983.
16. Fleisher LA, Beckman JA, Brown KA, et al: 2009 ACCF/AHA focused update on perioperative beta blockade incorporated into the ACC/AHA 2007 guidelines on perioperative cardiovascular evaluation and care for noncardiac surgery: A report of the American College of Cardiology Foundation/American Heart Association Task Force on practice guidelines, *Circulation* 120:e169-e276, 2009.
17. Mehta SR, Yusuf S, Peters RJ, et al: Effects of pretreatment with clopidogrel and aspirin followed by long-term therapy in patients undergoing percutaneous coronary intervention: The PCI-CURE study, *Lancet* 358:527-533, 2001.
18. King SB III, Smith SC Jr, Hirshfeld JW Jr, et al: 2007 focused update of the ACC/AHA/SCAI 2005 guideline update for percutaneous coronary intervention: A report of the American College of Cardiology Foundation/American Heart Association Task Force on practice guidelines, *J Am Coll Cardiol* 51:172-209, 2008.
19. Hertzer NR, Beven EG, Young JR, et al: Coronary artery disease in peripheral vascular patients. A classification of 1000 coronary angiograms and results of surgical management, *Ann Surg* 199:223-233, 1984.
20. Eagle KA, Berger PB, Calkins H, et al: ACC/AHA guideline update for perioperative cardiovascular evaluation for noncardiac surgery: Executive summary, *Circulation* 105:1257-1267, 2002.
21. Fleisher LA, Beckman JA, Brown KA, et al: ACC/AHA 2007 guidelines on perioperative cardiovascular evaluation and care for noncardiac surgery: A report of the American College of Cardiology Foundation/American Heart Association Task Force on practice guidelines, *Circulation* 116:e418-e499, 2007.
22. Bauer SM, Cayne NS, Veith FJ: New developments in the preoperative evaluation and perioperative management of coronary artery disease in patients undergoing vascular surgery, *J Vasc Surg* 51:242-251, 2010.
23. Motarjeme A, Gordon GI, Bodenhagen K: Thrombolysis and angioplasty of chronic iliac artery occlusions, *J Vasc Interv Radiol* 6:S66-S72, 1995.
24. Duc SR, Schoch E, Pfyffer M, et al: Recanalization of acute and subacute femoropopliteal artery occlusions with the rotarex catheter: One year follow-up, single center experience, *Cardiovasc Inter Rad* 28:603-610, 2005.
25. Simons PC, Nawijn AA, Bruijninckx CM, et al: Long-term results of primary stent placement to treat infrarenal aortic stenosis, *Eur J Vasc Endovasc Surg* 32:627-633, 2006.
26. Klein WM, van der Graaf Y, Seegers J, et al: Dutch iliac stent trial: Long-term results in patients randomized for primary or selective stent placement, *Radiology* 238:734-744, 2006.
27. Moise MA, Alvarez-Tostado JA, Clair DG, et al: Endovascular management of chronic infrarenal aortic occlusion, *J Endovasc Ther* 16:84-92, 2009.
28. Powell RJ, Rzucidlo EM. Aortoiliac disease: Endovascular treatment. In Rutherford RB, editor: *Vascular surgery*, ed 7, Philadelphia, 2010, Saunders, pp 1667-1681.
29. Alvarez-Tostado JA, Moise MA, Bena JF, et al: The brachial artery: A critical access for endovascular procedures, *J Vasc Surg* 49:378-385, 2009.

32 Spine Exposure

JEFFREY L. BALLARD

Historical Background

Anterior intervertebral body fusion was described in 1932 by Carpenter[1] and promoted by Hodgson and Stock[2] in 1956 as a definitive treatment of anteriorly oriented spine pathology while avoiding posterior element injury. Anterior discectomy, decompression, and intervertebral fusion are usually combined with supplemental posterior fixation to increase the rate of complete spinal fusion. Spine exposure for lumbosacral (LS) pathology was originally performed through an open retroperitoneal exposure using a large incision, with extensive tissue manipulation and significant patient morbidity.[3] The anterior retroperitoneal approach is currently performed using a miniature open technique with minimal tissue manipulation, taking advantage of the space between the peritoneal contents and kidney anteriorly and the quadratus lumbar and psoas muscles posteriorly to afford excellent anterior spine exposure. Other recently described surgical approaches, such as an endoscopic retroperitoneal exposure and endoscopic lateral transpsoas exposure, capitalize on the retroperitoneal approach without compromising anterior spine exposure.[3-16] Laparoscopic transperitoneal spine exposure also has it proponents.[6,8,9,11] Regardless of the preferred technique, all surgical approaches necessitate dissection and mobilization of the thoracic aorta, abdominal aorta, or iliac arteries with the accompanying vena cava and iliac veins depending upon the disc levels that require fusion.

Notwithstanding the potential for major arterial or venous injury during anterior spine exposure, significant injury to other vulnerable structures may also occur during spine exposure.[4] Recognition of these possible complications has led most centers of excellence to develop a two-team approach, consisting of vascular surgery and either orthopedic surgery or neurosurgery, to minimize morbidity and to maximize optimal operative exposure for reconstructive spine surgery. Advantages of the anterior spine exposure include preservation of posterior elements, decreased incidence of nerve injury, and avoidance of epidural scarring.[3] From the perspective of the vascular surgeon, the key to success is providing the spine surgeon with adequate exposure so that discectomy, decompression, and partial corpectomy can be safely performed from vertebra side to side and implants accurately inserted based on the center of the disc space.

Preoperative Preparation

- **Risk assessment.** Patients who need spine exposure are often younger, have few to no risk factors for coronary or peripheral arterial disease, and are frequently overweight because of inactivity. Patients often have chronic back pain with radiculopathy and a long-standing pain syndrome that is managed by multiple specialists. Many have had a work-related injury. Older patients may need preoperative cardiac stress testing or pulmonary function studies, particularly if the procedure requires thoracic spine exposure.

- **Peripheral vascular examination.** LS spine exposure involves extensive mobilization of major arteries within the abdomen and pelvis, as well as their accompanying major veins. Therefore the presence of an abnormality in the peripheral pulse examination should prompt preoperative noninvasive testing and, if indicated, computed tomography (CT) angiography or formal arteriography for further evaluation. An accurate assessment of peripheral pulses before surgery is mandatory, because temporary vessel occlusion may occur during miniature open retroperitoneal anterior spine exposure.
- **Role of preoperative imaging.** Significant aortoiliac artery calcification increases the risk of arterial injury or dissection as a consequence of retractor placement. The extent of calcification can be evaluated with plain radiographs or CT imaging.
- **Surgical history.** In addition to peripheral pulse examination, assessment of the thorax, abdomen, and flank for signs of previous chest or abdominal procedures may influence the placement of the operative incision. For instance, the lower LS spine can be exposed via a right retroperitoneal approach if the procedure is a redo operative procedure in which adjacent proximal or distal disc levels are being exposed, or if there has been prior abdominal surgery in the left upper or lower quadrant.
- **Incision position and length.** The proposed incision should be discussed with the patient before surgery. Incision length may need to be extended to facilitate adequate spine exposure when there is significant calcific atherosclerotic disease or the patient has a large body habitus.
- **Obtaining consent.** Possible complications of surgery should be reviewed with the patient, including major artery or vein injury, bowel or ureter injury, deep vein thrombosis, wound infection or seroma, and nerve injury. In addition, the patient should be aware of the potential risk of erectile dysfunction, which usually consists of retrograde ejaculation, as opposed to impotence, due to disruption of the intermesenteric nerve plexus and superior hypogastric nerve plexus that course over the left common iliac artery origin.[4] Significant anterior spinal scarring is present in the setting of infection or a history of previous anterior or posterior laminectomy with an attendant increased risk of complication.

Pitfalls and Danger Points

- **Morbid obesity.** In a morbidly obese patient, the risks of surgery often exceed the benefits until significant weight loss has been achieved.
- **Redo surgery.** Redo operative procedures are always associated with significant scarring of the anterior spine, which results in adherent vessels and ureteral fixation. This is particularly true for explantation of previously placed artificial discs, which occasionally become displaced or have component failure. Alternate spine access strategies are often used for these potentially complicated cases.[17] Arteriorrhaphy or venorrhaphy with pledgeted polypropylene suture is recommended when an injury is encountered, because these vessels tend to be friable when redissected off the anterior spine surface. Large venous rents are best controlled with a side-biting vascular clamp, because it may not be possible to occlude the vein proximal and distal to the injury site without risking further injury.
- **Calcified arteries.** Calcified arteries present a unique problem because of the retraction required to expose the disc space. Even pliable vessels are frequently retracted at rather acute angles to limit dissection yet afford complete disc space exposure. Therefore the risk of arterial injury or dissection increases significantly when the vessel is heavily calcified. The best way to avoid calcified vessel injury is to mobilize more length of the artery proximal and distal to the disc levels of

interest, even if this requires extension of the incision or more mobilization of adjacent structures.

- **Vascular injury.** Significant arterial injury is rarely encountered during anterior spine exposure, but if it is noted, appropriate arterial reconstruction should be performed as needed, as opposed to risking acute arterial occlusion by applying multiple blindly directed sutures and pledgets to an injured vessel. To appropriately expose and securely repair a seemingly uncontrollable major venous injury, it is best to partially excise and subsequently repair the common iliac artery rather than risk exsanguinating hemorrhage by multiple failed attempts at vascular control.

- **L4-5 discectomy.** Although tempting in some cases, it is unwise to perform discectomy and spinal instrumentation at more than one disc space at a time. Attempting to expose multiple levels at once either occludes the aorta or common iliac artery or risks significant damage to the confluence of the common iliac veins and vena cava. This is especially true when the L4-5 disc space is involved, because there can be significant variability in the arterial and venous anatomy. In the usual scenario, the disc space is exposed after left-to-right mobilization of the aorta and left common iliac artery across the anterior spine. However, the left common iliac artery and vein occasionally need to be separated and retracted away from each other to fully expose the disc space without prolonged arterial occlusion or arterial injury. Less common dissection schemes occasionally need to be used at the L4-5 disc space, in cases with a high aortic bifurcation or duplicated vena cava. These alternate schemes are particularly helpful for redo cases, in which the iliac veins may be densely adherent to part of the anterior surface of the spine, or after previous posterior LS spine surgery, when significant scarring of the anterior spine surface may be encountered.

- **Right-sided discectomy.** Spine exposure performed from a right-sided miniature open retroperitoneal approach necessitates mobilization of the vena cava and to some extent the right common iliac vein for lower LS spine procedures. Retraction of the vena cava medially all the way across the anterior surface of the spine often occludes the vessel and results in significant decrease in preload, which is not well tolerated in elderly patients. Depending on arterial or venous anatomy, the disc spaces in these patients may be better exposed by dissecting between the vena cava and the abdominal aorta. There is less compression of each structure with lateral retraction away from the midline.

- **Self-retaining retractors.** Self-retaining renal vein retractors (Omni-Tract Surgical, Minneapolis) are used to maintain disc space exposure and to protect the adjacent vessels and peritoneal contents. These retractors are slightly angled forward at their tip, and this angled portion can usually be positioned to hug the disc space laterally, supplying the spine surgeon with just enough room to operate even in very large patients. These retractors should be placed with care to avoid excessive traction on the mobilized structures and positioned just medial to the sympathetic chains that course along the lateral aspects of the vertebra to protect this structure from inadvertent injury.

Operative Strategy

In most procedures the disc spaces of operative interest are exposed by dissection and mobilization of the overlying vessels from left to right across the midline via a left retroperitoneal approach for LS spine cases or from right to left across the midline via a right thoracotomy for most thoracic spine cases. No single approach lends itself to all circumstances; therefore it is wise to become comfortable with the relationship of the target disc levels to overlying skin and boney structures such as ribs, the costal margin, and the anterior superior iliac spine, because the appropriately placed incision minimizes soft tissue dissection and the extent of vessel mobilization. Palpation of pedal pulses before and after the procedure is also prudent, because temporary arterial occlusion often accompanies disc exposure and spinal instrumentation.

Thoracic spine exposure requires the least extent of vessel dissection, because the interbody implants are designed to be placed from a more lateral position as opposed to LS spine exposure, where the implants are usually positioned from a true anterior approach. Therefore a miniature, open, right or left thoracotomy with the lung deflated is commonly used for cases that are limited to the thoracic spine. Very proximal thoracic spine cases that involve disc pathology from T1 to T3 are usually approached posteriorly except in unusual circumstances that may require medial claviculectomy or ministernotomy. A limited right thoracotomy facilitates spine access and exposure from T3 to T8 or T9, and a limited left thoracotomy is usually used for cases that involve disc pathology from T9 or T10 to T12, although the surgeon can also obtain spine exposure through the L2 vertebra from a low thoracotomy approach if needed.

Thoracolumbar (T12-L2), lumbar (L2-L5), and LS (L5-S1) spine exposure necessitates more extensive mobilization of major abdominal and pelvic vessels and risks injury to other structures within the operative field.[4] Various surgical approaches, including miniature open retroperitoneal, laparoscopic transperitoneal, endoscopic retroperitoneal, and endoscopic lateral transpsoas exposure, have been used for anterior thoracolumbar and LS spine exposure to minimize vessel dissection and surgical morbidity without compromising anterior spine exposure.[4-16]

Transperitoneal LS spine exposure requires extensive mobilization of the mid- and hindgut out of the operative field. This can be a demanding exercise, particularly in obese patients or in those who have dense adhesions as a result of a prior abdominal procedure or inflammatory process. Furthermore, the transperitoneal approach is associated with prolonged postoperative ileus, third-space fluid sequestration, and increased risk of retrograde ejaculation in male patients.[6,12-15] Sasso and associates[15] found a tenfold increased risk of retrograde ejaculation when they compared transperitoneal with retroperitoneal L4 through S1 spine exposure. In addition, transperitoneal exposure risks adhesion formation and postoperative bowel obstruction. Miniature, open, anterior retroperitoneal LS spine exposure has advantages similar to those that have been described for retroperitoneal aortic vascular procedures.[18] This is particularly true in regard to length of hospital stay, postoperative ileus, and perioperative complications.

Operative Technique

THORACIC SPINE EXPOSURE

Thoracic spine exposure is optimized by placing the patient in either the left or the right lateral decubitus position after dual-lumen endotracheal intubation to facilitate lung deflation. A beanbag is useful to support the patient's position on the operating table, and the patient's flank should be positioned over the kidney rest. The free upper extremity can be passed across the upper chest and supported on a cushioned Mayo stand. Care should be taken to ensure appropriate padding of the lower extremities and to be sure that there is no external pressure on the feet or that the feet are severely plantar flexed. Transcranial motor-evoked potential monitoring and somatosensory-evoked potential (SSEP) monitoring of the posterior tibial nerve, with the ulnar nerve as control, are used for all thoracic spine cases.

The rib interspace to enter after the lung is deflated depends primarily on the extent of thoracic spine that is to be exposed. There is no need to divide the costal margin in most cases. In general, the best operating exposure for the spine surgeon is afforded by entering the chest two intercostal levels proximal to the disc level of interest. The lower rib is occasionally removed to facilitate multidisc level access and then morselized for use as a bone graft. However, removal of the rib facilitates spine visualization at the potential cost of increased postoperative pain. Intraoperative fluoroscopy is vital to identify the appropriate disc spaces and to limit the extent of surgical dissection. For proximal thoracic spine exposure via a right thoracotomy, incision of the parietal pleura along the lateral aspect of the thoracic vertebra and limited division of ipsilateral intercostal arteries or veins facilitate anterior exposure of the disc spaces as needed. Venous tributaries coursing into the azygous vein should be divided to prevent injury and troublesome bleeding. The preceding maneuvers are generally sufficient for proximal thoracic spine exposure, and the surgeon rarely encounters an esophagus or vagus nerve that courses parallel and medial to the azygous vein in the proximal chest.

From the left side, the approach for mid- to distal thoracic spine exposure is similar to that mentioned earlier except that the descending thoracic aorta is encountered as the surgeon dissects across the anterior surface of the thoracic vertebra and disc space. After limited division of ipsilateral intercostal arteries and veins, the descending thoracic aorta can be retracted medially with Omni-Tract renal vein retractors to minimize the risk of arterial injury. Preservation of the blood supply to the spinal cord is critical; therefore it is wise to ligate intercostal arteries close to the aorta to preserve potential collateral vessels. Brockstein and colleagues[19] have stressed the importance of the arteria radicularis magna or artery of Adamkiewicz in providing circulation to the anterior spinal artery. This vessel is a branch of either a distal intercostal or a proximal lumbar artery. It has been identified as proximal as T5 and as distal as L4.[19] However, the artery generally arises between the T8 and the L1 vertebra levels. Therefore it is unwise to ligate any large intercostal or proximal lumbar artery unless necessary for adequate disc space exposure. Finally, the diaphragm can be divided in a limited fashion just lateral to its central tendinous portion to extend the dissection distally and thus facilitate exposure through the L1-2 disc space.

T12 TO L2 EXPOSURE

For thoracolumbar (T12-L2) spine exposure, the patient is positioned on the operating table with the kidney rest at waist level and usually in a slightly opened right lateral decubitus position. The kidney rest can be elevated and the operating table can be gently flexed to open the space between the left anterior superior iliac spine and the costal margin. The free left upper extremity is positioned as described earlier. A limited flank incision is made over the anterior extent of the twelfth rib. This decreases the chance of injury to the main trunk of the intercostal nerve within the eleventh intercostal space. Abdominal and flank muscle fibers should be split in their respective orientations as opposed to transected. Resection of the twelfth rib facilitates safe entry into the retroperitoneal space, as well as an extraperitoneal plane of dissection. Alternatively, this limited thoracolumbar spine exposure can be obtained through the tenth or eleventh intercostal space as mentioned earlier, with dissection just lateral to the central tendinous portion of the diaphragm as opposed to inferior to the diaphragm, as described later.

Extraperitoneal entry into the upper left retroperitoneal space exposes the Gerota fascia with the contained left kidney and spleen, which can then be rotated inferomedially off the diaphragm and proximal psoas muscle. This maneuver facilitates exposure of the left diaphragmatic crus, which is divided to reveal the underlying vertebra and abdominal aorta. Limited ligation and division of intercostal and lumbar arteries as needed should be performed to preserve spinal blood flow. The Omni-Tract retraction system, with its multiple and varied blades, is critical for maintaining this exposure. The previously mentioned thoracolumbar spine exposure can also be readily performed from a right flank approach but requires mobilization of the right lobe of the liver and in some cases the vena cava. This limited thoracolumbar spine exposure has also been performed via a left upper quadrant paramedian incision, which affords the spine surgeon superb anterior spine exposure.

L2 TO S1 EXPOSURE

More distal LS spine exposure, typically from L2 through S1, is usually performed with the patient supine via small oblique or transverse left, and occasionally right, paramedian incisions. The lateral lumbar spine radiograph can be useful to determine the appropriate position of the incision for optimal disc exposure. The relationship of the palpable iliac wing, which is easily visualized on the lateral radiograph, to the lower lumbar disc levels provides an excellent determination of the incision level. Transverse incisions that are centered over or just between the target discs are useful for one- or two-level disc exposure cases, and oblique paramedian incisions facilitate multilevel disc exposure. Electromyography, in addition to SSEP monitoring, is used for these cases. A reduction in SSEP amplitude may signal diminished blood flow and ischemia to the affected limb.

In either orientation the incision is carried through the anterior layer of the rectus sheath to expose the rectus abdominis muscle. The muscle belly is dissected medially away from the rectus sheath and retracted laterally to expose the posterior layer of the rectus sheath or the transversalis fascia. These layers are incised to develop an extraperitoneal plane of dissection. Rotation of the peritoneal contents from inferolateral to superomedial opens the lower retroperitoneal space and exposes the major arteries and veins that overlay the spine. For higher levels of lumbar spine exposure, a retronephric, extraperitoneal plane of dissection can be used by rotating the kidney, as well as the peritoneal contents, medially off the psoas muscle. The spleen occasionally requires medial mobilization away from the psoas muscle and diaphragm to facilitate some types of thoracolumbar spine exposure.

These maneuvers, depending on their extent, facilitate exposure of the entire abdominal aorta and left common iliac artery with the accompanying left common iliac vein (Fig. 32-1). Mobilization of these vessels from left to right across the midline is usually required to anteriorly expose the spine and disc space from side to side (Fig. 32-2). The left ureter is generally swept medially with the posterior peritoneum and therefore out of harm's way. However, if the ureter appears to be under too much stretch and at risk for injury, it should be gently dissected away from the medially rotated posterior peritoneum. The ipsilateral vas deferens and testicular or ovarian vessels are gently dissected away from the posterior peritoneum to maintain their normal anatomic positions, and division of the round ligament in women occasionally facilitates medial rotation of the peritoneal contents. The vestigial ipsilateral umbilical artery that courses into the internal iliac artery can be divided with impunity. Careful division and secure ligation of the iliolumbar veins are critical to facilitate exposure of distal LS disc levels, particularly the L4-5 disc space (Fig. 32-3). Finally, and particularly in males, a concerted effort is made to protect the condensation of nerve elements consisting of the intermesenteric nerve plexus and superior hypogastric nerve plexus that course over the left common iliac artery origin (Fig. 32-4). The use of bipolar cautery in this area for small paraspinal bleeders also helps to decrease inadvertent nerve injury.

It is wise to assist the spine surgeon with discectomy, partial corpectomy, and spinal instrumentation to ensure swift recognition and repair of inadvertent vital structure injury. Meticulous hemostasis should be achieved throughout the operative site, and fibrin sealant (Tisseel, Baxter BioSurgery, Deerfield, Ill.) is typically sprayed over each operative disc site to effect complete hemostasis and, in theory, to decrease adhesions over the anterior spine surface.[20] The peritoneal contents are rotated back into place after confirming a palpable pulse in each common iliac artery. The wound should be closed in anatomic layers, and skin is routinely

398 THE ABDOMINAL AORTA AND ILIAC ARTERIES

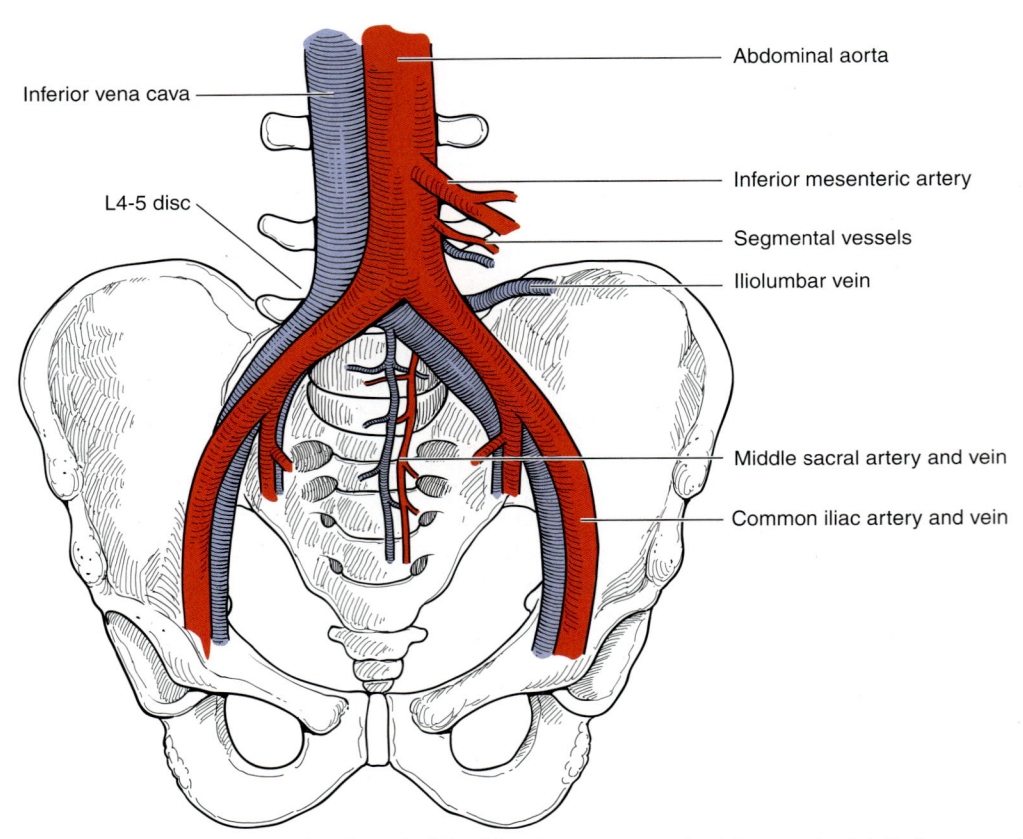

Figure 32-1. Arterial and venous anatomy that is typical for LS spine exposure. In this case the L4-5 disc space is underneath the terminal abdominal aorta and confluence of the common iliac veins.

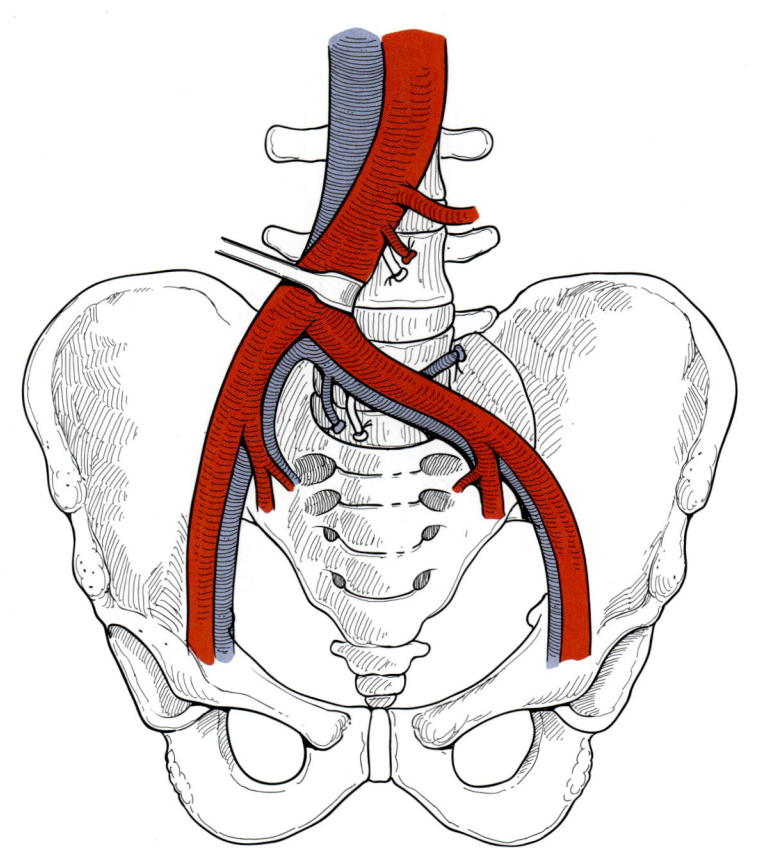

Figure 32-2. Left-to-right vessel mobilization is typically used to facilitate disc exposure.

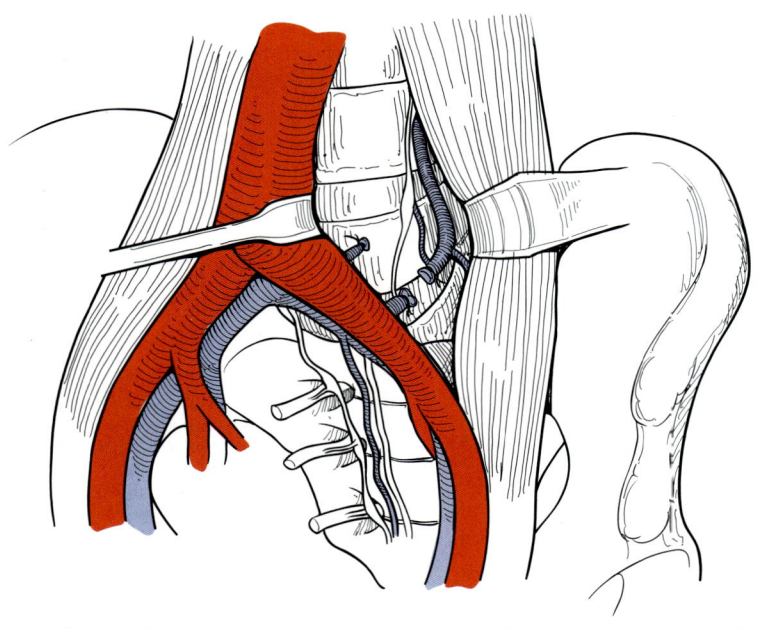

Figure 32-3. Division of the iliolumbar vein (or veins) is key for safe exposure of midlumbar and LS disc levels.

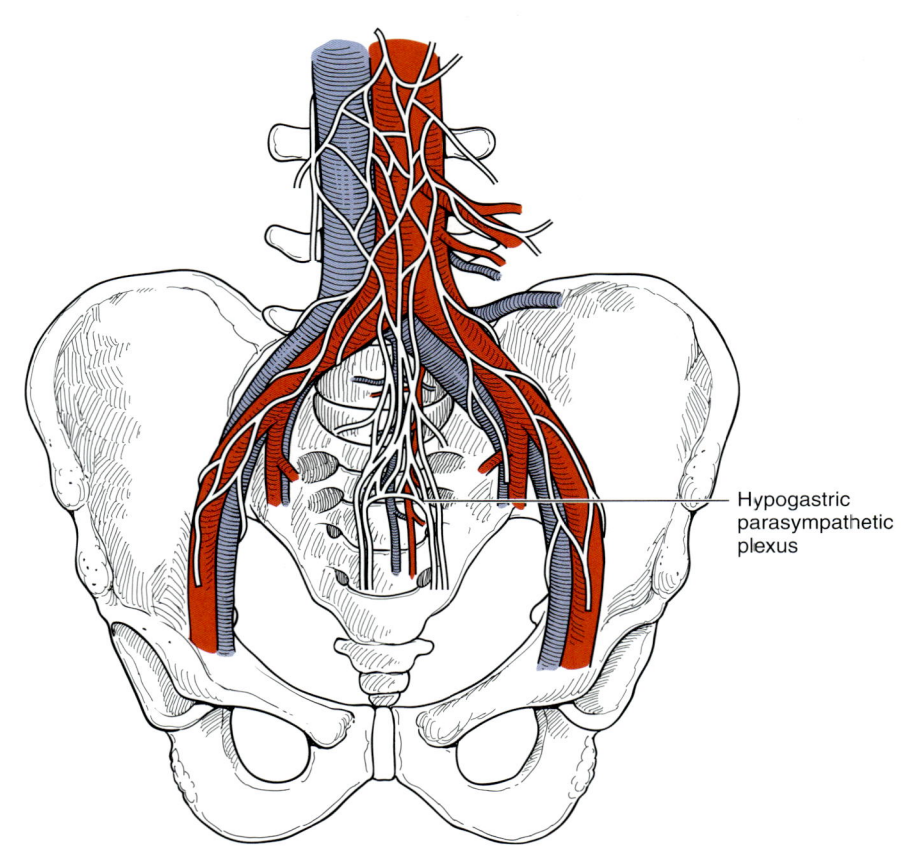

Figure 32-4. Relationship of the infrarenal parasympathetic nerves to the aorta and iliac arteries.

closed in a subcuticular manner. A 1-inch Steri-Strip applied longitudinally for the length of the incision completes the closure. Pedal pulses are confirmed to be present before the patient transfers to the recovery room.

Postoperative Care

- **Postoperative activity.** Patient activity is rapidly progressed during the early postoperative period, and most patients can be discharged to home in 4 or 5 days. The retroperitoneal approach for spine exposure facilitates early return

TABLE 32-1 Vascular Complications Associated With Anterior Retroperitoneal Spine Exposure

Author	Surgical Approach (no. patients)	Intraoperative (no. patients)	Perioperative (no. patients)
Bianchi et al.[4]	Miniature open retroperitoneal (72)	Major vein injury (1)	DVT (1)
Gumbs et al.[7]	Miniature open retroperitoneal (64)	Major vein injury (2) Ureter injury (1)	None
Zdeblick and David[8]	Miniature open retroperitoneal (25)	None	None
Kaiser et al.[9]	Miniature open retroperitoneal (51)	Major vein injury (2)	None
Brau[21]	Miniature open retroperitoneal (684)	Major arterial injury (6) Major vein injury (6)	DVT (7)

DVT, Deep vein thrombosis.

TABLE 32-2 Nonvascular Complications Associated With Anterior Retroperitoneal Spine Exposure

Author	Surgical Approach (no. patients)	Intraoperative (no. patients)	Perioperative (no. patients)
Bianchi et al.[4]	Miniature open retroperitoneal (72)	Small bowel injury (1)	Erectile dysfunction (2) LE paresis (1) Cholecystitis (1) Pneumonia (1) Myocardial infarction (1)
Gumbs et al.[7]	Miniature open retroperitoneal (64)	Scarring/case aborted (2)	Persistent fever (8) Spinal headache (2) Colitis (1)
Zdeblick and David[8]	Miniature open retroperitoneal (25)	None	Retroperitoneal hematoma (1)
Kaiser et al.[9]	Miniature open retroperitoneal (51)	Dural tear (1)	Ileus (1) Retroperitoneal hematoma (1) UTI (1) Wound infection (1) Worse radiculopathy (1)
Brau[21]	Miniature open retroperitoneal (684)	None	Erectile dysfunction (1) Ileus (4) Wound infection (3) Wound hernia (2) Compartment syndrome (2) Myocardial infarction (1) Death (1)

LE, Lower extremity; *UTI*, urinary tract infection.

of normal bowel function and minimizes pulmonary problems.[4] Paramedian and flank incisions are generally well tolerated, and subcuticular wound closure minimizes postoperative wound care.

- **Pain management.** Intercostal nerve block is often helpful in improving lung excursion, cough, and deep breathing for thoracic spine exposure cases. This maneuver has little downside for pneumothorax, because there is already an ipsilateral chest tube in place.
- **Vascular surveillance.** Vascular follow-up occurs as needed, because few to no long-term vascular problems require continued care except for the occasional patient who develops deep vein thrombosis or a chronic wound problem.

Complications

- The miniature, open thoracic, and retroperitoneal approaches are associated with rare intraoperative complications and few perioperative or long-term complications (Tables 32-1 and 32-2).
- Postoperative complications are more common in patients who present with a history of coronary artery disease or whose age is greater than 50 years at the time of surgery.
- Increased operative blood loss and an extended paramedian incision are associated with increased risk of perioperative complications.[4] An oblique paramedian incision is typically used for multilevel disc exposure, and these cases require significant surgical dissection and major vessel mobilization.

REFERENCES

1. Carpenter N: Spondylolisthesis, *Brit J Surg* 19:374-386, 1932.
2. Hodgson AR, Stock FE: Anterior spinal fusion a preliminary communication on the radical treatment of Pott's disease and Pott's paraplegia, *Brit J Surg* 44:266-275, 1956.
3. Foley KT, Holly LT, Schwender JD: Minimally invasive lumbar fusion, *Spine* 28:S26-S35, 2003.
4. Bianchi C, Ballard JL, Abou-Zamzam AM Jr, et al: Anterior retroperitoneal lumbosacral spine exposure: Operative technique and results, *Ann Vasc Surg* 17:137-142, 2003.
5. Bergey DL, Villavicencio AT, Goldstein T, et al: Endoscopic lateral transpsoas approach to the lumbar spine, *Spine* 29:1681-1688, 2004.
6. Kleeman TJ, Michael Ahn U, Clutterbuck WB, et al: Laparoscopic anterior lumbar interbody fusion at L4-L5: An anatomic evaluation and approach classification, *Spine* 27:1390-1395, 2002.
7. Gumbs AA, Shah RV, Yue JJ, et al: The open anterior paramedian retroperitoneal approach for spine procedures, *Arch Surg* 140:339-343, 2005.
8. Zdeblick TA, David SM: A prospective comparison of surgical approach for anterior L4-L5 fusion: Laparoscopic versus mini anterior lumbar interbody fusion, *Spine* 25:2682-2687, 2000.
9. Kaiser MG, Haid RW Jr, Subach BR, et al: Comparison of the mini-open versus laparoscopic approach for anterior lumbar interbody fusion: A retrospective review, *Neurosurgery* 51 97-103, 2002.
10. Gumbs AA, Bloom ND, Bitan FD, et al: Open anterior approaches for lumbar spine procedures, *Am J Surg* 194:98-102, 2007.
11. Shen FH, Samartzis D, Khanna AJ, et al: Minimally invasive techniques for lumbar interbody fusions, *Orthop Clin North Am* 38:373-386, 2007.
12. Tiusanen H, Seitsalo S, Osterman K: Retrograde ejaculation after anterior interbody lumbar fusion, *Eur Spine J* 4:339-342, 1995.
13. Rajaraman V, Vingan R, Roth P: Visceral and vascular complications resulting from anterior lumbar interbody fusion, *J Neurosurg* 91:S60-S64, 1999.
14. Cohn EB, Ignatoff JM, Keeler TC, et al: Exposure of the anterior spine: Technique and experience with 66 patients, *J Urol* 164:416-418, 2000.
15. Sasso RC, Burkus JK, LeHuec JC: Retrograde ejaculation after anterior lumbar interbody fusion: Transperitoneal versus retroperitoneal exposure, *Spine* 28:1023-1026, 2003.
16. Katkhouda N, Campos GM, Mavor E: Is laparoscopic approach to lumbar spine fusion worthwhile? *Am J Surg* 178:458-461, 1999.
17. Wagner WH, Regan JJ, Leary SP, et al: Access strategies for revision or explantation of the Charité lumbar artificial disc replacement, *J Vasc Surg* 44:1266-1272, 2006.
18. Ballard JL, Yonemoto H, Killeen JD: Cost effective aortic exposure: A retroperitoneal experience, *Ann Vasc Surg* 14:1-5, 2000.
19. Brockstein B, Johns L, Gewertz BL: Blood supply to the spinal cord: Anatomic and physiologic correlations, *Ann Vasc Surg* 8:394-399, 1994.
20. Amrani DL, Diorio JP, Delmotte Y: Wound healing: Role of commercial fibrin sealants, *Ann New York Acad of Sciences* 936:566-579, 2001.
21. Brau S: Mini-open approach to the spine for anterior lumbar interbody fusion: Description of the procedure, results and complications, *Spine J* 2:216-223, 2002.

Section 7

LATE AORTIC GRAFT COMPLICATIONS

33 Total Graft Excision and Extraanatomic Repair for Aortic Graft Infection

SUNITA SRIVASTAVA

Historical Background

Many early series recognized that aortic graft infection is difficult to diagnose, is associated with substantial amputation and mortality risks, and has a tendency to recur if inadequately treated.[1-3] It was recognized early on that inadequately treated aortic graft infection could lead to systemic sepsis or, in propagating to the anastomosis, could lead to pseudoaneurysm and hemorrhage from anastomotic disruption. The 0.2% to 2% incidence of aortic graft infection has remained remarkably constant over the last 4 decades, with an interval between initial graft implantation and symptomatic infection ranging between 41 and 62 months and amputation and mortality rates of 11% and 40%, respectively.[4-10]

Graft infection may occur at the time of initial surgery because of contamination from skin flora or exposure to bowel organisms through an unrecognized enterotomy during graft tunneling (Fig. 33-1). Other factors associated with the development of aortic graft infection include emergent repairs, lengthy procedures, development of wound complications, or perioperative bacteremia from a urinary tract infection, line sepsis, or pneumonia. Aortofemoral reconstructions are more prone to infection than aortoiliac bypasses, probably because of risk of groin wound necrosis or infection.[5] Although many aortic graft infections can be indolent, others can manifest with protean clinical symptoms of hemorrhage or systemic sepsis.

Graft infections have been categorized as early or late based upon time of presentation after implantation. Early aortic graft infections are often associated with more virulent organisms than those presenting late. Most common causative organisms are *Staphylococcus*, with *Staphylococcus aureus* often implicated in early infection and coagulase negative *Staphylococcus*, such as *Staphylococcus epidermis*, more prevalent in late infections.[11] *Enterococcus* organisms, gram-negative organisms, fungi, and anaerobes can also be cultured, especially in the presence of graft-enteric erosion. In many aortic graft infections, however, an organism is not identified because of lack of suitable specimens, because of inadequate culture methods, or because antimicrobial coverage was instituted before the collection of tissue for culture.

Early reports demonstrated that simultaneous graft excision and revascularization were associated with very high mortality, so delaying or omitting revascularization was initially advocated to decrease the magnitude of the procedure, even though it was practical for only a minority of patients.[12] Staged extraanatomic arterial reconstruction followed by graft excision was first reported by Elliott and colleagues in 1974.[13] Objections were initially raised to this approach because of concerns related to the presumed risk of bacterial seeding of the new prosthesis, thrombosis of the extraanatomic graft from competitive flow, and risk of interval hemorrhage

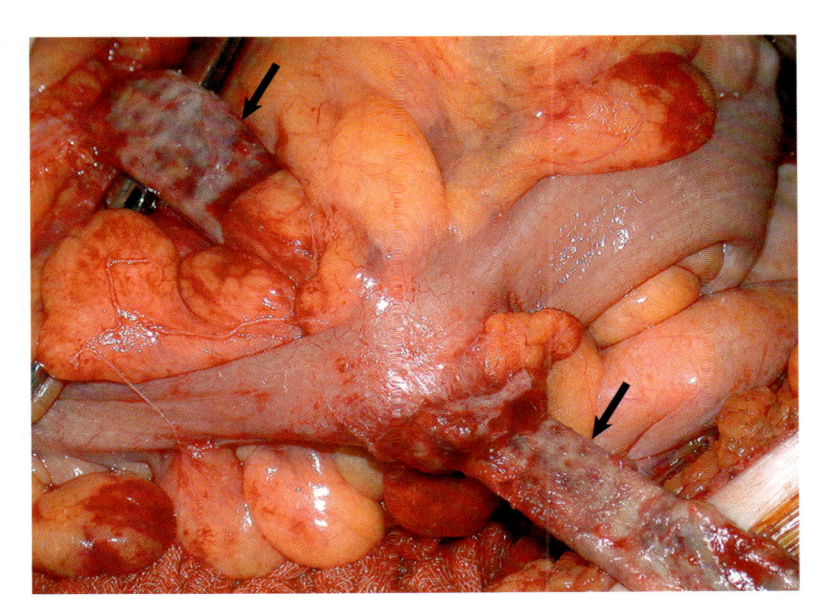

Figure 33-1. Intraoperative photograph of the left limb of an infected aortofemoral graft *(arrows)* tunneled through the sigmoid colon.

from the infected graft in the period prior to graft excision. Reilly and associates subsequently demonstrated in a large series that these concerns were unfounded with use of adequate antibiotic coverage and graft removal within 1 week of the initial extraanatomic bypass.[8,14]

Preoperative Preparation

- **Clinical manifestations.** The presentation of aortic graft infection can be variable, and early diagnosis is challenging. Patients with a history of prior aortic graft placement presenting with recurrent fever and chills, pain or pulsatile mass in the abdomen or groin, or evidence of wound infection should be suspected to have aortic graft infection, and those presenting with gastrointestinal hemorrhage, systemic sepsis and shock, or vertebral osteomyelitis usually have advanced infection. The spectrum of gastrointestinal hemorrhage is wide. Suture line fistula can lead to abrupt massive bleeding, whereas graft body erosion into the gastrointestinal tract typically results in low-grade bleeding from the intestinal mucosa. Early presentation of *S. aureus* or gram-negative infection in the setting of aortoenteric fistula is typically more virulent and can spread rapidly, leading to anastomotic breakdown and exsanguinating hemorrhage. Methicillin-resistant *S. aureus* has become recognized as a particularly dangerous pathogen because of its destructive characteristics that result in high mortality and risk of limb loss. Indolent, late prosthetic infections may present with limb thrombosis, pseudoaneurysm formation, or fluid collections around poorly incorporated grafts without systemic symptoms and typically involve *S. epidermis*. This organism secretes a glycoprotein biofilm, which makes its detection difficult unless broth culture and graft sonification are used to isolate the organism. Physical examination may reveal exposed graft material in a contaminated wound or abscess cavity. Graft thrombosis, anastomotic pseudoaneurysm, and septic emboli to the lower extremities are consistent with but not diagnostic of chronic graft infection.
- **Laboratory findings.** Leukocytosis, elevated inflammatory markers, positive blood cultures, and anemia may be present but are nonspecific findings.
- **Upper gastrointestinal endoscopy.** Gastroduodenoscopy to the fourth portion of the duodenum should be performed on patients with a history of aortic graft placement presenting with gastrointestinal bleeding to exclude an aortoenteric fistula. This is demonstrated by exposed graft material if a graft-enteric communication is present (Fig. 33-2).

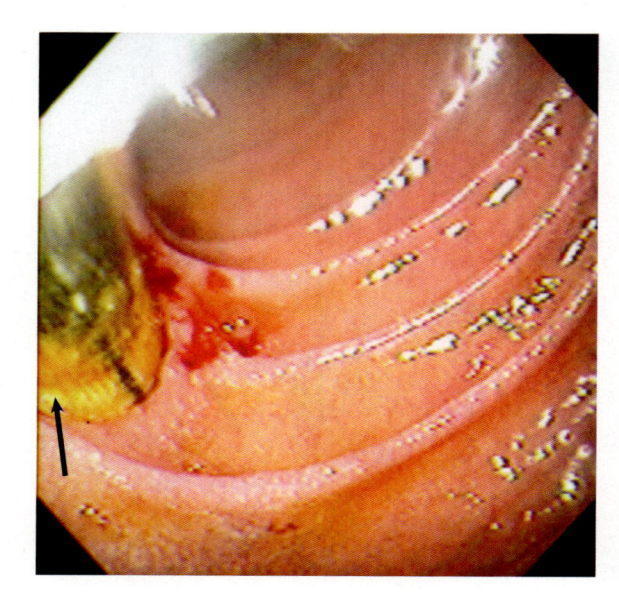

Figure 33-2. Endoscopic photograph taken during gastroduodenoscopy demonstrating an aortoenteric fistula. Note the black line in the synthetic graft and the bile staining of the graft material (arrow).

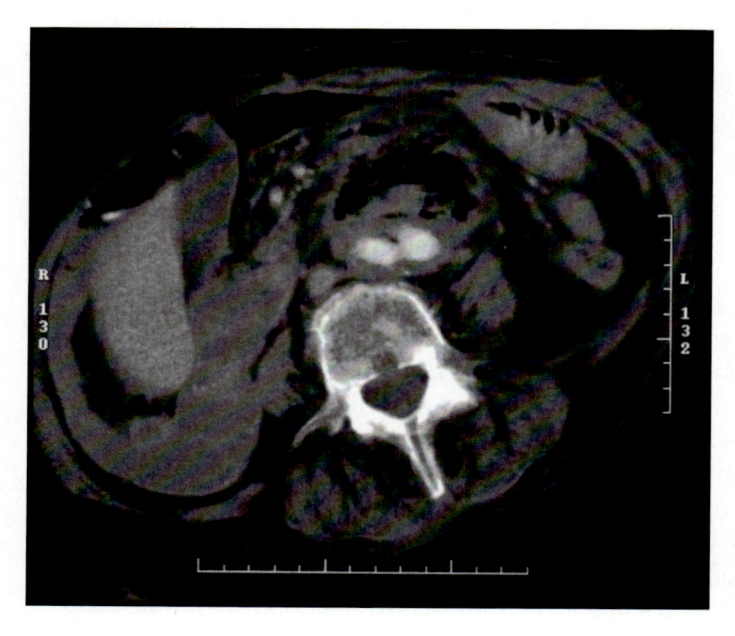

Figure 33-3. CT scan demonstrating gas in an aneurysm sac adjacent to an infected aortobiiliac synthetic graft.

- **Computed tomography (CT) imaging.** CT imaging is the initial diagnostic modality of choice, because it can assess of the extent of graft involvement, as well as provide percutaneous guidance if aspiration of a fluid collection for microbial analysis is required. CT scanning is reported to identify aortic graft infection with a sensitivity of 94% and a specificity of 85%.[15] Characteristic CT findings suggesting the presence of late aortic prosthetic graft infection include periprosthetic gas or fluid, soft tissue thickening, hydronephrosis, vertebral body degeneration, and bowel wall thickening.[16] Although the presence of fluid or loculated air around the graft is common in the early postoperative period after graft implantation, CT demonstration of perigraft gas more than 2 months after aortic reconstruction is suggestive of graft infection (Fig. 33-3).

- **Additional imaging studies.** Although radionuclide tagged white cell scanning has been used to identify aortic graft infection, its utility is limited by false-positive results because of uptake in other inflammatory beds. Duplex ultrasonography can identify fluid collections and the presence of a pseudoaneurysm, but its usefulness is limited by bowel gas and body habitus. Magnetic resonance imaging can evaluate inflammatory changes and soft tissue attenuation and can distinguish hematoma from other fluid collections in determining the extent of graft involvement, but it does not add information to that available through a CT scan. Recent studies have suggested that fused fluoro-2-deoxy-d-glucose positron emission tomography (FDG-PET)-CT imaging may improve the diagnostic accuracy of detecting graft infection.

- **Extent of graft infection.** Determination of the extent of graft infection is important to successful treatment planning. If the entire graft is involved, it will likely require removal in its entirety. However, if only one limb of an aortobifemoral graft is involved, it may be possible to remove only the infected portion and salvage the remaining uninfected graft. Complete graft excision is usually required in early infections, because the graft is not incorporated. However, late infections with solitary limb involvement can be treated with limited graft excision if the rest of the graft is well incorporated. Operative inspection of tissue incorporation into the graft and microbial identification can assist in determining the amount of graft that might be salvaged.

- **Assessment of lower extremity perfusion.** Preoperative assessment of lower extremity perfusion is necessary to plan treatment and may be based on physical examination and lower extremity noninvasive studies. If the infected prosthesis is occluded and the lower extremities are viable, excision of the infected graft material alone should be adequate. However, if lower extremity perfusion depends on the involved graft, extraanatomic bypass is required to avoid amputation once the infected graft is removed. CT or conventional arteriography can identify patent vessels available for revascularization of the lower extremities, if required once the infected graft is removed.

- **Nutritional assessment.** Patients with aortic graft infection are often elderly and debilitated, especially if the process is chronic. Adequate nutritional support is critical to meet the metabolic demands of sepsis and a prolonged operative and postoperative course. In the presence of aortoenteric fistula, enteral nutrition may be delayed for a lengthy period. The transition to enteral nutrition may be facilitated by the use of feeding gastrostomy or jejunostomy.

Pitfalls and Danger Points

- **Failure to control hemorrhage.** Careful preoperative planning should determine options for proximal and distal arterial control and assess the extent of possible involvement of neighboring venous structures.
- **Failure to control sepsis.** Removal of all infected grossly foreign material is mandatory to minimize the risk of persistent or recurrent infection. Careful management of the aortic stump with an omental flap and oversewn femoral vessels with a sartorius muscle flap after graft removal is a critical component of effective treatment.
- **Failure of revascularization.** Assessment of options for revascularization that bypass the infected field, including the need for an axillofemoral, axilloprofunda, or axillopopliteal bypass, is essential to ensure adequate lower extremity perfusion.

Operative Strategy

Critical concepts central to the treatment of aortic synthetic graft infection include excision of the infected graft material, debridement of infected tissue, provision of adequate drainage to control local sepsis, revascularization of critical vascular beds, and appropriate antibiotic therapy for primary infection and to prevent secondary infection in the aortic bed, as well as the extraanatomic bypass.[17]

CHOICE OF RECONSTRUCTION

Considerations influencing the choice of reconstruction after the diagnosis of late prosthetic graft infection include the extent of the graft infection, the infecting organism, the dependence of end-organ perfusion on the graft, and the presence of associated patient comorbidities. Because graft material can harbor organisms, which are excluded from the circulation and consequently are not affected by antibiotics delivered in the bloodstream, complete excision of all infected graft material is imperative to control the persisting sepsis. Continuation of appropriate, broad-spectrum antibiotic therapy is necessary to treat the underlying sepsis and prevent bacterial seeding of the new extraanatomic bypass. If the infected graft is patent and the limbs are depending upon the graft for adequate perfusion, then an alternative method of lower extremity perfusion must be provided when the infected graft is removed. Available options include extraanatomic bypass in clean tissue planes or in situ aortoiliac reconstruction. The latter may be performed using a cryopreserved allogeneic homograft or, in an unstable patient, a polytetrafluoroethylene graft or gelatin-impregnated prosthesis soaked in rifampin (45-60 mg/mL) for 15 minutes. Alternatively, in situ reconstruction can use autogenous deep femoral vein to fashion a neoaortoiliac system procedure, as described in the next chapter.

In general, placement of a synthetic graft in a grossly contaminated bed should be avoided because of the risk of recurrent or persistent graft infection, a situation associated with pseudoaneurysm formation and hemorrhage. However, in situ reconstruction with a synthetic Dacron graft soaked in an antibiotic solution, such as rifampin, may be an expeditious option for carefully selected patients with graft infections attributable to organisms of relatively low virulence, such as *Staphylococcus epidermidis*, in which the infecting organisms are confined to a biofilm on the graft. Important adjuncts to in situ reconstruction include debridement of the aneurysm sac, if present; interposition of healthy tissue, such as omentum around the new prosthesis; and lifelong antibiotic suppression. Extensive synthetic graft infections caused by virulent organisms, such as *Pseudomonas aeruginosa*, are probably better treated with the complete excision of all infected synthetic material followed by extraanatomic bypass placed in uninvolved tissue planes.

STAGING OF EXTRAANATOMIC RECONSTRUCTION AND GRAFT EXCISION

When excision of an infected aortic graft and extraanatomic bypass is planned, the sequence in which the procedures are performed may have important consequences. Several considerations are important when determining the optimal sequence for a particular patient. These include the presence of hemodynamic instability or the potential for rapid decompensation from hemorrhage or sepsis, uncertainty regarding the diagnosis and extent of graft infection, whether lower extremity perfusion depends on the infected graft, and the anticipated duration of the graft excision procedure, especially if additional measures, such as duodenal reconstruction, are likely to be required. Control of hemorrhage is the first priority, but minimizing the duration of lower extremity ischemia while adequately controlling the septic process is necessary for optimal management.

For stable patients in whom the diagnosis and extent of the underlying synthetic graft infection is clear, preliminary extraanatomic bypass is preferable to reduce lower extremity ischemia time. Furthermore, the second stage can sometimes be performed on another day with a fresh team. The theoretical risk of preliminary extraanatomic graft occlusion from competitive flow is usually not a major problem if the interval between stages is minimized. This approach has resulted in substantially higher limb salvage rates compared with simultaneous excision and bypass.[4,8]

If the patient is hemodynamically unstable, usually from active hemorrhage from an aortoenteric fistula or rupture of an anastomotic pseudoaneurysm and less commonly from overwhelming sepsis, then expeditious exploration with control of the hemorrhage, excision of the infected graft material, and adequate drainage is warranted as the initial procedure. Secondary extraanatomic bypass should be performed in clean surgical fields at the same sitting after reprepping and draping the patient and with a new set of instruments, if the lower extremities are severely ischemic.

SELECTION OF AN EXTRAANATOMIC BYPASS

The selection of an extraanatomic bypass depends upon the extent of the underlying graft infection, the extent of associated occlusive disease, and the type of aortic reconstruction requiring removal. If the patient has had a prior aortobiiliac graft and the entire graft is involved, then an axillobifemoral graft is the optimal selection to provide lower extremity perfusion (Fig. 33-4, A). The arm with the highest systolic blood pressure should be used for inflow for the extraanatomic bypass, but if both arm blood pressure measurements are equal, the right axillary artery is preferred, because right subclavian artery occlusive disease is less common than left subclavian artery involvement. This configuration also has the advantage of preserving the option to approach the aorta through the left retroperitoneal approach, if needed in the future. However, if the patient has an infected aortobifemoral graft requiring prosthetic removal from both femoral anastomotic sites, then bilateral axillofemoral bypass grafts tunneled through clean tissue planes to the superficial femoral or above-knee popliteal arteries may be necessary (Fig. 33-4, B). Extension to the popliteal artery can usually be accomplished through a lateral subcutaneous tunnel extending across the distal thigh that traverses medially to the popliteal space at a level above the knee. After graft removal, the resulting femoral arteriotomy sites in the groin incisions are closed with an autogenous patch, such as saphenous vein or endarterectomized superficial femoral artery, and if needed are covered with a sartorius muscle flap.

If only a single distal aortobifemoral graft limb is involved with a groin infection but the remaining graft is uninfected, initial division and ligation of the uninvolved proximal limb is performed through a clean retroperitoneal incision. The distal portion of the limb is left in the wound, unless an obturator bypass is considered, and the incision is closed. Limb perfusion is then be restored by constructing an axillosuperficial femoral artery synthetic bypass graft (Fig. 33-5, A). Alternatively, an obturator bypass graft is tunneled medially through the obturator foramen around the infected groin incision through uninvolved tissue planes (Fig. 33-5, B). After closure and placement of occlusive dressings over the extraanatomic bypass incisions, the infected graft material is then removed from the groin and the anastomotic site in the femoral artery is reconstructed using a patch angioplasty with autogenous material.

AVOIDANCE OF URETERAL INJURY

Because the ureters cross anterior to the iliac arteries, they are often adherent to the limbs of a bifurcated synthetic aortic graft in the anatomic tunnel. Consequently, they may be difficult to identify at the time of reoperation, especially in the presence of severe scarring or distortion from the phlegmon, which is often associated with the synthetic graft infection. To avoid ureteral injury or devascularization in this situation, cystoscopic placement of bilateral ureteral stents is indicated.

CONSIDERATIONS IN THE PRESENCE OF AN AORTOENTERIC FISTULA

It is generally acknowledged that the presence of a secondary aortoenteric fistula is associated with greater mortality and morbidity than is aortic graft infection alone.[4,18] Contamination of the aortic graft from gastrointestinal flora often mandates removal of the entire aortic graft, which typically exhibits bile staining in the region of the graft-enteric communication (Fig. 33-6). Closure of the aortic stump, appropriate drainage, and repair of the duodenum will likely require a fairly lengthy abdominal procedure. Preliminary extraanatomic bypass grafting, if

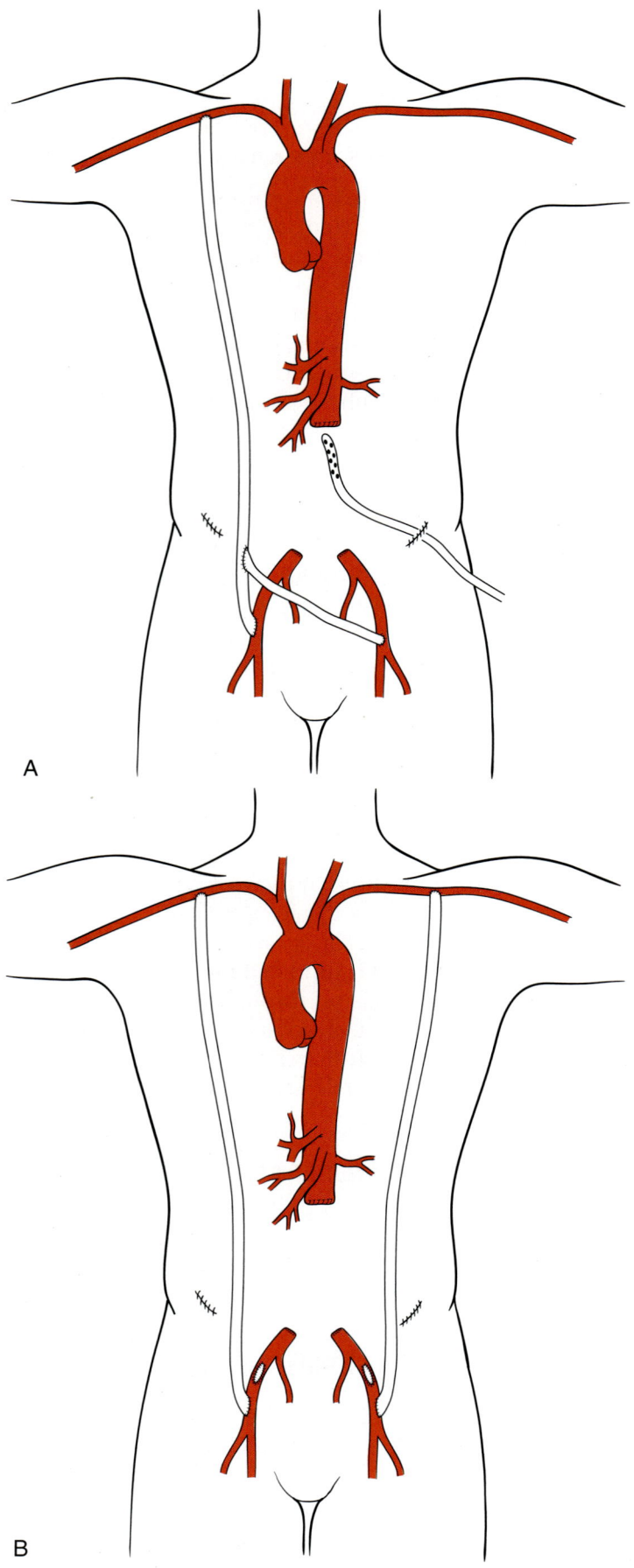

Figure 33-4. A, Right axillobifemoral extraanatomic bypass graft performed to provide lower extremity perfusion after removal of an infected aortobiiliac synthetic graft. Note the large sump drain placed in the aortic bed and brought out through the left flank. **B,** Bilateral axilloproximal superficial femoral artery extraanatomic bypass grafts performed to provide lower extremity perfusion after removal of an infected aortobifemoral synthetic graft. Note the autogenous patch angioplasties used to maintain femoral perfusion.

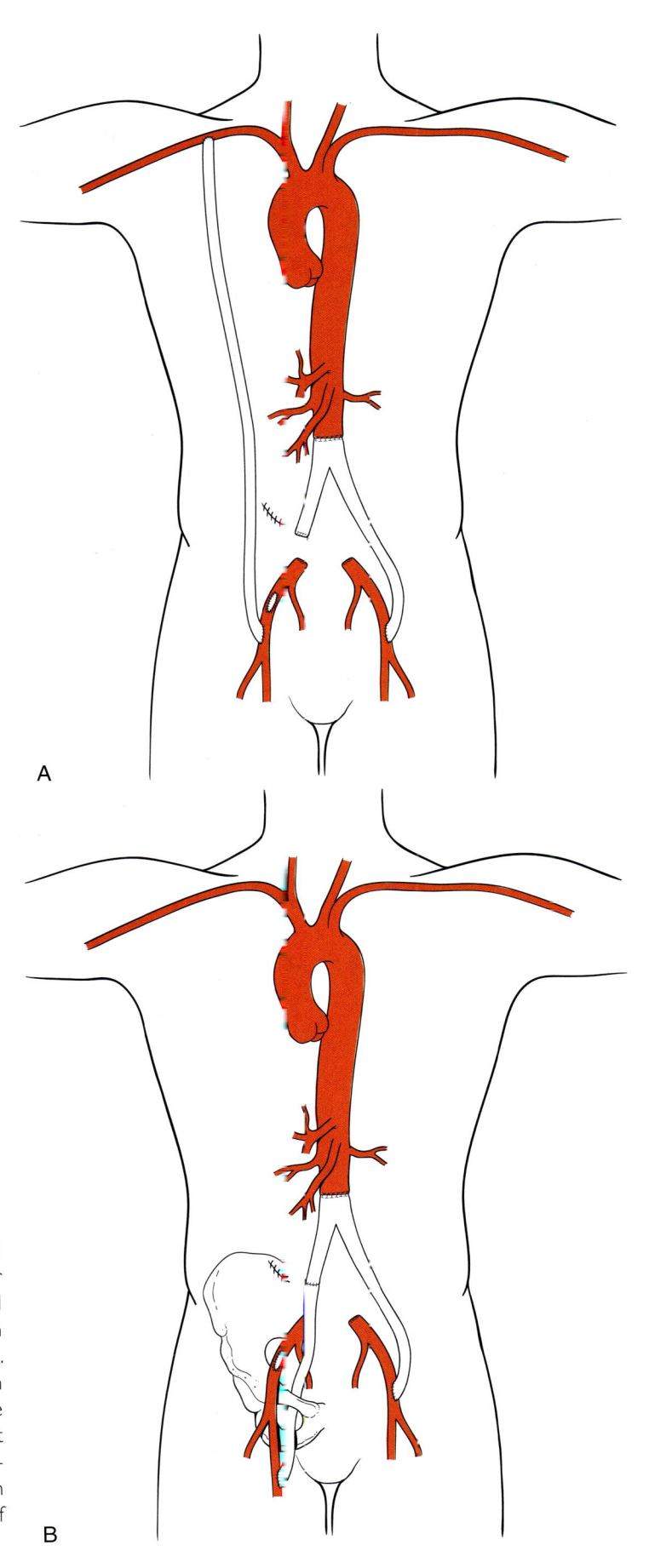

Figure 33-5. A, Right axilloproximal superficial femoral artery extraanatomic bypass graft performed to provide lower extremity perfusion after removal of an infected right distal limb of an aortobifemoral synthetic graft. The limb resection was performed through a clean right retroperitoneal approach. The rest of the original graft was not involved in the right groin infection. **B,** An obturator bypass graft is performed to provide lower extremity perfusion after removal of an infected right distal limb of an aortobifemoral synthetic graft. The limb resection and distal anastomosis are first performed through clean right retroperitoneal and proximal thigh incisions. The rest of the original graft was not involved in the right groin infection.

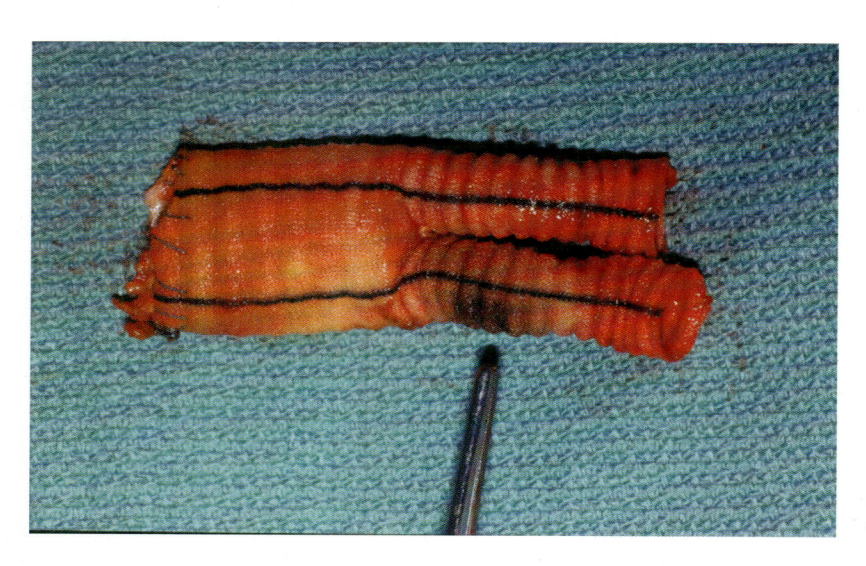

Figure 33-6. Photograph of a surgical specimen of infected synthetic graft removed during treatment of an aortoenteric graft erosion. Note the bile staining of the graft at the site of the communication with the duodenal lumen (forceps).

feasible, shortens the period of lower extremity ischemia and reduces the risk of amputation in this setting. However, if the patient is actively bleeding from the aortoenteric fistula, control of hemorrhage must take precedence over extraanatomic bypass, and urgent abdominal exploration is the priority. Depending upon the condition of the duodenal tissues, drainage or a diversion procedure may be required, but more often the duodenal defect is modest in size and primary closure is appropriate. An important technical point is wide mobilization of the duodenum away from the retroperitoneal phlegmon such that a precise, two-layer closure with 4-0 silk Lembert sutures is possible. A draining gastrostomy and feeding jejunostomy should be considered in this setting and may lessen the time during which intravenous hyperalimentation is required.

CONSIDERATIONS RELATED TO UNDERLYING ANEURYSMAL OR OCCLUSIVE DISEASE

After infected graft removal, involved arterial tissue should be resected back to normal, uninvolved tissue, which holds sutures to allow reliable closure of the remaining artery at the anastomotic sites and lessen the chance of late stump pseudoaneurysm formation. Removal of an infected synthetic graft, which had been originally placed to treat an aortic aneurysm, can be associated with difficult aortic stump closure, particularly in the presence of a short infrarenal neck. In this situation it may be necessary to isolate the suprarenal or supraceliac aorta at the diaphragm to achieve proximal control. Furthermore, in contrast to patients with predominately occlusive disease, the aortic tissue may be of much poorer quality. If the quality of the aortic stump is not good, autogenous pledgets of abdominal wall fascia or endarterectomized artery or saphenous vein may be useful to minimize the tendency for the sutures to tear through diseased artery.[19] If the proximal aortic stump is too short for adequate closure, additional length can sometimes be obtained by preliminary splenorenal or hepatorenal saphenous vein bypass to preserve at least one or possibly both kidneys and gain an additional centimeter of aorta for closure.

To minimize the risk of colonic ischemia after infected aortic graft excision, it is important to maintain adequate pelvic blood flow by preserving at least one hypogastric artery or the inferior mesenteric artery, which may be difficult to do in the presence of severe, associated occlusive disease. Usually pelvic perfusion is best maintained by means of retrograde perfusion via the extraanatomic bypass through the external iliac arteries to the hypogastric arteries. In the presence of severe external iliac occlusive disease, adjunctive measures such as endarterectomy or autogenous bypass may be required to prevent severe pelvic or colon ischemia. Creativity is often required to preserve hypogastric and profunda perfusion using autogenous tissue.

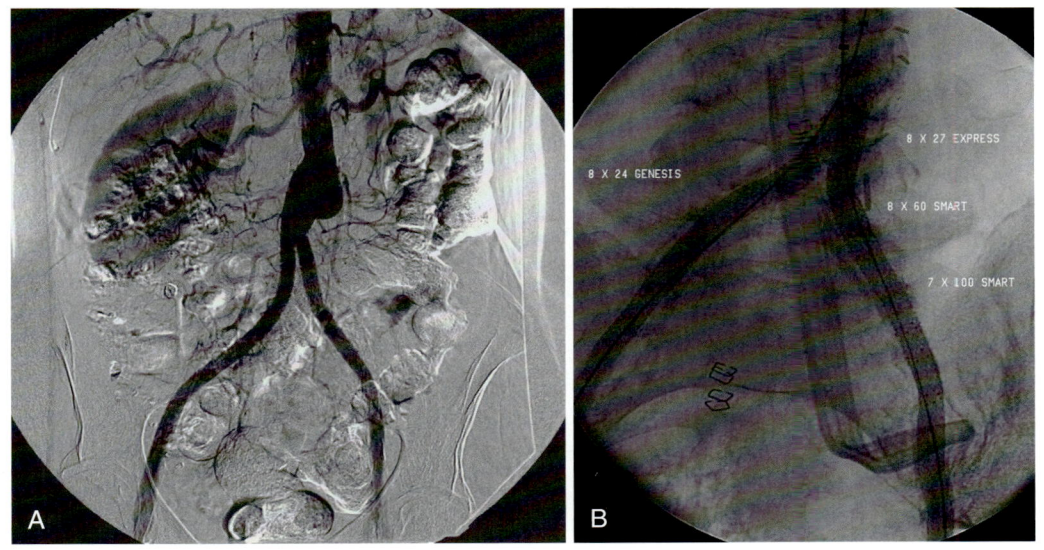

Figure 33-7. A, Aortogram in a patient with an infected aortobifemoral graft demonstrating end-to-side proximal anastomosis. **B,** Intraoperative aortogram after recanalization and stenting of previously occluded native iliac arteries. The aortobifemoral infected synthetic graft was subsequently excised with an autogenous patch closure.

ROLE OF ENDOVASCULAR THERAPY

Endovascular therapy has a limited but potentially valuable role in the treatment of aortic graft infection. Depending upon the extent and pattern of associated occlusive disease, percutaneous recanalization of stenotic or occluded outflow vessels may obviate the need for extraanatomic reconstruction or revascularization either before or after excision of an infected synthetic aortic graft (Fig. 33-7). Although endovascular intervention involving the placement of stents or stent grafts is subject to secondary infection and pseudoaneurysm formation, it may provide a temporary bridge to definitive open therapy in select critically ill or unstable patients.[20] In the clinical setting of hemorrhage secondary to aortoenteric fistula with hemodynamic instability, placement of a covered stent graft may be an expeditious and effective method to control bleeding and stabilize the patient long enough to facilitate controlled extraanatomic bypass, repair of the bowel, and graft excision.

Operative Technique

INCISION

If the clinical circumstances permit, the extraanatomic bypass is preferentially done first. The proximal incision for axillofemoral bypass is made parallel to and one fingerbreadth below the clavicle, and both common femoral arteries are exposed through longitudinal groin incisions, which allow exposure of the distal profunda femoris artery, if required. It is often possible to apply this strategy even in the case of infected aortobifemoral grafts by use of lateral inferior groin incisions to directly expose the profunda femoris arteries. The transpubic femoral-femoral tunnel is made in the clean tissue planes superficial to the fascia, and the axillofemoral tunnel is made deep to the pectoralis major muscle and continued in the subcutaneous plane just medial to the anterior superior iliac spine. This lessens the risk of graft occlusion by the iliac wing if it is tunneled more laterally. If a counterincision is required to complete the tunnel, it should be offset so that it does not lie directly over the extraanatomic graft, because breakdown of the counterincision may expose an underlying graft. If extension of the extraanatomic bypasses beyond the groin is required, lateral approaches to the popliteal or distal superficial femoral arteries may be used and the graft may be tunneled subcutaneously across the distal thigh.

When the extraanatomic bypass graft is completed, the incisions are excluded with sterile occlusive dressings. The aorta is exposed through the previous midline abdominal incision to facilitate exposure of the aorta and both iliac arteries, as well as the duodenum, if its repair is anticipated. If necessary, the aorta can be exposed through a left retroperitoneal incision, but care must be taken not to compress a right axillofemoral graft. This approach is not feasible if a left axillofemoral graft is required, and it provides less favorable exposure of the duodenum and the right iliac system.

EXPOSURE OF THE ABDOMINAL AORTA

At abdominal exploration, the initial goal is to obtain expeditious proximal control of the aorta, which may be difficult in the presence of extensive retroperitoneal inflammation. In many situations early supraceliac aortic control is the safest approach. With proximal control assured, exposure of the distal iliac arteries can proceed to facilitate graft excision and iliac artery closure, but potential iliac vein injury is a significant risk in a reoperative field. If inflammation or hemorrhage precludes direct distal control, intraluminal occlusion catheters may provide a useful alternative, because iliac artery backbleeding can be substantial if an axillofemoral graft has been placed. The placement of the stents in both ureters facilitates their identification in the presence of extensive retroperitoneal inflammation and scarring. With proximal and distal arterial control established, the retroperitoneal phlegmon can be entered and the infected graft can be located and excised.

EXPOSURE OF THE COMMON FEMORAL, SUPERFICIAL FEMORAL, AND PROFUNDA FEMORIS ARTERIES

When a prior aortobifemoral graft has become infected with involvement of both femoral anastomotic sites, preliminary bilateral axillosuperficial femoral or axillopopliteal artery bypass grafts placed distal to the involved femoral anastomoses are necessary. Once these extraanatomic bypass grafts are completed, the incisions are isolated with the occlusive dressings, and the aorta is exposed through the previous midline incision for excision of the infected aortic graft. The infected femoral incisions are then opened, and control of the infected graft, as well as the native common, superficial femoral, and profunda femoris arteries, is obtained. This exposure facilitates complete removal of the infected aortobifemoral graft and allows autogenous repair of the femoral anastomotic site.

GRAFT EXCISION

With leg perfusion maintained through an extraanatomic bypass and proximal and distal aortic control established, the retroperitoneal phlegmon is entered. The infected aortic graft identified and dissected proximally and distally to its arterial anastomoses. To avoid the risk of persistent or recurrent infection in the graft bed, the graft should be removed, including synthetic Teflon felt pledgets. A grossly infected graft is usually bathed in perigraft serous or milky fluid or pus, not incorporated within surrounding tissue, and easily exposed. After removal of the infected synthetic material in its entirety, the distal common iliac arteries should be closed with monofilament synthetic suture material. This allows retrograde perfusion of at least one hypogastric artery through the extraanatomic bypass, minimizing the risk of colon and pelvic ischemia. If the infected aortic graft limb extends to the femoral incision, drainage of the tunnel can be facilitated by suturing a large Penrose or sump drain to the limb, which can be used to draw the drain through the tunnel as the limb is removed.

CLOSURE OF THE PROXIMAL AORTIC STUMP AND OMENTAL PEDICLE FLAP

If the proximal anastomosis of the infected synthetic aortic graft has been constructed end to side, infrarenal aortic proximal control is usually straightforward. In addition, the aortic closure is simplified by utilization of an autogenous patch angioplasty consisting of vein or endarterectomized arterial tissue after the residual native vessel has been debrided back to healthy aortic tissue or, if needed,

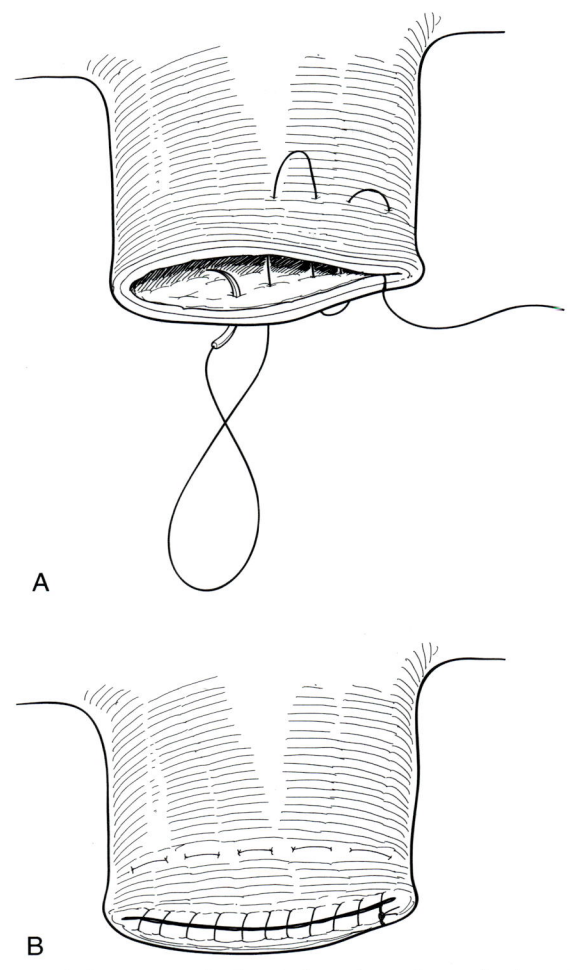

Figure 33-8. Closure of the aortic stump after removal of an infected aortic synthetic graft. **A,** The proximal layer is closed with a row of running or interrupted horizontal mattress sutures of a monofilament, nonabsorbable synthetic suture material. **B,** This is followed by a second row of running suture material of the same type.

simply oversewn. When the infected proximal anastomosis has been fashioned in an end-to-end configuration, such as required for aortic aneurysm repair, the proximal aortic stump should be debrided back to healthy aortic tissue and closed in two layers with a synthetic monofilament suture material, such as 2-0 or 3-0 polypropylene. The proximal suture line consists of a running or interrupted horizontal mattress layer followed by a second-layer closure of running monofilament synthetic suture (Fig. 33-8). If the aortic stump tissues are friable, they may be reinforced with autogenous tissue consisting of strips or pledgets of abdominal wall or prevertebral fascia, if available. Other autogenous materials, such as endarterectomized occluded aortoiliac or hypogastric arterial segments or saphenous vein pledgets, can be used to prevent the sutures from tearing through friable aortic tissue. Synthetic reinforcement material must be avoided to avoid persistent stump infection. If sufficient omental tissue is available, a pedicle of omentum should be fashioned and passed retrocolically through an avascular opening in the mesocolon into the aortic bed, to fill the dead space in the retroperitoneum, and over the site of aortic stump closure (Fig. 33-9).

MANAGEMENT OF THE DUODENAL STUMP

The defect in the duodenum can be closed primarily in the manner of a pyloroplasty if the quality of the duodenum is adequate. However, if the duodenal tissues are severely scarred or inflamed, a diversion procedure such as a Roux-en-Y bypass may be required. Adequate drainage, in accordance with general surgical principles, should be provided. If a prolonged ileus is anticipated, construction of a draining gastrostomy and a feeding jejunostomy are useful adjuncts.

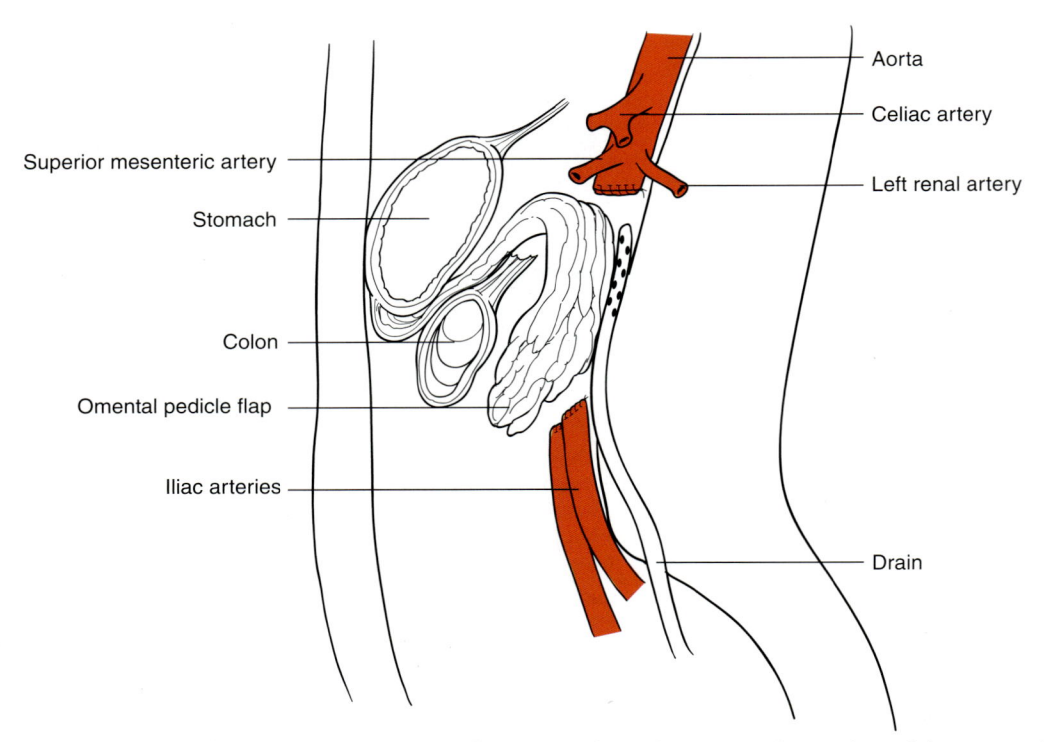

Figure 33-9. An omental pedicle flap is passed in a retrocolic manner through an avascular section of the mesocolon to cover the aortic stump. A large sump drain is placed in the retropperitoneal space.

CLOSURE OF THE FEMORAL ARTERIES

The femoral artery should be closed using autogenous tissue to maintain retrograde perfusion to the profunda femoris artery and at least one hypogastric artery through the external iliac artery. Depending upon the extent of associated occlusive disease, this may be accomplished using a saphenous vein patch, with or without an associated endarterectomy of the external iliac or femoral arteries. If adequate saphenous vein is not available, endarterectomized segments of occluded superficial femoral artery may be used for patch material.

SARTORIUS MUSCLE FLAP

If scarring or tissue destruction is severe, coverage of the femoral vessels can be provided by detaching the sartorius muscle laterally from its insertion onto the anterior superior iliac spine. The muscle is rotated medially as an autogenous muscle flap to cover the femoral reconstruction.[21]

DRAINS

Adequate drainage of the aortic bed, as well as the tunnels of the removed infected iliac limbs and site of duodenal closure, if applicable, is important to minimize the risk of continuing sepsis and aortic stump blowout. The need for the provision of ample drainage with large sump drains placed in the aortic bed and brought out through the flank or through the femoral incisions cannot be overemphasized.

CLOSURE

When the extraanatomic bypass has been placed before removal of the infected aortic graft, clean incisions are closed and isolated with sterile occlusive dressings. Depending upon the degree of contamination of the aortic and femoral wounds after removal of the infected prosthesis from these regions, primary closure with placement of drains may be adequate. However, a delayed primary closure of the skin may be necessary for more severely contaminated wounds. If circumstances require that the infected graft excision be carried out before extraanatomic bypass, the contaminated wounds are closed and isolated with occlusive dressings. The patient is prepared again and draped, and a new set of sterile operative instruments is used to perform the extraanatomic bypass.

Postoperative Care

- Patients require intensive care monitoring for respiratory and cardiac support, as well as volume resuscitation.
- Continuing assessment of lower extremity perfusion and neuromotor evaluation are critical. Fasciotomy is necessary if compartment syndrome develops.
- Antimicrobial therapy is guided by the results of intraoperative cultures from the resected graft material, as well as the aortic bed. Depending upon the organism, the extent of infection, and the presence of residual synthetic graft material, protracted antibiotic therapy may be recommended.

Complications

- **Persistent local sepsis.** Lack of adequate debridement or drainage may lead to aortic stump blowout (10%-20%), pseudoaneurysm formation, or infection of the extraanatomic prosthetic bypass (10%-40%).[7,8]
- **Amputation.** Lower extremity amputation has been reported in up to 20% of patients after removal of an infected aortic graft.
- **Inadequate pelvic perfusion.** Gluteal and colon ischemia with buttock or bowel necrosis may occur if there are inadequate pelvic collaterals or retrograde iliac artery perfusion from the femoral artery.
- **Deep vein thrombosis**
- **Myocardial infarction or arrhythmia**
- **Bleeding**
- **Renal failure**
- **Graft thrombosis**

REFERENCES

1. Fry WJ, Lindenauer SM: Infection complicating the use of plastic arterial implants, *Arch Surg* 94:600-609, 1967.
2. Jamieson GG, DeWeese JA, Rob CG: Infected arterial grafts, *Ann Surg* 181:850-852, 1975.
3. Liekweg WG, Greenfield LJ: Vascular prosthetic infections: Collected experience and results of treatment, *Surgery* 81:335-342, 1977.
4. O'Hara P, Hertzer N, Beven E, et al: Surgical management of infected abdominal aortic grafts: Review of a 25-year experience, *J Vasc Surg* 3:725-731, 1986.
5. Szilagyi D, Elliott J, Vrandecic M, et al: Infection in arterial reconstruction with synthetic grafts, *Ann Surg* 176:321-323, 1972.
6. Kieffer E, Sabatier J, Plissonnier D, et al: Prosthetic graft infection after descending thoracic/thoracoabdominal aortic aneurysmectomy: Management with in situ allografts, *J Vasc Surg* 33:671-678, 2001.
7. Seeger J, Petrus H, Welborn M, et al: Long term outcome after treatment of aortic graft infection with staged extraanatomic bypass grafting and aortic graft removal, *J Vasc Surg* 32:451-461, 2000.
8. Reilly L, Altman H, Lusby R, et al: Late results following surgical management of vascular graft infections, *J Vasc Surg* 1:36-44, 1984.
9. Vogel T, Symons R, Flum D: The incidence and factors associated with graft infection after aortic aneurysm repair, *J Vasc Surg* 47:264-269, 2008.
10. O'Connor S, Andrew P, Batt M, et al: A systemic review and meta-analysis of treatments for aortic graft infection, *J Vasc Surg* 44:38-45, 2006.
11. Fitzgerald S, Kelly C, Humphreys H: Diagnosis and treatment of prosthetic aortic graft infections: Confusion and inconsistency in the absence of evidence or consensus, *J Antimicrob Chemotherapy* 56:996-999, 2005.
12. Goldstone J, Moore WS: Infection in vascular prostheses: Clinical manifestations and surgical management, *Am J Surg* 128:225-233, 1974.
13. Elliott JP, Smith RF, Szilagyi DE: Aortoenteric and paraprosthetic-enteric fistulas, *Arch Surg* 108:479-490, 1974.

14. Reilly LM, Stoney RJ, Goldstone J, et al: Improved management of aortic graft infection: The influence of operation sequence and staging, *J Vasc Surg* 5:421-431, 1987.
15. Orton D, LeVeen R, Saigh J, et al: Aortic prosthetic graft infections: Radiographic manifestations and implications for management, *Radiographics* 20:977-993, 2000.
16. O'Hara P, Borkowski G, Hertzer N, et al: Natural history of periprosthetic air on computerized axial tomographic examination of the abdomen following abdominal aortic aneurysm repair, *J Vasc Surg* 1:429-433, 1984.
17. Bunt T: Synthetic vascular graft infections, *Surgery* 93:733-746, 1983.
18. Valentine R: Diagnosis and management of aortic graft infection, *Sem Vasc Surg* 14:292-301, 2001.
19. Sarac T, Augustinos P, Lyden S, et al: Use of fascia-peritoneum patch as a pledget for an infected aortic stump, *J Vasc Surg* 38:1404-1406, 2003.
20. Burks J, Faries P, Gravereaux E, et al: Endovascular repair of bleeding aortoenteric fistulas: A 5 year experience, *J Vasc Surg* 34:1055-1059, 2001.
21. Landry G, Carlson J, Liem T: The sartorius muscle flap: An important adjunct for complicated femoral wounds involving vascular grafts, *J Vasc Surg* 50:961, 2009.

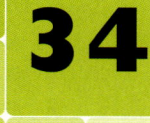

34 Neoaortoiliac System Procedure for Treatment of an Aortic Graft Infection

RYAN T. HAGINO • CHRISTOPHER A. DeMAIORIBUS

Historical Background

Dissatisfaction with traditional single-stage or multistage extraanatomic bypass followed by resection of infected aortic grafts arises from aortic stump blowout after excision of the infected graft and more importantly from compromised long-term performance of axillofemoral reconstructions.[1] Ehrenfeld and colleagues[2] reported their experience with in situ reconstruction of the aorta using endarterectomized arterial autografts in 1979. Limitations with available arterial conduit prevented widespread adoption of this technique. Early reports of in situ reconstruction after excision of infected aortic grafts using saphenous vein described a conduit plagued by diffuse intimal hyperplasia.[3,4] In 1981 Schulman and Badhey[5] used femoral popliteal vein (FPV) as an alternative conduit for infrainguinal revascularization. Separate reports published in 1993 described the use of FPV as an autogenous graft for aortic reconstruction,[4,6] and the term neoaortoiliac system (NAIS) was used to describe the reconstructed vessels using FPV.[4] The large caliber of the FPV lends itself to direct anastomosis with the aorta, and concerns of late aneurysmal degeneration or graft blowout were not realized. Long-term follow-up suggests that clinically significant venous complications are infrequent.[7-9] Excellent patency, limb salvage rate, and lack of recurrent infection make the NAIS procedure an often preferred method of treatment.[10-13]

Preoperative Preparation

- The initial care of the patient with an aortic graft infection should be directed toward treatment of systemic or local sepsis. If possible, culture-directed systemic antibiotic therapy should be initiated. Hemodynamic instability related to sepsis may require aggressive intravenous hydration or resuscitation, invasive monitoring, and vasoactive medication. Extensive preoperative evaluation of cardiac risk is often unnecessary given the life-threatening nature of aortic graft infection and the need for expeditious surgical therapy.
- Duplex ultrasound, computed tomography angiography, magnetic resonance imaging, conventional arteriography, nuclear imaging, and positron emission tomography scanning aid in defining the extent of graft infection and arterial-graft anastomotic integrity. In instances of subacute biofilm infection, imaging studies may be inadequate and operative graft exploration may be necessary to confirm an infectious etiology as a cause for an anastomotic pseudoaneurysm. Preoperative imaging also provides information regarding the original procedure and arterial anatomy. The location and configuration of the aortic anastomosis and anastomotic pseudoaneurysms, and the presence of prior lower extremity arterial reconstructions can be accurately assessed. This knowledge is of great value if infrainguinal revascularization for ischemia is required after

aortic reconstruction. Finally, radiographic studies define associated abscess or involvement of surrounding viscera.
- Both lower extremities should be evaluated with venous duplex imaging. The lower extremity veins should be evaluated for (1) patency and caliber of the FPV, (2) absence of deep vein thrombosis, (3) presence of duplicated FPVs, and (4) presence or absence of the great saphenous veins.

Pitfalls and Danger Points

- Hemorrhage from conduit
- Acute limb ischemia
- Compartment syndrome
- Deep vein thrombosis and venous hypertension

Operative Strategy

SELECTION OF CONDUIT FOR IN SITU REPAIR

Preoperative imaging of the FPV is used to confirm the absence of deep vein thromboses, assess conduit size, and identify duplication of the deep venous system. In the latter situation removal of the larger-caliber FPV and preservation of its duplicate may reduce complications related to chronic swelling or venous hypertension after complete harvest. Full reconstruction of an aortobifemoral configuration usually requires complete use of bilateral FPVs. However, reconstructions after partial graft excisions ("hemi-NAIS" procedures) or removal of aortic or aortoiliac grafts may require considerably shorter lengths.

STAGING THE NEOAORTOILIAC SYSTEM PROCEDURE

Clinical stability in a patient may afford some logistic flexibility. Staging FPV harvest as a separate procedure can save the more difficult graft excision and reconstruction for a second operation on a different day without an increase in overall operative time or complication rate.[14] In such patients the veins are mobilized and left in situ, maintaining axial venous continuity and flow. The wounds are temporarily closed, and standard prophylactic antithrombotic therapy is initiated. When ready, the patient returns to the operating room, the veins are removed, and the definitive procedure is completed.

Operative Technique

HARVESTING FEMORAL POPLITEAL VEIN

Full lower extremity circumferential preparation is required, and the limbs are positioned in a frog-leg manner. The incision is made over the sartorius muscle, from the groin to the medial knee (Video 34-1 and Fig. 34-1, *A*). The sartorius is reflected medially, allowing exposure of the Hunter canal. This area represents the division between the anterior and the medial adductor compartments of the thigh; its contents include the femoral artery and vein and the saphenous nerve. The overlying aponeurosis is opened, and the vein is the first visible vascular structure. Mobilization of the vein begins with exposure of its anterior surface. Dissection of the femoral vein is carried centrally to its confluence with the deep femoral vein. Branches of the mobilized femoral vein are doubly ligated flush with the main vein rather than at a distance from the vein often described for saphenous vein harvest. This flush ligation pulls in adventitia, adding strength to the ligature, and does not result in significant impingement of the large lumen. If the full length of FPV is needed, exposure and dissection of the popliteal vein requires division of the adductor longus insertion at the adductor hiatus (Fig. 34-1, *B*). Up to 15 cm of usable popliteal vein may be obtained in continuity with the femoral vein, but care should be taken to preserve major popliteal venous branches and at least one

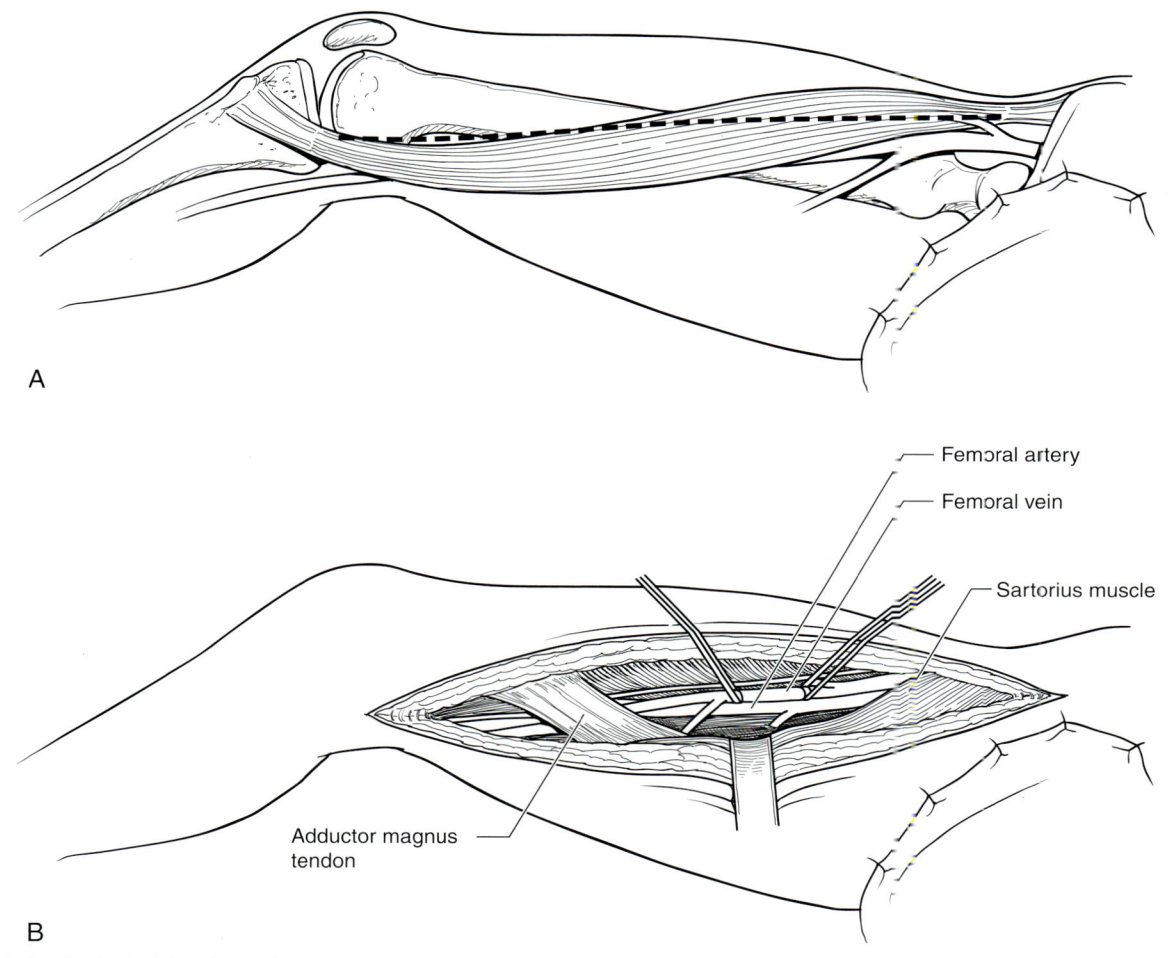

Figure 34-1. A, An incision is made over the sartorius muscle (dashed line). After medial reflection of the sartorius muscle, the FPV, superficial femoral artery, and saphenous nerve are exposed. **B,** The adductor hiatus is usually opened to expose the popliteal vein.

popliteal valve in the residual stump, thus preserving venous collaterals after graft excision and preventing excessive venous hypertension.[15]

After exposure of the infected graft, the vein harvest can be completed. The popliteal end of the graft is ligated and divided. The cephalad end of the conduit is divided flush with the deep femoral vein, and the divided vein is oversewn with nonabsorbable monofilament suture. This allows avoidance of a femoral vein stump and provides a smooth transition from deep femoral vein to common femoral vein. A vein stump at this location may provide a nidus for postoperative deep vein thrombosis and pulmonary embolus.

A nonreversed configuration of vein graft is usually preferred for size-match considerations. Rather than using a valvulotome to lyse the valves, which may leave residual flow-limiting valve leaflets, the vein is easily intussuscepted, turned inside out to allow valve excision under direct vision, and then returned to its native state by reverting the conduit (Fig. 34-2).

CONSTRUCTION OF THE NEOAORTOILIAC SYSTEM

The configuration of the reconstruction can be tailored according to clinical circumstances, available conduit, anatomic requirements for replacement of the infected graft, and best size match. For aortobifemoral reconstructions, if adequate length of FPV is available to create a true bifurcated graft, the proximal segments of the two veins can be spatulated and sewn together to form a pantaloon graft (Fig. 34-3). If a conduit is limited or clinical circumstances preclude a true in situ aortobifemoral reconstruction, other configurations are possible. For instance, it may be advisable to avoid retunneling a new vein graft through a pelvic or retroperitoneal abscess,

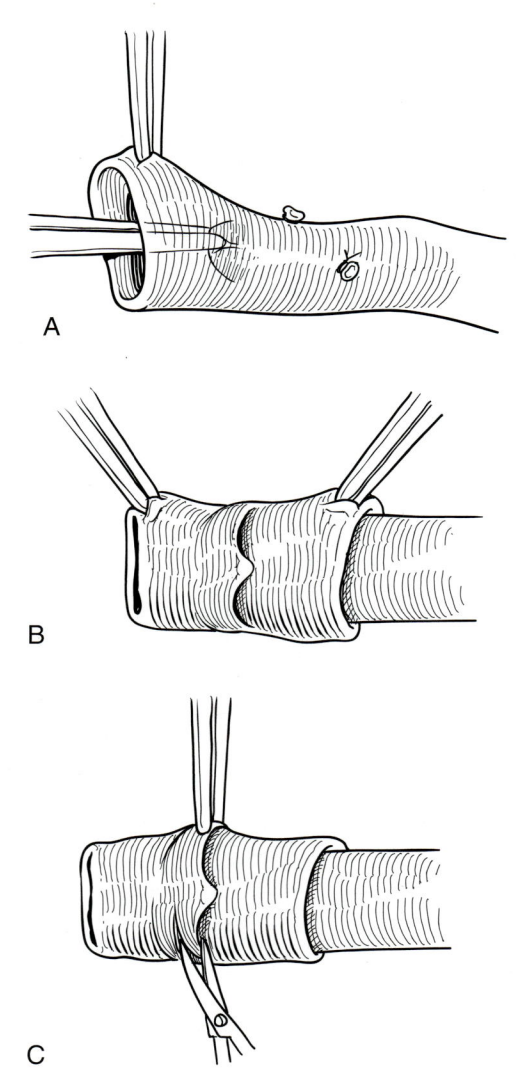

Figure 34-2. After explant of the vein, the vein is easily turned inside out by grasping the interior surface with forceps (**A**) while pulling the outer surface over the instrument with other forceps (**B**). **C,** This allows direct visualization of the valve leaflets and allows valve excision, which is preferred over valve lysis strategies typically applied to the saphenous vein.

in which case a unilateral aortofemoral reconstruction away from the abscess with a cross-femoral graft is a safe option. Vein grafts should be passed through the new tunnels while nondistended, reducing the possibility of dragging ligated side branches in the tunnel, tie avulsion, or graft hemorrhage.

PROXIMAL ANASTOMOSIS

Despite the large caliber of the FPV, there frequently remains a size mismatch between the conduit and the native aorta. Good end-to-end anastomosis can be achieved without significant "purse stringing" if the anastomosis is constructed with at least four quadrant, nonabsorbable, 4-0 monofilament anchoring sutures run together rather than a single running suture. This technique allows more precise suture placement to evenly distribute the vein over the circumference of the anastomosis to the aorta.

DISTAL ANASTOMOSIS

Direct distal anastomoses are usually created to preexisting anastomotic sites after arterial wall debridement. Limitations in conduit length often preclude anastomoses at surgically clean sites distal to the original reconstruction. Rarely, an anastomosis is created proximal to the old one and the old anastomotic site is closed with a vein patch. Care must be taken to remove all residual prosthetic material and infected arterial wall. Sometimes an end-to-end femoral anastomosis is

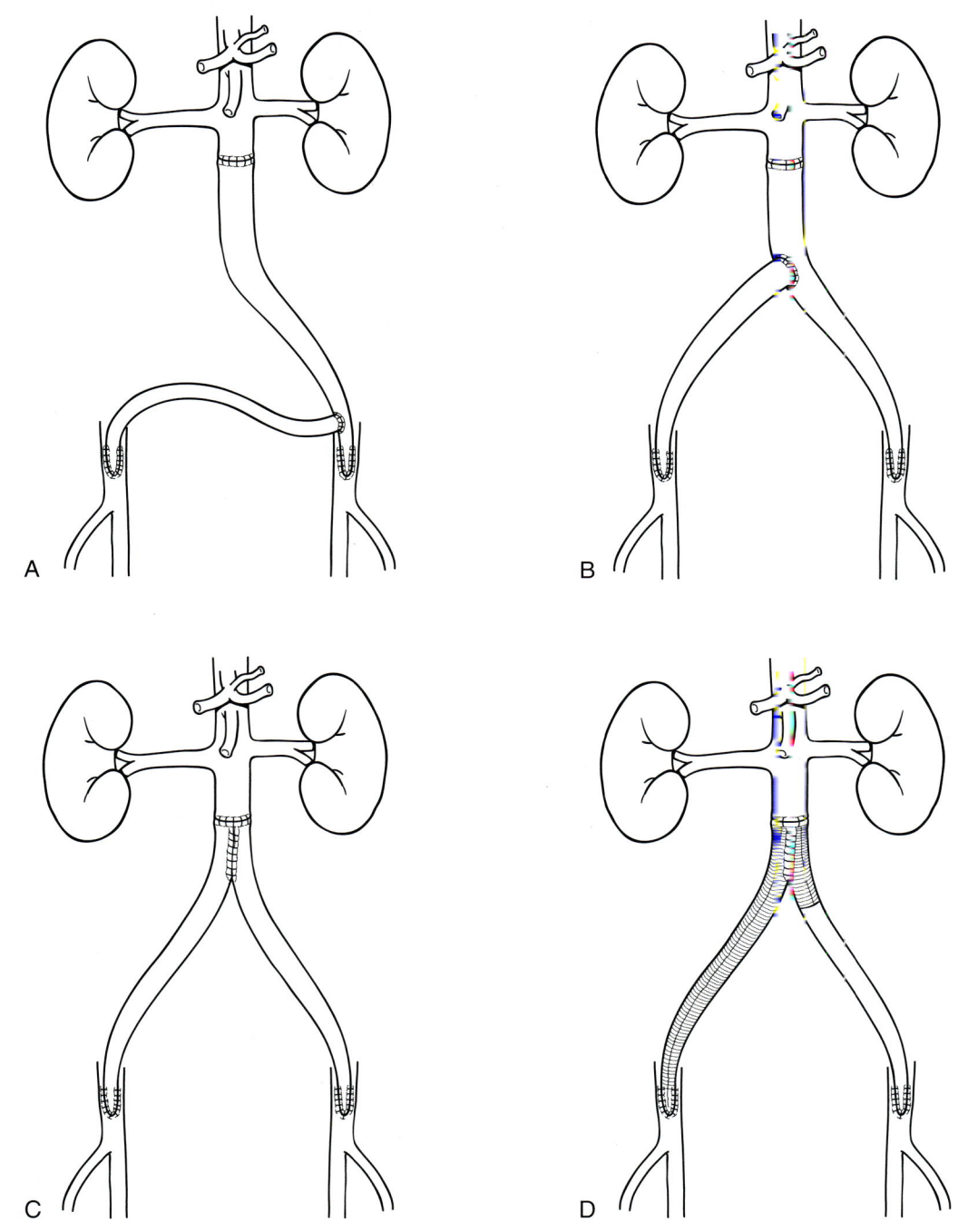

Figure 34-3. Four graft configurations are generally used in the NAIS procedure: aortounifemoral with femoral-femoral crossover graft (**A**), aortounifemoral with contralateral iliofemoral graft (**B**), aortobifemoral graft (**C**), and single limb replacement (hemi-NAIS; **D**).

required after aggressive arterial debridement, which precludes retrograde pelvic flow. This is acceptable, but resultant pelvic ischemia is a concern.

FLAP COVERAGE

Flap coverage is not universally required. However, extensive retroperitoneal contamination may require an additional measure to prevent recurrent infection. An omental pedicle flap is an excellent, liberally used option. The omentum is mobilized from the transverse colon in the avascular plane. The gastroepiploic arcade is preserved, and the omentum is detached from the gastric wall, creating a pedicle flap. The flap is passed retrocolic through a window created in the transverse mesocolon, allowing apposition to the contaminated area in the inframesocolic retroperitoneum. The flap is secured around the aortic anastomosis and graft. The gap in the mesocolon around the tunneled pedicle is loosely closed to prevent retraction or internal herniation.

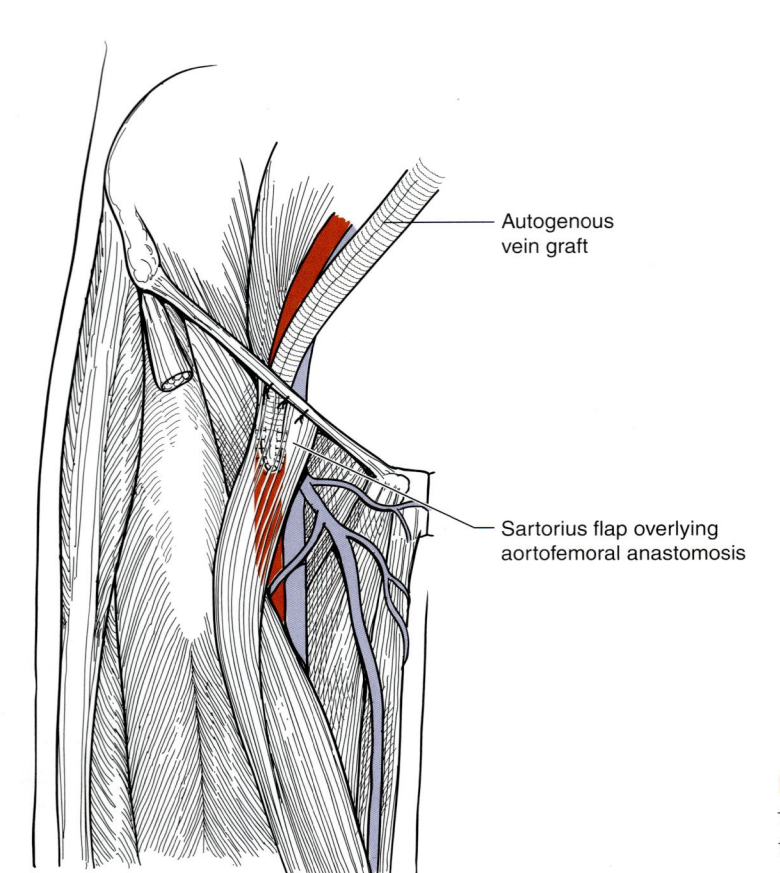

Figure 34-4. Sartorius myoplasty. The muscle's origin at the anterior superior iliac spine is divided, and the muscle is flipped over the femoral vessels rather than transposing the muscle en bloc.

Femoral incisions often require extensive debridement to clear contamination. These large cavities defy closure, and muscle flap coverage is required. This is usually accomplished with a sartorius muscle rotational flap or myoplasty. To perform a myoplasty, the lateral border of the sartorius muscle is dissected proximally toward its origin at the anterior-superior iliac spine. Adequate exposure may require a lateral counterincision. The blood supply to the muscle is segmental, arising medially. The first vascular pedicle is approximately 6 to 7 cm from the origin of the muscle and should be preserved to avoid flap necrosis. After mobilization, the origin of the muscle is divided through its tendinous portion, and the muscle is flipped over from lateral to medial rather than shifted en masse (Fig. 34-4). The muscle is then secured over the femoral vessels. If skin coverage cannot be achieved without undue tension, then a vacuum-assisted wound closure device can be used over the myoplasty.

Postoperative Care

- Venous hypertension, stasis in the popliteal venous stump, and a significant amount of damaged venous intima in the vein closure sites necessitate postoperative antithrombotic therapy with prophylactic doses of unfractionated heparin or low-molecular-weight heparin. Lower extremity compression pumps can be used, as well as foot pumps in patients with fasciotomies.
- Frequent neurovascular examination of the lower extremities is paramount in detecting early compartment syndrome or ischemia.
- Compression garments should be used to limit lower extremity swelling.

Complications

- **Hemorrhage.** Early bleeding from the conduit is usually related to inadequately ligated side branches. Late bleeding is usually caused by recurrent or progressive infection. Graft blowouts are rare but catastrophic. Factors associated with NAIS graft infection include chronic malnutrition, immunosuppression, and polymicrobial and fungal infections.

- **Compartment syndrome.** Acute venous hypertension, in combination with prolonged ischemia with reperfusion, can lead to postoperative compartment syndrome. Patients with prior or concurrent saphenectomy, prolonged clamp times, preexisting arterial insufficiency, or hemodynamic instability should probably undergo prophylactic fasciotomy. In these cases closure is often accomplished during the index hospitalization.

- **Acute limb ischemia.** Division of collaterals arising from the femoral-popliteal arteries during FPV harvest can result in limb ischemia, particularly in patients with preexisting atherosclerotic occlusive disease. This disappointing complication often requires the addition of infrainguinal revascularization after an already lengthy operation.

- **Recurrent infection.** Although reinfection rates are low, inadequate mechanical debridement of infected graft material, native arteries, and soft tissues contribute to recurrent infection. Infectious morbidity associated with graft-enteric erosions and secondary arterial-enteric fistulae are largely a result of intestinal contamination and bowel-related complications.

- **Postoperative neuropathy.** Extensive groin dissection and debridement may result in edema or injury to cutaneous branches of the femoral nerve. This results in anterior and lateral thigh dysesthesia that, although bothersome to the patient, is often self-limited. In addition, the saphenous nerve lies close to the femoral vein within the Hunter canal. Injury to the nerve during femoral vein mobilization can result in saphenous neuralgia.

- **Late stenosis.** The incidence of restenosis in these grafts is low. Published reports suggest no predilection for a juxtaanastomotic location compared with midgraft lesions. Direct valve resection, as described earlier, is a means of reducing hyperplastic lesions at residual valve leaflets in nonreversed conduits.[12,13]

- **Chronic venous insufficiency or venous hypertension.** Some degree of lower limb swelling after FPV harvest is inevitable. Physiologic data confirm a high incidence of venous outflow obstruction after FPV removal, but clinically significant venous complications are uncommon.[8,9] The development of late venous complications is related primarily to the presence or absence of valvular competence and collaterals in the remaining popliteal venous segment. The absence of the great saphenous venous system before FPV harvest does not correlate strongly with these complications. Therefore previous removal or saphenous vein harvest concurrent with FPV removal should not be considered a contraindication to FPV harvest.[9]

REFERENCES

1. O'Connor S, Andrew P, Batt M: A systematic review and meta-analysis of treatments for aortic graft infection, *J Vasc Surg* 44:38-45, 2006.
2. Ehrenfeld WK, Wilbur BG, Olcott CN, et al: Autogenous tissue reconstruction in the management of infected prosthetic grafts, *Surgery* 85:82-92, 1979.
3. Seeger JM, Wheeler JR, Gregory RT, et al: Autogenous graft replacement of infected prosthetic grafts in the femoral position, *Surgery* 93:39-45, 1983.
4. Clagett GP, Bowers BL, Lopez-Viego MA, et al: Creation of a neo-aortoiliac system from lower extremity deep and superficial veins, *Ann Surg* 218:239-249, 1993.
5. Schulman ML, Badhey MR: Deep veins of the leg as femoropopliteal bypass grafts, *Arch Surg* 116:1141-1145, 1981.
6. Nevelsteen A, Lacroix H, Suy R: The superficial femoral vein as autogenous conduit in the treatment of prosthetic arterial infection, *Ann Vasc Surg* 7:556-560, 1993.
7. Schanzer H, Chiang K, Mabrouk M, et al: Use of lower extremity deep veins as arterial substitutes: Functional status of the donor leg, *J Vasc Surg* 14:624-527, 1991.
8. Wells JK, Hagino RT, Bargmann KM, et al: Venous morbidity after superficial femoral-popliteal vein harvest, *J Vasc Surg* 29:282-291, 1999.

9. Modrall JG, Hocking JA, Timaran CH, et al: Late incidence of chronic venous insufficiency after deep vein harvest, *J Vasc Surg* 46:520-525, 2007.
10. Clagett GP, Valentine RJ, Hagino RT: Autogenous aortoiliac/femoral reconstruction from superficial femoral-popliteal veins: Feasibility and durability, *J Vasc Surg* 25:255-270, 1997.
11. Daenens K, Fourneau I, Nevelsteen A: Ten-year experience in autogenous reconstruction with the femoral vein in the treatment of aortofemoral prosthetic infection, *E J Vasc Endovasc Surg* 25:240-245, 2003.
12. Beck AW, Murphy EH, Hocking JA, et al: Aortic reconstruction with femoral-popliteal vein: Graft stenosis incidence, risk and reintervention, *J Vasc Surg* 47:36-44, 2008.
13. Faulk J, Dattilo JB, Guzman RJ, et al: Neoaortic reconstruction for aortic graft infection: Need for endovascular adjunctive therapies? *Ann Vasc Surg* 19:774-781, 2005.
14. Ali AT, Mcleod N, Kalapatapu VR, et al: Staging the neoaortoiliac system: Feasibility and short-term outcomes, *J Vasc Surg* 48:1125-1131, 2008.
15. Santilli SM, Lee ES, Wernsing SE, et al: Superficial femoral popliteal vein: An anatomic study, *J Vasc Surg* 31:450-455, 2000.

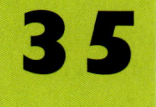

35 Surgical Treatment of Pseudoaneurysm of the Femoral Artery

WILLIAM D. JORDAN, JR. • MICHAEL J. GAFFUD

Historical Background

The development of prosthetic grafts has extended the vascular surgeon's ability to replace or bypass diseased arterial segments. However, the risk of infection, although small, constantly looms over a patient with an indwelling prosthetic graft, and preventive measures remain the most effective means of infection control. When infection occurs, subsequent degeneration of the anastomosis with arterial bleeding is potentially both limb and life threatening. Few attempts at drainage and sterilization can clear the infection when a foreign material remains in proximity, and infection involving the anastomosis inevitably leads to hemorrhage.[1] The principles of management of an infected prosthetic have two objectives: removal of infected prosthesis and restoration of blood flow to the affected extremity.[2] Although historical teaching mandates complete removal of the infected prosthetic with revascularization using a new conduit placed in an alternative, noninfected route, recent data have suggested that in situ reconstruction with an autogenous conduit or even a prosthetic conduit may provide an alternate treatment option in select patients.[3] In 1963 the obturator bypass was described by Shaw and Baue,[4] which proved to be a durable option for lower extremity revascularization. Although infection complicates the management of femoral pseudoaneurysm, most such lesions are degenerative without associated infection. In prior practice suture breakdown was an important etiology, whereas arterial degeneration is responsible in the modern era.

Indications

- All anastomotic femoral aneurysms require treatment, because they are at risk for continued enlargement and rupture. This posture is, or course, tempered in patients with limited longevity.

Preoperative Preparation

- The physical findings and time interval from initial operation can direct the extent of evaluation that is required before surgical intervention. Hemorrhage or a draining abscess are emergent conditions that are best managed in the operating room. Chronic infection or degenerative processes allow time for comprehensive evaluation.
- Abscesses or wounds should not be probed at the bedside because of the risk of disruption of a loose clot that could lead to extensive bleeding.
- If infection is suspected, blood cultures should be obtained and empirical antibiotics should be initiated.
- Echocardiography should be considered to exclude valvular vegetations that may alter clinical management, antibiotic choice, and duration of treatment.

- If infection manifests as a chronic process, thorough evaluation of vasculature with ultrasound, as well as conventional, computed tomography (CT) or magnetic resonance angiography, can be performed. Sinus tracts may be identified between the skin or bowel and the graft. Although normal in the postoperative period, perigraft fluid or soft tissue attenuation is suggestive of infection. Ultrasound- or CT-guided drainage of fluid may be diagnostic and suggest direct antibiotic therapy. Although rarely necessary, a tagged leukocyte study can also be obtained.

Pitfalls and Danger Points

- Shaw and Baue advised that "a bold and well conceived surgical approach to this problem is much preferred over timid, unjustifiably hopeful procrastination and half measures."[4] The greatest pitfall with an infectious process is to be conservative, which inevitably leads to limb loss or death.
- All infected graft should ideally be removed, but the physiologic condition of the patient sometimes mandates a less aggressive approach. Close monitoring of any residual prosthesis is mandatory because it remains at risk for infection.
- Preservation of retrograde iliac artery flow may be difficult to achieve at the time of vascular reconstruction. Therefore the status of both hypogastric arteries must be appreciated on preoperative studies to ensure adequate pelvic perfusion.

Operative Technique for a Noninfected Anastomotic Femoral Artery Pseudoaneurysm

INCISION

Sterile preparation to include the abdomen and the legs circumferentially gives the opportunity to assess distal perfusion after repair. Regardless of whether the femoral artery functions as inflow or outflow, this preparation allows complete control and evaluation of the concerned vasculature, entry into the abdomen for proximal control if needed, and inspection of the lower extremity. The previous vertical or transverse incision can be used and extended proximally for dissection in a fresh plane.

EXPOSURE AND VASCULAR CONTROL

The dissection begins with identifying the superior portion of the proximal graft and the proximal common femoral artery. If there is a concern that complete dissection of the common femoral artery is precarious because of scar tissue, control may be best obtained with a balloon occlusion catheter or by treating the artery and the graft as one vascular "unit" and placing a vascular clamp across them both. The inguinal ligament can be incised if needed to provide adequate exposure. The proximal graft and femoral artery should be dissected free from the surrounding scar and encircled with vessel loops or umbilical tape. Sharp dissection continues on the lateral and medial sides of the common femoral artery to identify the bifurcation, the superficial femoral artery, and the profunda femoris artery. Each vessel can be dissected completely to be encircled with vessel loops for control or handling in preparation of placing clamps.

If the scar tissue is too severe to safely dissect, a retroperitoneal or midline incision should be considered to expose the abdominal component of the graft for proximal control. Distal control can be obtained through an incision lateral to the sartorius muscle. Mobilizing the sartorius medially and incising the deep fascia exposes the superficial femoral and the profunda femoris arteries. Another alternative for distal vascular control is to open the aneurysm and place balloon occlusion catheters in the distal vessel lumen (Fig. 35-1).

VASCULAR RECONSTRUCTION

An appropriately sized graft should be selected to closely match the diameter of the native arteries, typically a 6- or 8-mm ringed polytetrafluoroethylene graft or Dacron graft. After heparinization, clamps are applied and the aneurysm is incised along the

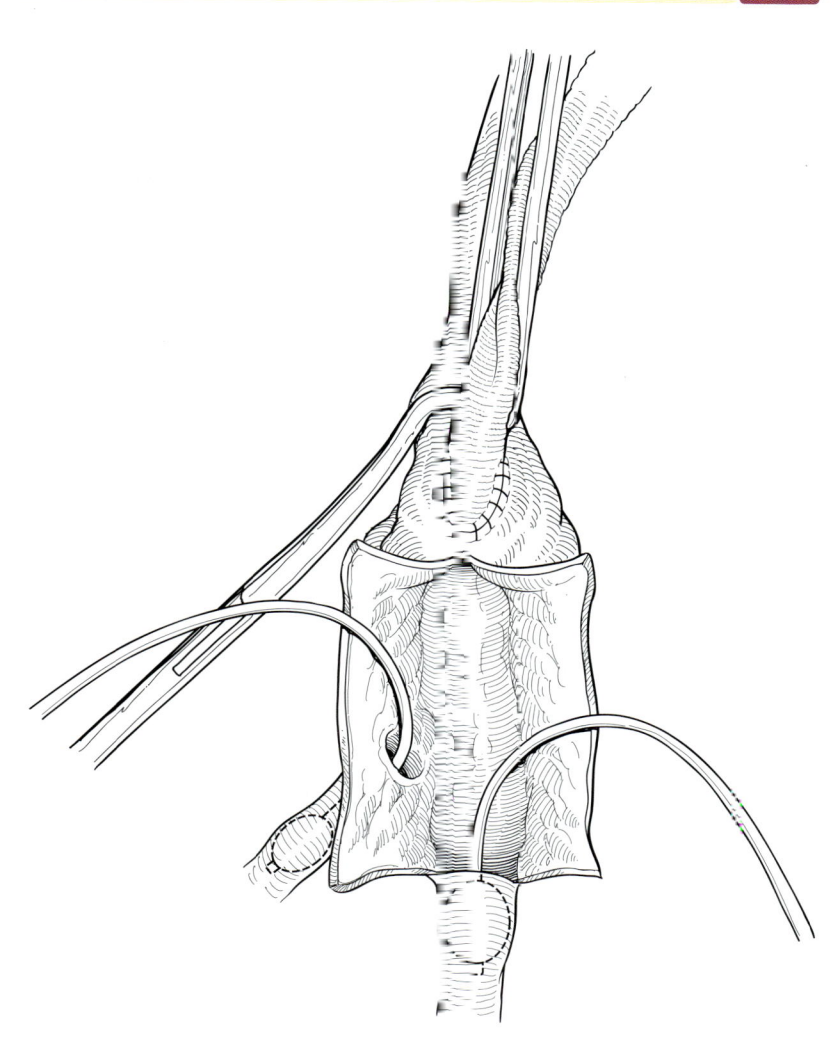

Figure 35-1. Vascular control of a noninfected anastomotic common femoral artery. Inflammation and scar tissue may prohibit control with clamps alone. This illustration demonstrates proximal clamps on the common femoral artery and graft limb, and the aneurysm is opened. Balloon occlusion catheters have been placed in the superficial femoral and profunda femoris arteries for control.

top. The thrombus is removed, and the lumen is inspected for bleeding. The remaining lumen is inspected for adequacy to sew the distal anastomosis with attention toward an endoaneurysmorrhaphy. Endarterectomy is performed as indicated. Interposition of a new tubular prosthesis, bifurcated prosthesis, or patch angioplasty repair is dictated by the availability of healthy arterial tissue. Preservation of retrograde flow in the native system may be challenging or impossible. Therefore the status of both hypogastric arteries must be appreciated preoperatively to aid clinical decision making. Flow in the common femoral, superficial femoral, and profunda femoris arteries is evaluated for adequate backbleeding. The superficial femoral artery or common femoral artery can be disconnected if completely occluded. Proximal and distal anastomoses are performed, flow in the superficial femoral and profunda femoris arteries is assessed by Doppler examination, and the foot is inspected for adequate perfusion and absence of distal embolization. Arteriography can be performed as needed.

CLOSURE

Closure typically requires multiple layers. If the inguinal ligament was divided, it should be repaired with permanent suture. The subcutaneous tissues are closed to remove dead space and thus prevent seroma or fluid accumulation near the graft. Skin can be closed with staples, interrupted nylon, or subcuticular suture. Prophylactic perioperative antibiotics are administered for 24 hours.

Operative Technique for an Infected Femoral Artery Pseudoaneurysm

INCISION

In the presence of an infected femoral pseudoaneurysm, revascularization should most often be done separate from the infected anatomic field. Sterile preparation excludes the infected groin to prevent contamination of the new bypass graft and includes the entire abdomen and the bilateral circumferential lower extremities. Depending on the suspected extent of infection, a midline incision or oblique flank incision is used. The oblique flank incision begins lateral to the border of the rectus muscle, 3 cm above the inguinal ligament, and continues to the midaxillary line between the iliac crest and the costal margin. The oblique flank incision allows retroperitoneal access. During dissection of the graft and iliac artery, the ureter should be identified and protected, usually with medial mobilization so that the graft can be accessed lateral to the ureter. Incorporation of surrounding tissue into the graft and absence of perigraft fluid is evidence that infection does not involve the limb at this level. The affected distal graft limb needs to be fully mobilized distally in the abdomen so that it can be completely excised, subsequently from the groin incision.

DISTAL EXPOSURE AND VASCULAR CONTROL

Distal dissection depends on available outflow options, as identified by angiography. An incision is made in an uninfected area of the thigh to expose the superficial femoral or popliteal artery. With appropriate proximal and distal points, tunneling through the obturator foramen is performed. The obturator membrane is palpated behind the superior pubic ramus and inguinal canal. Sweeping a finger along the membrane, the small foramen where the obturator artery and nerve perforate the membrane posterolaterally can be palpated. The tunnel begins with sharp dissection or cautery through the tough membrane in an anteromedial position, and then a standard tunneling device is passed into the thigh (Fig. 35-2). If there is concern about infection in the pelvis, a red rubber catheter can be placed in the tunnel rather than the graft until the extent of infection has been determined.

After establishing uninfected points of inflow and outflow, heparin is administered. The original limb of the graft is divided proximal to the inguinal ligament for creation of an end-to-end proximal anastomosis. The distal portion of the

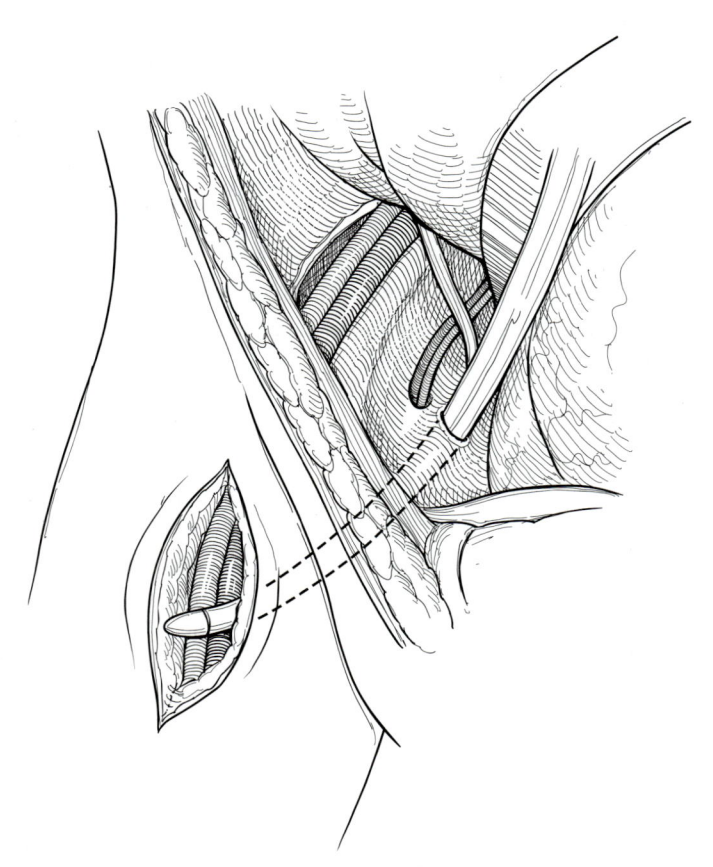

Figure 35-2. A curvilinear retroperitoneal incision exposes the obturator foramen. With the obturator foramen exposed, a tunneling device passes through the obturator foramen into the midthigh for access to the superficial femoral artery.

graft limb is fully mobilized so that it can be subsequently removed from the groin. A small sample of the presumably uninfected distal graft is sent for culture to assess for the presence of subclinical infection that may direct later antibiotic therapy. Proximal and distal anastomoses are then performed (Fig. 35-3). The wounds are then closed and covered with an occlusive barrier dressing before the infected groin is exposed.

REMOVAL OF THE INFECTED GRAFT

The infection source is addressed with direct dissection of the groin. Although the main arterial inflow source has been disconnected, there remains risk of hemorrhage. For example, collaterals may provide residual prograde flow to the external iliac artery, and backbleeding is likely from the superficial femoral and profunda femoris arteries. In an abscess cavity the femoral vein is also at risk for injury. Control of the common femoral, superficial femoral, and profunda femoris arteries should be obtained, or balloon occlusion catheters should be readily available. The pseudoaneurysm cavity is entered, the disconnected infected portion of the distal graft is identified, and the remaining proximal portion of the graft is

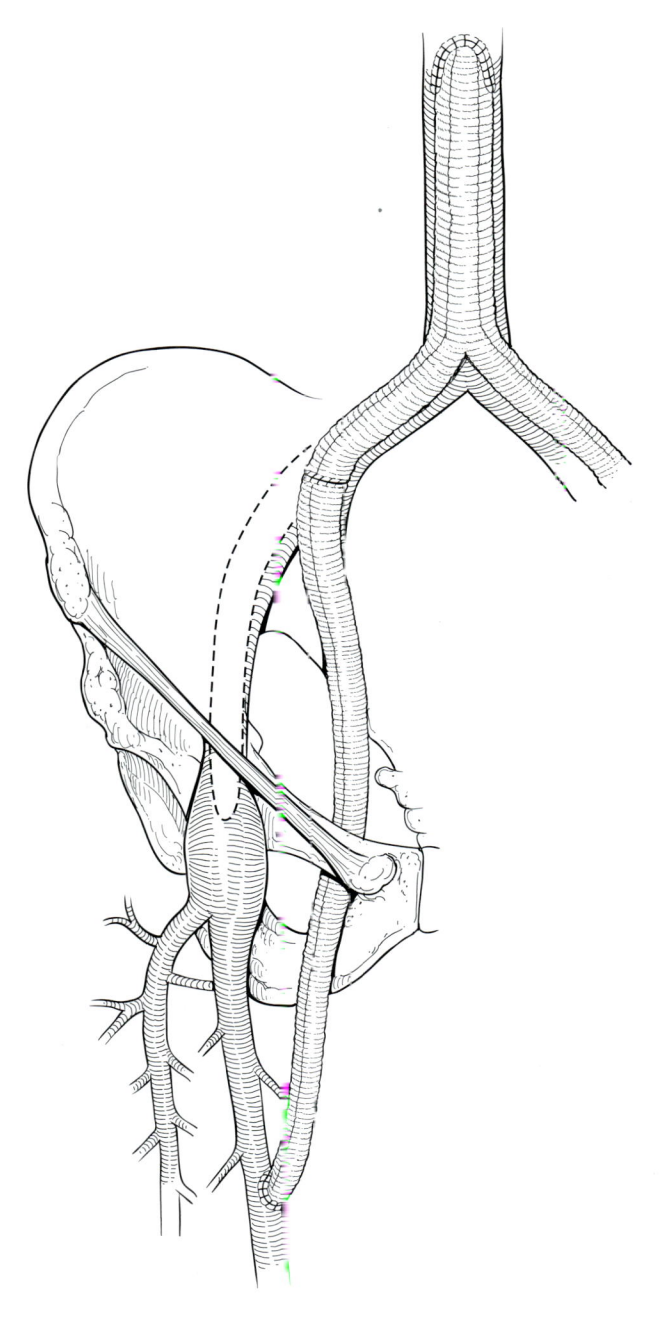

Figure 35-3. Anatomic location of the obturator foramen bypass, passing through the pelvis to the medial thigh to avoid the septic process in the femoral triangle.

mobilized from beneath the inguinal ligament and removed. Both fluid from the abscess cavity and a portion of the infected graft should be sent for culture. The ligament can be cut if needed to safely remove the graft. The proximal common femoral artery can be oversewn to simplify the reconstruction if pelvic perfusion from the contralateral femoral artery is adequate. Profunda femoris artery flow should be preserved if possible. Patch angioplasty using vein or bovine pericardium can be used if the defect in the common femoral artery is minimal. Other techniques to maintain profunda femoris artery flow include anastomosing the superficial femoral artery to the profunda femoris artery or using the divided proximal portion of the common femoral artery as a patch over the more distal junction between the profunda femoris and the superficial femoral arteries. Both approaches depend on the patent superficial femoral artery to provide retrograde flow to the profunda femoris artery. If the infection process is too great, the superficial femoral and profunda femoris arteries can be ligated. Once vascular control is complete, the field should be aggressively debrided and copiously irrigated, preferably with a pulse irrigation device.

CLOSURE

Although no graft is in the field, the ligated vessels often require soft tissue coverage. The best option is the sartorius myoplasty.[5] Raising a minimal flap to identify the tendinous insertion at the anterior superior iliac spine, the muscle is completely mobilized and the tendinous portion is transected. The muscle is sutured securely over the vessels with stitches, eliminating potential space between the muscle and the soft tissue bed. Mattress stitches in a U configuration are helpful in securing the sartorius muscle to the femoral sheath. Depending on habitus and tissue availability, closure of remaining tissue is over closed suction drains with the skin left open; alternatively, the wound can be left open to close by secondary intention. Vacuum-assisted dressings have expedited healing of these open wounds.

Endovascular Options for Anastomotic and Infected Pseudoaneurysms

Use of stent grafts in the femoral artery is limited to case reports with ongoing concerns for stent fracture and occlusion of the profunda femoris artery. Brountzos and colleagues[6] reported stent-graft placement in a degenerative pseudoaneurysm when patient comorbidities precluded general anesthesia, with graft patency at 6 months. Klonaris and associates[7] temporized ruptured infected anastomotic pseudoaneurysms with a stent graft in six patients, four of whom had lower extremity bypasses and two of whom had dialysis access grafts. Debridement was performed during the same admission, occluded grafts were removed, and stent grafts, if encountered, were covered with a sartorius myoplasty. All patients were placed on long-term antibiotics.

Placement of an endovascular graft may be considered a temporizing maneuver when the clinical condition mandates. However, stent-graft placement risks occlusion of the profunda femoris or superficial femoral artery, and the endoprosthesis is at high risk for infection with continued arterial destruction.

Endovascular Treatment of an Iatrogenic Femoral Artery Pseudoaneurysm

Iatrogenic femoral artery pseudoaneurysms have increased with catheter-based interventions, especially those relying on larger sheaths for complex interventions, with a reported frequency between 0.05% and 4%.[8] Until 1991 open surgical repair was the gold standard treatment, when ultrasound scan–guided compression was introduced as a nonsurgical intervention.[9] Although helpful, ultrasound scan–guided compression can be painful for the patient, time consuming, and subject to recurrent pseudoaneurysm. Ultrasound-guided thrombin injection was introduced in 1986.[10] Initial concerns regarding intraarterial injection and immunogenic complications proved to be unfounded with proper technique and patient selection.[8,11,12] Khoury and associates[13] noted greater patient satisfaction, shorter thrombosis time, and a higher success rate with thrombin injection (96%) than with ultrasound guided compression (75%).

Indications

- All iatrogenic femoral pseudoaneurysms larger than 2 cm in diameter should be surgically repaired or undergo thrombin injection.
- The presence of an arteriovenous fistula and poor visualization of the neck of the pseudoaneurysm are contraindications to ultrasound-guided thrombin injection.
- If a patient is not on anticoagulation, a small pseudoaneurysm (<1 cm) can be observed with a high rate of spontaneous thrombosis. Follow-up imaging should be performed within 2 weeks.
- If superficial infection, expanding hematoma, skin necrosis, distal ischemia, or sensory and motor findings suggestive of femoral nerve compression are present, surgical repair is recommended.
- Severe pain often necessitates evacuation of a large hematoma for patient comfort.

Preoperative Care

- Evaluation of the patient includes history and physical examination, duplex ultrasound imaging, and an ankle-brachial index.
- Careful note should be made of anticoagulation status.

Endovascular Technique

Thrombin injection can be done at the bedside with portable ultrasound. Recommended needle sizes range from 19 to 25 Ga. Concentrations for injection have progressively decreased and adequate doses of thrombin now range from 20 to 100 International Units. After infiltration with local anesthesia, thrombin injection is performed with ultrasound guidance. A 1 mL tuberculin syringe and 25 Ga needle are most convenient. The needle should access the pseudoaneurysm as far from the neck as possible. When multilobed pseudoaneurysms are present, beginning at the lobe closest to the parent artery may thrombose all components of the aneurysm. Otherwise, individual injections are appropriate. After injection, ultrasound should confirm persistent flow in the artery and vein.[12]

Postoperative Care

- Bed rest is not required after injection, but the patient is reevaluated in 6 hours and duplex ultrasound is repeated within 24 hours to confirm persistent thrombosis of the pseudoaneurysm.
- After discharge, the patient is evaluated in 1 month with duplex ultrasound and ankle-brachial indices.

REFERENCES

1. Schramel RJ, Creech O: Effects of infection and exposure on synthetic arterial prostheses, *Arch Surg* 78:271-279, 1959.
2. Fry WJ, Lindenauer SM: Infection complicating the use of plastic arterial implants, *Arch Surg* 94:600-609, 1967.
3. O'Connor S, Andrew P, Batt M, et al: A systematic review and meta-analysis of treatments for aortic graft infection, *J Vasc Surg* 44:38-45, 2006.
4. Shaw RS, Baue AE: Management of sepsis complicating arterial reconstructive surgery, *Surgery* 53:75-86, 1963.

5. Landry GJ, Carlson JR, Liem TK, et al: The Sartorius muscle flap: An important adjunct for complicated femoral wounds involving vascular grafts, *Am J Surg* 197:655-659, 2009.
6. Brountzos EN, Malagari K, Gougoulakis A, et al: Common femoral artery anastomotic pseudoaneurysm: Endovascular treatment with Hemobahn stent grafts, *JVIR* 11:1179-1183, 2000.
7. Klonaris C, Katsagyris A, Vasileiou I, et al: Hybrid repair of ruptured infected anastomotic femoral pseudoaneurysms: Emergent stent-graft implantation and secondary surgical debridement, *J Vasc Surg* 49:938-945, 2009.
8. Olsen DM, Rodriguez JA, Vranic M, et al: A prospective study of ultrasound scan-guided thrombin injection of femoral pseudoaneurysm: A trend toward minimal medication, *J Vasc Surg* 36:779-783, 2002.
9. Fellmeth BD, Roberts AC, Bookstein JJ, et al: Postangiographic femoral artery injuries: Nonsurgical repair with ultrasound guided compression, *Radiology* 178:671-675, 1991.
10. Cope C, Zeit R: Coagulation of aneurysms by direct percutaneous thrombin injection, *AJR Am J Roentgenol* 147:383-387, 1986.
11. Sheiman RG, Brophy DP: Treatment of iatrogenic femoral pseudoaneurysms with percutaneous thrombin injection: Experience in 54 patients, *Radiology* 219:123-127, 2001.
12. Hanson JM, Atri M, Power N: Ultrasound-guided thrombin injection of iatrogenic groin pseudoaneurysm: Doppler features and technical tips, *Br J Radiol* 81:154-163, 2009.
13. Khoury M, Rebecca A, Greene K, et al: Duplex scanning-guided thrombin injection for the treatment of iatrogenic pseudoaneurysms, *J Vasc Surg* 35:517-521, 2002.

Section 8

RENAL ARTERY DISEASE

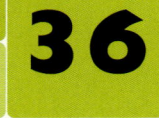

36 Direct Surgical Repair of Renovascular Disease

KIMBERLEY J. HANSEN • CHRISTOPHER J. GODSHALL

Historical Background

In 1937 Goldblatt[1] demonstrated that renal artery constriction produced atrophy of the kidney and systemic hypertension in a canine model. His elegant experiments defined a causal relationship between renovascular disease and hypertension. Leadbetter and Burkland[2] are credited with the first successful treatment of renovascular hypertension. A 5-year-old child was cured of severe hypertension after removal of an ischemic kidney. After Leadbetter and Burkland's 1938 report, nephrectomy was performed for patients based on the presence of hypertension associated with a small kidney as demonstrated by intravenous pyelography. In a 1956 review of 575 nephrectomies, Smith[3] found that only 25% of patients were cured of hypertension.

In 1954 Freeman and colleagues[4] performed the first direct surgical repair of renovascular disease—a transaortic bilateral renal artery thromboendarterectomy. His treatment represented the first cure of hypertension by direct surgical repair. This success was accompanied by widespread aortography and direct renovascular repair for presumed blood pressure benefit. However, in the early 1960s it was recognized that repair of renovascular disease in all hypertensive patients benefited less than half of individuals.[5]

Morris, DeBakey, and Cooley[6] reported in 1962 on eight azotemic patients who had improved blood pressure and renal function after direct surgical repair of renovascular disease. This report marked a shift in focus from renovascular hypertension to renovascular renal insufficiency or ischemic nephrectomy. Since that time other groups have found a similar beneficial function response in select patients with global renal ischemia.[7,8]

Indications

Natural history studies of atherosclerotic renovascular disease among patients with hypertension demonstrated anatomic progression of renal artery stenosis with concomitant decline in kidney size and function.[9-11] However, more recent studies suggest that anatomic progression is rare in the absence of severe hypertension.[12,13] After a mean follow-up of 8 years, the rate of progression to more severe renal artery stenosis or occlusion among independent, elderly subjects was estimated at 0.5% per year.[12] Among 434 hypertensive patients, 6% to 9% demonstrated progression of stenosis and 2.3% progressed to occlusion over follow-up of 3.2 years.[13] Progression of disease correlated with renal length but not with renal function. Consequently, in the absence of hypertension, renovascular intervention is not recommended as either isolated repair or renal artery repair in combination with aortic reconstruction.

In the absence of positive physiologic studies, such as select renal vein assays, the most important clinical characteristic of significant renovascular disease is severe hypertension. Severe hypertension is strongly associated with blood pressure benefit and improved renal function when ischemic nephropathy is present. However, severity of hypertension is estimated by untreated blood pressure, not by the number of antihypertensive medications prescribed. The highest recorded blood pressure is a useful surrogate for severity of hypertension.

Preoperative Preparation

- Patients with severe hypertension requiring large doses of multiple medications often have requirements reduced when placed on bed rest. Otherwise, hypertension medications are reduced to the minimum necessary for blood pressure control during the preoperative period. If the blood pressure remains in excess of the 95th percentile for age and length in children or greater than 120 mm Hg diastolic in adults, surgical repair should be postponed until blood pressure is brought under control.
- The combination of an intravenous calcium channel-blocking agent, such as nicardipine, and selective beta-adrenergic blocking agents, such as esmolol or metoprolol, is administered in an intensive care setting.

Pitfalls and Danger Points

- **Renal atheroembolism.** During renal artery exposure tissues are dissected away from the aorta and renal artery. Systemic heparinization is confirmed by activated clotting time. The distal renal artery or its branches are controlled with atraumatic clamps before proximal aortic or proximal renal artery control. Arterial reconstructions are flushed vigorously with heparinized saline. Renal artery control is released as the final step after reconstruction.
- **Criteria for renal endarterectomy.** Successful endarterectomy requires that the aortic atheroma end within 1 or 1.5 cm of the renal artery origin. In addition, preaneurysmal degenerative change of the aorta and transmural calcific atheroma must be excluded before endarterectomy.

Operative Strategy for Renovascular Occlusive Disease

UNILATERAL OR BILATERAL RENAL ARTERY REPAIR

The rationale for treatment of renovascular disease is to improve event-free survival. Best evidence suggests that adults cured of severe hypertension and patients with renal insufficiency who demonstrate incremental increase in excretory renal function have improved dialysis-free survival.[7,8] In the absence of hypertension or renal insufficiency, prophylactic renal artery intervention is not recommended by either direct surgical repair or endovascular intervention.

In contrast to prophylactic intervention, empiric renal artery repair implies that hypertension, excretory renal dysfunction, or both are present even though a causal relationship between renovascular disease and clinical sequelae has not been established. Direct surgical repair of a unilateral renal artery lesion is performed when hypertension remains severe and uncontrollable, despite maximum drug therapy in a young patient without significant risk factors for repair. When a patient has bilateral renovascular disease and hypertension, the decision for direct surgical repair is based on the severity of the hypertension and the severity of the renal artery lesions. When severe stenosis of one renal artery exists with mild to moderate contralateral disease, the patient is treated for a unilateral lesion. When both renal artery lesions are moderately severe (60%-80%), direct repair is undertaking only if the associated hypertension or renal insufficiency is severe. When both renal arteries display severe stenosis (>80%) and are associated with severe hypertension, bilateral renal revascularization is performed.

RENAL ARTERY ANATOMY

The renal arteries may vary in location and number. Renal arteries may arise from any portion of the abdominal aorta or iliac system. Single renal arteries to each kidney are found in 80% to 85% of patients. These renal artery origins are usually at the body of the L2 vertebra. The right artery arises from the anterolateral aspect of the aorta, whereas the left artery usually originates from the posterolateral aorta. Between 15% and 20% of patients demonstrate multiple renal arteries. On the right, inferior polar renal arteries frequently course anterior to the inferior vena cava, and all such vessels should be presumed to be renal branches. In the presence of severe occlusive lesions, collateral vessels are prominent, especially in childhood.

EXPOSURE OF THE PARARENAL AORTA

Exposure of the pararenal aorta is facilitated by complete mobilization of the left renal vein from caval origin to renal hilum. The adrenal, gonadal, and renal lumbar branches are identified, ligated, and divided if necessary for exposure. The renal vein may then be retracted superiorly or inferiorly as needed. The right renal artery can be exposed in its entire retrocaval course. This usually does not require division of lumbar veins. Dissection of the neural plexus surrounding the renal arteries is performed with electrocoagulation to minimize blood loss.

SELECTION OF A METHOD FOR DIRECT SURGICAL REPAIR

No single direct surgical repair provides optimal reconstruction for all renovascular diseases. Of the three direct techniques—aortorenal bypass, thromboendarterectomy, and renal artery implantation—aortorenal bypass is the most versatile technique. In the atherosclerotic adult, saphenous vein is the preferred conduit, whereas autogenous artery repair is preferred for children. When a conduit is necessary in a child, the hypogastric artery is preferred; however, if the renal artery demonstrates sufficient redundancy, reimplantation is particularly useful in children. In cases of ostial atherosclerotic renovascular disease involving both renal arteries or in the presence of multiple renal arteries, transaortic renal endarterectomy may be preferred. However, successful endarterectomy requires that the aortic atheroma end within 1 or 1.5 cm of the renal artery origin. In addition, preaneurysmal degenerative change of the aorta and transmural calcific atheroma must be excluded before endarterectomy.

SOURCE OF INFLOW

Direct surgical repair is selected over indirect methods for most patients. Concomitant celiac stenosis occurs in 40% of adult patients, and bilateral renovascular repair is required in half.[8] The infrarenal aorta is the preferred inflow source; however, when patient anatomy precludes this site, the supraceliac aorta is used for inflow. To avoid compromise associated with progressive atherosclerosis, the iliac vessels are avoided as a source of inflow. To minimize renal ischemia during renal artery bypass, the proximal aortorenal anastomosis is performed first, followed by the distal anastomoses.

INTRAOPERATIVE ASSESSMENT OF RENOVASCULAR REPAIR

Regardless of the method of direct surgical repair, each reconstruction is evaluated at completion with renal duplex sonography. Images are obtained from sites of arterial exposure, control, and reconstruction with associated Doppler-shifted signals and Doppler spectrum analysis. Major B-scan defects, with a peak systolic velocity of at least 180 cm/sec, have been noted in 12% of all direct repairs. A disproportionate number of major defects occur in association with thromboendarterectomy. When direct surgical repair of renovascular disease is associated with normal completion duplex sonography, a 95% long-term primary patency of reconstruction has been observed.

Operative Strategy for a Renal Artery Aneurysm

RENAL PROTECTION

Branch renal artery involvement in association with renal artery aneurysm disease because of atherosclerosis or dissection may be complex, with exposure of branch anatomy often obscured by associated renal veins. When more than 40 minutes of warm renal ischemia are anticipated for direct repair, measures to protect renal function should be used.

Of the methods and techniques purposed for renal protection, the use of hypothermia seems to be most important. Intermittent hypothermic perfusion is preferred, with intracellular electrolyte composition supplemented by topical cooling with ice slush. If exposure is sufficient for branch renal artery repair, the ipsilateral renal vein is left intact and controlled in its caval origin and a small venotomy is made for the drainage of perfusate. If exposure is inadequate, a partial occluding clamp is placed at the origin of the renal vein, and the vein is divided with a cuff of vena cava. In either instance the perfusate is supplemented with topical ice slush, and the kidney is returned to an orthotopic location after repair.

For both in situ and ex vivo perfusion preservation, the ureter is controlled with a doubly passed vessel loop to control periureteric collaterals. Care is taken to mobilize the ureter with an abundant amount of periureteric soft tissue. For ex vivo reconstruction the ureter is mobilized to the level of the pelvic brim, allowing elevation of the kidney.

SELECTION OF A METHOD FOR DIRECT SURGICAL REPAIR

A number of techniques have been described for direct surgical repair of renal artery aneurysms. Branch renal reconstruction with syndactyly is preferred to patch angioplasty. In the course of dissection each major and segmental branch of the renal artery is exposed, and the aneurysm is opened at a point remote from the branches. This allows the direct assessment of each branch origin and the elimination of associated stenosis when present.

Operative Technique for Aortorenal Bypass

INCISION

For bilateral renovascular repair and combined aortorenal reconstruction, a midline abdominal incision is preferred (Fig. 36-1). With the patient positioned supine and the table break at the level of the umbilicus, the operating table is flexed 10 to 15 degrees. To expose the upper abdominal aorta through a midline incision, it is important that the superior aspect of the wound extend 1 to 2 cm to one side of the xiphoid. Extended flank and subcostal incisions are used for direct unilateral branch reconstruction or for indirect repair. In both instances a fixed mechanical retractor is advantageous.

EXPOSURE OF THE PARARENAL AORTA

When the midline incision is used, the posterior peritoneum overlying the aorta is incised longitudinally (Fig. 36-1). The duodenum is mobilized at the ligament of Treitz. This maneuver can be facilitated by the division of the inferior mesentery vein after excluding visceral collaterals, which may course at this level. The duodenum is reflected to the right, and the posterior peritoneal incision is extended along the left renal vein. This creates a plane along the inferior border of the pancreas, which can be retracted superiorly to expose the left renal hilum (Fig. 36-2, *A*). The left renal artery lies posterior to the vein, which is retracted

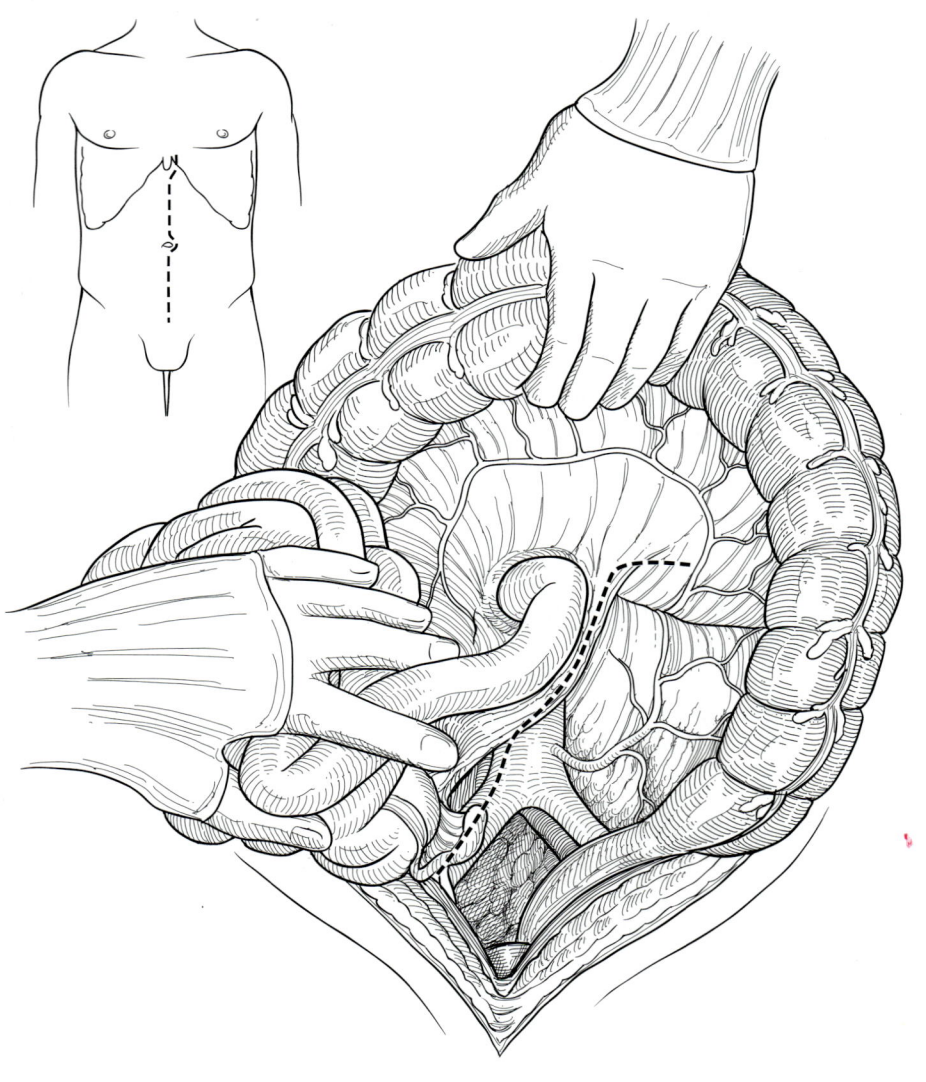

Figure 36-1. Exposure of the aorta and left renal hilum through the base of the mesentery. Extension of the posterior peritoneal incision to the left, along the inferior border of the pancreas, provides entry to an avascular plane posterior to the pancreas. This allows excellent exposure of the entire left renal vein and hilum, as well as the proximal right renal artery. *(Adapted from Benjamin ME, Dean RH: Techniques in renal artery reconstruction: Part I, Ann Vasc Surg 10:306-314, 1996.)*

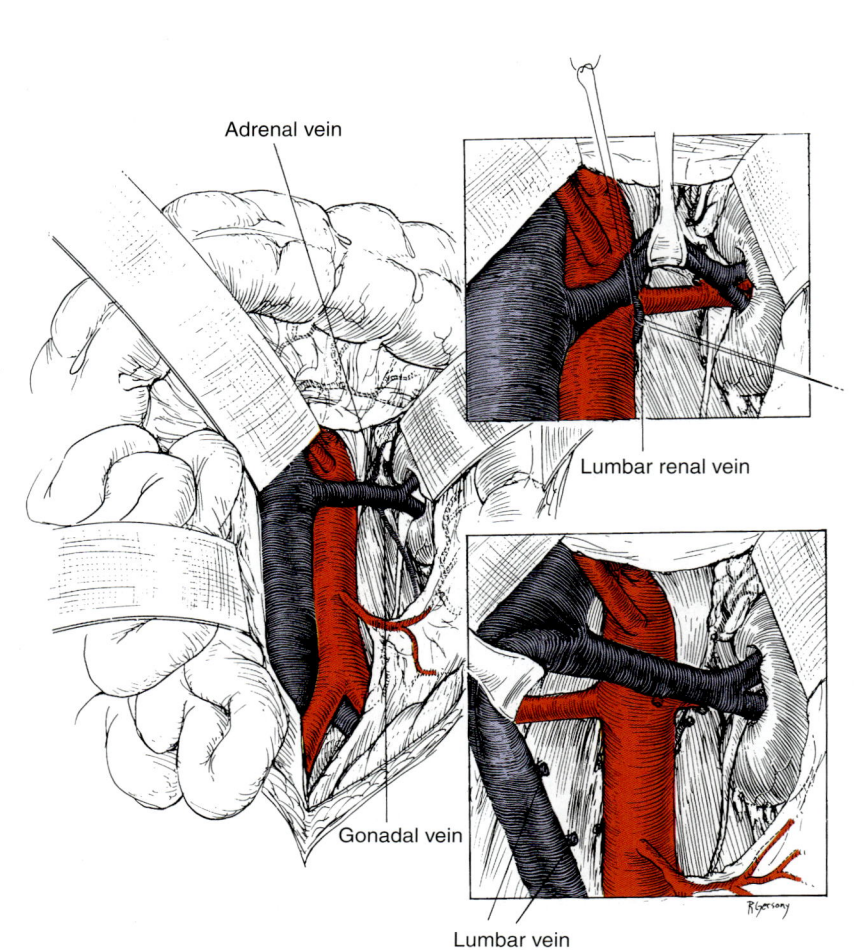

Figure 36-2. Exposure of the proximal right renal artery through the base of the mesentery. Mobilization of the left renal vein by ligation and division of the adrenal and gonadal veins, as well as the renal lumbar vein, allows exposure of the entire left renal artery to the hilum (*inset, top*). Lumbar veins are occasionally ligated and divided to allow retraction of the vena cava to the right (*inset, bottom*). Often, adequate exposure of the proximal renal artery disease can be obtained without this maneuver. *(From Benjamin ME, Dean RH: Techniques in renal artery reconstruction: Part I, Ann Vasc Surg 10:306-314, 1996.)*

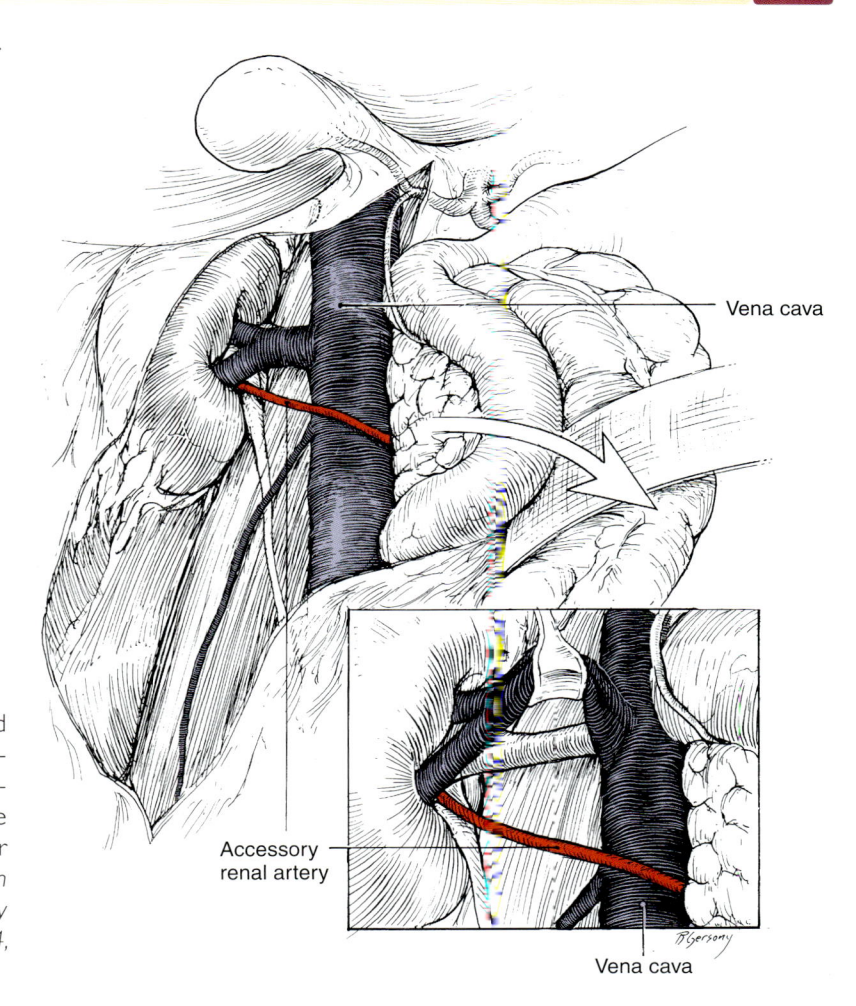

Figure 36-3. A Kocher maneuver was performed to expose the right renal hilum. Arteries encountered anterior to the vena cava should be considered accessory renal arteries and preserved. The right renal vein is typically mobilized superiorly for exposure of the distal right renal artery (*inset*). (*From Benjamin ME, Dean RH: Techniques in renal artery reconstruction: Part I, Ann Vasc Surg 10:306-314, 1996.*)

to expose the artery (Fig. 36-2, *B*). A lumbar vein frequently exits the posterior wall of the left renal vein, and special care should be taken to avoid injury to this structure. The proximal right renal artery can be visualized in its entire retrocaval course (Fig. 36-2, *C*). The hilar portion of the right renal artery is best exposed by mobilizing the hepatic flexure of the colon, in combination with a wide Kocher maneuver (Fig. 36-3, *A*). This exposes 3 to 4 cm of the infrarenal aorta, preserving associated lumbar arteries.

RENAL ARTERY BYPASS

Systemic heparinization is verified by clotting time, and the infrarenal aorta is controlled segmentally. On the left, a lateral aortotomy is preferred; on the right, the aortotomy may originate from the anterior or posterior lateral aorta depending on whether the bypass is routed anterior or posterior to the vena cava. This latter bypass route may require division of one or more pairs of lumbar veins. An aortotomy is made with two or three applications of a 4.8-mm aortic punch. Creation of this elliptical aortotomy is especially important in the atherosclerotic aorta. The conduit for bypass is then spatulated three times its diameter to allow proximal anastomosis without stenosis using continuous 6-0 polypropylene sutures (Fig. 36-4). It is important to create a bypass of correct length that allows a tension-free anastomosis without the kinking associated with redundancy. This is best accomplished by placing the bypass conduit and native renal artery on gentle tension and selecting a length for spatulation of each structure three times their diameters. The distal anastomosis is created with continuous 7-0 polypropylene suture. Before completing the anastomosis, the conduit is flushed of air and debris, and the distal native circulation is allowed to backbleed.

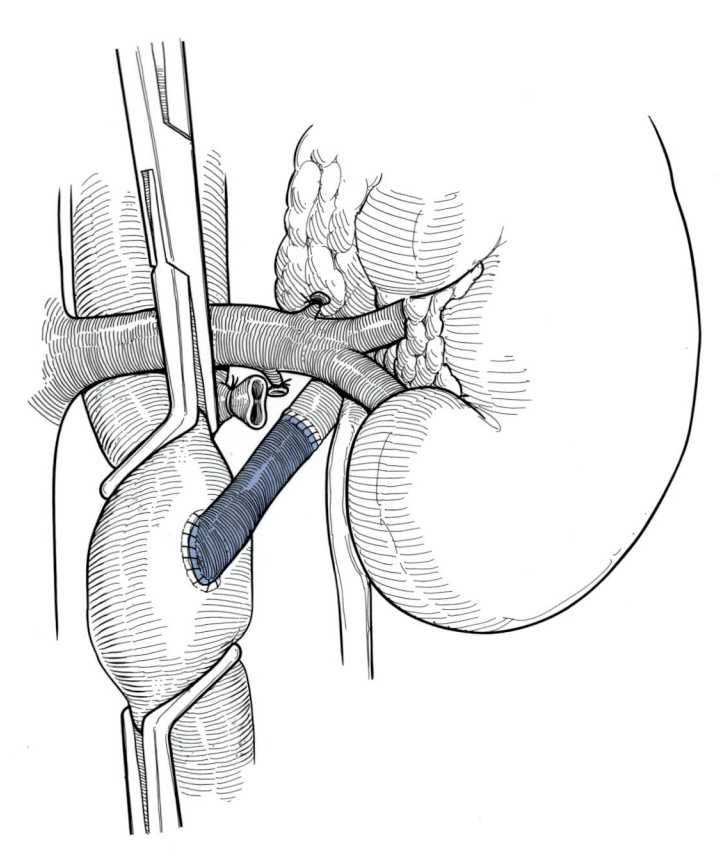

Figure 36-4. Technique for end-to-end aortorenal saphenous vein bypass grafting. The length of arteriotomy is at least three times the diameter of the artery to prevent recurrent anastomotic stenosis. For the anastomosis, 6-0 or 7-0 monofilament polypropylene sutures are used continuously with loupe magnification. If the apex sutures of the distal anastomosis are placed too deeply or with excess advancement, stenosis can be created, posing a risk of late graft thrombosis. *(Adapted from Benjamin ME, Dean RH: Techniques in renal artery reconstruction: Part I, Ann Vasc Surg 10:306-314, 1996.)*

Operative Technique for Renal Artery Endarterectomy

EXPOSURE OF THE PARARENAL AORTA

Patient positioning, surgical incision, and infrarenal aortic and renal artery exposure are the same as for bypass. However, endarterectomy requires more extensive aortic exposure proximal to the superior mesenteric artery. This is facilitated by dissection of the dense periaortic neural plexus present at this level and partial division of the right and left aortic crura (Fig. 36-5, *A*). The origin of the superior mesenteric artery is exposed for subsequent control.

TRANSAORTIC RENAL ARTERY ENDARTERECTOMY

After exposure has been obtained and systemic heparin anticoagulation has been established and verified, the superior mesenteric artery is controlled with a doubly passed elastic loop. The renal arteries are controlled with atraumatic spring bulldog clamps, well distal to the endpoint of atherosclerotic disease. Aortic control is initially obtained, proximal to the superior mesenteric artery, followed by infrarenal aortic control. Intervening lumbar arteries are controlled with curved bulldog clamps. A longitudinal arteriotomy is made extending from the base of the superior mesenteric artery 2 cm inferior to the lowest renal artery origin (Fig. 36-5, *B*).

The endarterectomy plane is best initiated at the site of most advanced, calcific disease. A sleeve endarterectomy of the aorta is performed first, extending above both renal arteries to the base of the superior mesenteric artery, where the atherosclerotic plaque is divided flush with the residual adventitia using scissors. The distal atheroma is divided similarly, tacking the distal intima with 5-0 polypropylene suture.

With the endarterectomy of the aorta completed, transaortic endarterectomy of the renal artery is performed last. This portion of the procedure is facilitated by the eversion of the renal artery into the aortic lumen by the assistant (Fig. 36-5, *C*). The endarterectomy is best performed with gentle pressure on the undiseased outer arterial layer, pushing this layer from the atherosclerotic plaque. When the

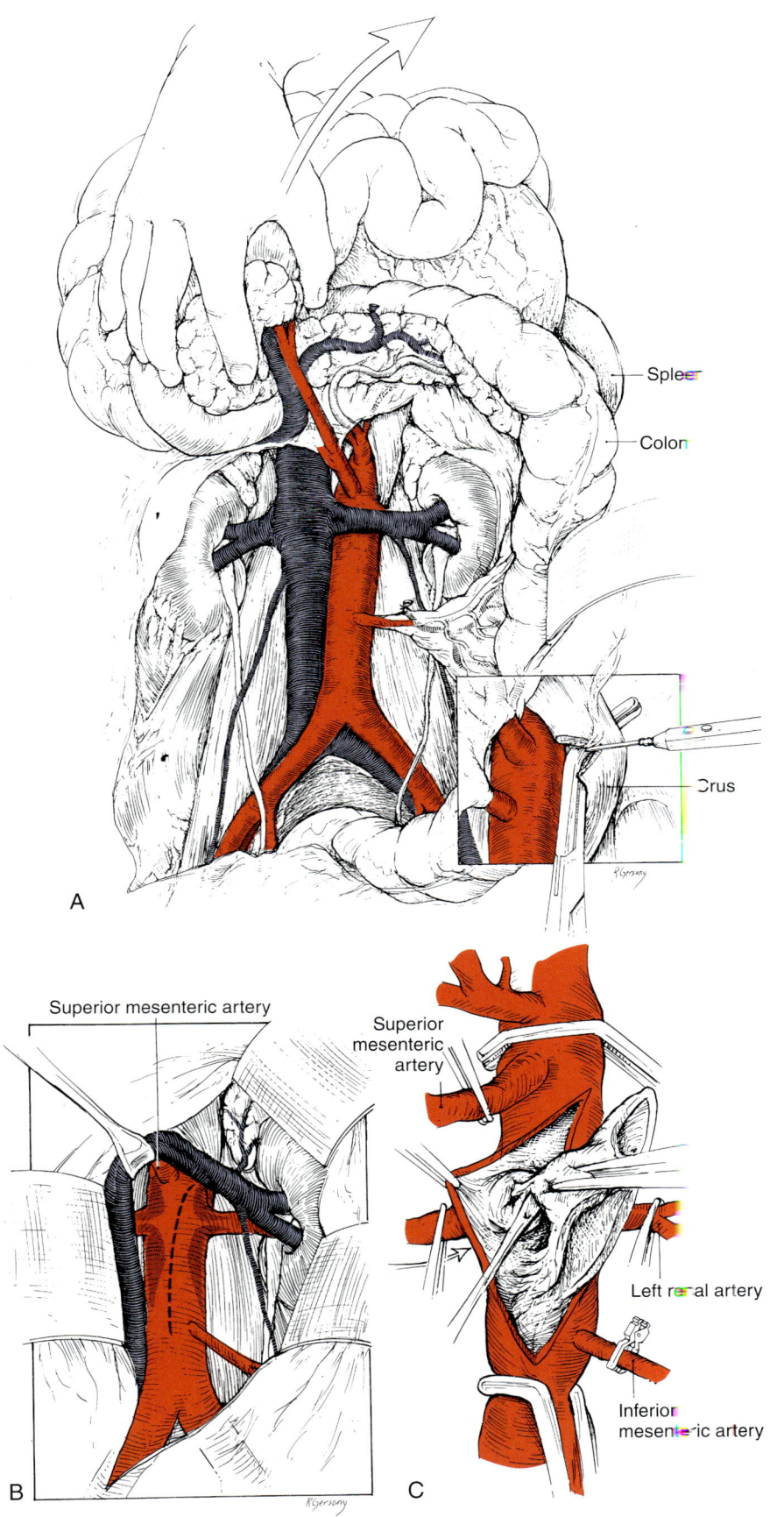

Figure 36-5. A, For bilateral renal artery reconstruction, combined with aortic repair, extended exposure can be obtained using a right-side medial visceral rotation with mobilization of the cecum and ascending colon. The entire small bowel and right colon are then mobilized to the right upper quadrant and retracted superiorly. Partial division of the diaphragmatic crura exposes the origin of the mesenteric vessels (*inset*). **B** and **C,** Exposure for a longitudinal transaortic endarterectomy by a standard transperitoneal approach in which the duodenum has been mobilized at the ligament of Treitz in a standard fashion. If more complete exposure is desired, the ascending colon and small bowel can be mobilized. **B,** The dotted line shows the location of the aortotomy. **C,** The plaque is transected sharply, and with eversion of the renal arteries, the atherosclerotic plaque is removed from each renal ostium. The aortotomy is typically closed with a running 4-0 or 5-0 polypropylene suture. (*From Benjamin ME, Dean RH: Techniques in renal artery reconstruction: Part I,* Ann Vasc Surg *10:306-314, 1996.*)

444 RENAL ARTERY DISEASE

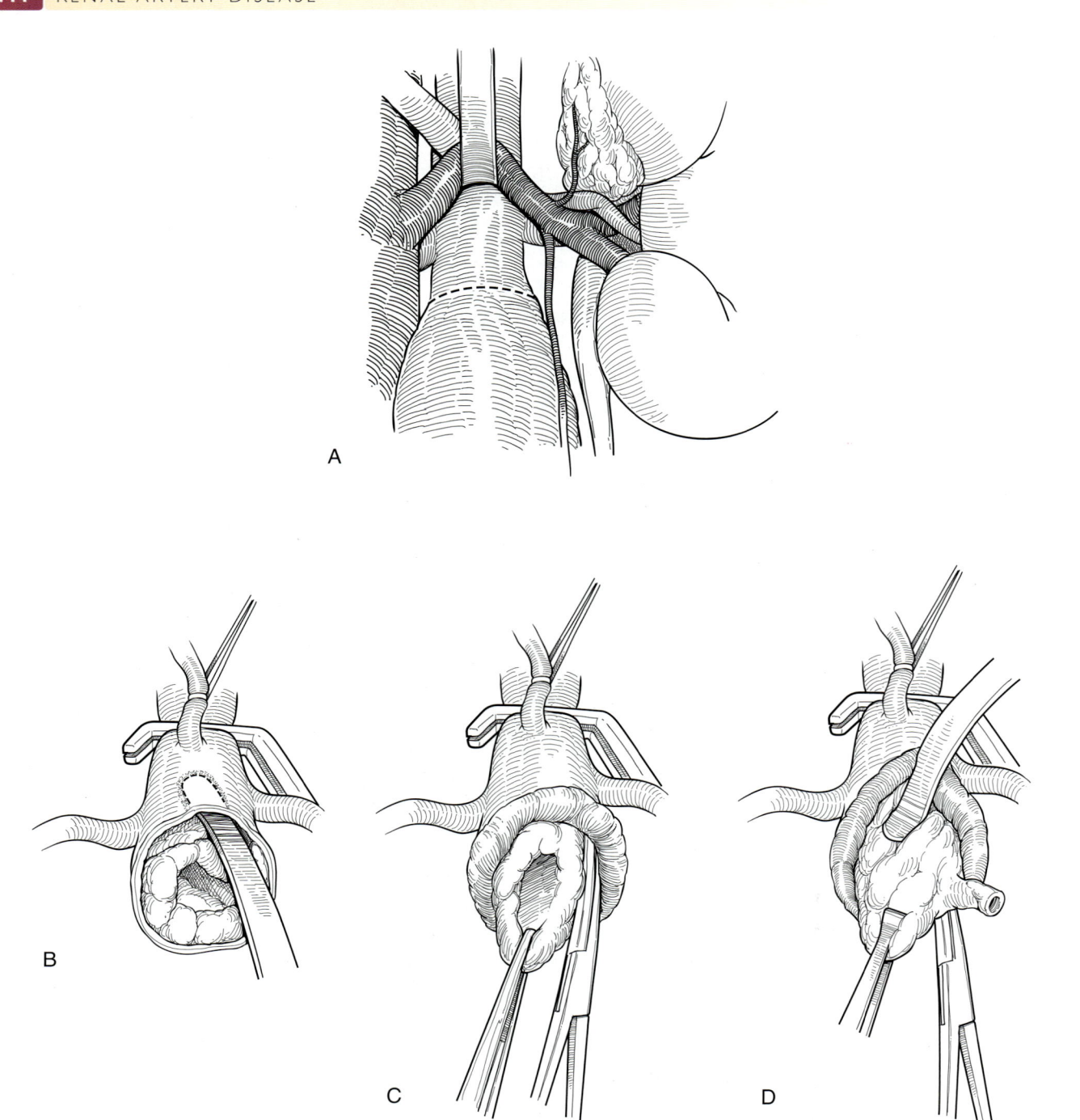

Figure 36-6. A, Renal artery occlusive disease is present in association with a juxtarenal aortic aneurysm. **B** and **C,** After transection of the aortic neck a sleeve endarterectomy is created, and the plaque is divided just distal to the superior mesenteric artery origin. **D,** Eversion endarterectomy of the renal arteries is performed through the divided aorta.

anatomy is properly selected for endarterectomy, the endpoint of the endarterectomy can be visualized directly using the eversion technique. After removal of the surgical specimen, the site of endarterectomy is irrigated vigorously with heparinized saline and the arteriotomy is closed using running 5-0 polypropylene suture. Blood flow is first established to the distal native circulation with external compression of the femoral arteries. The superior mesenteric artery and both renal arteries are then released.

When transaortic renal artery endarterectomy is combined with aortic reconstruction, the endarterectomy is performed through the divided aorta (Fig. 36-6, *A*). A sleeve endarterectomy is created, and the plaque divided just distal to the superior mesenteric artery origin (see Fig. 36-6, *B* and *C*). Eversion endarterectomy of the renal arteries is performed through the divided aorta (see Fig. 36-6, *D*).

Operative Technique for Branch Repair Using In Situ and Ex Vivo Techniques

INCISION

When isolated branch renal artery repair is performed, an extended flank incision is used (Video 36-1). The patient is positioned on the operating table with the ipsilateral flank elevated using folded sheets. The ipsilateral arm is padded and tucked to the side with sheets, allowing the arm to rest posteriorly. With the break in the table positioned at the level of the umbilicus, the table is flexed 15 degrees. For extensive aortic exposure the incision maybe extended to the contralateral semilunar line, but for most repairs the incision extends only to the midline. To facilitate anatomic closure of the wound after direct repair, the musculofascial layers of the abdominal wall are clearly identified.

EXPOSURE OF THE DISTAL RIGHT RENAL ARTERY

Right renal artery reconstruction is facilitated by complete division of the falciform ligament. On both the left and right, it is key to identify the correct plane of dissection between the mesentery and Gerota fascia. After mobilization of the hepatic and splenic attachments of the right and left colon, the renal vein serves as an important landmark. On the right, adhesions between the right lobe of the liver and the posterior peritoneum are divided to allow cephalad retraction of the liver. The colon is mobilized at the lateral peritoneal reflection, and a wide Kocher maneuver of the duodenum is performed. The vena cava and right renal vein are identified, and care is taken to avoid injury to the gonadal vein arising from the anterior cava. An in situ repair of the renal artery without cold perfusion preservation requires no further exposure. However, if performed, cold perfusion preservation requires complete mobilization of the kidney and dissection of the renal hilum. This is accomplished after a cruciate incision is made in Gerota fascia. A dissection plane within Gerota space is created. A key to the complete mobilization of the kidney is dissection of the superior pole first, which allows inferior retraction of the kidney and facilitates posterior exposure. At the inferior pole of the kidney, care should be taken to identify the ureter. The ureter is mobilized with an abundant amount of periureteric soft tissue to the level of pelvic brim. The renal hilum is skeletonized, exposing the proximal renal vein and retrocaval renal artery circumferentially.

EXPOSURE OF THE DISTAL LEFT RENAL ARTERY

On the left, exposure of the kidney requires dissection of the avascular plane posterior to the pancreas. Attachments between the left colon and the spleen must be divided carefully. This allows superior retraction of the pancreas and spleen. On exposing the superior pole of the left kidney, care should be taken to avoid injury of the left adrenal. As in right renal artery exposure, early identification of the left renal vein is key. The adrenal, gonadal, and renal lumbar branches are ligated and divided, and the renal artery is exposed from its aorta origin to the level of hilar disease.

RENAL PROTECTION

Pathologies that require branch exposure and reconstruction may require complex repair associated with prolonged renal ischemia, using the same methods given earlier for renal artery aneurysm. Otherwise, steps that are common to branch renal artery reconstruction include small repeated intravenous doses of mannitol during branch exposure and before renal reperfusion.

If exposure is satisfactory without division of the renal vein, the vein is controlled with an atraumatic clamp, a venotomy is made for the egress of cold perfusate, and the renal artery is doubly ligated and divided. The kidney is perfused with perfusate chilled to 39.2°F (4°C) and elevated 1 to 2 m above the kidney. The

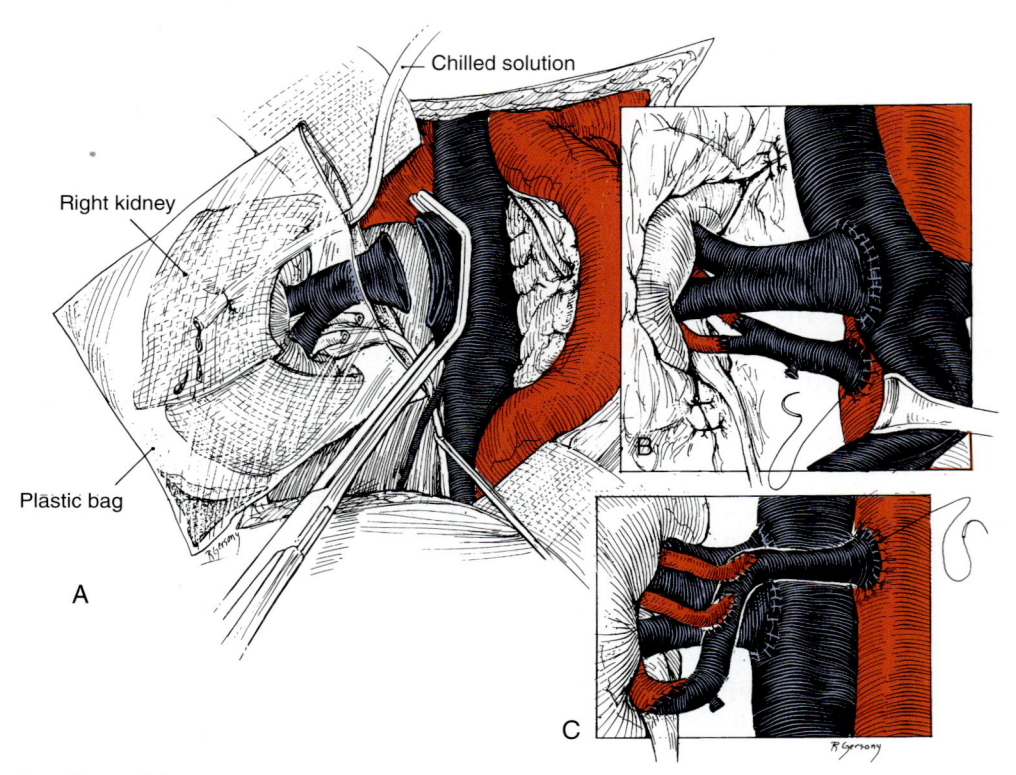

Figure 36-7. A, An ellipse of the vena cava containing the renal vein origin is excised after placement of a large partially occluding clamp to obtain a sizable vein cuff so as to minimize the risk of anastomotic stricture. After ex vivo branch arterial repair, the kidney is returned in its native bed. **B,** Arterial branch reconstruction can be accomplished via end-to-end anastomoses after syndactylizing distal branch or can be combined with end-to-side anastomoses. In this case a bifurcated vein graft is used for arterial branch reconstruction. The renal vein can then be reattached. **C,** Gerota fascia is reapproximated to provide stability to the repaired kidney. *(From Benjamin ME, Dean RH: Techniques in renal artery reconstruction: Part II, Ann Vasc Surg 10:409-414, 1996.)*

volume of initial perfusion ranges between 300 and 500 mL, at which point the venous efferent should be clear. The kidney is placed on a plastic barrier drape and immersed in ice slush (Fig. 36-7, A). To provide more extensive hilar exposure, the renal vein is controlled at its caval junction with a partial occluding clamp and divided with a cuff of vena cava. The kidney can then be elevated into the surgical wound on a plastic barrier drape and immersed in ice slush. The final branch hilar dissection is performed after cold perfusion. After the arterial dissection is complete, the kidney is perfused with 200 to 300 mL of chilled perfusate. To assess for venous injuries made during the dissection, the vein is temporarily occluded with a spring bulldog clamp during perfusion.

RENAL ANEURYSM REPAIR

For treatment of renal artery aneurysm it is preferred to syndactylize the individual branches for one or two distal anastomoses rather than to perform multiple anastomoses. The distal branch reconstruction is performed with continuous 7-0 polypropylene sutures (see Fig. 36-7, B and C). In branch reconstructions, saphenous vein is the conduit of choice in adults. The vein is spatulated at least three times its diameter and sewn end to end to the artery using continuous 7-0 polypropylene suture.

After completion of the distal arterial reconstruction, the kidney is returned to Gerota space and covered with ice slush, and the vein is reattached at its caval origin (see Fig. 36-7, B). This is accomplished with 5-0 polypropylene suture. The continuous posterior suture line is performed first, followed by anterior closure. After vein reattachment, the renal vein is controlled with a bulldog clamp, the partial occluding clamp on the cava is removed, and the venous anastomosis is inspected for hemostasis.

The proximal arterial anastomosis to the aorta is completed last. On the right, the route preferred for the saphenous vein is posterior to the vena cava (Fig. 36-7, B). Techniques for proximal arterial anastomosis are the same as described for aorta renal bypass.

CLOSURE

After vascular reconstruction is completed and repair is free of major defects as defined by renal duplex sonography, Gerota fascia is reapproximated with running 3-0 polydioxanone. The musculofascial layers of the abdominal wall are closed anatomically with 1-0 polydioxanone suture.

Postoperative Care

- Immediate postoperative care is delivered in a surgical intensive care unit setting. Surgical stress and volume expansion associated with direct repair frequently aggravate hypertension in the early postoperative period. Intravenous calcium channel-blocking agents, such as nicardipine, are preferred over other agents. In adults, select beta-adrenergic blocking agents, including esmolol or metoprolol, may be administered intravenously to maintain heart rate below 80 beats per minute.
- Early ambulation is recommended for all patients except those who have undergone ex vivo repair. In this instance the patient is kept at bed rest for 24 to 48 hours after complete mobilization of the kidney and division of the renal hilum.
- Determination of blood pressure response to repair is assessed 8 weeks after the operation. During this time, converting enzyme inhibitors and angiotensin receptor blockers are avoided. Patients are requested to maintain a daily blood pressure diary at random times using an upper arm oscillometer. This latter method correlates well with continuous ambulatory blood pressure measures.

Complications

- **Prerenal oliguria.** Prerenal causes are the most frequent source of acute renal dysfunction after repair. This may go unrecognized in the absence of oliguria after multiple doses of intravenous mannitol are administered during the operation. Oliguria unresponsive to physiologic fluid challenge should be evaluated by determination of filling pressures and urine studies. The latter includes urinalysis, urine sodium, urea and creatinine concentrations, urea osmolarity, and calculation of fractional excretion of sodium.
- **Acute tubular necrosis.** Renal parenchymal causes of acute dysfunction pose the greatest risk for permanent compromise of renal function. Among direct repairs, ischemic acute tubular necrosis and renal parenchymal atheroembolism are particularly relevant. Recovery of renal function varies with the duration of ischemia, preexisting renal dysfunction, and patient age. Generally, 20 minutes of renal ischemia is well tolerated, and most direct surgical repair should be accomplished within this time interval. In addition, 20 to 40 minutes of ischemia is associated with renal tubular damage that is usually reversible. However, greater than 40 minutes of ischemia can be expected to cause varying degrees of permanent damage.
- **Atheroembolism-related renal dysfunction.** Atheroembolism can cause postoperative acute renal dysfunction progressing to permanent dialysis dependence. The diagnosis is suggested in a patient who demonstrates other manifestations of atheroembolism, such as skin involvement, eosinophils on urinalysis, and eosinophilia on peripheral blood smear. Because treatment is supportive, prevention constitutes the most important consideration.

REFERENCES

1. Goldblatt H: Studies on experimental hypertension, *J Exp Med* 59:346, 1934.
2. Leadbetter WFG, Burkland CE: Hypertension in unilateral renal disease, *J Urol* 39:611, 1938.
3. Smith HW: Unilateral nephrectomy in hypertensive disease, *J Urol* 76:685, 1956.
4. Freeman NL, Leeds FH, Elliott WG, et al: Thromboendarterectomy for hypertension due to renal artery occlusion, *JAMA* 156:1077-1079, 1954.
5. Morris GC, Cooley DA, Crawford ES, et al: Renal revascularization for hypertension. Clinical and physiological studies in 32 cases, *Surgery* 48:95-110, 1960.
6. Morris GC, DeBakey ME, Cooley DA: Surgical treatment of renal failure of renovascular origin, *JAMA* 182:609, 1962.
7. Hansen KJ, Cherr GS, Craven TE, et al: Management of ischemic nephropathy: Dialysis-free survival after surgical repair, *J Vasc Surg* 32:472-481, 2000.
8. Cherr GS, Hansen KJ, Craven TE, et al: Surgical management of atherosclerotic renovascular disease, *J Vasc Surg* 35:236-245, 2002.
9. Dean RH, Kieffer RW, Smith BM, et al: Renovascular hypertension: Anatomic and renal function changes during drug therapy, *Arch Surg* 116:1408-1415, 1981.
10. Zierler RE, Bergelin RO, Isaacson JA, et al: Natural history of atherosclerotic renal artery stenosis: A prospective study with duplex ultrasonography, *J Vasc Surg* 19:250-257, 1994.
11. Zierler RE, Bergelin RO, Davidson RC, et al: A prospective study of disease progression in patients with atherosclerotic renal artery stenosis, *Am J Hypertens* 9:1055-1061, 1996.
12. Pearce JD, Craven BL, Craven TE, et al: Progression of atherosclerotic renovascular disease: A prospective population-based study, *J Vasc Surg* 44:955-963, 2006.
13. Davis RP, Pearce JD, Craven TE, et al: Atherosclerotic renovascular disease among hypertensive adults, *J Vasc Surg* 50:564-571, 2009.

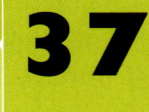

37 Extraanatomic Repair for Renovascular Disease

MOUNIR J. HAURANI • MARK F. CONRAD

Historical Background

Extraanatomic revascularization of the renal arteries using the splenic or hepatic branches of the celiac trunk for inflow generally yields inferior results when compared with traditional aortorenal bypass. These procedures are usually reserved for patients in whom exposure of the aorta is considered difficult or dangerous. Splenorenal revascularization was initially described by Thompson and Smithwick[1] in 1952 as a splenic artery transposition in a patient with hypertension secondary to unilateral renal disease, and successful bypass with autogenous grafts was reported later in the same decade.[2,3] The use of the hepatic circulation for revascularization of the right renal artery was not described until 1977,[4] and since then, there have been several larger series detailing both procedures.[5-10] Extraanatomic renal artery bypasses continue to be used as component hybrid endovascular approaches to abdominal aortic aneurysm repair where revascularization of the renal arteries from the hepatic and splenic circulation allowed extension of an endovascular seal zone to the superior mesenteric artery.[11,12] In addition, extraanatomic renal artery bypass has been described as a salvage maneuver for inadvertent coverage of the renal arteries during endovascular aneurysm repair.

Preoperative Preparation

- **Imaging.** Variable anatomy of the arterial branches of the celiac artery and, in particular, the hepatic arterial circulation is observed in up to 40% of patients, making preoperative imaging essential.[13,14] The increased fidelity of fine-cut helical computed tomography or magnetic resonance angiography has led to these modalities being used as first-line studies.[15,16]
- **Renal insufficiency.** The presence of renal insufficiency as determined by a low glomerular filtration rate may preclude the use of gadolinium-based contrast agents, and hydration with sodium bicarbonate may be necessary to decrease the risk of contrast nephropathy.[17]

Pitfalls and Danger Points

- An anomalous origin of the right hepatic artery off the gastroduodenal artery precludes the sacrifice or use of the gastroduodenal artery during right renal artery revascularization.
- The gastroduodenal artery is a critical collateral in patients with occlusive disease or superior mesenteric artery disease and cannot be used for right renal artery revascularization.
- Significant occlusive disease at the origin of the celiac artery precludes splenorenal or hepatorenal bypass.

- A heavily calcified splenic artery cannot be easily mobilized, and a tortuous splenic artery may be subject to kinking during transposition. A bypass graft with an end-to-side anastomosis off the splenic artery is an alternate approach.
- Hepatic insufficiency precludes the use of the hepatic artery for right renal artery revascularization. Despite hepatic blood supply from the portal vein, diversion of even a fraction of hepatic artery flow may prove detrimental.
- The common hepatic artery lies anterior to the portal vein and to the left of the bile duct. Both the vein and the duct, as well as the duodenum, are at risk of injury during exposure of the hepatic artery.
- The splenic artery travels along the superior border of the pancreas, where it gives off multiple small-branch vessels. The pancreas is at risk of injury during mobilization of the splenic artery.
- The spleen is at risk of injury during a splenorenal bypass.

Operative Strategy

SURGICAL ANATOMY OF THE HEPATIC AND SPLENIC ARTERIES

The celiac trunk originates from the anterior surface of the aorta at the T12-L1 interspace and consists of three branches: the left gastric artery, the splenic artery, and the common hepatic artery. The common hepatic artery courses anterior of and to the right along the superior border of the pancreas. It then runs along the right side of the lesser omentum, entering the hepatoduodenal ligament cranial to the pylorus. The common hepatic artery almost always lies anterior to the portal vein and to the left of the bile duct. Because it courses toward the hilum of the liver, it gives off the gastroduodenal artery, which is an important collateral between the celiac and the superior mesenteric artery circulation. The hepatic artery travels toward the liver, superior and cephalad to the common bile duct, and terminates at the liver hilum as the right and left hepatic arteries. The splenic artery travels along the superior border of the pancreas, where it gives off the dorsal pancreatic artery and several small branches and terminates at the spleen (Fig. 37-1).

SELECTION OF CONDUIT

For hepatorenal bypasses, a reversed saphenous vein is preferred. Because this bypass lies close to the duodenum, an autogenous conduit should be more resistant to infection. However, when the saphenous vein is less than 4 mm in caliber or absent, a 6-mm polytetrafluoroethylene or polyester graft can be used. For splenorenal bypasses, transposition of the splenic artery is preferred; alternatively, a saphenous vein graft or, if necessary, a synthetic graft can be used.

Operative Technique of Hepatorenal Bypass

INCISION

The patient is supine, and a roll is placed longitudinally to elevate the right flank. The right arm is extended on an arm board. The abdomen and thigh are prepped and draped. A right subcostal incision, two finger's breadths or 4 to 5 cm below and parallel to the inferior costal margin that extends from the midline to the eleventh rib, affords access to both arteries and limits bowel manipulation. This incision can be extended across the midline to improve exposure in larger patients. The three muscle layers of the abdomen are divided, the peritoneum is entered, and a self-retaining retractor is placed. In most patients adequate exposure can be obtained with minimal or no division of the rectus muscle (Fig. 37-2, A).

EXPOSURE OF THE RIGHT RENAL ARTERY

The small intestines are wrapped in a moist towel and packed inferiorly and to the left. The right colon is then freed from its lateral peritoneal attachments in an avascular

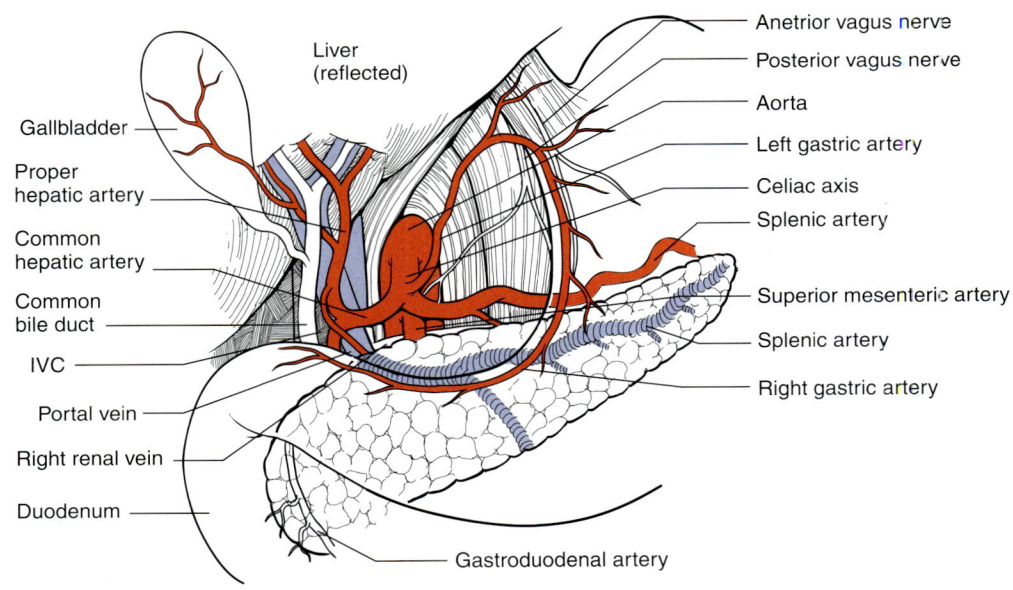

EXTRAANATOMIC REPAIR FOR RENOVASCULAR DISEASE 451

Figure 37-1. Anatomy of the celiac trunk and its branches. *IVC,* Inferior vena cava.

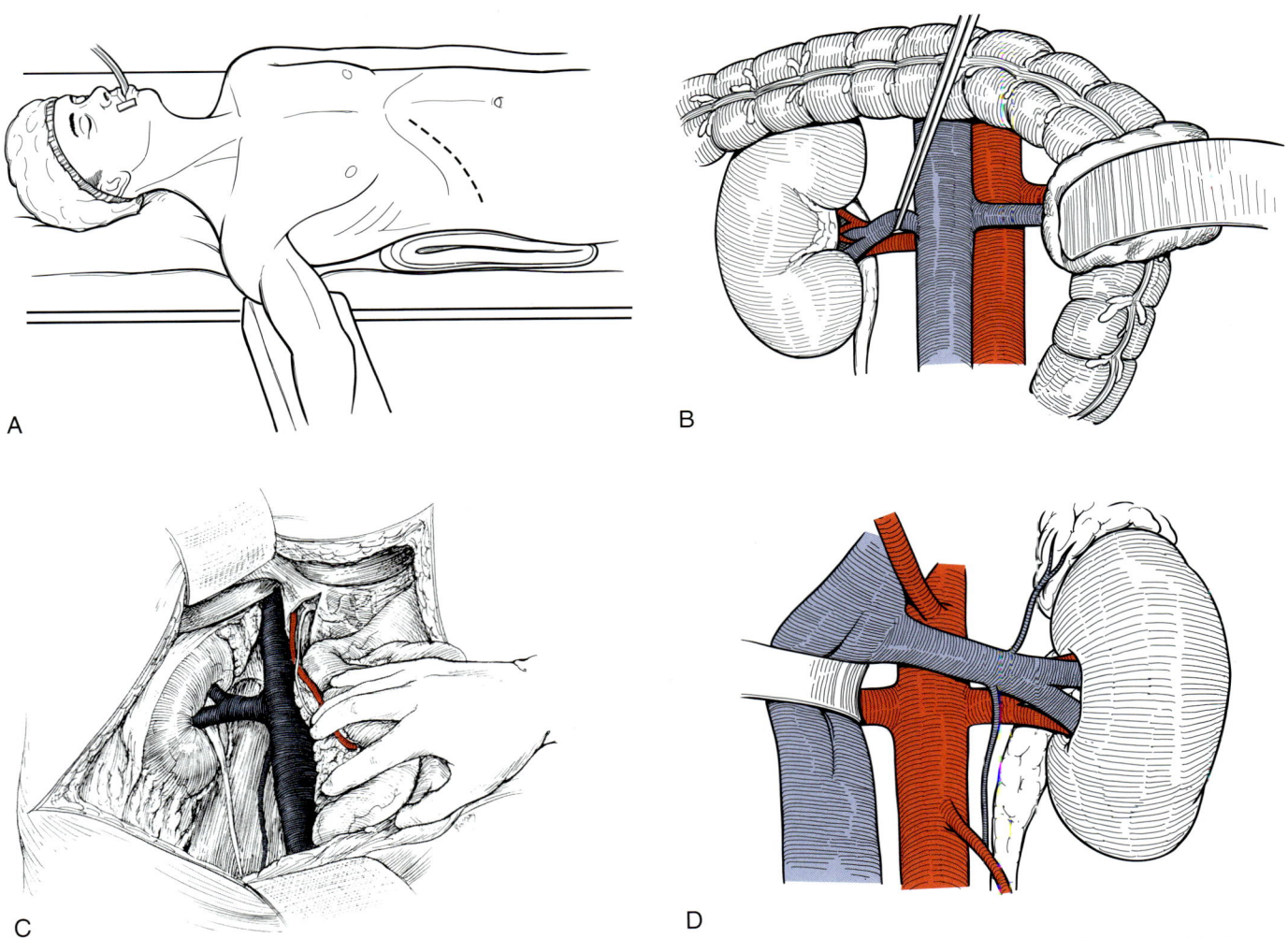

Figure 37-2. Exposure for a hepatorenal bypass. **A,** Patient positioning for a right subcostal incision. **B** through **D,** Exposure of the hepatic and right renal arteries for hepatorenal bypass. (**C,** *From Benjamin ME, Dean RH: Techniques in renal artery reconstruction: Part II, Ann Vasc Surg 10:409-414, 1996.*)

plane from the hepatic flexure to the cecum. The mobilized colon and mesentery can then be retracted to an inferior and medial position. The second portion of the duodenum is mobilized with an extended Kocher maneuver, and the duodenum and pancreas are reflected to the left. This exposes the inferior vena cava and the right renal vein, which is anterior to the artery in this position. The right renal vein is dissected free and circled with a vessel loop or thin Penrose drain. The inferior vena cava should be mobilized at the level of the renal artery to allow access to the origin of artery at the aorta. This occasionally requires ligation of a lumbar vein to ensure safe mobility in both directions. The gonadal vein enters the inferior vena cava on the anterior surface, inferior to the renal veins, and care should be taken to avoid avulsion during inferior vena cava mobilization. The right renal vein can be retracted either superiorly or inferiorly to expose the underlying renal artery. The renal artery should be freed from its aortic origin to the first renal branch of surrounding nerve and lymphatic tissue, which can be quite thick. Gentle rightward traction of the inferior vena cava allows direct access to the aorta and right renal artery origin (see Fig. 37-2, *D*).

EXPOSURE OF THE HEPATIC ARTERY

The right lobe of the liver is gently retracted superiorly to expose the hepatoduodenal ligament. The hepatic artery can be located by dividing the lesser omentum and is located to the left of the common duct. The common hepatic, gastroduodenal, and proper hepatic arteries are circled with vessel loops.

PROXIMAL ANASTOMOSIS

After systemic administration of heparin, the proximal and distal hepatic arteries are controlled with small, atraumatic clamps. The anastomosis to the hepatic artery is performed from end to side. The location of the anastomosis depends on the patient's anatomy and the need to avoid graft kinking. An inferior arteriotomy either proximal or distal to the gastroduodenal artery is generally used, and the gastroduodenal artery may be sacrificed if it is not an important collateral. The conduit is spatulated to provide a generous opening for the anastomosis, and the graft should be oriented with the heel toward the patient's right. The running anastomosis is created with 5-0 or 6-0 polypropylene, and it is technically easier to begin the suture line in the center of the back wall of the arteriotomy and run the inferior suture line in both directions (Fig. 37-3, *A*). In some instances the right renal artery may be of adequate length to anastomose directly to the hepatic artery, thus avoiding the need for a conduit.

DISTAL ANASTOMOSIS

Heparinization is maintained until after the distal anastomosis is completed. The distal renal artery is controlled with an atraumatic clamp such as a bulldog, and the proximal renal artery is controlled as close to the aorta as possible. The artery is transected, and the renal stump on the aorta can be initially controlled with a large clip. After completion of the distal anastomosis, the renal stump is oversewn with one or two doubly pledgeted 3-0 polypropylene sutures. If desired, cold renal protection can be initiated with a bolus of 250 mL of renal preservation fluid, consisting of 39.2°F (4°C) lactated Ringer solution with 25 g of mannitol and 1 g of methylprednisolone per liter, into the renal artery. The bypass graft is brought behind the duodenum and measured so that it reaches the right renal artery without kinking or tension. The distal anastomosis is usually performed from end to end, with both vessels spatulated to ensure a widely patent connection (see Fig. 37-3, *B*). If an accessory renal artery is present, the gastroduodenal artery can be used as a conduit connected from end to end. The graft is flushed before completion of the suture line, and adequacy of flow can be confirmed by manual palpation and duplex ultrasound.

CLOSURE

Hemostasis should be assessed including all anastomoses, as well as the mobilized inferior vena cava. The graft should lie without tension or kinking. A drain can be placed if necessary and is removed after 24 hours. The abdominal wall muscles are reapproximated with fascial sutures that can be either interrupted or running, and the skin is closed.

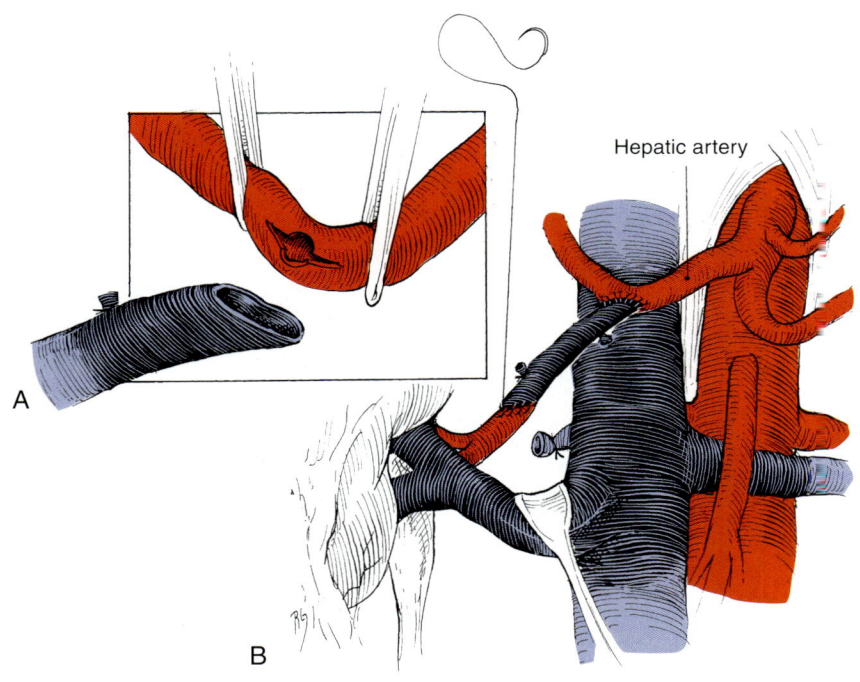

Figure 37-3. The hepatorenal bypass is completed from end to side to the hepatic artery (**A**) and from end to end to the right renal artery (**B**). *(From Benjamin ME, Dean RH: Techniques in renal artery reconstruction: Part II, Ann Vasc Surg 10:409-414, 1996.)*

Operative Techniques of Splenorenal Bypass

INCISION

The patient is placed in a modified right lateral decubitus position with the left flank elevated 45 degrees by a beanbag. The right inner thigh is exposed for vein harvest. The abdomen, chest, and leg are prepared and draped. A flank incision is made in the tenth interspace above the eleventh rib and extended to the left lateral border of the rectus sheath parallel to the rib. The intercostal muscles are detached from the superior border of the eleventh rib. The incision continues through the abdominal wall musculature, dividing the left rectus muscle as needed for exposure (Fig. 37-4, A).

EXPOSURE OF THE SPLENIC ARTERY

The descending colon is mobilized along the avascular white line of Toldt from the splenic flexure distally, and a plane is developed above Gerota fascia, because the colon is retracted caudally and to the right. This allows the pancreas to be approached along the inferior margin. The posterior surface of the pancreas is exposed by turning the inferior margin anteriorly while leaving the spleen in its normal location. The avascular plane between the posterior surface of the pancreas and Gerota fascia is then developed, and the splenic artery is identified. It is located close to the left renal artery, which is posterior and caudal. The splenic artery is controlled immediately proximal to the left gastroepiploic artery origin, and the proximal splenic artery is carefully separated from the pancreas. Branches at this level are ligated and divided. This dissection often leads to arterial spasm, which can be reduced by a papavarine-soaked sponge (see Fig. 37-4, B).

EXPOSURE OF THE LEFT RENAL ARTERY

Gerota fascia overlying the left renal hilum is incised, and the left renal vein is exposed as it crosses anterior to the aorta. The vein is mobilized by ligating and dividing the gonadal, adrenal, and renal lumbar venous branches. The left renal vein is then encircled with a vessel loop for easy retraction. The left renal artery lies directly beneath the anterior border of the left renal vein and should be dissected from its origin at the aorta to the first major renal branch (see Fig. 37-4, B and C).

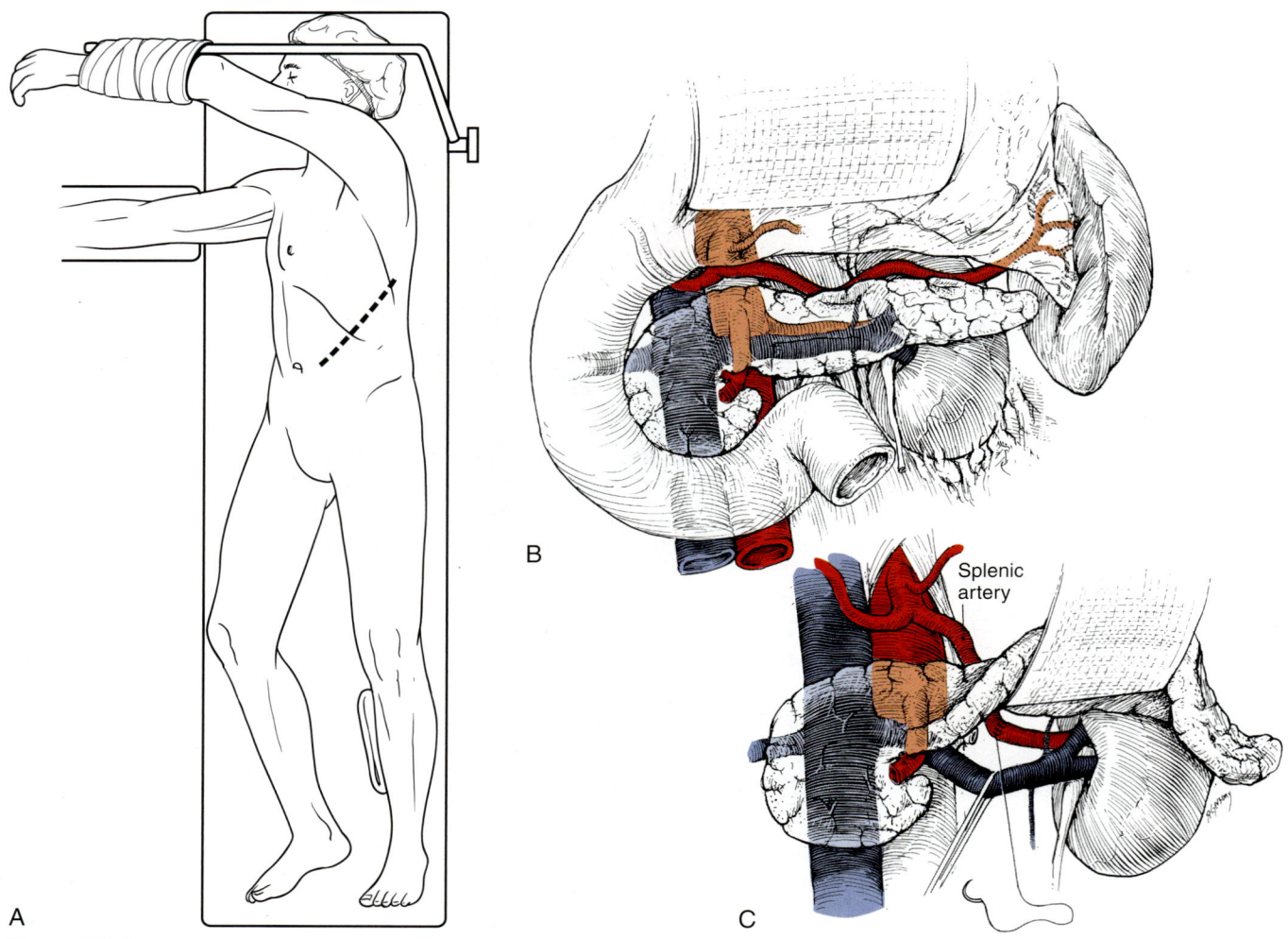

Figure 37-4. Exposure for a splenorenal bypass. **A,** Patient positioning for a retroperitoneal approach. **B,** Exposure of the hilum of the left kidney. The pancreas is mobilized along its inferior border and retracted superiorly. **C,** The transected splenic artery is anastomosed end to end to the left renal artery. (**B** and **C,** From Benjamin ME, Dean RH: Techniques in renal artery reconstruction: Part II, Ann Vasc Surg 10:409-414, 1996.)

SPLENORENAL ANASTOMOSIS

Systemic heparin is administered, and the splenic artery is controlled proximally with an atraumatic bulldog clamp. The splenic artery is divided proximal to the left gastroepiploic artery, and the distal splenic artery is oversewn. The spleen has a rich blood supply, and splenectomy is rarely necessary. The artery is spatulated on its inferior surface and is then directed toward the renal artery. In most cases 5 cm or less of freed splenic artery is needed to perform a direct anastomosis to the renal artery. If the splenic artery is small or the length is inadequate, saphenous vein can be harvested and used as a conduit. The renal artery is controlled at the aorta with a clamp, the artery is transected, and the renal stump on the aorta is oversewn with one or two doubly pledgeted 3-0 polypropylene sutures. If desired, cold renal preservation fluid can be administered, as described earlier. The end of the renal artery is spatulated on the anterior surface, and an oblique end-to-end anastomosis is created between the splenic and the left renal arteries using 5-0 or 6-0 polypropylene. Three interrupted sutures can be placed at the toe of the splenic artery to avoid narrowing the anastomosis.

CLOSURE

Hemostasis is assured at the level of the aorta and the anastomosis. The spleen is inspected for capsular tears that could lead to bleeding during the postoperative period, and a drain is placed if desired. The abdominal wall musculature is closed. If the chest was entered, the diaphragm is reapproximated and the pleura are closed over a chest tube.

Complications

- **Mortality.** Several large studies have shown that extraanatomic renal artery bypass can be performed with a mortality rate of 2% to 6% largely related to cardiac events.[6-10] Long-term survival is similar to that of patients undergoing aortorenal revascularization, with most late deaths caused by cardiac disease.[18]
- **Morbidity.** Respiratory failure, pulmonary embolism, congestive heart failure, splenic or pancreatic abscess, and wound infection have been described with overall morbidity of 20%.
- **Graft thrombosis.** Early graft thrombosis is rare, occurring in 3% to 6% of patients.[6-10] Although graft thrombosis can be managed with both endovascular and open surgical approaches, the risk of dialysis dependence increases substantially.[19]
- **Renal function.** For patients who present with renovascular hypertension, the cure rate is low (11%-27%). However, the majority of patients demonstrate some improvement in symptoms, with only 9% to 18% experiencing no benefit from bypass. Most patients who have not demonstrated benefit are found to have a thrombosed graft on surveillance imaging.[6,9]
- **Hepatic and splenic ischemia.** Ischemia to the end organs from which donor blood flow is obtained, such as the liver or spleen, is rare, especially if care is taken to preserve collateral flow to the spleen and avoid hilar dissection.

REFERENCES

1. Thompson JE, Smithwick RH: Human hypertension due to unilateral renal disease with special reference to renal artery lesions, *Angiology* 3:493-505, 1952.
2. Abelson DS, Haimovici H, Hurwitt ES, et al: Splenorenal arterial anastomoses, *Circulation* 14:532-539, 1956.
3. Decamp PT, Snyder CH, Bost RB: Severe hypertension due to congenital stenosis of artery to solitary kidney; correction by splenorenal arterial anastomosis, *Arch Surg* 75:1023-1026, 1957.
4. Novick AC, Banowsky LH, Stewart BH, et al: Splenorenal bypass in the treatment of stenosis of the renal artery, *Surg Gynecol Obstet* 144:891-898, 1977.
5. Chibaro EA, Libertino JA, Novick AC: Use of the hepatic circulation for renal revascularization, *Ann Surg* 199:406-411, 1984.
6. Khauli RB, Novick AC, Ziegelbaum M: Splenorenal bypass in the treatment of renal artery stenosis: Experience with sixty-nine cases, *J Vasc Surg* 2:547-551, 1985.
7. Geroulakos G, Wright JG, Tober JC, et al: Use of the splenic and hepatic artery for renal revascularization in patients with atherosclerotic renal artery disease, *Ann Vasc Surg* 11:85-89, 1997.
8. Fergany A, Kolettis P, Novick AC: The contemporary role of extra-anatomical surgical renal revascularization in patients with atherosclerotic renal artery disease, *J Urol* 153:1798-1801, 1995.
9. Moncure AC, Brewster DC, Darling RC, et al: Use of the splenic and hepatic arteries for renal revascularization, *J Vasc Surg* 3:196-203, 1986.
10. Brewster DC, Darling RC: Splenorenal arterial anastomosis for renovascular hypertension, *Ann Surg* 189:353-358, 1979.
11. Fulton JJ, Farber MA, Marston WA, et al: Endovascular stent-graft repair of pararenal and type IV thoracoabdominal aortic aneurysms with adjunctive visceral reconstruction, *J Vasc Surg* 41:191-198, 2005.
12. Kabbani LS, Criado E, Upchurch GR II, et al: Hybrid repair of aortic aneurysms involving the visceral and renal vessels, *Ann Vasc Surg* 24:219-224, 2010.
13. Ugurel MS, Battal B, Bozlar U, et al: Anatomical variations of hepatic arterial system, coeliac trunk and renal arteries: An analysis with multidetector CT angiography, *Br J Radiol* 83:661-667, 2010.
14. Covey AM, Brody LA, Maluccio MA, et al: Variant hepatic arterial anatomy revisited: Digital subtraction angiography performed in 600 patients, *Radiology* 224:542-547, 2002.
15. Cikrit DF, Harris VJ, Hemmer CG, et al: Comparison of spiral CT scan and arteriography for evaluation of renal and visceral arteries, *Ann Vasc Surg* 10:109-115, 1996.
16. Cambria RP, Kaufman JL, Brewster DC, et al: Surgical renal artery reconstruction without contrast arteriography: The role of clinical profiling and magnetic resonance angiography, *J Vasc Surg* 29:1012-1021, 1999.
17. Martin DR, Semelka RC, Chapman A, et al: Nephrogenic systemic fibrosis versus contrast-induced nephropathy: Risks and benefits of contrast-enhanced MR and CT in renally impaired patients, *J Magn Reson Imaging* 30:1350-1356, 2009.
18. Cambria RP, Brewster DC, L'Italien GJ, et al: Renal artery reconstruction for the preservation of renal function, *J Vasc Surg* 24:371-380, 1996.
19. Hansen KJ, Deitch JS, Oskin TC, et al: Renal artery repair: Consequence of operative failures, *Ann Surg* 227:678-689, 1998.

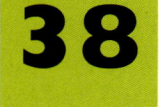

38 Endovascular Treatment of Renal Artery Stenosis

MATTHEW S. EDWARDS • JOEL K. DEONANAN • THOMAS CONLEE

Historical Background

In 1978 Grüntzig and colleagues[1] were the first to describe angioplasty for the treatment of atherosclerotic renal artery disease, and in 1991 early experience with balloon-expandable and self-expanding stents for treatment of renal artery stenosis was reported.[2-4] Stent placement was subsequently demonstrated to be superior to primary angioplasty and has lead to a marked increase in the number of patients treated for renal artery disease, with more than 90% of all contemporary renal artery revascularization procedures being performed by endovascular techniques.[5-7] In 2001 the use of a distal embolic protection device was introduced as an adjunct to renal angioplasty and stenting to decrease the adverse effects of atheroemboli.[8]

Indications

Recent randomized clinical trials have demonstrated no benefit in renal function retrieval, blood pressure control, or survival when renal artery stent placement was compared with medical therapy alone. However, these trials were limited by inclusion and exclusion criteria that likely resulted in study groups with significant numbers of patients with only moderate renal artery stenosis and patients unlikely to benefit from revascularization.[9-12] Furthermore, those data are limited in their power to examine selected patient groups thought by many experts to be more likely to receive benefit from renal artery revascularization. A significant amount of existing nonrandomized clinical trial data suggests that patients with high-grade renal artery stenosis and truly refractory hypertension, renal insufficiency with concomitant severe hypertension, and flash pulmonary edema or other cardiac disturbance syndrome may benefit from restoring renal perfusion.

Preoperative Preparation

- Warfarin is held for at least 72 hours before renal artery stenting, and intravenous bridging heparin is used as needed.
- Clopidogrel therapy is initiated 1 week before renal artery stenting and continued for at least 4 weeks after revascularization. For those who cannot tolerate clopidogrel, aspirin is used at a daily dosage of 81 or 325 mg. Data demonstrate that antiplatelet therapy reduces renal artery embolization during renal artery stenting.[13,14]
- 3-Hydroxy-3-methylglutaryl coenzyme A reductase inhibitors, or statins, are prescribed to all patients who do not have a documented history of adverse reaction. Evidence suggests that statin therapy reduces restenosis after renal artery stenting.[15]
- Patients should not ingest food or fluids after midnight the evening before the procedure but should shower with chlorhexidine.

- Iodinated contrast agents can lead to impaired renal function, especially in patients with diabetes, dehydration, and chronic renal insufficiency. Preoperative administration of N-acetylcysteine, vitamin C, and normal saline hydration are recommended. Sodium bicarbonate hydration is used in lieu of normal saline for patients with severe preexisting renal insufficiency, with an estimated glomerular filtration rate of less than 45 mL/min. These measures may decrease the risk of contrast-induced nephropathy.[16-18]

- At the time of admission, nonsteroidal antiinflammatory, diuretics, and metformin are held to minimize the risk of deterioration in renal function.

- Agents that target the renin-angiotensin system, such as angiotensin-converting enzyme inhibitors and angiotensin receptor antagonists, are discontinued on the day of renal artery stenting and reinitiated 1 week later to minimize deleterious intrarenal vascular shunting in the setting of a hyperemic kidney after revascularization.

- Routine antihypertensive medications are taken on the morning of the procedure with a sip of water.

- A first-generation cephalosporin antibiotic, or vancomycin if the patient is allergic, is administered intravenously 30 minutes before the procedure.

Pitfalls and Danger Points

- **The decision to intervene.** Some anatomic variants are best treated by means other than renal artery angioplasty and stenting, including congenital renal artery stenosis, branch level renal artery disease, and disease involving multiple, small renal arteries. Initial technical success can often be achieved in these situations; however, the response to treatment both clinically and anatomically is often short lived, and renal artery angioplasty and stenting may complicate the secondary application of surgery to definitively correct the problem.

- **Wire access.** Translesion crossing must be intraluminal, and subintimal crossing must be avoided. This can best be accomplished by avoiding doubling back of the wire and avoidance of treating occluded renal arteries with stenting in all but the most highly select situations. Once the lesion is crossed, maintenance of guidewire position is critical until the procedure is complete. The terminal renal arteries and parenchyma are soft, and wires can easily perforate these tissues if they are allowed to migrate distally. Furthermore, angioplasty and stenting are occasionally complicated by dissection of the distal renal artery. This complication can usually be treated by additional stent placement but may be impossible to remedy if guidewire access is lost. Finally, once a stent is positioned with extension into the aorta, reaccess of the stent orifice can be challenging, making proper treatment of inadequate stent results difficult if access is lost before satisfactory completion of the procedure.

- **Stent deployment.** Inaccurate stent deployment can lead to permanent loss of access and occlusion of major renal artery branches if distal deployment occurs. This is best avoided by frequent angiography to optimally position the stent before deployment. The risk of inaccurate stent deployment is greatest if the lesion is nonostial or if the main renal artery is short.

Endovascular Strategy

ANGIOGRAPHIC ANATOMY

Angiographic visualization of arterial anatomy is a fundamental element of both diagnosis and endovascular treatment of atherosclerotic renovascular disease. Initial anteroposterior (AP) images of the visceral aorta are obtained using power injections of contrast through a multiside-holed flush catheter positioned just beneath the diaphragm at the level of the first lumbar vertebra. In patients with severe renal insufficiency, initial localizing views can be performed using carbon dioxide. Dilute

(50%) iodinated contrast can be used for imaging purposes in the vast majority of cases. Initial AP views provide an overview of the renal artery and perivisceral aortic anatomy (Fig. 38-1). Further nonselective images of the renal arteries should be obtained after repositioning the catheter to a location below the origin of the superior mesenteric artery to prevent contrast opacification of the visceral vessels that may obscure anatomic details of the renal arteries, especially the ostia. Care must be taken to identify accessory renal arteries, which may be present in up to 18% of kidneys and may not be identified during screening renal duplex sonography.

The ostia of the renal arteries usually arise from the anterolateral or posterolateral aspect of the aorta. Therefore lesions within the renal ostia are frequently not seen or may appear insignificant in an AP aortogram. Oblique aortography or oblique selective renal arteriography projects these portions of the vessel in profile and often better identifies lesions. The most useful projections to visualize the renal ostia are usually moderate ipsilateral anterior oblique views, although contralateral oblique views may also be necessary. Previously obtained axial images of the renal origins via computed tomography imaging may assist in estimating the required obliquity and thereby decrease iodinated contrast and ionizing radiation.

Lesions within the body of the renal artery may require selective arteriographic views for full delineation. Selective cannulation is usually performed using an angled catheter, such as a Cobra, Sos, renal double-curved, or inferior mesenteric catheter, in combination with a directional guidewire. Before selective renal artery cannulation, intravenous heparin is administered. Once the guidewire and catheter are gently advanced into the renal artery ostia, a hand injection of contrast should be performed to ensure an intraluminal position. Selective images can then be obtained using hand-injected angiographic images. The proximal third of the left renal artery usually courses anteriorly, the middle third courses transversely, and the distal third courses posteriorly, whereas the right renal artery pursues a more consistent posterior course. Oblique and cranial-caudad rotated images may be necessary to fully delineate lesions in these various segments.

UNFAVORABLE ANATOMIC FEATURES FOR RENAL ARTERY ANGIOPLASTY AND STENTING

Branch renal artery stenosis is often poorly suited for endovascular treatment because of anatomic constraints and compromised durability. Surgical revascularization is also preferred in patients requiring operative aortic repair of aneurysms, aortoiliac occlusive disease, and coral reef atheromas. Addition of renal revascularization in these patients does not require significant modification of surgical exposure, allows treatment of both pathologies in a single procedural setting, and avoids the potential for ostial stent occlusion or fracture during subsequent aortic manipulation. Endovascular treatment is not absolutely contraindicated, but it has distinct technical challenges and compromised durability when compared with open surgical revascularization in patients with disease involving multiple, small-caliber renal arteries or in children with hypoplastic renal artery lesions.

CONSIDERATIONS IN THE TREATMENT OF BRANCH VESSEL DISEASE

Potential problems in dealing with branch vessels must be recognized when considering renovascular disease that affects a very short main renal artery, the distal main renal artery, or the branches themselves (Fig. 38-2). Specifically, the risk of covering or excluding a major branch ostium is significant and must be avoided.

CONSIDERATIONS IN THE PRESENCE OF A SOLITARY KIDNEY

Treatment of a solitary kidney involves a risk to the entirety of a patient's functional renal mass. This does not preclude endovascular treatment of a solitary

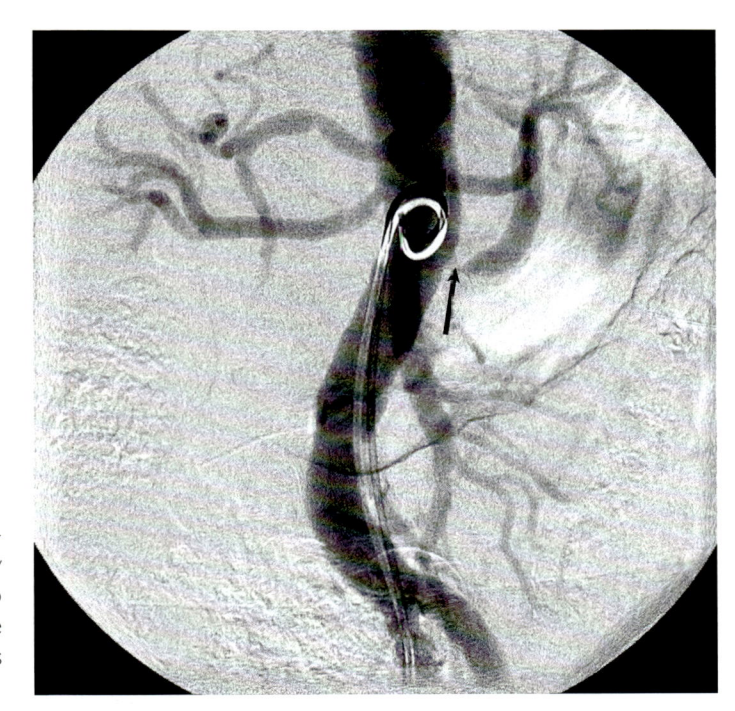

Figure 38-1. Digital subtraction aortogram via a flush catheter positioned at the level of the renal takeoffs. This clearly demonstrates the essential regional anatomy and relationship between two right renal arteries, two left renal arteries, and the superior mesenteric artery. A high-grade proximal stenosis is noted within the inferior left renal artery.

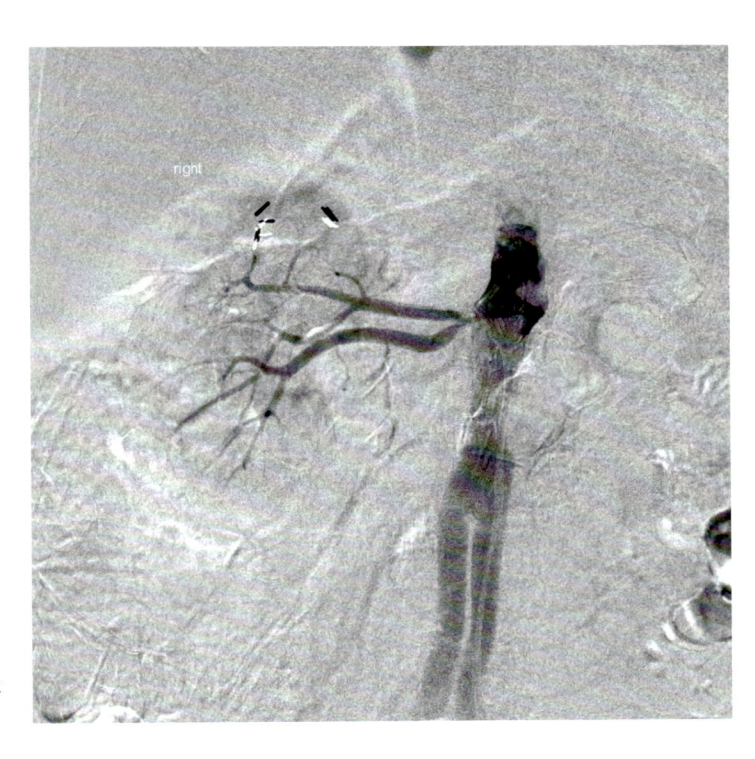

Figure 38-2. Arteriogram demonstrating a short right main renal artery with a high-grade stenosis just proximal to arterial bifurcation, highlighting the potential risk of segmental renal ischemia if a substantial renal branch is covered with a stent or stent graft.

kidney, but it should lead to circumspection in the presence of anatomic factors that increase risk or adversely affect long-term durability. Such conditions include multiple small renal arteries, branch level disease, or a short main renal artery.

SELECTION OF ANTEGRADE OR RETROGRADE AORTIC ACCESS FOR TREATMENT

Common femoral artery access is safe and versatile, and this artery is the most common access site for renal angioplasty and stenting. When selective renal artery cannulation is planned, selection of the femoral artery contralateral to the targeted renal artery for access facilitates ostial cannulation through a tendency of the catheter to preferentially track along the contralateral aortic wall (Fig. 38-3).

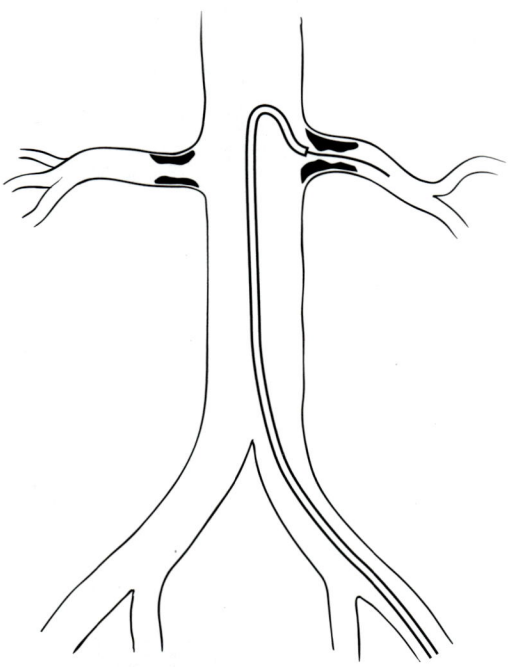

Figure 38-3. Selective cannulation of the left renal artery through a right femoral artery approach. This approach illustrates the tendency of the selective catheter placed from the ipsilateral femoral artery to track along the contralateral wall of the aorta.

The brachial artery is an alternative access site that may be preferred in patients with aortoiliac occlusive disease, in patients with renal arteries with significant inferior angulation relative to the main axis of the aorta, or when selective cannulation via a femoral approach has been unsuccessful. Compared with the femoral artery, disadvantages of brachial access include higher incidence of access-related complications and limitations of catheter and sheath size.

COAXIAL OR MONORAIL BALLOON CATHETER DESIGNS

Coaxial (over the wire) and monorail (rapid exchange) systems are both available for angioplasty and delivery of balloon-mounted stents for renal artery revascularization. Coaxial systems offer a theoretical advantage in terms of the surgeon's ability to track across lesions by advancing along the path of the wire, with a longitudinal column of support increasing "pushability." Monorail systems offer the ability to have a single operator in control of the balloon catheter and the guidewire, minimizing loss of wire control.

ROLE OF BALLOON PREDILATION

Predilation of lesions should be limited to situations in which stent delivery devices cannot be advanced across the lesion but guidewire access has been achieved. Predilation can also be used, when necessary, to facilitate the crossing of an embolic protection device. In both instances the smallest available balloon size should be used, such as a 2.5- or 3-mm-diameter coronary balloon.

ANGIOPLASTY VERSUS PRIMARY STENTING

Although primary angioplasty is considered appropriate endovascular management for renal artery fibromuscular dysplasia, primary endoluminal stenting for treatment of ostial atherosclerotic renovascular disease is associated with superior technical success and a lower incidence of recurrent stenosis. Contemporary endovascular management of ostial atherosclerotic renovascular disease therefore consists of percutaneous angioplasty with primary endoluminal stenting. Primary angioplasty is more commonly used for management of recurrent disease. Nonostial atherosclerotic lesions may also respond well to angioplasty alone, but secondary stent placement should be considered if primary angioplasty is unsuccessful because of elastic recoil, residual stenosis, persistent pressure gradient, or arterial dissection.

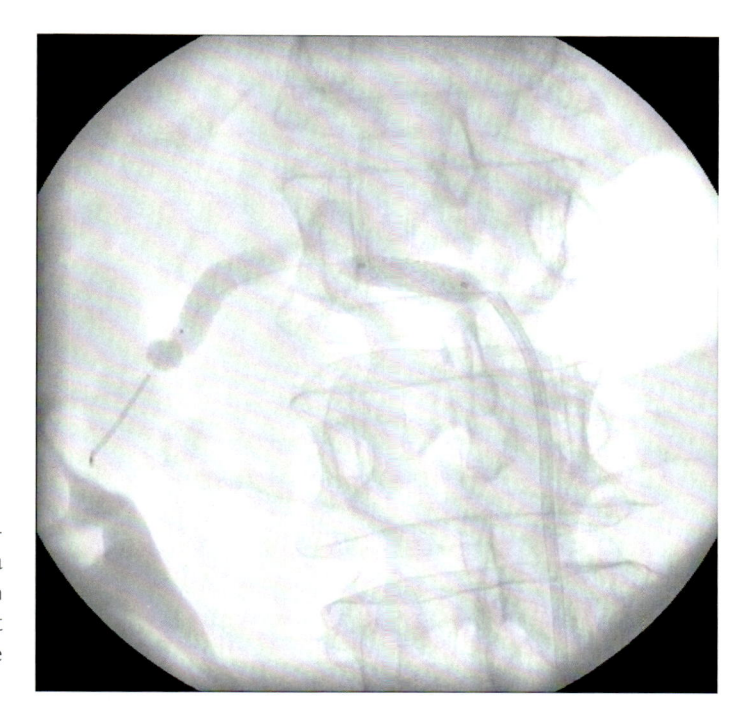

Figure 38-4. Digital subtraction angiography demonstrating deployment of a right renal artery stent with the use of a distal embolic protection device. The distal embolic protection balloon is inflated, demonstrating a static column of contrast between the distal occlusion balloon and the balloon-inflatable stent during deployment.

SELECTION OF A STENT

Balloon-expandable and self-expanding stents are available in an array of sizes appropriate for renal artery use. Balloon-expandable stents possess greater inherent accuracy of deployment and radial strength relative to self-expanding stents. Therefore balloon-expandable stents are the most common choice for atherosclerotic renal artery stenosis. There are theoretical advantages to open and closed cell designs; the potential to decrease embolization or to increase conformability to the arterial wall is associated with closed and open cell designs, respectively. However, these advantages are as yet unproven.

USE OF EMBOLIC PROTECTION

Although atheroembolization occurs during renal angioplasty and stenting and may affect renal function response to intervention,[19,20] a distal embolic protection device for use in the renal circulation has not been approved by the U.S. Food and Drug Administration (FDA). If distal embolic protection is used, a guidewire system incorporating an occlusion balloon or filter is used for crossing the lesion and is subsequently deployed distally. If an occlusion balloon is used, complete renal artery occlusion is confirmed by hand injection of contrast (Fig. 38-4). Angioplasty and stenting is then performed, followed by aspiration of the static column of blood distal to the treated lesion, irrigation with heparinized saline, and repeat aspiration. The distal occlusion balloon is then deflated, and completion angiography is performed. Filter devices permit ongoing distal renal artery flow in their deployed configurations and use a porous membrane to trap embolic material. If a filter design device is used, the filter is collapsed back into its nondeployed state after the stent procedure is completed to trap captured embolic material before device withdrawal.

TREATMENT OF RECURRENT STENOSIS

Recurrent disease complicates up to 50% of renal angioplasty and stenting procedures within 12 months.[15] In-stent lesions are the most common form of recurrence and represent a particularly challenging problem (Fig. 38-5, *A*). Because the etiology of this lesion is most often intimal hyperplasia, repeat balloon angioplasty often does little to improve the lesion. For recurrent lesions, initial dilatation with a "cutting" balloon is extremely useful to release fibrous scar tissue of the restenotic lesion and allows subsequent dilatation with a larger-diameter balloon. The cutting balloon (Boston Scientific, Natick, Mass.) consists of a noncompliant

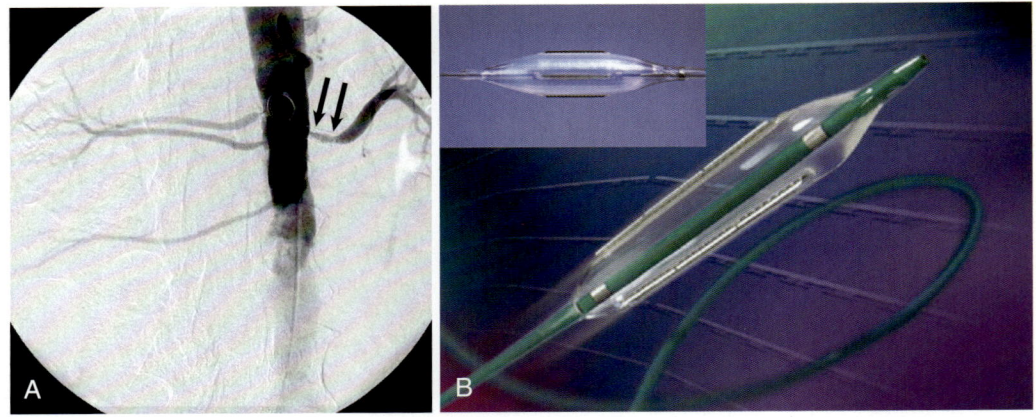

Figure 38-5. A, Angiogram demonstrating recurrent stenosis after stenting (*arrows*) of the left renal artery. **B,** A cutting balloon can be used to dilate recurrent renal artery stenosis (in-stent stenosis). (**B,** *Courtesy Boston Scientific, Natick, Mass. Reprinted from Cronenwett JL, Johnston KW, editors.* Rutherford's vascular surgery, *ed 7. Philadelphia, 2010, Saunders, p 1279, Fig. 85-2A.*)

balloon with three or four atherotomes or microsurgical blades mounted longitudinally or in a spiral configuration on its outer surface (Fig. 38-5, *B*). When the cutting balloon is inflated, the atherotomes score the intimal hyperplasia within the stent. The balloon is then rotated and reinflated to score the lesion in multiple planes. This technology has been best described in coronary arteries, but its use has also been studied with renal artery in-stent restenosis.[21]

Endovascular Technique for Treatment of a Renal Artery Stenosis

APPROACHES FOR ANTEGRADE OR RETROGRADE ACCESS

Retrograde common femoral artery access is preferred whenever feasible. Selection of the femoral location contralateral to the targeted renal artery for access facilitates ostial cannulation through a tendency for the catheter to preferentially track along the contralateral aortic wall. The technique for access includes preaccess localization of the femoral head using fluoroscopy to ensure puncture in an area that can be compressed against a firm structure for hemostasis. Ultrasound can be used to ensure puncture of the common femoral artery, and manual compression can be applied for at least 15 minutes at the end of the procedure, with reversal of the heparin effect by administration of protamine sulfate. Arterial closure devices can also be employed according to their FDA-approved instructions for use.

The brachial artery offers an alternative access site that may be preferred in patients with aortoiliac occlusive disease, prior aortofemoral or infrainguinal bypass grafting, or renal arteries with significant inferior angulation relative to the main axis of the aorta, as well as when selective cannulation via a femoral approach has been unsuccessful. Open brachial artery access facilitates the procedure if a 6-Fr or larger sheath is required, as is the case for most renal angioplasty and stenting procedures.

SHEATH PLACEMENT FOR PLANNED INTERVENTION

Initially a 4- or 5-Fr sheath and diagnostic catheter system are placed after accessing the femoral or brachial artery. Small diagnostic catheters are ample to provide initial diagnostic images that confirm suspected anatomy and the intention to proceed with intervention. Once the decision to intervene is confirmed, a 6-Fr sheath is required, and shaped 6-Fr guide catheters can be used to engage the renal artery for intervention. These guide catheters are available in the usual diagnostic shapes, including renal double curved, inferior mesenteric, and cobra head, and are routinely used to cannulate the renal arteries and allow guidewire access, device placement, and angiography. They also allow repeat angiography with devices in place to ensure optimal positioning. Alternatively, the surgeon may access the renal artery using shaped diagnostic catheters, cross the lesion with a wire, and then follow with a 6-Fr shaped sheath for secure renal access. This latter approach can be complicated, because the tracking of these sheaths to the renal artery often requires a significant degree of wire support. Use of a guide catheter allows lesion crossing as a single maneuver using smaller 0.014-inch guidewires intended for intervention.

CROSSING A LESION

Intravenous heparin is administered prior to crossing a stenotic renal artery lesion. Once the guide catheter has engaged the ostia, the lesion is crossed with a 0.014-inch guidewire. The wire is advanced in line, avoiding doubling back of the wire that indicates subintimal crossing. If this platform will not cross, extrasupportive 0.014-inch guidewires can be used. On occasion 0.035-inch hydrophilic wires are required for crossing, with subsequent catheter exchange for a smaller 0.014- or 0.018-inch guidewire for device delivery.

IN SITU PHYSIOLOGIC ASSESSMENT USING THE RADI WIRE

The Radi pressure wire (St. Jude Medical, St. Paul) allows simultaneous measurement of aortic and renal pressures distal to a stenotic lesion using two separate pressure sensors in the distal portion of a hydrophilic 0.014-inch guidewire. This wire is FDA approved for use in the coronary arteries and its use has been described in determining the physiologic significance of a renal artery stenosis and the efficacy of renal angioplasty and stenting.[22] The major benefit is the ability to gain this information without giving up wire access across the lesion postintervention, which is necessary for traditional catheter pullback pressure measurement. Another means to accomplish pressure gradient measures without losing wire access is through the use of a monorail aspiration catheter such as the Medtronic Export catheter (Medtronic, Minneapolis). The aspiration catheter can be used to aspirate debris after renal angioplasty and stenting with a distal occlusion balloon and then used to perform pullback pressure measures over the 0.014-inch balloon-tipped guidewire after balloon deflation.

ANGIOPLASTY

Angioplasty is a reasonable stand-alone therapy for renal artery fibromuscular dysplasia lesions, mid–renal artery atherosclerosis, or recurrent in-stent stenosis. To perform renal artery angioplasty, the balloon catheter is advanced and centered across the lesion over a 0.014-inch guidewire and is positioned with minimal extension of the balloon into the distal normal renal artery. The balloon is then inflated to its nominal pressure to dilate the target lesion. It is of paramount importance to maintain guidewire access across the lesion while removing the angioplasty balloon and to perform completion arteriography to assess technical success, as well as the potential of dissection, pseudoaneurysm, or rupture (Video 38-1).

STENT PLACEMENT

Balloon-mounted stents are the treatment of choice for atherosclerotic ostial renovascular disease, which is the predominant form of renal artery stenosis encountered in contemporary clinical practice. The shortest possible balloon-mounted stent size is chosen to cover the entire lesion with 1 to 2 mm of extension into the aorta, with a diameter matching the distal normal-appearing renal artery. The stent is advanced across the lesion over a 0.014-inch guidewire and positioned with 1 to 2 mm of extension into the aorta. Frequent hand injection of contrast through the guide catheter allows precise placement of the stent and helps avoid misdeployment. Placement of a stent too far into the artery does not support the true renal orifice and is prone to residual or recurrent disease. Because recurrent disease is frequent and may not respond to further endovascular intervention, the shortest possible stent needed to support the lesion should be used. A stent that extends well out into the distal renal artery can make later surgical options more difficult and carry a higher failure rate. Once the optimal location is defined, the guide catheter is retracted and the delivery balloon is inflated to its nominal pressure, deploying the stent. Prolonged inflation is not necessary with stent placement. A spot radiographic examination can be made to examine the contour of the deployed stent. The delivery balloon can be carefully removed, paying attention to maintaining guidewire access, followed by completion arteriography.

Lesions in proximity to the renal artery bifurcation are not uncommon. Several techniques have been reported for dealing with this situation, including the use of "buddy" wires to protect branch vessels, as well as the use of kissing balloons and stents. For lesions of the main renal artery challenged by the proximity of the bifurcation, these may be appropriate in a medically compromised patient. Otherwise, these problems should be treated with open repair as a safe and durable solution, avoiding the risks of major branch vessel occlusion and restenosis that are so common in the treatment of small renal vessels.

COMPLETION STUDIES

After a stent is deployed, residual narrowing within the stent—visible upon fluoroscopic evaluation of the stent or detected during selective renal angiography—may require balloon dilatation. Identification of renal artery dissection, rupture, thrombosis, and pseudoaneurysm may also be treated with additional stents, covered stents, or administration of thrombolytic agents as appropriate. After all therapeutic measures are complete, pressure gradients or intravascular ultrasound is performed to assess the technical result. If satisfactory, guidewire and sheath access may be removed and hemostasis secured. Renal duplex sonography can also be performed as an additional measure to ensure an adequate hemodynamic result.

Postoperative Care

- After intervention, patients are monitored overnight for access site problems or hemodynamic instability.
- Serum creatinine and a complete blood count are measured the morning of discharge.
- Clopidogrel is continued for a minimum of 30 days, whereas aspirin and statin therapy are maintained indefinitely.
- Clinical follow-up with surveillance renal duplex ultrasonography is performed at 1 month, subsequently at 6-month intervals for 2 years, and annually thereafter. A renal artery peak systolic velocity of more than 180 cm/sec is suggestive of recurrent stenosis.
- For patients with recurrent stenosis in the setting of normal blood pressure and renal function, increased frequency of clinical follow-up and imaging surveillance is appropriate, with reintervention reserved should renal function deteriorate.

Complications

- **Morbidity.** Contemporary large clinical trials of renal angioplasty and stenting have reported complications in 9% of patients.[11]
- **Bleeding.** Hemodynamic instability should prompt computed tomography imaging to assess for retroperitoneal or perinephric hematoma, often not detectable on physical examination.[23] Bleeding because of renal artery perforation can often be managed with a covered stent.
- **Renal artery dissection.** Procedure-related renal artery dissection is frequently manageable with additional stent deployment.
- **Renal artery thrombosis.** Thrombolysis has been described in the treatment of renal artery thrombosis.
- **Acute renal failure**
- **Atheroembolization**

REFERENCES

1. Grüntzig A, Kuhlmann U, Vetter W, et al: Treatment of renovascular hypertension with percutaneous transluminal dilatation of a renal artery stenosis, *Lancet* 1:801-802, 1978.
2. Wilms GE, Peene PT, Baert AL, et al: Renal artery stent placement with use of the Wallstent endoprosthesis, *Radiology* 179:457-462, 1991.
3. Kuhn FP, Kutkuhn B, Torsello G, et al: Renal artery stenosis: Preliminary results of treatment with the Strecker stent, *Radiology* 180:367-372, 1991.
4. Rees CR, Palmaz JC, Becker GJ, et al: Palmaz stent in atherosclerotic stenoses involving the ostia of the renal arteries: Preliminary report of a multicenter study, *Radiology* 181:507-514, 1991.
5. van de Ven PJ, Kaatee R, Beutler JJ, et al: Arterial stenting and balloon angioplasty in ostial atherosclerotic renovascular disease: A randomised trial, *Lancet* 353:282-286, 1999.
6. Centers for Medicare and Medicaid Services. Percutaneous transluminal angioplasty (PTA) and stenting of the renal arteries. Baltimore, 2007, Centers for Medicare and Medicaid Services.
7. Textor SC: Atherosclerotic renal artery stenosis: Overtreated but underrated? *J Am Soc Nephrol* 19:656-659, 2008.
8. Henry M, Klonaris C, Henry I, et al: Protected renal stenting with the PercuSurge GuardWire device: A pilot study, *J Endovasc Therapy* 8:227-237, 2001.
9. Ziakka S, Ursu M, Poulikakos D, et al: Predictive factors and therapeutic approach of renovascular disease: Four years' follow up, *Ren Fail* 30:965-970, 2008.
10. Bax L, Woittiez AJ, Kouwenberg HJ, et al: Stent placement in patients with atherosclerotic renal artery stenosis and impaired renal function: A randomized trial, *Ann Intern Med* 150:840-848, 2009.
11. ASTRAL Investigators, Wheatley K, Ives N, et al: Revascularization versus medical therapy for renal-artery stenosis, *N Engl J Med* 361:1953-1962, 2009.
12. Steichen O, Amar L, Plouin PF: Primary stenting for atherosclerotic renal artery stenosis, *J Vasc Surg* 51:1574-1580, 2010.
13. Cooper CJ, Haller ST, Colyer W, et al: Embolic protection and platelet inhibition during renal artery stenting, *Circulation* 117:2752-2760, 2008.
14. Edwards MS, Corriere MA, Craven TE, et al: Atheroembolism during percutaneous renal artery revascularization, *J Vasc Surg* 46:55-61, 2007.
15. Corriere MA, Edwards MS, Pearce JD, et al: Restenosis after renal artery angioplasty and stenting: Incidence and risk factors, *J Vasc Surg* 50:813-819, 2009.
16. Aspelin P, Aubry P, Fransson SG, et al: Nephrotoxic effects in high-risk patients undergoing angiography, *N Engl J Med* 348:491-499, 2003.
17. Pannu N, Wiebe N, Tonelli M: Prophylaxis strategies for contrast-induced nephropathy, *JAMA* 295:2765-2779, 2006.
18. Sharma SK, Kini A: Effect of nonionic radiocontrast agents on the occurrence of contrast-induced nephropathy in patients with mild-moderate chronic renal insufficiency: Pooled analysis of the randomized trials, *Catheter Cardiovasc Interv* 65:386-393, 2005
19. Cooper CJ, Haller ST, Colyer W, et al: Embolic protection and platelet inhibition during renal artery stenting, *Circulation* 117:2752-2760, 2008.
20. Edwards MS, Corriere MA, Craven TE, et al: Atheroembolism during percutaneous renal artery revascularization, *J Vasc Surg* 46:55-61, 2007.
21. Munneke GJ, Engelke C, Morgan RA, et al: Cutting balloon angioplasty for resistant renal artery in-stent restenosis, *J Vasc Interv Radiol* 13:327-331, 2002.
22. Drieghe B, Madaric J, Sarno G, et al: Assessment of renal artery stenosis: Side-by-side comparison of angiography and duplex ultrasound with pressure gradient measurements, *Europ Heart J* 29:517-524, 2008.
23. Axelrod DJ, Freeman H, Pukin L, et al: Guide wire perforation leading to fatal perirenal hemorrhage from transcortical collaterals after renal artery stent placement, *J Vasc Interv Radiol* 15:985-987, 2004.

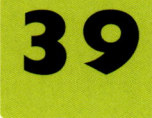

39 Endovascular Treatment of Renal Artery Aneurysms

CHRISTOPHER J. KWOLEK • MOUNIR J. HAURANI

Historical Background

Although renal artery aneurysms located in a distal branch can be sacrificed with little consequence to renal function, centrally located aneurysms posed an initial challenge for the development of successful endovascular treatment options. In 1995 Bui and colleagues[1] described the treatment of a renal artery aneurysm with a stent graft. Although a useful strategy in carefully selected patients, covered stents could not be used for aneurysms located at a bifurcation point, in tortuous vessels, or at more peripheral sites. Indeed, renal artery aneurysms occur predominantly at the renal bifurcation or in the first-order renal artery branches.[2] Moreover, because most renal artery aneurysms are large necked or fusiform, traditional coil embolization is associated with significant potential for coil migration and occlusion of the parent artery. In response to this challenge, stent-assisted embolization, in which coils are delivered to the aneurysm through the struts of a stent in the parent vessel, was first described in 2008 for the treatment of renal aneurysms.[3] Endovascular repair is the predominant treatment for renal artery aneurysms.[4] Although current data suggest that both short- and intermediate-term outcomes of endovascular interventions are excellent, long-term durability remains to be determined.

Indications

Aneurysms of the renal artery and its branches are uncommon, occurring in less than 0.1% of the general population and are often discovered incidentally through computed tomography (CT) imaging.[5] Renal aneurysms may present more frequently among women in the sixth decade of life and may be related to fibromuscular dysplasia, atherosclerosis, trauma, or mycotic infection. Renal aneurysms are also observed with vasculitis, such as Takayasu or Behçet disease and Marfan syndrome or neurofibromatosis. Rupture is the main complication.

Aneurysms larger than 2 cm and all renal aneurysms in women considering future pregnancy or in a solitary kidney are considered appropriate for repair due to the risk of rupture. Although 2 cm has been used as the threshold for treatment, even smaller aneurysms can rupture or may cause renovascular hypertension by direct compression of the main renal artery or branch vessel. Renal aneurysms may also embolize to terminal vessels, causing renal infarcts with pain, or may be associated with an arteriovenous fistula.

Preoperative Preparation

- Patients are symptomatic in fewer than 50% of cases undergoing repair.[2,6]
- Preoperative imaging is critical in determining the type of endovascular repair that can be performed. Three-dimensional (3D) CT angiography or magnetic resonance angiography can define the relationship of the aneurysm to the surrounding branch vessels or the surrounding renal parenchyma. CT angiography

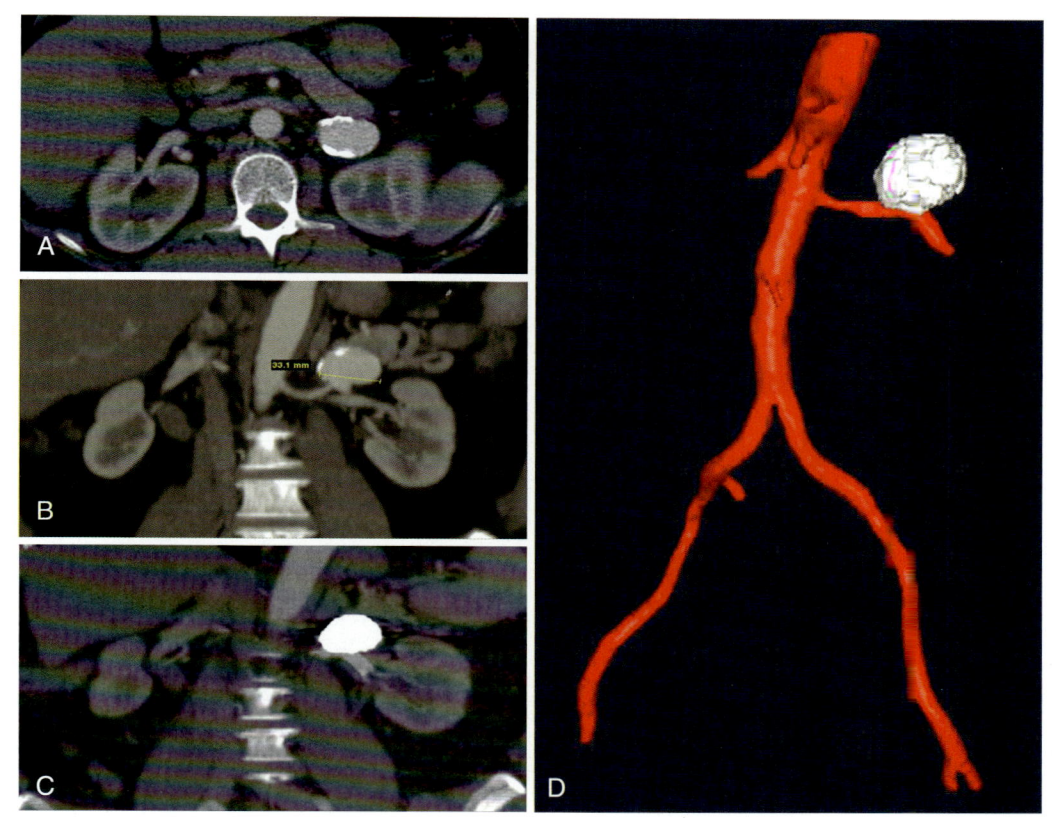

Figure 39-1. **A** and **B,** Axial CT images and coronal reconstruction revealing a saccular left renal artery aneurysm. **C** and **D,** Coronal and 3D CT imaging after coil embolization and stenting of the renal artery aneurysm.

can also reveal the extent of calcification in the aneurysm sac and adjacent arteries. Once occlusion coils or stents have been placed, artifact may limit the ability of CT angiography or magnetic resonance angiography to evaluate aneurysm exclusion (Fig. 39-1).

- Conventional angiography may provide additional information, such as the association of the renal artery aneurysm with an arteriovenous fistulae, or define entry site tears in patients with renal artery dissection associated with aneurysmal dilatation (Fig. 39-2).

Pitfalls and Danger Points

- A brachial approach may be needed in severely caudally angulated renal arteries. Many devices needed for treating renal aneurysms require a 7-Fr sheath with open repair of the brachial artery.
- Ipsilateral oblique images are critical for identifying occult ostial stenosis and for ensuring that the aneurysm does not obscure the true length or the neck of the aneurysm.
- Care must be taken when crossing the aneurysm to avoid rupture of the vessel or embolization of mural thrombus.
- Renal artery aneurysms occur predominantly at the renal bifurcation or in the first-order renal artery branches (Fig. 39-3).[2] This precludes placement of a covered stent and requires repair with a combination of coil or glue embolization and stenting.[7]
- Renal artery aneurysms that arise as a poststenotic dilation, often seen in patients with fibromuscular dysplasia, may benefit from stent grafting to address both the stenosis and the aneurysm.[8-10]
- Peripheral renal artery aneurysms may be treated with distal coil embolization, sacrificing a small amount of renal parenchyma (Fig. 39-4).

468 RENAL ARTERY DISEASE

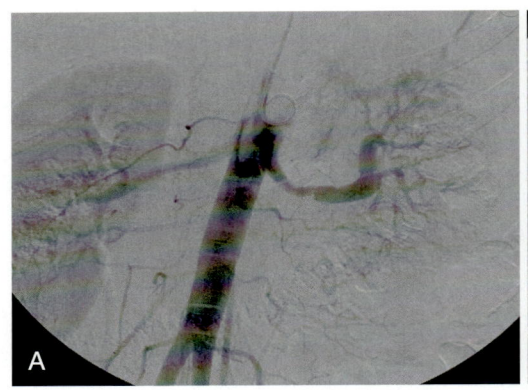

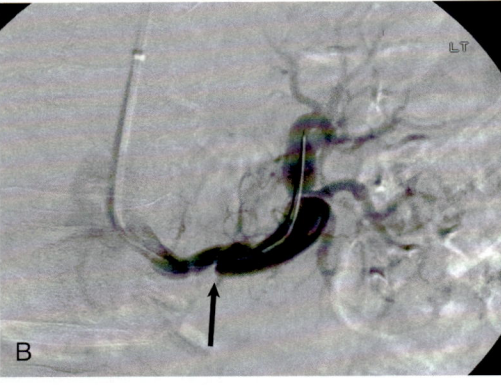

Figure 39-2. A, Aneurysmal dilatation of the left renal artery after arterial dissection. **B,** The entry tear to the false lumen is revealed by the presence of an intimal defect *(arrow)*.

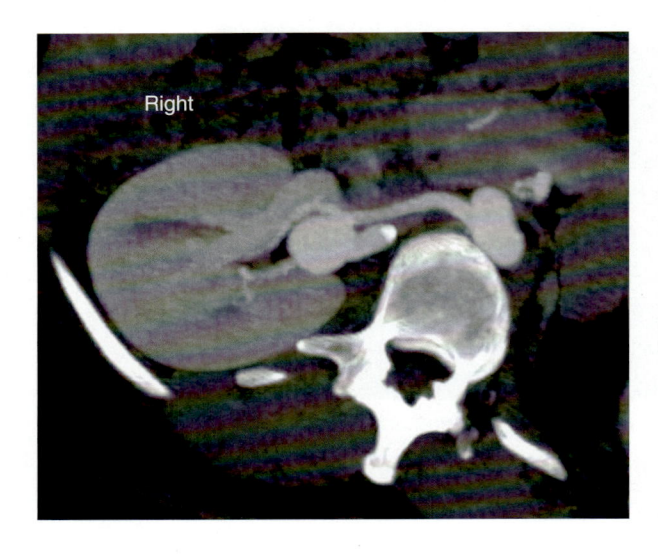

Figure 39-3. CT angiogram demonstrating a renal artery aneurysm at a distal branch point of the main renal artery.

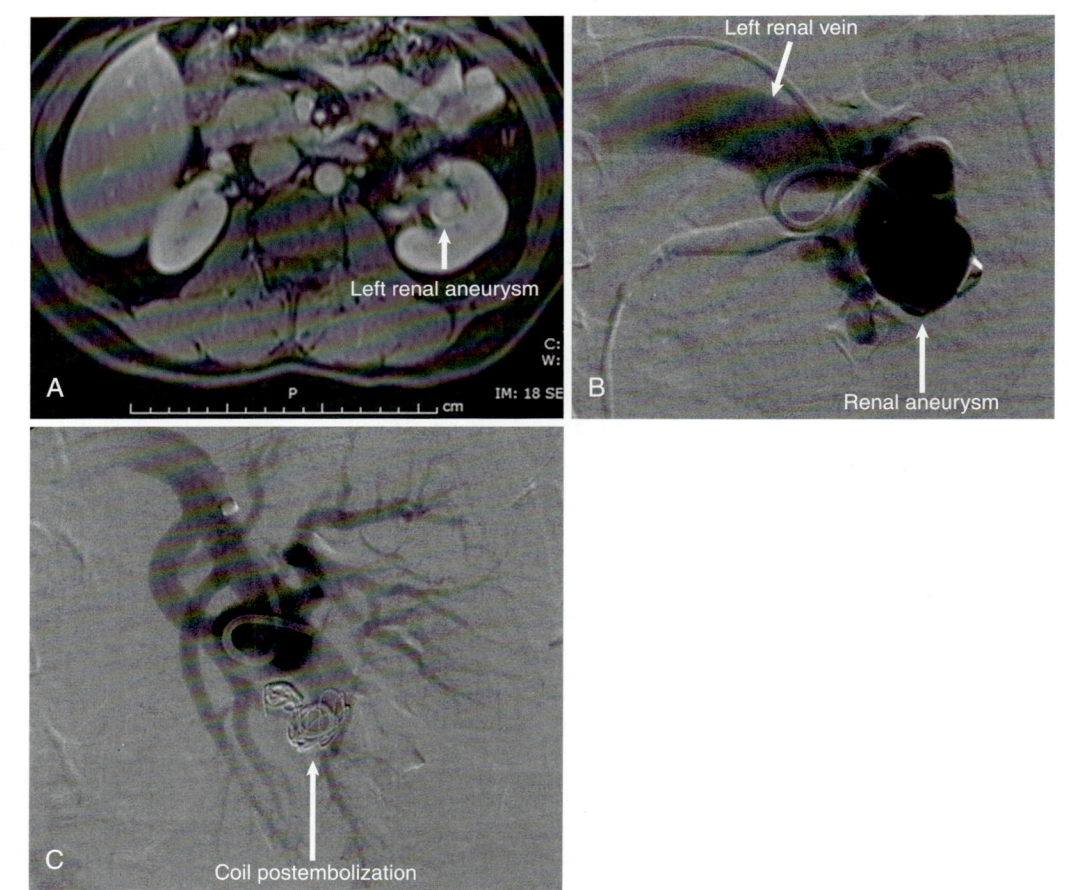

Figure 39-4. A, Magnetic resonance angiogram of a distal left renal artery aneurysm. **B,** Angiogram of the distal renal aneurysm revealing filling of the left renal vein and the presence of an arteriovenous fistula. **C,** Status post coil embolization of the left renal artery aneurysm with obliteration of the arteriovenous fistula.

Endovascular Strategy

Initial angiography should be performed with a flush catheter at the level of the renal arteries. Avoid placement of the catheter in the visceral segment of the aorta, as the superior mesenteric artery often obscures the origin of the left renal artery. A visceral selective, Cobra 2, or renal double-curved (RDC) catheter can be used to select the renal artery to be treated. In general there are four methods described for the endovascular management of renal artery aneurysms: use of bare stents or stent grafts, coil or glue occlusion of the aneurysm sac, stent-assisted embolization of the aneurysm sac, and occlusion of the inflow and outflow vessels of the portion of the renal artery supplying the aneurysm. If there are multiple aneurysms, or if the aneurysm involves a major branch point, endovascular repair may not be possible.

Endovascular Technique

Techniques used to gain access to the renal arteries are similar to those used for the treatment of renal artery occlusive disease.[11] Retrograde femoral access can be used with either a 6- or 7-Fr, 45- to 55-cm sheath and 5-Fr diagnostic catheter, such as Cobra 2 or a visceral selective catheter. Additionally, a 7- or 8-Fr sheath with a compatible guide catheter may be used (left internal mammary artery or RDC). Retrograde brachial access may provide a better approach to access severely angulated renal arteries. The advent of 0.014- and 0.018-inch guidewires, catheters, and balloons has also allowed easier access to these vessels.

DEPLOYMENT OF A BARE STENT

Renal artery aneurysms best suited for stenting alone are those that arise secondary to dissection.[12] Newer stent technologies that implement multiple braided layers may allow continued perfusion of side branches while changing flow dynamics within the aneurysm sac to increase the propensity of thrombosis.[13]

DEPLOYMENT OF A STENT GRAFT

Given that most renal aneurysms tend to be saccular as opposed to fusiform, use of a covered stent works well for excluding the aneurysms.[1,14] An endoleak is not likely given that there are few collaterals. Another advantage of stent grafting is immediate resolution of flow within the aneurysm, as opposed to coil embolization, which may not lead to immediate thrombosis. Nonetheless, of the three available self-expanding stent grafts, Viabahn (W.L. Gore and Associates, Newark, Del.), Fluency (Bard Medical, Covington, Ga.), and Wallgraft (Boston Scientific, Natick, Mass.), and the two balloon-expandable stent grafts, iCast (Atrium Medical, Hudson, N.H.) and Jostent (Abbott Vascular, Abbott Park, Ill.), none is approved in the United States for use in renal arteries (Table 39-1). These stent grafts tend to be bulkier and have less trackability compared with bare metal stents and microcatheters. The smallest inner diameter needed to deliver any of these stent grafts is 6 Fr, with the majority requiring a 7- or 8-Fr sheath. This should be considered if a brachial approach is planned and a direct cutdown should be performed.

TABLE 39-1 Types of Covered Stents

Name (coating material)	Company	Diameters/Lengths	Type	Delivery Sheath
Jostent (PTFE)	Abbott Vascular	3-5 mm/12-26 mm	Balloon expandable	6-Fr sheath
iCast (PTFE)	Atrium Medical	5-10 mm/16-59 mm	Balloon expandable	6- or 7-Fr sheath
Viabahn (PTFE)	W.L. Gore and Associates	5-10 mm/2.5, 5, 10 cm	Self-expanding	6- or 7-Fr sheath
Fluency (PTFE)	Bard Medical	5-10 mm/20, 40, 60, 80 mm	Self-expanding	8- or 9-Fr bareback
Wallgraft (Silastic*)	Boston Scientific	8-10 mm/40, 60, 80 mm	Self-expanding	8-Fr bareback

PTFE, Polytetrafluoroethylene.
*Silastic is a trademark for silicone elastomer.

Renal aneurysms often occur in the main branch or at the bifurcation of the main renal artery, with about 90% of aneurysms being extraparenchymal. Thus an effective seal of the aneurysm may require sacrifice of renal artery branches and a significant portion of renal parenchyma. In a patient with compromised renal function, loss of renal parenchyma may increase the risk of renal failure.

EMBOLIZATION

There are several methods for embolizing renal artery aneurysms, including coiling, using prothrombotic agents, using liquid polymers, and combining these with bare metal stenting. Perhaps the most widely described method is coil embolization. The basic premise is that platinum or stainless steel coils are delivered into the aneurysm sac. In addition to Guglielmi coils, newer microcoils now incorporate procoagulant fibers or coatings, which are activated once in contact with blood. These fibers and coating effectively increase the surface area of the coils, improving their ability to induced thrombosis. Newer controlled-release, detachable coils allow safer deployment with less risk for distal embolization.

Coil embolization has been described for both narrow- and wide-mouthed aneurysms of the main renal artery occurring at branch points and even for intraparenchymal aneurysms. Unlike stent grafting, coil embolization can be performed through a smaller delivery system. Many coils can be delivered via a catheter with an inner diameter as small as 0.018 inches, and neurovascular coils can be delivered through catheters with a lumen of 0.010 inches.

A disadvantage of coil embolization is the potential for coils to migrate or protrude into the main lumen of the nonaneurysmal vessel. It may also be difficult to stabilize a catheter within the aneurysm sac for effective deployment of the coils. Several methods have been developed to overcome this issue. One method is the use of a distal occlusion balloon to reduce flow beyond the aneurysm while coils are being deployed. Another method involves caging the coils within the aneurysm. The origin of the aneurysm is covered using a bare metal stent, and a microcatheter is passed through the interstices of the stent to embolize the sac. The potential for the coils to migrate or protrude into the lumen of the vessel is thus reduced (Fig. 39-5).

Another variation of this technique involves the placement of a microcatheter within the aneurysm sac followed by deployment of a nitinol stent across the neck of the aneurysm sac, trapping the catheter in place. After the occlusion coils are used to pack the aneurysm sac, the catheter is removed. The disadvantage of this technique is that it requires the simultaneous placement of two working catheters, which often requires dual arterial access.

Use of an ethylene vinyl alcohol (EVOH) copolymer (Onyx, eV3-Covidien, Plymouth, Minn.) has recently been described for treatment of renal artery aneurysms.[15-17] Of note is an off-label use of Onyx, which is approved for presurgical embolization of intracerebral vascular malformations. The method for delivering the polymer involves using a microcatheter that is compatible with the dimethyl sulfoxide (DMSO) solvent used for the EVOH. The Onyx material is delivered as a liquid, but upon contact with blood, DMSO rapidly diffuses, allowing the polymer to precipitate and form a radiopaque embolus. Care has to be taken when delivering the Onyx to prevent distal embolization. The balloon occlusion method has been described as one way to control flow beyond the aneurysm to minimize this risk. The outflow vessel is temporarily occluded as a small volume of the polymer is deployed in the sac, with flow restored intermittently until the sac is filled. The polymer makes a cast of the sac, including outflow vessels, increasing the likelihood of aneurysm thrombosis. In addition, it resurfaces the vessel lumen as it fills in the aneurysm sac.[15-17]

ENDOVASCULAR TREATMENT OF RENAL ARTERY ANEURYSMS 471

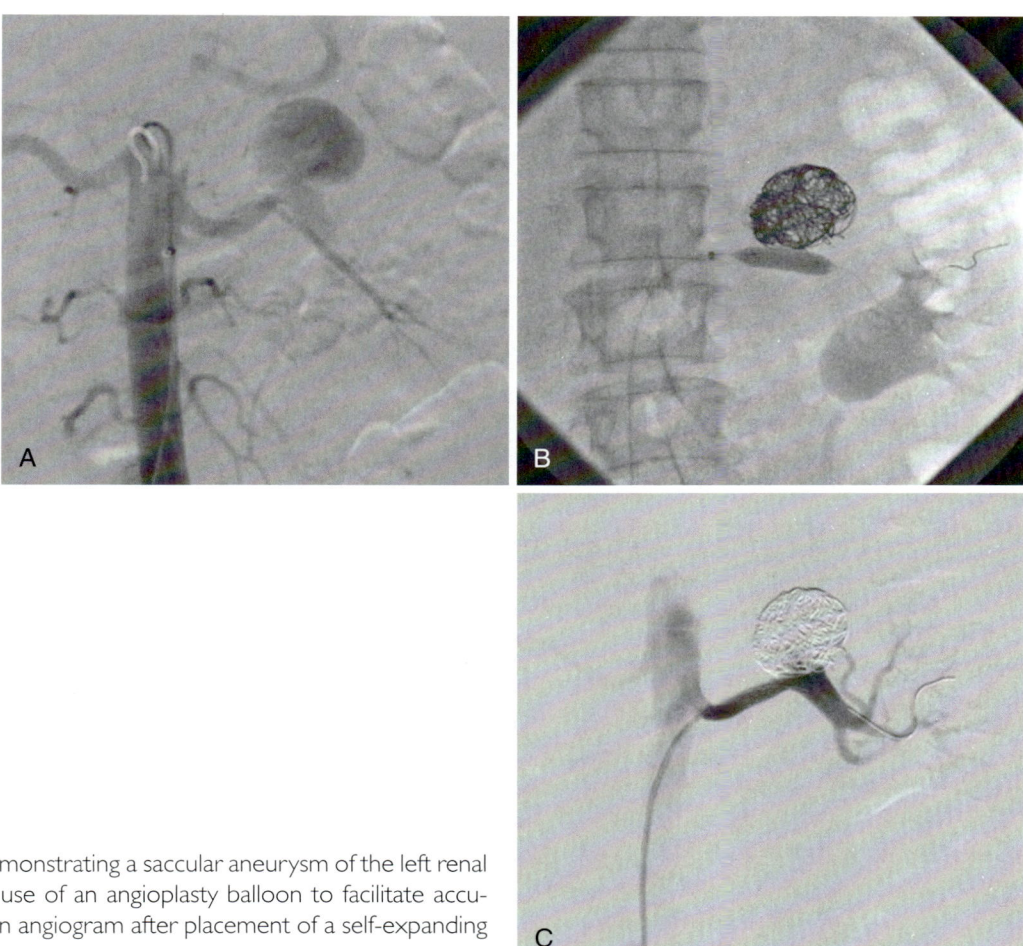

Figure 39-5. A, Angiography demonstrating a saccular aneurysm of the left renal artery. **B,** Coil embolization with use of an angioplasty balloon to facilitate accurate coil placement. **C,** Completion angiogram after placement of a self-expanding stent to prevent coil migration.

OCCLUSION OF THE RENAL ARTERY

Occlusion of the renal artery is a final method used to treat renal artery aneurysms and can be used when there is bleeding from either a traumatic injury or a spontaneous rupture. This technique is useful in high-risk patients who are not candidates for open repair.

Pseudoaneurysms of the renal artery secondary to iatrogenic injury have also been described. If located in the main segment of the renal artery, they may be successfully treated with a covered stent (Fig. 39-6). However, when there has been extensive damage to the arterial wall from trauma or life-threatening bleeding, temporary control may be obtained with balloon occlusion of the aorta or the renal artery origin, with subsequent embolization of the renal artery using coils or an Amplatzer occluder plug (St. Jude Medical, St. Paul; Fig. 39-7). Because the renal artery is an end organ, the surgeon can also occlude this vessel by covering the renal artery orifice directly with an aortic stent graft, assuming that adequate flow can be preserved to the contralateral kidney. If needed, a fenestrated stent graft can be used to preserve flow to one renal artery while occluding the contralateral vessel (Fig. 39-8).

Postoperative Care

- After intervention, patients are monitored overnight for access site problems or hemodynamic instability.
- Serum creatinine, blood urea nitrogen, and a complete blood count are measured the morning of discharge.

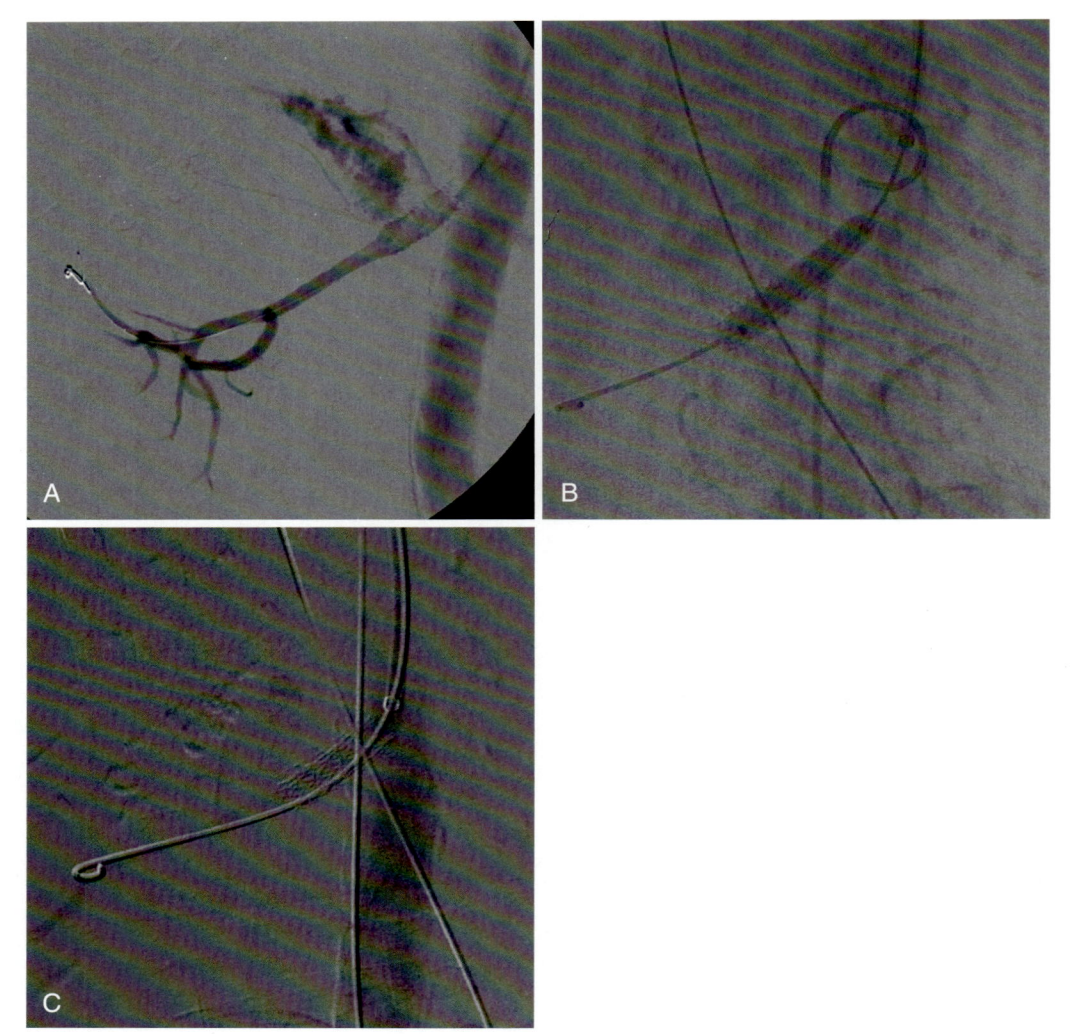

Figure 39-6. **A,** Rupture of the right renal artery with extravasation of contrast after placement of a bare metal stent. **B,** Control of perforation with an angioplasty balloon. **C,** A polytetrafluoroethylene-covered stent was used to treat the perforation.

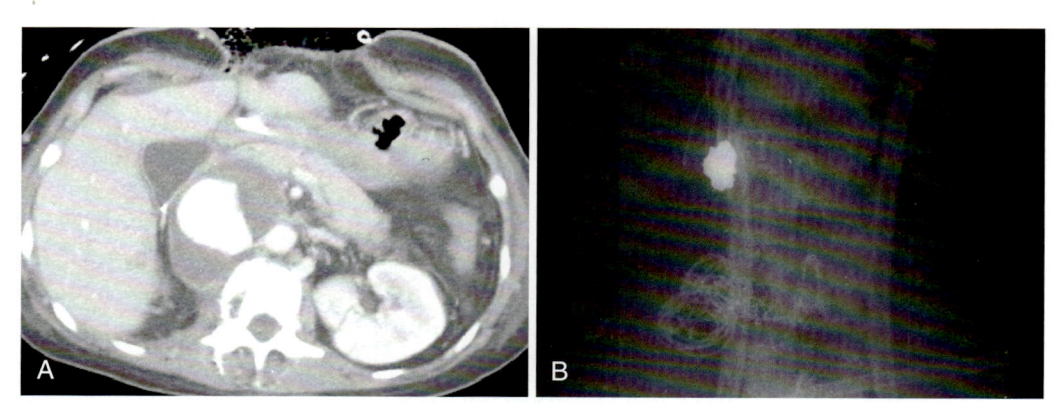

Figure 39-7. **A,** Right renal artery pseudoaneurysm present on CT imaging after a gunshot wound to the abdomen. **B,** Coils have been placed to occlude the pseudoaneurysm. A retained bullet fragment is seen superiorly.

- Clopidogrel is continued for a minimum of 30 days. Aspirin is maintained indefinitely.
- Clinical follow-up with CT imaging and surveillance renal duplex ultrasonography is performed at 1 month, subsequently at 6-month intervals for 2 years, and annually thereafter. A renal artery peak systolic velocity of more than 180 cm/sec suggests stenosis. If the aneurysm is stable or regresses in size, ultrasound can be used for surveillance.

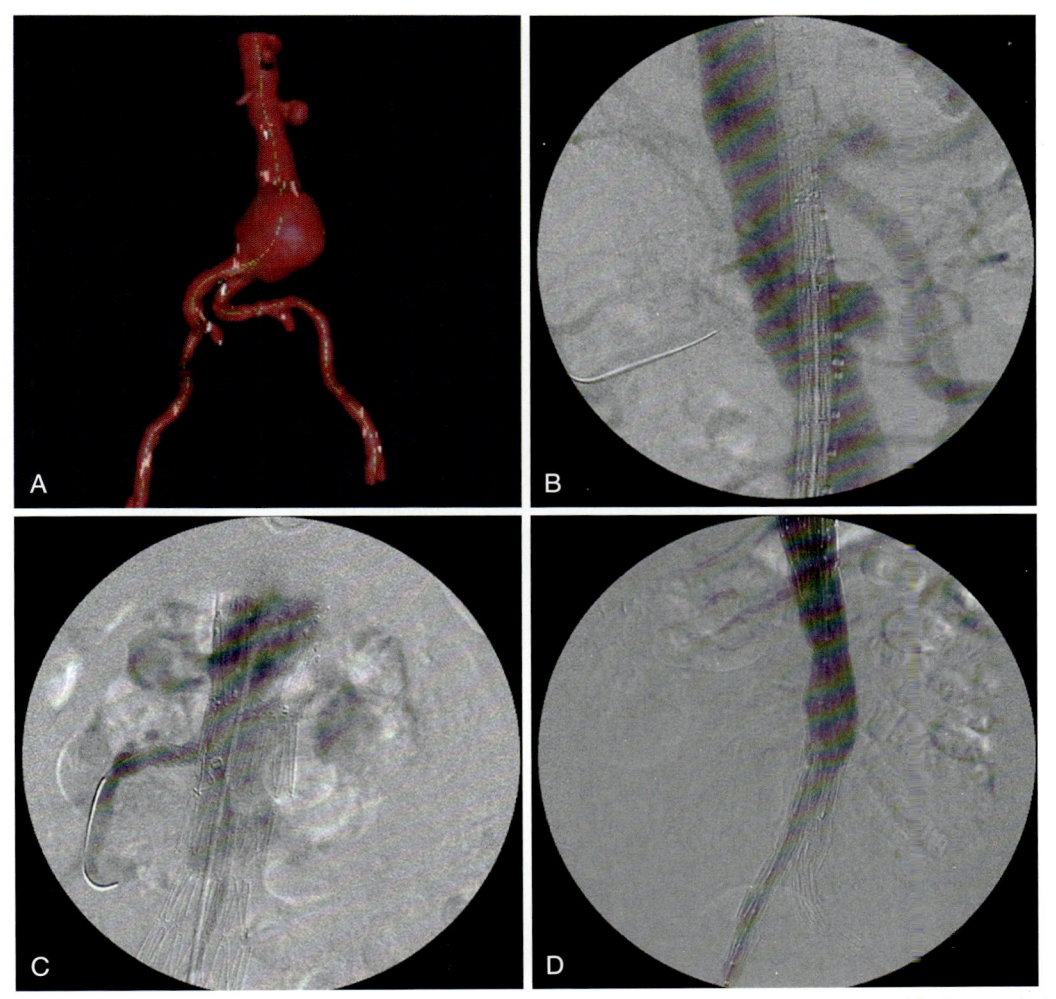

Figure 39-8. **A,** 3D reconstruction of CT angiogram revealing a left renal artery aneurysm and infrarenal abdominal aortic aneurysm. **B,** Intraoperative angiogram demonstrating the aneurysmal origin of the left renal artery and atrophic left kidney. **C,** A fenestrated aortic endograft was placed with stenting of the right renal artery and coverage of the left renal artery. **D,** Completion angiography demonstrates successful exclusion of the aortic aneurysm and left renal artery aneurysm and preservation of flow to the right renal artery.

Complications

- **Embolization.** Embolization may not be readily apparent but may manifest as renal dysfunction and urine eosinophils. Treatment is largely supportive.
- **Stent fractures.** Stents may fracture and lead to stenosis or inadequate treatment of the renal artery aneurysm. Repeat angioplasty or stenting may be necessary.
- **Thrombosis of the stent graft.** Thrombosis can lead to loss of the kidney and deterioration of renal function if not discovered acutely.

REFERENCES

1. Bui BT, Oliva VL, Leclerc G, et al: Renal artery aneurysm: Treatment with percutaneous placement of a stent-graft, *Radiology* 195:181-182, 1995.
2. Tham G, Ekelund L, Herrlin K, et al: Renal artery aneurysms: Natural history and prognosis, *Ann Surg* 197:348-352, 1983.
3. Manninen HI, Berg M, Vanninen RL: Stent-assisted coil embolization of wide-necked renal artery bifurcation aneurysms, *J Vasc Intervent Radiol* 19:487-492, 2008.
4. Hislop SJ, Patel SA, Abt PL, et al: Therapy of renal artery aneurysms in New York state: Outcomes of patients undergoing open and endovascular repair, *Ann Vasc Surg* 23:194-200, 2009.
5. Stanley J, Rhodes EL, Gewertz BL, et al: Renal artery aneurysms: Significance of macroaneurysms exclusive of dissections and fibrodysplastic mural dilatations, *Arch Surg* 110:1327-1333, 1973.
6. Henke PK, Cardenau JD, Welling TH, et al: Renal artery aneurysms: A 35 year clinical experience with 252 aneurysms in 168 patients, *Ann Surg* 234:454-463, 2001.

7. Eskandari MK, Resnick SA: Aneurysms of the renal artery, *Semin Vasc Surg* 18:202-208, 2005.
8. Bisschops RH, Popma JJ, Meyerovitz MF: Treatment of fibromuscular dysplasia and renal artery aneurysm with use of a stent-graft, *J Vasc Interv Radiol* 12:757-760, 2001.
9. Sciacca L, Ciocca RG, Eslami MH, et al: Endovascular treatment of renal artery aneurysm secondary to fibromuscular dysplasia: A case report, *Ann Vasc Surg* 23(536):e9-e12, 2009.
10. Serter S, Oran I, Parildar M, et al: Fibromuscular dysplasia-related renal artery stenosis associated with aneurysm: Successive endovascular therapy, *Cardiovasc Intervent Radiol* 30:297-299, 2007.
11. Kwolek CJ: Endovascular management of renal artery stenosis: Current techniques and results, *Perspectives in Vascular Surgery and Endovascular Therapy* 16:261-279, 2004.
12. Mali WP, Geyskes GG, Thalman R: Dissecting renal artery aneurysm: Treatment with an endovascular stent, *AJR Am J Roentgenol* 153:623-624, 1989.
13. Henry M, Polydorou A, Frid N, et al: Treatment of renal artery aneurysm with the multilayer stent, *J Endovasc Ther* 15:231-236, 2008.
14. Tan WA, Chough S, Saito J, et al: Covered stent for renal artery aneurysm, *Catheter Cardiovasc Interv* 52:106-109, 2001.
15. Lupattelli T, Abubacker Z, Morgan R, et al: Embolization of a renal artery aneurysm using ethylene vinyl alcohol copolymer (Onyx), *J Endovasc Ther* 10:366-370, 2003.
16. Rautio R, Haapanen A: Transcatheter embolization of a renal artery aneurysm using ethylene vinyl alcohol copolymer, *Cardiovasc Intervent Radiol* 30:300-303, 2007.
17. Abath C, Andrade G, Cavalcanti D, et al: Complex renal artery aneurysms: Liquids or coils? *Tech Vasc Interv Radiol* 10:299-307, 2007.

Section 9

SUPERIOR MESENTERIC AND CELIAC ARTERY DISEASE

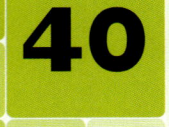

40 Direct Surgical Repair for Celiac Axis and Superior Mesenteric Artery Occlusive Disease

THOMAS S. HUBER

Historical Background

Embolectomy of the superior mesenteric artery for acute mesenteric ischemia was suggested by Ryvlin in 1943[1] and Klass in 1951,[2] with the first successful embolectomy reported by Shaw and Rutledge in 1957.[3] The feasibility of performing synchronous superior mesenteric artery embolectomy and small bowel resection was described a year later.[4]

The manifestation of occlusive disease of the superior mesenteric artery and celiac axis as chronic abdominal pain and intestinal ischemia was recognized by Klein in 1921.[5] Although a variety of surgical procedures were described for treatment of chronic mesenteric ischemia during the 1950s, including transection and reimplantation of the superior mesenteric artery[6] and superior mesenteric artery endarterectomy,[7] an aortomesenteric bypass for chronic mesenteric ischemia was first reported by Morris and DeBakey[8] in 1961, with construction of Dacron bypass grafts to the superior mesenteric and hepatic arteries. A larger series of patients with chronic mesenteric ischemia treated with surgical bypass was published in 1962.[9] The first case of an ileomesenteric bypass for chronic mesenteric ischemia was also reported in 1962 by Mavor and Lyall.[10]

Indications

In the setting of acute mesenteric ischemia, impaired intestinal perfusion leads to mucosal ischemia, which can progress to bowel infarction with perforation and peritonitis. Emergent revascularization is warranted. Likewise, all patients with chronic mesenteric ischemia should undergo elective revascularization to prevent bowel infraction and by resolving characteristic food avoidance restoring normal nutritional status. There is no role for chronic parenteral alimentation and noninterventional therapies, even among patients at high risk for revascularization. The indication for revascularization in asymptomatic patients with visceral arterial occlusive disease remains unresolved. Thomas and associates[11] reported that patients with significant occlusive disease in all three visceral vessels represent a "high-risk" group for bowel infarction, whereas other reports have documented adverse outcomes after aortic reconstruction among patients with untreated occlusive disease of the celiac axis and superior and inferior mesenteric arteries.

Endovascular therapy has evolved over the past several years and has become the first line of therapy for patients with chronic mesenteric ischemia in most institutions. An endovascular approach offers the advantages of a shorter length of hospital stay, reduced morbidity and mortality, and improved quality of life. However, long-term vessel patency is inferior to open revascularization with a requirement for secondary procedures. Nonetheless, recurrent stenosis after endovascular treatment does not necessarily equate to recurrence of symptoms, nor does it appear to precipitate acute mesenteric ischemia. The role of endovascular treatment for acute mesenteric ischemia has been limited by the need to assess the integrity of the bowel, as well as by an increased risk of embolization when recanalizing an acute embolic or thrombotic occlusion. However, a combined open and endovascular approach may be feasible, with endovascular revascularization performed at the time of laparotomy.

Preoperative Preparation

ACUTE MESENTERIC ISCHEMIA

- Patients with acute mesenteric ischemia from embolus or in situ thrombosis require emergent definitive treatment. Extensive preoperative evaluation is potentially harmful because of the narrow window for salvaging the bowel. There is no role for nonoperative treatment.
- Heparin anticoagulation should be initiated to limit clot propagation and broad spectrum antibiotics administered that are effective against enteric organisms.
- Patients are frequently hypovolemic, and resuscitation should be initiated before the induction of anesthesia.

CHRONIC MESENTERIC ISCHEMIA

- Patients with chronic mesenteric ischemia should undergo expeditious medical and cardiac evaluation. However, a careful preoperative assessment is required to exclude other potential causes of chronic abdominal pain.
- Operative planning is facilitated by a computed tomography (CT) angiogram of the aorta and visceral vessels. Imaging is obtained to identify the extent of atherosclerotic occlusive disease, as well as the suitability of the supraceliac aorta as a site to originate an antegrade bypass, if required.
- Ankle-brachial indices and duplex imaging of the saphenous and femoral veins as potential conduits should be obtained.
- Patients with minimal postprandial pain should be counseled to avoid large meals or the specific food types that exacerbate their symptoms. Those with continuous abdominal pain should avoid oral intake with the exception of medications. Although the operative procedure should not be delayed in an attempt to replete nutritional stores, malnourished patients may be started on total parenteral nutrition if a somewhat prolonged preoperative course is anticipated.
- Preoperative bowel preparation is unnecessary.

Pitfalls and Danger Points

- Both acute and chronic mesenteric ischemia are life-threatening problems frequently associated with diagnostic delays before referral to a surgeon. A high index of suspicion and an expedited evaluation are mandatory to reduce adverse outcome.
- Acute mesenteric ischemia may be the first manifestation of visceral artery occlusive disease.
- Major operative procedures, particularly aortic reconstructions, can precipitate acute mesenteric ischemia in patients with visceral artery occlusive disease. Preemptive visceral revascularization of the asymptomatic patient may be indicated selected patients.
- Preoperative evaluation should include a CT angiogram and lower extremity duplex vein survey to assess the supraceliac aorta and variability in visceral vessel configuration, as well as the saphenous and femoral veins, respectively.

- Adequate exposure of the supraceliac aorta is mandatory during antegrade bypass to avoid injuring the esophagus and to assure precise suture placement.
- Caution should be exercised while creating the retropancreatic tunnel during antegrade bypass to avoid injuring the splenic vein.
- A retrograde aorto–superior mesenteric artery bypass courses both caudal to cephalad and posterior to anterior. The propensity of this bypass to kink may be reduced by using an externally supported graft.
- Resection of ischemic bowel that is not infarcted should be delayed until after revascularization. A "second look" operation the following day is warranted should there be any doubt regarding the viability of the bowel.
- The postoperative course after visceral vessel revascularization may be complicated by multiple organ dysfunction, which requires supportive therapy.
- Acute mesenteric ischemia secondary to an early graft occlusion can be confused with multiple organ dysfunction. A high index of suspicion will necessitate imaging of the bypass graft.

Operative Strategy

SURGICAL ANATOMY

There is an extensive collateral network among the celiac axis, superior mesenteric artery, inferior mesenteric artery, and internal iliac arteries. The celiac axis and superior mesenteric artery collateralize through the superior and inferior pancreaticoduodenal arteries, respectively, with the direction of flow contingent on the location of the stenosis. The superior and inferior mesenteric arteries collateralize through both the meandering artery and the marginal artery of Drummond. The meandering artery is the most significant collateral vessel and connects the ascending branch of the left colic artery with the middle branch of the middle colic artery. It lies at the base of the mesentery and is at risk of being ligated along with the inferior mesenteric vein during exposure of the infrarenal aorta. The inferior mesenteric artery communicates with the internal iliac artery via the hemorrhoidal branches and may represent a more important collateral than originally appreciated. This collateral pathway may be disrupted during sigmoid colectomy or infrarenal aortic aneurysm repair.

A significant amount of variability exists in the configuration of the visceral vessels. The "classic" three-vessel pattern for the celiac axis, consisting of the splenic, left gastric, and common hepatic arteries, occurs in approximately 75% of patients. Replaced or accessory hepatic arteries can originate from the superior mesenteric artery, and the left hepatic artery can arise off of the left gastric artery and course through the gastrohepatic ligament. A thorough review of preoperative imaging studies should be performed because both exposure and surgical planning for revascularization can be affected.

ACUTE MESENTERIC ISCHEMIA SECONDARY TO EMBOLIZATION, IN SITU THROMBOSIS, AND DISSECTION

Emboli responsible for acute mesenteric ischemia originate in the heart, usually as a result of atrial fibrillation, an acute myocardial infarction, or a ventricular aneurysm, and lodge in the superior mesenteric artery. Patients frequently have had a history of prior embolic events. Notably, an embolism to the superior mesenteric artery is quite large, in contrast to the micron-sized atheroembolic particles that cause blue toe syndrome. As a consequence, flow is easily restored in most situations by superior mesenteric artery embolectomy.

Acute mesenteric ischemia secondary to in situ thrombosis is superimposed upon the symptoms of chronic mesenteric ischemia in more than 50% of the patients.[12] Patients with acute mesenteric ischemia secondary to in situ thrombosis require a mesenteric bypass. Although antegrade and retrograde bypasses are both options, retrograde bypass from the infrarenal aorta or iliac artery is the optimal procedure in the acute setting because of the ease of exposing the inflow source.

Dissections can occur in visceral vessels as an extension of an aortic dissection or, less commonly, as an isolated event. Mesenteric revascularization may be appropriate for patients with an acute aortic dissection and visceral malperfusion, but this approach is complicated by the underlying aortic pathology. Isolated or spontaneous dissections can occur in any visceral vessel although the superior mesenteric artery appears to be the most common. The underlying cause or etiology remains unknown, although atherosclerosis, medial degeneration, trauma, fibromuscular disease, pregnancy, and a host of arteriopathies have been implicated. Patients' symptoms may include abdominal pain. However, in one of the largest series in the literature, most patients were asymptomatic.[13] The optimal treatment for an isolated dissection remains unresolved. Intervention is indicated for mesenteric ischemia, aneurysmal degeneration, and rupture. Both open and endovascular treatments have been reported, although the latter may be optimal given that the dissection can extend distally within the vessel. Expectant, conservative treatment with anticoagulation is likely adequate for asymptomatic or minimally symptomatic patients. Patients should be followed with serial CT imaging because of the risk of late aneurysmal degeneration. Similar to other vascular beds, these dissections can "heal" or resolve over time.

SELECTION OF AN INFLOW SOURCE

Mesenteric bypass, either antegrade from the supraceliac aorta or retrograde from the infrarenal aorta or common iliac artery, is indicated for patients with chronic mesenteric ischemia and those with acute mesenteric ischemia secondary to in situ thrombosis. The advantages of an antegrade bypass include the observation that the supraceliac aorta is usually free of atherosclerosis and the graft limbs follow a direct path while maintaining prograde flow. However, a retrograde bypass from the infrarenal aorta and common iliac artery is easier and faster to perform. Furthermore, although it is possible to partially occlude the supraceliac aorta while performing the proximal anastomosis of an antegrade bypass, the hemodynamic and ischemic impact of clamping the infrarenal aorta or iliac artery is minimal. One major disadvantage of a retrograde bypass is its potential to kink, which is particularly problematic for venous conduits. The graft must transition from the aorta that sits posterior in the abdomen to the superior mesenteric artery that sits more anterior. A ringed expanded polytetrafluoroethylene (ePTFE) conduit is a preferred choice. However, should a vein graft be required in the setting of enteric contamination, a relatively short conduit originating from the aorta, which is positioned to account for the normal lie of the superior mesenteric artery, should be considered.

Inherent to the debate about the type of bypass procedure is the number of vessels to be revascularized. Multivessel revascularization offers the advantage that if one graft limb occludes; the patient will not necessarily develop recurrent symptoms or acute mesenteric ischemia. Indeed, Hollier and colleagues[14] reported that the rate of recurrent symptoms after open revascularization was inversely related to the number of vessels revascularized. Proponents of an isolated retrograde bypass to the superior mesenteric artery emphasize that the procedure revascularizes the primary vessel of concern, multivessel reconstruction significantly increases the complexity of the procedure, and more recent series have not demonstrated a clinical advantage for multivessel bypass.

SELECTION OF THE CELIAC ARTERY OUTFLOW SITE: MAIN CELIAC TRUNK OR COMMON HEPATIC ARTERY

Either the main celiac artery trunk or the common hepatic artery may be used as the outflow site for an antegrade bypass. The atherosclerotic occlusive process is essentially "aortic spillover" disease that affects the proximal portion of the vessel and usually extends to the first branch. Both options have relative advantages and disadvantages. Using the main celiac trunk facilitates an end-to-end anastomosis with a generous anastomosis given its larger size. In contrast, the common hepatic is more superficial to expose, although it is more difficult to orient the graft and the artery to configure the anastomosis.

APPROACH TO THE SUPERIOR MESENTERIC ARTERY

The superior mesenteric artery may be exposed using one of three approaches as dictated by the underlying etiology and the planned configuration of the bypass (Fig. 40-1). First, it may be exposed caudal to the inferior border of the pancreas by entering the lesser sac and incising the retroperitoneum (Fig. 40-1, *A*). Second, it may be exposed at the transverse base of the mesocolon by elevating this segment of the colon and incising the proximal mesentery horizontally (Fig. 40-1, *B*). Lastly, the superior mesenteric artery can be approached laterally by completely mobilizing the fourth portion of the duodenum after incising the ligament of Treitz and the other peritoneal attachments (Fig. 40-1, *C*). The approaches through the lesser sac and the base of the transverse mesocolon are useful for antegrade

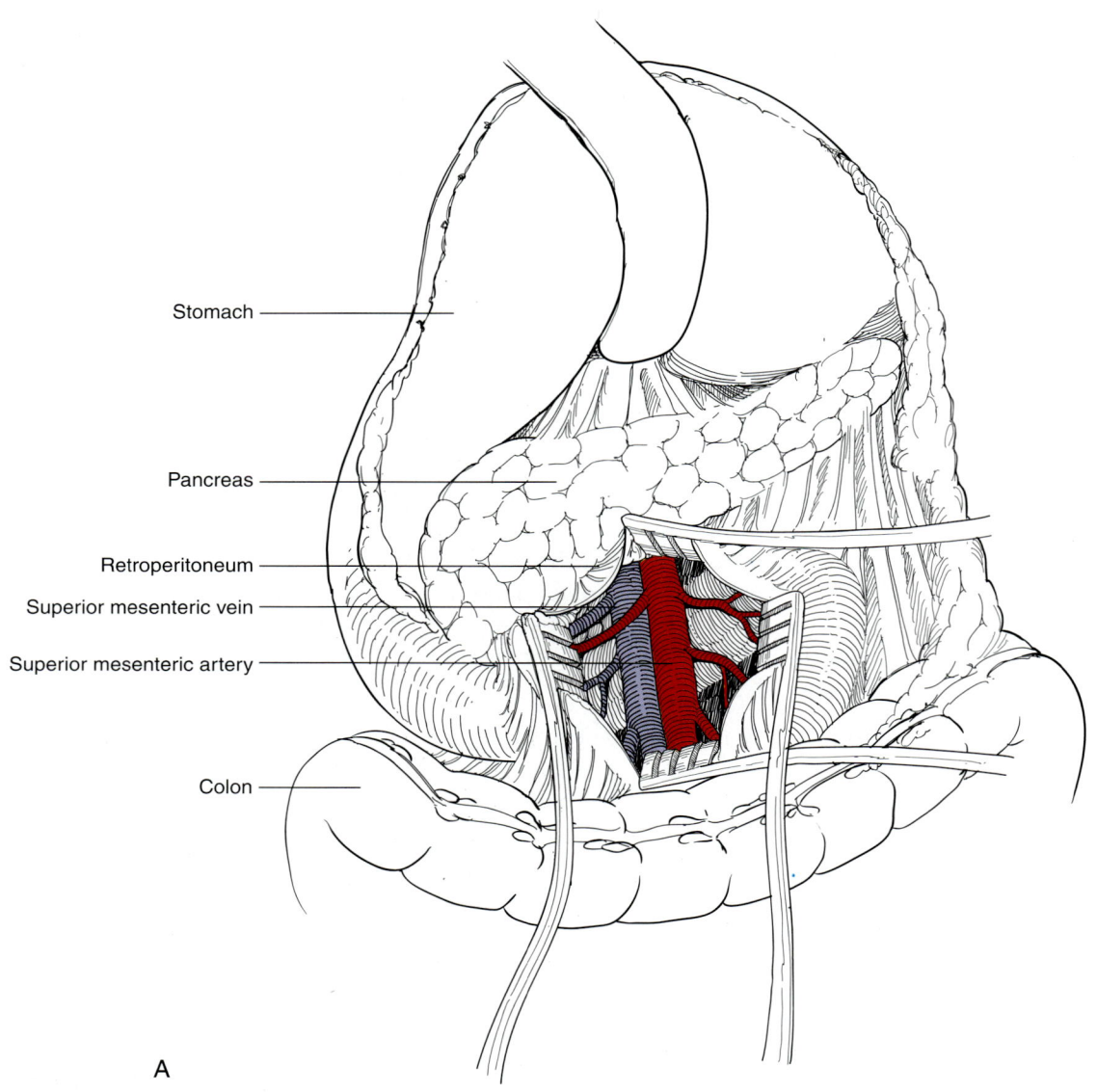

Figure 40-1. A, The superior mesenteric artery is exposed through a longitudinal midline incision in the retroperitoneal tissue immediately inferior to the border of the pancreas. The stomach is retracted superiorly, and the small bowel and colon are retracted inferiorly. Two Weitlander retractors have been used to separate the retroperitoneal fat and further facilitate the exposure of the artery. The adjacent superior mesenteric vein, which lies to the right of the superior mesenetric artery, can be used as a landmark to help identify the artery. There are relatively few crossing veins that require division and ligation during exposure of the superior mesenteric artery.

DIRECT SURGICAL REPAIR FOR CELIAC AXIS AND SUPERIOR MESENTERIC ARTERY OCCLUSIVE DISEASE

bypass, whereas the lateral approach is preferred when a retrograde bypass is contemplated. An embolectomy can be performed most expeditiously by exposing the superior mesenteric artery at the base of the transverse mesocolon.

SELECTION OF A CONDUIT

Both prosthetic and autogenous conduits have been used to construct a mesenteric bypass. Kihara and associates[15] reported lower patency rates for vein grafts than for prosthetic grafts, but multivariate analysis demonstrated that gender rather than type of conduit was responsible for the observed difference. Modrall and

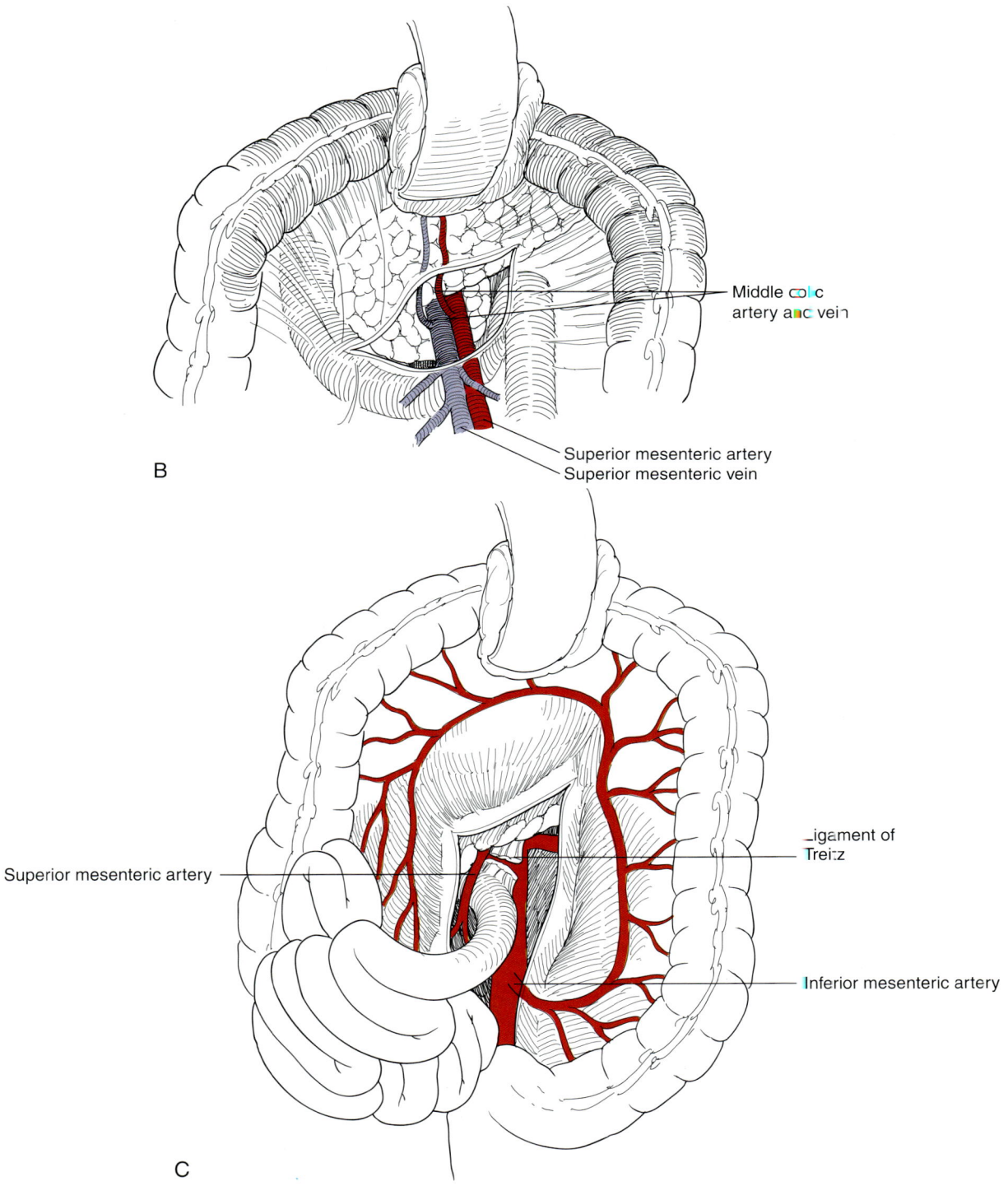

Figure 40-1, cont'd B, The superior mesenteric artery is exposed at the base of the transverse mesocolon through a horizontal incision in the mesentery. **C,** The superior mesenteric artery is exposed above the superior margin of the duodenum by completely mobilizing the fourth portion of the duodenum after incising the ligament of Treitz and the other peritoneal attachments.

colleagues[16] reported that symptom recurrence after mesenteric bypass was lower in patients who underwent reconstruction using femoral vein rather than saphenous vein. The femoral vein may represent an ideal conduit when a prosthetic conduit is contraindicated due to enteric contamination or bowel infarction, given a mean diameter of 7 mm and a relatively thick wall.[17] However, harvesting the femoral vein adds substantial time and complexity to the procedure.

Operative Technique for Antegrade Bypass

POSITION

For antegrade aortoceliac or aortosuperior mesenteric artery bypass, the patient is positioned supine. The distal pulses are interrogated with continuous wave Doppler, and the operative field, including the chest, abdomen, groin and both lower extremities, is prepared in the standard fashion.

INCISION

Either a midline or a bilateral subcostal incision can be used, because the anatomic structures that need to be exposed during the procedure are all along the axial skeleton. The major advantage of the midline incision is that it is somewhat easier and faster to close. The major advantage of the bilateral subcostal incision is that it provides the most optimal exposure to the upper abdomen and is helpful in larger individuals.

EXPOSURE OF THE AORTA

The supraceliac aorta is exposed by incising the left triangular ligament of the liver (Fig. 40-2). Care should be exercised during this step to avoid injuring the vena cava or hepatic veins that serve as the lateral extent of the dissection. The left lateral segment of the liver is then folded back and retracted to the patient's right. Exposure is facilitated by using a self-retaining Bookwalter retractor with a large round ring and by positioning four medium or deep right-angled retractor blades throughout the length of the bilateral subcostal incision. Placing the patient in a significant amount of reverse Trendelenburg also facilitates exposure by allowing the visceral structures to "fall away" from the operative field. The gastrohepatic ligament is then incised. Care should be exercised, because a replaced left hepatic artery from the left gastric artery may course through the ligament. The esophagus and stomach are then retracted to the patient's left with the assistance of a retractor blade. The esophagus can usually be identified by the presence of a nasogastric tube or transesophageal echocardiography probe. The median arcuate ligament is subsequently incised along the longitudinal axis of the aorta, and both lateral crus of the diaphragm are incised horizontally. The pleural cavity is occasionally entered, which necessitates a chest radiograph in the immediate postoperative period to confirm that the lungs are fully expanded. The posterior peritoneum is then incised, and the supraceliac aorta exposed. Approximately 6 cm of the supraceliac aorta should be dissected free to facilitate aortic clamping. It is not necessary to dissect the aorta circumferentially.

EXPOSURE OF THE CELIAC AXIS

The celiac axis is exposed by dissecting caudal along the anterior surface of the aorta (Fig. 40-2). This requires incising the remaining fibers of the diaphragm and the dense, fibrous neural tissue know as the celiac ganglion that surrounds the proximal celiac artery. This is facilitated by incising the fibers with electrocautery between the jaws of a right-angled clamp. The stomach and viscera can be retracted inferiorly either manually or with a malleable retractor. The preferred technique is to dissect the origin of the celiac axis and its proximal branches circumferentially. Approximately 3 cm of the celiac artery along with its proximal branches should be exposed to facilitate constructing an end-to-end anastomosis

DIRECT SURGICAL REPAIR FOR CELIAC AXIS AND SUPERIOR MESENTERIC ARTERY OCCLUSIVE DISEASE

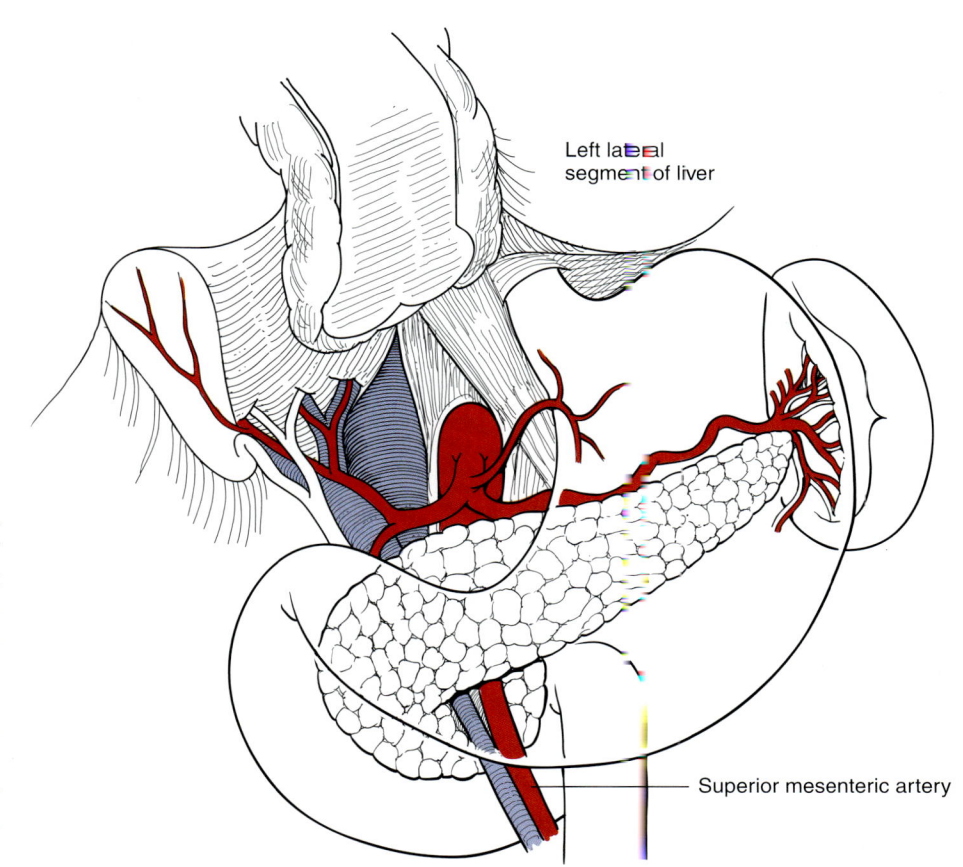

Figure 40-2. The exposure of the supraceliac aorta and the celiac axis. The left lateral segment of the liver has been mobilized and reflected back using a self-retaining retractor blade. The median arcuate ligament, the crus of the diaphragm, and the dense neural tissue encasing the aorta have been incised to facilitate exposure. After the supraceliac aorta is exposed, the dissection is advanced caudally along the anterior aspect of the aorta to completely expose the celiac axis and its proximal branches.

and oversewing the proximal remnant, after the vessel is transected. The proximal branches of the celiac artery, including the splenic and left gastric arteries, occasionally need to be sacrificed to facilitate the anastomosis. This is rarely of clinical significance since the orifice of the celiac artery was already occluded or severely stenotic, and because the stomach and spleen have a rich collateral network. Alternatively, the distal anastomosis can be performed to the common hepatic artery in an end-to-side manner. This is facilitated by dissecting the common hepatic, proper hepatic, and gastroduodenal arteries circumferentially along the lesser curve of the stomach in the proximal porta hepatis. Although the dissection is somewhat easier, it is more difficult to properly orient the graft.

EXPOSURE OF THE SUPERIOR MESENTERIC ARTERY

A suitable segment of the superior mesenteric artery can be exposed using a variety of techniques, as detailed previously. In a preferred approach, the artery is dissected immediately caudal to the inferior border of the pancreas (see Fig. 40-1, A). The vessel is approached either through the lesser sac by incising the gastrocolic ligament or through the gastrohepatic ligament by retracting the lesser curve of the stomach inferiorly. A longitudinal incision is made in the retroperitoneum immediately below the inferior border of the pancreas to expose the artery. This can be facilitated by retracting the stomach superiorly and the small bowel and transverse colon inferiorly using the malleable retractor blades. The retroperitoneal tissue overlying the superior mesenteric artery and vein can be retracted with two Weitlander self-retaining retractors oriented at 90 degrees relative to each other. It can be somewhat challenging to find the superior mesenteric artery in patients with a significant amount of retroperitoneal fat. Identifying the adjacent superior mesenteric vein or tracing the middle colic artery retrograde can be helpful. Approximately 2 cm of the artery should be exposed to facilitate construction of the anastomosis, but caution should be exercised because multiple branches of the artery at this level are easily injured. Alternatively, the superior mesenteric artery can be exposed at the root of the transverse mesocolon (see Fig. 40-1, *B*). The transverse colon is elevated, and the proximal mesentery incised horizontally. Finally, the superior mesenteric artery can be approached along its left lateral surface. The ligament of Treitz and other peritoneal attachments are incised (see Fig. 40-1, *C*), followed by completely mobilization of the duodenum's fourth portion. The superior mesenteric artery is surrounded by fatty tissue at this level. Arterial or venous branches will rarely be encountered when the artery is approached along its left lateral surface.

TUNNELING THE BYPASS GRAFT

After the superior mesenteric artery is exposed, a retropancreatic tunnel is created using gentle, bimanual finger dissection between the exposed supraceliac aorta and the superior mesenteric artery. This step should be performed with caution, because the tunnel courses adjacent to the superior mesenteric vein, deep to the splenic vein, and near their confluence with the portal vein. A straight aortic clamp or red rubber catheter can be passed through the tunnel and left in place until it is necessary to pass the limb.

PROXIMAL AORTIC ANASTOMOSIS

The proximal anastomosis to the supraceliac aorta is performed as the next step (Fig. 40-3). Before occluding the aorta, the patient is systemically heparinized (100 units per kilogram of body weight) and given 25 g of mannitol as both an antioxidant and a diuretic. A bifurcated Dacron graft with a body diameter of 12 mm and limb diameters of 7 mm may be used. However, grafts of this size are not universally available and can be substituted with those measuring 12 × 6 or 14 × 7 mm. Both ePTFE and autogenous femoral vein are acceptable substitutes. Aortic control can usually be achieved with a partial occluding clamp, such as a Lambert-Kay clamp that has been modified with a locking device that secures the tips. When it is not possible to partially occlude the aorta because of calcification or atherosclerotic involvement, two straight aortic clamps can be used. Completely occluding the aorta is less optimal, although the time to complete the anastomosis is usually less than 15 minutes.

An arteriotomy is made along the longitudinal axis of the aorta, and the graft is spatulated so that the limbs of the graft are oriented on top of each other, in contrast to the case of an aortobifemoral graft in which the limbs are oriented side by side. The anastomosis is performed with a 3-0 nonabsorbable, monofilament suture, and 5-0 sutures with felt pledgets are used as necessary for suture line bleeding. The body of the graft should be as short as possible, with the heel of the anastomosis essentially being the start of the inferior limb to the superior mesenteric artery. A short graft body is necessary because the distance between the aortic anastomosis and the celiac anastomosis is quite short. A limited endarterectomy of the aorta is occasionally necessary, but creating an aorta that is thin and will not hold sutures should be avoided. The proximal anastomosis can be challenging in large patients. Exposure of a large segment of aorta is helpful, as is the placement of retracting stay sutures in the aortotomy, parachuting the anastomosis or placing interrupted sutures.

DISTAL ANASTOMOSES

The anastomoses to the celiac artery and the superior mesenteric artery are performed in sequence. The cephalad limb of the graft is used for the celiac anastomosis, whereas the caudal limb is tunneled deep to the pancreas. Vascular control of the branches of the celiac artery is obtained with microvascular clamps or vessel loops, whereas proximal control of the celiac artery is obtained with a right-angled clamp. The celiac artery is transected, and the stump is oversewn with a 4-0 nonabsorbable, monofilament suture. The distal celiac artery is spatulated to account for any size discrepancy between the native artery and

DIRECT SURGICAL REPAIR FOR CELIAC AXIS AND SUPERIOR MESENTERIC ARTERY OCCLUSIVE DISEASE

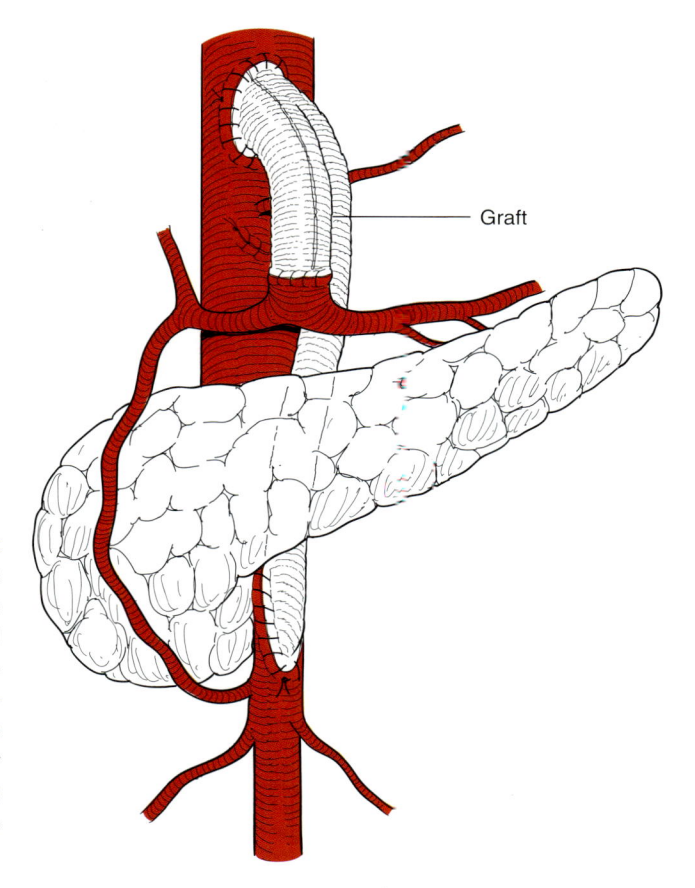

Figure 40-3. A completed antegrade bypass from the supraceliac aorta to the celiac axis and the superior mesenteric artery. The limbs of the graft are oriented on top of each other (anteroposterior) in contrast to the side-by-side configuration used for an aortobifemoral graft. The anastomosis to the celiac axis is performed in an end-to-end manner, whereas the distal anastomosis to the superior mesenteric artery is constructed using an end-to-side configuration. The body of the bifurcated graft is very short because of the proximity of the aorta and the celiac axis. The caudal limb of the graft forms the heel of the aortic anastomosis so that it can be tunneled deep to the pancreas.

graft, and the anastomosis performed using a 5-0 suture. The anastomosis to the superior mesenteric artery is configured in an end-to-side manner using a 5-0 suture. Upon completion of the anastomoses, the target arteries and their branches are interrogated with continuous wave Doppler to confirm adequacy of visceral perfusion.

CLOSURE

The retroperitoneal tissue over the superior mesenteric artery anastomosis is closed with interrupted 3-0 absorbable sutures, whereas the proximal aortic anastomosis is not covered. The bilateral subcostal or midline incision is then closed using standard technique.

Operative Technique for Retrograde Bypass

The principles and approaches outlined for antegrade bypass are relevant to retrograde aortosuperior mesenteric artery bypass (Fig. 40-4). However, several technical points merit further comment.

EXPOSURE OF THE AORTA OR COMMON ILIAC ARTERY

The proximal anastomosis can be positioned on the proximal right common iliac artery, the infrarenal aorta, or the proximal left common iliac artery. The preference is to position the heel of the graft on the distal aorta and the toe on the right common iliac artery. However, the choice is contingent on the anatomic course of the graft and the degree of atherosclerotic involvement in the vessels. The inflow vessels are exposed by incising the retroperitoneal tissue over the midinfrarenal aorta and extending the incision over the course of the designated common iliac artery. The inflow vessels are dissected to allow clamp application, and it is not necessary to circumferentially dissect the aorta or common iliac vessels. Although the proximal anastomosis is performed in an end-to-side fashion, it may not be possible to use a partial occluding vascular clamp.

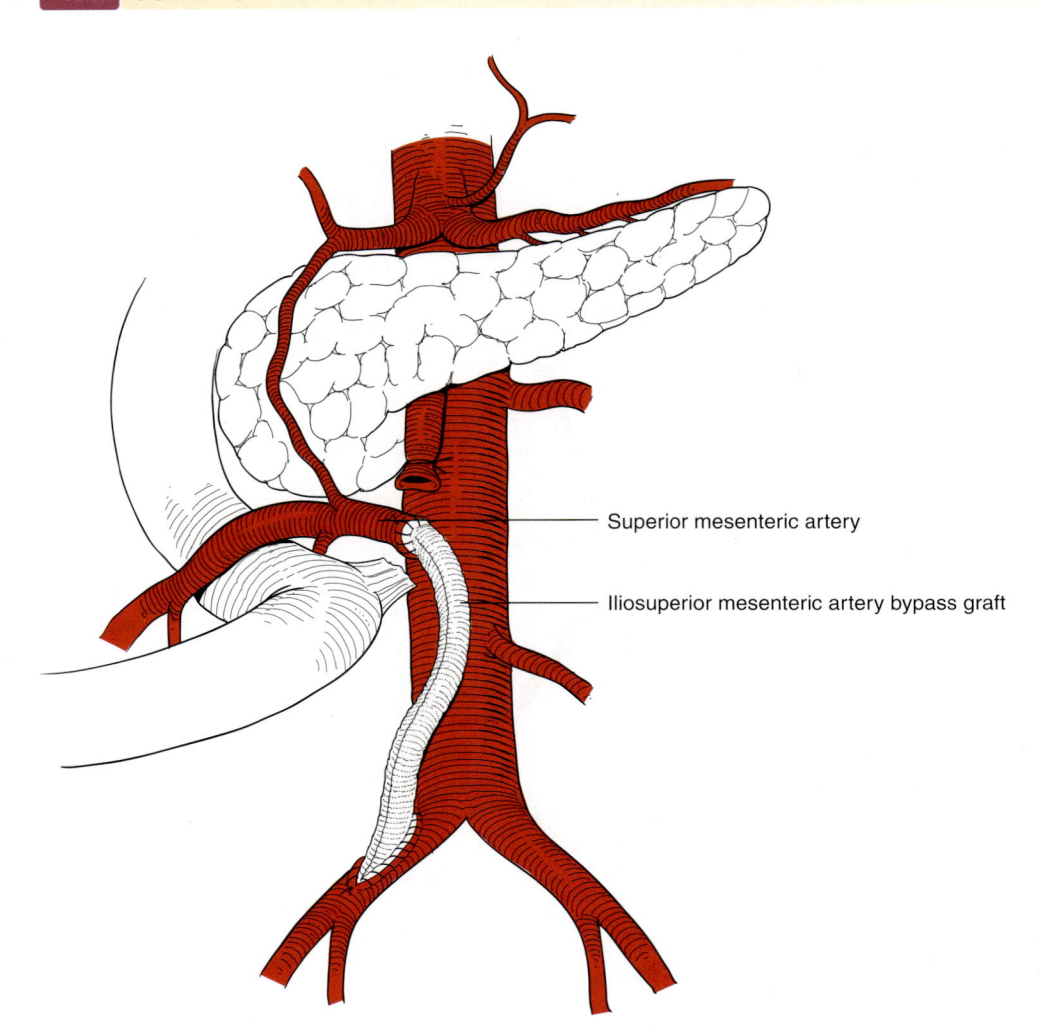

Figure 40-4. A completed retrograde bypass from the terminal aorta and proximal right common iliac artery to the superior mesenteric artery. The proximal anastomosis is performed in an end-to-side manner, whereas the distal anastomosis may be constructed in either an end-to-side or, as illustrated in this figure, in an end-to-end manner. The bypass graft should be positioned to take a gentle curve or C loop as it transitions posterior to anterior and caudal to cephalad.

EXPOSURE OF THE SUPERIOR MESENTERIC ARTERY

The superior mesenteric artery is exposed by incising the ligament of Treitz and the other peritoneal attachments and then retracting the duodenum to the patient's right side (see Fig. 40-1, C). As the base of the mesentery is dissected laterally from left to right, the superior mesenteric artery is the first structure to be encountered and is a sizable vessel.

TUNNELING THE BYPASS GRAFT AND ANASTOMOSES

Either a 6- or a 7-mm-diameter Dacron graft is a suitable conduit, although a comparable externally supported ePTFE graft is a reasonable alternative to minimize the risk of kinking. The proximal anastomosis is usually performed first, although some surgeons have proposed the opposite to simplify the process of tunneling the graft and to obtain the optimal configuration. The distal anastomosis can be performed in either an end-to-end or end-to-side fashion, but the anatomic course of the graft may be more favorable if distal anastomosis is performed in an end-to-end manner. The graft should be tunneled so that it forms a gentle curve or C loop between the two anastomoses as it traverses caudal to cephalad and posterior to anterior. It is imperative that the graft does not kink and that the anastomoses are tension free.

CLOSURE

The retroperitoneal tissue over the aorta, the ligament of Treitz, and the peritoneum over the superior mesenteric artery are reapproximated to exclude the graft from contact with the intestine. In addition, a segment of the omentum can be mobilized to cover the graft.

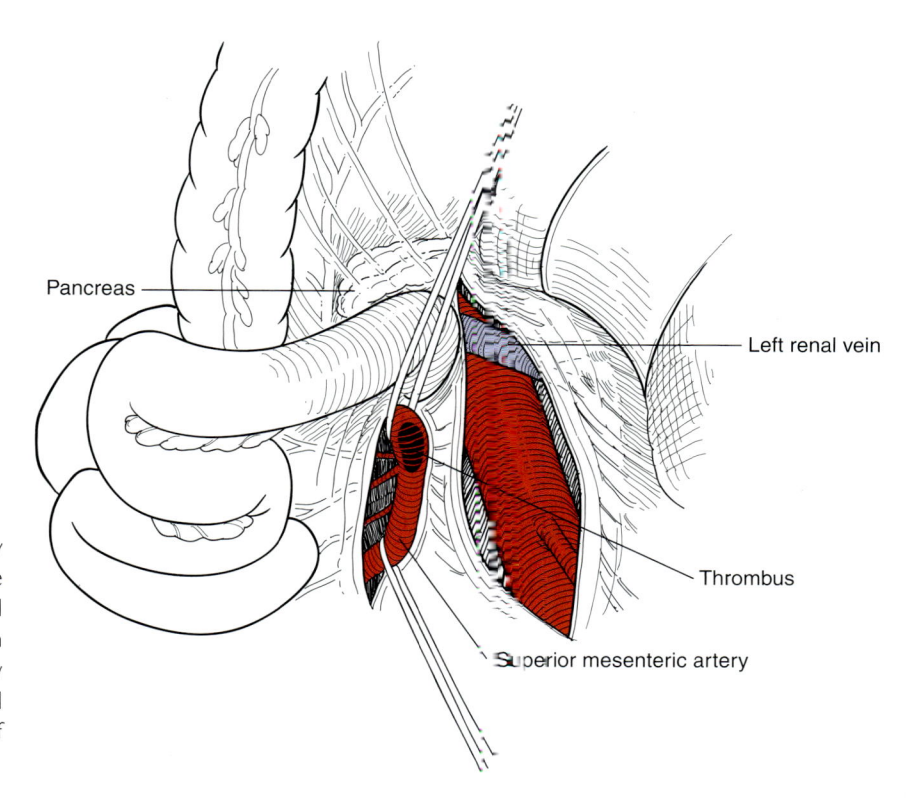

DIRECT SURGICAL REPAIR FOR CELIAC AXIS AND SUPERIOR MESENTERIC ARTERY OCCLUSIVE DISEASE

Figure 40-5. The superior mesenteric artery has been exposed by elevating the transverse colon cephalad and displacing the small bowel to the patient's right. The visceral peritoneum overlying the superior mesenteric artery below the third portion of the duodenum is incised to expose the vessel for thrombectomy or, if required, bypass.

Operative Technique for Superior Mesenteric Artery Embolectomy

Antegrade and retrograde bypass principles and approaches are pertinent to superior mesenteric artery embolectomy (Fig. 40-5). In addition, a few technical points require explanation.

EMBOLECTOMY

The diagnosis of acute mesenteric ischemia from an embolus is usually confirmed by the distribution of the ischemic or infarcted bowel that extends from the proximal jejunum to the transverse colon. Although a palpable pulse or Doppler signal in the superior mesenteric artery may be noted, clinical suspicion warrants exploration of the vessel. It is possible to be misled by a water hammer pulse above the level of occlusion, and a Doppler signal does not exclude the presence of a thrombus or embolus. The embolus may be extracted from the superior mesenteric artery using a Fogarty embolectomy catheter. The simplest approach to the superior mesenteric artery is through the base of the transverse mesocolon (see Fig. 40-1 B). The transverse mesocolon should be retracted superiorly and the small bowel displaced inferiorly, and a horizontal incision made at the base of the mesocolon. Alternatively, the small bowel can be retracted to the patient's right and the peritoneum incised over the superior mesenteric artery just below the inferior margin of the duodenum (see Fig. 40-5). The arteriotomy in the superior mesenteric artery may be performed either longitudinally or horizontally. Although the longitudinal arteriotomy may need to be closed with a saphenous vein patch to prevent narrowing the lumen, it affords greater flexibility if a bypass is required. Notably, it can be difficult to differentiate acute mesenteric ischemia secondary to an embolus from that secondary to in situ thrombus. If a horizontal arteriotomy was initially performed and an anastomosis required, a vertical arteriotomy can be created. The horizontal extensions can then be approximated with a running 5-0 polypropylene incision prior to performing the anastomosis.

MESENTERIC INFARCTION

Revascularization should precede bowel resection with the exception of obviously necrotic bowel. It is impressive how marginally appearing bowel improves after revascularization. Furthermore, there is little downside to deferring bowel resection until after revascularization unless there is gross spillage of enteric contents. Differentiating viable from nonviable bowel may be challenging. Simple adjuncts include visual inspection for peristalsis, use of continuous wave Doppler to detect arterial signals within the mesentery, and intravenous fluorescein in combination with a Wood's lamp. A second-look operation 24 to 48 hours after the index procedure can be helpful to further assess the viability of the bowel, and the decision to perform this second procedure should be made at the time of the original operation. The construction of abdominal wall stomas is preferred over a primary anastomosis with marginal-appearing bowel. Admittedly, this commits patients to an additional procedure to restore intestinal continuity. However, the viability of the stoma and the bowel can be assessed at the bedside, and the potential for disruption of an intestinal anastomosis can be avoided. Indeed, breakdown of a bowel anastomosis is potentially catastrophic, because diagnosis can be delayed or confounded by multiple organ dysfunction, which is a common sequela of ischemia-reperfusion injury. Revascularization should be performed using an autogenous conduit in the presence of dead bowel.

Postoperative Care

- The immediate postoperative course for patients undergoing open revascularization for both acute and chronic mesenteric ischemia is frequently complicated by the development of multiple organ dysfunction, which likely accounts for prolonged hospitalization, and is a leading cause of death.[18,19] The optimal management strategy is to support the individual organ systems until dysfunction resolves.
- Patients may be extubated in the early postoperative period when they satisfy the standard weaning criteria.
- Thrombocytopenia and coagulopathy are managed with platelets, plasma, or both. Harward and colleagues[18] emphasize that coagulopathy after mesenteric revascularization is not responsive to vitamin K.
- Patients should be maintained on total parenteral nutrition throughout the postoperative period until their bowel function returns. A prolonged ileus is common.
- The bypass should be interrogated with either a mesenteric duplex or a CT angiogram before discharge. Any change in clinical status should prompt imaging to confirm that bypasses are patent.
- Patients should be seen frequently in the early postoperative period until all active issues resolve and at 6-month intervals thereafter for a mesenteric duplex examination. Recurrent symptoms merit evaluation with duplex ultrasound or a CT angiogram.

Complications

- **Morbidity and mortality from acute mesenteric ischemia.** The mortality rate for patients with acute mesenteric ischemia is approximately 70%, which has changed little over the past several decades.[20] A recent systematic review by Schoots and associates[21] reported that the mortality rate after an acute mesenteric embolus was lower than after an in situ thrombosus. Aggregate mortality rates included embolus (54%), nonocclusive mesenteric ischemia (74%), and in situ thrombosis (77%). Factors associated with mortality include, age, time to definitive surgery, shock, acidosis, leukocytosis, cardiac status, and coagulopathy.[22,23]

- **Morbidity and mortality from chronic mesenteric ischemia.** The corresponding aggregate morbidity and mortality rates after open revascularization for treatment of chronic mesenteric ischemia are approximately 30% and 8%, respectively,[19,24,25] with 45% complication and 15% mortality rates reported for a large population-based analysis.[26] Mateo and colleagues[27] observed that mortality and complication rates after open repair were increased by simultaneous aortic reconstruction, complete revascularization, and the presence of preoperative renal insufficiency.

- **Postoperative diarrhea.** Diarrhea is a common complaint after open revascularization and can persist for several months. It is more common in patients with preoperative diarrhea and can necessitate total parenteral nutrition. Jimenez and colleagues[19] reported that 33% of the patients in their series experienced significant postoperative diarrhea, which persisted for more than 6 months in 24%. Kihara and associates[15] reported that patients had almost two stools daily (1.9 ± 0.4) after revascularization for chronic mesenteric ischemia. The etiology of diarrhea may be related to intestinal atrophy, bacterial overgrowth, or disruption of the mesenteric neuroplexus.

- **Durability of revascularization.** Open revascularization for chronic mesenteric ischemia provides durable relief of symptoms. Jimenez and colleagues[19] noted a gain of 103% of ideal body weight at 6 months. The 5-year primary patency ranged from 57% to 92%, with the corresponding primary assisted patency ranging from 89% to 96%.[19,24,28,29] Survival approached 75% at 5 years after open revascularization for chronic mesenteric ischemia.[19,24,28-30]

REFERENCES

1. Wilson GSM, Block J: Mesenteric vascular occlusion, *Arch Surg* 73:330-345, 1956.
2. Klass AA: Embolectomy in acute mesenteric occlusion, *Ann Surg* 134:913-917, 1951.
3. Shaw RS, Rutledge RH: Superior mesenteric-artery embolectomy in treatment of massive mesenteric infarction, *NEJM* 257:595-598, 1957.
4. Miller HI, DiMare SI: Mesenteric infarction: Report of a case of superior-mesenteric-artery embolectomy and small-bowel resection, with recovery, *NEJM* 259:512-515, 1958.
5. Klein E: Embolism and thrombosis of superior mesenteric artery, *Surg Gynec Obstet* 33:385-405, 1921.
6. Mikkelsen WP: Intestinal angina: Its surgical significance, *Am J Surg* 94:262-269, 1957.
7. Shaw RS, Maynard EP III: Acute and chronic thrombosis of mesenteric arteries associated with malabsorption: Report of two cases successfully treated by thromboendarterectomy, *NEJM* 258:874-878, 1958.
8. Morris GC Jr, DeBakey ME: Abdominal angina: Diagnosis and surgical treatment, *JAMA* 176:89-92, 1961.
9. Morris GC, Crawford ES, Cooley DA, et al: Revascularization of the celiac and superior mesenteric arteries, *Arch Surg* 84:95-107, 1962.
10. Mavor GE, Lyall AD: Superior mesenteric-artery stenosis treated by iliac-mesenteric arterial bypass, *Lancet* 7266:1143-1146, 1962.
11. Thomas JH, Blake K, Pierce GE, et al: The clinical course of asymptomatic mesenteric arterial stenosis, *J Vasc Surg* 27:840-844, 1998.
12. Kaleya RN, Sammartano RJ, Boley SJ: Aggressive approach to acute mesenteric ischemia, *Surg Clin North Am* 72:157-182, 1992.
13. Takayama T, Miyata T, Shirakawa M, et al: Isolated spontaneous dissection of the splanchnic arteries, *J Vasc Surg* 48:329-333, 2008.
14. Hollier LH, Bernatz PE, Pairolero PC, et al: Surgical management of chronic intestinal ischemia: A reappraisal, *Surgery* 90:940-946, 1981.
15. Kihara TK, Blebea J, Anderson KM, et al: Risk factors and outcomes following revascularization for chronic mesenteric ischemia, *Ann Vasc Surg* 13:37-44, 1999.
16. Modrall JG, Sadjadi J, Joiner DR, et al: Comparison of superficial femoral vein and saphenous vein as conduits for mesenteric arterial bypass, *J Vasc Surg* 37:362-366, 2003.
17. Hertzberg BS, Kliewer MA, DeLong DM, et al: Sonographic assessment of lower limb vein diameters: Implications for the diagnosis and characterization of deep venous thrombosis, *AJR Am J Roentgenol* 168:1253-1257, 1997.
18. Harward TR, Brooks DL, Flynn TC, et al: Multiple organ dysfunction after mesenteric artery revascularization, *J Vasc Surg* 18:459-467, 1993.
19. Jimenez JG, Huber TS, Ozaki CK, et al: Durability of antegrade synthetic aortomesenteric bypass for chronic mesenteric ischemia, *J Vasc Surg* 35:1078-1084, 2002.

20. Moore EM, Endean EC: Treatment of acute intestinal ischemia caused by arterial occlusions. In Rutherford RB, editor: *Vascular Surgery*, ed 6, Philadelphia, 2005, Saunders, pp 1718-1727.
21. Schoots IG, Koffeman GI, Legemate DA, et al: Systematic review of survival after acute mesenteric ischaemia according to disease aetiology, *Br J Surg* 91:17-27, 2004.
22. Costa-Merida MA, Marchena-Gomez J, Hemmersbach-Miller M, et al: Identification of risk factors for perioperative mortality in acute mesenteric ischemia, *World J Surg* 30:1579-1585, 2006.
23. Yasuhara H, Niwa H, Takenoue T, et al: Factors influencing mortality of acute intestinal infarction associated with SIRS, *Hepatogastroenterology* 52:1474-1478, 2005.
24. Atkins MD, Kwolek CJ, LaMuraglia GM, et al: Surgical revascularization versus endovascular therapy for chronic mesenteric ischemia: A comparative experience, *J Vasc Surg* 45:1162-1171, 2007.
25. Park WM, Cherry KJ II, Chua HK, et al: Current results of open revascularization for chronic mesenteric ischemia: A standard for comparison, *J Vasc Surg* 35:853-859, 2002.
26. Derrow AE, Seeger JM, Dame DA, et al: The outcome in the United States after thoracoabdominal aortic aneurysm repair, renal artery bypass, and mesenteric revascularization, *J Vasc Surg* 34:54-61, 2001.
27. Mateo RB, O'Hara PJ, Hertzer NR, et al: Elective surgical treatment of symptomatic chronic mesenteric occlusive disease: Early results and late outcomes, *J Vasc Surg* 29:821-831, 1999.
28. Cho JS, Carr JA, Jacobsen G, et al: Long-term outcome after mesenteric artery reconstruction: A 37-year experience, *J Vasc Surg* 35:453-460, 2002.
29. Kruger AJ, Walker PJ, Foster WJ, et al: Open surgery for atherosclerotic chronic mesenteric ischemia, *J Vasc Surg* 46:941-945, 2007.
30. Norgren L, Hiatt WR, Dormandy JA, et al: Inter-society consensus for the management of peripheral arterial disease (TASC II), *J Vasc Surg* 45:S5-S67, 2007.

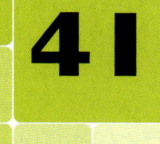

41 Endovascular Treatment of Occlusive Superior Mesenteric Artery Disease

ARASH BORNAK • ROSS MILNER

Historical Background

Traditionally, the preferred treatment to restore adequate blood flow to the visceral organs was open surgical bypass. This treatment resulted in significant morbidity and mortality rates, ranging from 12% to 33% and 2% to 15%, respectively.[1-4] In 1980 Furrer and colleagues[5] were the first to report a successful angioplasty of a superior mesenteric artery stenosis. The role of percutaneous mesenteric revascularization has since expanded and in most circumstances has become the initial treatment of choice for chronic superior mesenteric artery occlusive disease. A recent examination of a nationwide database in the period between 2000 and 2006 that included 5583 chronic mesenteric ischemia patients estimated that 69% of patients with chronic mesenteric ischemia were treated by percutaneous transluminal angioplasty with or without stent placement (PTA/S).[6] Despite a higher proportion of elderly patients with medical comorbidities undergoing PTA/S, mortality and morbidity rates were 3.7% and 20%, respectively, compared with 13% and 38%, respectively, after surgical bypass. Admittedly, endovascular treatment is associated with lower long-term patency and a greater likelihood of repeat interventions.

Indications

Chronic mesenteric ischemia is usually related to atherosclerosis, with symptoms occurring over a period of weeks to months. Postprandial intestinal angina appears when perfusion of visceral organs fails to meet normal metabolic requirements. A dull, colicky pain typically starts within 15 to 30 minutes of food intake and can persist 5 to 6 hours. The abdominal pain is commonly misdiagnosed as another gastrointestinal disorder.

Food phobia results in malnourishment, with an average weight loss of 20 to 30 pounds.[7] In addition, stenotic arteries harbor a risk of atherosclerotic plaque rupture and focal thrombosis or embolization, which can result in acute mesenteric ischemia and bowel infarction. One third of patients with multiple mesenteric vessel involvement and symptoms may progress to acute mesenteric ischemia and intestinal infarction, with a mortality rate of more than 50%.[8-10] Nonatherosclerotic causes of chronic mesenteric ischemia include radiation arteritis, chronic aortic dissection, fibromuscular dysplasia, median arcuate ligament syndrome, or vasculitis, such as Takayasu disease, Buerger disease, and polyarteritis nodosum. Most symptomatic patients have an atherosclerotic occlusion or more than 70% stenosis of the superior mesenteric artery combined with occlusion or stenosis of at least one other mesenteric vessel. Symptomatic mesenteric artery stenosis is an indication for intervention. Endovascular therapy is the preferred initial approach in patients with chronic mesenteric ischemia, whereas open revascularization is reserved for early or late failures.[11] In principle, PTA/S also allows correction of malnourishment should subsequent open revascularization be required.[12]

The presence of an asymptomatic mesenteric artery stenosis is not automatically associated with subsequent acute or chronic mesenteric ischemia and is a frequent finding among elderly patients. Asymptomatic disease of the celiac axis or superior mesenteric artery may be safely observed, and prophylactic intervention is not warranted.[13] However, in certain circumstances, a symptomatic patients with significant three-vessel disease may benefit from revascularization, particularly if aortic or colonic resection is planned. That type of surgery can compromise the collateral vascular network and result in acute mesenteric ischemia.[14]

Preoperative Preparation

- Patients experiencing postprandial pain and weight loss should have an extensive diagnostic workup to rule out other gastrointestinal disorders, including hepatobiliary disease and gastric, colonic, or pancreatic malignancy.

- The initial diagnostic study to evaluate for the presence of chronic mesenteric ischemia is a duplex flow study of the superior mesenteric artery (Fig. 41-1). It is noninvasive and usually easy to perform because patients are often thin; however, bowel gas and arterial calcifications may limit accurate determination of flow velocity.

- If the symptom complex and duplex findings are consistent with chronic mesenteric ischemia, an angiogram and intervention can be offered. Preoperative computed tomography (CT) angiography imaging can be obtained for procedure planning but is not mandatory (Figs. 41-2 and 41-3). Major collateral pathways exist between the celiac artery and the superior mesenteric artery through the gastroduodenal and pancreaticoduodenal arcade, between the superior and inferior mesenteric arteries through the meandering artery and the marginal artery of Drummond, and between the inferior mesenteric artery and the hypogastric arteries through the hemmorrhoidal arteries (Fig. 41-4). Patients with severe three-vessel disease often display increased lumbar, phrenic, and pelvic collaterals. Whereas lateral angiography can reveal the degree of stenosis, anteroposterior views are necessary to assess the collateral pathways.

- If symptoms or mesenteric duplex imaging are equivocal, additional imaging should be obtained. CT angiography has very high sensitivity and specificity for mesenteric stenosis and can detect other intraabdominal pathologies. Moreover, CT angiography allows the surgeon to assess the angulation of the mesenteric artery in relation to the aorta, multifocal arterial stenosis, thrombus, and collateral pathways, as well as tortuosity, stenosis, or aneurysmal disease in the aorta or iliac arteries. All of this helps in procedural planning. When the diagnosis of chronic mesenteric ischemia is in question, such as in the case of single-vessel disease, gastric and jejunal exercise tonometry has been reported as an aid in diagnosis.[15] Such studies are available in only a minority of centers.

- When providing consent, patients should be made aware that percutaneous mesenteric revascularization carries a risk of acute bowel ischemia because of distal embolization or arterial dissection. The operator should be prepared for an emergent open procedure if either of these problems occurs and cannot be corrected.

- Risk factor modification, such as smoking cessation, should be encouraged. Antiplatelet therapy with aspirin or clopidogrel should be initiated, and patients should begin statin therapy.[16] Nutritional status should be assessed and improved.

- Laboratory workup should include albumin, prealbumin, vitamin B_{12}, folate, coagulation parameters, a complete blood cell count, and serum creatinine. If a patient is on metformin, it should be discontinued the day of procedure and restarted 48 hours after contrast infusion if the glomerular filtration rate has not deteriorated. Preprocedural antibiotics are recommended.

ENDOVASCULAR TREATMENT OF OCCLUSIVE SUPERIOR MESENTERIC ARTERY DISEASE

Pitfalls and Danger Points

- **Identification and access.** Most patients with mesenteric occlusive disease, symptomatic or not, have stenosis or short-segment (2 cm) occlusions at or within the first few centimeters of the origin of the mesenteric vessels. Lesions are frequently associated with aortic atherosclerosis and atheroma, with an attendant risk of embolization during percutaneous revascularization. If occluded, the ostium of the artery may not be easily identified and gaining access to the vessel may be difficult,

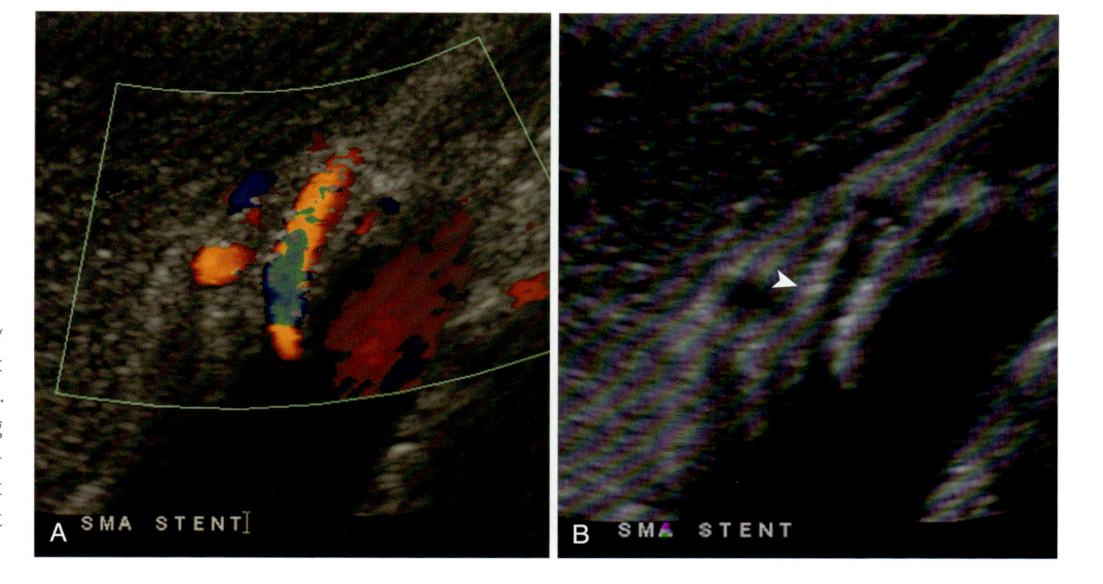

Figure 41-1. Duplex flow study of the superior mesenteric artery after stent placement. **A,** Color flow duplex imaging of the stent. **B,** B-mode imaging of the superior mesenteric artery (*arrowhead*) after stent placement.

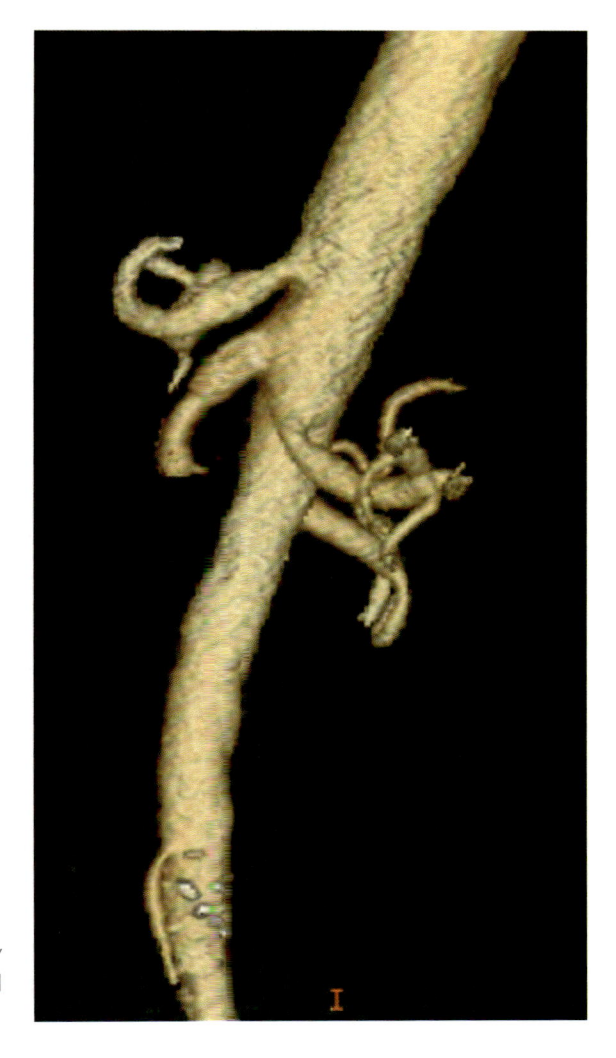

Figure 41-2. Computed tomography angiogram demonstrating patency of the proximal portions of the celiac artery, superior mesenteric artery, and inferior mesenteric artery.

particularly if an occluded celiac artery precludes retrograde filling of the superior mesenteric artery (Fig. 41-5).

- **Excessive manipulation.** Excessive endovascular manipulation can result in arterial dissection, perforation, or embolization. Ideally, a short stump of the patent artery is necessary to gain wire access. At least one report has suggested that endovascular treatment of short-segment occlusions and stenoses are associated with comparable patency rates.[17]

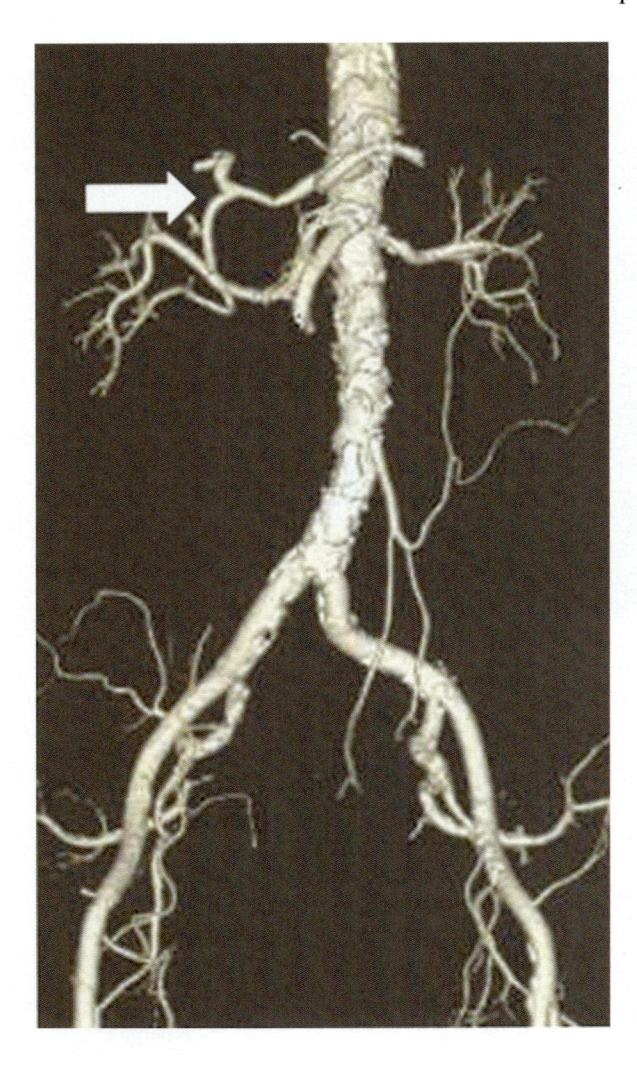

Figure 41-3. CT angiogram demonstrating patency of the celiac artery, superior mesenteric artery, and inferior mesenteric artery, as well as a large gastroduodenal collateral artery (arrow).

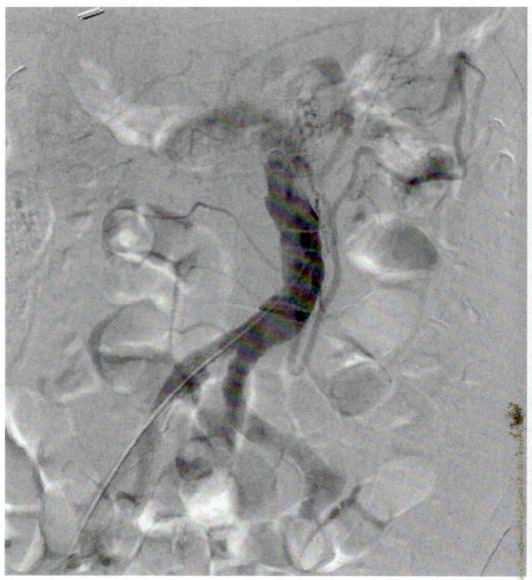

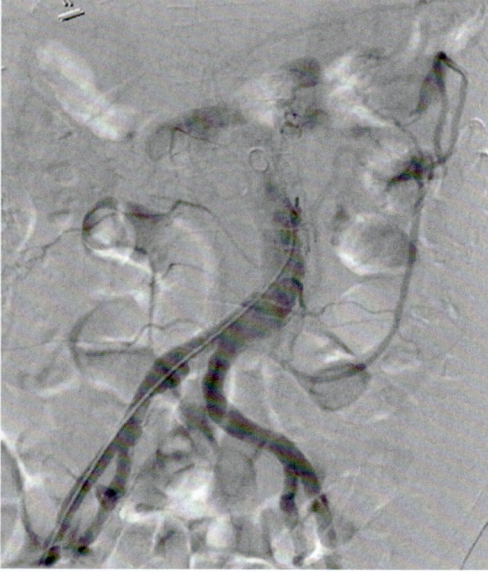

Figure 41-4. Angiographic images demonstrating a large meandering collateral artery providing arterial blood supply from the inferior mesenteric artery to the superior mesenteric artery.

- **Calcification.** Severely calcified or long lesions and small-diameter mesenteric arteries are also associated with an increased risk of distal embolization and restenosis. An embolic protection device may be considered in the presence of a large thrombus burden.

Endovascular Strategy

There is no evidence that treatment of both the celiac artery and the superior mesenteric artery yields improved outcomes when compared with treatment of the superior mesenteric artery alone.[18,19] Recanalization of the celiac artery is performed if superior mesenteric artery intervention is too risky or fails or if symptoms do not improve.

A severe stenosis should be predilated with a 1.5- to 2.5-mm angioplasty balloon to facilitate placement of a larger-profile balloon and stent. If the lesion cannot be crossed directly, retrograde revascularization may be considered if a large collateral vessel is present.[20] In highly calcified, thrombotic, occlusive, or dissected lesions, primary stenting is favored.

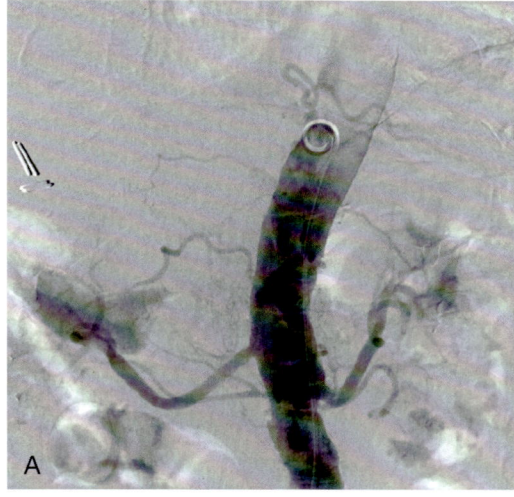

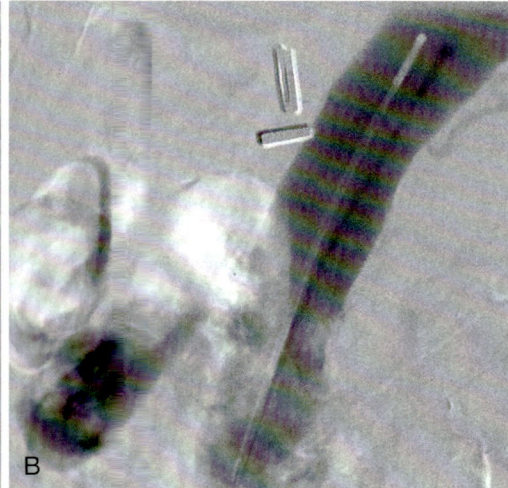

Figure 41-5. Neither the celiac artery nor the superior mesenteric artery is visualized on anteroposterior (**A**) or lateral aortograms (**B**).

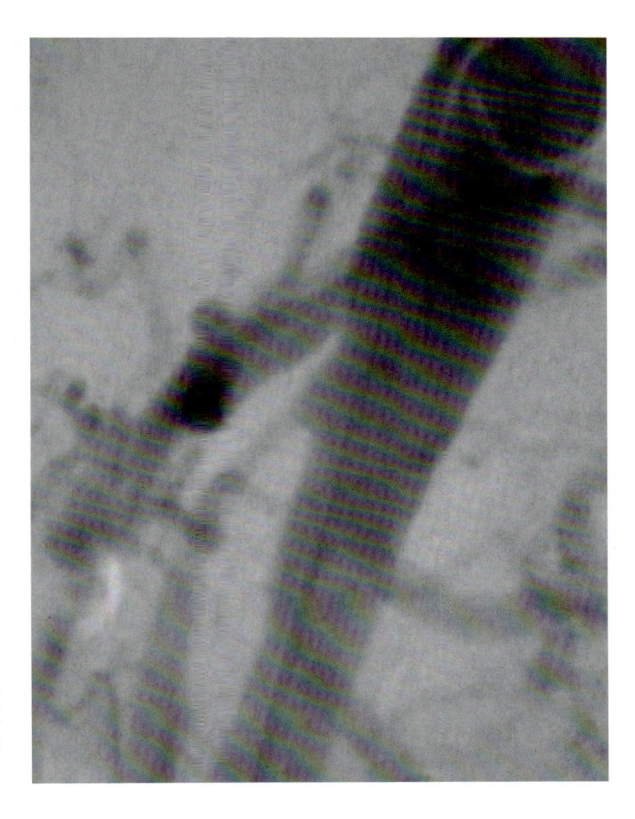

Figure 41-6. Lateral aortogram demonstrating the superior mesenteric artery after treatment with a covered stent (6 × 22 mm iCast). Recurrent in-stent stenosis was noted 6 months after initial treatment using a bare metal stent.

Balloon-expandable bare metal or covered stents (iCast, Atrium Medical, Lebanon, N.H.) are preferred to treat ostial lesions (Figs. 41-6 through 41-8). Self-expandable stents should be considered for longer lesions within the more distal portion of the vessel. The role of embolic protection devices is not well defined but may be of value if preprocedural imaging demonstrates thrombus.

Endovascular Technique

In most cases access to the superior mesenteric artery can be gained through a retrograde femoral approach. Antegrade left brachial artery access is favored for an acutely angulated mesenteric artery, an excessively narrow or tortuous distal aorta or iliac arteries, or occlusive and long segment lesions of the visceral vessels (Figs. 41-7 and 41-8). Some studies have reported more frequent stent dislodgement[21] and mortality[22] through a femoral approach because of greater catheter manipulation.

A 5-Fr introducer sheath is first placed in the access artery, and a pigtail catheter is used to perform an aortogram. A lateral view demonstrates the origins of the celiac artery and the superior mesenteric artery and the presence and extent of stenosis. Anteroposterior views are used to assess the collateral circulation, as well as the origin of the inferior mesenteric artery. Selective magnified views complete the initial angiogram.

If endovascular treatment is selected, the 5-Fr sheath is exchanged for a long guiding 6-Fr sheath to allow better support and pushability to catheterize and cross the lesion. A brachial artery cutdown can be performed if a larger sheath is required to prevent access site complications. Systemic heparin (80-100 units per kilogram of body weight) is given, and an activated clotting time greater than 240 sec is maintained during the procedure. From a femoral approach the target vessel may be accessed using a hydrophilic 0.035-inch angled wire and a preshaped catheter such as a Cobra 2 or Sos II. At times a simple angled glide catheter will suffice. If the lesion is difficult to cross, 0.018- or 0.014-inch wires should be considered. After the wire placement has crossed the lesion, the catheter is advanced beyond the lesion and its position within the lumen is confirmed by an angiogram performed through the catheter. The extent of the lesion is assessed, and distal embolization and arterial dissection are excluded.

When the severity of stenosis is uncertain, a mean pressure gradient can be measured across the lesion to confirm a hemodynamically significant lesion (>10 mm Hg). If the lesion is occlusive or nearly occlusive, predilation should be performed with a 1.5- to 2.5-mm coronary balloon. In severely calcified or eccentric lesions with thrombus, a distal embolic protection device can be deployed.

A stiff wire, such as an Amplatz wire (Cook Medical, Bloomington, Ind.) is then placed across the lesion to track larger balloons or stents. Severely calcified, eccentric, occlusive, or dissected lesions are primarily stented. Ostial lesions should be stented using a balloon-expandable stent (5- to 7-mm diameter) with 1 to 2 mm extending into the aorta. A simple angioplasty can be performed on straightforward atherosclerotic lesions, and a stent can be placed for residual stenosis (>30%) or a residual pressure gradient.

Completion angiography in lateral and anteroposterior views is performed. Occasionally, because of wire or catheter manipulation, vasospasm may be present, and selective intraarterial infusion of nitroglycerin (200 mcg) or papaverine (30 mg) is used to reverse the spasm. The presence of dissection or embolization is also assessed, and if present, an attempt to retrieve the embolic particles can be made using a suction export catheter. If unsuccessful, focal thrombolytic therapy should be pursued. Emergent open revascularization should be pursued if ischemic bowel is suspected. Delay in treatment results in propagation of a clot and progressive intestinal infarction. Vessel rupture can also occur, particularly if the vessel is severely calcified. A covered stent, such as the iCast, can be used to seal the rupture site. Dislodged or fractured stents should be removed using a snare or grasping forceps, followed by an angiogram to rule out traumatic vessel dissection or perforation.

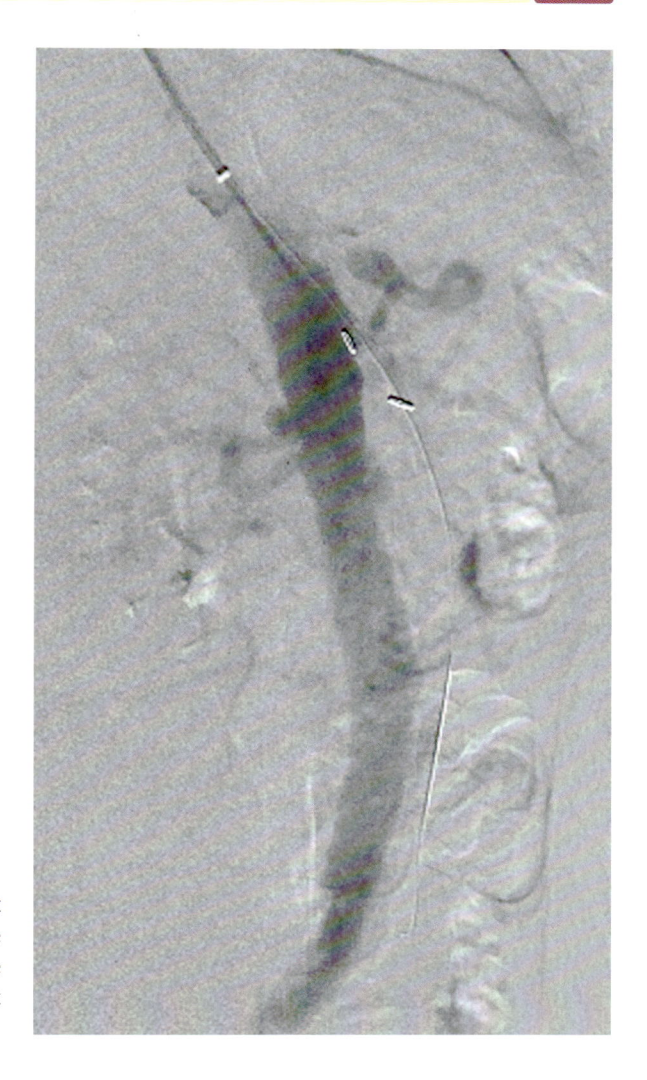

Figure 41-7. Left brachial artery approach to the superior mesenteric artery. A 6-Fr sheath has been placed in the abdominal aorta, and a wire has been passed into the superior mesenteric artery. Because of the severe stenosis, there is poor visualization of the superior mesenteric artery.

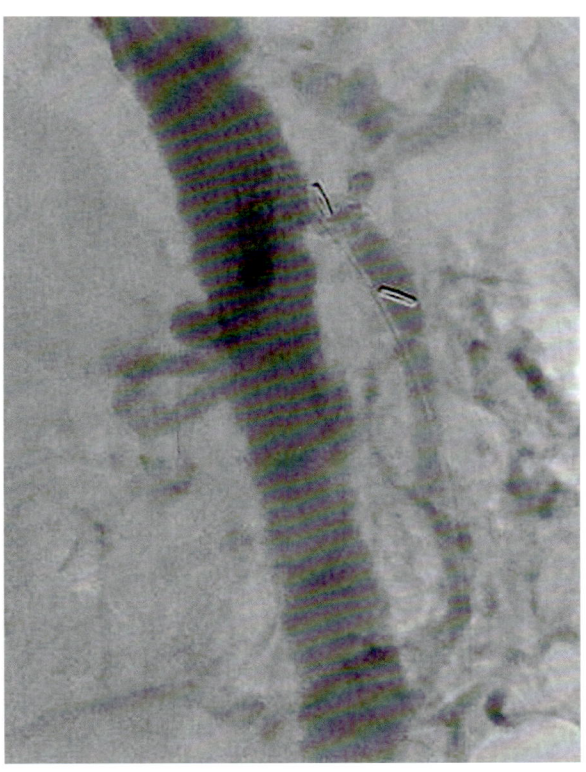

Figure 41-8. Successful treatment of an occlusive lesion of the superior mesenteric artery by primary stenting. The stent protrudes slightly into the abdominal aorta, which is the desired location.

Postoperative Care

- Procedure-related complications range from 0% to 29%.[23] Therefore all patients should be admitted for 24-hour observation and hydration after angioplasty and stenting of the superior mesenteric or celiac artery.
- Clopidogrel should be initiated at an oral loading dose of 300 mg and continued at 75 mg daily for 1 month. Daily aspirin (81 or 325 mg) should be initiated and continued indefinitely.
- Complaint of abdominal pain or tenderness should be assessed with duplex or computed tomography imaging.
- Urine output and creatinine should be monitored, because renal embolization can occur during the procedure.
- Patients can be fed the day after the procedure.
- A baseline duplex of the treated vessel should be obtained before discharge, every 6 months for 1 year, and annually thereafter.

Complications

- **Morbidity and mortality.** Over the last 10 years, numerous reports have documented excellent technical results (82%-100%) with low morbidity and 30-day mortality rates of less than 5%.[23]
- **Access site complications.** Most common early complications are related to the access site, including a hematoma or pseudoaneurysm, brachial sheath hematoma, access artery thrombosis, or retroperitoneal hematoma. A recent report of local complications of percutaneous brachial access noted a local complication rate of 6.5%, although complications occurred more frequently in females (11.5% vs 2.7%).[24,25] Aspirin lowered the risk, whereas oral anticoagulation was associated with an increased risk of hematoma.
- **Embolization.** Wire and catheter manipulation during the procedure can result in particle embolization into the renal arteries or lower extremities, and splenic infarction has been reported after celiac artery intervention.[26]
- **Acute superior mesenteric artery thrombosis.** Early complications can result in acute mesenteric ischemia, including symptomatic thrombotic occlusion because of unrecognized arterial dissection or arterial injury and stent thrombosis.[27] Reperfusion hemorrhage is rare.[28]
- **Long-term patency.** Cumulative patency over 3 years is reported between 44% and 88%. Sarac and associates reported a 1-year patency, a primary assisted patency, and a secondary patency of 65%, 97%, and 99%, respectively.[22] Atkins and colleagues reported a primary patency of 58% and a primary assisted patency of 65% at 1 year.[29] The most recent report of midterm patency notes a 3-year primary patency of 57% and a secondary patency of 92%.[24]
- **Recurrent stenosis.** Patients with recurrent stenosis may be treated with repeat angioplasty and stenting. The use of cutting balloons has not been shown to be superior in the treatment of restenosis. Although longitudinal follow-up is necessary, the use of covered stents provides an alternate treatment strategy (see Fig. 41-6).

REFERENCES

1. Kruger AJ, Walker PJ, Foster WJ, et al: Open surgery for atherosclerotic chronic mesenteric ischemia, *J Vasc Surg* 46:941-945, 2007.
2. Mateo RB, O'Hara PJ, Hertzer NR, et al: Elective surgical treatment of symptomatic chronic mesenteric occlusive disease: Early results and late outcomes, *J Vasc Surg* 29:821-831, 1999.
3. Park WM, Cherry KJ II, Chua HK, et al: Current results of open revascularization for chronic mesenteric ischemia: A standard for comparison, *J Vasc Surg* 35:853-859, 2002.

4. Kasirajan K, O'Hara PJ, Gray BH, et al: Chronic mesenteric ischemia: Open surgery versus percutaneous angioplasty and stenting, *J Vasc Surg* 33:63-71, 2001.
5. Furrer J, Grüntzig A, Kugelmeier J, et al: Treatment of abdominal angina with percutaneous dilatation of an arteria mesenterica superior stenosis: Preliminary communication, *Cardiovasc Intervent Radiol* 3:43-44, 1980.
6. Schermerhorn ML, Giles KA, Hamdan AD, et al: Mesenteric revascularization: Management and outcomes in the United States, 1988-2006, *J Vasc Surg* 50:341-348, 2009.
7. Johnston KW, Lindsay TF, Walker PM, et al: Mesenteric arterial bypass grafts: Early and late results and suggested surgical approach for chronic and acute mesenteric ischemia, *Surgery* 118:1-7, 1995.
8. Kolkman JJ, Mensink PB, van Petersen AS, et al: Clinical approach to chronic gastrointestinal ischaemia: From "intestinal angina" to the spectrum of chronic splanchnic disease, *Scand J Gastroenterol Suppl.* 241:9-16, 2004.
9. Cho JS, Carr JA, Jacobsen G, et al: Long-term outcome after mesenteric artery reconstruction: A 37-year experience, *J Vasc Surg* 35:453-460, 2002.
10. Kougias P, Lau D, El Sayed HF, et al: Determinants of mortality and treatment outcome following surgical interventions for acute mesenteric ischemia, *J Vasc Surg* 46:467-474, 2007.
11. Fioole B, van de Rest HJ, Meijer JR, et al: Percutaneous transluminal angioplasty and stenting as first-choice treatment in patients with chronic mesenteric ischemia, *J Vasc Surg* 51:386-391, 2010.
12. Biebl M, Oldenburg WA, Paz-Fumagalli R, et al: Endovascular treatment as a bridge to successful surgical revascularization for chronic mesenteric ischemia, *Am Surg* 70:994-998, 2004.
13. Wilson DB, Mostafavi K, Craven TE, et al: Clinical course of mesenteric artery stenosis in elderly Americans, *Arch Intern Med* 166:2095-2100, 2006.
14. Thomas JH, Blake K, Pierce GE, et al: The clinical course of asymptomatic mesenteric arterial stenosis, *J Vasc Surg* 27:840-844, 1998.
15. Otte JA, Huisman AB, Geelkerken RH, et al: Jejunal tonometry for the diagnosis of gastrointestinal ischemia: Feasibility, normal values and comparison of jejunal with gastric tonometry exercise testing, *Eur J Gastroenterol Hepatol* 20:62-67, 2008.
16. Perler BA: The effect of statin medications on perioperative and long-term outcomes following carotid endarterectomy or stenting, *Semin Vasc Surg* 20:252-258, 2007.
17. Sarac TP, Altinel O, Kashyap V, et al: Endovascular treatment of stenotic and occluded visceral arteries for chronic mesenteric ischemia, *J Vasc Surg* 47:485-491, 2008.
18. Steinmetz E, Tatou E, Favier-Blavoux C, et al: Endovascular treatment as first choice in chronic intestinal ischemia, *Ann Vasc Surg* 16:693-699, 2002.
19. Malgor RD, Oderich GS, McKusick MA, et al: Results of single- and two-vessel mesenteric artery stents for chronic mesenteric ischemia, *Ann Vasc Surg* 24:1094-1101, 2010.
20. Stephens JC, Cardenas G, Safian RD: Percutaneous retrograde revascularization of the superior mesenteric artery via the celiac artery for chronic mesenteric ischemia, *Catheter Cardiovasc Interv* 76:222-228, 2010.
21. Oderich GS, Bower TC, Sullivan TM, Bjarnason H, Cha S, Gloviczki P: Open versus endovascular revascularization for chronic mesenteric ischemia: Risk-stratified outcomes, *J Vasc Surg* 49:1472-1479, 2009.
22. Sarac TP, Altinel O, Kashyap V, et al: Endovascular treatment of stenotic and occluded visceral arteries for chronic mesenteric ischemia, *J Vasc Surg* 47:485-491, 2008.
23. Loffroy R, Guiu B, Cercueil JP, et al: Chronic mesenteric ischemia: Efficacy and outcome of endovascular therapy, *Abdom Imaging* 35:306-314, 2010.
24. Kennedy AM, Grocott M, Schwartz MS, et al: Median nerve injury: An underrecognised complication of brachial artery cardiac catheterisation? *J Neurol Neurosurg Psychiatry* 63:542-546, 1997.
25. Alvarez-Tostado JA, Moise MA, Bena JF, et al: The brachial artery: A critical access for endovascular procedures, *J Vasc Surg* 49:378-385, 2009.
26. Almeida JA, Riordan SM: Splenic infarction complicating percutaneous transluminal coeliac artery stenting for chronic mesenteric ischaemia: A case report, *J Med Case Reports* 2:261, 2008.
27. Allen RC, Martin GH, Rees CR, et al: Mesenteric angioplasty in the treatment of chronic intestinal ischemia, *J Vasc Surg* 24:415-421, 1996.
28. Moore M, McSweeney S, Fulton G, et al: Reperfusion hemorrhage following superior mesenteric artery stenting, *Cardiovasc Intervent Radiol* 31:S57-S61, 2008.
29. Atkins MD, Kwolek CJ, LaMuraglia GM, et al: Surgical revascularization versus endovascular therapy for chronic mesenteric ischemia: A comparative experience, *J Vasc Surg* 45:1162-1171, 2007.

42 Direct Surgical Repair of Visceral Artery Aneurysms

CARON B. ROCKMAN • THOMAS S. MALDONADO

Historical Background

Visceral artery aneurysms are a rare but clinically important vascular condition and have been recognized for more than 200 years. As of 2002, there were about 3000 cases reported in the literature, and the incidence of visceral artery aneurysms in the general population has been estimated at 0.1% to 2%.[1,2] The first successful surgical repair of a visceral aneurysm, the repair of a mycotic aneurysm of the superior mesenteric artery, was reported by DeBakey and Cooley in 1953, and in 1954 Williams and Harris reported the first successful resection of a splenic artery aneurysm.[3,4] The natural history of visceral artery aneurysms and their potential for rupture are poorly defined because of their overall scarcity. Visceral artery aneurysms encompass intraabdominal aneurysms, which are not part of the aortoiliac system, and lesions of the celiac artery, the superior and inferior mesenteric arteries, and their branches. The etiologies associated with these lesions are diverse, and there is a spectrum of anatomic locations within the visceral vasculature. One third of visceral artery aneurysms may be associated with other aneurysmal diseases that occur, in order of decreasing frequency, in the thoracic aorta, abdominal aorta, renal arteries, iliac arteries, lower extremity arteries, and intracranial arteries.[5]

Visceral artery aneurysms include true aneurysms and false aneurysms, or pseudoaneurysms. True visceral artery aneurysms are typically degenerative or atherosclerotic, with histology demonstrating reduced smooth muscle, disruption of elastic fibers, and deficiency of the arterial media. Other conditions associated with true visceral artery aneurysms include fibromuscular dysplasia, collagen vascular diseases, inflammatory conditions, and rare inherited illnesses such as Ehlers-Danlos syndrome. In contrast to true aneurysms of the visceral vessels, splanchnic artery pseudoaneurysms are most commonly related to trauma, iatrogenic injury, local inflammatory processes, or infection.

Indications

Visceral artery aneurysms are managed with either serial observation or repair, depending on their size, the underlying clinical scenario, and the anatomic location of the lesion.[6] Asymptomatic splenic artery aneurysms larger than 2 to 2.5 cm should be considered for repair, particularly in patient subgroups that appear to have a propensity for rupture, such as patients undergoing liver transplantation and women of childbearing age. A similar size criterion is used for hepatic and celiac artery aneurysms. All symptomatic aneurysms should be repaired, and all visceral artery pseudoaneurysms should be considered for repair regardless of size because of their increased risk of rupture. Small asymptomatic visceral artery aneurysms have a slow growth rate (0.2 mm/yr) and can be observed. Open surgical options are increasingly reserved for patients who have failed or are not candidates for endovascular approaches. Surgical options include aneurysm exclusion or ligation, aneurysmectomy, and aneurysmorrhaphy, with or without concomitant revascularization. The necessity of revascularization depends on the location of the lesion and the collateral vascular anatomy. In areas of the splanchnic circulation with an abundance of collateral flow, proximal and distal ligation of the aneurysm segment is a viable surgical option, and revascularization is often not necessary.[6]

For a ruptured visceral artery aneurysm discovered at laparotomy, ligation of the aneurysm without vascular reconstruction is the preferred treatment. Patients with ruptured splenic artery aneurysms are usually treated with concomitant splenectomy. Ligation without revascularization can generally be performed for common hepatic artery aneurysms proximal to a patent gastroduodenal artery (GDA). Emergency surgical therapy of mesenteric branch artery aneurysms may require simultaneous intestinal resection for bowel ischemia or infarction.

Preoperative Preparation

- The most critical aspect of appropriate preoperative planning is the exact delineation of the anatomy of the lesion. This can be done with formal arteriography, magnetic resonance arteriography, or computed tomography (CT) arteriography. Magnetic resonance arteriography and CT arteriography postprocessing using volume rendering techniques allows excellent three-dimensional reconstruction of the aneurysm in relation to its afferent and efferent branches, whereas axial images enable the surgeon to visualize mural thrombus that may not be apparent on conventional angiography. If CT arteriography or magnetic resonance arteriography cannot provide adequate details, formal arteriography should be performed and may demonstrate the feasibility of an endovascular approach.

- Many patients with an idiopathic visceral artery aneurysm are younger than the typical patient who undergoes an abdominal vascular operation, and they do not have associated atherosclerotic precursors. In these patients no particular preoperative medical or cardiac workup other than routine laboratory testing, a chest radiographic examination, and an electrocardiogram is warranted. However, an older patient with medical comorbidities that may require extensive abdominal vascular reconstruction, with possible aortic clamping during the procedure, deserves a more complete preoperative medical workup, with cardiac stress testing and echocardiography as dictated by the clinical situation.

- In patients with multiple or unusual visceral aneurysms, the surgeon must consider the possibility of an underlying condition such as an infectious or inflammatory process, periarteritis nodosa, or Ehlers-Danlos syndrome. Although rare, the proper diagnosis of these conditions may have significant implications before undertaking operation. For example, in patients with periarteritis nodosa, regression of these aneurysms after pharmacologic management with immunosuppressive or cytotoxic agents is well documented.[7] Visceral aneurysms in patients with Ehlers-Danlos syndrome appear to be equally distributed among the hepatic, splenic, renal, and celiac arteries. Surgical repair in these patients is exceedingly difficult, and ligation is preferred to vascular reconstruction when possible.

- A ruptured visceral artery aneurysm is typically not diagnosed until laparotomy is performed for an abdominal catastrophe. These patients are often in hypovolemic shock, and massive hemoperitoneum can be encountered. Aggressive resuscitation with blood products must be instituted, and temporary clamping of the supraceliac aorta at the level of the diaphragm may be necessary. Packing and exploration of the abdomen to localize the area of pathology are then performed. These patients typically have not had detailed preoperative imaging studies, and localization of the area of pathology can be challenging. The surgeon must use careful judgment in deciding whether ligation or arterial reconstruction is appropriate. This is based on both the location of the aneurysm and the underlying condition of the patient.

- In the specific case of ruptured splenic artery aneurysms, a vascular surgeon is occasionally called by an obstetric team when a pregnant patient has been explored for a presumed obstetric calamity. This is an extremely difficult situation, because the obstetrician typically has explored the patient through a Pfannenstiel incision or lower abdominal situation. This must be rapidly converted to a midline laparotomy for adequate visualization of the upper abdominal cavity.

Pitfalls and Danger Points

- Careful review of detailed preoperative imaging studies is necessary to delineate the anatomy and location of the aneurysm and the adequacy of collateral circulation to avoid end-organ ischemia if ligation without revascularization is planned.
- Careful review of detailed preoperative imaging studies is required to identify associated variations in the mesenteric circulation, such as stenoses or vascular anomalies, that may dictate the need for revascularization as opposed to ligation.
- Awareness is necessary of the possibility of associated medical and surgical conditions, such as pancreatitis, infection, collagen vascular disease, or collagen production disorders, that may complicate open surgical repair.
- The surgeon should be aware of multiple options for aneurysm treatment if revascularization is required, including aneurysm plication, aneurysmorrhaphy, and interposition bypass grafting.
- Awareness of alternative inflow sources for revascularization, such as the supraceliac aorta, is important should technical issues arise.
- The surgeon should avoid kinking of autologous bypass grafts.
- Injury to associated venous and visceral structures should be avoided.
- Careful monitoring is necessary in the postoperative period for hemorrhage or signs of end-organ ischemia that could indicate bypass thrombosis.

Operative Strategy

The celiac artery is typically a short, thick trunk that arises from the anterior surface of the abdominal aorta, just below the diaphragmatic hiatus. It typically divides into three large branches: the left gastric artery, the hepatic artery, and the splenic artery (Fig. 42-1). The hepatic artery is directed toward the right and forms the lower boundary of the foramen of Winslow. A large branch, the GDA, descends from the hepatic artery and subsequently divides into the right gastroepiploic and superior pancreaticoduodenal arteries. The GDA functions as an important collateral between the celiac artery and the superior mesenteric artery. The portion of the hepatic artery proximal to the GDA is termed the common hepatic artery, and the portion distal to the GDA is called the proper hepatic artery. The proper hepatic artery lies in relation to the common bile duct and portal vein and subsequently divides into the right and left hepatic arteries.

The splenic artery is usually the largest branch of the celiac artery and often is notable for marked tortuosity. It passes to the left side, behind the stomach, and along the upper border of the pancreas, where it gives rise to numerous pancreatic branches. The other branches of the splenic artery before its termination in the splenic hilum are the short gastric and left gastroepiploic arteries.

Operative Technique for Splenic Artery Aneurysm Repair

Splenic artery aneurysms comprise 60% of all visceral aneurysms (Fig. 42-1). They are often saccular, usually less than 2 cm in diameter, and most are located in the

DIRECT SURGICAL REPAIR OF VISCERAL ARTERY ANEURYSMS **503**

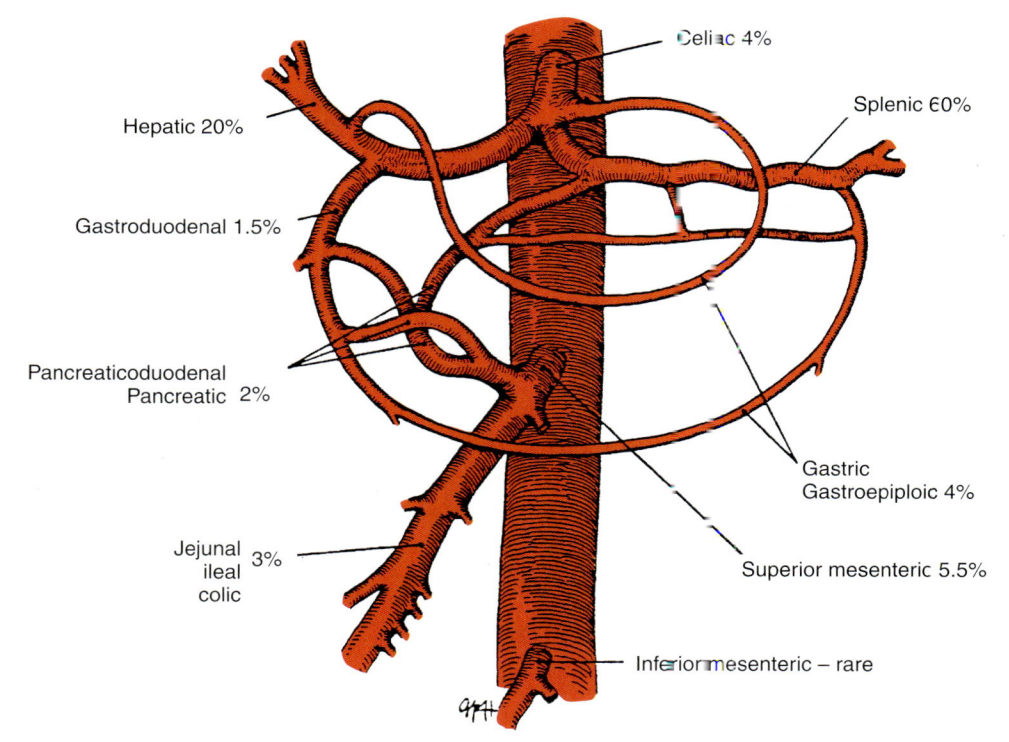

Figure 42-1. Schematic representation of the visceral artery anatomy as it arises from the aorta, showing the nature of the collateral circulation between the celiac and the superior mesenteric artery vascular distributions. Percentages next to the named vessels indicate the prevalence of aneurysms in the distribution of the particular artery. *(From Rutherford RB, editor: Vascular surgery, ed 6. Philadelphia, 2005, Saunders, p 1566, Fig. 107-1.)*

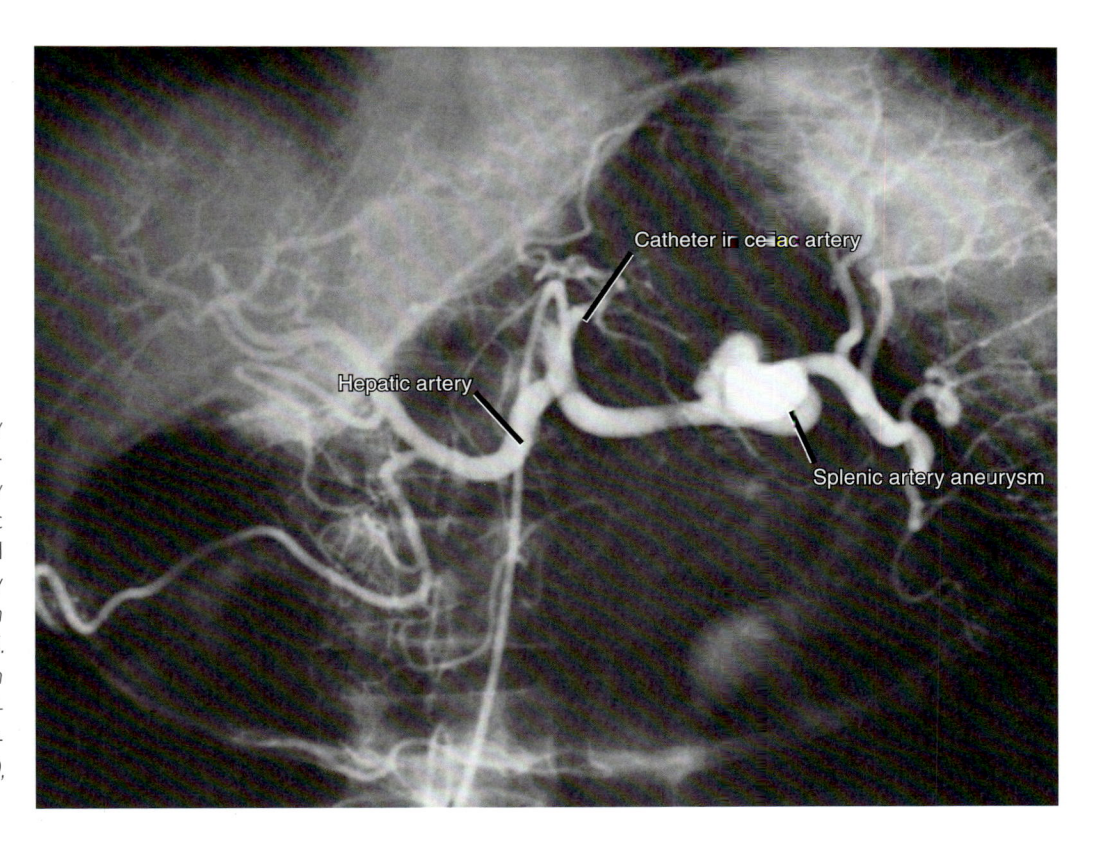

Figure 42-2. Celiac artery injection revealing the typical location of a splenic artery aneurysm in the midsplenic artery. The hepatic artery and the catheter in the celiac artery are clearly visualized. *(From Rockman CB, Maldonado TS. Splanchnic artery aneurysms. In Cronenwett JL, Johnston KW, editors: Rutherford's vascular surgery. ed 7. Philadelphia, 2010, Saunders, p 2145, Fig. 138-4.)*

mid- or distal splenic artery (Fig. 42-2).[2,8] Most splenic artery aneurysms are found incidentally during unrelated abdominal imaging. When rupture occurs, patients usually experience acute left-sided abdominal pain and shock. However, an initial contained rupture into the lesser sac may occur, providing a window of opportunity for treatment. This "double rupture" phenomenon may be seen in 20% to 30% of cases. Splenic artery aneurysms may occasionally rupture into adjacent structures, including the gastrointestinal tract, pancreatic ducts, or splenic vein. Splenic artery pseudoaneurysms secondary to pancreatitis may rupture into a pancreatic pseudocyst or into the pancreatic duct, a condition called hemosuccus pancreaticus.

The overall mortality rate of ruptured splenic artery aneurysms is as high as 25%. Rupture of a splenic artery aneurysm during pregnancy, which usually occurs during the third trimester, has devastating maternal and fetal mortality rates of 80% and 90%, respectively.[9,10] The frequent occurrence of rupture in the third trimester, and the presentation of abdominal pain and shock, often leads to misdiagnosis as an obstetric emergency.

Splenic artery aneurysms that are ruptured or symptomatic require urgent treatment, and aneurysms in pregnant women or in women of childbearing age also warrant intervention. Less stringent indications for treatment include aneurysms that are enlarging or those more than 2 cm in diameter, but these size criteria are not absolute. The traditional surgical management of splenic artery aneurysms consists of proximal and distal ligation or aneurysmectomy for lesions in the proximal or middle portion of the splenic artery. Revascularization of the distal splenic artery is generally not warranted, because collateral flow to the spleen is maintained by the short gastric arteries. For more distal lesions adjacent to the splenic hilum, splenectomy has been the most commonly performed operation.

INCISION

The appropriate incision for open surgical treatment of an aneurysm in the middle portion of the splenic artery is either a midline laparotomy or a bilateral subcostal approach. An aneurysm in the distal portion of the splenic artery can be approached from either a left subcostal or a midline abdominal incision.

EXPOSURE OF THE SPLENIC ARTERY

After initial exploration of the abdominal cavity, the greater omentum is reflected upward while downward traction is maintained on the transverse colon. The omentum is separated using sharp dissection, and the lesser sac is entered. The posterior gastric wall is swept away from the underlying pancreas, and the entire pancreas is exposed from its head to the hilum of the spleen. The splenic artery and vein are located as they run along the superior surface of the body and tail of the pancreas. An incision in the posterior peritoneum allows direct exposure of the origin and middle portion of splenic artery, where most splenic artery aneurysms are located.

If the aneurysm is located in the distal splenic artery or adjacent to the splenic hilum and concomitant splenectomy is planned, the lesser sac may be entered via the gastrosplenic ligament using medial traction on the stomach. The distal portion of the splenic artery can be palpated after its course along the upper margin of the pancreas. The peritoneum overlying the vessel is incised, proximal vascular control is gained, and the artery, along with the splenic vein, is ligated. Splenectomy with the distally located aneurysm can then be performed en bloc.

LIGATION OF THE SPLENIC ARTERY ANEURYSM

The operative treatment of splenic artery aneurysms almost never requires formal vascular reconstruction. There is a rich collateral network of blood vessels supplying the spleen and emanating from the short gastric arteries, and splenic infarction is rare. When the aneurysm is located in the distal splenic artery, adjacent to the splenic hilum, splenectomy is performed. When the aneurysm is located in the middle portion of the splenic artery, formal ligation of the splenic artery both proximal and distal to the aneurysm is the preferred treatment (Fig. 42-3). Although some authors have reported performing excision of the aneurysm, if small, with a primary end-to-end anastomosis to reestablish flow in the splenic artery, this is not clinically necessary to maintain adequate perfusion of the spleen. After the aneurysm has been located and confirmed by palpation within the lesser sac, gentle dissection of the proximal splenic artery is performed close

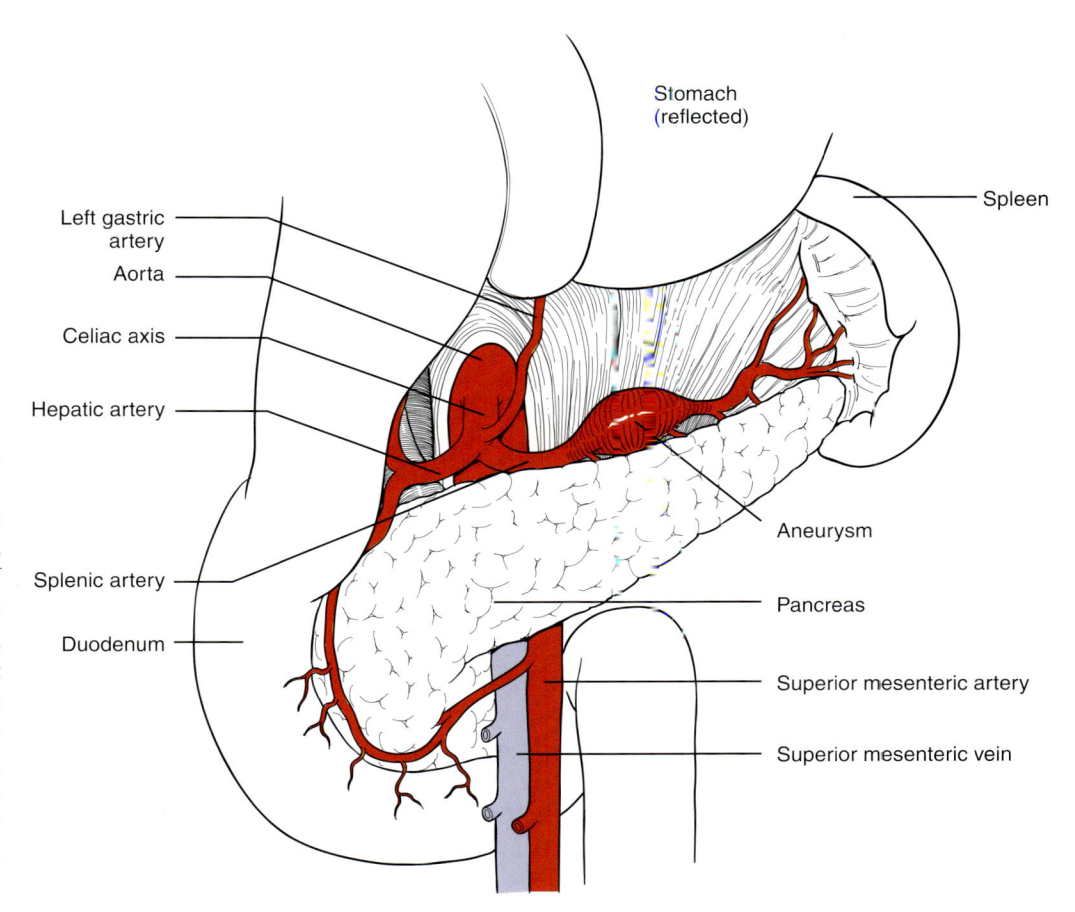

Figure 42-3. After identification of the splenic artery in the lesser sac running along the upper border of the pancreas, proximal and distal control of the splenic artery aneurysm is obtained. The artery is clamped, and the aneurysm is explored; ligation of the small pancreatic branches supplying the aneurysm is performed. The splenic artery proximal and distal to the aneurysm is then formally ligated using running monofilament suture.

to its origin from the celiac artery trunk; the artery is mobilized and encircled with a vessel loop. Similarly, dissection of the splenic artery distal to the aneurysm is performed. When the aneurysm is relatively small, this is relatively simple to accomplish. However, when an extremely large or "giant" splenic artery aneurysm is present, location of the normal proximal and distal splenic artery may be difficult, with visualization compromised by the large aneurysm. Once control of the splenic artery proximal and distal to the aneurysm has been obtained, the vessels may be clamped and the aneurysm may be opened. If small pancreatic branches are bleeding from within the aneurysm sac, these may be ligated from within. A portion of the aneurysm wall may be excised for pathology if this is deemed necessary, but it is not necessary to remove the aneurysm sac. The proximal and distal arteries are then ligated using running monofilament suture.

Operative Technique for Hepatic Artery Aneurysm Repair

The hepatic artery is the second most common location for aneurysmal degeneration in the visceral circulation (see Fig. 42-1). Approximately 80% of hepatic artery aneurysms are extrahepatic, with 63% located in the common hepatic artery.[11,12] Although many hepatic artery aneurysms are asymptomatic and found incidentally, they have the highest rate of rupture among all visceral artery aneurysms and frequently become symptomatic.[13] Symptoms can include epigastric or right upper quadrant pain and subsequent gastrointestinal hemorrhage and jaundice. The classic triad of Quincke consisting of abdominal pain, hematobilia, and obstructive jaundice is seen in less than one third of cases.[14,15]

Intervention for hepatic artery aneurysms should be considered in all patients who are symptomatic and in those asymptomatic patients who have true aneurysms more than 2 cm in diameter or who demonstrate rapid growth on serial imaging studies. Intrahepatic pseudoaneurysms, which may be seen after iatrogenic injury or trauma, should be considered for repair irrespective of size. Treatment options depend on the location and morphology of the hepatic artery aneurysm and the presence of associated liver disease. Common hepatic artery aneurysms can usually be treated with ligation, because the GDA generally provides sufficient collateral flow to the liver. When the GDA is diminutive or inadequate, arterial revascularization may be necessary to preserve hepatic arterial flow. Hepatic artery ligation should never be performed in the presence of cirrhosis or other of liver disease, because even a slight degree of ischemic compromise can be catastrophic. Aneurysms distal to the GDA arising in the proper hepatic artery generally require arterial reconstruction. Intrahepatic aneurysms or pseudoaneurysms are ideal candidates for endovascular embolization.

INCISION

The appropriate incision for open surgical treatment of an aneurysm of the hepatic artery is either a midline laparotomy or a bilateral subcostal approach.

EXPOSURE OF THE HEPATIC ARTERY

The lesser sac is entered, and the common hepatic artery and proximal portion of the proper hepatic artery are easily palpated in the lesser omentum. The proper hepatic artery is located more distally within the porta hepatis, just medial to the common bile duct. The area of the hepatoduodenal ligament is exposed by retraction of the right lobe of the liver superiorly. An incision is made transversely into the hepatoduodenal ligament, and the artery is localized by palpation of the pulse. The junction of the common and proper hepatic arteries is located at the origin of the GDA. To achieve more proximal exposure of the origin of the hepatic artery from the celiac trunk, the stomach is elevated and the remainder of the lesser sac is exposed by separating the leaves of omentum, as described in the approach to the midsplenic artery. Depending on the location of the aneurysm and its morphology, either aneurysmorrhaphy or interposition grafting can be performed (Figs. 42-4 and 42-5).

ROUTING THE BYPASS

Once proximal and distal exposure and control of the vessels have been obtained, the patient is systemically heparinized, and the hepatic artery is clamped. The aneurysm is entered and explored. Small bleeding vessels may be ligated from within the aneurysm sac. An assessment of the extent of the aneurysm is performed, and areas of normal nonaneurysmal hepatic artery both proximal and distal to the aneurysm are located. Appropriate areas are then chosen for performing an interposition graft, using either reversed saphenous vein or prosthetic material as deemed appropriate to the clinical situation. The bypass can typically be performed entirely from within the lesser sac so that no formal tunneling is required. However, in the case of a more proximal common hepatic artery aneurysm adjacent to the origin of the vessel from the celiac axis, the supraceliac aorta may be used as an inflow source. In this case the proximal common hepatic artery is ligated, and an aortic to distal hepatic artery bypass is performed. When an aneurysm of the hepatic artery involves the origin of the GDA, this vessel can be ligated if the superior mesenteric artery is patent or reimplanted onto the bypass if concern exists regarding collateral flows. A common hepatic to proper hepatic bypass is then performed to maintain perfusion to the liver.

The use of reversed autologous vein may be preferred in cases of concomitant infection because of associated inflammatory disease, such as pancreatitis, or when the aneurysm or pseudoaneurysm is felt to be mycotic in origin. However, autologous mesenteric bypasses may kink within the abdominal cavity or retroperitoneum, particularly when the length of the bypass is relatively long. Prosthetic bypasses have the disadvantage of being more prone to infection but are relatively resistant to kinking and obstruction.

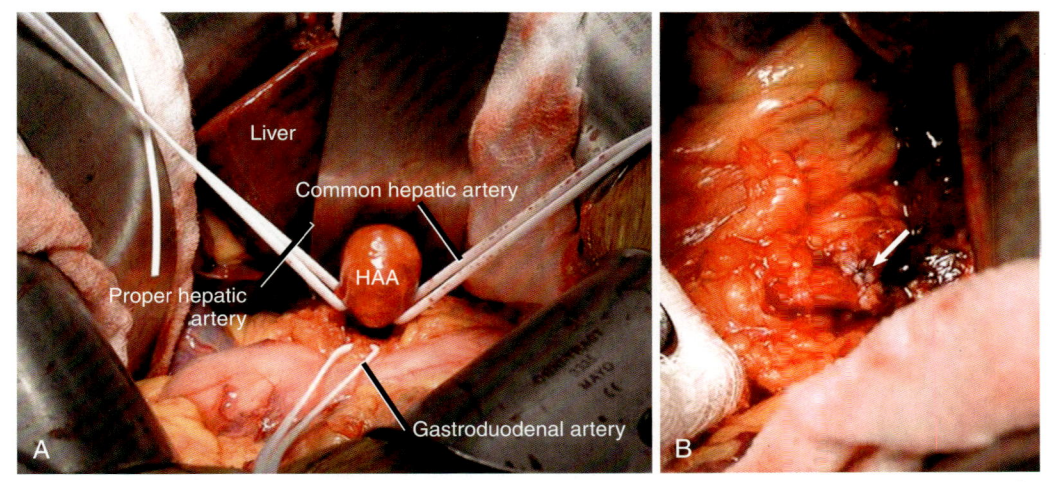

Figure 42-4. Intraoperative photographs revealing a hepatic artery aneurysm. **A,** Proximal and distal control of the hepatic artery and the gastroduodenal artery have been obtained with vessel loops. *HAA,* Hepatic artery aneurysm. **B,** Completed reconstruction after excision of the aneurysm and simple plication or aneurysmorrhaphy, revealing suture line on the anterior vessel wall (*arrow*). (**A,** From Rockman CB, Maldonado TS. Splanchnic artery aneurysms. In Cronenwett JL, Johnston KW, editors: Rutherford's vascular surgery. ed 7. Philadelphia, 2010, Saunders, p 2148, Fig. 138-10.)

Figure 42-5. Aneurysms of the hepatic artery are often treated with interposition grafting. After identification of the hepatic artery aneurysm in the lesser sac and localization of the gastroduodenal artery (GDA), proximal and distal control of the hepatic artery is obtained. The proximal and distal arteries are clamped, and the aneurysm is explored. Interposition grafting can be performed with reversed saphenous vein or with a prosthetic graft. The proximal anastomosis is typically performed to the common hepatic artery, and the distal anastomosis is performed to the proper hepatic artery within the lesser sac. The GDA may be ligated if the superior mesenteric artery is normal or reimplanted onto the hepatic artery bypass if concern regarding adequate collateral circulation exists.

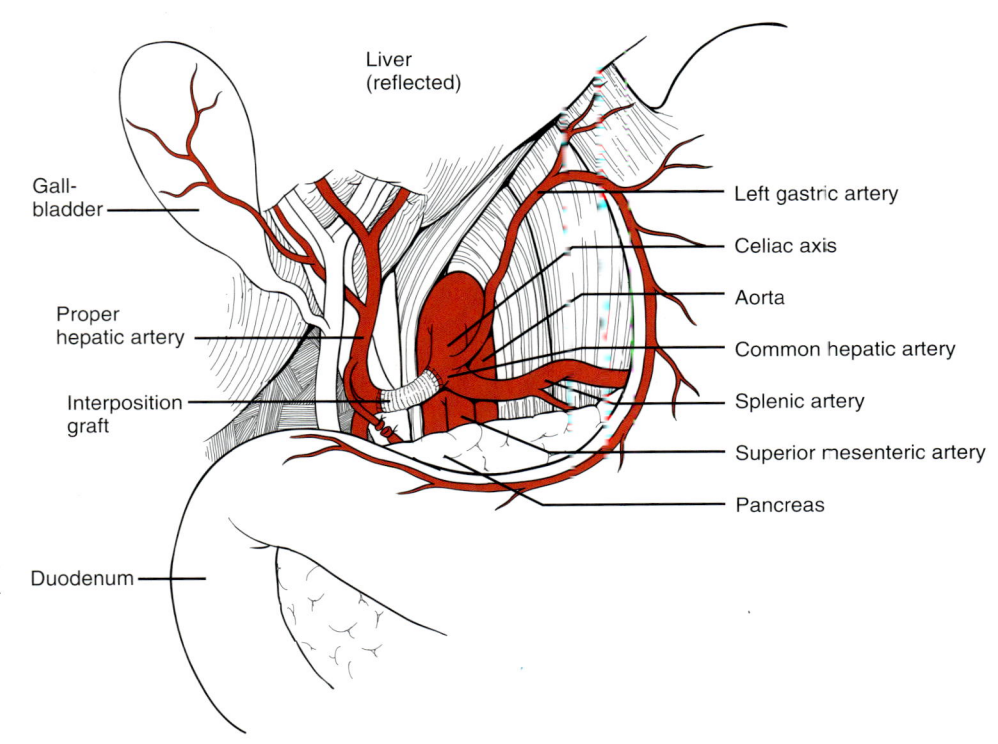

PROXIMAL ANASTOMOSIS

If the aneurysm is located in the proper hepatic artery, the proximal anastomosis can be performed at the level of the more proximal common hepatic artery from within the lesser sac (see Fig. 42-5). This is typically performed from end to end using running monofilament suture. If the aneurysm is located in the common hepatic artery but proximal and distal ligation is judged to be unsafe, then it may be necessary to perform the proximal anastomosis at the supraceliac aorta. The surgical approach to the supraceliac aorta is described in the section detailing surgical repair of celiac artery aneurysms. In a more urgent situation the proximal anastomosis may be performed from the common iliac artery to avoid the systemic consequences of interrupting aortic and mesenteric flow. An iliac to hepatic artery bypass requires tunneling through the transverse mesocolon.

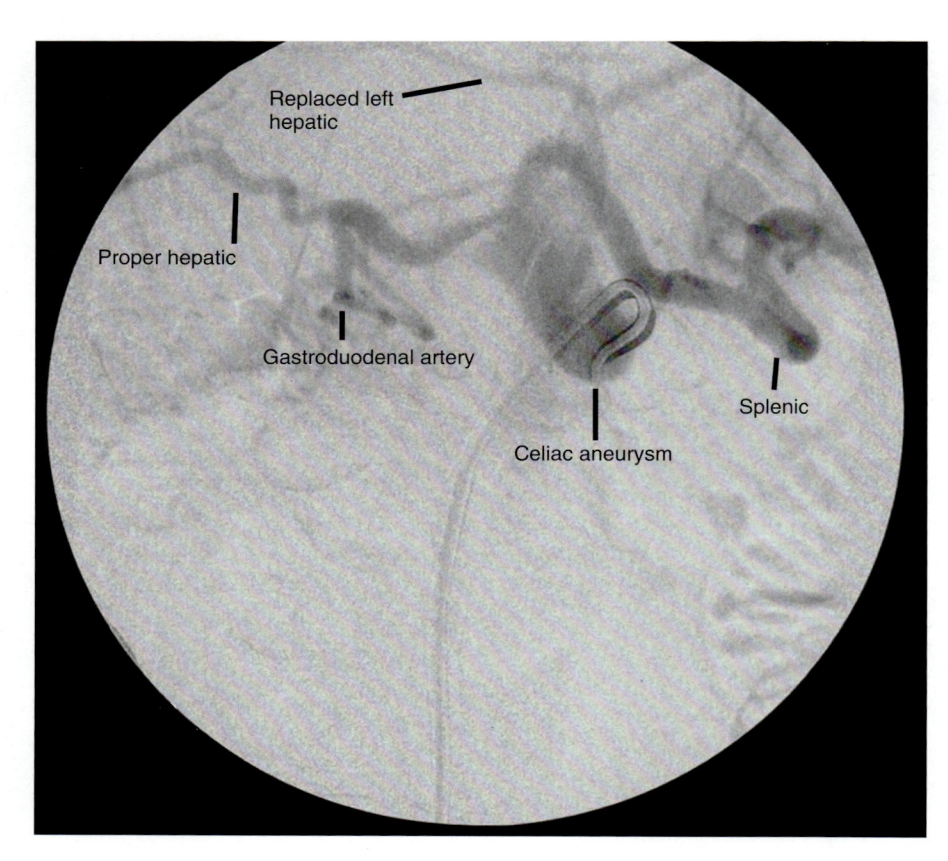

Figure 42-6. Celiac artery angiogram revealing an aneurysm of the celiac artery trunk. The catheter in the celiac artery, splenic artery, proper hepatic artery, and gastroduodenal artery is marked. Note the replaced left hepatic artery originating from the left gastric artery. In this case endovascular repair was not feasible because of the presence of the replaced left hepatic artery.

DISTAL ANASTOMOSIS

The distal anastomosis is performed to the most proximal area of nonaneurysmal hepatic artery from end to end, again using running monofilament suture. Intraoperative assessment of the adequacy of revascularization can be performed using a Doppler probe, duplex examination, and gross assessment of the liver.

Operative Technique for Celiac Artery Aneurysm Repair

Celiac artery aneurysms account for approximately 5% of all visceral artery aneurysms and have a strong tendency to rupture with a high mortality rate.[16] Symptoms related to celiac artery aneurysms can include epigastric abdominal pain or hemorrhagic shock related to rupture. Like splenic artery aneurysms, celiac artery aneurysms may rupture initially into the lesser sac, causing localized epigastric pain and mild hypovolemia. This "double rupture" sequence may occur in up to 25% of cases.[17]

Considering the high mortality rate with rupture, it is reasonable to consider treatment for all patients in whom a large or symptomatic celiac artery aneurysm is diagnosed. The decision to treat is based on size, anatomy, and etiology, as well as the potential morbidity of the proposed procedure. Occult coexisting visceral artery occlusive disease is an important factor in determining whether revascularization is warranted (Fig. 42-6). Other anatomic features, including the presence of a suitable proximal aneurysm neck, may weigh into the consideration of endovascular options for treatment.

Historically, surgical treatment has been the only feasible option for management. Ligation of the celiac artery is usually well tolerated except in patients with underlying hepatic disease. Standard surgical revascularization involves celiac aneurysmectomy with aortoceliac bypass grafting, most commonly using a prosthetic graft (Figs. 42-7 and 42-8). Aneurysmorrhaphy for isolated saccular lesions of the celiac artery has also been reported.

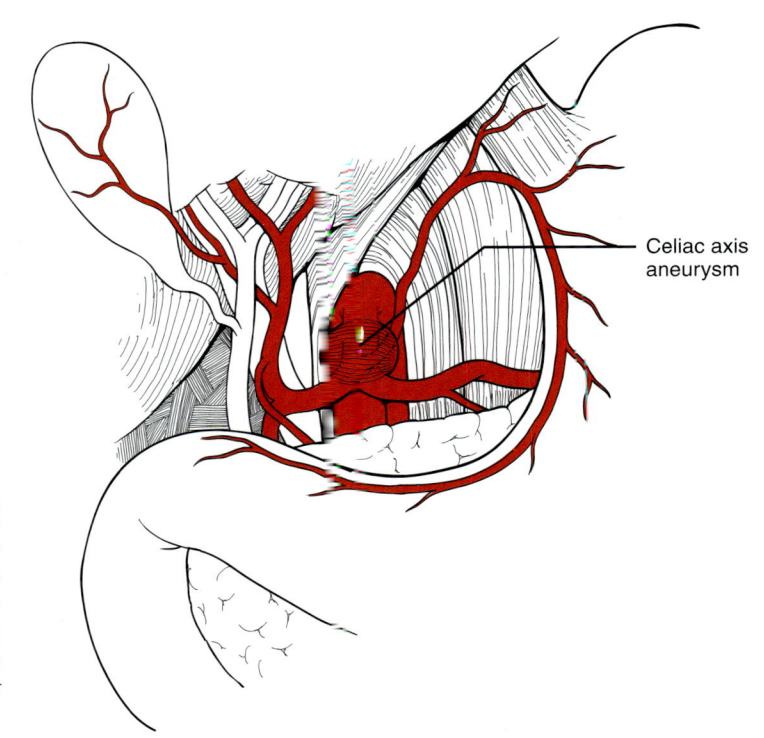

Figure 42-7. An aneurysm of the celiac artery involving the origins of all three major branches (splenic, left gastric, and hepatic). When a less extensive aneurysm is present, ligation of the celiac artery proximal and distal to the aneurysm may be performed without vascular reconstruction and is often well tolerated. If the aneurysm is small, celiac artery aneurysmorrhaphy or a short interposition graft of the celiac artery may be an option.

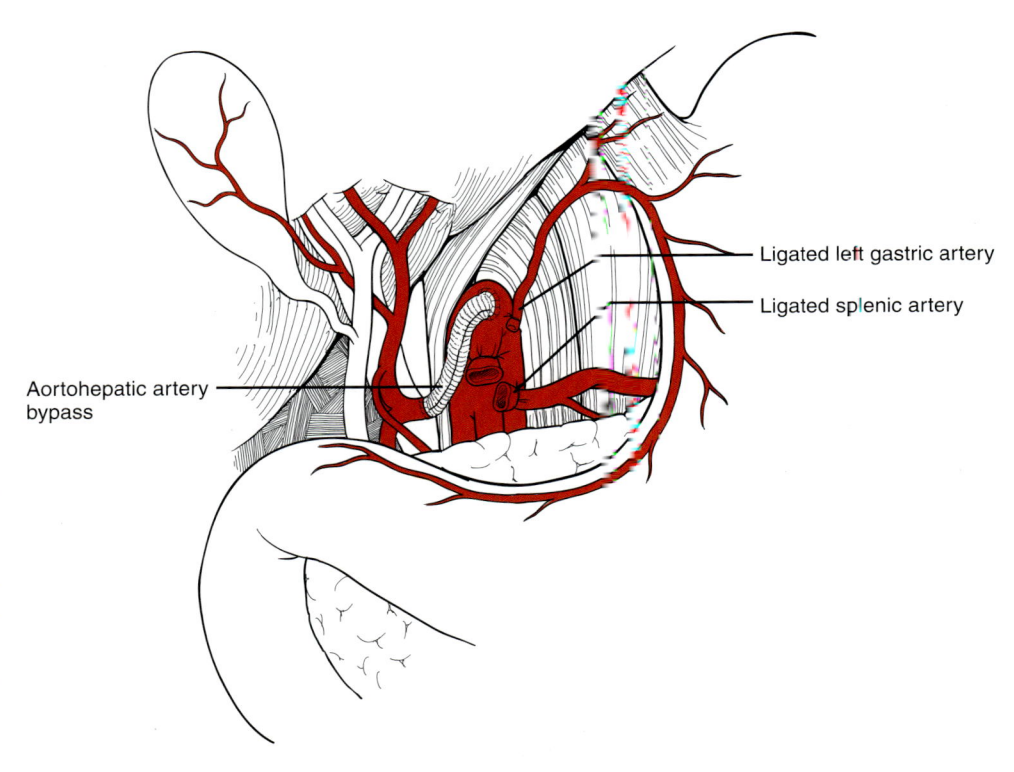

Figure 42-8. The standard approach to a large celiac artery aneurysm that involves all major branches is an aortohepatic artery bypass originating from the supraceliac aorta. The origins of the splenic artery and left gastric artery are typically ligated, because sufficient collateral circulation exists to maintain end-organ perfusion to the stomach and spleen. The bypass is performed to the common hepatic artery to avoid end-organ ischemia of the liver.

INCISION

The celiac artery can be approached anteriorly via a longitudinal incision in the upper midline or bilateral subcostal incisions. Alternatively, a thoracoabdominal incision extending from the left midaxillary line within the seventh intercostal space, across the costal margin, and inferiorly along the midline to the edge of the rectus sheath may be preferable in cases of ruptured celiac aneurysms or in the setting of a "hostile" abdomen. The retroperitoneal approach may allow better exposure of the thoracic aorta when the supraceliac abdominal aorta is heavily calcified and suboptimal for sewing a proximal anastomosis. However, this approach may make access to the hepatic artery difficult.

EXPOSURE OF THE AORTA

When using an anterior midline or bilateral subcostal approach, the patient is placed in the supine position. The small bowel is packed into the lower half of the abdomen, and the greater omentum and transverse colon are retracted caudally. The left triangular ligament is incised to permit for mobilization and retraction of the left hepatic lobe superiorly and to the patient's right. The gastrohepatic ligament is incised longitudinally, allowing access to the lesser sac. Care is taken to avoid injury to vagus nerve fibers coursing along the lesser curvature of the stomach, as well as to an anomalous replaced left hepatic artery. The supraceliac aorta can be easily palpated overlying the spine and is best exposed by retracting the stomach and esophagus to the left. Manual identification of the esophagus is facilitated by placement of a nasogastric tube. The aorta is best controlled at the level of the diaphragm, where it is usually free of atherosclerotic disease and amenable to safe clamping. This portion of the supraceliac aorta is exposed by incising the thin layer of posterior peritoneum and incising the median arcuate ligament, as well as the right crus of the diaphragm. Circumferential dissection of the aorta is unnecessary and potentially hazardous because of the limited exposure of the thoracic aorta when using the anterior abdominal approach. Instead, gentle blunt dissection using finger dissection can be performed medially and laterally to allow placement of an occlusion clamp.

EXPOSURE OF THE CELIAC ARTERY

After exposure of the aorta proximally by dividing the arcuate ligament and right crus, the celiac artery can be identified as it lies perpendicular to the aorta and is bordered by the pancreas inferiorly. Careful dissection is required to properly expose the origin of the celiac trunk, because it is often enveloped by a fibrous tissue consisting of the celiac ganglion. The three major outflow branches are then identified and controlled. Larger aneurysms can displace surrounding organs and make identification of outflow branches difficult. Often such aneurysms are best approached from within, because obtaining proximal celiac control may be treacherous. In such cases the proximal celiac is oversewn and a bypass is performed to the distal celiac artery. When an aneurysm involves the trifurcation of the celiac trunk, the splenic and left gastric arteries can be sacrificed and an aortohepatic bypass can be performed preserving flow to the liver (Fig. 42-8).

ROUTING THE BYPASS

Either an autogenous or a prosthetic conduit can be used for arterial reconstructions after celiac artery aneurysmectomy. For proximal celiac artery aneurysms, bypass requires a proximal aortic anastomosis. Aneurysms confined to the midportion of the celiac trunk can be repaired with a short interposition graft, if technically feasible, either with saphenous vein or with a short, small-diameter prosthetic graft. The conduit does not require tunneling. Care should be taken to avoid kinking, especially when a vein graft is used.

PROXIMAL ANASTOMOSIS

After systemic heparinization the aorta is clamped proximally and distally. Alternatively, a partially occlusive side-biting clamp can be used. The graft is beveled appropriately, and an aortic anastomosis is constructed using a standard four-quadrant suture technique with either 3-0 or 4-0 monofilament suture.

DISTAL ANASTOMOSIS

The distal anastomosis can be fashioned either to normal distal celiac artery or more commonly to the hepatic artery, because this is often more easily accessible. Ligation of the other branches of the celiac trunk is acceptable because of the presence of rich collateral circulation. Doppler evaluation of the anastomosis, as well as the distal hepatic artery, should be performed. The liver and bowel should be inspected for signs of ischemia, especially if a celiac artery aneurysm has been treated with ligation and exclusion.

Postoperative Care

- Patients should be monitored in an intensive care unit or step-down–type unit with close observation of blood pressure, hemodynamic parameters, urine output, and hematocrit levels. Most surgeons advocate the use of a nasogastric tube until the return of bowel function, and venous thromboembolic prophylaxis should be used.
- Patients who undergo visceral revascularization do not routinely require postoperative anticoagulation or antiplatelet agents to maintain bypass patency. However, patients who have undergone hepatic or celiac revascularization procedures should be monitored carefully for signs of bypass thrombosis, which can initially be subtle. Any rise in liver enzymes, or other signs of hepatic ischemia, should prompt an evaluation of the bypass with either duplex scanning or arteriography if necessary.

Complications

- **Bleeding.** Because extensive dissection in the retroperitoneum is required in many open visceral artery aneurysm repairs, postoperative hemorrhage must be considered as a potential cause of hemodynamic instability.
- **Myocardial infarction.** Elderly patients with degenerative visceral artery aneurysms may have coexisting coronary artery disease, and perioperative myocardial ischemia or infarction is a complication of these complex surgical procedures.
- **Ileus or small bowel obstruction.** Extensive intraperitoneal and/or retroperitoneal dissection required in open visceral artery aneurysm repairs may result in postoperative ileus or small bowel obstruction.
- **Pancreatitis.** Revascularization is not typically performed for splenic artery aneurysms, and monitoring for splenic infarction is not necessary. However, patients may develop pancreatitis if extensive dissection is performed in this area or if the tail of the pancreas is traumatized during splenectomy.
- **Bypass thrombosis.** Hepatic or celiac revascularization can be complicated by bypass thrombosis and hepatic ischemia. If this occurs early in the postoperative period, it is most likely because of technical error, and thrombectomy and bypass revision are performed.

REFERENCES

1. Messina LM, Shanley CJ: Visceral artery aneurysms, *Surg Clin North Am* 77:425-442, 1997.
2. Stanley JC, Wakefield TW, Graham LM, et al: Clinical importance and management of splanchnic artery aneurysms, *J Vasc Surg* 3:836-840, 1986.
3. DeBakey ME, Cooley DA: Successful resection of mycotic aneurysm of superior mesenteric artery: Case report and review of literature, *Am Surg* 19:202-212, 1953.
4. Williams RW, Harris RB: Successful resection of splenic artery aneurysm: Suggestion as to technique in surgical management, *Arch Surg* 69:530-532, 1954.
5. Carr SC, Mahvi DM, Hoch JR, et al: Visceral artery aneurysm rupture, *J Vasc Surg* 33:806-811, 2001.
6. Rockman CB, Maldonado TS: Splanchnic artery aneurysms. In Cronenwett JL, Johnston KW, editors: *Rutherford's vascular surgery*, ed 7, Philadelphia, 2010, Saunders, pp 2140-2155.
7. Mogle P, Halperin Y, Kobrin I, et al: Rapid regression of aneurysms in polyarteritis nodosa, *Br J Radiol* 55:536-538, 1982.
8. Dave SP, Reis ED, Hossain A, et al: Splenic artery aneurysm in the 1990s, *Ann Vasc Surg* 14:223-229, 2000.
9. Holdsworth RJ, Gunn A: Ruptured splenic artery aneurysm in pregnancy: A review, *Br J Obstet Gynaecol* 99:595-597, 1992.
10. Barrett JM, Van Hooydonk JE, Boehm FH: Pregnancy-related rupture of arterial aneurysms, *Obstet Gynecol Survey* 37:557-566, 1982.
11. Luebke T, Heckenkamp J, Gawenda M, et al: Combined endovascular-open surgical procedure in a great hepatic artery aneurysm, *Ann Vasc Surg* 21:807-812, 2007.
12. Abbas MA, Fowl RJ, Stone WM, et al: Hepatic artery aneurysm Factors that predict complications, *J Vasc Surg* 38:41-45, 2003.

13. Zachary K, Geier S, Pellecchia C, et al: Jaundice secondary to hepatic artery aneurysm: Radiological appearance and clinical features, *Am J Gastroenterol* 81:295-298, 1986.
14. Harlaftis NN, Akin JT: Hemobilia from ruptured hepatic artery aneurysm: Report of a case and review of the literature, *Am J Surg* 133:229-232, 1977.
15. Berceli SA: Hepatic and splenic artery aneurysms, *Semin Vasc Surg* 18:196-201, 2005.
16. Graham LM, Stanley JC, Whitehouse WM II, et al: Celiac artery aneurysms: Historic (1745-1949) versus contemporary (1950-1984) differences in etiology and clinical importance, *J Vasc Surg* 2:757-764, 1985.
17. Wagner WH, Allins AD, Treiman RL, et al: Ruptured visceral artery aneurysms, *Ann Vasc Surg* 11:342-347, 1997.

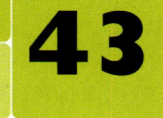

43 Endovascular Treatment of Hepatic, Gastroduodenal, Pancreaticoduodenal, and Splenic Artery Aneurysms

JAVIER E. ANAYA-AYALA • WAEL SAAD • MARK G. DAVIES • ALAN B. LUMSDEN

Historical Background

Hepatic artery aneurysms are the second most common type of visceral aneurysms after those of the splenic artery.[1] In 1809 Wilson[2] first described a hepatic artery aneurysm as the "size and shape of a heart involving the left hepatic artery," and in 1903 Kehr[3] reported the first successful ligation of a hepatic artery aneurysm. Hepatic artery aneurysms comprise 20% of visceral artery aneurysms,[3] and although still not well defined, the natural history of the hepatic artery aneurysm typically results in enlargement, rupture, and life-threatening hemorrhage.[4] The optimal management of hepatic artery aneurysms remains controversial, and the risk-benefit ratio of treating asymptomatic cases is difficult to assess.[5]

True aneurysms involving the gastroduodenal artery (GDA) or the pancreaticoduodenal artery (PDA) are extremely rare, accounting for only 3.5% of all visceral artery aneurysms (PDA = 2%, GDA = 1.5%).[6] The first PDA aneurysm was reported by Ferguson[7] in 1895, and fewer than 100 cases have been reported in the literature.[8] These types of aneurysms are primarily caused by arterial injury during surgery on surrounding organs, autoimmune disease, or pancreatic inflammation.[9] GDA aneurysms are significant because of their high associated risks of rupture and death.

First reported by Beaussier in 1770,[10] splenic artery aneurysm (SAA) is the most commonly reported visceral aneurysm, accounting for up to 60% of such lesions.[11] The vast majority are smaller than 2 cm and are saccular, and more than 80% are located in the midsplenic or distal splenic artery.[6] SAAs are found in women four times more frequently than in men, and the reported risk of rupture ranges from 3.0% to 9.6%.[12] Approximately 70% of SSAs are true aneurysms and occur at the bifurcation within the splenic hilum.[13] Most frequently asymptomatic, these aneurysms are usually identified as an incidental finding. A curvilinear or signet ring-shaped calcification may be observed in the left upper quadrant of an abdominal radiographic examination. Symptomatic patients present with left upper quadrant or epigastric pain that radiates to the left shoulder. Rupture of the aneurysm, which may manifest as hypovolemic shock, occurs in less than 2% of patients.[14]

Common causes for SAAs include atherosclerosis, portal hypertension, and pancreatitis, which may cause pseudoaneurysms.[15] Less common etiologies include idiopathic dissection, septic emboli, essential hypertension,[16] polyarteritis nodosa, and systemic lupus erythematosus.[17] Pseudoaneurysms of the splenic artery are most often caused by chronic pancreatitis or trauma.[18] The incidence of SAAs is higher in multiparous women with, on average, 4.5 pregnancies[19] and in patients with splenomegaly or those who have undergone orthotopic liver transplantation.[20]

Indications

Most authors have recommended repair of hepatic artery aneurysms, whether symptomatic or not, because of the associated risk of rupture and death. Intervention is indicated for all nonatherosclerotic aneurysms and for multiple hepatic aneurysms because of the higher incidence of eventual symptoms and rupture. For asymptomatic atherosclerotic hepatic artery aneurysms, which are 2 to 5 cm in diameter, treatment options are more controversial in patients with marginal health. Intervention should be reserved for those aneurysms that enlarge or become symptomatic.

The literature includes only case reports and small case series. A definitive study evaluating the natural history of both GDA and PDA aneurysms or the preferred method for treatment has not been conducted.[21] The risk of rupture of GDAs and PDAs is unrelated to size, and any aneurysm should be considered for definitive treatment.[9,22]

Treatment for an SAA is recommended for any symptomatic patient, as well as for asymptomatic pregnant women, women of childbearing age who may subsequently become pregnant, patients who may undergo liver transplantation, and those who present with a pseudoaneurysm associated with an inflammatory process. Patients with aneurysms larger than 2 to 2.5 cm should be considered for treatment. With the advent of endovascular techniques, percutaneous transcatheter embolization or stent-graft placement has become a preferred option.

Preoperative Preparation

- Nothing should be taken by mouth after midnight except regular medications. If the patient is diabetic, half the insulin dose should be given and sulfonylureas should be held.
- Coumadin should be discontinued, and heparin bridge therapy should be used as appropriate. Enteric-coated acetylsalicylic acid (aspirin) may be taken the day of the procedure.
- In the presence of renal insufficiency (serum creatinine > 1.5 mg/dL), normal saline should be administered to prevent contrast nephropathy. Alternatively, dextrose with sodium bicarbonate (150 mEq/L) should be infused at 3 mL/kg for 1 hour before contrast load and 1 mL/kg/hr for 6 hours after contrast load. Six doses of *N*-acetylcysteine (600 or 1200 mg) should be administered twice daily beginning 12 hours preoperatively.
- In the presence of a contrast allergy, oral prednisone (50 mg) should be prescribed 13, 7, and 1 hour before contrast load and both ranitidine (50 mg intravenously), and diphenhydramine (50 mg intravenously) should be administered 1 hour before contrast load.

Pitfalls and Danger Points

- Arterial injury, including dissection, rupture, and pseudoaneurysm
- Occlusion of the main vessel while attempting to preserve it
- Loss of access during the procedure, including force buildup with recoil resulting in the stent system inadvertently displacing the guide catheter
- Access angle to the celiac axis that may require a change in primary access from femoral to brachial artery, or vice versa
- Organ infarction because of occlusion of the main splenic or proper hepatic arteries without sufficient collateral vessels or in the presence of liver disease
- Errant coil and stent deployment
- Stent-graft foreshortening with type I or II endoleak

Endovascular Strategy

Two strategies are available for the endovascular treatment of visceral aneurysms. The first entails excluding the aneurysm and its donor artery and relying on collateral arterial pathways to reconstitute blood supply to the spleen or liver. The second involves excluding the aneurysm while maintaining arterial flow through the donor artery. The first strategy requires embolization, and the second requires stent-graft placement with or without coil embolization of collateral branches to prevent backbleeding (type II endoleak).

Rarely, upper celiac, hepatic, splenic, gastroduodenal, or pancreaticoduodenal aneurysms are inaccessible using transcatheter techniques. In these instances direct percutaneous puncture of the aneurysm can be performed, embolizing the aneurysm with coils or by thrombin injection. Another alternative is to perform a "hybrid procedure" that involves a laparotomy, dissection, and surgical cutdown for isolation of vessels that lead directly to the aneurysm for access combined with cannulation and transcatheter techniques for management of the aneurysm.

Endovascular Technique

ACCESS AND GUIDING SHEATH PLACEMENT

Arterial access to the celiac axis is typically performed via a femoral artery approach, although a brachial approach can be considered in the event of severe aortoiliac occlusive disease or aortoiliac aneurysm or tortuous anatomy, or if the preoperative computed tomography (CT) scan or magnetic resonance angiography demonstrates a downward-angled vessel. Once the introducer sheath is placed in the femoral artery, an anteroposterior aortogram can be obtained, with a pigtail catheter placed in the suprarenal aorta at or above the T10 level to best visualize the origin of the celiac trunk and its branches. A lateral projection can be of significant benefit if visualization or easy cannulation of the celiac axis is not achieved. The initial catheterization of the celiac artery can be performed using a variety of selective angled catheters, including Cobra 2; Simmons 1, 2, or 3; Sos Omni, renal double-curved; or RC-2 catheters.

Once the celiac axis is accessed, a celiac angiogram is performed (5-6 mL/sec for 25-36 mL, low rise, 800 psi). A guidewire is advanced into the hepatic artery, GDA, or splenic artery, and after catheter placement a selective angiogram is performed. Once the specific artery is identified, a 0.035-inch wire, a transitional wire, or smaller-profile (down to 0.014-inch) guidewire is used to cross the aneurysm. Once wire traversal is achieved, a longer 45- to 55-cm sheath or guide catheter is placed to improve stability of access for planned intervention. The selection of sheath type and size is based on preprocedural planning and whether a stent-graft or coil embolization is required for treatment. Stent grafts require a sheath of up to 8 Fr, whereas a 5-Fr catheter with a coaxially placed microcatheter may suffice for microcoil embolization. To reduce the possibility of rupture, it is important to maintain distal wire position during the placement of the guiding sheath, without movement into secondary and tertiary branches. The definitive procedure may be initiated once the guiding sheath or catheter is advanced into the splenic or hepatic artery.

ANGIOGRAPHIC IMAGING

Digital subtraction angiography allows multidirectional angiographic acquisitions with a single injection of contrast medium. Three-dimensional rotational angiography is generally used in the anatomic and morphologic assessment of aneurysms.

Endovascular Treatment of Hepatic Artery Aneurysm

HEPATIC ARTERY EMBOLIZATION

Embolization is the accepted treatment for intrahepatic hepatic artery aneurysms. This technique is usually performed using coil embolization. A 3-Fr microcatheter uses the sheath of a normal-sized 5-Fr catheter and is inserted into the aneurysm, followed by deployment of appropriately sized coils. Embolization distal and proximal to the aneurysm should be achieved to prevent reconstitution of the aneurysm from backbleeding from the distal artery because of intrahepatic collaterals. Intrahepatic collaterals may not be seen on the original angiogram and may form later because of the proximal artery embolization. Therefore all hepatic aneurysms should be embolized proximally and distally, if technically feasible. In the central, main hepatic artery, and in main branch hepatic aneurysms, care must be taken to avoid displacement of the coils into the proper hepatic artery and to avoid occlusion of the GDA. This can be achieved by a remodeling technique, which involves placement of an occluding balloon across to the neck of the aneurysm to minimize coil protrusion into the donor artery. When embolizing major branches of the hepatic artery, it is important to be aware of conditions that increase the susceptibility of hepatic parenchyma to ischemia or infarction, including advanced cirrhosis, liver transplants, and hereditary hemorrhagic telangiectasia (Osler-Weber-Rendu disease).

HEPATIC ARTERY STENT PLACEMENT

Stents can be delivered over a 0.014- or 0.018-inch guidewire system, with a preference for balloon-mounted stent grafts, because these are more precisely deployed. Contrast can be given through the guiding sheath to ensure appropriate stent position before deployment. The stent is deployed, and additional overlapping stent grafts may be required to exclude the aneurysm (Fig. 43-1).

Endovascular Treatment of Gastroduodenal and Pancreaticoduodenal Aneurysms

Transarterial catheter embolization is the most common treatment option, and the presence of collateral flow is documented with preoperative imaging. Because of the abundance of collaterals, all upper gastrointestinal arteries should be embolized proximal and distal to the aneurysm. In the case of GDA aneurysms, the entire GDA is embolized from the pancreaticoduodenal arcades to the hepatic artery. Coil embolization remains a common approach; however, deployment of Amplatzer plugs has been described.[23] Celiac artery, superior mesenteric artery, or both types of angiography is required to ensure that no other feeding vessels supply the aneurysm or pseudoaneurysm (Figs. 43-2 and 43-3), especially in the presence of pancreatitis or abdominal trauma.

Stent-graft exclusion is a less feasible treatment option because of smaller and tortuous vessels. Embolization is effective and without ischemic sequelae in most cases. If stent grafts are used, balloon-mounted ones are preferable. Contrast injection through the guiding sheath ensures appropriate position of the covered stent and that there are no overlooked feeding vessels supplying the aneurysm or pseudoaneurysm.

Endovascular Treatment of Splenic Artery Aneurysms

ENDOVASCULAR STRATEGY

Catheter selection for initial access to the splenic artery depends on the patient's anatomy, but most visceral aneurysms can be easily accessed with a selective catheter. Injudicious guidewire advancement can lead to vessel rupture. Therefore the tip of the wire should maintain a fixed position throughout the procedure. Sheath and guidewire compatibility for the intended stent system, as well as balloon compliance and rated burst pressure, should be reviewed during the course of case planning. Special care must be taken to avoid overdilation and rupture the artery.

HEPATIC, GASTRODUODENAL, PANCREATICODUODENAL, AND SPLENIC ARTERY ANEURYSMS 517

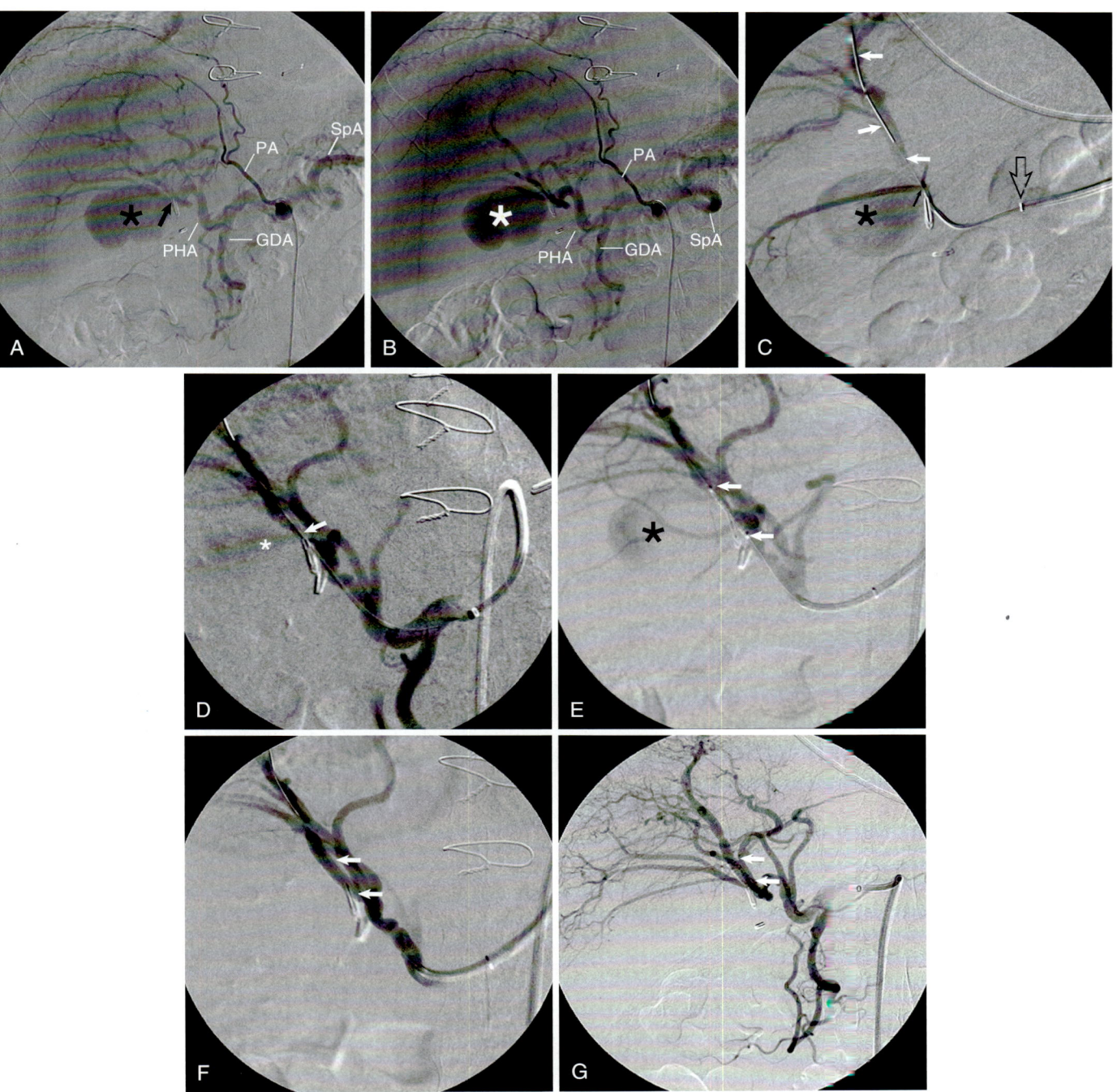

Figure 43-1. Hepatic artery aneurysm stent-graft exclusion. **A** and **B,** The patient is stable after laparoscopic cholecystectomy with intraabdominal bleeding. Two sequential images of an angiogram of the celiac axis through a 5-Fr catheter demonstrate a hepatic artery pseudoaneurysm (*asterisk*) off one of the right hepatic artery branches adjacent to a laparoscopic surgical clip (*arrow*). **C,** Superselective angiogram through a 4-Fr catheter around a 0.018-inch wire (*white arrows*). The solid black arrow points to the site of injury with associated pseudoaneurysm (*asterisk*). The 4-Fr catheter has been coaxially advanced through a 5-Fr sheath (*hollow black arrow*). The 4-Fr catheter helped select the injured arterial branch with the 0.018-inch wire. **D,** An angiogram through the 5-Fr sheath around the 0.018-inch wire. The white arrow points to the site of injury, with contrast jetting out into the pseudoaneurysm (*asterisk*). **E,** An angiogram through the 5-Fr sheath around the 0.018-inch wire. An undeployed stent graft (*between arrows*) is advanced into position over the 0.018-inch wire. Contrast is seen on the more peripheral or lateral wall of the pseudoaneurysm (*asterisk*). **F** and **G,** Two images in series of an angiogram through the 5-Fr sheath after stent-graft (*between arrows*) deployment demonstrating complete exclusion of the pseudoaneurysm. *GDA,* Gastroduodenal artery; *PA,* phrenic artery; *PHA,* proper hepatic artery; *SpA,* splenic artery.

SPLENIC ARTERY EMBOLIZATION

Coil embolization requires positioning a microcatheter in the distal artery and coil occlusion of the outflow tract (Video 43-1). Significant branches of the aneurysm should be coiled before coil exclusion of the aneurysm and the inflow vessel. The splenic artery and its branches should be embolized proximal and distal to the

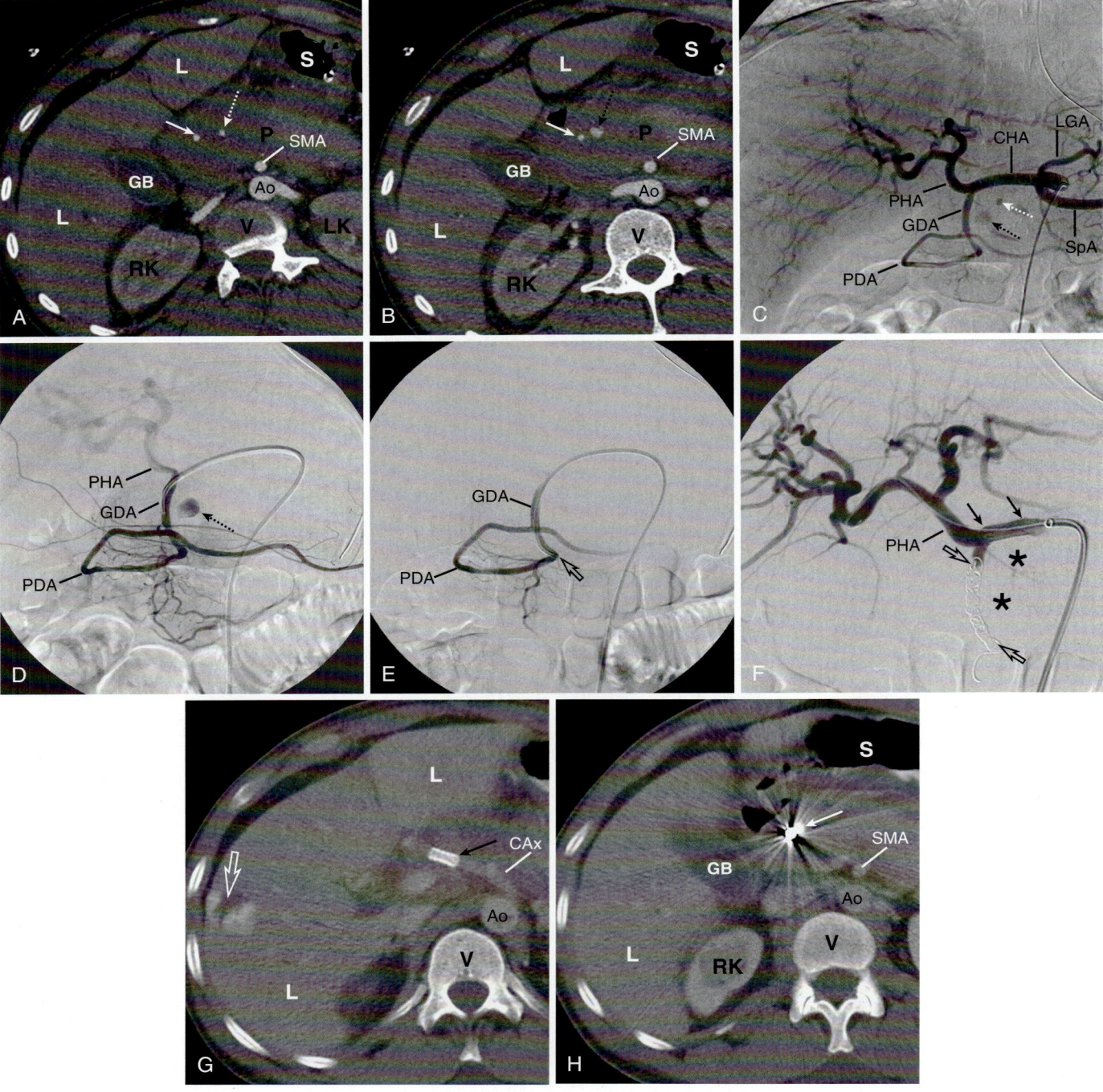

Figure 43-2. Gastroduodenal artery (GDA) embolization with hepatic artery stent-graft placement. **A** and **B,** Axial contrast-enhanced computed tomography (CT) images in sequence (**A** cephalad to **B**) in a patient with focal pancreatitis of the pancreatic head and upper gastrointestinal bleeding. Notice the relatively low attenuation of the pancreatic head and neck compared with the pancreatic body. The pancreas (P) is positioned at the interface between the pancreatic head and the pancreatic body. There are two foci of contrast pooling in the pancreatic head, consistent with two separate pseudoaneurysms. **A,** The smaller pseudoaneurysm (*white dotted arrow*) is just inferior to the common hepatic artery (CHA) and medial to the GDA. **B,** The larger pseudoaneurysm (*black dotted arrow*) is closer to the GDA (*white arrow*). **C,** Angiogram of the celiac axis demonstrating the two foci of contrast pooling in the vicinity of the pancreatic head, consistent with two separate pseudoaneurysms and correlating well with the CT findings (**A** and **B**). Again noted is the smaller, more cephalad pseudoaneurysm (*dotted white arrow*, **A** and **C**) and the larger, more caudad pseudoaneurysm (*dotted black arrow*, **B** and **C**). **D,** Image from a selective angiogram of the GDA demonstrating the GDA pseudoaneurysm (*dotted black arrow*). **E,** Limited selective angiogram of the more distal GDA. The tip of the 5-Fr Cobra 2 catheter (*hollow arrow*) is in the very distal (cephalad) aspect of the GDA. This is the position where the operator has decided to start coil embolizing the GDA from its most caudad aspect, back to the hepatic artery (its most cephalad aspect), and across the origin of the GDA pseudoaneurysm. **F,** Completion angiogram of the CHA after stent-graft placement (*solid arrows*) in the CHA and coil embolization (*hollow arrows*) of the GDA. Both pseudoaneurysms are now treated. The asterisks demarcate their prior locations. The proper hepatic artery (PHA) and its branches are patent. **G** and **H,** Axial contrast-enhanced CT images in sequence (**G** cephalad to **H**) after GDA coil embolization (*white arrow*, **H**) and stent-graft placement (*black arrow*, **G**). Compare with the CT images (**A** and **B**). The hollow arrow points to an incidental finding of a small arterioportal vein fistula, with the resultant enhancement of the parenchyma of the liver region supplied by the involved portal vein branch. *Ao,* Abdominal aorta; *CAx,* celiac axis; *GB,* gallbladder; *L,* liver; *LGA,* left gastric artery; *LK,* left kidney; *RK,* right kidney; *S,* stomach; *SMA,* superior mesenteric artery; *V,* vertebral column.

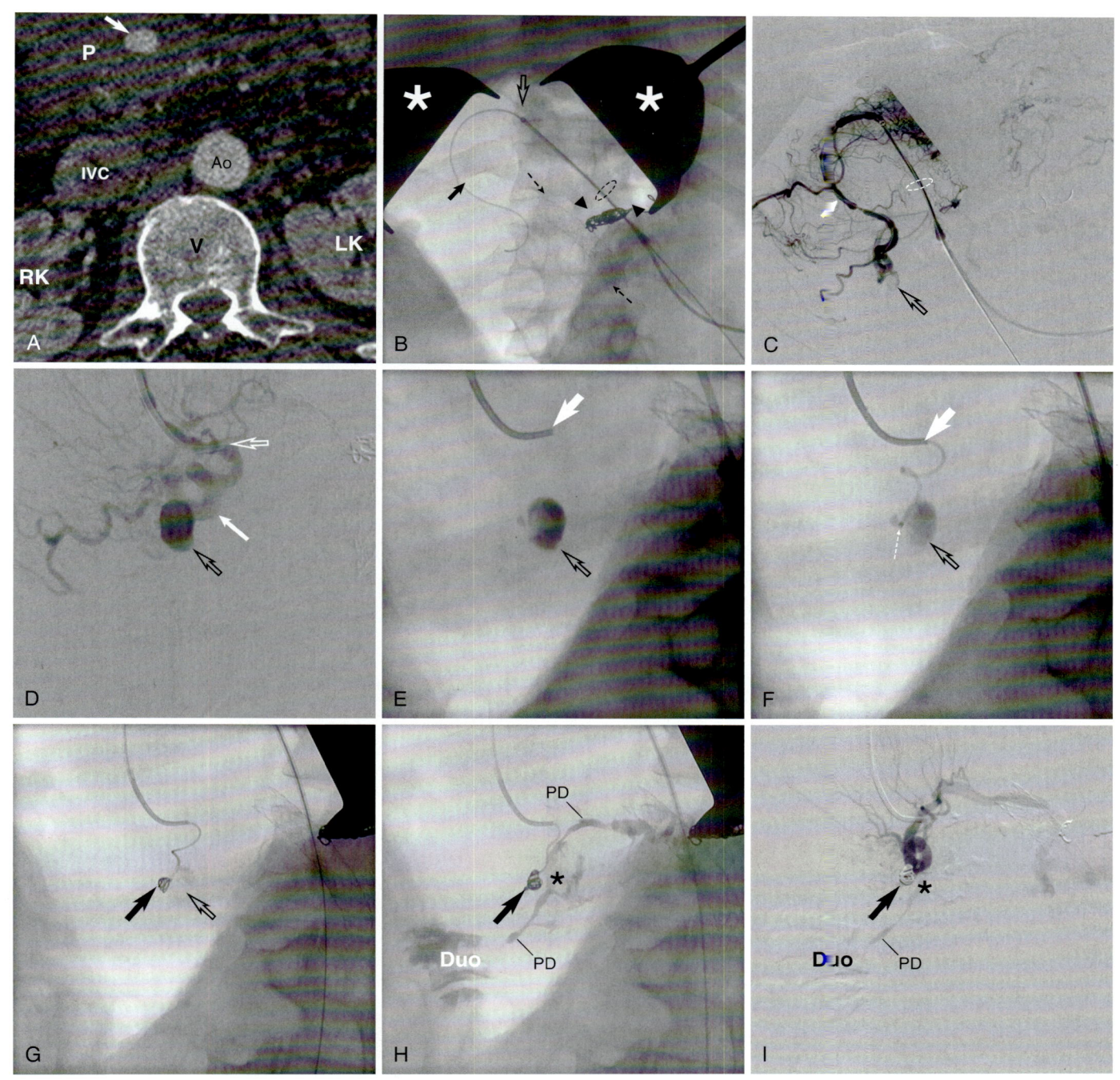

Figure 43-3. Pancreaticoduodenal artery (PDA) embolization with a hybrid procedure (laparotomy, cutdown over vessel, and transcatheter embolization) combined with direct aneurysm puncture and embolization. **A,** Axial contrast-enhanced computed tomography (CT) image in a patient with upper gastrointestinal bleeding. There is a focus of contrast pooling in the pancreatic head, consistent with pancreaticoduodenal pseudoaneurysms (*arrow*). The patient had undergone endovascular management in which coil embolization of the spleen and stent-graft placement across the gastroduodenal artery were performed. However, the patient continued to have gastrointestinal bleeding and a persistent pseudoaneurysm. Multiple endovascular attempts at accessing the pancreaticoduodenal pseudoaneurysm from the superior mesenteric artery side failed. **B,** Fluoroscopic image after an upper abdominal midline incision exposing the distal stomach. Exposure has been gained with retractors (*asterisks*). The gastroepiploic artery has been dissected, isolated, and cannulated by a 5-Fr sheath (*hollow arrow*). The dashed ellipse marks the area where the gastroepiploic artery has been cannulated on the greater curvature of the stomach. A 0.035-inch wire (*solid arrow*) has been passed through the gastroepiploic artery and into the PDAs. The previously placed stent graft (between *dashed arrows*) and the coils in the splenic artery (between *arrowheads*) are noted. **C,** An angiogram through the sheath in the gastroepiploic artery demonstrating the pseudoaneurysm (*hollow arrow*). The dashed ellipse again marks where the gastroepiploic artery has been cannulated, and the solid white arrow indicates the presence of a 5-Fr catheter in the artery. **D,** Magnified angiogram through a 5-Fr catheter (*hollow white arrow*) placed within the gastroepiploic artery (*solid arrow*) demonstrating the pseudoaneurysm (*hollow black arrow*). **E,** Magnified fluoroscopic projection after the angiogram. The image demonstrates persistent contrast pooling in the pseudoaneurysm (*hollow black arrow*). The solid white arrow points to the 5-Fr catheter tip, which is in the gastroepiploic artery. **F,** Magnified fluoroscopic projection during an attempt to catheterize the pseudoaneurysm. A microcatheter (*dashed arrow* at microcatheter tip) is seen at the opening of the pseudoaneurysm. The microcatheter is being passed coaxially through the 5-Fr catheter tip (*solid arrow*). Attempts to access the pseudoaneurysm itself failed. **G** and **H,** Magnified fluoroscopic projection after a microcoil (*solid arrow*) has been deployed in the vessel, leading to the pseudoaneurysm (*hollow arrow*). **H,** Continued contrast injection shows contrast extending into the area of bleeding or focal inflammation and pseudoaneurysm (*asterisk*) amid the pancreatic duct (PD). Contrast is seen emptying into the duodenum (Duo) via the ampulla (*dashed arrow*). **I,** Angiogram from the gastroepiploic artery not demonstrating the pseudoaneurysm. The coils (*arrow*) block the pseudoaneurysm from its cephalad aspect. Coincidentally, contrast is seen passing through the PD and into the Duo. The asterisk marks the area of the pseudoaneurysm, which does not fill with contrast.

Continued

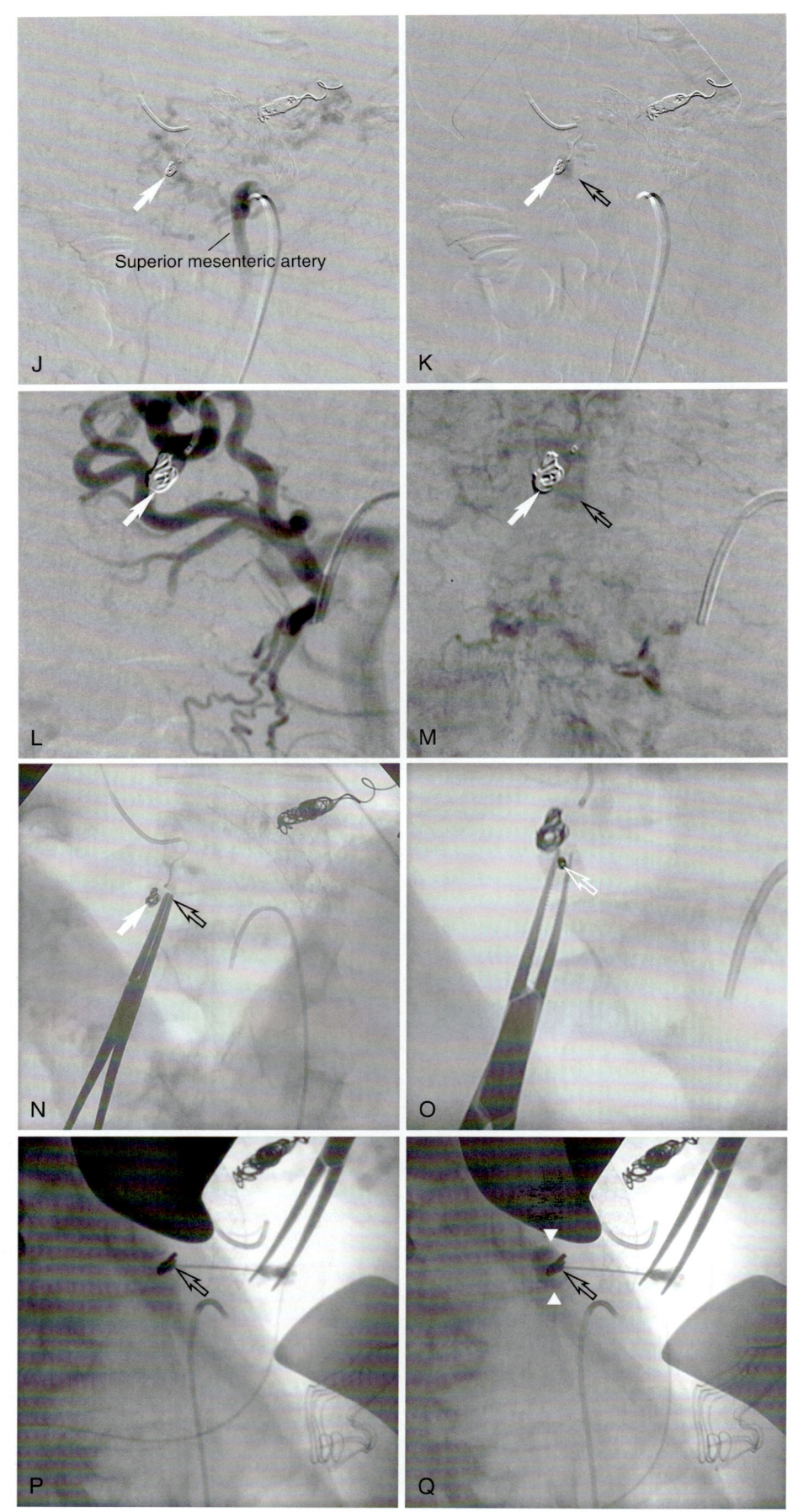

Figure 43-3, cont'd. J and **K,** Two images from an angiogram of the superior mesenteric artery. Newly deployed coils (*white arrows*) are noted on the cephalad side of the pseudoaneurysm (*hollow arrow*, **K**). **L** and **M,** Two magnified views of an angiogram of the superior mesenteric artery. Coils deployed on the cephalad side of the pseudoaneurysm are noted. The pseudoaneurysm (*hollow arrow*) continues to be visualized, especially in the delayed image (**M**). **N-Q,** Four fluoroscopic images in series during a direct needle puncture of the pseudoaneurysm. **N,** First, the operator passes a Kelly clamp so that its tip projects over the pseudoaneurysm (*hollow arrow*). The solid arrow points to the adjacent coils placed by the microcatheter. **O,** Next, a 21-gauge needle is held under fluoroscopy. The needle (*hollow arrow*) is held in the clamp, with its longitudinal axis and shaft running parallel to the image intensifier. **P,** An oblique image is obtained orthogonal to the projection (**O**). This projection helps gauge the depth of the needle as it punctures the pseudoaneurysm. The needle tip (*hollow arrow*) is in the pseudoaneurysm. **Q,** To confirm this, the operator injects contrast through the needle. The image confirms that the needle tip (*hollow arrow*) is in the pseudoaneurysm (between *arrowheads*).

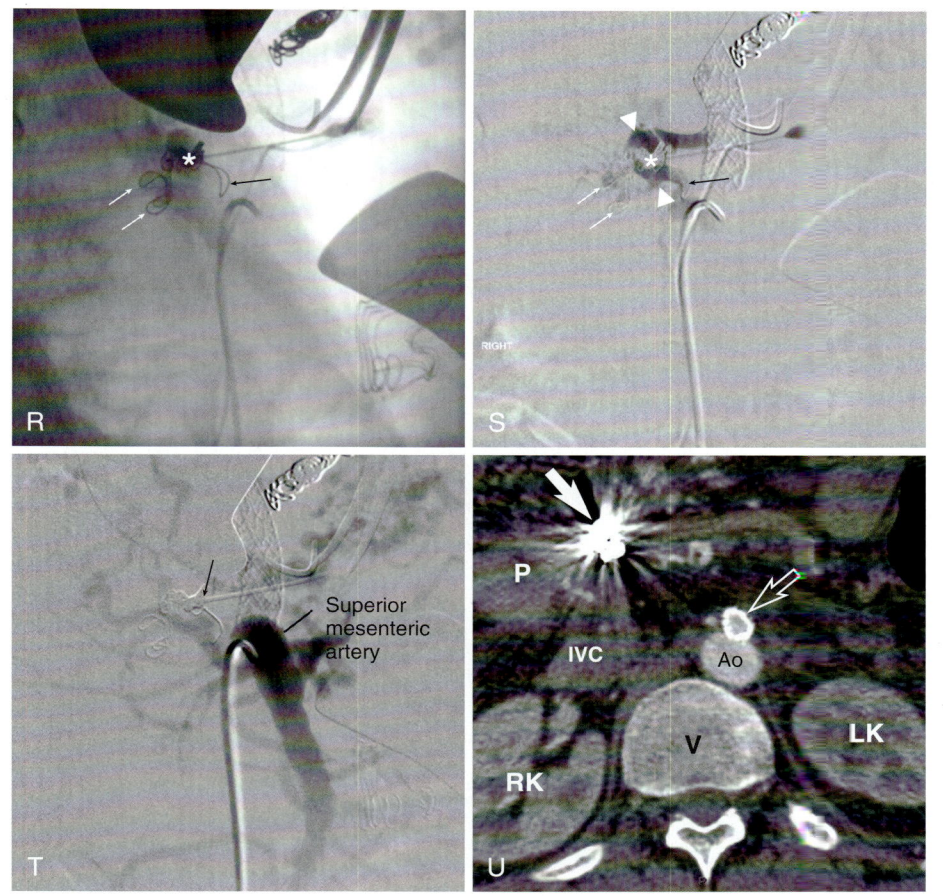

Figure 43-3, cont'd. R and **S,** Two images of the same exact projection and magnification after coil embolization through the direct access needle: a fluoroscopic image (**R**) and a digital subtraction angiogram (**S**) with contrast injected through the needle. The main nest of coils (*asterisk*) is located in the pseudoaneurysm. However, some coil loops extend out of the pseudoaneurysm. One loop extends into the feeding artery (*black arrow*), and that is good. Two loops (*solid white arrows*) extend outside of the pseudoaneurysm and probably outside of the vessels (in the surrounding pancreatic tissue). There is still a residual pseudoaneurysm that has not been obliterated (*arrowheads*). At this point, the operator injected thrombin to obliterate the aneurysm. **T,** Completion angiogram of the superior mesenteric artery. The needle is still in the obliterated pseudoaneurysm (*arrow*). There is no longer filling of the pseudoaneurysm. **U,** Axial contrast-enhanced CT image after pseudoaneurysm obliteration with coils and thrombin (*solid arrow*). The patient had no other upper gastrointestinal bleeding. The hollow arrow points to the celiac axis stent graft placed previously. *IVC,* Inferior vena cava.

aneurysm to prevent retrograde filling from the distal splenic artery branches. Embolic materials include metal coils, *n*-butyl cyanoacrylate, and Onyx (ev3 Endovascular, Plymouth, Minn.). In the presence of portal hypertension, transcatheter embolization may be preferred because of the higher likelihood of collateral vessels.

SPLENIC ARTERY STENT-GRAFT PLACEMENT

Covered stents require a sufficient landing zone proximal and distal to the aneurysm. If there is a branch point off the aneurysm or in the landing zones, coil embolization of the arterial branch is required to ensure that a type II endoleak does not occur. Stent tracking is facilitated by careful positioning of the guiding sheath or catheter. However, celiac axis angulation, splenic arterial tortuosity, and distal aneurysms may pose significant technical challenges. Stent grafts can be positioned over 0.014- or 0.018-inch guidewire systems. If overlapping stent grafts are required to exclude the aneurysm, the smaller-diameter stent graft should be deployed first. As an alternative technique, multiple, overlapping bare metal stents with narrow interstices can be used with or without deployment of coils through the interstices into the aneurysm. This approach is useful in the presence of excessive tortuosity and angulations where the larger and stiffer stent grafts may be more difficult to track (Fig. 43-4).

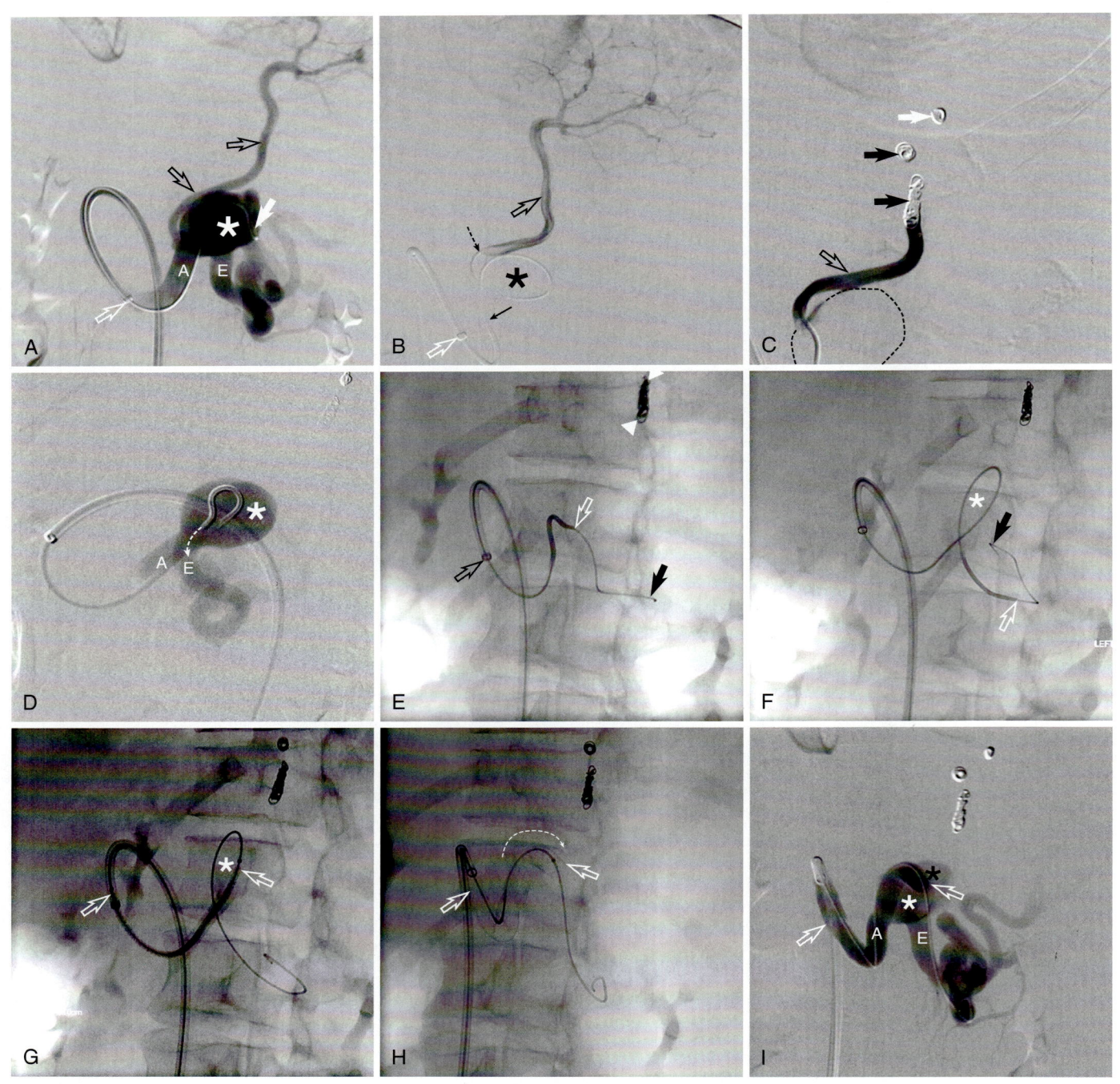

Figure 43-4. Splenic artery aneurysm (SAA) stent-graft exclusion and branch embolization. **A,** Selective splenic artery angiogram through an 8-Fr sheath (*hollow white arrow*) at an oblique projection demonstrating the SAA (*asterisk*) with its afferent limb (A, proximal splenic artery) and its efferent limb (E, distal splenic artery). A 0.035-inch Rosen wire is in the aneurysm maintaining access (*solid white arrow* at wire tip). The superior splenic pole branch (*hollow black arrows*) is seen arising off the most proximal aspect of the aneurysm. **B,** Superselective superior splenic artery branch angiogram through a microcatheter (*dashed black arrow*) placed coaxially through a 5-Fr Cobra 2 catheter (*solid black arrow*). The microcatheter is looped in the aneurysm (*asterisk*). This was technically required to selectively catheterize the superior branch (*hollow black arrow*). Embolizing the branch was necessary to prevent backbleeding (type II) endoleak after stent-graft placement. **C,** Postembolization superior splenic artery branch angiogram through the microcatheter showing successful occlusion (stagnation of the contrast) of the superior splenic artery branch (*hollow arrow*) right at the properly sized coils (*solid black arrow*). Undersized coils are also seen distally (*solid white arrow*). The SAA (*asterisk*) is outlined with a dotted line for orientation. **D,** Limited angiogram through a 5-Fr Omni Flush catheter that is in the aneurysm (*asterisk*). The angiogram shows the sharp, double-backed relationship between A and E limbs of the splenic artery. The sharp reverse-curved catheter (Omni Flush) was chosen to help select the E limb with a Glidewire (*dotted white arrow*). **E,** Fluoroscopic spot image after the 0.035-inch Glidewire (*black arrow*) has been passed through the A limb through the 5-Fr Omni Flush catheter (*hollow white arrow*), which is placed through the 8-Fr sheath. Coils (*between arrowheads*) are noted in the superior pole branch. **F,** Fluoroscopic spot image after exchanging the 5-Fr Omni Flush catheter for a 5-Fr hydrophilic catheter (*hollow white arrow*) over the 0.035-inch Glidewire (*black arrow*). The wire and catheter are looped in the aneurysm (*asterisk*). The loop was not resolved with multiple catheter and wire maneuvers. **G,** Fluoroscopic spot image as a Viabahn (W.L. Gore and Associates, Newark, Del.) stent graft 8 mm in diameter and 10 cm long is advanced into the aneurysm (*asterisk*). The Viabahn stent (*between arrows*) could not be advanced all the way into the E limb. The sharp turn inside the aneurysm impeded the stiff platform (wire and stent delivery system). **H,** Fluoroscopic spot image after the 8-mm Viabahn stent graft has been deployed (*between arrows*) proximally. This "opened up" the angle (*dotted line*) in the aneurysm (see wire angulation in **G** in same projection or image intensifier angle). This is unconventional; when deploying two stents of the same size, the operator usually deploys distally and then proximally across the aneurysm. However, because the stent graft could not be deployed farther, it was deployed with the hope that it would help open the angle and facilitate placement of a more distally placed stent graft. **I,** Digitally subtracted angiogram through the 8-Fr vascular sheath. The stent graft is fully deployed (*between hollow arrows*). The aneurysm (*asterisk*) is not completely excluded. The stent graft covers the A limb and does not bridge to the E limb.

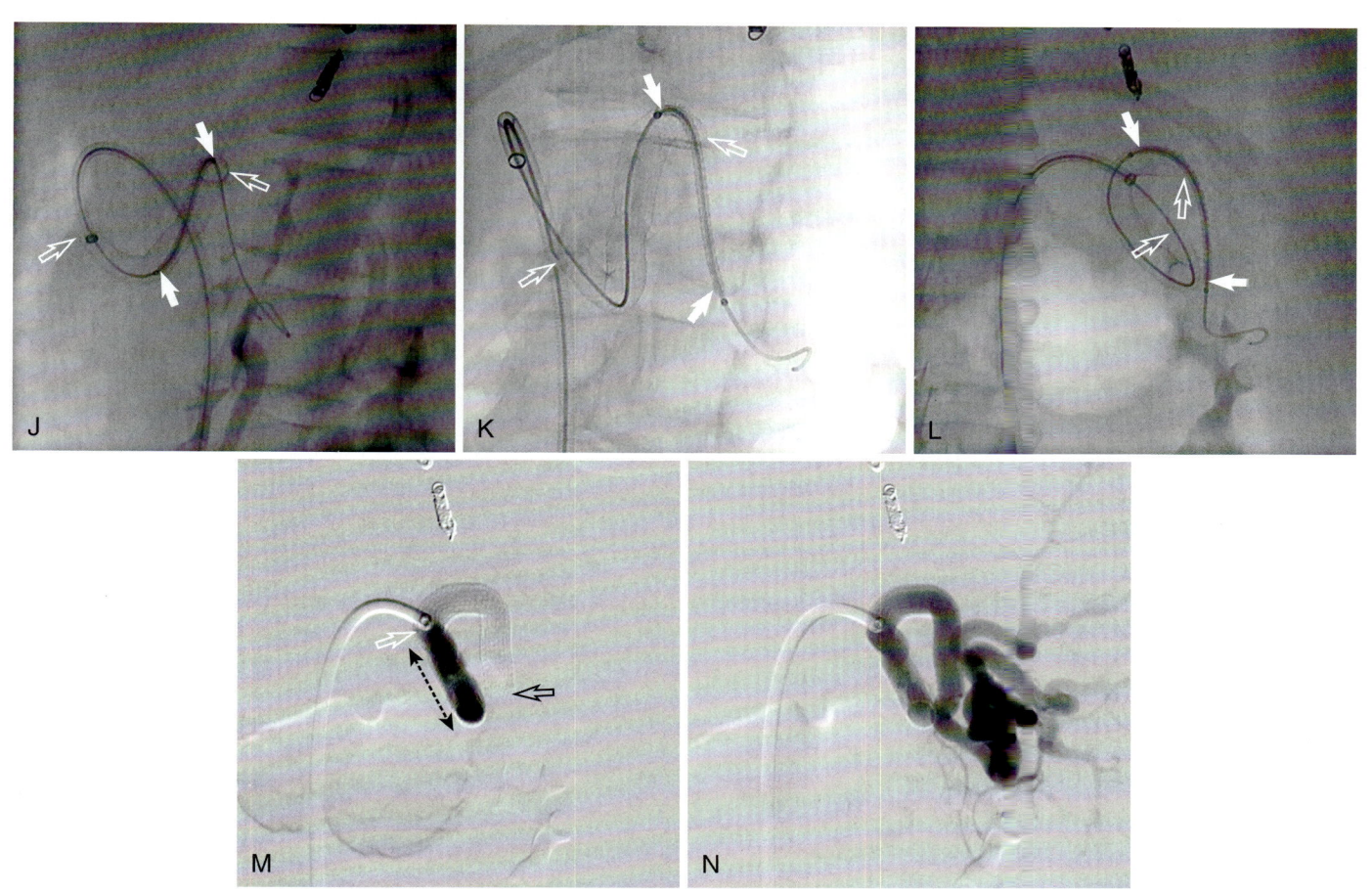

HEPATIC, GASTRODUODENAL, PANCREATICODUODENAL, AND SPLENIC ARTERY ANEURYSMS 523

Figure 43-4, cont'd. J-L, Sequential fluoroscopic spot images as a second 8 mm × 5 cm Viabahn stent graft (between *solid arrows*) is advanced coaxially through the deployed 8 mm × 10 cm proximal Viabahn (between *hollow arrows*). **M** and **N,** Sequential images after the second 8 mm × 5 cm Viabahn stent graft has been deployed, excluding the splenic aneurysm. **M,** The bidirectional dashed arrow runs along the double-backed proximal stent graft. The distal stent graft lies between the hollow arrows. **N,** The aneurysm is completely excluded, and the stent grafts bridge the splenic artery from its A to E limbs relative to the aneurysm.

COMPLETION ANGIOGRAM

After aneurysm exclusion and before removal of the guidewire and sheath, a completion angiogram is performed. A small volume of contrast administered via hand injection through the sheath may be warranted. However, these images have less detail when compared with a flush aortogram or a formal celiac angiogram. If a flush aortogram is indicated, it is preferable to use a tandem wire technique to maintain wire access across the recently stented lesion. The sheath is withdrawn into the infrarenal aorta while maintaining the guidewire position across the stented segment of splenic artery, and a second wire is advanced into the supradiaphragmatic aorta. Over the second wire and through the guide sheath, a 4-Fr pigtail catheter is placed in the suprarenal position. A power injection is performed. If secondary intervention is indicated, the 0.014- or 0.018-inch wire that remains in its original position is used to cross the lesion.

Postoperative Care

- Serial postoperative imaging with duplex ultrasound or CT scanning should be obtained at 1, 6, and 12 months to confirm durable exclusion or obliteration of blood flow within the aneurysm with the absence of end-organ ischemia.
- Duplex ultrasound or CT scan imaging should be obtained annually.

REFERENCES

1. O'Driscoll D, Olliff SP, Olliff JFC: Hepatic artery aneurysm, *Br J Radiol* 72:1018-1025, 1999.
2. Guida PM, Moore SW: Aneurysm of the hepatic artery: Report of five cases with brief review of the previously reported cases, *Surgery* 60:299-310, 1966.
3. Lumsden AB, Mattar SG, Allen RC, et al: Hepatic artery aneurysms: The management of 22 patients, *J Surg Res* 60:345-350, 1996.
4. Countryman D, Norwood S, Register D, et al: Hepatic artery aneurysm: Report of an unusual case and review of the literature, *Am Surg* 49:51-54, 1983.
5. Abbas MA, Fowl RJ, Stone WM, et al: Hepatic artery aneurysm: Factors that predict complications, *J Vasc Surg* 38:41-45, 2003.
6. Shanley CJ, Shah NL, Messina L: Common splanchnic artery aneurysm: Splenic, hepatic and celiac, *Ann Vasc Surg* 10:315-322, 1996.
7. Ferguson F: Aneurysm of the superior pancreaticoduodenal artery, *Proc NY Pathol Soc* 24:45-49, 1895.
8. Chong WW, Tan SG, Htoo MM: Endovascular treatment of gastroduodenal artery aneurysm, *Asian Cardiovasc Thorac Ann* 16:68-72, 2008.
9. Ducasse E, Roy F, Chevalier J, et al: Aneurysm of the pancreaticoduodenal arteries with a celiac trunk lesion: Current management, *J Vasc Surg* 39:906-911, 2004.
10. Beaussier M: Sur un aneurisme de l'artere splenique dont les parois se sont ossifiees, *J Med Clin et Pharm Paris* 32:157, 1770.
11. Stanley JC, Thompson NW, Fry WJ: Splanchnic artery aneurysm, *Arch Surg* 101:689-697, 1970.
12. Messina LM, Shanley CJ: Visceral artery aneurysms, *Surg Clin North Am* 77:425-442, 1997.
13. Carr SC, Pearce WH, Vogelzang RL, et al: Current management of visceral artery aneurysms, *Surgery* 120:627-633, 1996.
14. Trastek VF, Pairolero PC, Joyce JW, et al: Splenic artery aneurysm, *Surgery* 91:694-699, 1982.
15. Abbas MA, Stone WM, Fowl RJ, et al: Splenic artery aneurysm: Two decades experience at Mayo Clinic, *Ann Vasc Surg* 16:442-449, 2002.
16. Lee PC, Rhee RY, Gordon RY, et al: Management of splenic artery aneurysm: The significance of portal and essential hypertension, *J Am Coll Surg* 189:483-490, 1999.
17. Tazawa K, Shimoda M, Nagata T, et al: Splenic artery aneurysm associated with systemic lupus erythematosus: Report of a case, *Surg Today* 29:76-79, 1999.
18. Tessier DJ, Stone WM, Fowl RJ, et al: Clinical features and management of splenic artery pseudoaneurysm: Case series and cumulative review of the literature, *J Vasc Surg* 38:969-974, 2003.
19. Busuttil RW, Brin BJ: The diagnosis and management of visceral aneurysm, *Surgery* 88:619-624, 1980.
20. Kobori L, Van der Kolk MJ, de Jong KP, et al: Liver Transplant Group. Splenic artery aneurysm in liver transplant patients, *J Hepatol* 27:890-893, 1997.
21. Takao H, Nojo T, Ohtomo K: True pancreaticoduodenal artery aneurysms: A decision analysis, *Eur J Radiol* 75:110-113, 2010.
22. Katsura M, Gushimiyagi M, Takara H, et al: True aneurysm of the pancreaticoduodenal arteries: A single institution experience, *J Gastrointest Surg* 14:1409-1413, 2010.
23. Pech M, Kraetsch A, Wieners G, et al: Embolization of the gastroduodenal artery before selective internal radiotherapy: A prospectively randomized trial comparing platinum-fibered microcoils with the Amplatzer Vascular Plug II, *Cardiovasc Intervent Radiol* 32:455-461, 2009.

Section 10

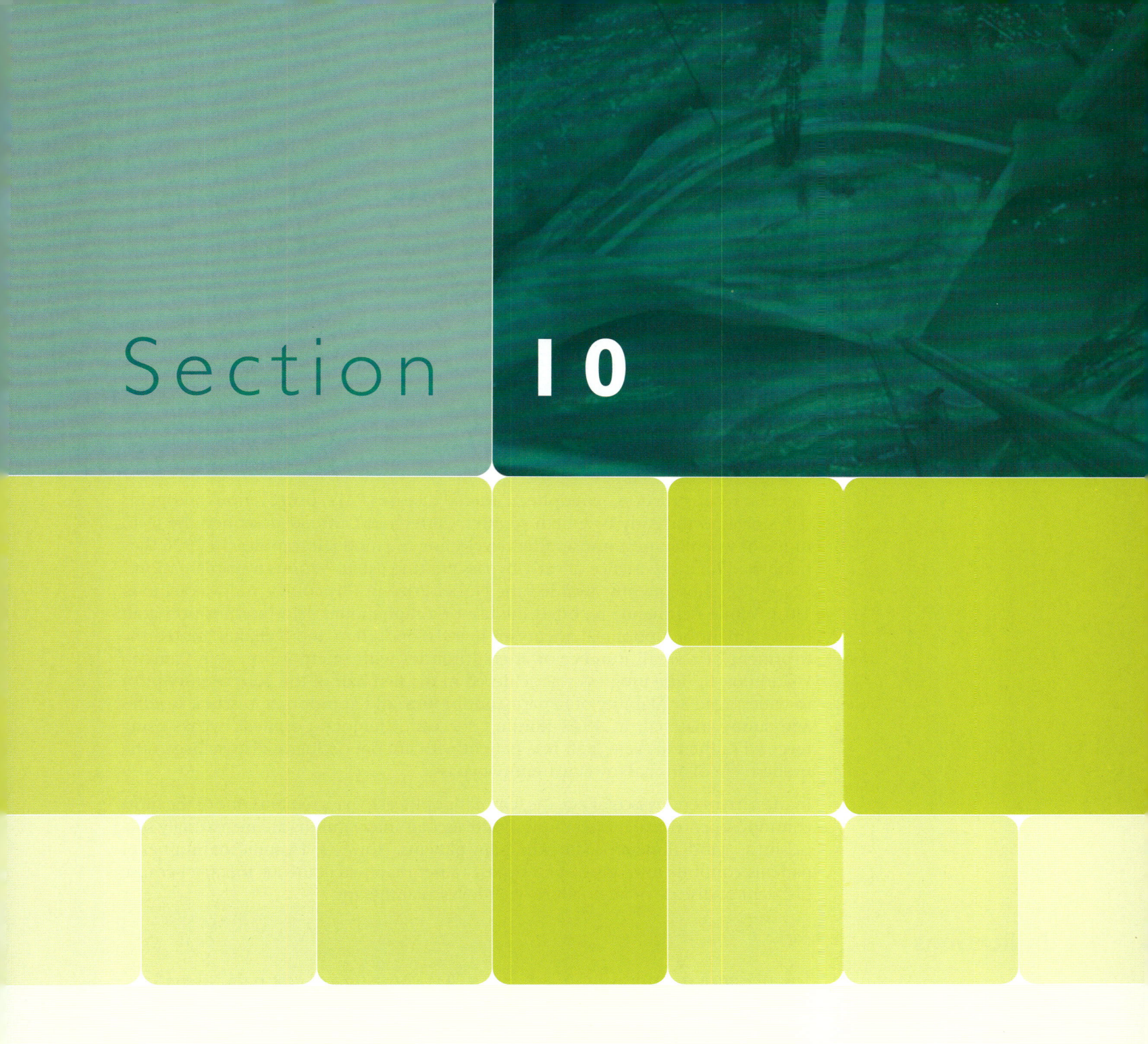

LOWER EXTREMITY ARTERIAL DISEASE

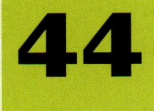

44 Open Surgical Bypass of Femoral-Popliteal Arterial Occlusive Disease

LAYLA C. LUCAS • KAORU R. GOSHIMA • JOSEPH L. MILLS, SR.

Historical Background

Vascular reconstruction of peripheral arterial disease (PAD) using venous autografts dates back to the early twentieth century. Carrel and Guthrie[1] described the technique of vascular anastomosis after developing the model in canines. In 1906 they published their experience of early bypass grafting using "venous transplantation." Carrel was subsequently awarded the Nobel Prize in Physiology and Medicine in 1912. While Bernheim[2] reported the use of a saphenoues vein interposition graft for treatment of a popliteal aneurysm in 1916 and Elkin and DeBakey[3] noted the treatment of a small number of arterial injuries with interposition vein grafts in World War II, little progress was achieved in the first half of the 20th century prior to widespread availability of heparin, antibiotics, and appropriate vascular needles and suture material. In 1948 Kunlin's successful femoral-popliteal bypass using reversed saphenous vein graft in a patient with arterial occlusive disease began the modern era of arterial lower extremity bypass.[4]

In the current endovascular era, the femoral-popliteal bypass remains one of the most common open vascular operations. Endovascular interventions are increasingly successful as stand-alone procedures in many patients. However, a significant number of patients continue to require open bypass rather than percutaneous therapy because of extent of disease or after failure of endovascular therapy.

Indications

The presence of critical limb ischemia (CLI) consisting of rest pain, tissue loss, or gangrene is a mandatory indication for intervention, whereas lifestyle-limiting intermittent claudication is a relative indication for intervention.

Preoperative Preparation

- **History and physical examination.** A complete history and a physical examination usually establish PAD as the source of symptoms. Patients with intermittent claudication typically describe exertional, muscular pain in the calves, thighs, or buttocks that is burning or cramping, resolves with rest, and is reproducible at a specific distance. Nocturnal pain, commonly in the forefoot, that occurs with the leg flat or elevated and resolves after placing the limb in a dependent position is typical of ischemic rest pain. Patients with CLI have symptoms including rest pain, tissue loss, or gangrene or develop nonhealing ulcers that arise spontaneously or after minor trauma. Gangrene is a late sign of CLI. PAD patients also often have a personal and family history of cardiovascular, cerebrovascular, or both diseases. Pertinent physical findings include absent pulses, trophic changes, and often, dependent rubor and pallor on elevation. Gangrene and nonhealing ulcers typically appear on the toes, forefoot, or areas of foot trauma.

- **Noninvasive vascular laboratory testing.** Vascular laboratory studies are required to confirm the degree of limb ischemia, determine the anatomic site or sites of involvement, and differentiate stenotic lesions from total occlusions. An ankle-brachial index (ABI) of less than 0.9 is diagnostic for hemodynamically significant occlusive disease and has been found to be 95% sensitive in identifying angiographically confirmed PAD.[5] Claudicants with proximal PAD may only show a reduction in ABI after exercise. A 20% or greater reduction in ABI after exercise is abnormal.[6] Arterial waveform patterns, toe waveforms and Doppler-derived pressures, and transcutaneous oxygen saturations are useful when the ABI cannot be measured because of incompressibility of calcified vessels (suprasystolic ABI), a frequent finding in individuals with diabetes mellitus or renal failure. Arterial duplex demonstrates sites of arterial occlusion or stenosis with color flow changes (mosaic color pattern) and elevated peak systolic velocities.

- **Imaging studies.** In patients who have diminished or absent femoral pulses, computed tomography or magnetic resonance imaging defines the length and extent of aortoiliac disease, factors with important implications in selecting the optimal intervention. Percutaneous angiography is the final step in assessing the anatomy of the arterial supply to the lower extremities, either serving as the immediate prelude to endovascular therapy or providing a road map for open bypass.

- **Cardiovascular risk factor modification.** PAD is a manifestation of a systemic disease process that affects the arterial circulation throughout the body. The incidence of nonfatal myocardial infarction, stroke, and vascular death is reported to be 5% to 7% per year for PAD patients.[7] Mortality in patients with PAD averages 2% per year.[7] PAD should be considered a coronary artery disease equivalent. Optimizing medical therapy is mandatory in all PAD patients, regardless of whether intervention is planned, and consists of risk factor modification to halt the progression of arterial disease not only in the lower extremities but in the body as a whole. Trans-Atlantic Inter-Society Consensus document II regarding the treatment of PAD outlines evidence-based recommendations for the medical management of PAD risk factors.[7] Smoking is an independent risk factor for PAD development and progression. Smokers are three to five times more likely to have an amputation than are nonsmokers. Tobacco cessation rates can be improved with physician advice, group counseling, nicotine replacement, and a variety of pharmacologic adjuncts. Hyperlipidemia, a common independent risk factor for PAD, is preferentially controlled with a statin drug and dietary modification. Goals to achieve are a low-density lipoprotein level of less than 70 mg/dL in patients with coronary disease and a level of less than 100 mg/dL in those without. Fibrates, niacin, or both are useful in raising high-density lipoprotein levels and lowering triglyceride levels. Elevated serum homocysteine levels can be lowered with dietary supplementation of vitamin B_{12}, vitamin B_6, and folate, although beneficial effects of such therapy on PAD are not well substantiated. Hypertension is an additional strong risk factor for PAD. Blood pressure control can reduce PAD events by 22% to 26%, as well as significantly reduce the subsequent occurrence of cardiovascular and cerebrovascular events.

- **Diabetes management.** Large-scale studies[8] have shown that intensive diabetes management reduces diabetes-related myocardial infarcts and other diabetes-related endpoints. The target hemoglobin A1c is less than 7.0%.

- **Antiplatelet therapy.** Antiplatelet therapy is a mainstay in the reduction of future cardiovascular and cerebrovascular events. Patients with cardiovascular disease experience a 25% odds reduction in further cardiovascular events by taking daily aspirin.

- **Cardiopulmonary status.** A chest radiograph and electrocardiogram should be performed as part of the preoperative evaluation. Further cardiopulmonary evaluation or optimization is recommended if the patient has unstable angina, significant arrhythmias, or symptoms of congestive heart failure or shortness of breath.

Pitfalls and Danger Points

- **Inadequate vein conduit.** Most vein conduit problems can be anticipated preoperatively if proper duplex vein mapping is performed. When vein problems are encountered unexpectedly during the intraoperative preparation of the vein, options are available to preserve the vein graft conduit. If a focal vein abnormality is found, it may be resected and a venovenostomy may be performed. Care is taken to spatulate the ends to create a wide anastomosis. If long segments of the vein are unusable, consideration should be given to harvesting from an alternate site: the contralateral great saphenous vein, the small saphenous vein, or spliced arm veins. Creating the proximal anastomosis to the profunda femoris artery or superficial femoral artery can allow utilization of shorter segments of vein.

- **Small-caliber vein.** At times, there is a size mismatch between the small-caliber reversed vein and a larger, thick-walled artery at the proximal anastomosis. If possible, a large branch at the distal end of the great saphenous vein should be preserved during harvest (Fig. 44-1, A). The venotomy can incorporate this branch to create a heel that sits away from the artery. Anastomosis of the vein graft to a Linton vein patch can also remedy a size mismatch, particularly if an endarterectomy has been performed.

- **Unexpected inflow disease.** Perioperative angiography helps the surgeon anticipate the presence of inflow disease. Atherosclerotic disease of the common femoral artery and profunda femoris artery can be addressed with an endarterectomy. This may entail partial division of the inguinal ligament to allow

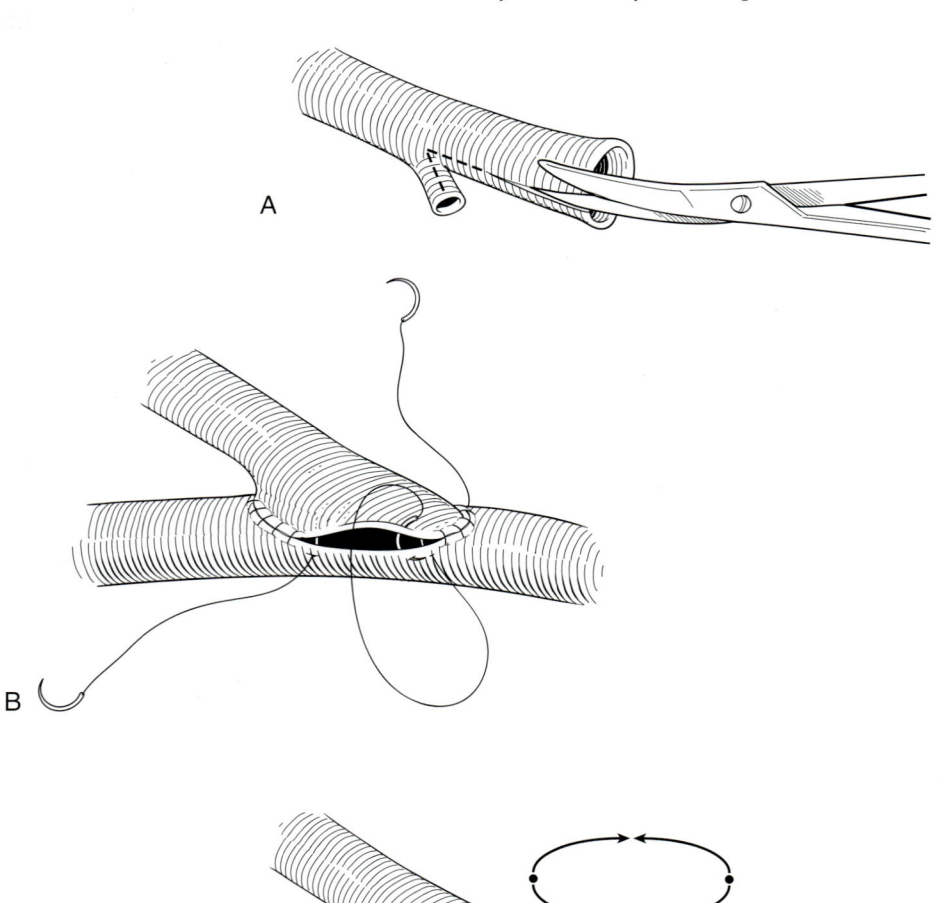

Figure 44-1. A, A vein tributary is incorporated into the venotomy to create a wider and slightly elevated anastomosis. This help prevents stenosis at heel of the graft. **B,** The first suture typically begins at the heel. The sutures are sewn continuously to a point halfway along the anastomosis, and then the second suture is started at the toe and sewn to the first suture. **C,** The two sutures are sewn continuously toward each other. The use of two separate sutures ensures symmetry and prevents "purse stringing," as noted in the circular schematic.

clamp placement on the nondiseased external iliac artery. A long venotomy can be used for the anastomosis if the conduit is of adequate caliber. Otherwise, the arteriotomy may require a vein patch with subsequent anastomosis of the bypass conduit to the patch. Alternatively, a segment of occluded superficial femoral artery can be endarterectomized and used to patch the arteriotomy.

- **Unexpected outflow disease.** The distal target for a femoral-popliteal bypass graft is an area free of disease with at least one continuous runoff artery to the foot. Unexpected hemodynamically significant popliteal disease may require direct bypass to more distal tibial or pedal target vessels. Intraoperative angiography is used to locate the most proximal segment of tibial or peroneal artery that is continuous with the foot. The distal bypass is performed to this site. Sequential bypass is useful for situations in which an isolated patent popliteal artery exists between severely diseased superficial femoral artery and proximal tibial arteries. A bypass graft from the thigh is connected to the proximal portion of the popliteal island. A separate bypass graft uses the distal popliteal segment as inflow and connects to a tibial or pedal vessel that has continuity with the foot. The advantage of this technique is that it allows shorter bypass segments and avoids creation of long, spliced vein conduits.

- **Tunneling problems.** It is recommended that an experienced member of the operative team perform the tunneling of the conduit. Passing the conduit through a large-bore tunneler protects it from tearing or shearing as it is pulled into place. Tunneling should always be undertaken along muscles and not through dense fascia or the belly of a muscle. The vein conduit should always be fully distended as it is passed through the tunnel to avoid twisting and kinking. After tunneling, if the proximal anastomosis has not yet been constructed, irrigation through the proximal end of the graft should produce vigorous flow through the distal anastomosis. Upon completion of the proximal anastomosis, the graft should have pulsatile flow. If not observed, the graft should be retunneled.

- **Anastomotic stenosis.** Prevention is the key to avoiding anastomotic stenoses. Diligence in tailoring the graft during the anastomosis often precludes this problem. When a size mismatch exists between the vein conduit and the artery, branches of the vein graft should be incorporated into the venotomy or a modified Linton patch should be used. Adequate vein length should always be measured with the knee extended before tailoring the vein for the distal anastomosis, because tension on the vein either proximally or distally results in vein stenosis just distal or proximal to the anastomosis. Clamp injury of the artery may also result in an anastomotic stenosis by plaque disruption. Completion angiography, intraoperative Doppler, or duplex ultrasound identifies anastomotic stenoses that occur despite careful operative technique. If a stenosis occurs, the anastomosis is examined and the trapped adventitia is freed or disrupted plaque is excised or tacked down. If this does not help, the heel of the graft requires a vein patch to widen the anastomosis.

- **Reoperative bypass.** The reoperative bypass is a taxing, time-consuming operation, even for the most experienced surgeon. In general, all efforts are taken to use autogenous vein to provide optimal long-term patency. Meticulous preparation of the conduit is paramount, especially if the primary bypass failed because of technical error. If possible, the surgeon should avoid previously operated fields and consider alternative inflow and outflow sources; these approaches may require exposure of the distal profunda femoris artery, the superficial femoral artery, and tibial or pedal vessels.

Operative Strategy

SURGICAL ANATOMY OF THE FEMORAL AND POPLITEAL ARTERIES

The femoral triangle is the anatomic space bordered by the inguinal ligament superiorly, the sartorius muscle laterally, and the adductor magnus muscle medially

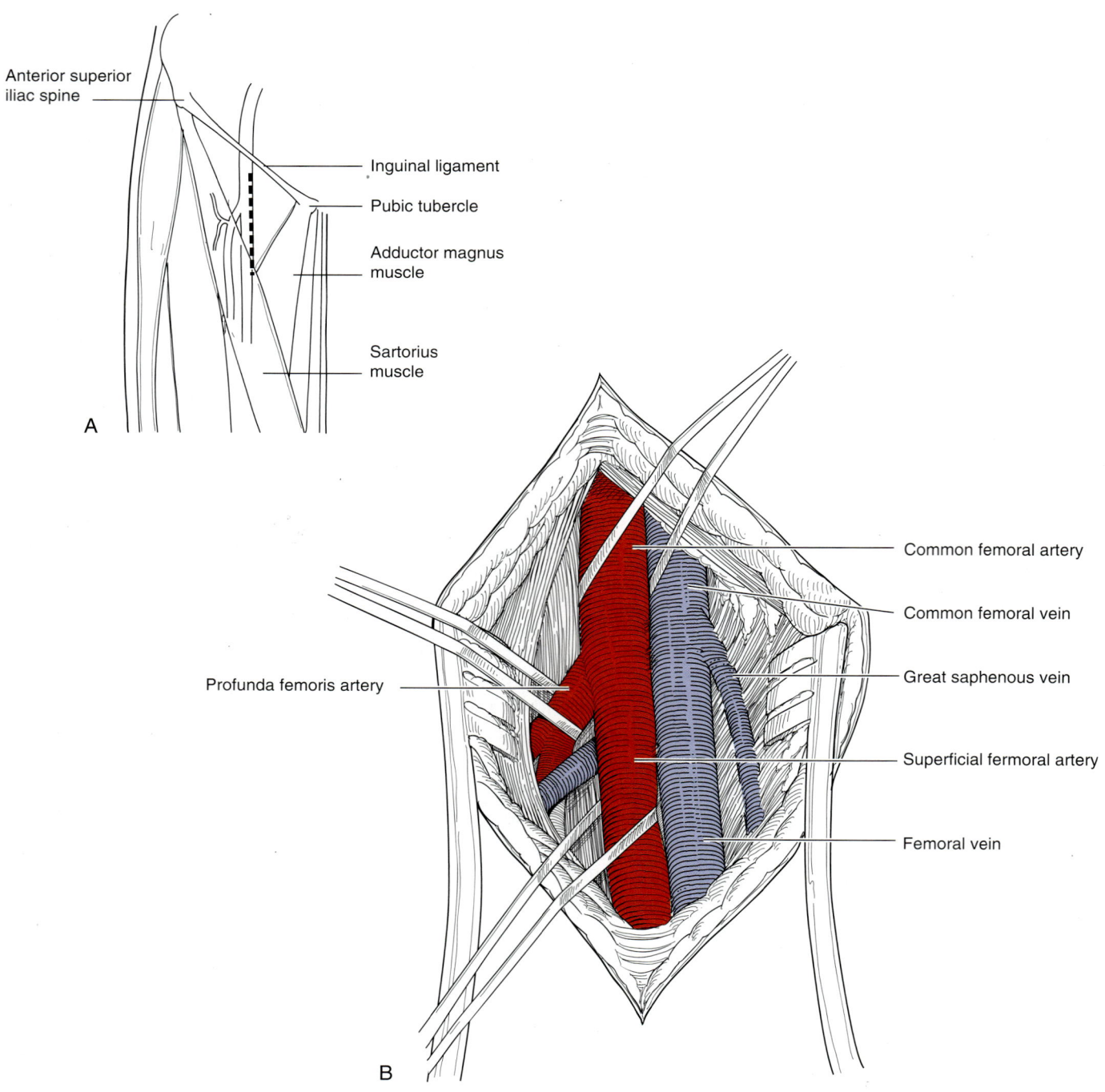

Figure 44-2. A, The femoral triangle is bordered by the inguinal ligament and the adductor magnus and sartorius muscles. The dashed line is the proposed skin incision for exposure of the common femoral artery and proximal superficial fermoral artery and profunda femoris artery. **B,** The common femoral artery lies laterally to the common femoral vein. The profunda femoris artery exits posterolaterally. The great saphenous vein enters anteromedially.

(Fig. 44-2, *A*). The floor of the femoral triangle contains four muscles: the iliacus, psoas major, pectineus, and adductor magnus. A fascial covering called the femoral sheath contains the major vascular structures in the femoral triangle. The common femoral artery is the continuation of the external iliac artery below the inguinal ligament. In the femoral triangle, the common femoral artery divides into two major branches (Fig. 44-2, *B*). The profunda femoris artery is most commonly a posterolateral branch, not only providing blood to the thigh but also serving as the major collateral to the lower extremity in patients with occlusion of the superficial femoral artery. The superficial femoral artery is the continuation of the common femoral artery and carries blood to the lower leg. Exiting the femoral triangle, the superficial femoral artery proceeds distally on its course into the adductor canal.

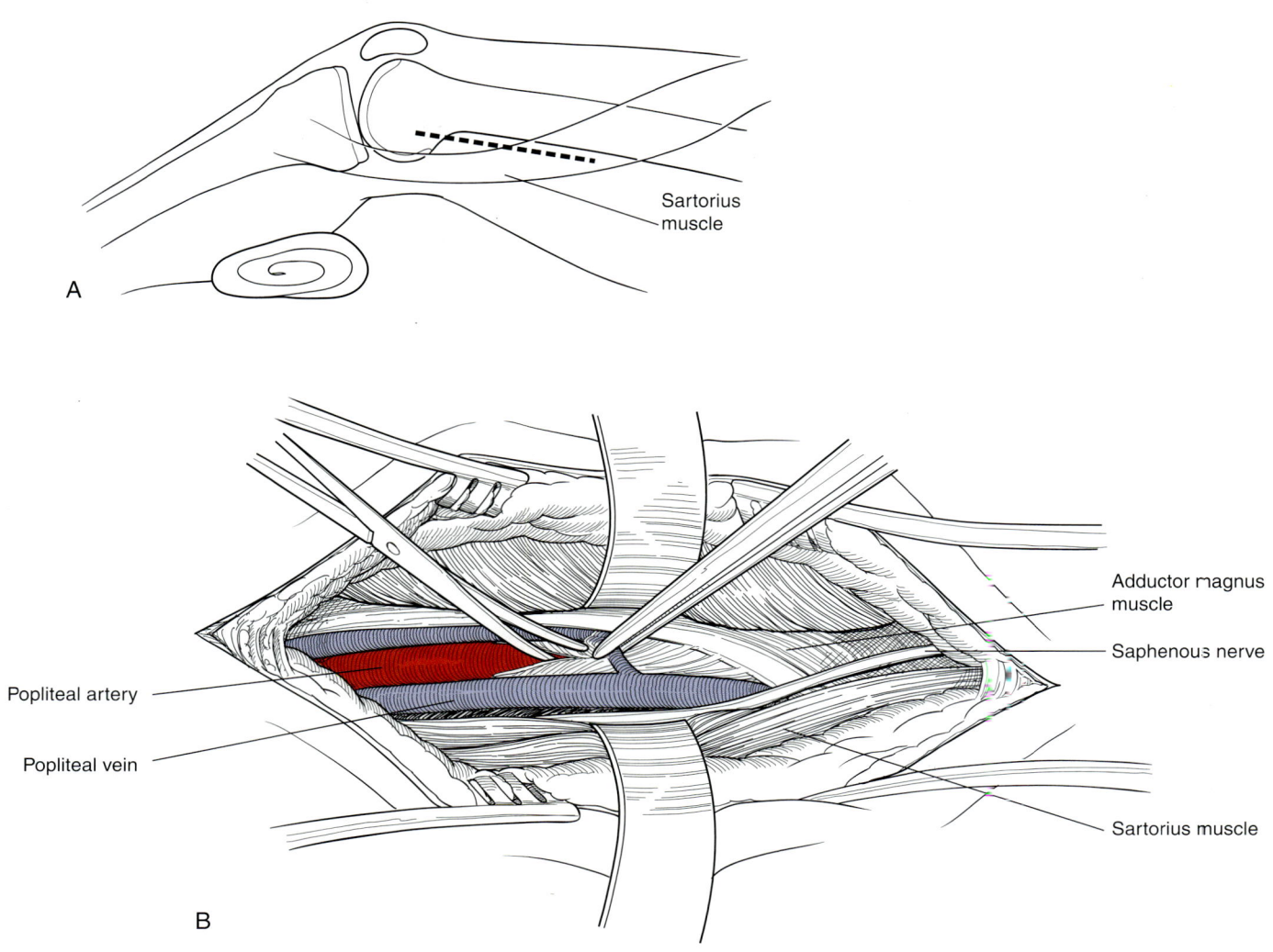

OPEN SURGICAL BYPASS OF FEMORAL-POPLITEAL ARTERIAL OCCLUSIVE DISEASE   531

Figure 44-3. A, The dashed line anterior to the sartorius muscle marks the skin incision for exposure of the above-knee popliteal artery. Placing a stack of towels beneath the knee facilitates this exposure. **B,** The above-knee popliteal artery is seen exiting the adductor magnus tendon (Hunter canal). The popliteal artery is encased in a fibrous sheath and closely surrounded by paired popliteal veins.

The common femoral vein is located just medially to the common femoral artery in the triangle (Fig. 44-2, *B*). The great saphenous vein enters the common femoral vein at the fossa ovalis. Other important structures in the femoral triangle include the femoral nerve. The nerve is lateral to the artery and provides motor and sensory function primarily to the thigh. Medial to the common femoral vein are the lymphatic structures draining interstitial fluid from the leg.

The popliteal fossa is another anatomic area of significance in lower extremity revascularization. It is a diamond-shaped space defined anteriorly by the femur, upper tibia, and popliteus muscle; posteriorly by the skin, subcutaneous tissue, and fascia; laterally by biceps femoris and gastrocnemius muscles; and medially by semitendinosus and semimembranosus muscles. Figures 44-3 and 44-4 illustrate the common surgical exposures for the above- and below-knee portions of the popliteal artery, respectively. The superficial femoral artery exits the adductor canal at the apex of the popliteal fossa, where it becomes the popliteal artery. Paired popliteal veins are closely adjacent. Below the knee, at variable areas in the distal popliteal fossa, the popliteal artery divides into the anterior tibial artery and the tibioperoneal trunk. The anterior tibial artery exits laterally above the interosseous membrane and enters the anterior compartment of the lower leg. The tibioperoneal trunk continues and divides into the posterior tibial artery and the peroneal artery. These two vessels enter the deep posterior compartment of the lower leg.

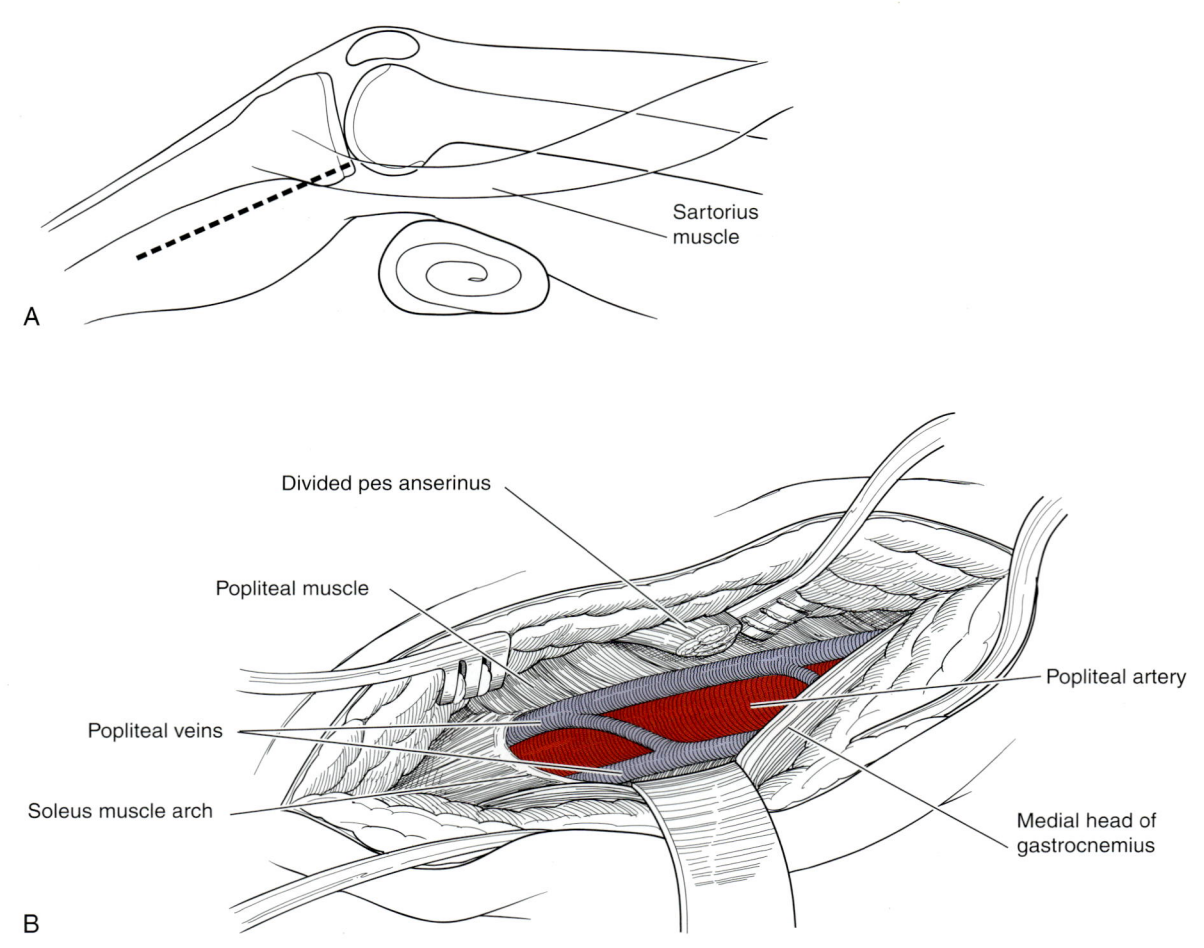

Figure 44-4. A, The dashed line marks the skin incision for exposure of the below-knee popliteal artery. The same incision is used for harvesting the great saphenous vein in this location. **B,** The popliteal fossa below the knee is exposed by dividing the fascia and mobilizing the medial head of the gastrocnemius muscle posteriorly. The pes anserinus tendon, which is the conjoined tendon of the sartorius, gracilis, and semitendinosus muscles that inserts on the anteromedial surface of the tibia, may be divided to facilitate this exposure. The popliteal artery is closely surrounded by paired popliteal veins. Care is taken not to injure the tibial nerve.

SELECTION AND ASSESSMENT OF INFLOW

The inflow target for femoral-popliteal bypass is selected preoperatively by imaging studies or on-table angiography. Hemodynamically significant inflow lesions of the iliac arteries should be addressed before or in conjunction with an infrainguinal bypass procedure. Typically, the common femoral artery is the inflow vessel of choice for bypass, although distal origin sites, when appropriately selected, are equally effective, especially if vein conduit is limited. If the common femoral artery exhibits significant atherosclerotic disease, consideration of common femoral artery endarterectomy, to include the profunda femoris artery origin if it is also involved, is a prudent adjunct. Access to the common femoral artery may be prohibitive in reoperative procedures or obese patients. The profunda femoris artery or superficial femoral artery can often serve as an alternate inflow source.

SELECTION AND ASSESSMENT OF OUTFLOW

The distal target vessel in a femoral-popliteal bypass should be of normal caliber, free of stenosis, and continuous with at least one of the arteries supplying the foot. The above-knee popliteal artery has a higher incidence of atherosclerotic disease extending from the superficial femoral artery. Therefore the below-knee popliteal artery is more commonly used for femoral-popliteal bypass. Improper selection of the outflow target artery causes graft failure and potentially jeopardizes limb viability. As with the assessment of inflow, preoperative imaging, often complemented with angiography, is essential in selecting the most appropriate outflow or target artery.

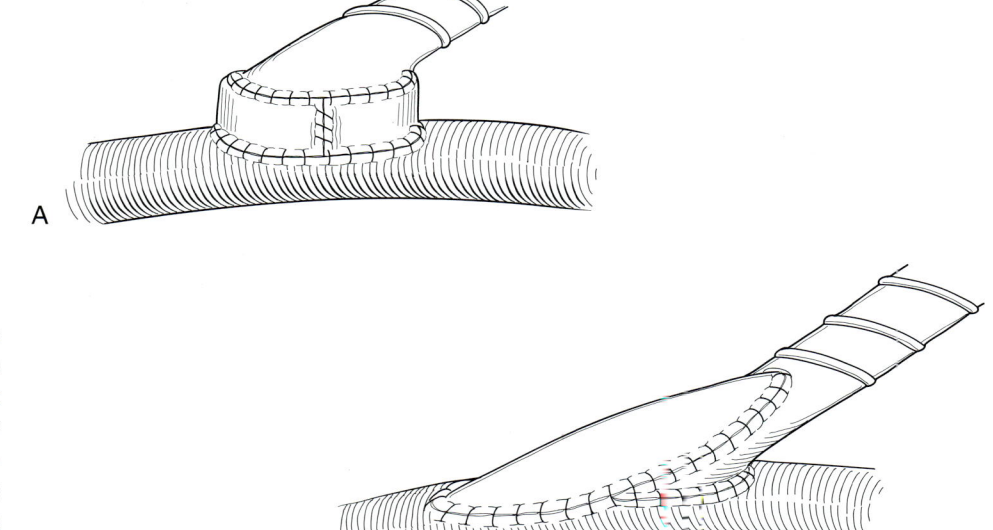

Figure 44-5. A, An autogenous vein cuff (Miller cuff) is attached to the distal portion of a prosthetic graft when this conduit is used below the knee. **B,** Alternatively, an autogenous vein patch (Taylor patch) can be applied to the distal portion of a prosthetic graft when this conduit is used below the knee.

PREOPERATIVE ASSESSMENT OF VEIN QUALITY

A complete history and a physical examination often reveal whether the great saphenous veins have been used for coronary bypass, used for previous lower extremity revascularization, or stripped for varicosities. Vein mapping via venous duplex imaging should be done if there is any question as to the presence or quality of the vein conduit. If the great saphenous vein is unavailable or appears inadequate, vein mapping should include the cephalic, basilic, and small saphenous veins. The venous duplex study should evaluate the diameter, compressibility, wall thickness and flow through the proposed conduit. The diameter of the vein conduit should be at least 3 mm to optimize patency. If mapping is done perioperatively, the location of the vein should be marked on the skin to facilitate harvest and minimize creation of skin flaps during vein harvest.

SELECTION OF CONDUIT

Autogenous vein grafts provide the best patency for use in arterial bypass for all infrainguinal reconstructions, regardless of distal target.[9,10] The conduit of choice for a femoral-popliteal bypass is therefore ipsilateral great saphenous vein. Reversed and in situ configurations are equally effective[1,12] but reversed vein is applicable to more patients and generally simpler to use. Although reversed vein is generally preferred, some groups have achieved equivalent success with in situ vein conduits.[11,12] If ipsilateral great saphenous vein is inadequate or unavailable, contralateral great saphenous vein is the second-best choice, provided the extremity does not have significant arterial compromise. Splicing the small saphenous veins and cephalic or basilic veins from the arms often provides enough length for bypass in the absence of suitable leg vein.

Nonautogenous options exist for those patients who have no suitable vein conduit. The most commonly used prosthetic conduit for femoral-popliteal bypass is expanded polytetrafluoroethylene (ePTFE). Varieties of ePTFE grafts may be coated with heparin or impregnated with carbon, but their long-term patency is similar to that of untreated ePTFE grafts. In femoral above-knee popliteal bypass, ePTFE grafts have the same patency as reversed great saphenous vein for the first 2 to 3 years, but vein is superior thereafter and therefore is preferred.[5,10,13] Prosthetic bypasses to the below-knee popliteal and tibial arteries have uniformly poor patency rates. The patency of the latter can be improved by the use of an adjunctive Miller or St. Mary's vein cuff (Fig. 44-5, *A*) or Taylor vein patch (Fig. 44-5, *B*).[14-16] Cryopreserved cadaveric vein grafts have exceedingly poor patencies and should be reserved for limb salvage indications[17]; they may also have a niche in the management of transplant patients or those with infected prosthetic grafts.[17]

IN SITU OR REVERSED GREAT SAPHENOUS VEIN

The main advantage of the in situ conduit is a better size match between the artery and the vein; prior claims of biologic superiority of the in situ technique have been disproved, because nearly all randomized trials have shown equivalent results for in situ and reversed vein.[11,12] Small veins seem to perform poorly regardless of technique. Patency and limb survival are generally equivalent. Reversed vein conduits are more user-friendly and more readily adaptable to a variety of potential intraoperative situations; a flexible approach takes advantage of either technique.

Operative Techniques for Harvest of Great or Small Saphenous Vein and Arm Veins

OPEN VEIN HARVEST

The great saphenous vein can be found medially in the femoral triangle using the same incision for exposing the common femoral artery, although care should be taken to orient the initial incision obliquely along the course of the saphenous vein. Preoperative skin marking at the time of duplex vein mapping is helpful, especially in obese patients. Skin incisions should be made directly over the vein to avoid undermined, subcutaneous flaps that are prone to necrosis. The great saphenous vein can be identified in the fossa ovalis as it enters the common femoral vein. Circumferential dissection is facilitated with silicone elastomer (Silastic) loops to avoid direct grasping of the vein with forceps. Gentle retraction provides exposure as the periadventitial tissue is dissected from the vein. Small tributaries must be ligated with silk suture. When tying close to the vein the surgeon must leave a short stump of the divided branch. Failure to do so may result in a stenosis of the vein graft. Dissection is continued distally until an adequate length of great saphenous vein has been acquired. Skip incisions are preferred to provide skin bridges and minimize wound complications. A small clamp is then placed flush with the common femoral vein to maximize length of the conduit. The great saphenous vein is divided proximally, and the stump is oversewn in two layers with monofilament suture. Trauma to the great saphenous vein should be minimized during the harvest.

The great saphenous vein graft is then prepared for use as a conduit. The graft is placed in a bath of heparinized saline. A small bulldog clamp is placed at the proximal end of the vein. Heparinized saline is flushed under gentle pressure from the distal end to identify tears or small, untied branches. These are repaired with 7-0 polypropylene suture, again ensuring that kinks or stenoses are not created. The vein should be soft and distend fully, but overdistention of the vein should be avoided. Irrigant should readily pass through the prepared conduit. If focal areas of sclerosis are present, they should be resected. Once prepared, the vein is stored in chilled, autologous heparinized blood on a back table until creation of the tunnel.

The small saphenous vein is best harvested with the patient in the prone position. A longitudinal incision is created on the posterior aspect of the calf. The subcutaneous tissue is carefully divided with scissors until the vein is identified. Small branches are carefully tied away from the vein to prevent stenoses. The sural nerve runs along the course of the small saphenous vein and must be protected during harvest.

The cephalic and basilic veins are useful conduits when they are of good caliber and not traumatized by previous venipunctures. Vein mapping helps identify potential conduits. The cephalic and basilic veins originate at the wrist and extend to the shoulder. They may be joined at the elbow by the median antecubital vein. Multiple configurations of the arm and forearm components of both veins can be used to create a conduit for femoral-popliteal bypass. If the two segments are connected by the median antecubital vein, the nonreversed segment needs valvulotomy. Segments of arm vein that are not in direct continuity need to be spliced together.

ENDOSCOPIC VEIN HARVEST

Endoscopic great saphenous vein harvest has become a routine part of coronary artery bypass grafting. A large metaanalysis of endoscopic great saphenous vein harvest for coronary artery bypass grafting suggests that the technique affords significantly fewer overall complications, wound infections, and wound dehiscences.[18] However, some studies have suggested inferior performance in the coronary circulation for endoscopically harvested vein grafts. This technique has crossed over into lower extremity bypass grafting, although it remains controversial whether outcomes are equivalent to open harvest. The potential benefits of endoscopic vein harvest can only be enjoyed once the surgeon has overcome the steep learning curve associated with this technique. It is particularly useful when harvesting the contralateral great saphenous vein to the extremity undergoing the bypass.

A longitudinal 2-cm incision is made over the great saphenous vein at the knee. The vein is dissected circumferentially, and a subcutaneous pocket is created. A commercially available endoscope with a conical dissecting tip is then placed in the pocket. The pocket is enlarged with further dissection via the scope until the port can be advanced into the incision. The port is inflated to create an airtight seal. Carbon dioxide is then insufflated through the port. By keeping the endoscope close to the great saphenous vein a tunnel is created around the vein, allowing the remaining tissues to fall away. Dissection continues toward the saphenofemoral junction. A ringed retractor is used to gently expose tributaries of the great saphenous vein which are then divided with clips or cautery. Once enough length has been mobilized, a small incision is created over the proximal extent of the vein. The proximal segment of the great saphenous vein is carefully exteriorized and ligated. The port is then removed. The great saphenous vein is ligated distally at the port incision. The conduit is then prepared on the back table, as described previously.

CONSTRUCTION OF A SPLICED VEIN BYPASS

Short segments of vein can be connected via venovenostomies to create a conduit of sufficient length for the intended bypass. These spliced vein conduits are particularly useful when using segments of arm vein for bypass. The ends of both veins are spatulated to accommodate size mismatches and to help create a wide oval anastomosis. Although interrupted fine polypropylene sutures are recommended to avoid purse stringing the spliced veins with the potential of stenosis of the vein conduit, use of a two-suture running technique, with sutures placed at the heel and toe of the venovenostomy, is an acceptable alternative. Arm veins frequently harbor sclerotic segments or valve abnormalities and should be assessed by either angioscopy or completion duplex imaging.

IN SITU VALVE LYSIS

In situ vein grafts require preparation that differs from the traditional reversed great saphenous vein. Various techniques have evolved to prepare in situ vein grafts, but the key steps remain the same: division of the first venous valves under direct visualization, lysis of the remaining valves with a valvulotome, and closure of venous tributaries. Once the great saphenous vein has been mobilized for 5 to 10 cm, the saphenofemoral junction is divided and the first venous valves are excised using Potts scissors. If the entire great saphenous vein is exposed, the proximal anastomosis is performed. A variety of retrograde valvulotomes are then advanced from the distal great saphenous vein. Arterial blood can be seen flowing through the graft once the valves have been successfully lysed. Alternatively, the valves can be lysed under angioscopic guidance. After excising the first valves, a 1.9-mm angioscope is advanced into the great saphenous vein. Irrigation from

Operative Technique for Femoral to Above-Knee Popliteal Bypass

The common femoral artery is the inflow vessel most frequently used for above-knee popliteal bypass. The pulse of the common femoral artery is palpated midway between the pubic tubercle and the anterior superior iliac spine below the inguinal ligament. A vertical incision is made directly over this pulsation (see Fig. 44-2, A). The soft tissue is dissected with electrocautery down to the level of the femoral sheath, with self-retaining retractors providing adequate exposure. The common femoral artery is dissected proximally to the inguinal ligament (see Fig. 44-2, B). Distally, the dissection is carried out onto the proximal superficial femoral artery. The profunda femoris artery is identified and exposed. A blunt, right-angled clamp is used to place medium Silastic vessel loops around each vessel. This step facilitates subsequent clamp placement or vessel loop use for control of the superficial femoral artery and profunda femoris artery if the arteries are soft and nondiseased.

The above-knee popliteal is exposed from the medial thigh (see Fig. 44-3, A). A longitudinal incision is carried out anterior to the sartorius muscle above the knee. The soft tissue is divided with electrocautery, allowing the sartorius muscle to be retracted posterolaterally. The deep fascia overlying the adductor canal is then visible. The fascia is divided sharply with Metzenbaum scissors, exposing the popliteal fossa (see Fig. 44-3, B). The popliteal artery is dissected from the surrounding fatty tissue. Palpation is used to identify a healthy segment of artery for the distal anastomosis. The artery is carefully mobilized from the popliteal vein to ensure that adequate length is available for the anastomosis. Vessel loops are placed proximally, distally, and around side branches. A duplicate popliteal vein or high confluence of the tibial veins may be observed.

Once proximal and distal arterial targets have been properly prepared, the conduit can be tunneled. A long, hollow-bore, curved tunneling device with a removable blunt tip is passed from the groin incision beneath the sartorius muscle to the popliteal fossa. The prepared vein conduit is again checked for leaks. It is distended with heparinized saline, allowing all twists and kinks to resolve. The vein is marked along its length to check its orientation once it has been tunneled. The proximal end of the vein conduit is attached to the obturator of the tunneler and pulled into position. The tunneler is then removed, and the orientation of the vein is rechecked.

The proximal anastomosis is typically performed first. Heparin is administered systemically and allowed to circulate for 5 minutes before arterial clamp placement. If the distal vein was divided at a branch point, an incision is made through both branches to spatulate the end (see Fig. 44-1, A). Otherwise, a longitudinal incision is made in the vein 1.5 times its diameter and tailored to create a spatulation. The inflow vessels are clamped. An arteriotomy is created with a No. 11 blade scalpel on the anterior wall of the common femoral artery and extended proximally and distally with Potts scissors to a size appropriate for the vein graft. Typically, running 5-0 polypropylene suture is used to create the end-to-side anastomosis. The heel of the graft is secured first, and the graft is sutured continuously to a point halfway toward the toe of the graft (see Fig. 44-1, B). A second suture is started at the toe and continued toward the first stitch. With each stitch attention is paid to creating an everted symmetric anastomosis (see Fig. 44-1, C). After flushing, the clamps are released and a surgical hemostatic agent with gentle pressure is applied to the anastomosis. Single repair sutures of 6-0 polypropylene are used if bleeding between running sutures is encountered. A soft bulldog clamp is placed on the vein graft proximally until the distal anastomosis is complete.

The distal anastomosis is performed in a similar fashion. The above-knee popliteal is most often controlled with vessel loops or clamps. A long arteriotomy is again performed at a length 1.5 times the diameter of the graft. Fogarty catheters can be used for control of the arteriotomy if clamps cannot be used because excessive calcification is present. The vein graft orientation is rechecked; release of the bulldog clamp should result in highly pulsatile flow through the graft. The vein is tailored appropriately for the end-to-side anastomosis. The heel is secured with a running 6-0 polypropylene suture and continued toward the toe. A second suture starting from the toe is sewn until it meets the first suture. Before completing the anastomosis, the artery and vein graft are flushed, the anastomosis is completed, and the clamps or vessel loops are released to reconstitute flow.

Operative Technique for Femoral to Below-Knee Popliteal Bypass

Exposure of the below-knee popliteal is made using a longitudinal incision 1 to 2 cm posterior to the medial edge of the tibia (see Fig. 44-4, A) or along the course of the harvested great saphenous vein. Care must be undertaken not to injure the great saphenous vein. The subcutaneous tissue is divided with electrocautery. The pes anserinus tendon is divided. The posterior fascia is identified and divided longitudinally. The medial head of the gastrocnemius muscle is bluntly mobilized and retracted posteriorly, exposing the popliteal fossa. Gentle dissection through the fatty tissue is performed until the neurovascular contents of the fossa are identified. Self-retaining retractors are replaced to hold the soft tissue posteriorly. A fascial sheath around the vessels is entered with Metzenbaum or tenotomy scissors. The popliteal veins are adherent to the artery (see Fig. 44-4, B). The veins are carefully dissected from the artery, and the venae comitantes are divided with 4-0 silk sutures to expose the artery. Proximal and distal control with large vessel loops is carefully performed. The tunneling device is advanced from the popliteal fossa between the medial and lateral heads of the gastrocnemius muscle and in the subsartorial space to the groin incision. Alternatively, the tunnel can be created sequentially in two steps after the proximal anastomosis is created. The conduit can be first passed through the tunnel, making sure the orientation is correct from the groin to the above-knee popliteal fossa and, subsequently, from the above-knee popliteal fossa to the below-knee popliteal fossa. The anastomoses proceed in the same fashion as for the femoral to above-knee popliteal bypass.

Intraoperative Assessment of Femoral-Popliteal Bypass

Intraoperative assessment of the graft confirms patency, establishes the integrity of the conduit, confirms the adequacy of the outflow tree, and identifies potential conduit or anastomotic defects and technical errors that may predispose a patient to early thrombosis. A sterile Doppler probe is the simplest way to assess graft flow and the presence and quality of the flow in the foot. Intraoperative duplex imaging can also be used to analyze changes in velocity or spectral broadening and detect technical or intrinsic conduit defects. If there is concern for stenosis or outflow obstruction, an angiogram should be performed; some centers routinely perform completion arteriography. Typically, a 21-Ga butterfly needle connected to a three-way stopcock is used to inject contrast into the hood of the proximal anastomosis, generally through a side branch left long to accommodate the procedure. Digital subtraction angiography is performed from the proximal graft down to the foot. Angioscopy is helpful in evaluating the quality of the conduit, especially when using in situ vein or arm vein conduits.

Wound Closure

Once the bypass has been deemed a success and hemostasis is achieved with or without partial reversal of the heparin, the wounds can be closed. The fascia is reapproximated using absorbable suture, taking care not to anatomically close the deep fascia of the popliteal fossa. The subcutaneous tissue is closed in layers with absorbable suture, which obliterates dead space. In elective procedures the skin can be closed subcuticularly. In patients with significant edema, the skin should be closed in an interrupted fashion with nylon mattress sutures. Closed suction drains may be placed in the groin incision if there is a concern for lymphatic leak, especially in reoperative procedures or if postoperative anticoagulation is planned. Sterile dry gauze or skin glue is then used to cover the incisions.

Alternate Inflow Sources

Length of available vein may be insufficient to allow bypass origin from the common femoral artery, or common femoral artery exposure may be difficult because of scarring from previous revascularization. The profunda femoris artery may serve as a useful alternative inflow source when it is free of proximal obstructive disease (Fig. 44-6). The mid-profunda femoris artery or distal profunda femoris artery is typically exposed by a longitudinal incision on the upper thigh, lateral to the sartorius muscle (Fig. 44-6, *A*). The soft tissue is dissected until the sartorius muscle can be retracted medially. The superficial femoral artery is visualized and retracted medially as well. Dissection is carried out between the adductor magnus and the vastus medialis to expose the profunda femoris artery (Fig. 44-6, *B*). Division of the lateral femoral circumflex vein overlying the profunda femoris artery may be necessary to provide adequate exposure. Silastic vessel loops are placed to control the branches of the profunda femoris artery. The proximal anastomosis is carried out as described previously on the common femoral artery.

The superficial femoral artery may be used as an alternate inflow source, provided it is free of proximal obstructive disease. If a vertical incision has been made in the groin, this can be extended distally. The sartorius muscle is retracted laterally to further expose the superficial femoral artery. The mid-superficial femoral artery and distal superficial femoral artery may be approached via a near vertical incision on the medial thigh near the posterior border of the sartorius muscle (Fig. 44-7, *A*). The subcutaneous tissue is dissected, the fascia is divided, and the sartorius muscle is retracted anteriomedially. The superficial femoral artery is mobilized within the Hunter canal (Fig. 44-7, *B*). The proximal anastomosis proceeds in the same fashion as the common femoral artery.

Femoral-Popliteal Thromboembolectomy

Early graft thrombosis is most often the result of technical error and poor inflow or outflow and may not be accompanied by dramatic symptoms. An agreed-upon strategy to following the status of the reconstruction should be in place. Indeed, early loss of an initial strongly palpable pulse, despite the persistence of a Doppler signal, may suggest early graft thrombosis. Early failure of bypasses occurs in 5% to 10% of cases and requires immediate transfer to the operating room. A reversed great saphenous vein bypass presents a challenge for thromboembolectomy because of the presence of valves. The incision for the popliteal exposure is reopened, and the distal anastomosis is controlled. A dose of intravenous heparin is given. A longitudinal venotomy is made over the hood of the graft. Any visible clot in the graft is removed. An embolectomy catheter is then passed distally to treat the runoff vessels. An attempt is made

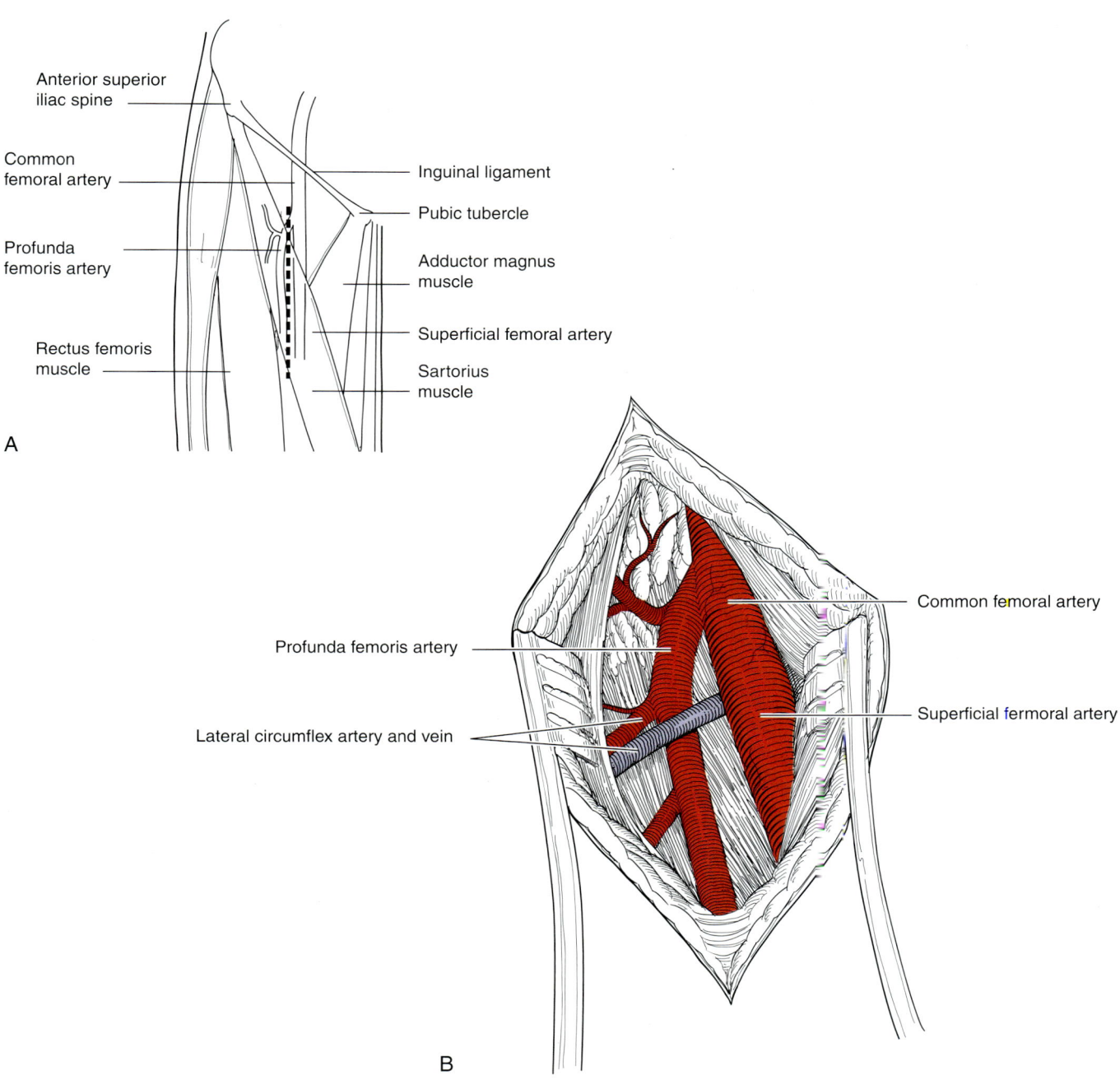

OPEN SURGICAL BYPASS OF FEMORAL-POPLITEAL ARTERIAL OCCLUSIVE DISEASE | 539

Figure 44-6. **A,** The proximal profunda femoris artery can be accessed with the same incision used for common femoral artery exposure. The mid-profunda femoris artery or distal profunda femoris artery is exposed through a more distal incision (*dashed line*), and the dissection is lateral to the sartorius muscle. **B,** The proximal profunda femoris artery is exposed. Unlike the superficial femoral artery, the profunda femoris artery has multiple branches that must be controlled. Care is taken to ligate the circumflex femoral vein to avoid inadvertent injury.

to pass the embolectomy catheter proximally and continue the thrombectomy. If the valves prevent passage of the catheter, the proximal incision can be reopened, exposing the anastomosis. Once control of the vessels is obtained, an incision is made in the hood of the graft. The embolectomy catheter is passed proximally to distally. A suture is attached to the tip of the catheter. A separate embolectomy catheter is attached to the distal aspect of the suture, allowing it to be pulled against the valves toward the groin. The balloon is then inflated, and the thrombus can be brought out through the distal incision. Completion angiography should be performed to assess adequacy of thromboembolectomy. As with any case of acute limb ischemia, if there is concern for reperfusion syndrome, a four-compartment fasciotomy should be considered (see Chapter 53).

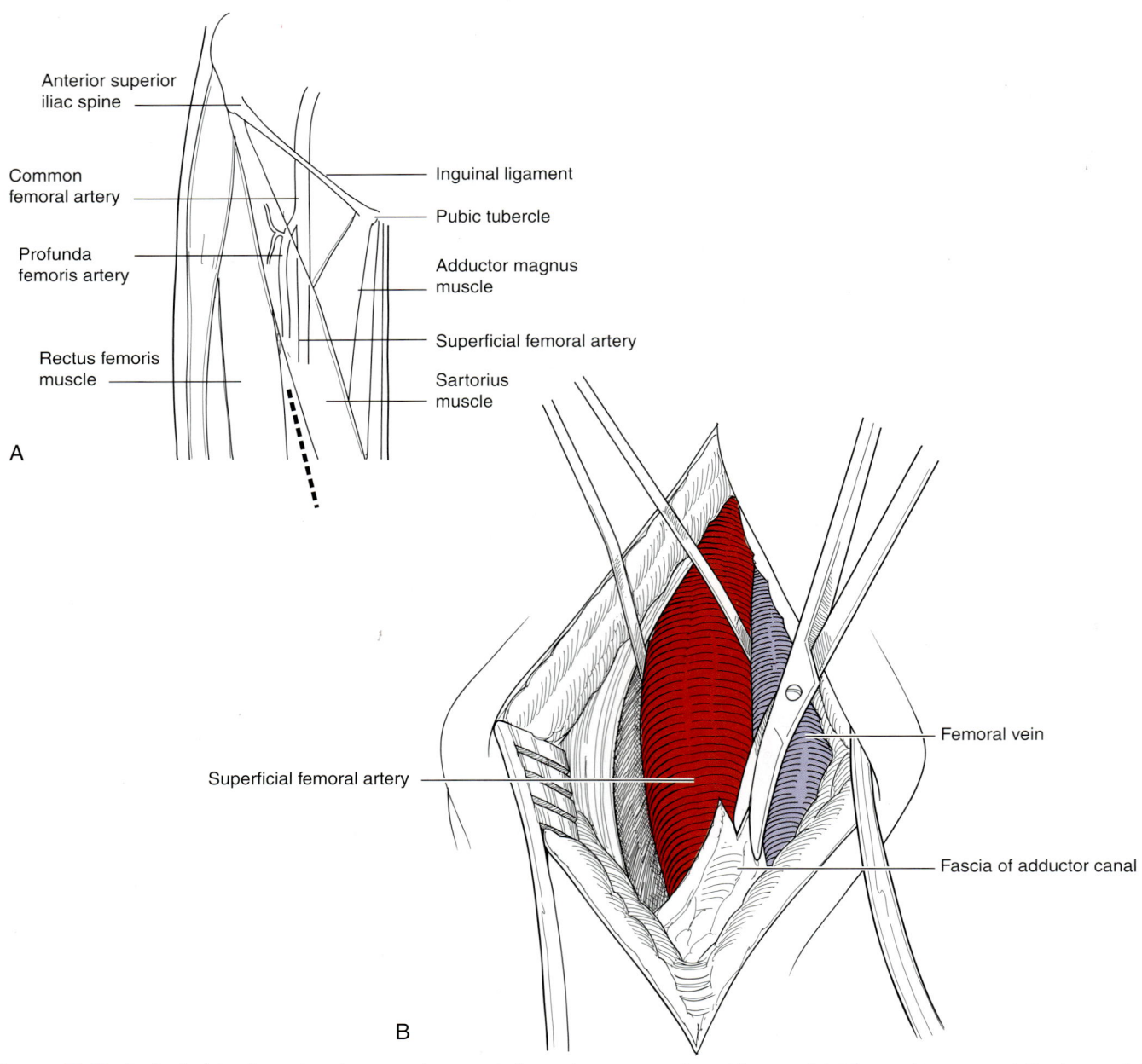

Figure 44-7. A, An incision lateral to the sartorius muscle is used to expose the mid- superficial femoral artery and distal superficial femoral artery. **B,** The superficial femoral artery travels in the adductor canal (Hunter canal) and is close to the femoral vein.

Postoperative Care

- Frequent neurovascular assessment is mandatory, and a change in neurovascular status should initiate evaluation of graft patency. In the event of early graft thrombosis, prompt return to the operating room is indicated to correct technical errors. Continued clinical assessment for compartment syndrome should not be overlooked.
- PAD patients often suffer from concomitant cardiac disease, and cardiac-related symptoms should be thoroughly evaluated.
- Diet can usually be resumed in the early postoperative period, unless the patient suffers from an adverse reaction to the anesthetic.
- Pain control should be adequate to allow early mobilization and thus prevent other complications related to immobility, such as deep vein thrombosis or generalized deconditioning. Physical therapy should be involved to optimize early rehabilitation, especially in elderly patients.
- Antiplatelet therapy has been shown to improve graft patency and should be continued.

Complications

- **Early graft thrombosis (<30 days).** Perioperative graft failure is most often attributed to errors in technique or errors in judgment. Poor selection of inflow and outflow sites, as well as technical errors at the anastomosis, including plaque disruption, backwalling, or intimal flaps, can cause graft thrombosis. Kinking or twisting of the graft during tunneling creates a functional stenosis or occlusion, leading to graft thrombosis. Once early graft thrombosis occurs, the patient should be taken immediately back to the operating room. Angiography after thrombectomy usually identifies the problem. The graft can be thrombectomized, and measures to correct the culprit lesion can be performed. Patient factors associated with early graft thrombosis include age less than 60 years, African American race, and bypass to tibial vessels. It is important to inform such patients of their increased risk of early graft thrombosis.[19]

- **Late graft thrombosis (>30 days).** Late graft thrombosis is usually related to intimal hyperplasia. Cytokines activate smooth muscle proliferation in the vein graft, and subsequent matrix deposition eventually creates a stenosis. Routine duplex surveillance can identify areas of narrowing in vein grafts. Early percutaneous or open intervention can improve the primary assisted patency of the graft.

- **Bleeding.** Meticulous hemostasis during the dissection is mandatory. When harvesting vein grafts, all small side branches must be ligated. Hemostatic clips on the vein graft may become dislodged during tunneling and should be avoided. Careful inspection of the vein on the back table is time well spent. Bleeding of the vein graft in the tunnel can be repaired by direct cut down onto the area of concern. Focal bleeding from the anastomosis usually requires placing single repair sutures. Severe bleeding from the anastomosis may be the result of improper technique, failure to include all layers of the arterial wall when suturing, poor vessel wall integrity, or excessive tension. The anastomosis may need to be redone if this occurs.

- **Infection.** If infection of the foot was present immediately before the bypass, the patient should be receiving systemic antibiotics, and if appropriate, adequate drainage should have been performed before bypass. In the absence of preoperative infection, a perioperative dose of antibiotics to cover skin flora should be adequate. Surgical site infections may be superficial; these can be treated with simple dressing changes and antibiotics. Deep wound infections may lead to graft exposure and require aggressive debridement and muscle flap closure. Prosthetic graft infection is devastating and typically requires complete graft removal with or without extraanatomic revascularization with autologous or cryopreserved vein conduit.

- **Lymphatic complications.** Lymphocele or lymphatic leak may cause significant morbidity and lead to late infection of graft, especially if a prosthetic has been used. Prevention is often the best solution. These complications result from the disruption of the lymph channels, particularly in the groin. Longitudinal dissection in the femoral sheath and careful ligation of lymphatics during the initial operation can help prevent lymphatic leak. However, reoperative procedures in the groin are prone to the formation of lymphoceles, and lymph leaks and drains can be placed if anticipated. If a lymphocele or lymph leak is present, operative exploration to oversew leaking lymphatics is prudent.

REFERENCES

1. Carrel A, Guthrie CC: Uniterminal and biterminal transplantation of veins, *Am J Med Sci* 132:415, 1906.
2. Bernheim BM: The ideal operation for aneurysms of the extremity: Report of a case, *Johns Hopkins Hosp Bull* 27:1, 1916.
3. Elkin DC, DeBakey ME, editors: *Vascular surgery in World War II*, Washington, DC, 1955, Office of the Surgeon General, Department of the Army.
4. Kunlin J: Le traitement de l'ischemie arteritique par la greffe veineuse longue, *Rev Chir Paris* 70:206-236, 1951.

5. Murphy TP, Dhangana R, Pencina MJ, D'Agostino RB Sr: Ankle-brachial index and cardiovascular risk prediction: An analysis of 11,594 individuals with 10-year follow-up, *Atherosclerosis* 220:160-167, 2012.
6. Peach G, Griffin M, Jones KG, et al: Diagnosis and management of peripheral arterial disease, *BMJ* 345:e5208, 2012.
7. Norgren L, Hiatt WR, Dormandy JA, et al: Inter-society consensus for the management of peripheral arterial disease (TASC II), *J Vasc Surg* 45(Suppl S):S5-S67, 2007.
8. Brown A, Reynolds LR, Bruemmer D: Intensive glycemic control and cardiovascular disease: An update, *Nat Rev Cardiol* 7:369-375, 2010.
9. Klinkert P, Schepers A, Burger DHC, et al: Vein versus polytetrafluoroethylene in above-knee femoropopliteal bypass grafting: Five-year results of a randomized controlled trial, *J Vasc Surg* 37:149-155, 2003.
10. Pereira CE, Albers M, Romiti M, et al: Meta-analysis of femoropopliteal bypass grafts for lower extremity arterial insufficiency, *J Vasc Surg* 44:510-517, 2006.
11. Harris PL, Veith FJ, Shanik GD, et al: Prospective randomized comparison of in situ and reversed infrapopliteal vein grafts, *Br J Surg* 80:173-176, 1993.
12. Watelet J, Soury P, Menard JF, et al: Femoropopliteal bypass: In situ or reversed vein grafts? Ten-year results of a randomized prospective study, *Ann Vasc Surg* 18:149-157, 1999.
13. Mills JL Sr: *P* values may lack power: The choice of conduit for above-knee femoropopliteal bypass graft, *J Vasc Surg* 32:402-405, 2000.
14. Yeung KK, Mills JL Sr, Hughes JD, et al: Improved patency of infrainguinal polytetrafluoroethylene bypass grafts using a distal Taylor vein patch, *Am J Surg* 182:578-583, 2001.
15. Taylor RS, Loh A, McFarland RJ, et al: Improved technique for polytetrafluoroethylene bypass grafting: Long-term results using anastomotic vein patches, *Br J Surg* 79:348-354, 1992.
16. Stonebridge PA, Prescott RJ, Ruckley CV: Randomized trial comparing infrainguinal polytetrafluoroethylene bypass grafting with and without vein interposition cuff at the distal anastomosis, *J Vasc Surg* 26:543-550, 1997.
17. Fujitani RM, Bassiouny HS, Gewertz BL, et al: Cryopreserved saphenous vein allogenic homografts: An alternative conduit in lower extremity arterial reconstruction in infected fields, *J Vasc Surg* 15:519-526, 1992.
18. Cadwallader RA, Walsh SR, Cooper DG, et al: Great saphenous vein harvesting: A systematic review and meta-analysis of open versus endoscopic techniques, *Vasc Endovasc Surg* 43:561-566, 2009.
19. Singh N, Sidawy AN, DeZee KJ, et al: Factors associated with early failure of infrainguinal lower extremity bypass, *J Vasc Surg* 47:556-561, 2008.

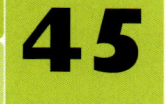

45 Direct Surgical Repair of Tibial-Peroneal Arterial Occlusive Disease

RENEE C. MINJAREZ • GREGORY L. MONETA

Historical Background

The feasibility of arterial reconstruction was first realized in the early 1900s through pioneering early studies performed by Carrell and Guthrie[1] at the University of Chicago, as well as Bernheim[2] at Johns Hopkins University. The availability of a safe heparin formulation, as developed by Best[3] at the University of Toronto by the late 1940s, enabled arterial bypass grafting to be a practical intervention for the treatment of limb ischemia. In 1951 Kunlin[4] reported using reversed great saphenous vein for femoral popliteal artery bypass grafting to successfully treat foot gangrene. In describing his experience with 17 vein bypass graft procedures, Kunlin was the first to introduce the end-to-side anastomosis as a means of preserving collateral branches near the thrombotic zone. He advocated a two-suture technique with separate heel and toe sutures. Heparin was administered and maintained postoperatively, followed by coumadin anticoagulation. Whereas a small number of vein grafts were performed for treatment of vascular injuries in World War II, during the Korean and Vietnam wars traumatic arterial injuries treated with vein bypass emerged as an alternative treatment to simple ligation or amputation.[5,6] Likewise, in the 1950s case series replicated Kunlin's approach with reports of excellent results with vein bypass grafting to treat chronic limb ischemia.[7] By the end of the 1960s arterial bypass with venous conduit was a well-accepted treatment for symptomatic limb ischemia. Although endovascular techniques have emerged as an option for infrainguinal revascularization, arterial bypass grafting with venous conduit is still regarded as the gold standard with which endovascular techniques are compared with regard to efficacy and durability in the treatment of lower extremity ischemia.[8]

Indications

Tibial and peroneal artery bypass procedures are indicated for the treatment of ischemic rest pain, chronic ischemic ulcerations, gangrene of the foot, and highly selected patients with short distance claudication. Patients with critical limb ischemia (CLI) however, comprise the vast majority of patients for whom distal revascularization procedures are performed; many vascular surgeons only consider tibial level bypass grafting for CLI.

Preoperative Preparation

- **Coronary artery disease.** Patients undergoing tibial artery bypass are more likely to have vascular disease and comorbidities of greater severity than those undergoing more proximal bypass.[9] Given the ubiquitous presence of coronary artery disease in patients with peripheral arterial disease, patients with CLI should be considered for assessment of cardiac status before vascular reconstruction. In addition to a preoperative electrocardiogram, an echocardiogram and noninvasive cardiac stress testing with cardiac imaging are often selectively used to assist with preoperative risk stratification. This information can also be useful in postoperative management. According to American College of Cardiology/American Heart Association guidelines, coronary revascularization is not indicated in patients with stable coronary artery disease undergoing vascular surgery, including lower extremity arterial reconstruction.[10]

- **Risk factor modification.** Medical therapy should be optimized before lower extremity revascularization. Specifically, hypertension and diabetes should be under good control. Smoking cessation is encouraged. Beta-blockers should be continued through the perioperative period, and consideration should be given to initiation of beta-blockers in select beta-blocker naïve patients.[11] Patients should be on a statin medication preoperatively. Statin use has been shown to decrease the rate of perioperative myocardial infarction and cerebral ischemic events in vascular surgical patients and may increase vein graft patency.[12-14]

- **Antiplatelet therapy.** All patients with peripheral arterial disease, including those undergoing lower extremity bypasses, should be on antiplatelet medication, preferably aspirin (81-325 mg/day) or clopidogrel (75 mg/day).

- **Imaging.** Digital subtraction arterial angiography is the preoperative imaging modality of choice to determine revascularization targets for tibial artery bypass. Detailed views of the foot and lower leg, including a lateral view, are needed to best identify patent arteries to determine the best distal target for the bypass.

Pitfalls and Danger Points

- **Conduit selection.** The quality of the conduit is the most important factor in the success of a lower extremity bypass procedure. Great saphenous vein is the conduit of choice in leg bypass grafts, particularly when the reconstruction is carried to tibial and pedal vessels. Ultrasound vein mapping should be performed preoperatively to identify optimal venous conduit.

- **Wounds.** Operative planning must take into account the location of chronic or infected wounds when deciding where to place incisions. Before lower extremity revascularization, active infection should be controlled by antibiotics and aggressive wound care should be initiated.

- **Tunneling.** For reversed vein bypass grafts, the graft should be tunneled while maintaining proper orientation and with the graft fully distended to avoid kinking or twisting.

- **Working with small-caliber arteries.** Surgical loupes are required for accuracy. Delicate handling and fine instrumentation are needed to avoid unnecessary trauma or vasospasm; strategies such as tourniquet control and intraluminal occlusion may be applied in circumstances of highly calcified recipient vessels.

- **Limited outflow.** A distal arteriovenous fistula may increase graft patency. Long-term anticoagulation with warfarin may increase graft patency when prosthetic grafts are used.

Operative Stratmegy

SELECTION OF CONDUIT

Selection of conduit for tibial bypass is of paramount importance. The best conduit is great saphenous vein, but when not available, another source of vein should be obtained. As such, preoperative vein mapping using duplex ultrasound should be performed before tibial bypass to identify the optimal venous conduit. In general, thin-walled veins, 3 to 5 mm in diameter, serve as good conduits.

Failure rates are high with use of an inadequate conduit.[15] The ipsilateral great saphenous vein is preferred, but if unavailable or inadequate, adequate contralateral great saphenous vein is the next best choice. Saving a contralateral great saphenous vein for a possible future coronary or contralateral lower extremity bypass is a fallacious argument. The best available vein should be used for the current operation and not saved for a future potential operation. If adequate great saphenous vein is not available, single-segment arm vein is preferred, usually cephalic vein for tibial bypass, followed by spliced, composite vein composed of the best available venous conduits.

Prosthetic conduits are inferior for tibial bypass. However, if reasonable autogenous conduit is not available, a prosthetic conduit can be used for tibial bypass. Adjuncts, such as heparin-impregnated grafts and Linton patch angioplasty, at the distal anastomotic site have been advocated to improve results. Acceptable short-term results have been reported.[16,17]

SELECTION AND ASSESSMENT OF A SITE FOR INFLOW

The selection of an adequate inflow site is dictated by the preoperative imaging studies and the amount of available conduit. Preferably, the inflow pulse should be strong and not distal to known high-grade stenoses. Depending on conduit availability, preoperative angiographic assessment may allow correction, either by angioplasty or stenting, of proximal lesions to potential inflow sites. At operation, the inflow artery is palpated to assess pulsatility, plaque presence and location, and its suitability for clamping and anastomosis. Arteries suitable for inflow to the tibials are the common femoral artery, profunda femoris artery, superficial femoral artery and the above- and below-knee popliteal arteries.[18] Occasionally, proximal tibial vessels can also be used as inflow sources. The more distal the inflow source, the shorter the length of conduit required, and in general, shorter conduits are preferred over longer conduits.

Should there be any question regarding the adequacy of inflow of the selected artery for the proximal anastomosis, a pressure gradient can be measured at that location by comparing the measured pressure with the systemic pressure. Some surgeons recheck the pressure after intraarterial administration of a vasodilator at the site, such as 200 mcg of nitroglycerine or 30 mg of papaverine. After the administration of a vasodilator, a gradient of 15 to 20 mm Hg systolic pressure is considered significant.

SELECTION AND ASSESSMENT OF A SITE FOR DISTAL ANASTOMOSIS

The outflow target vessel for receipt of the bypass should be in continuity with the pedal vessels. However, the peroneal artery is an acceptable target vessel, despite the lack of direct communication to the pedal circulation.[19] Arteries distal to the outflow target should be free of hemodynamically significant stenoses.

Heavily calcified tibial arteries encountered at operation should not preclude anastomosis provided the lumen is patent. Modified cutting "armor piercing" needles may be helpful in constructing the anastomosis in these circumstances, in addition to the strategies noted earlier.

CONSIDERATIONS IN THE PRESENCE OF AN OPEN ULCER

Open wounds pose a risk of contamination to the operative field, potentially exposing the vascular graft to infection and increasing the risk of a wound infection. Preoperative incision planning needs to take into account open wounds in the lower extremity. In addition, the operative sites should be chosen so that the graft is adequately covered with viable tissue. Incisions should be made as far away from open wounds as feasible. Grossly infected or large wounds are excluded from the operative field by first scrubbing with a povidone-iodine preparation (Betadine) and then isolating the wound with an Ioban (3M, St. Paul), iodophor-impregnated adhesive occlusive dressing. A piece of gauze may be left in the wound bed to soak up drainage. Feet are routinely covered with sterile bags to also help limit contamination.

INSTRUMENTATION AND TUNNELERS

Dissection of tibial vessels should be done with minimal handling to avoid vasospasm. A combination of sharp and blunt dissection using fine-tipped tonsil dissectors or mosquito-type clamps with fine Metzenbaum scissors or tenotomy scissors works well. Self-retaining retractors are used to provide exposure. Dissection-induced vasospasm can be relieved by topical application of papaverine.

Tunneling the graft requires a rigid tunneling device that allows passage of the vein graft from the inflow site to the outflow artery without twisting or kinking. Tunneling is performed before heparinization and may be anatomic or subcutaneous.

PROXIMAL AND DISTAL CONTROL

Vascular clamps are preferably placed on soft portions of the artery. A Wylie subclavian clamp is a reliable choice for control of the common femoral artery. Its jaws can be oriented anterior or posterior to the long axis of the artery, compressing the usually soft anterior artery wall flat against the posterior plaque. Clamping the artery walls side to side, fractures the posterior plaque along its length in an uncontrolled manner. If suitable, the superficial femoral artery and profunda femoris artery can be controlled with small vascular clamps or vessels loops. Balloon occlusion with a Fogarty embolectomy catheter inflated with heparinized saline can also effectively control inflow arteries unsuitable for clamping. In operative sites where the artery is deep, tightened vessel loops can help raise the artery into the wound, easing the awkwardness of "working in a hole."

Vascular control of smaller arteries can be achieved with double-looped, tightened vessel loops, small vascular clamps, Fogarty balloon catheters or intraluminal vessel occluder, such as the Flo-rester (Synovis Surgical Innovations, St. Paul). The vessels are rarely unable to be locally controlled in the incision; however, a sterile tourniquet may also be used to provide proximal vascular control. The use of the tourniquet obviates the need for complete circumferential dissection of the artery, which facilitates the procedure when significant inflammatory changes exist between the artery and the vein. A tourniquet is used after the proximal anastomsis has been completed and the vein graft tunneled to the site of the distal anastomosis. With the patient fully heparinized, the foot and leg are elevated and exsanguinated with an Esmarch bandage, followed by the inflation of a low thigh tourniquet to 300 mm Hg. Placement of a tourniquet around the upper calf should be avoided because of the potential risk of injury to the peroneal nerve as it crosses the head of the fibula. Complications are uncommon with tourniquet times of less than 1 hour.

ANASTOMOTIC TECHNIQUE

Because of the long length of venous conduit required to perform distal bypasses, the distal diameter of the conduit, which serves as the inflow end of a reversed vein graft, may be small when compared with the inflow artery. The venous hood can be augmented by incorporating a venous side branch into the heel of the hood configuration (Figs. 45-1 and 45-2). The in situ or nonreversed vein bypass technique provides a method for optimal size matching of the vein conduit to the inflow and outflow arteries, which is preferred by some surgeons for tibial bypass grafting.

The distal anastomosis is performed with either 6-0 or 7-0 double-armed, nonabsorbable monofilament suture. Heel and toe stitches are placed to anchor the anastomosis, and then the sutures are run toward the midportion of the anastomosis. Another method that is useful in small, visually constrained fields is to "parachute" the heel stitches. This allows the graft to float above the field, providing an

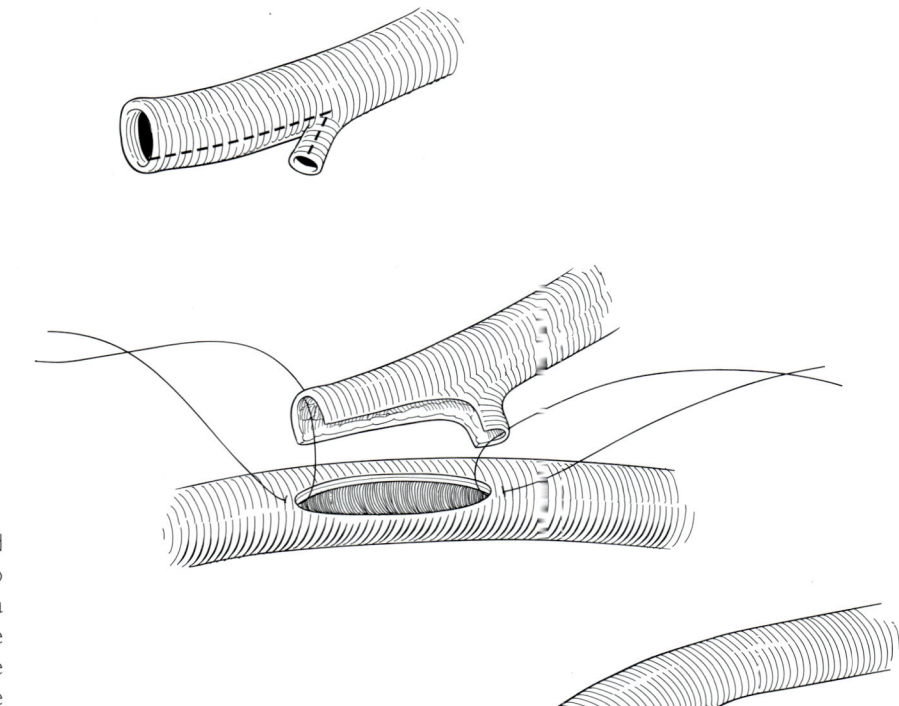

Figure 45-1. The inflow end of the reversed great saphenous vein graft can be tailored to provide a wide anastomosis by preserving a side branch that is then incorporated into the anastomosis. The vein is incised in line with the lumen of the side branch. Potts scissors are used to hook into the side branch, opening it as the terminal portion of the spatulated end of the graft, producing a flange on the heel of the graft.

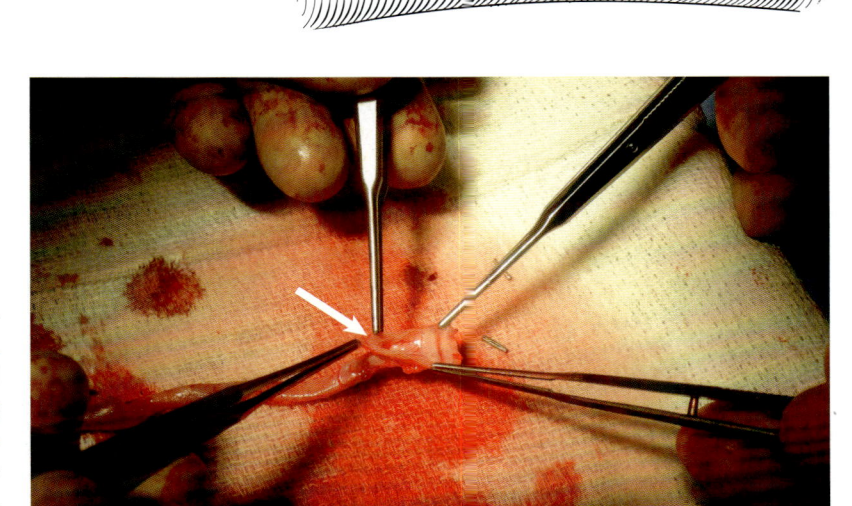

Figure 45-2. Intraoperative photograph of a tailored inflow end of a reverse saphenous vein graft. By incorporating a side branch (*arrow*) into the heel of the proximal anastomosis, there is less crimping of the heel of the graft at the proximal anastomosis. The technique is particularly useful if the inflow artery is somewhat thickened at the site of the proximal anastomosis.

unobstructed field of view within which to place heel sutures. Once the heel sutures are placed, the anastomosis can be pulled down and completed in the standard fashion.

Operative Technique for Femoral Distal Artery-Vein Bypass Grafting

POSITIONING AND DRAPING

The patient is positioned supine on the operating room table. Gel pads are placed under pressure points, including the heels. Body hair is clipped in the operating room. Infected or large wounds are scrubbed with antiseptic and covered with occlusive dressings such as an Ioban, iodophor-impregnated adhesive drape. A Foley catheter is placed and taped to the table to limit slack and brought out behind a thigh to rest on the floor. If the patient has a large pannus, it should be retracted and secured with tape to aid exposure of the groin. The patient is prepped with chlorhexidine from the level of the umbilicus to the toes, laterally "table to table," and circumferentially around both legs. The genitals are prepped and then covered with a folded operating room towel, which is secured to the skin with staples. The feet are covered with sterile clear bags.

Draping should allow the legs free movement for changes in position intraoperatively. The lower abdomen below the navel should also be draped to allow access to the iliac arteries when more proximal inflow is unexpectedly needed or the operative plan changes. A sterile "bump" can be made of bound bundled towels and is essential for positioning. The bump is placed under the thigh with the knee slightly externally rotated in a "frog leg" position to allow the proximal calf to float between the knee and the foot. With the musculature relaxed, exposure of the popliteal and tibial arteries is facilitated. When placed below the knee, the bump allows the distal thigh musculature to relax, aiding access to the distal superficial femoral artery and above-knee popliteal artery.

VEIN HARVEST TECHNIQUE AND PREPARATION

There are a variety of techniques for vein preparation, including in situ grafting with or without exposure of the entire vein, endoscopic harvest as frequently used in coronary artery bypass grafting, and conventional harvest for reversed vein grafting, which is preferred. Harvesting of great saphenous vein is aided by skin markings placed during preoperative ultrasound vein mapping. Incisions are kept directly over the vein, minimizing large tissue flaps that may contribute to poor wound healing or infection. The vein is gently dissected free. Vein branches are ligated with 4-0 silk, taking care not to narrow the lumen. Distal side branches on the venous conduit are temporarily controlled with clips, preserving the length of the side branch in anticipation of incorporation into the heel of the anastomosis. Once removed, the vein is stored in a chilled solution composed of 50 mL of the patient's blood, 3000 units of heparin, 30 mg of papaverine, 2 mL of 1% lidocaine without epinephrine, and 500 mL of normal saline. The vein is fully distended with the storage solution to identify holes or side branches requiring repair or ligation. Suboptimal venous segments that are thick walled, calcified, not distensible, or less than 3 mm in diameter should be replaced with alternate venous segments.

Inflow Exposure at the Femoral and Popliteal Arteries

GENERAL EXPOSURE AT THE GROIN

A longitudinal incision is most often made over the pulse in the groin, which is located just medial to the line of bisection of the inguinal ligament. Alternatively, a transverse incision is an option if the longitudinal length of the arterial dissection is not anticipated to be extensive. Along the lines of the incision, dissection is carried down through the fascia lata, keeping medial to the sartorius muscle. The sartorius is reflected laterally to expose the femoral sheath, which is incised along its length to reveal the common femoral artery. Dissection proceeds along the long axis of the vessels. Every attempt should be made to avoid devascularized tissue flaps or failure to ligate lymphatics during the groin dissection.

The superior limit of the groin dissection is the inguinal ligament. It can be retracted superiorly with a bed-mounted self-retaining retractor, such as the Iron Intern (Automated Medical Products, Edison, N.J.), if exposure of the distal external iliac artery is required to locate a soft spot for clamping or if the patient is obese. The inguinal ligament may be divided if more proximal exposure is necessary but should be reapproximated at the end of the operation.

Routine groin exposure includes isolating the common femoral artery, profunda femoris artery, and superficial femoral artery. The proximal common femoral artery is dissected and looped with either an umbilical tape or a large vessel loop. The

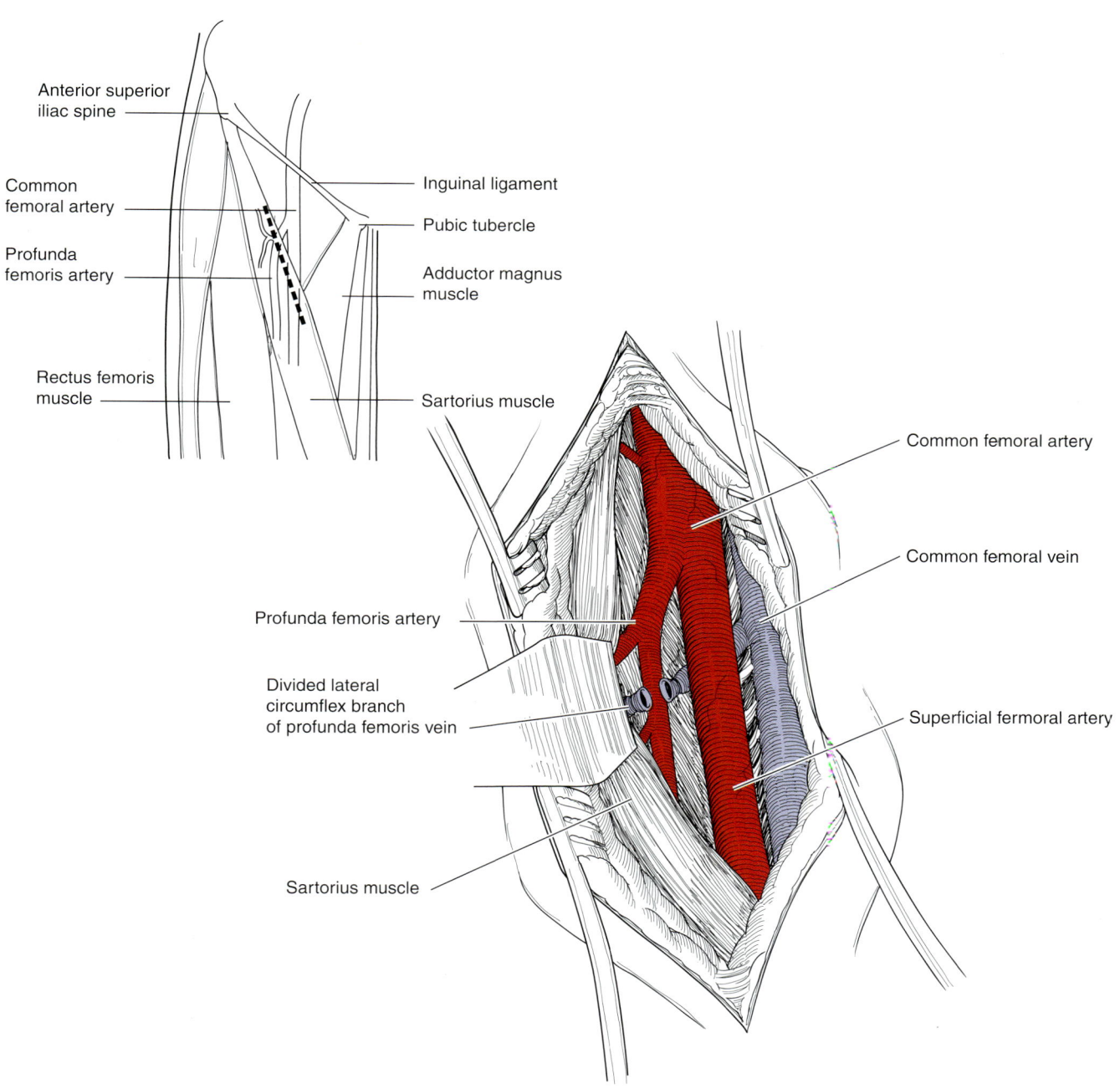

DIRECT SURGICAL REPAIR OF TIBIAL-PERONEAL ARTERIAL OCCLUSIVE DISEASE

Figure 45-3. Exposure of the profunda femoris artery medial to the sartorius muscle can be accomplished as an extension of the groin dissection by retracting the sartorius muscle medially. The lateral circumflex branch of the femoral vein must be divided to expose the mid- and distal profunda femoris artery.

bifurcation of the femoral artery is often marked by a subtle bulge in the common femoral artery as the profunda femoris artery branches posterolaterally. On occasion there may be more than one major profunda femoris artery, with additional vessels arising from the posterior aspect of the common femoral artery. The common femoral artery tapers slightly to become the superficial femoral artery.

PROFUNDA FEMORIS ARTERY

The profunda femoris artery, which may be branched at its origin, dives deep to adductor fascia, which is divided to reveal the deep lateral circumflex femoral vein lying atop the proximal profunda femoris artery. This vein can be quite large but can be divided without reservation for exposure of the profunda femoris artery beyond its origin (Fig. 45-3). If more distal exposure of the profunda femoris artery is needed, dissection proceeds along the length of the profunda femoris artery to expose and control perforator branches. The adductor longus muscle may be

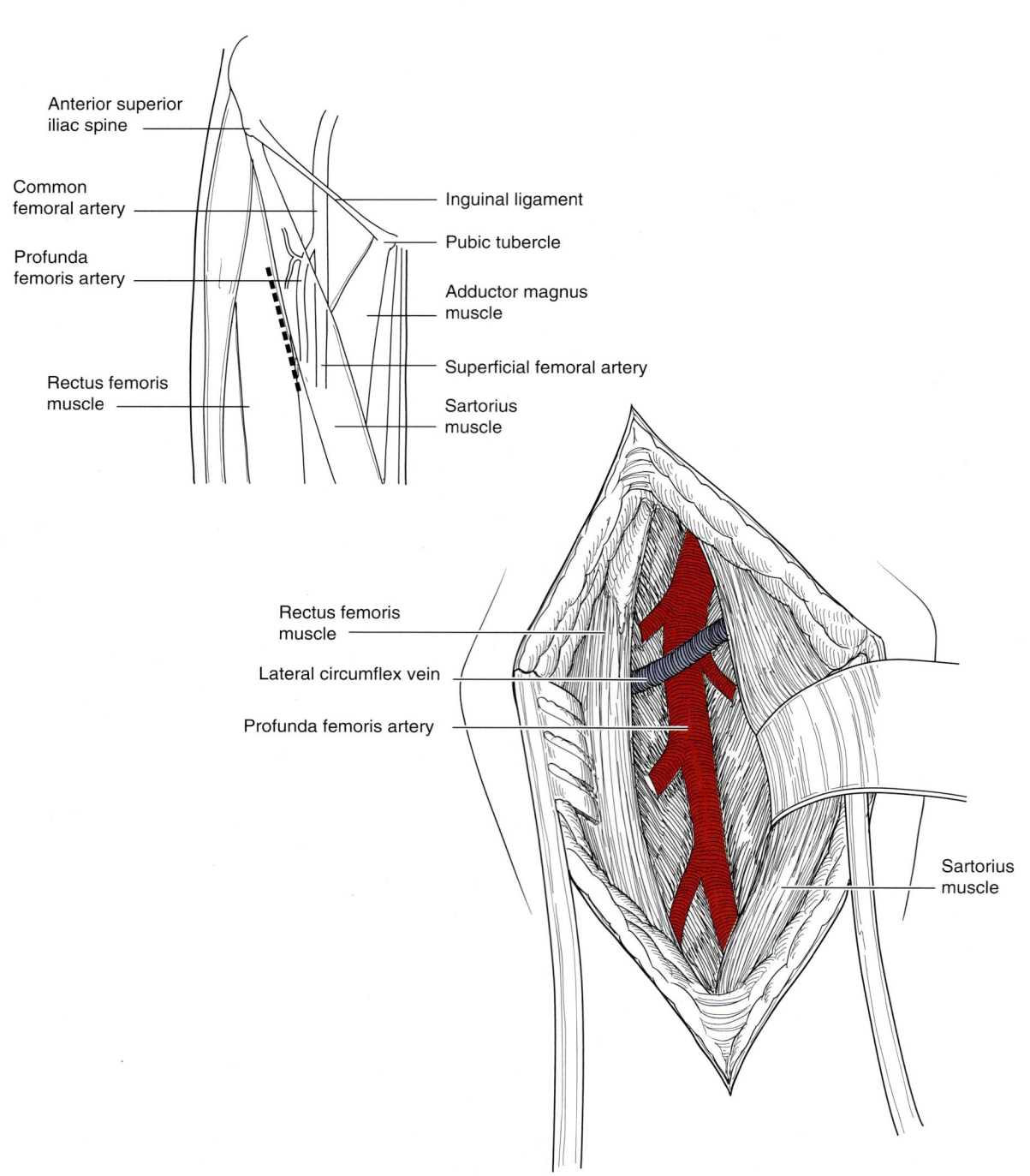

Figure 45-4. The profunda femoris artery can be isolated lateral to the sartorius muscle by incising along the lateral aspect of the course of the sartorius and reflecting the muscle medially. The artery is found deep to the vastus medialis and rectus femoris muscles, which can be retracted laterally. The vastus medialis lies a bit deeper than the rectus femoris muscle and is obscured by the rectus femoris when looking from above with the muscles retracted as shown.

divided distally to obtain additional exposure. Mobilization of the superficial femoral artery upward and medially facilitates distal profunda femoris artery exposure.

PROFUNDA FEMORIS ARTERY LATERAL APPROACH

The profunda femoris artery can also be approached laterally. Although the common femoral and superficial femoral arteries are not available for anatomic orientation, the lateral approach is useful when the groin is scarred or there is infection within the femoral triangle. The incision is made lateral to the sartorius muscle. The sartorius muscle is retracted medially to expose the rectus femoris and vastus medialis muscles. These muscles are then retracted laterally to expose the profunda femoris artery (Fig. 45-4).

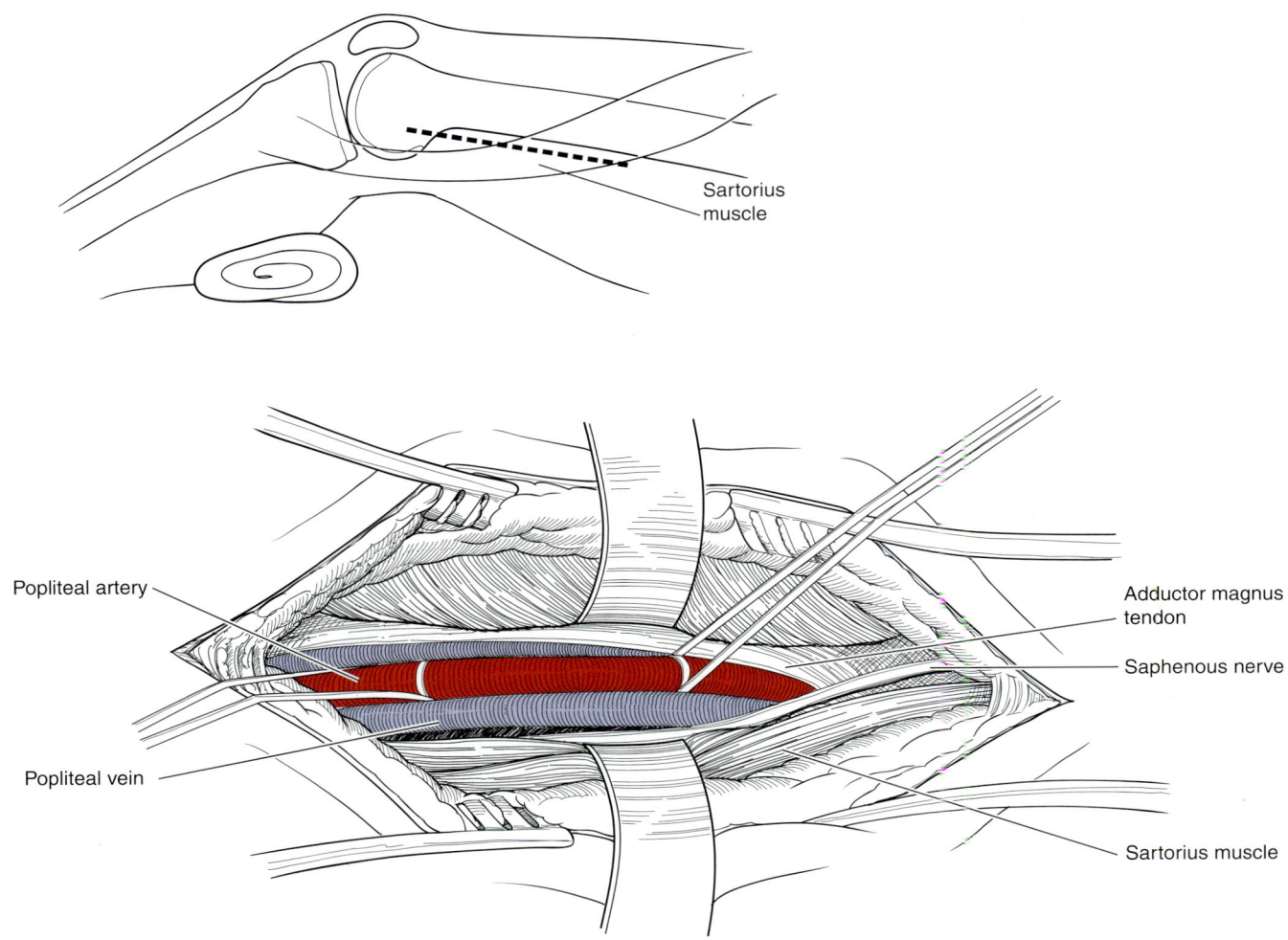

Figure 45-5. Exposures of the superficial femoral artery and above-knee popliteal artery are performed via a medial longitudinal distal thigh incision superior to the sartorius muscle. The sartorius is retracted inferiorly, and the adductor muscle group is reflected superiorly to expose a pocket of fatty tissue that is bluntly retracted inferiorly. The above-knee popliteal artery can be located as it exits the adductor hiatus, immediately posterior to the femur.

SUPERFICIAL FEMORAL ARTERY AND ABOVE-KNEE POPLITEAL ARTERY

The proximal or mid-superficial femoral artery can be exposed with a longitudinal incision in the anterior medial thigh over the anticipated site of anastomosis. The sartorius muscle is retracted superiorly. Once the sartorius muscle reaches the midthigh, it can be retracted inferiorly to allow access to the distal superficial femoral artery.

For exposure of the distal superficial femoral artery, a distal longitudinal medial thigh incision is used. The sartorius muscle is retracted inferiorly, and the adductor magnus muscle is retracted superiorly. The neurovascular bundle is found immediately posterior to the femur (Fig. 45-5).

BELOW-KNEE POPLITEAL ARTERY

The incision to approach the below-knee popliteal artery is made on the medial upper calf, posterior to the tibia. The great saphenous vein and saphenous nerve lie superficial in this area and should be preserved. The crural fascia is incised, exposing the medial head of the gastrocnemius muscle, which is retracted posteriorly. The conjoined tendons of the semitendinosus, gracilis, and semimembranosus muscle group insert on the proximal tibia as the pes anserinus and can be divided to facilitate more proximal exposure. The vascular bundle is surrounded by fatty tissue and lies directly posterior to the tibia (Figs. 45-6 and 45-7).

552 LOWER EXTREMITY ARTERIAL DISEASE

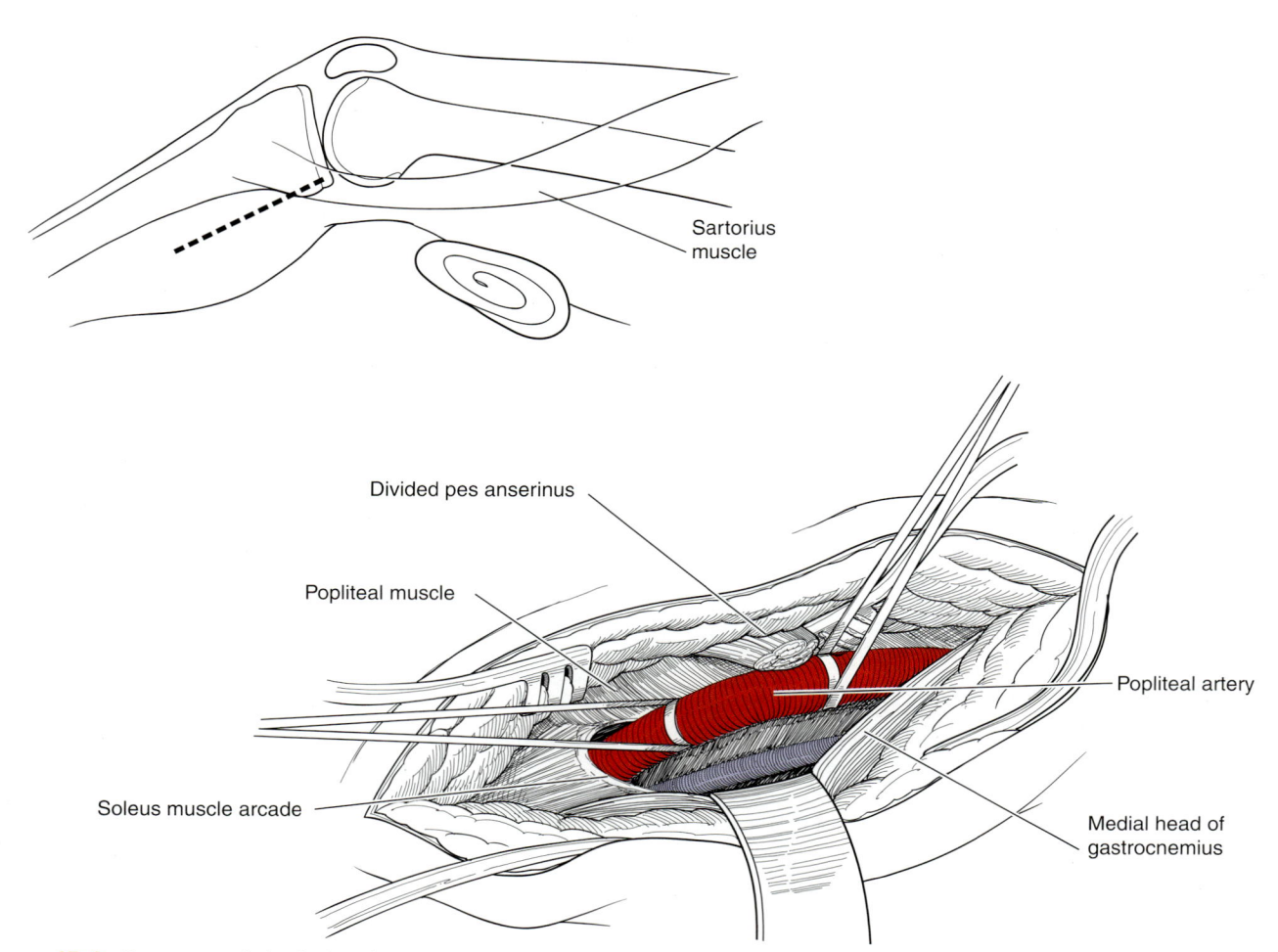

Figure 45-6. Exposure of the below-knee popliteal artery is performed via a longitudinal medial calf incision. The gastrocnemius muscle is retracted inferiorly to expose the fatty tissue surrounding the popliteal space. This fatty tissue is retracted inferiorly to demonstrate the vascular bundle lying immediately posterior to the tibia. The popliteal vein (typically paired) always lies immediately on the artery, necessitating its dissection off and inferior to the artery.

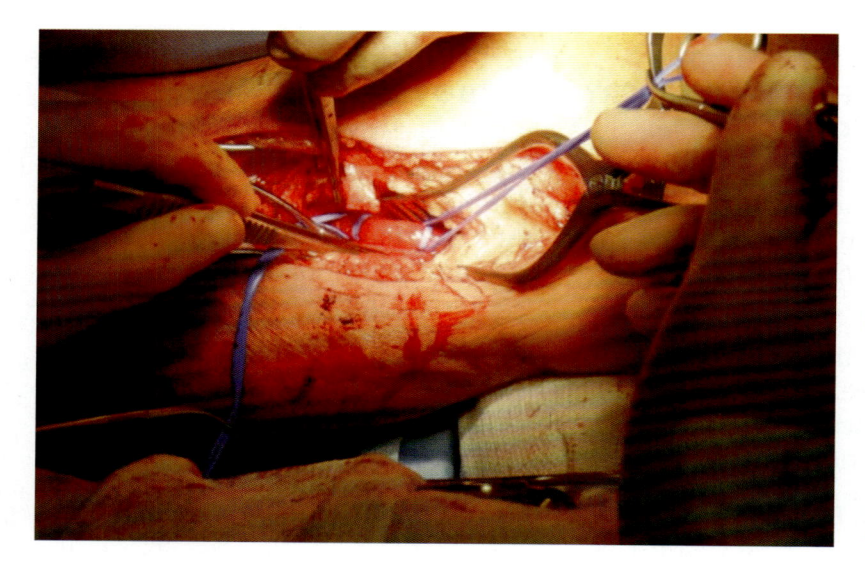

Figure 45-7. Intraoperative photograph of exposure and control of the below-knee popliteal artery. The below-knee popliteal artery is a good source of inflow to a tibial graft if the proximal vasculature is free of hemodynamically significant stenoses. The artery can be easily controlled with silicone elastomer (Silastic) vessel loops and gently retracted toward the wound opening to facilitate the anastomosis.

Distal Artery Exposures and Bypass Graft Configurations

FEMORAL-ANTERIOR TIBIAL ARTERY BYPASS

A vertical incision is made in the anterolateral lower leg, midway between the tibia and the fibula. The incision is brought down to the crural fascia, which is incised along the lateral border of the tibialis anterior muscle. A plane is bluntly developed between the tibialis anterior muscle and the extensor digitorum longus

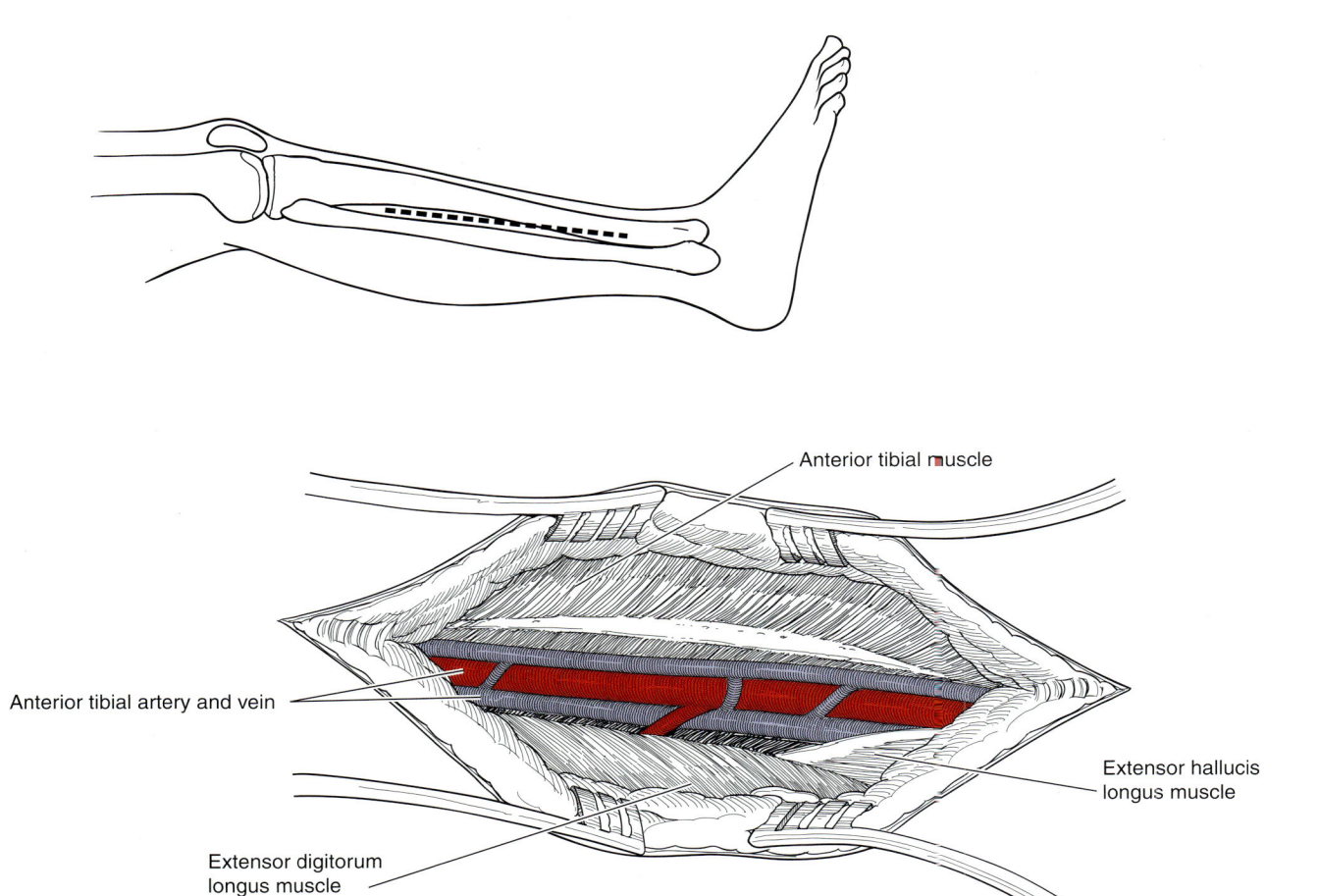

DIRECT SURGICAL REPAIR OF TIBIAL-PERONEAL ARTERIAL OCCLUSIVE DISEASE 553

Figure 45-8. Anterolateral exposure of the anterior tibial artery. A plane is bluntly developed between the tibialis anterior muscle and the extensor digitorum longus muscle to expose the anterior tibial artery, which is immediately above the interosseous membrane.

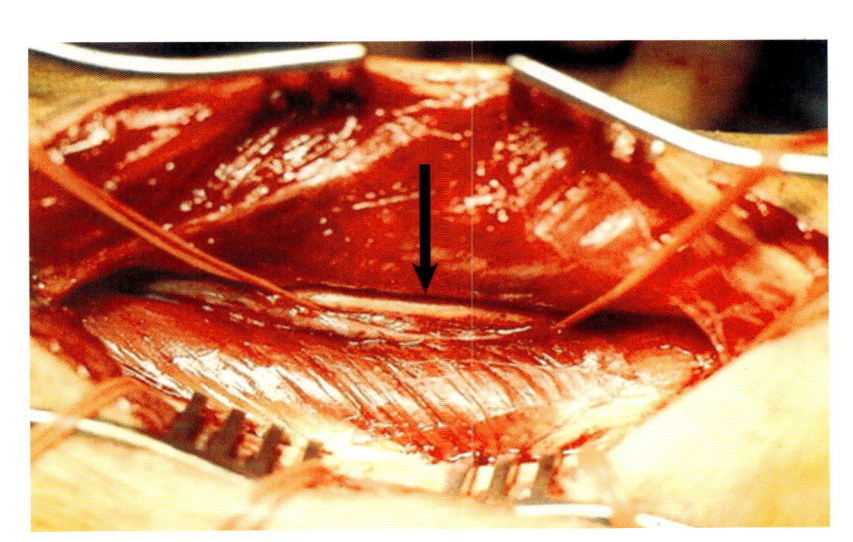

Figure 45-9. Intraoperative photograph of exposure of the anterior tibial artery (*arrow*). Vessel loops are sufficient for vascular control under most circumstances.

muscle to expose the anterior tibial vessels lying immediately above the interosseous membrane (Figs. 45-8 and 45-9).

Anatomic Tunneling

In most cases of reversed vein bypass grafts, anatomic tunneling is preferred. Anatomic tunneling permits the use of shorter grafts, and the vein graft is protected against exposure from wound breakdown. The proximal tunneling is done subsartorially as is done for a femoral to popliteal bypass graft. A medial calf exposure of the popliteal fossa, as described for the below-knee popliteal artery, is

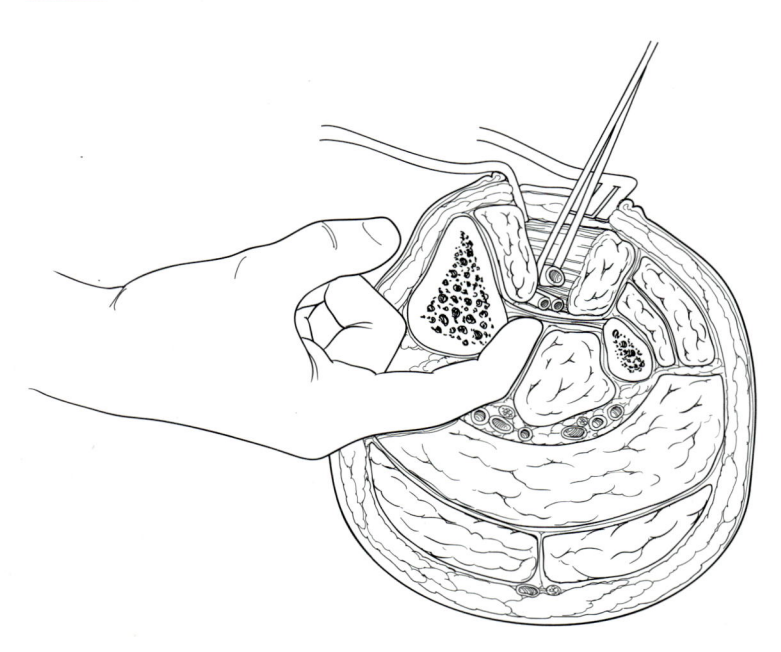

Figure 45-10. The interosseous membrane is incised with a knife proximal to the anticipated anastomotic site to the anterior tibial artery. The membrane is then widened with a hemostat or large aortic clamp. An aortic clamp is then directed proximally from the lateral exposure of the anterior tibial artery to the below-knee popliteal exposure. Once the tough membrane is traversed, it is dilated to prevent ledges that can kink the graft. With an aortic clamp, the graft is then drawn from medial to lateral into the anterior compartment for anastomosis to the anterior tibial artery.

used to route the tunneler to the groin exposure. A space in the popliteal fossa between the femoral condyles and between the two heads of the gastrocnemius muscle is bluntly developed. The tunneler is passed into this space with the curved portion pointing toward the ceiling. The tunneler is then directed toward the groin, keeping the course subsartorial until the tip exits in the groin. Taut fascial bands at the extremes of the tunnel are divided to prevent impingement on the graft. If needed, the tunnel can be passed in two steps from the below to the above knee popliteal fossa and from the above knee popliteal fossa, subsartorially, to the groin. At each stage 16 Fr red rubber catheters can be placed and secured by Kelly clamps.

For in situ grafts, the vein graft is directed into the popliteal fossa below the knee through the crural fascia, between the medial and lateral heads of the gastrocnemius muscle into the popliteal space. From there, the vein graft is directed to the anterior tibial artery, which lies in the anterior compartment of the leg in the same manner as for a reversed vein bypass.

From the popliteal fossa to the anterior tibial artery, the graft is tunneled through the interosseous membrane to reach the anterior tibial artery (Fig. 45-10). From the lateral lower leg exposure, a cruciate incision is made in the interosseous membrane 2 cm proximal to the planned anastomosis site. The opening is widened with a hemostat so that the vein graft can lie in a smooth path without impingement from a fascial edge. A long, gently curved vascular clamp, passed lateral to medial, is used to grasp the graft from the popliteal space and pull it into the anterolateral incision for the distal anastomosis to the anterior tibial artery.

Lateral Tunneling

For grafts traveling from the proximal femoral vessels to the anterior tibial artery, a subcutaneous course that traverses the midthigh may be used. Beginning at the distal arterial exposure on the anterolateral calf, the tunneler is directed subcutaneously, crossing the knee at the midpoint of the lateral femoral condyle. If the graft is tunneled too anterior, flexion of the knee results in stretching, compression, and ultimately failure of the graft. Care must be taken to avoid the area around the fibular head and thus prevent injury to the peroneal nerve. The tunneler is redirected toward the medial thigh, over the sartorius muscle emerging in the groin exposure. A counterincision is sometimes needed at the distal lateral thigh to smoothly redirect the tunneler medially.

FEMORAL-POSTERIOR TIBIAL ARTERY BYPASS

Exposure of the Proximal Posterior Tibial Artery

For exposure of the proximal portion of the tibioperoneal trunk and the posterior tibial artery, an extension of the medial calf exposure of the below-knee popliteal artery is used. A 10-cm longitudinal incision is placed 2 cm posterior to the medial edge of the tibia. Dissection is carried down through the crural fascia to the medial head of the gastrocnemius muscle, which is reflected posteriorly to expose the soleus muscle. Soleus muscle fibers originating on the posterior aspect of the tibia are divided using a right-angled clamp to protect the underlying arteries and veins. Highly branched, crossing tibial veins lie close to the tibioperoneal trunk and proximal posterior tibial and peroneal arteries. Meticulous dissection is required to avoid bleeding and vascular injury at this level.

Exposure of the Midportion of the Posterior Tibial Artery

In the midportion of the leg, the posterior tibial artery is approached with a medial calf incision 2 cm posterior to the tibial edge. The soleus muscle is mobilized off the edge of the tibia, as well as off of the anterior aponeurosis attached to the tibia, and is retracted posteriorly. A plane is then developed between the flexor digitorum longus, which lies along the undersurface of the tibia, and the soleus muscles to expose the posterior tibial artery and veins (Fig. 45-11). Care should be taken not to inadvertently mobilize the flexor digitorum longus muscle off of the tibia. The posterior tibial artery is often first identified by the visualization of perforating branches of the tibial veins, which perforate through the anterior aponeurosis.

Tunneling

Grafts to the posterior tibial artery are tunneled anatomically through the popliteal fossa. A skin bridge can be maintained between the incision used to expose the posterior tibial artery and the below-knee popliteal artery incision.

FEMORAL-PERONEAL ARTERY BYPASS

Medial Exposure of the Peroneal Artery

A longitudinal incision 2 cm posterior to the medial edge of the tibia in the midportion of the calf is made for a length of 10 cm. Dissection is carried down through the crural fascia until the soleus muscle fibers are exposed. The soleus muscle is mobilized off the tibia and off of the anterior aponeurosis and is reflected posteriorly to reveal the flexor digitorum longus muscle posterior to the tibia. The fascia of the flexor digitorum longus muscle is incised to enter into the deep posterior fascial compartment. Often the posterior tibial vessels are initially seen when dissecting the peroneal artery. They should be retracted inferiorly, with dissection continued medially to the peroneal artery. The peroneal vascular bundle is encountered on the anterior surface of the flexor hallucis longus muscle overlying the fibula.

Tunneling

Grafts are tunneled anatomically and carried down under the skin bridge to the peroneal artery for the distal anastomosis.

Groin Wound Closure

Groin wound healing complications such as seroma, hematoma, and infection vary in severity from nuisance wounds to placing the vascular graft at risk for failure with the possibility of limb loss. Therefore groin wounds are meticulously closed in multiple layers. Wounds are first generously irrigated with antibiotic solution. Fascia and soft tissues are reapproximated in at least three layers to obliterate dead spaces where fluid collections may form. Either a running or an interrupted braided absorbable suture is advisable. The skin is approximated with staples or monofilament absorbable subcuticular sutures, and a dry dressing is applied. Skin adhesive, such as Dermabond, is also acceptable as a skin sealant. Drains are not used routinely, but may be considered if postoperative heparinization is planned.

Calf Incision Closure

The fascia of the lower leg incision can be closed loosely if compartment syndrome is not a concern. The crural fascia can be closed with a running Vicryl suture in the case of an anatomically tunneled graft. If an in situ graft is placed, then the crural

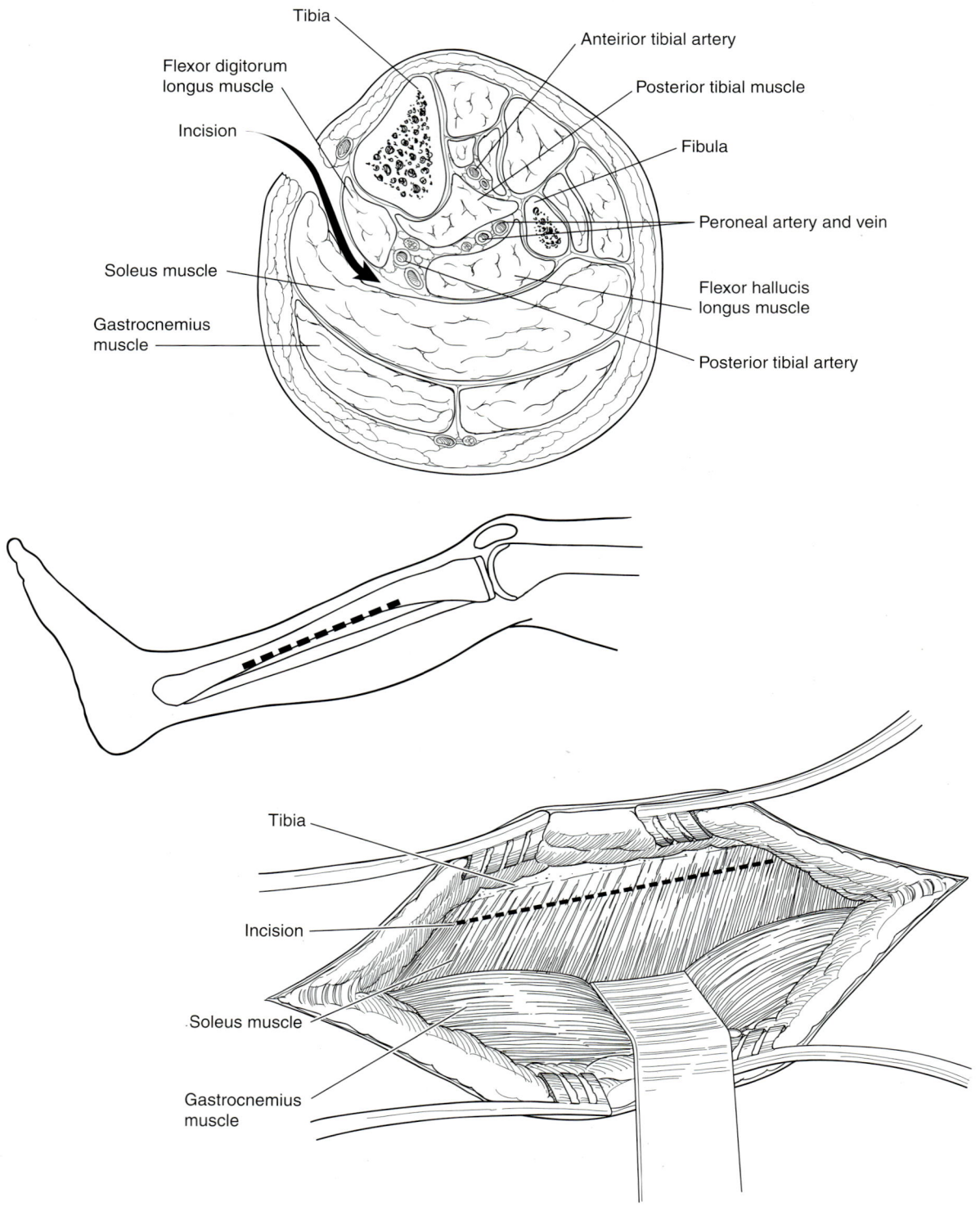

Figure 45-11. Exposures of both the peroneal and the posterior tibial arteries are performed via a medial calf incision. The posterior tibial artery is encountered between the soleus muscle and the flexor digitorum longus muscle. The peroneal artery is encountered deeper in the wound on the anterior surface of the flexor hallucis longus muscle as depicted.

fascia is best left open where the graft dives down into the popliteal space to prevent scar tissue from impinging on the bypass graft. Subcutaneous tissues are also reapproximated with Vicryl sutures. Skin dehiscence from stretching because of postoperative edema and lack of redundant tissue in the lower leg discourages the use of fine subcuticular sutures in favor of stronger materials. Nylon interrupted vertical mattress sutures or staples are preferred.

Adjunctive Techniques for Distal Bypasses

A distal arteriovenous fistula can be used as an adjunct to increase flow in "at risk" vein grafts or prosthetic grafts supplying highly diseased vascular beds, but efficacy in improving graft patency is unproved.[20] Additional adjuncts for increasing patency rates of prosthetic tibial bypass grafts include vein cuffs and patches. Incorporation of a venous interface between prosthetic material and small-caliber arteries is thought to decrease the growth of intimal hyperplasia by reducing compliance mismatch.[21] A Taylor patch, Miller cuff Linton patch, as well as a graft that has a preincorporated mini-cuff (Dista-low, Bard Peripheral Vascular, Inc., Tempe, Ariz.) or heparinized surface (Propaten, W.L. Gore & Associates Inc., Newark, Del.), are well-described options.

Postoperative anticoagulation is used to increase patency rates in prosthetic and at-risk vein grafts, including vein grafts with multiple prior revisions and patients with a history of prior graft thrombosis without a clear anatomic etiology, poor outflow, or a suspected or confirmed hypercoagulable state.[22] All prosthetic grafts to tibial arteries should receive long-term anticoagulation. Postoperatively, the

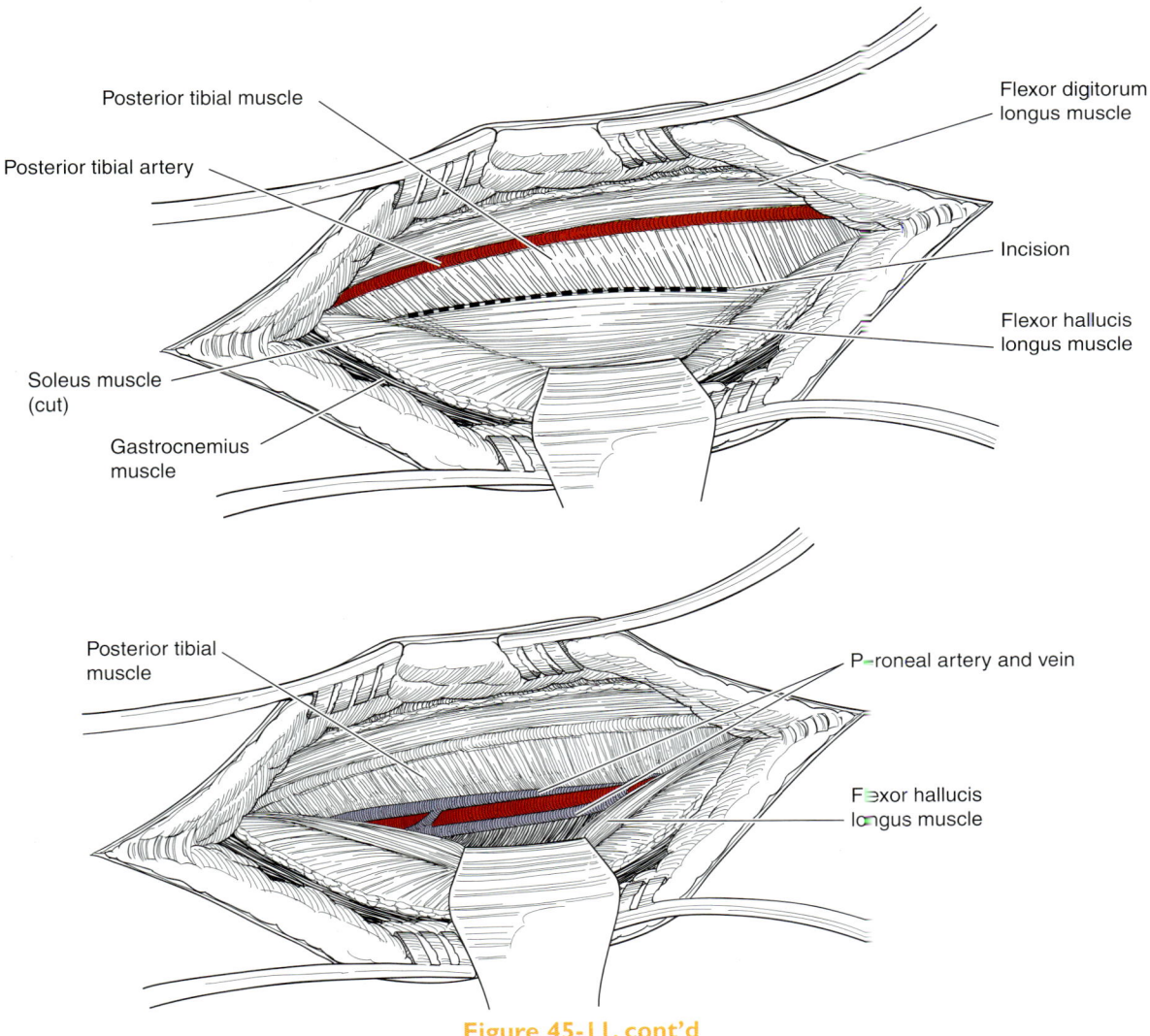

Figure 45-11, cont'd

patient is started on a therapeutic heparin drip as a bridge to Coumadin with a target international normalized ratio of 2 to 3. Drains are more liberally used in patients requiring uninterrupted anticoagulation after bypass surgery in anticipation of possible wound hematoma. If possible, a delay of several hours after skin closure to beginning anticoagulation appears to decrease the incidence of wound hematoma. In addition, careful monitoring of partial thromboplastin time (PTT) levels is essential. Markedly elevated PTT levels in the early postoperative period increase the risk of wound hematoma.

LOWER EXTREMITY FASCIOTOMY

Acute onset of ischemia, prolonged ischemia, and prolonged operative revascularization are predisposing factors for the development of compartment syndrome.[23] A low threshold for performing fasciotomies is prudent.[24]

Postoperative Care

- **Wound care.** Operative dressings are removed on the second postoperative day, and incisions are left open to air if there is no evidence of drainage. Draining wounds are covered with gauze dressings, which are changed as needed. Groin wounds are kept covered with dry gauze to prevent accumulation of moisture or perineal soilage, especially if the patient is obese with pannus overlying the wounds.
- **Leg edema.** Compression devices such as CircAids (CircAid, San Diego) and compression hose, combined with leg elevation, are the mainstays of treatment to reduce edema and tension on wounds, which is frequently present after tibial bypass and can lead to dehiscence. Sitting with the legs dependent and without leg compression is discouraged. Rooke boots (Osborn Medical, Utica, Minn.) or similar protective boots are supplied to all patients to help protect wounds and heels. Early mobilization is encouraged, with involvement of physical therapists as needed.
- **Prophylaxis for venous thromboembolism.** Prophylactic doses of subcutaneous heparin are used routinely during hospitalization until the patient is mobilized and walking. Pneumatic compression devices are not routinely used.
- **Blood glucose.** Blood glucose levels are monitored and are maintained below 150 mg/dL with supplementary insulin as needed.
- **Prophylactic antibiotics.** Postoperative antibiotics are continued for patients who have established infections.
- **Associated need for foot surgery.** Foot surgery (i.e., amputations and debridements) is not performed concurrently with lower extremity revascularization, particularly if there is gross infection. Waiting 2 to 3 days after revascularization to perform needed foot surgery reduces the risk of contamination of operative sites while allowing time for questionably viable tissue to fully demarcate.
- **Risk factor modification.** All patients are maintained on aspirin and statins unless they are intolerant to these medications.
- **Graft surveillance.** A duplex ultrasound graft flow study is performed before discharge to serve as a baseline examination, confirm the success of the operation, and screen for early technical problems that can be immediately addressed. Patients are examined in the clinic 2 weeks after discharge for a wound check and then every 3 months for graft surveillance by duplex ultrasound. If no abnormalities are found at 1 year, surveillance intervals are increased to every 6 months.

Complications

- **Systemic complications.** The common association of comorbidities among patients who undergo lower distal bypass may lead to a variety of postoperative complications, including myocardial infarction, renal failure, pneumonia, respiratory failure, delirium, and stroke.

- **Wound complications.** Wound complications range from simple skin dehiscence, leading to poorly healing wounds, to overt groin or deep leg sepsis. Groin seroma can also be troublesome. Rotation of a sartorius flap into the wound can be used to cover the graft after treatment of significant seromas or persistent lymph leaks. Wound hematomas are evacuated surgically with drain placement to decompress the overlying skin.
- **Early graft failure.** Early graft failures are uncommon but may result from a variety of factors, mostly technical, that include an imperfect anastomosis, kinking or compression of the graft from adventitial bands, graft redundancy, and fibrotic valve leaflets that may produce stenosis. Unrecognized hypercoagulable states may lead to graft thrombosis without an identifiable flow-limiting lesion. Low flow states such as shock may also cause early graft thrombosis. Poor outflow can also contribute to early graft failure. Rarely, the cause of graft failure is unidentifiable.

REFERENCES

1. Stephenson HE, Kimpton RS: Americas First Nobel Prize in medicine or physiology: The story of Guthrie and Carrel, Boston, 2001, Midwestern Vascular Surgical Society.
2. Bernheim BM: Notebooks on vascular anastomosis, 1908-1909. The Alan Mason Chesney Medical Archives of The Johns Hopkins Medical Institutions. Available at http://www.medicalarchives.jhmi.edu/papers/bernheim.html. Accessed November 2013.
3. Wardrop D, Keeling D: The story of the discovery of heparin and warfarin, *Brit J Haemat* 141:757-763, 2008.
4. Kunlin J: Long vein transplantation in treatment of ischemia caused by arteritis, *Rev Chir* 70: 206-235, 1951.
5. Hughes CW: Arterial repair during the Korean War, *Ann Surg* 147:555-561, 1958.
6. Levitsky S, James PM, Anderson RW, et al: Vascular trauma in Vietnam battle casualties: An analysis of 55 consecutive cases, *Ann Surg* 168:831-836, 1968.
7. Szilagyi DE, Smith RF, Whitcomb JG: Contribution of angioplastic surgery to therapy of peripheral occlusive arteriopathy: Critical evaluation of 8 years' experience, *Ann Surg* 152:660-677, 1960.
8. Beard JD: Which is the best revascularization for critical limb ischemia: Endovascular or open surgery? *J Vasc Surg* 48:11S-16S, 2008.
9. Goodney PP, Nolan BW, Schanzer A, et al: Factors associated with death 1 year after lower extremity bypass in northern New England, *J Vasc Surg* 51:71-78, 2010.
10. Fleisher LA, Beckman JA, Brown KA, et al: ACC/AHA 2007 guidelines on perioperative cardiovascular evaluation and care for noncardiac surgery: A report of the American College of Cardiology/American Heart Association Task Force on Practice Guidelines, *Circulation* 116:e418-499, 2007.
11. Bauer SM, Cayne NS, Veith FJ: New developments in the preoperative evaluation and perioperative management of coronary artery disease in patients undergoing vascular surgery, *J Vasc Surg* 51:242-251, 2010.
12. Schanzer A, Hevelone N, Owens CD, et al: Statins are independently associated with reduced mortality in patients undergoing infrainguinal bypass graft surgery for critical limb ischemia, *J Vasc Surg* 47:774-781, 2008.
13. Feringa HH, Schouten O, Karagiannis SE, et al: Intensity of statin therapy in relation to myocardial ischemia, troponin T release, and clinical cardiac outcome in patients undergoing major vascular surgery, *J Am Coll Cardiol* 50:1649-1656, 2007.
14. Abbruzzese TA, Havens J, Belkin M, et al: Statin therapy is associated with improved patency of autogenous infrainguinal bypass grafts, *J Vasc Surg* 39:1178-1185, 2004.
15. Schanzer A, Hevelone N, Owens CD, et al: Technical factors affecting autogenous vein graft failure: Observations from a large multicenter trial, *J Vasc Surg* 46:1180-1190, 2007.
16. Dorrucci V, Griselli F, Petralia G, et al: Heparin-bonded expanded polytetrafluoroethylene grafts for infragenicular bypass in patients with critical limb ischemia: 2-year results, *J Cardiovasc Surg (Torino)* 49:145-149, 2008.
17. Losel-Sadee H, Alefelder C: Heparin-bonded expanded polytetrafluoroethylene graft for infragenicular bypass: Five-year results, *J Cardiovasc Surg (Torino)* 50:339-343, 2009.
18. Probst H, Saucy F, Dusmet M, et al: Clinical results of autologous infrainguinal revascularization using grafts originating distal to the femoral bifurcation in patients with mild inflow disease, *J Cardiovasc Surg (Torino)* 47:437-443, 2006.
19. Darling RC III, Shah DM, Chang BB, et al: Arterial reconstruction for limb salvage: Is the terminal peroneal artery a disadvantaged outflow tract? *Surgery* 118:763-767, 1995.
20. Laurila K, Lepäntalo M, Teittinen K, et al: Does an adjuvant AV-fistula improve the patency of a femorocrural PTFE bypass with distal vein cuff in critical leg ischaemia? A prospective randomised multicentre trial, *Eur J Vasc Endovasc Surg* 27:180-185, 2004.

21. Neville RF, Tempesta B, Sidway AN: Tibial bypass for limb salvage using polytetrafluoroethylene and a distal vein patch, *J Vasc Surg* 33:266-271, 2001. discussion 271–272.
22. Brumberg RS, Back MR, Armstrong PA, et al: The relative importance of graft surveillance and warfarin therapy in infrainguinal prosthetic bypass failure, *J Vasc Surg* 46:1160-1166, 2007.
23. Jensen SL, Sandermann J: Compartment syndrome and fasciotomy in vascular surgery: A review of 57 cases, *Eur J Vasc Endovasc Surg* 13:48-53, 1997.
24. Rush DS, Frame SB, Bell RM, et al: Does open fasciotomy contribute to morbidity and mortality after acute lower extremity ischemia and revascularization? *J Vasc Surg* 10:343-350, 1989.

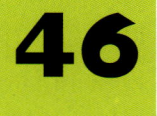

46 Direct Surgical Repair of Popliteal Artery Aneurysm

FRANK B. POMPOSELLI • MARK C. WYERS

Historical Background

In 1785 Hunter successfully ligated the popliteal artery of a coachman with a large popliteal aneurysm, relying on collateral circulation to maintain the viability of the limb.[1] In 1916, while working at Johns Hopkins, Bertram Bernheim[2] was the first to report the use of a saphenous vein interposition graft for treatment of a popliteal aneurysm. As a proponent of aneurysm ligation, Halsted did not support Bernheim's work. Halsted presumed that interposition grafts would be at high risk of thrombosis, which would extend proximally and distally and interfere with natural collaterals. This work was not pursued and only some four decades later did Bernheim's pioneering work finally enter mainstream clinical medicine as standard of care. Modern surgical treatment combines arterial bypass with ligation or interposition grafting and remains the gold standard for treatment. In addition, endovascular stent grafting has become an alternative treatment option in carefully selected patients. This chapter focuses only on the open surgical approaches.

Popliteal aneurysms may manifest as an asymptomatic pulsating mass behind the knee or with symptoms of either chronic or acute ischemia. A minority of patients experience pain or pressure behind the knee or with compressive symptoms involving the popliteal vein or peroneal nerve. Rupture is an unusual complication, occurring in 0% to 7% of published series with an average of about 2%.[3] Acute limb ischemia is the most feared complication of popliteal aneurysms. Its occurrence can complicate treatment and is associated with significant risk of limb loss. In recent years the liberal use of thrombolytic therapy coupled with distal arterial reconstructive surgery has decreased the likelihood of major limb amputation with acute ischemia; however it remains a significant problem.

Indications

Any symptomatic popliteal aneurysm, regardless of size, should be repaired. In most series, however, only 60% to 70% of patients treated had symptoms at the time of presentation.[4,5] For asymptomatic aneurysms, controversy remains regarding which need to be repaired or safely followed. For bypasses done to repair small, asymptomatic aneurysms, long-term graft patency and limb salvage is usually greater than 95%. Corresponding perioperative mortality with treatment is low, usually around 1% to 2%. Mortality rates can be three to four times higher in patients treated with critical limb ischemia. Aggressive recommendations for repair of asymptomatic aneurysms more than 2 cm in diameter have been proposed,[6] especially in European centers, based on poor outcomes once thromboembolic complication occurs. Some reports have instead suggested that popliteal aneurysms smaller than 3 cm can be carefully watched.[7,8] Mitigating features that further justify observation include the absence of intraluminal thrombus, normal runoff, and poor overall patient condition. Conversely, in good risk patients even small aneurysms with absent pulses suggesting occult embolization should be repaired, because 86% develop ischemic complications if left untreated. The advent of endovascular stent-graft treatment of popliteal aneurysms and better lytic therapy to improve runoff may also affect individual decision making.

An acceptable approach is to offer elective repair for all asymptomatic aneurysms that are 2.5 cm or greater unless the physician feels the risks of treatment are excessive because of the health status of the patient. For frail patients in poor health or with limited life expectancy the physician should observe even larger aneurysms provided that the estimated risk of complications is low, assuming minimal intraluminal thrombus, palpable distal pulses, and no evidence of continued expansion.

Preoperative Preparation

- An ankle-brachial index, Doppler waveforms, and pulsed volume recordings or toe pressures are advisable to evaluate for silent distal embolization.
- Computed tomography (CT) angiography (Fig. 46-1) or magnetic resonance angiography can be used to determine the extent of the aneurysm and to

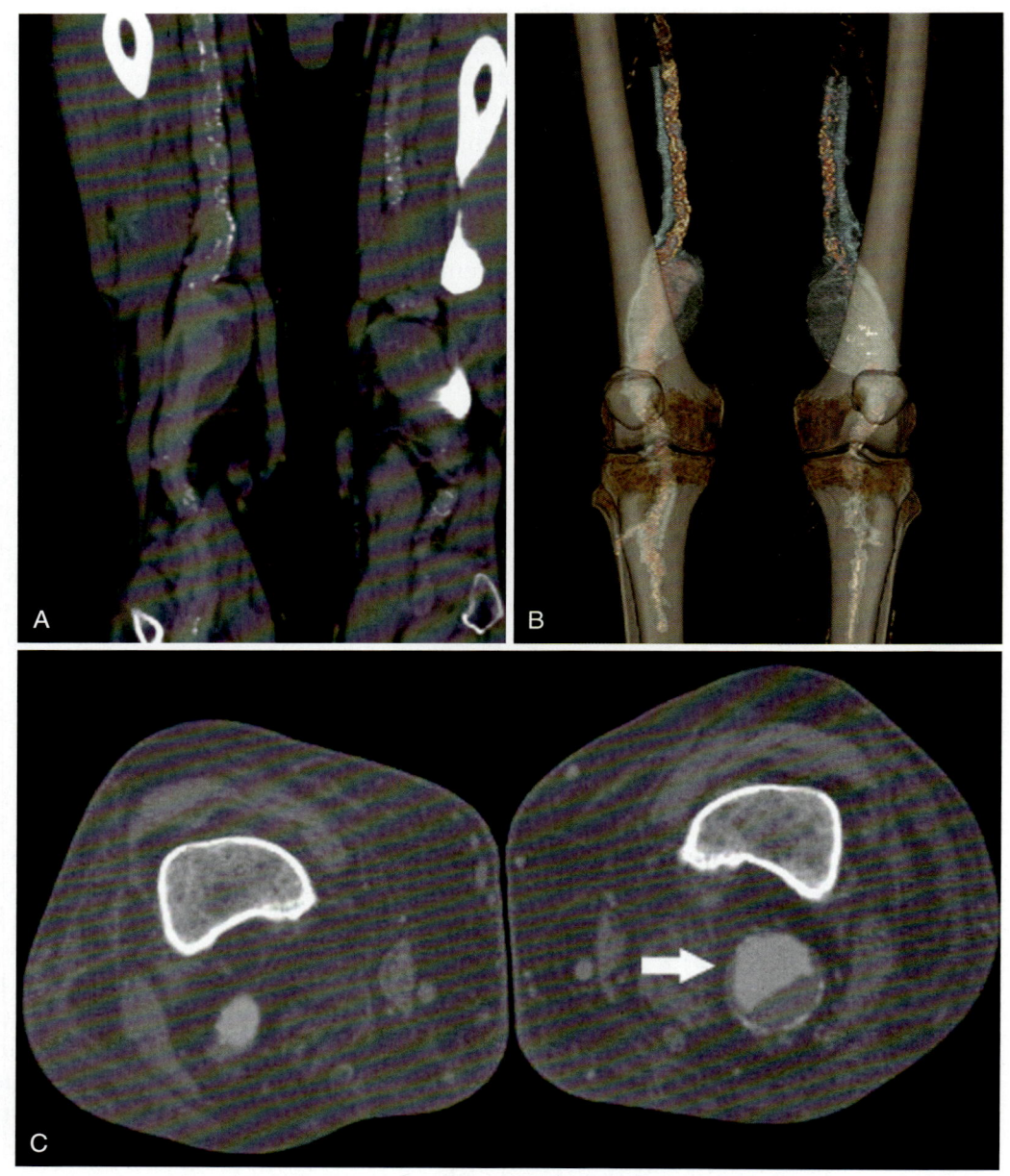

Figure 46-1. A, Multiplanar reformatted computed tomography angiogram demonstrating the size and extent of a large popliteal aneurysm. **B,** Surface-shaded computed tomography representation of bilateral aneurysms. Blood flow is modeled in red and thrombus in green. The left popliteal aneurysm is thombosed. **C,** Axial computed tomography angiogram demonstrating smaller, bilateral aneurysms with thrombus.

select inflow and outflow targets for bypass in patients with no evidence of distal embolization on clinical or noninvasive testing. CT angiography, because of its ability to evaluate calcification, is complementary to angiography.

- Arteriography remains important for evaluating outflow, especially when there is thrombosis or evidence of distal embolization. Angiography can be combined with preoperative lytic therapies in the setting of acute thrombosis without a suitable bypass target. In the elective evaluation of asymptomatic patients, high-quality CT angiography or magnetic resonance angiography may obviate the need for arteriography, especially with demonstrable normal runoff vessel anatomy.
- Preoperative vein mapping, including great and small saphenous veins, should always be performed before popliteal aneurysm repair. Vein location should be marked on the skin and is used for planning the location of the incision. The small saphenous vein is rarely large enough to be a suitable conduit.
- As with any peripheral bypass, low-dose aspirin should be initiated preoperatively and continued indefinitely.
- Anticoagulation is not required for asymptomatic aneurysms but is advisable for evidence of embolization.
- Clinical perioperative cardiac risk assessment is routine with selective use of noninvasive stress testing.
- Screening for a contralateral popliteal artery aneurysm and for an aneurysm of the abdominal aorta should be performed. Bilateral popliteal aneurysms are present in approximately 50% of patients, and the combined incidence of aortic and popliteal aneurysm ranges from 40% to 70%.[3,9]

Pitfalls and Danger Points

- Avoid excessive manipulation of aneurysms containing thrombus to minimize the risk of distal embolization.
- Poor preoperative runoff may require bypass to a distal target artery at the ankle or on the foot. Vein conduit is mandatory for these procedures.
- Posterior vertical incision across the popliteal fossa should be avoided. The lazy S-shaped incision (Figs. 46-2 and 46-3) should be used, with the horizontal portion across the flexion crease to avoid wound dehiscence and contracture. Even when done well, the posterior approach is associated with local wound swelling and can be associated with significant incisional discomfort.
- Ligation of the aneurysm should be performed proximally and distally, as close as possible to the aneurysmal sac. Jones and associates[10] demonstrated that proximal ligature alone or ligating the inflow and outflow arteries remotely from

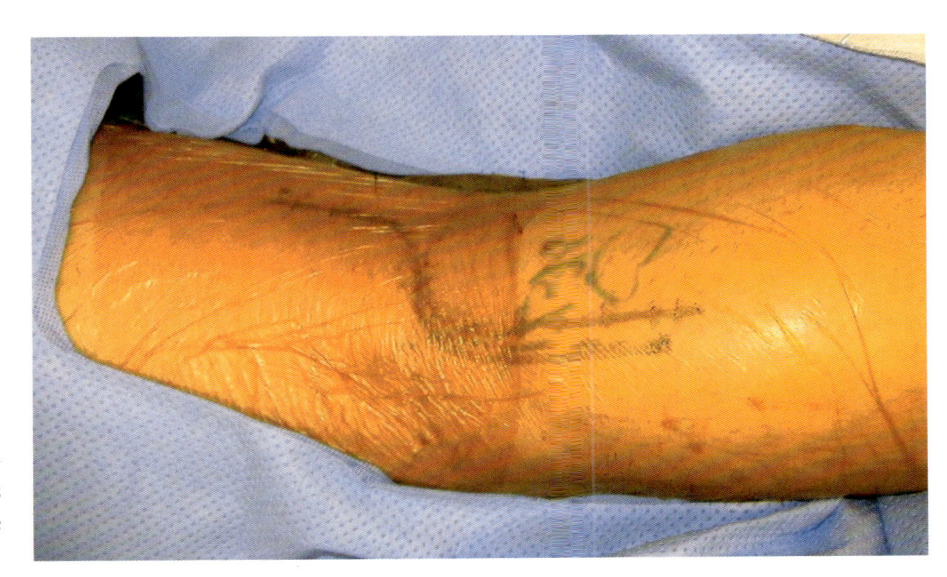

Figure 46-2. Orientation of the posterior lazy S incision. The patient's left leg is pictured, with the calf to the right of the photograph.

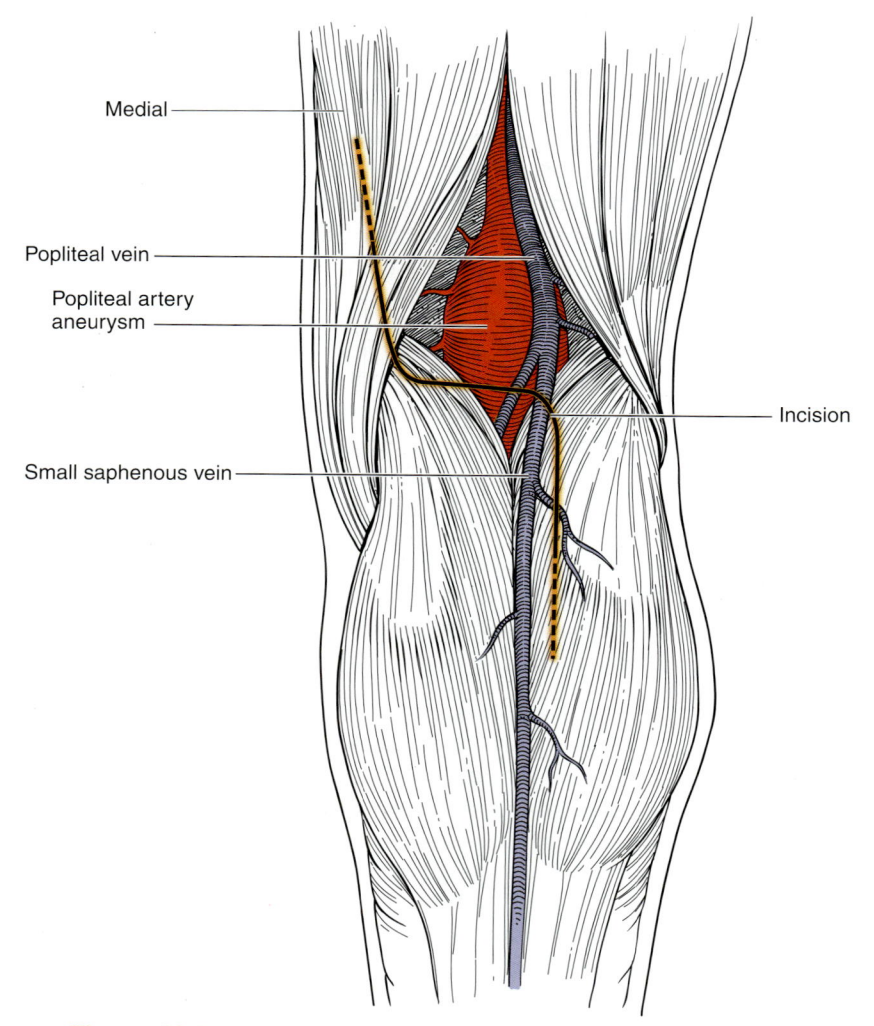

Figure 46-3. Incision for a posterior approach to the popliteal fossa.

the aneurysmal sac increases the likelihood of continued aneurysm expansion. Numerous studies have shown that even with proximal and distal ligation, as many as 30% of aneurysms do not thrombose and may continue to enlarge if collateral blood flow into the aneurysmal sac persists in a situation analogous to that of a type II endoleak with endovascular aneurysm repair.[11,12] Continued expansion can result in pain, compression symptoms, and even rupture.[13]

- In patients with simultaneous aortic and popliteal aneurysms, treatment of the abdominal aneurysm may precipitate popliteal aneurysm thrombosis.[6] In the posterior approach, care must be taken to avoid injury to the medial cutaneous sural, tibial, and peroneal nerves (Fig. 46-4).
- Compressive symptoms created by the aneurysm, such as leg edema, local pain, or weakness, require decompression of the aneurysmal sac.
- Arterial exposure of the above- or below-knee popliteal artery can be difficult with large aneurysms or in the presence of arteriomegaly. Extensive kinking, tortuosity, and lateral displacement, especially of the distal popliteal artery, can occasionally make exposure and separation from the adjacent structures challenging.

Operative Strategy

SELECTION OF APPROACH

Small or fusiform aneurysms are best approached medially by conventional bypass with aneurysm ligation. For large aneurysms limited to the popliteal fossa,

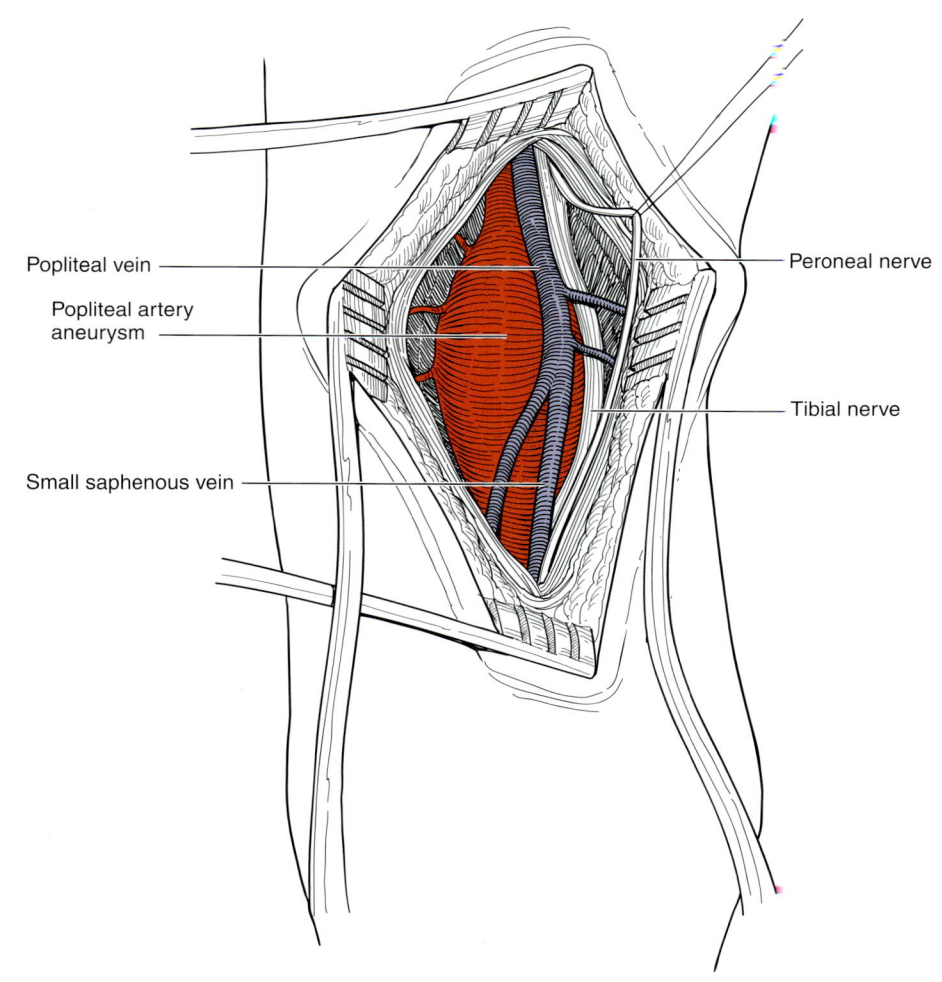

Figure 46-4. Posterior popliteal exposure.

especially with symptoms attributable to compression of adjacent structures, direct exposure from the posterior approach with interposition grafting from within the aneurysmal sac is preferable, unless the aneurysm extends too far proximally. The posterior approach is also advantageous to decompress an aneurysm that has continued to enlarge after bypass and ligation, because of backfilling from geniculate branches.

The medial approach is the preferred technique for most popliteal aneurysm repairs and the only logical option for bypass grafts that need to extend to distal tibial or pedal vessels. The medial approach has the advantages of being familiar to all vascular surgeons and providing easy access to the entire great saphenous vein. Virtually all of the procedure is performed some distance from the aneurysm, reducing the likelihood of operative injury to structures adherent to the surface popliteal aneurysm. The principal disadvantage of the medial approach is that access to the aneurysm is limited, making decompression of the sac difficult.

CONDUIT SELECTION

Vein conduit, as with peripheral bypasses performed for occlusive disease, is preferred for most reconstructions. Some surgeons prefer the routine use of prosthetic conduits for the posterior approach, because these posterior grafts are quite short, the diameter of the graft can be closely matched to the diameter of the popliteal artery, and their use avoids the complications of vein harvest. Excellent short-term results with prosthetic popliteal bypass have been reported, especially when good outflow exists.[14]

SURGICAL ANATOMY (SEE FIG. 46-4)

Avoiding Nerve Injury

- The saphenous nerve must be protected in the medial approach to the above-knee popliteal artery as it exits the adductor hiatus and during harvest of the below-knee great saphenous vein.
- The sural nerve is the terminal synthesis of the medial cutaneous sural nerve and cutaneous branches of the lateral sural nerve. In the lower calf, it is closely associated with the small saphenous vein.
- The medial cutaneous sural nerve is located deep to the fascia and is the first nerve encountered in the posterior approach. It, like the tibial and peroneal nerves, is best retracted laterally in exposing the popliteal artery.
- The tibial nerve is lateral and superficial within the popliteal fossa. It is large and easily identified. In distal posterior approaches a small branch to the medial gastrocnemius muscle may need to be sacrificed but is usually well tolerated by older patients.
- The peroneal nerve is the lateralmost nerve in the popliteal fossa and is retracted laterally with the tibial nerve.

Avoiding Venous Injury

- The great and small saphenous veins are best protected from inadvertent injury by preoperative vein mapping, marking their location on the overlying skin.
- The popliteal vein anatomy is variable, commonly duplicated, and easily distorted or compressed by larger popliteal aneurysms. To limit venous injury, it is advisable to perform essential dissection only, until the artery is controlled and can be decompressed. From the posterior approach, the vein is best mobilized lateral to the artery. As described later, the medial infrageniculate approach requires both anterior (distal popliteal or tibial) and posterior (proximal below-knee popliteal) mobilization of the vein relative to the artery.

SELECTION AND ASSESSMENT OF INFLOW AND DISTAL OUTFLOW

As with any lower extremity arterial reconstruction, proper treatment requires careful planning and a comprehensive arteriogram of the entire extremity from the groin to the toes. Alternatively, this information can be obtained with magnetic resonance angiography or spiral CT angiography. Duplex ultrasonography is useful for vein mapping in preparation for bypass. The information obtained from contrast angiography or magnetic resonance angiography is used to determine the location of the proximal and distal anastomotic sites and to determine the size, shape, and extent of the aneurysm for selection of the medial or posterior approach.

CONSIDERATIONS IN THE PRESENCE OF ACUTE THROMBOSIS

- *Anticoagulation.* Patients presenting with acute limb ischemia require urgent intervention to avoid amputation. In patients having a viable limb and no symptoms of sensory or motor dysfunction, intravenous heparin can be administrated to stabilize the patient.
- *Arteriography.* Surgery and arteriography are performed during the same admission. If the aneurysm is fully occluded and a patent distal outflow vessel is identified on arteriography, a vein bypass is performed. Exploration of the below-knee popliteal artery, the tibioperoneal trunk, or both combined with catheter thrombectomy may be indicated to select the optimal graft recipient artery.

- *Preoperative thrombolysis.* If an outflow vessel is not identified and the patient's limb is not immediately threatened, intraarterial thrombolysis is initiated to restore flow to potential outflow target vessels.
- *Thromboembolectomy.* When the patient's limb is immediately in jeopardy with sensory and motor dysfunction and there is no time for thrombolysis, surgery should be immediately performed. If no outflow vessel was identified on the arteriogram, thromboembolectomy of the distal popliteal, tibial, or both types of vessels should be attempted. Embolectomy or thrombectomy of the popliteal artery is relatively straightforward and is best approached from the below-knee popliteal artery. For embolectomy of individual tibial arteries, blind passage of embolectomy catheters from the popliteal artery usually fails and is ill advised. The region of the trifurcation of the popliteal artery should be exposed to gain access to all three arteries. A No. 2 Fogarty balloon embolectomy catheter can then be passed into each of the three tibial vessels. This must be done with utmost care to avoid potential intimal injury, perforation, or rupture. Alternatively, tibial vessels can be exposed at the ankle and retrograde passage of Fogarty catheters can be attempted.[15] Bypass grafts can then be extended to this level using the same arteriotomy, or a patch angioplasty with vein can be performed of the distal arteriotomy with bypass to the more proximal portion of the artery.
- *Intraarterial thrombolysis.* Use of an intraoperative lytic, in conjunction with bypass and embolectomy, has been described to further clear residual thrombus from outflow vessels.[16,17]
- *Compartment syndrome.* After bypass, signs of reperfusion injury, including rhabdomyolysis, may be present and may require fasciotomy. Prolonged thrombolysis before revascularization increases the risk of this complication.

Operative Technique

MEDIAL APPROACH

Position and Incision

The patient is positioned supine with the leg externally rotated, and a small bolster is placed under the knee, just as would be done for a lower extremity bypass. The saphenous vein is exposed as the first step in the procedure, starting in the groin, midthigh, or ankle depending on the inflow, distal target, and quality of available vein conduit. Once the vein has been mobilized and harvested, the same incision can be used to expose the popliteal artery above and below the knee joint in a fashion identical to a femoral-popliteal bypass. Similarly, the same incision can be used to expose the posterior tibial or proximal peroneal artery. When the anterior tibial, distal peroneal, or pedal arteries are the best distal targets, separate incisions are required.

Proximal Exposure

The medial above-knee incision is made longitudinally between the vastus medialis anteriorly and the sartorius muscle posteriorly. The deep fascia is divided in line with the intermuscular septum. The upper popliteal artery often can be palpated against the posterior femur. It is easily exposed at the point where it exits the Hunter canal just distal to the overlying adductor magnus tendon. In obese patients' dissection through the adipose tissue of the popliteal fossa can be accomplished bluntly. The saphenous nerve can be seen exiting with the artery from the adductor hiatus and should be preserved. The popliteal vein is usually located behind the artery, but anatomy may be distorted with large or tortuous aneurysms. A nonaneurysmal popliteal or distal superficial femoral artery is isolated and controlled with silicone rubber vessel loops, as are any geniculate branches arising from a nonaneurysmal artery. Easily accessible branches from the aneurysmal segment should be ligated externally before opening the vessel to minimize backbleeding once the artery is opened.

Distal Exposure

The deep fascia is incised longitudinally, approximately 1 cm posterior to the tibia, to gain entrance to the deep posterior compartment by retracting the medial head of the gastrocnemius muscle posteriorly. Blunt dissection can be used to locate the upper portion of the below-knee popliteal artery. In the more proximal exposure of the below-knee popliteal artery, the vein is best retracted posteriorly. To expose the distal popliteal artery, the upper soleus muscle fibers are divided with cautery. The popliteal vein in this distal portion of the dissection is encountered, with the tibial nerve located superior and deeper within the wound. This distal exposure is best facilitated by retracting the popliteal vein anteriorly and, frequently, by mobilization of the anterior tibial vein and division of the tributaries from the soleus veins.

Tunneling

In most cases, a tunnel is created from the above- to below-knee popliteal space between the medial and lateral heads of the gastrocnemius muscle. This may be difficult in patients with large popliteal aneurysms filling most of the popliteal space. Decompression of the aneurysmal sac and endoaneurysmorrhaphy may be required before tunneling can be safely performed.

Anastomosis

Intravenous heparin is administered at a dose of 80 to 100 units per kilogram of body weight or at a dose to prolong the activated clotting time to 250 to 300 seconds. Arterial bypass performed in the standard fashion with either end-to-side or end-to-end anastomoses. There is frequently a size discrepancy between the vein grafts and the popliteal arteries, especially above the knee, making the end-to-side anastomosis preferable. Either reversed or nonreversed vein grafts can be used depending on surgeon preference and experience. In bypasses extending from the common femoral artery to a distal tibial vessel, in situ bypass is an alternative. For occluded aneurysms, the procedure is conducted like any other lower extremity arterial bypass.

Aneurysm Ligation

If the aneurysm is patent, ligation must be performed in conjunction with the bypass procedure. The inflow and outflow arteries to the aneurysmal sac should be ligated as close to the aneurysm as possible. In focal aneurysms confined to the proximal and midpopliteal artery, the aneurysm is ligated just distal to the proximal anastomosis and just proximal to the distal arterial anastomosis. If an in situ bypass to a more distal target is performed, separate exposure of the two points of ligation is required. The aneurysm should always be ligated both proximally and distally as close to the aneurysmal sac as possible to promote aneurysm thrombosis and decrease the likelihood of continued expansion from collateral filling. Depending on the size of the popliteal artery, ligation using a horizontal mattress suture with an anterior and posterior felt buttress may be needed to ensure secure occlusion of the artery. Most authors are proponents of opening all but the smallest popliteal aneurysms to suture ligated backbleeding side branches. This can usually be done from the above- or below-knee popliteal space. A thigh tourniquet can decrease bleeding from collaterals once the aneurysmal sac is opened.[9] In some cases, it may be necessary to divide the tendon of the medial head of the gastrocnemius muscle to facilitate access to the popliteal aneurysm, but this maneuver is associated with significant postoperative pain. The tendon can then be reattached after decompression using a heavy-gauge monofilament suture. Completion arteriography, angioscopy, or duplex ultrasonography is performed before closure.

POSTERIOR APPROACH

Position and Incision

For large aneurysms confined to the popliteal space and causing symptoms from compression or for aneurysms causing distortion and displacement of normal anatomy from tortuosity, elongation, and kinking, the posterior approach is preferred. This is also an appropriate approach for smaller aneurysms, but it is not applicable to aneurysms that extend proximally beyond the popliteal space.

The patient is placed prone. An S-shaped incision is made, with the superior end starting on the medial side of the thigh to expose the proximal popliteal artery and great saphenous vein. The incision extends laterally across the flexion crease of the knee and ends on the lateral aspects of the proximal calf directly over the proximal small saphenous vein (see Figs. 46-2 and 46-3). If the small saphenous vein is of adequate size for bypass, the incision can be continued for harvest of the vein.

Exposure

The route to the popliteal artery is fairly direct (see Fig. 46-4) and proceeds just medial to the small saphenous vein, where the deep fascia is incised vertically. The medial sural nerve is located deep to the fascia, over the lateral head of the gastrocnemius muscle, and is best retracted laterally. The small saphenous vein can be used as a useful landmark and traced to its junction with the popliteal vein. The popliteal artery lies medially in the sheath and slightly deep to the vein. One or two popliteal venous tributaries will likely require division to allow full mobilization of the artery. The vein is best retracted laterally. The proximal popliteal artery is identified by palpation distal to the adductor canal and exposed by separating the semimembranosus and semitendinosus muscles medially from the long head of the biceps femoris laterally. Circumferential control is obtained with silicone rubber vessel loops. Dissection is continued distally on the anterior surface of the aneurysm to avoid injury to the tibial and peroneal nerves, which may be encountered coursing lateral to the aneurysm. These nerves are best retracted laterally, and care must be taken to avoid direct compression or traction of the nerves with retractors. The distal popliteal artery is identified after dissection between the two heads of the gastrocnemius muscle. Occasionally there is a tibial nerve branch to the medial head of the gastrocnemius that must be sacrificed for more distal exposure. If exposure of tibioperoneal trunk or proximal tibial vessels is required, access from this approach is possible by division of muscular sling created by the medial attachments of the soleus muscle.

Bypass or Interposition Grafting

After administration of intravenous heparin, proximal and distal control is obtained and the aneurysmal sac is opened. Thrombus is removed, and backbleeding geniculate collaterals are oversewn from within, analogous to the approach used in aortic aneurysms (Fig. 46-5, A). Circulation can be restored by either bypass or interposition graft. If an interposition vein graft is planned, the graft can be beveled to facilitate an end-to-end anastomosis to the transected popliteal artery (Fig. 46-5). Alternatively, a standard end-to-side bypass can be performed and is preferable when there is a significant size discrepancy between the popliteal artery and the bypass graft, which commonly occurs when using a vein conduit. For interposition prosthetic grafts, an end-to-end anastomosis can be created from within the aneurysmal sac using the graft inclusion technique. This approach has the advantage of requiring less dissection of the popliteal artery.

Closure

Closure is performed in multiple layers and is facilitated by the placement of cross-hatch skin marks before the initial skin incision. Nylon or polypropylene interrupted skin sutures are preferred because of significant swelling, which is common.

Postoperative Care

- Compressive bandages help to decrease postoperative edema.
- The use of aspirin is adequate postoperative anticoagulation for vein bypasses and short prosthetic grafts behind the knee. Considerations can be made for

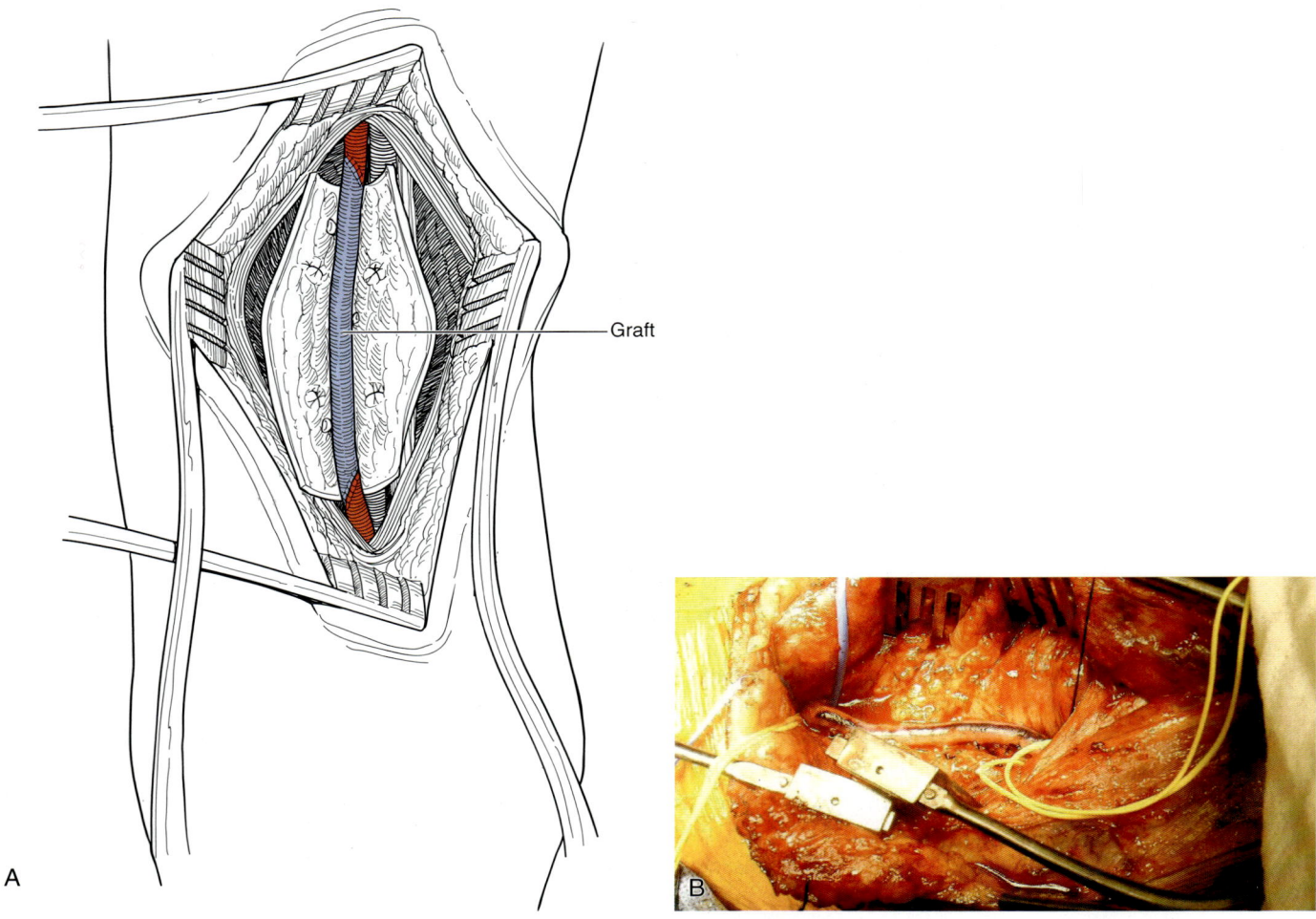

Figure 46-5. A, Posterior popliteal artery aneurysm repair. **B,** Interposition vein graft restores popliteal artery flow.

short-term anticoagulation for patients who have undergone thrombolysis to recruit occluded outflow vessels or patients with severely disadvantaged runoff secondary to chronic embolization.
- Patient are ambulated the next day.
- Assessment of popliteal or bypass hemodynamics must be performed to verify patency in the postoperative period.

Complications

- Edema is common in patients with a popliteal incision secondary to the interruption of popliteal and other vein branches and lymphatics.
- Nerve injury can be minimized by careful dissection of the nerves as delineated and with careful placement of retraction.
- Posterior popliteal incisions have more pain and inflammation than medial incisions to the popliteal.

REFERENCES

1. Perry MO: John Hunter—triumph and tragedy, *J Vasc Surg* 17:7-14, 1993.
2. Bernheim BM: The ideal operation for aneurysms of the extremity: Report of a case, *Johns Hopkins Hosp Bull* 27:1, 1916.
3. Dawson I, Sie RB, van Bockel JH: Atherosclerotic popliteal aneurysm, *Br J Surg* 84:293-299, 1997.
4. Galland RB, Magee TR: Popliteal aneurysms: Distortion and size related to symptoms, *Eur J Vasc Endovasc Surg* 30:534-538, 2005.

5. Varga ZA, Locke-Edmunds JC, Baird RN: A multicenter study of popliteal aneurysms. Joint Vascular Research Group, *J Vasc Surg* 20:171-177, 1994.
6. Dawson I, Sie R, van Baalen JM, et al: Asymptomatic popliteal aneurysm: Elective operation versus conservative follow-up, *Br J Surg* 81:1504-1507, 1994.
7. Bowyer RC, Cawthorn SJ, Walker WJ, et al: Conservative management of asymptomatic popliteal aneurysm, *Br J Surg* 77:1132-1135, 1990.
8. Schellack J, Smith RB III, Perdue GD: Nonoperative management of selected popliteal aneurysms, *Arch Surg* 122:372-375, 1987.
9. Huang Y, Gloviczki P, Noel AA, et al: Early complications and long-term outcome after open surgical treatment of popliteal artery aneurysms: Is exclusion with saphenous vein bypass still the gold standard? *J Vasc Surg* 45:706-713, 2007. discussion 13-15.
10. Jones WT III, Hagino RT, Chiou AC, et al: Graft patency is not the only clinical predictor of success after exclusion and bypass of popliteal artery aneurysms, *J Vasc Surg* 37:392-398, 2003.
11. Ebaugh JL, Morasch MD, Matsumura JS, et al: Fate of excluded popliteal artery aneurysms, *J Vasc Surg* 37:954-959, 2003.
12. Mehta M, Champagne B, Darling RC III, et al: Outcome of popliteal artery aneurysms after exclusion and bypass: Significance of residual patent branches mimicking type II endoleaks, *J Vasc Surg* 40:886-890, 2004.
13. van Santvoort HC, de Vries JP, van de Mortel R, et al: Rupture of a popliteal artery aneurysm 10 years after surgical repair, *Vascular* 14:227-230, 2006.
14. Beseth BD, Moore WS: The posterior approach for repair of popliteal artery aneurysms, *J Vasc Surg* 43:940-944, 2006. discussion 4-5.
15. Mahmood A, Hardy R, Garnham A, et al: Microtibial embolectomy, *Eur J Vasc Endovasc Surg* 25:35-39, 2003.
16. Ravn H, Bjorck M: Popliteal artery aneurysm with acute ischemia in 229 patients. Outcome after thrombolytic and surgical therapy, *Eur J Vasc Endovasc Surg* 33:690-695, 2007.
17. Thompson JF, Beard J, Scott DJ, et al: Intraoperative thrombolysis in the management of thrombosed popliteal aneurysm, *Br J Surg* 80:858-859, 1993.

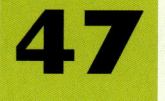

47 Direct Surgical Repair of Popliteal Entrapment

JEREMY R. HARRIS • THOMAS L. FORBES

Historical Background

Popliteal artery entrapment is a congenital anomaly in which the popliteal artery passes medial to and beneath the medial head of the gastrocnemius muscle or a slip of that muscle, with consequent compression or functional occlusion of the artery. Popliteal artery entrapment was first noted in 1879 by Stuart, an Edinburgh medical student, who described an anatomic variant of the popliteal artery dissected from a gangrenous limb.[1] The significance of this anomaly was not recognized until 1959, when Hamming at the University of Leyden reported a case of a 12-year-old boy with claudication and thrombosis of the popliteal artery with the same anatomic abnormality as initially described by Stuart.[2,3] Treatment included thrombectomy with division of the gastrocnemius muscle. In 1962 Servello[4] at the University of Padua described the case of a 28-year-old farmer who had an 8-year history of leg pain, medial displacement of the popliteal artery, and a small popliteal aneurysm. The medial head of the gastrocnemius muscle was divided, and an aneurysmorrhaphy performed. In 1965 Love and Whelan[5] described this anatomic variant as a cause of calf claudication in two young adults in the U.S. military.

The incidence of popliteal artery entrapment ranges from 0.17% in a review of 20,000 asymptomatic Greek soldiers to 3.5% in a study of autopsy specimens, suggesting that most cases are asymptomatic.[6,7] The concomitant entrapment of the popliteal vein with the artery has been reported in only 7.6% of cases.[8] Popliteal artery entrapment is more common in males and more than half the cases have been reported in patients younger than 30 years of age.[9] The anatomic variant causing the entrapment occurs bilaterally in up to two thirds of cases, although it may be asymptomatic in the contralateral limb.[10]

Preoperative Preparation

- The diagnosis of popliteal artery entrapment should be considered in any young adult with calf claudication, especially in the absence of atherosclerotic risk factors.
- The diagnosis of popliteal artery entrapment is confirmed by demonstrating a decrease in the ankle-brachial index and elevated popliteal artery velocities on duplex scanning in association with active plantar flexion of the ankle with the knee in full extension.[11] There is a high rate of false-positive results, especially in athletes.
- Computed tomography or magnetic resonance imaging displays both the vascular abnormality and the musculotendinous variation, as well as other pathology that may mimic entrapment syndrome, such as an adventitial cyst.[12]
- Conventional angiography should confirm medial displacement of the popliteal artery and extrinsic compression on active plantar flexion of the ankle. In up to 50% of patients, occlusion of the popliteal artery may be present.

Irregularity of the wall of the popliteal artery in an otherwise normal arterial tree may also be observed, along with prestenotic or poststenotic dilatation.

- Six variants of popliteal artery entrapment have been described that are related to variations in the embryologic development of the gastrocnemius muscle (Fig. 47-1).[12] In type I and type II entrapment the artery is displaced medially. In type I the gastrocnemius muscle is normally situated, whereas in type II the medial head of the gastrocnemius muscle has a variable attachment on the lateral aspect of the medial femoral condyle or intercondylar area. In type III entrapment a portion of the gastrocnemius muscle remains posterior to the artery, leaving an abnormal slip or band compressing the artery. Type IV entrapment describes a scenario in which the popliteal artery is situated deep to the popliteus muscle or fibrous bands. Type V entrapment can involve any of the previously mentioned abnormalities but also involves both the popliteal artery and the popliteal vein. Type VI entrapment is a functional form of entrapment without clear anatomic abnormality. This condition, termed physiologic popliteal artery entrapment syndrome, may be seen in high-performance athletes because of a hypertrophied gastrocnemius, soleus, plantaris, or semimembranosus muscle that causes vascular compression.[13] It may be confused with chronic recurrent exertional compartment syndrome that can occur in the same population.

Pitfalls and Danger Points

- **Exposure of the popliteal artery.** Most vascular surgeons are more familiar with the medial approach to the popliteal artery than with the direct, or posterior, approach.[14] Nonetheless, the posterior approach to the popliteal fossa provides excellent visualization of the anatomic abnormalities but can be limited if a bypass onto the tibioperoneal trunk or selected tibial vessels is required. The posterior approach to a patient with popliteal artery entrapment is preferably used in types III to VI, with standard medial exposure reserved for type I and type II entrapment.[15]
- **Accessibility of a venous conduit.** Although the small saphenous vein is readily accessible via the posterior approach, it may be unsuitable for use based on caliber or quality. If the cephalad portion of the S-shaped incision for the posterior approach is extended along the medial aspect of the thigh, the great saphenous vein is accessible. Nonetheless, it can be awkward to harvest the great saphenous vein in the prone position.

Operative Strategy

SURGICAL ANATOMY OF THE POPLITEAL FOSSA

The popliteal fossa is a diamond-shaped depression that is bordered by the semimembranosus muscle superomedially, the biceps femoris tendon superolaterally, and the medial and lateral heads of the gastrocnemius muscle inferiorly. The small saphenous vein, as well as the sural nerve, may be encountered as superficial structures in the popliteal fossa. The popliteal artery, popliteal vein, and posterior tibial nerve course between the medial and the lateral heads of gastrocnemius muscle.

AVOIDING NERVE INJURY

The two nerves that can be encountered during dissection are the sural nerve and the posterior tibial nerve. The sural nerve can be avoided by placing the skin incision lateral to the small saphenous vein and avoiding excessive traction with fixed retractors. Dissection continues deeper into the popliteal fossa, usually medial to the posterior tibial nerve. A branch to the medial head of the gastrocnemius muscle can be encountered and may be difficult to preserve, especially if extended exposure is necessary. Division of this branch of the posterior tibila nerve has minimal sequelae.

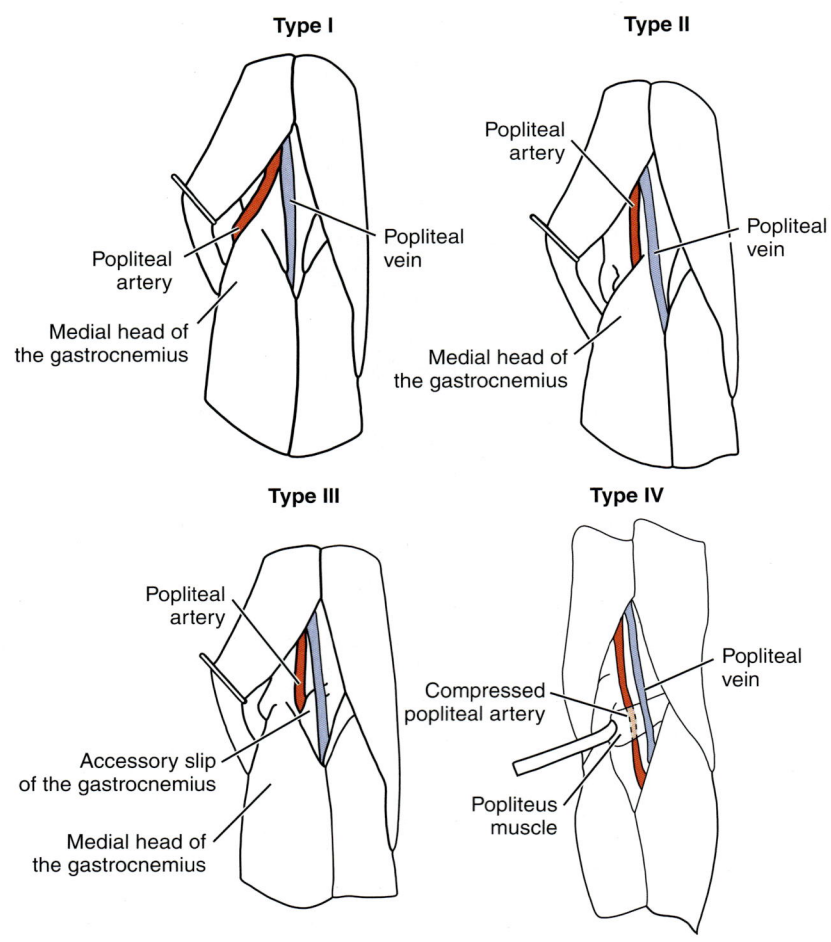

Figure 47-1. Types of popliteal artery entrapment syndrome. *(From Pillal J: A current interpretation of popliteal vascular entrapment, J Vasc Surg 48:61S-65S, 2008, Fig. 1.)*

AVOIDING VENOUS INJURY

The incision is placed lateral to the small saphenous vein to preserve this vein as a conduit should arterial repair be required. The popliteal artery lies medial to the popliteal vein, but tributaries of the popliteal vein may require ligation and division to allow adequate arterial exposure. Care must also be taken with the superior extent of the S-shaped incision to avoid injury to the great saphenous vein.

CONSIDERATIONS IN THE PRESENCE OF AN ARTERIAL LESION

Release of the musculotendinous abnormality is initially performed in the course of exposing the popliteal artery, followed by arterial repair, as required. Short-segment bypass with exclusion of the diseased popliteal artery or inline reconstruction with interposition grafting are acceptable options. When faced with poststenotic dilatation, arterial replacement with vein is performed. An autogenous conduit is preferred.

Operative Technique

INCISION

The patient is placed in the prone position. An S-shaped incision is performed, which begins as a midcalf vertical incision that is placed just lateral to the course of the small saphenous vein and sural nerve. The incision courses transversely at the level of the popliteal crease and then turns upward along the course of the great saphenous vein (Fig. 47-2).

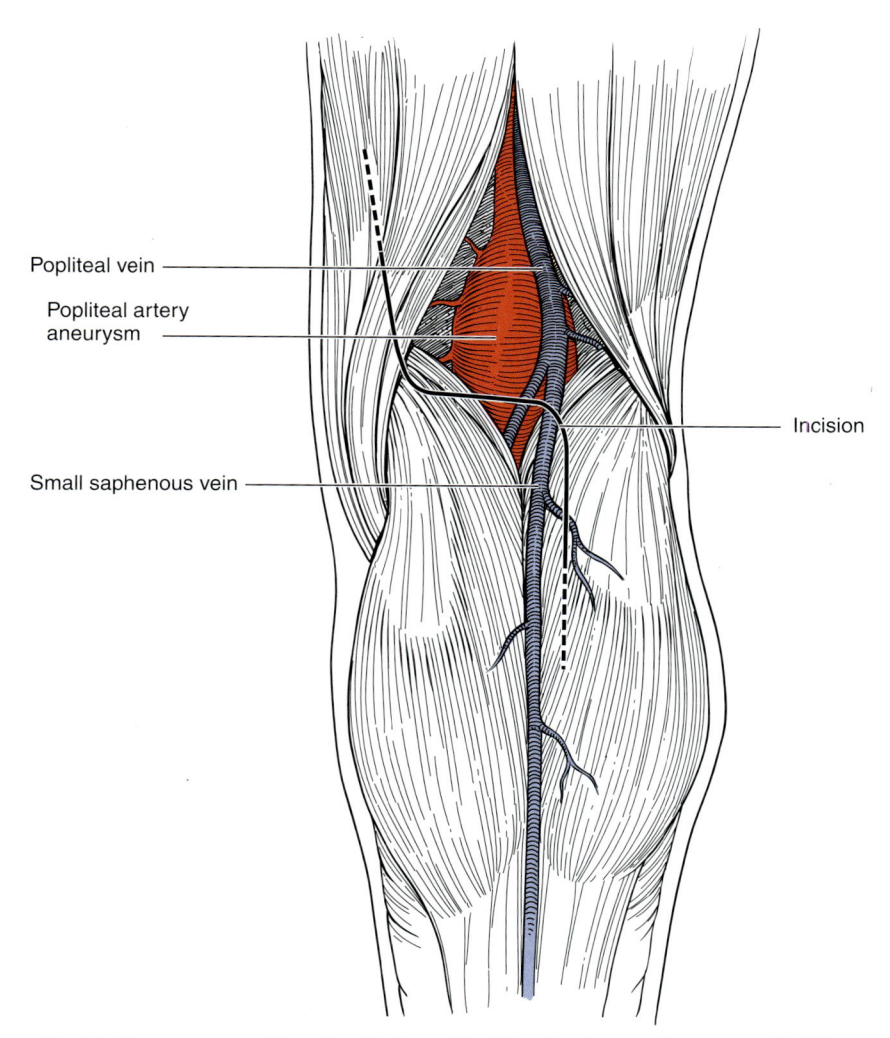

Figure 47-2. With the patient in the prone position, the S-shaped incision begins as a transverse incision across the popliteal crease, extending laterally below the crease, and then extending upward medially along the course of the great saphenous vein. The posterior approach may be used for exposure and surgical treatment of a popliteal artery aneurysm or entrapment. The incision below the popliteal crease usually lies lateral to the small saphenous vein and sural nerve. *(Redrawn from Rutherford RB, editor: Rutherford's atlas of vascular surgery, basic techniques and exposures. Philadelphia, 1993, Saunders, p 141, Fig. 77-A.)*

EXPOSURE OF THE POPLITEAL ARTERY

The posterior approach begins with the patient positioned prone on the operating room table and the knee slightly flexed. An S-shaped incision is made, with the upper portion of the incision along the posteromedial lower thigh, the transverse portion across the knee flexion crease, and the inferior portion lateral to midline and extending down the proximal calf (Fig. 47-2). Subcutaneous flaps are raised as necessary, and the small saphenous vein is identified and preserved. The deep fascia is divided in the midline, and the popliteal fossa is entered. The diamond-shaped popliteal fossa is bordered by the two heads of the gastrocnemius muscle inferiorly and the hamstring muscles superiorly. The first structure identified is the medial sural nerve, which should be isolated and retracted laterally. The tibial nerve is then identified, lying somewhat lateral and posterior to the popliteal vessels. It should be isolated and gently retracted laterally. The common peroneal nerve runs laterally with the tendon of the biceps femoris muscle toward the head of the fibula. At this level, the popliteal artery will lie medial to the popliteal vein (Fig. 47-3).

DIVISION OF FASCIAL AND MUSCULAR BANDS

The abnormal musculotendinous anatomy is appreciated in most cases, but may be more difficult to discern in patients with type I, type II, and type V entrapment.

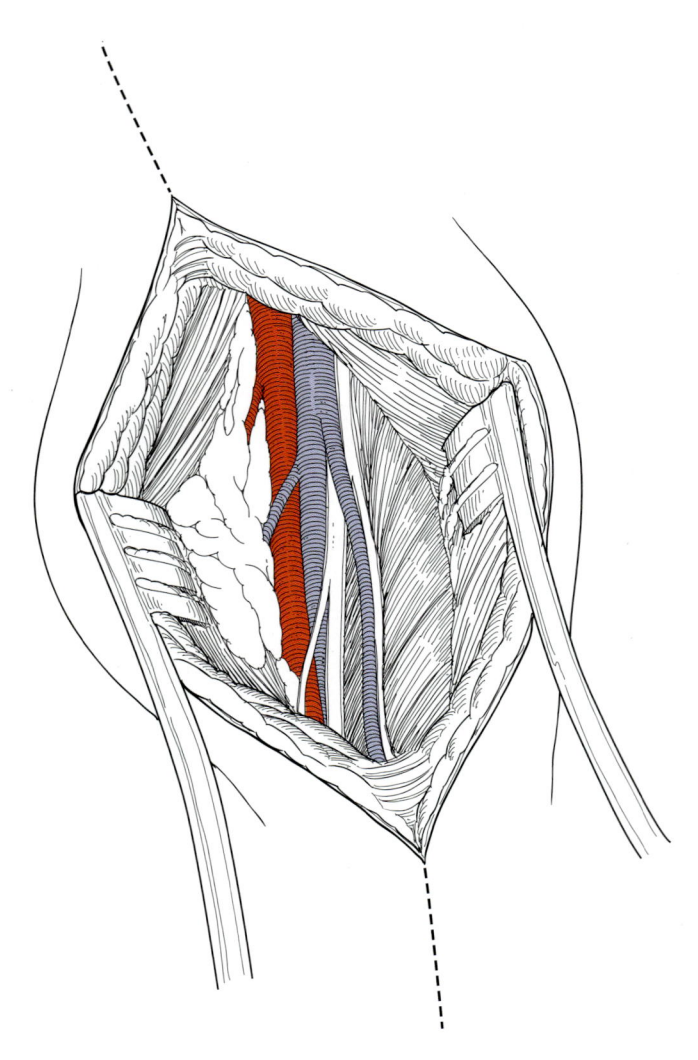

Figure 47-3. Exposure of the popliteal artery and vein along with the posterior tibial nerve in the depths of the popliteal fossa via the direct posterior approach. Division of some tributaries of the popliteal vein allows better exposure of the artery. *(Redrawn from Rutherford RB, editor: Rutherford's atlas of vascular surgery, basic techniques and exposures. Philadelphia, 1993, Saunders, p 142, Fig. 77-c.)*

Division of the medial head of the gastrocnemius muscle, accessory slips of muscle, or the popliteus muscle is straightforward once critical neurovascular structures are identified and protected.

CLOSURE

Wound closure can be undertaken using multiple layers culminating in a subcuticular stitch or skin staples. The S-shaped incision should minimize the wound contracture that might otherwise occur with a vertical incision across the highly mobile knee joint.

Complications

- **Edema.** The posterior calf can become more swollen because of the disruption of lymphatics and superficial veins, and there can be additional incisional discomfort when the knee is flexed.
- **Nerve injury.** The posterior tibial, sural, or peroneal nerve can be injured if they are not adequately visualized in the dissection, but are most likely injured if they are retracted, especially with self-retaining retractors that inadvertently incorporate the nerves.
- **Flexion contracture.** It is important to mobilize patients early with full flexion and extension of the knee. If this is not adequately done, immobility of the knee after dissection of the popliteal fossa can result in some flexion contracture.

REFERENCES

1. Stuart TPA: Note on a variation in the course of the popliteal artery, *J Anat Physiol* 13:162-165, 1879.
2. Hamming JJ: Intermittent claudication at an early age, due to an anomalous course of the popliteal artery, *Angiology* 10:369, 1959.
3. Hamming JJ, Vink M: Obstruction of the popliteal artery at an early age, *J Cardiov Surg* 6:516-524, 1965.
4. Servello M: Clinical syndrome of an anomalous position of the popliteal artery: Differentiation from juvenile arteriopathy, *Circulation* 16:885, 1962.
5. Love JW, Whelan TJ: Popliteal artery entrapment syndrome, *Am J Surg* 109:620-624, 1965.
6. Bouhoutsos J, Daskalakis E: Muscular abnormalities affecting the popliteal vessels, *Br J Surg* 68:501-506, 1981.
7. Gibson MHL, Mills JG, Johnson GE, et al: Popliteal entrapment syndrome, *Ann Surg* 185:341-348, 1977.
8. Persky JM, Kempezinski RF, Fowl RJ: Entrapment of the popliteal artery, *Surg Gynecol Obstet* 173:84-90, 1991.
9. Henry MF, Wilkins DC, Lambert AW: Popliteal artery entrapment syndrome, *Curr Treat Options Cardiovasc Med* 6:113-120, 2004.
10. Levien LJ, Veller MG: Popliteal artery entrapment syndrome: More common than previously recognized, *J Vasc Surg* 30:587-598, 1999.
11. di Marzo L, Cavallaro A, Sciacca V, et al: Diagnosis of popliteal artery entrapment syndrome: The role of duplex scanning, *J Vasc Surg* 13:434-438, 1991.
12. Forbes TL: Non-atheromatous popliteal artery disease. In Cronenwett JL, Johnston KW, editors: *Rutherford's Textbook of Vascular Surgery*, 7 ed, Philadelphia, 2010, Saunders, pp 1721-1734.
13. Turnipseed WD: Functional popliteal artery entrapment syndrome: A poorly understood and often missed diagnosis that is frequently mistreated, *J Vasc Surg* 49:1189-1195, 2009.
14. Beseth BD, Moore WS: The posterior approach for repair of popliteal artery aneurysms, *J Vasc Surg* 43:940-944, 2006.
15. di Marzo L, Cavallaro A, Sciacca V, et al: Surgical treatment of popliteal artery entrapment syndrome: A ten-year experience, *Eur J Vasc Surg* 5:59-64, 1991.

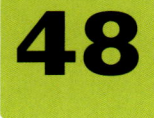

48 Endovascular Treatment of Femoral-Popliteal Arterial Occlusive Disease

MATTHEW J. ALEF • ZHEN S. HUANG • MARC L. SCHERMERHORN

Historical Background

Dotter and Judkins[1] first described percutaneous transluminal angioplasty (PTA) using a rigid catheter in 1964. By March 1977 approximately 1800 patients with femoral-popliteal arterial occlusions and stenoses had been treated using this technique, as reported in an international congress that included 12 European centers, to which Dotter[2] contributed 322 cases. Grüntzig and Hopff[3] introduced a high pressure balloon angioplasty catheter in 1974, and in 1979 Grüntzig and Kumpe[4] reported a 2-year patency rate of 86% in 188 patients with femoral-popliteal arterial lesions that had been treated by balloon angioplasty.

The occurence of immediate recoil, dissection, and occlusion after angioplasty, as well as high rates of early recurrent stenosis, led to the development of intravascular stents. In 1987 Sigwart and colleagues[5] described the earliest clinical experience with stenting for treatment of superficial femoral artery disease. Self-expanding stents were deployed for treatment of three patients with stenotic lesions of the superficial femoral artery and one patient after recanalization of a complete occlusion. The technique of subintimal angioplasty for recanalization of occlusions of the femoral and popliteal arteries was introduced by Bolia[6] in 1990. This initial experience with 71 limbs was followed by a report[7] detailing a 3-year experience in the treatment of 200 occlusions. Use of a polyester-covered stent-graft system for treatment of femoral-popliteal artery disease in 67 patients was described in 1996 by Henry.[8] In 2000 Lammer and associates[9] were the first to describe the use of a PTFE-covered stent-graft for treatment of superficial femoral artery disease. In 2005 the BASIL trial[10] demonstrated that balloon-angioplasty was associated with similar amputation-free survival as surgery for patients presenting with severe limb ischemia resulting from infrainguinal arterial occlusive disease.

Indications

Endovascular treatment is the preferred approach for patients presenting with intermittent claudication or critical limb ischemia and Trans-Atlantic Inter-Society Consensus (TASC) class A and B femoral-popliteal lesions of up to 15 cm in length but not involving the popliteal artery (Table 48-1 and Box 48-1).[11] Although surgery is preferred for treatment of TASC C and D lesions, endovascular therapy may be considered for the high-risk symptomatic patient who is otherwise an unsuitable operative candidate.

Preoperative Preparation

- **History, physical examination, and non invasive vascular studies.** History, physical examination, and noninvasive diagnostic evaluation should be performed for all patients who present with intermittent claudication, rest pain, or

TABLE 48-1 Trans-Atlantic Inter-Society Consensus Classification of Femoral-Popliteal Arterial Lesions

Lesion Type	Guidelines
A	• Single stenosis ≤ 10 cm in length
	• Single occlusion ≤ 5 cm in length
B	• Multiple lesions (stenoses or occlusions), each ≤ 5 cm
	• Single stenosis or occlusion ≤ 15 cm not involving the infrageniculate popliteal artery
	• Single or multiple lesions in the absence of continuous tibial vessels to improve inflow for a distal bypass
	• Heavily calcified occlusion ≤ 5 cm in length
	• Single popliteal stenosis
C	• Multiple stenosis or occlusions totaling >15 cm with or without heavy calcification
	• Recurrent stenosis or occlusions that need treatment after two endovascular interventions
D	• Chronic total occlusions of the CFA or SFA (>20 cm) involving the popliteal artery
	• Chronic total occlusion of the popliteal artery and proximal trifurcation vessels

CFA, Common femoral artery; *SFA,* superficial femoral artery.

Box 48-1 TRANS-ATLANTIC INTER-SOCIETY CONSENSUS TREATMENT RECOMMENDATIONS FOR FEMORAL-POPLITEAL ARTERIAL LESIONS

- TASC A. Endovascular therapy is the treatment of choice.
- TASC B. Endovascular treatment is the preferred treatment.
- TASC C. Surgery is preferred for patients with low operative risk.
- TASC D. Surgery is the treatment of choice.

---

gangrene of the forefoot., Acuity, clinical severity, and anatomic extent of arterial occlusive disease, as well as prior surgical or endovascular interventions, medical comorbidities, and current functional status, all influence the decision to intervene and the best method of treatment. Noninvasive vascular studies should include segmental lower extremity pressures, pulse volume recordings (PVRs), ankle-brachial index (ABI), and toe pressures. In patients with calcified, noncompressible, infrageniculate arteries, toe pressures are required for determining the severity of the underlying arterial occlusive disease.

- **Duplex ultrasound.** Duplex ultrasound is useful for determining the location and the severity of arterial disease. In addition, the absence of a suitable vein conduit as determined by a venous duplex study will likely influence the decision to perform a catheter-based intervention.
- **CT angiography.** If physical examination or other studies suggest the presence of inflow disease, computed tomography angiography can be used to assess aortoiliac disease and help plan intervention, such as the selection of an access site and potential need for femoral endarterectomy.
- **Perioperative medications.** All patients should be on aspirin and statin therapy before intervention, with initiation of clopidogrel when endovascular intervention is likely and the need for surgery is low.

Pitfalls and Danger Points

- **Access site complications.** Access site complications, including bleeding, pseudoaneurysm, or arteriovenous fistula, may be averted by using ultrasound guidance to aid in localizing and assessing the common femoral artery (CFA) with real-time visualization during access.
- **Arterial dissection or rupture.** The risk of arterial dissection or rupture may be minimized by avoiding excessive oversizing of angioplasty balloons. Dissections are treated with low-pressure, prolonged, repeat angioplasty or stenting, whereas rupture is treated with a stent graft.

- **Distal arterial embolization.** Gentle passage of wires and catheters minimizes the risk of distal arterial embolization. Embolic protection may be used for high-risk lesions.
- **Acute arterial thrombosis.** Ensure adequate heparinization before instrumentation of the lesion. Observation and careful control of the wire tip during delivery and retrieval of guidance and treatment catheters is essential.

Endovascular Strategy

ANGIOGRAPHIC ANATOMY AND COMMON COLLATERAL PATHWAYS

The femoral artery is the direct continuation of the external iliac artery and begins at the inguinal ligament and at the level of the femoral head. It passes down the anterior medial aspect of the thigh and ends in approximately the lower third of the thigh, where it passes through the adductor magnus to become the popliteal artery (Fig. 48-1). As documented by Lippert and Pabst,[12] variants in femoral artery branching exist and primarily involve variable origins of the profunda femoris and circumflex branches.[13] If the common femoral artery is severely diseased, the main collateral pathways include anastomoses between branches of the hypogastric artery and profunda femoris artery and between branches of the external iliac artery and femoral tributaries. Branches from the profunda femoris artery provide a collateral route to the medial and lateral superior geniculate arteries in the event of superficial femoral artery occlusive disease.

UNFAVORABLE ANATOMIC FEATURES FOR INTERVENTIONS ON THE SUPERFICIAL FEMORAL AND POPLITEAL ARTERIES

Innate anatomic factors unique to the femoral-popliteal arterial segment adversely affect long-term patency after endovascular intervention. This arterial segment is subjected to recurrent mechanical forces that cause vessel deformation.[14,15] Dynamic knee flexion and rotational and longitudinal compression of the SFA within the adductor hiatus may compromise outcomes after stenting.[16] In addition, long or eccentric calcified lesions, multifocal stenoses, occlusions, and poor distal runoff are associated with poor endovascular treatment outcomes.

ACCESS SITE SELECTION

Percutaneous access sites for femoral or popliteal artery disease include the femoral, popliteal, and pedal arteries. Brachial artery access has limited applicability because of available catheter lengths. The safest and most convenient site for most diagnostic and therapeutic interventions is the common femoral artery, which may be accessed in either an ipsilateral antegrade or a contralateral retrograde fashion. Retrograde access of the contralateral common femoral artery is typically the best approach for the initial study. From this access site, a therapeutic intervention may be performed on any lesion between the contralateral mid-common iliac artery and the peroneal or tibial vessels.

The ipsilateral antegrade femoral approach is technically more demanding, may increases radiation exposure to the operator, and is associated with an increased risk of local vascular complications.[17] However, the presence of a contralateral infrainguinal bypass, endovascular aneurysm repair, or extreme tortuosity of the iliac system may preclude the use of a contralateral femoral artery access site. Both of these approaches may be of limited utility for the recanalization of a superficial femoral artery, when occluded flush with the profunda femoris artery. In this case, retrograde popliteal or pedal artery access provides an alternate option.[18,19]

STENT SELECTION

Self-expanding stents are preferred in the femoral-popliteal region because of the proclivity of balloon-expandable stents to deform from external compression and

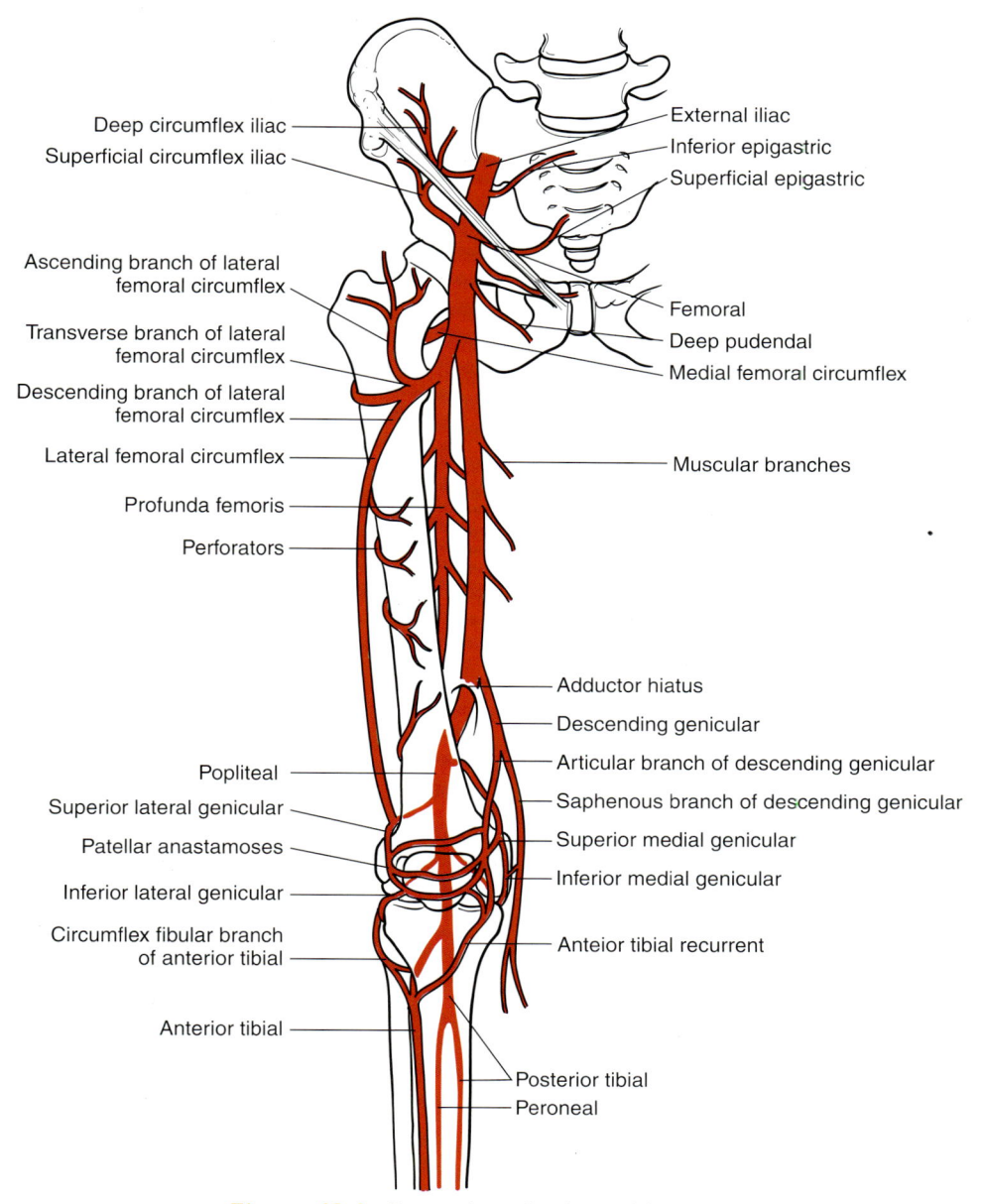

Figure 48-1. Femoral-popliteal arterial anatomy.

dynamic movement. Early randomized trials examining short femoral-popliteal lesions demonstrated no improvement after primary balloon-expandable stenting compared with PTA alone.[20,21] Recent data has suggested that nitinol stents may lead to improved primary patency for lesions of moderate length.[22-25]

Drug eluting stents have been evaluated for the treatment of superficial femoral artery disease. Although promising early results[26-28] were reported for sirolimus-eluting stents, little long-term benefit could be demonstrated. Superior 2-year primary patency has been recently reported[29,30] for pacliaxel eluting stents as compared to bare metal stents (drug eluting stent, n = 61 vs. bare metal stent, n = 59). Paclitaxel-coated balloons have also been used to reduce restenosis, but the clinical effectiveness of this technology remains an area of active study.[31]

Endovascular Technique

RETROGRADE AND ANTEGRADE APPROACHES FOR ARTERIAL ACCESS

With the patient supine on the fluoroscopic table, both groins are prepared and exposed for possible access. Percutaneous needle entry into the artery is performed with ultrasound guidance. Ultrasound guidance assists with precise placement of the puncture needle, facilitates an anterior wall puncture, allows the operator to note and avoid disease within the common femoral artery, enables access of a pulseless artery, and may assist in determining whether a percutaneous closure device should be used at the conclusion of the procedure.

For retrograde common femoral artery access, the ultrasound probe is first used transversely to clearly identify the bifurcation of the common femoral artery into the superficial femoral artery and profunda femoris artery and to scan through the course of the common femoral artery. Once the bifurcation is identified, the probe is turned longitudinally and followed cephalad until the femoral head is located while maintaining visualization of the bifurcation distally. This ensures common femoral artery access below the inguinal ligament. Sites with substantial anterior or posterior calcification should be avoided. Lidocaine is injected into the skin and the subcutaneous tissue, a small nick in the skin is made with a scalpel, and a hemostat is used to develop a tract. Antegrade common femoral artery access is performed in a similar manner.

A 21-Ga needle is visualized as it punctures the anterior wall of the artery, and a short 0.018-inch wire is inserted. Fluoroscopic confirmation is performed to document puncture over the femoral head and confirm wire placement in the external iliac artery. The wire is advanced, and a 3-Fr microsheath is placed, followed by exchange to a 0.035-inch wire and a 4-Fr short introducer sheath.

ANGIOGRAPHY OF THE LOWER EXTREMITY

An Omni Flush diagnostic catheter is advanced over the wire to the L1 vertebra, and an abdominal aortogram is obtained. The Omni Flush catheter can then be used to obtain contralateral access or, if unsuccessful, an angled Glidecath, Rösch inferior mesenteric, or Sos selective catheter may be used. Once a catheter is advanced into the contralateral external iliac artery, angiography of the affected limb is performed. Visualizing the common femoral artery bifurcation requires positioning the image intensifier in an ipsilateral oblique angle of 20 to 30 degrees. Below the bifurcation, femoral-popliteal disease is well visualized in an anteroposterior projection, although occasionally oblique views may be necessary. Tibial and pedal runoff vessels are imaged before intervention and at completion of the procedure.

ENDOVASCULAR TREATMENT OF FEMORAL-POPLITEAL ARTERY STENOSIS

A long interventional sheath is inserted once the target lesion is identified. A stiff, 0.035-inch, angled Glidewire is inserted through a diagnostic catheter and into the artery or bypass graft to be treated. The length and diameter of the sheath are determined by the anticipated intervention, with a 5- or 6-Fr sheath of 45 to 70 cm in length most commonly used. A 5-Fr sheath may be used if the lesion is less than 8 cm in length, since self-expanding stents of up to 8 cm in length are available for 5-Fr systems. However, for treatment of longer lesions, a 6-Fr system should be used. The sheath is passed over the stiff Glidewire and positioned approximately 10 cm proximal to the lesion. The sheath should be placed beyond the common femoral artery bifurcation when feasible to avoid the need for repeated selection of the superficial femoral artery.

After sheath placement, heparin (100 units per kilogram of body weight) is administered to achieve an activated clotting time (ACT) of 250 seconds. The stiff Glidewire is exchanged for a 0.014-inch wire to traverse the lesion. A hydrophilic-coated wire tip, such as the ChoICE PT Extra Support (Boston Scientific, Natick, Mass.), is preferred for stenoses, and a braided wire with a weighted tip, such as the ASAHI MiracleBros 6 (Abbott Vascular, Abbott Park, Ill.), is preferred when crossing an arterial occlusion is anticipated. The wire may be supported by a 0.018-inch angioplasty balloon catheter selected to treat the lesion. For complete occlusions, a 0.018-inch

Quick-Cross catheter (Spectranetics, Colorado Springs, Colo.) may be used to support the wire, facilitate passage across severely diseased segments, and facilitate exchange for a stiffer wire if one is needed to deliver the balloon or stent. If the 0.018-inch catheter crosses the lesion, the balloon catheter will most likely cross as well. If the 0.018-inch catheter is unable to traverse the lesion, a 0.014-inch catheter may be used, but predilation of the lesion with a 0.014-inch balloon will likely be necessary. The wire is advanced beyond the lesion to support the treatment, keeping the wire tip in view to avoid inadvertent injury to the distal vasculature. An appropriately sized balloon catheter is advanced over the wire with sizing based on an adjacent healthy vessel, lesion characteristics, and sheath size (Fig. 48-2). Once placed, the balloon catheter is inflated to profile, typically to 10 to 14 atm of pressure, with inflation maintained for 1 minute. Although the average diameters of the superficial femoral artery and popliteal artery are approximately 6 mm, these vessels may range from 4.5 to 7 mm in diameter.[32]

After deflation, a posttreatment angiogram is performed (Fig. 48-3, *A-D*). If a residual stenosis remains, options include retreatment with the same balloon at higher inflation pressure or upsizing the balloon diameter if appropriate. Stent placement may be considered if a flow-limiting dissection, intraluminal flap, or persistent stenosis remains after angioplasty. Low-pressure, prolonged inflation is often adequate treatment for dissection.

Self-expanding nitinol stents are selected with diameters that are 1 to 2 mm larger than the vessel diameter. Although the shortest stent length to treat the lesion is preferred, a single stent is favored over the use of multiple, overlapping stents. After stent deployment, postdilation is performed to ensure full expansion (Fig. 48-3, *E* and *F*) and a completion angiogram that includes tibial and pedal runoff should be obtained.

Although not commonly used, an embolic protection device or atherectomy may be considered under certain circumstances. For example, bulky calcific disease in the presence of a single patent tibial vessel or lesions that have previously embolized may be a relative indication for insertion of a filter. Devices allowing separate passage of a wire before delivery of the filter are preferred. Although the usefulness of atherectomy in the treatment of femoral-popliteal disease remains equivocal,

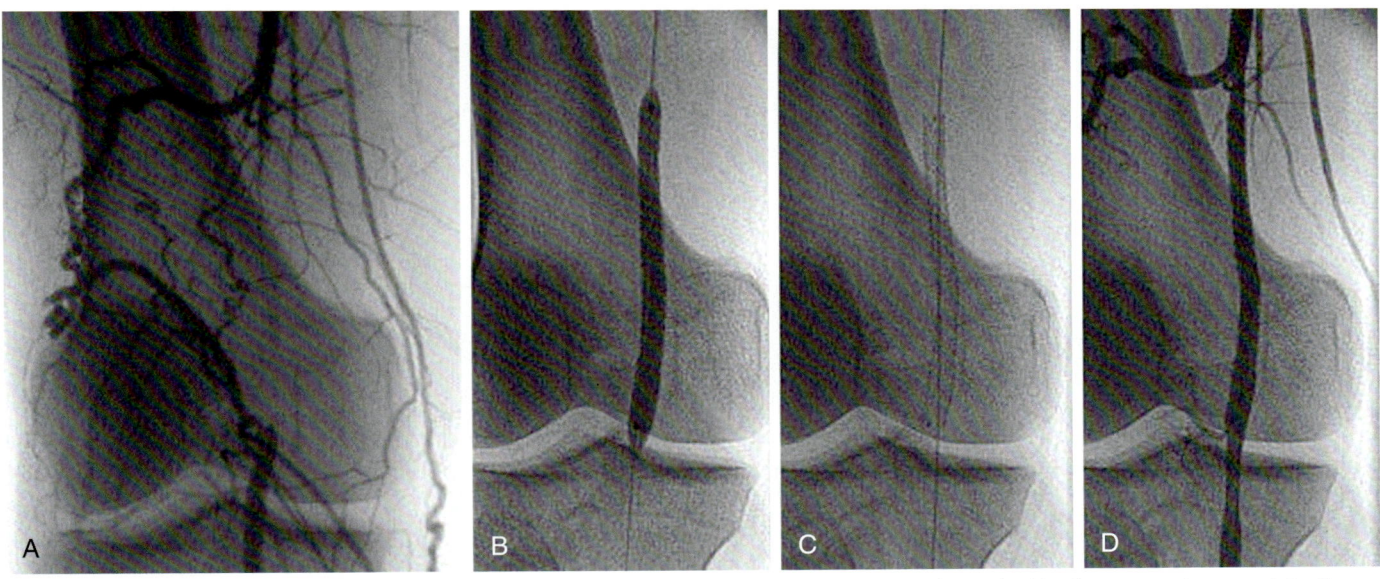

Figure 48-2. Deployment of a self-expanding stent. Self-expanding nitinol stents are selected with diameters that are 1 to 2 mm larger than the vessel diameter. A single stent is favored over the use of multiple, overlapping stents. Self-expanding stents are mounted on a carrier device and constrained by an outer sheath. The introducer sheath does not need to cross the lesion. After the lesion is identified (**A**) and balloon angioplasty is performed (**B**), stent deployment is achieved by holding the carrier device with one hand while retracting the outer sheath with the other in a pin-pull manner (**C**). An angiogram is subsequently performed to assess the presence of residual stenosis, dissection, or embolization(**D**).

584 LOWER EXTREMITY ARTERIAL DISEASE

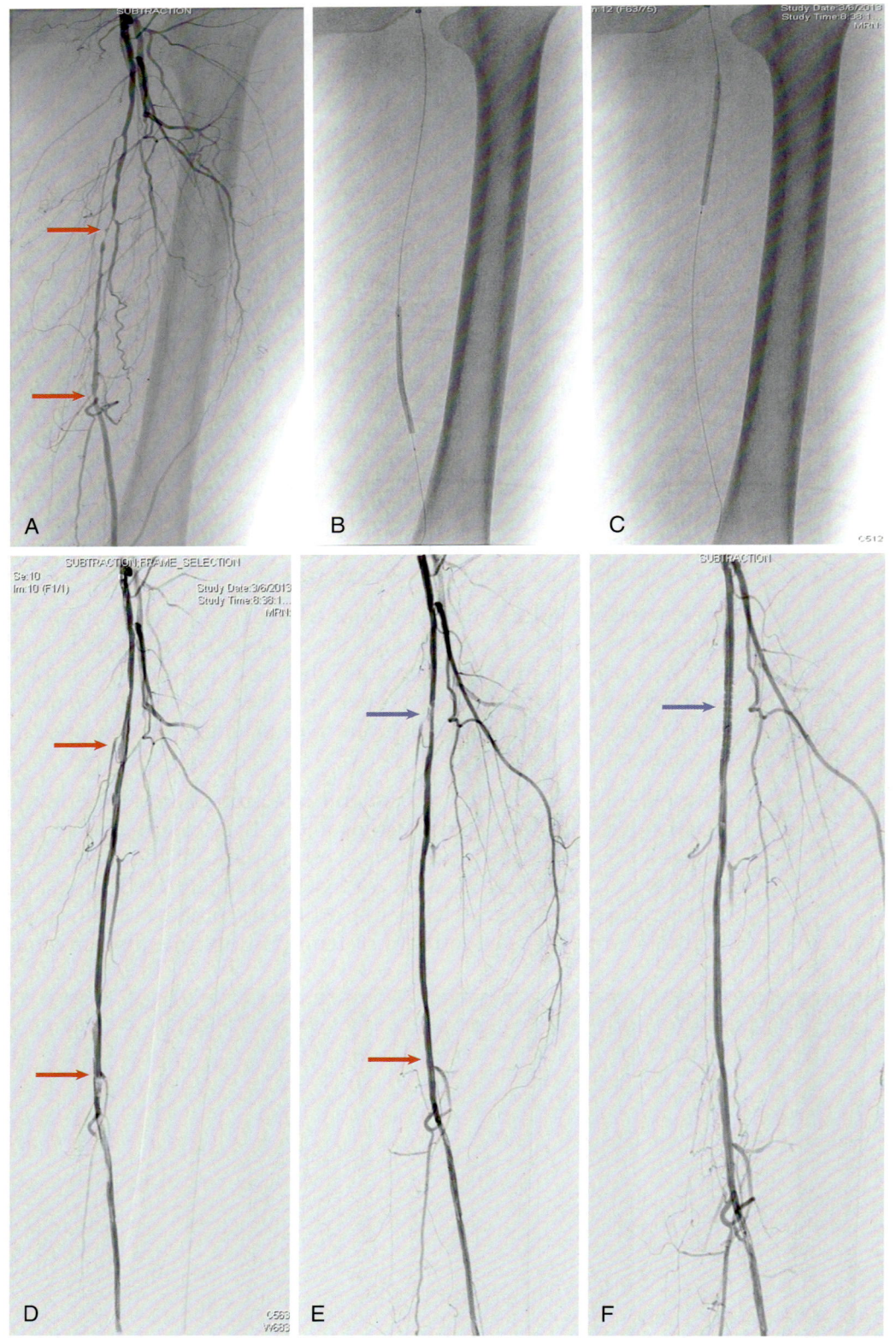

Figure 48-3. Endovascular therapy of diffuse occlusive disease of the superficial femoral artery. **A,** Two lesions are identified in the superficial femoral artery. **B** to **C,** Initial angioplasty of the distal and proximal lesions is performed. **D,** Flow-limiting dissections are noted at both angioplasty sites *(red arrows)*. Both were first treated with a second 2-minute angioplasty. **E,** The distal dissection *(red arrow)* improved, whereas the proximal dissection *(blue arrow)* did not. **F,** A self-expanding stent was used to treat the proximal dissection *(blue arrow)*.

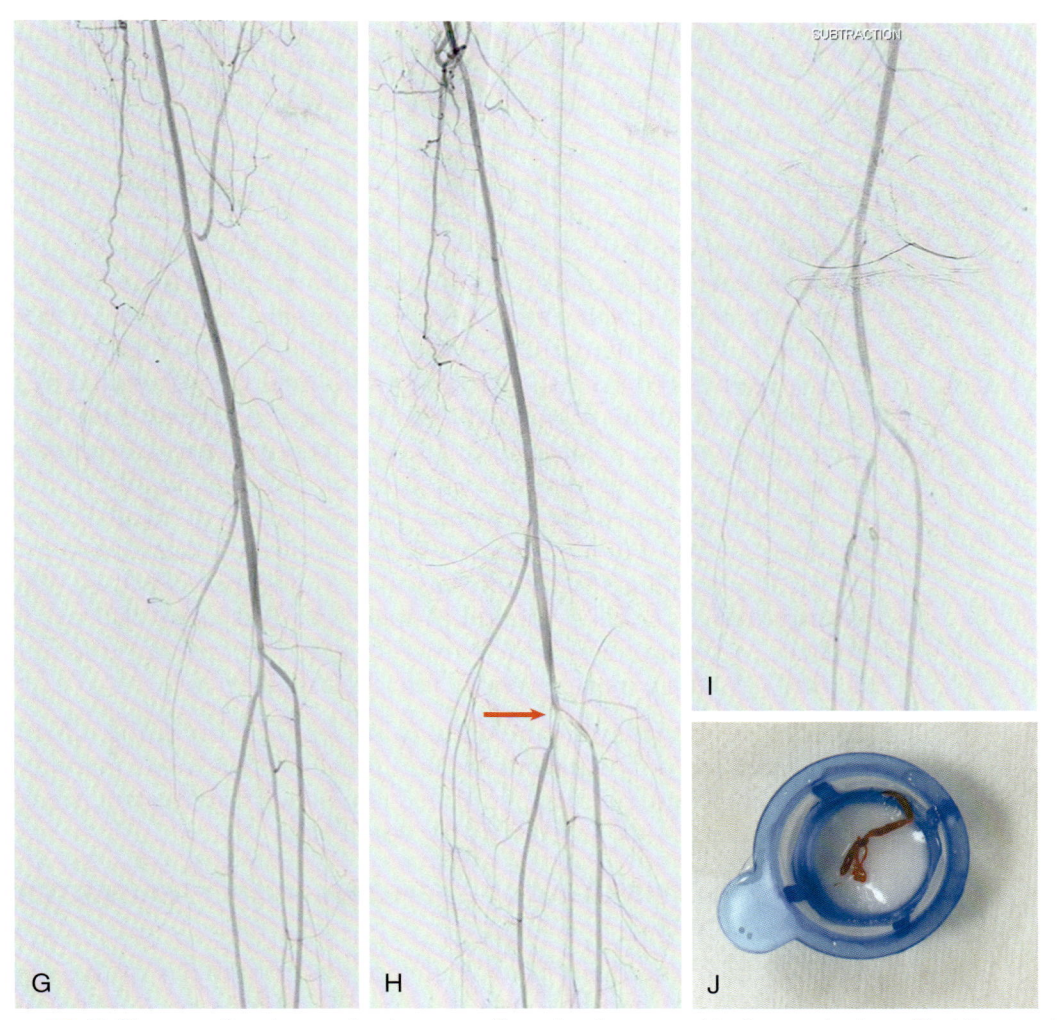

Figure 48-3, cont'd **G,** The runoff at the popliteal artery trifurcation is assessed before angioplasty. **H,** After treating the superficial femoral artery, a flow-limiting thrombus *(red arrow)* is observed at the trifurcation. **I,** Suction thrombectomy is performed at the trifurcation, with improvement demonstrated on a subsequent angiogram. **J,** Thrombus is removed by aspiration embolectomy with the suction catheter.

atherectomy may have a role for bulky lesions in the common femoral artery or popliteal artery, where stenting should be avoided.

After hemostasis is obtained, patients in whom suture-mediated closure was successful lie flat for 2 hours, whereas those who had manual pressure are kept supine, as a rule, 1 hour for each French size of the introducer sheath.

ENDOVASCULAR TREATMENT OF FEMORAL-POPLITEAL ARTERY OCCLUSIONS

Femoral-popliteal occlusions may be crossed via intimal or subintimal techniques. Intimal traversal uses the tip of the wire to steer through the occlusion. Intimal treatment results in the angioplasty displaying the typical "waist" at the lesion site. The proximal end of an occlusion typically has a fibrous cap that can be difficult to penetrate with a guidewire and is facilitated with the use of a braided wire with a weighted tip, such as the ASAHI MiracleBros 6 (Abbott Vascular, Abbott Park, Ill.).

Endovascular treatment of occlusions follows the previously described technique for treatment of stenosis up to the point of crossing the lesion. Once the sheath is placed and the patient is systemically anticoagulated, either a 0.014- or a 0.018-inch wire with a 0.018-inch Quick-Cross catheter is advanced to the fibrous cap of the occlusion. Intimal crossing begins with anchoring the catheter tip at the fibrous cap. The wire is then forcefully and deliberately drilled into the cap using a torque device. The wire and catheter are sequentially advanced until the lesion is crossed. After the catheter appears to be in the postocclusion lumen, the wire is removed and blood return, along with angiography, is used to confirm intraluminal location.

If intimal crossing fails, then a subintimal technique is used. A floppy 0.035-inch Glidewire and 0.035-inch angled-tip catheter are placed 2 cm proximal to the lesion. The wire is then forcefully pushed against the fibrous cap until a wire loop appears and advances. The loop is advanced past the occlusion subintimally, with sequential advancement of the accompanying catheter. Once the wire and catheter are past the occlusion, the wire is pulled back to remove the loop and gently readvanced until the wire is intraluminal, demonstrated by free passage of the wire tip without a loop. A new wire may be needed if the tip was deformed during subintimal passage. Spontaneous reentry occurs in approximately 80% of cases and is confirmed with blood return and angiography.[33] If reentry fails to occur spontaneously, then a reentry device, such as the Outback catheter (Cordis, Bridgewater, N.J.) or a device that includes intravascular ultrasound (IVUS), such as the Pioneer Plus (Medtronic Vascular, Minneapolis) is used. The Pioneer Plus reentry device travels over a 0.014-inch wire and uses IVUS to identify the true lumen. A constrained needle is then oriented toward the true lumen and is deployed, and the wire is advanced into the true lumen.

After crossing the lesion and confirming the location of the lumen, an appropriately sized balloon is introduced and inflated. Inflation is maintained for 1 minute. An angiogram is then performed, and a decision to stent is based on residual stenosis, dissection, or recoil of the vessel wall.

THROMBOLYSIS OF ACUTE FEMORAL-POPLITEAL ARTERY OCCLUSIONS

Endovascular treatment of an acute arterial thrombosis of the femoral-popliteal arteries follows the previously described technique for treatment of stenosis up to the point of crossing the lesion. Once the site of acute thrombosis is identified on an angiogram, a stiff, angled Glidewire is advanced through the flush catheter and a long 6-Fr sheath is inserted. The length and position of the sheath are determined by the level of the thrombus and may be placed anywhere from the common iliac artery to the distal superficial femoral artery.

The thrombus is then crossed with a floppy or stiff, 0.035-inch, angled Glidewire in combination with an angled hydrophilic catheter. For more distal lesions 0.014-inch wires are used in combination with a Quick-Cross catheter. An infusion of tissue plasminogen activator (tPA) proximal to the occlusion occasionally softens the thrombus sufficiently to allow it to be crossed.

Once the thrombus is successfully crossed with a wire, mechanical thrombectomy is performed using an AngioJet rheolytic catheter (Possis). Although eight percutaneous mechanical thrombectomy devices have been approved for hemodialysis grafts, only the AngioJet is approved in the United States for peripheral arterial occlusions. The power pulse setting allows infusion of a lytic agent, such as tPA (10 mg), directly into the thrombus, followed by a 15-minute incubation period and aspiration into the catheter. This technique rapidly lyses the thrombus and reestablishes some distal flow immediately. If a flow-limiting lesion is identified after AngioJet lysis, then angioplasty with or without stenting may be performed before instituting continuous infusion of tPA. Residual thrombus often remains and is treated with overnight lytic infusion followed by repeat angiography the next day. A multi-sidehole infusion catheter long enough to cover the length of the thrombus, such as a Cragg-McNamara (4-5 Fr diameter, 5-50 cm infusion length; EV3, Plymouth, Minn.) is placed across the remaining thrombus, and tPA is infused at 1 mg/hour. A MicroMewi microcatheter (2.9 Fr diameter, 5-10 cm infusion length; Covidien, Mansfield, Mass.) may be used for smaller vessels, and a Katzen infusion wire (Boston Scientific) may be used for very small arteries or to provide additional length beyond the maximum (50 cm) infusion length of most infusion catheters. Simultaneous intraarterial heparin infusion at 500 unit/hour is delivered through the sheath to prevent thrombosis around the catheter.

An angiogram is performed within 12 to 24 hours to assess the effectiveness of lysis. With long thrombotic occlusions, it may be necessary to advance the infusion catheter and continue lysis for another 12 to 24 hours of infusion. If an underlying stenotic lesion is identified, it is immediately treated percutaneously.

Postoperative Care

- **Sheath management.** The sheath is removed after the ACT is less than 180 seconds for those in whom a closure device has not been used and manual compression planned.
- **Antiplatelet therapy.** If not started preoperatively, a 300-mg oral loading dose of clopidogrel is administered in the recovery room and continued at an oral dosage of 75 mg daily for 1 month, along with lifelong aspirin therapy.
- **Postoperative surveillance.** Patients are evaluated with ABIs and duplex examination of the treated arterial segment at 1 month, every 6 months for 2 years, and annually thereafter. Angiographic assessment is indicated for an in-stent stenosis of more than 80%, as suggested by a peak systolic velocity (PSV) of at least 275 cm/sec and PSV ratio (PSV within the stent to PSV within the disease-free proximal superficial femoral artery) of at least 3.50, particularly in association with recurrent symptoms.

Complications

- **Arterial dissection.** Once a flow-limiting arterial dissection is diagnosed, management begins with confirmation that the guidewire is within the true lumen. Care should be taken to maintain the wire within the true lumen until stenting of the dissection has been performed. If the wire has been withdrawn, angiography and/or IVUS are used to assure that the wire is advanced within the true lumen.
- **Embolization and occlusion.** Treatment options for embolization and occlusion include suction thrombectomy with an Export aspiration catheter (Medtronic Vascular); rheolytic thrombectomy with or without a thrombolytic agent, such as tPA; or angioplasty with or without stenting (Fig. 48-3, G-J).
- **Arterial rupture.** Maintaining the wire within the true lumen distal to the ruptured arterial segment is essential. Initial control of active extravasation is performed with inflation of the initial treatment balloon. The wire is exchanged for a stiff 0.035-inch wire, such as an Amplatz wire, to facilitate upsizing of the sheath so that a stent graft may be deployed for definitive control. The stent graft is gently postdilated, and a completion angiogram is obtained.
- **Access site complications.** Bleeding from a high puncture in the external iliac artery requires surgical intervention; alternatively, stent-graft placement may be considered from contralateral femoral access. A femoral artery pseudoaneurysm may be observed if less than 1 cm in diameter, but treatment with thrombin injection or surgery is required if larger than 1 cm in diameter. An arteriovenous fistula may be managed conservatively, but surgical repair required if a large fistula persists.

REFERENCES

1. Dotter CT, Judkins MP: Transluminal treatment of arteriosclerotic obstruction. Description of a new technique and a preliminary report of its application, *Circulation* 30:654-670, 1964.

2. Zeitler E, Grüntzig A, Schoop W, et al: *Percutaneous vascular recanalization: Technique, applications, clinical results*, New York, 1979, Springer.
3. Grüntzig A, Hopff H: Perkutane rekanalisation chronischer arterieller verschlüsse mit einem neuen dilatationskatheter. Modifikation der Dotter-technik, *Dtsch Med Wochenschr* 99:2502-2505, 1974.
4. Grüntzig A, Kumpe DA: Technique of percutaneous trans-luminal angioplasty with the Grüntzig balloon catheter, *Am J Roentgenol* 132:547-552, 1979.
5. Sigwart V, Puel J, Mirkovitch V, Joffre F, Kappenberger L: Intravascular stents to prevent occlusion and restenosis after transluminal angioplasty, *N Engl J Med* 6:701-706, 1987.
6. Bolia A, Miles KA, Brennan J, Bell PRF: Percutaneous transluminal angioplasty of occlusions of the femoral and popliteal arteries by subintimal dissection, *Cardiovasc Intervent Radiol* 13: 357-363, 1990.
7. London NJM, Srinivasan R, Naylor AR, et al: Subintimal angioplasty of femoropopliteal artery occlusions. The long-term results, *Euro J Vasc Surg* 8:148-155, 1994.
8. Henry M, Amor M, Cragg A, et al: Occlusive and aneurysmal peripheral arterial disease: Assessment of a stent-graft system, *Radiology* 201:717-724, 1996.
9. Lammer J, Dake MD, Bleyn J, et al: Peripheral arterial obstruction: Prospective study of treatment with a transluminally placed self-expanding stent-graft, *Radiology* 217:95-104, 2000.
10. Adam DJ, Beard JD, Cleveland T, et al: Bypass versus angioplasty in severe ischaemia of the leg (BASIL): Multicentre, randomised controlled trial, *Lancet* 366(9501):1925-1934, 2005.
11. Norgren L, Hiatt WR, Dormandy JA, et al: Inter-society consensus for the management of peripheral arterial disease (TASC II), *J Vasc Surg* 45(Suppl S):S5-S67, 2007.
12. Lippert H, Pabst R: *Arterial variations in man: Classification and frequency*, New York, 1985, Springer Verlag.
13. Massoud TF, Fletcher EW: Anatomical variants of the profunda femoris artery: An angiographic study, *Surg Radiol Anat* 19:99-103, 1997.
14. Brown R, Nguyen TD, Spincemaille P, et al: In vivo quantification of femoral-popliteal compression during isometric thigh contraction: Assessment using MR angiography, *J Magn Reson Imaging* 29:1116-1124, 2009.
15. Wood NB, Zhao SZ, Zambanini A, et al: Curvature and tortuosity of the superficial femoral artery: A possible risk factor for peripheral arterial disease, *J Appl Physiol* 101:1412-1418, 2006.
16. Nikanorov A, Smouse HB, Osman K, et al: Fracture of self-expanding nitinol stents stressed in vitro under simulated intravascular conditions, *J Vasc Surg* 48:435-440, 2008.
17. Biondi-Zoccai GG, Agostoni P, Sangiorgi G, et al: Mastering the antegrade femoral artery access in patients with symptomatic lower limb ischemia: Learning curve, complications, and technical tips and tricks, *Catheter Cardiovasc Interv* 68:835-842, 2006.
18. Tønnesen KH, Sager P, Karle A, Henriksen L, Jørgensen B: Percutaneous transluminal angioplasty of the superficial femoral artery by retrograde catheterization via the popliteal artery, *Cardiovasc Intervent Radiol* 11:127-131, 1988.
19. Montero-Baker M, Schmidt A, Bräunlich S, et al: Retrograde approach for complex popliteal and tibioperoneal occlusions, *J Endovasc Therapy* 15:594-604, 2008.
20. Vroegingeweij D, Vos LD, Tielbeek AV, et al: Balloon angioplasty combined with primary stenting versus balloon angioplasty alone in femoropopliteal obstructions: A comparative randomized study, *Cardiovasc Intervent Radiol* 20:420-425, 1997.
21. Cejna M, Thurnher S, Illiasch H, et al: PTA versus Palmaz stent placement in femoropopliteal artery obstructions: A multicenter prospective randomized study, *J Vasc Interv Radiol* 12:23-31, 2001.
22. Schillinger M, Sabeti S, Loewe C, et al: Balloon angioplasty versus implantation of nitinol stents in the superficial femoral artery, *N Engl J Med* 354:1879-1888, 2006.
23. Schillinger M, Sabeti S, Dick P, et al: Sustained benefit at 2 years of primary femoropopliteal stenting compared with balloon angioplasty with optional stenting, *Circulation* 115:2745-2749, 2007.
24. Dick P, Wallner H, Sabeti S, et al: Balloon angioplasty versus stenting with nitinol stents in intermediate length superficial femoral artery lesions, *Catheter Cardiovasc Intervent* 74: 1090-1095, 2009.
25. Laird JR, Katzen BT, Scheinert D, et al: Nitinol stent implantation vs. balloon angioplasty for lesions in the superficial femoral and proximal popliteal arteries of patients with claudication: Three-year follow-up from the RESILIENT randomized trial, *J Endovasc Therapy* 19:1-9, 2012.
26. Duda SH, Pusich B, Richter G, et al: Sirolimus-eluting stents for the treatment of obstructive superficial femoral artery disease, *Circulation* 106:1505-1509, 2002.
27. Duda SH, Bosiers M, Lammer J, et al: Sirolimus-eluting versus bare nitinol stent for obstructive superficial femoral artery disease: The SIROCCO II trial, *J Vasc Interven Radiol* 16:331-338, 2005.
28. Duda SH, Bosiers M, Lammer J, et al: Drug-eluting and bare nitinol stents for the treatment of atherosclerotic lesions in the superficial femoral artery: Long-term results from the SIROCCO trial, *J Endovasc Therapy* 13:701-710, 2006.
29. Dake MD, Ansel GM, Jaff MR, et al: Paclitaxel-eluting stents show superiority to balloon angioplasty and bare metal stents in femoropopliteal disease: Twelve-month Zilver PTX randomized study results, *Circulation-Cardiovasc Intervent* 4:495-504, 2011.

30. Dake MD, Ansel GM, Jaff MR, et al: Sustained safety and effectiveness of paclitaxel-eluting stents for femoropopliteal lesions 2-year follow-up from the Zilver PTX randomized and single-arm clinical studies, *J Am Coll Cardiol* 61:2417-2427, 2013.
31. Tepe G, Zeller T, Albrecht T, et al: Local delivery of paclitaxel to inhibit restenosis during angioplasty of the leg, *N Eng J Med* 358:689-699, 2008.
32. Kröger K, Buss C, Goyen M, Santosa F, Rudofsky G: Diameter of occluded superficial femoral arteries limits percutaneous recanalization: Preliminary results, *J Endovasc Ther* 9:369-374, 2002.
33. London NJM, Srinivasan R, Naylor AR, et al: Subintimal angioplasty of femoropopliteal artery occlusions. The long-term results, *Europ J Vasc Surg* 8:148-155, 1994.

49 Endovascular Treatment of Tibial-Peroneal Arterial Occlusive Disease

TEJAS R. SHAH • PETER L. FARIES

Historical Background

Initial series demonstrating the feasibility of infrapopliteal angioplasty were reported in the late 1980s and early 1990s concomitant with the development of increasingly small, strong, low-profile balloons; steerable hydrophilic guidewires; and improved road-mapping techniques. These reports, largely for the treatment of critical limb ischemia, described acceptable technical success rates and promising short-term patency and clinical outcomes.[1-4]

The technique of subintimal angioplasty, first reported in 1990 by Bolia and colleagues[5] for treatment of occlusions in the femoral-popliteal artery, was subsequently extended for treatment of occlusions of the tibial and peroneal arteries, as reported in 1997.[6] Laser angioplasty for lower extremity atherosclerotic disease was first described in 1984, but was initially associated with unacceptably high complication rates of vessel perforation.[7] Subsequent technical improvements led to promising results for limb salvage in poor candidates for surgical revascularization.[8] Serino and associates[9] reported 2-year patency rates of 83% and limb salvage of 94% for laser-assisted balloon angioplasty in which the laser is coaxial to the balloon to increase the vessel diameter.

Feiring and co-workers[10] were among the first to describe primary stenting of tibial lesions using coronary stents, and the first randomized trial evaluating the use of bare metal stents to treat infrapopliteal disease was conducted by Rand and colleagues.[11] Subsequent studies have observed limb salvage rates of 89.3% with a 12-month primary patency rate of 62.8%.[12] The Chromis Deep stent (Invatec, Roncadelle, Italy) designed for treatment of infrapopliteal lesions was found to have a 91.5% limb salvage rate with a primary patency of 52.9% at 12 months.[13] In 2005 the first small series to use a drug-eluting, sirolimus stent for tibial occlusive disease described improved 6-month outcomes, with an in-segment restenosis rate of 32% compared with 66% for bare metal stents.[14]

Indications

In an effort to guide recommendations for treatment and standardize methodology for reporting anatomic-specific outcomes, lesion morphology has been classified in a Trans-Atlantic Inter-Society Consensus document.[15] Recent recommendations suggest that catheter-based interventions for infrapopliteal disease are most suitable for patients with critical limb ischemia in association with significant medical comorbidities.

Preoperative Preparation

- **History and assessment of risk factors.** Patients with a history of significant coronary or pulmonary disease may be better served by an endovascular intervention. However, renal insufficiency increases the risk of contrast-induced nephropathy. Minimizing known atherosclerotic risk factors through smoking cessation, treatment of diabetes or hypertension, and use of statins can reduce morbidity and improve outcomes. Patients should be placed on an antiplatelet regimen, such as aspirin and clopidogrel.

- **Physical examination.** A complete pulse examination should be performed, along with an assessment of skin integrity in the lower extremities, including the presence of web space ulcers, open wounds, and gangrene.
- **Noninvasive vascular laboratory studies.** The ankle-brachial index (ABI) and pulse volume recordings provide an objective analysis of both the location and the severity of peripheral arterial disease (PAD). ABI of less than 0.9 is indicative of PAD, whereas an ABI of less than 0.4 is consistent with critical limb ischemia. Treadmill exercise testing may help identify underlying PAD, particularly in those patients with appropriate symptoms and normal ABIs at rest. Duplex ultrasonography can be performed to determine the presence and extent of arterial disease and to evaluate potential target points for arterial reconstruction.
- **Imaging studies.** Computed tomography angiography or magnetic resonance angiography may help to characterize the location and severity of arterial lesions and the presence of calcification.

Pitfalls and Danger Points

- Rupture
- Arterial dissection
- Embolization
- Acute arterial occlusion
- Restenosis

Endovascular Strategy

ANGIOGRAPHIC ANATOMY AND COMMON COLLATERAL PATHWAYS

The anatomy of the infrageniculate vasculature begins at the adductor hiatus, where the superficial femoral artery (SFA) transitions to the popliteal artery, which tracks caudally through the popliteal fossa and down to the bifurcation of the anterior tibial artery and the tibioperoneal trunk. The popliteal artery occasionally bifurcates into its terminal branches in the popliteal fossa behind the knee, leading to a high takeoff of the anterior or posterior tibial artery. The popliteal artery rarely divides into the anterior tibial, posterior tibial, and peroneal arteries without the formation of a tibioperoneal trunk.

The popliteal artery gives rise to several branches, including the superior and inferior sural muscular branches, the cutaneous branches, the medial and lateral superior genicular arteries, a middle genicular artery, and the medial and lateral inferior genicular arteries. Rich collateralization is found around the patella, which becomes pronounced in patients with popliteal or distal SFA occlusions.

The anterior tibial artery commences at the popliteal bifurcation and extends to the dorsalis pedis artery, giving off several muscular branches, as well as the malleolar arteries, which supply the ankle joint. The posterior tibial artery extends from the tibioperoneal trunk and travels obliquely down behind the medial malleolus. Muscular, communicating, and nutrient branches arise from the posterior tibial along its course to the foot, where it divides into the medial and lateral plantar arteries. Finally, the peroneal artery arises at the bifurcation of the tibioperoneal trunk below the popliteus muscle and traverses along the posteromedial fibula to the level of the calcaneus.

UNFAVORABLE ANATOMIC AND PHYSIOLOGIC FEATURES FOR INTERVENTIONS ON THE TIBIAL OR PERONEAL VESSELS

Several anatomic features of tibioperoneal disease have increased the technical challenges and reduced the long-term durability associated with endovascular intervention, including densely calcified arteries, long-segment disease, serial stenoses or occlusions, small-diameter vessels, and compromised runoff beds.

SELECTION OF ANTEGRADE OR RETROGRADE ACCESS

Balloon angioplasty and stent placement of infrageniculate arteries are performed either through the ipsilateral femoral artery in an antegrade approach or through the contralateral femoral artery using an up-and-over approach. The advantages of the antegrade approach include better guidewire and catheter control; the ability to reach distal lesions with shorter wire lengths, which occasionally cannot be reached using the up-and-over approach; and avoidance of tortuous aortoiliac vessels. Nonetheless, the up-and-over approach permits the use of a simple retrograde femoral puncture and evaluation of the aortoiliac and femoral arteries before treatment of infrageniculate lesions. Both groins are always prepared in case an alternative approach is required during the procedure.

SELECTION OF A STENT

Percutaneous transluminal angioplasty (PTA) remains the treatment of choice for infrapopliteal disease, with stent implantation restricted to suboptimal outcomes after PTA. In the absence of an approved tibial stent, coronary stents have been used.

Endovascular Technique

TIBIAL ARTERY ANGIOPLASTY AND STENTING

Positioning

After lying the patient supine on a fluoroscopic table, the patient is positioned with the hip externally rotated and knee slightly flexed. The foot is padded and taped in the lateral position to maximize visibility of tibial runoff.

Arterial Access

Antegrade femoral access is preferred, because it allows easier guidewire and catheter control and "pushability," along with the opportunity to reach distal lesions with a shorter wire. Access is obtained using a 21-Ga needle and a 0.018-inch wire commonly found in a micropuncture kit. The needle and 0.018-inch guidewire are exchanged for a 3-Fr sheath, and sheath placement in the SFA is confirmed by intraluminal injection of contrast (Fig. 49-1). A 0.035-inch guidewire is advanced, and the 3-Fr sheath exchanged for a 5-Fr sheath. Once the sheath is secured, serial angiograms with runoff are performed in the anteroposterior projection to better characterize the inflow, pinpoint the lesion, and assess collateralization and outflow.

Identifying the Lesion

After the target lesion is identified, the 5-Fr sheath is exchanged for a long sheath, suitable for the planned intervention. The sheath should be advanced to within 10 cm of the target lesion. Placing the sheath tip close to the lesion improves catheter mechanics and allows performance of multiple angiograms without removing the wire.

Crossing the Lesion

The 0.035-inch guidewire is exchanged for a working wire, with selection determined by wire hydrophilicity, support, and size. The WhisperWire (Abbott Laboratories, Abbott Park, Ill.) is a hydrophilic, floppy, 0.014-inch-diameter wire and suitable for

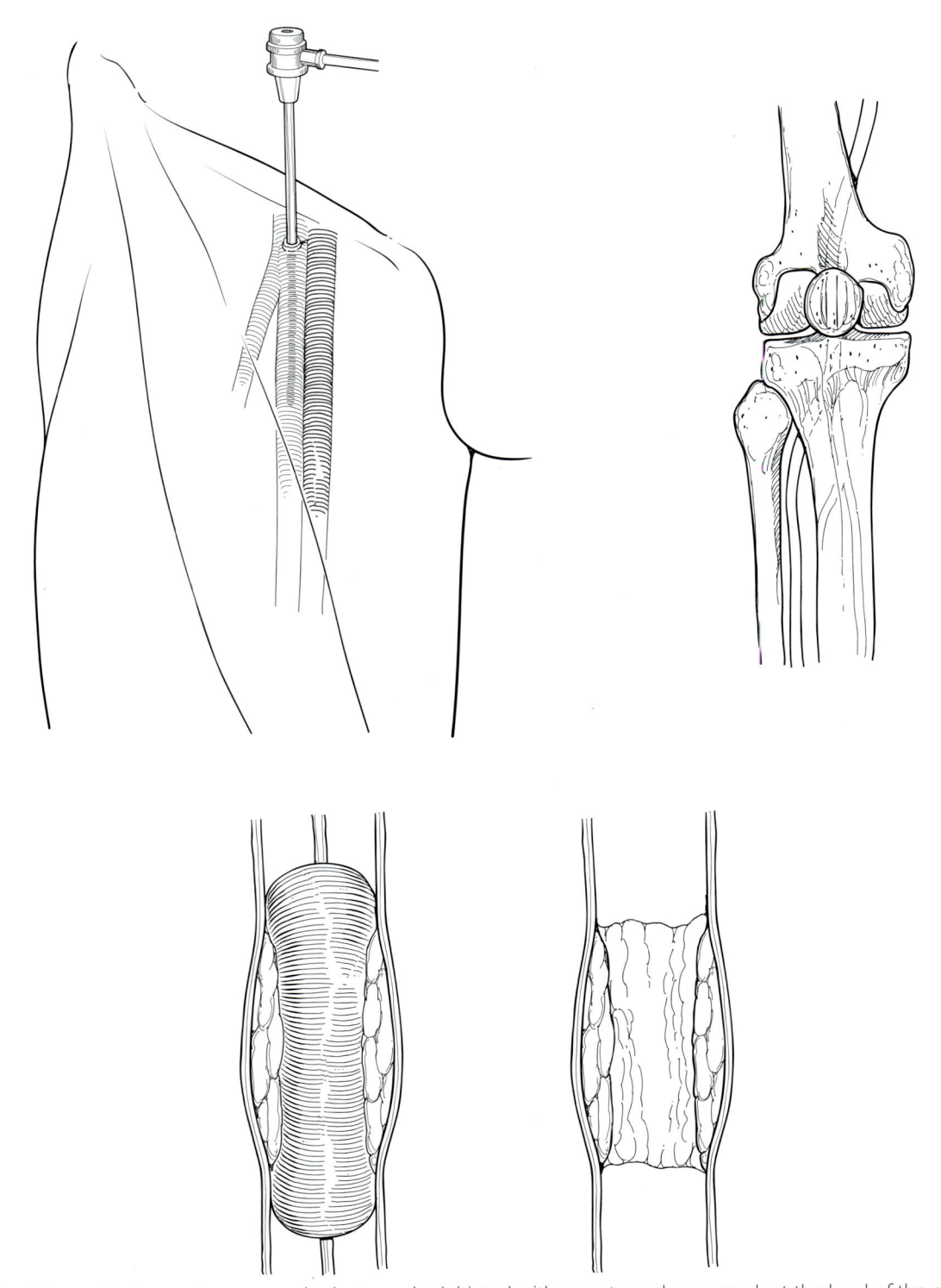

Figure 49-1. Infrapopliteal percutaneous angioplasty can be initiated with an antegrade approach at the level of the common femoral artery. The lesion is crossed with a selective, hydrophilic wire (e.g., Glidewire), which is advanced beyond the lesion to facilitate the subsequent steps. An appropriately sized angioplasty balloon (usually 5-6 mm in diameter for an SFA or popliteal artery and 3-4 mm for infrapopliteal vessels) is positioned and insufflated. A completion arteriogram can be obtained through the sheath to show complete effacement of the lesion.

most interventions. For lesions not traversable with the WhisperWire, an exchange is made for a stiffer wire. Alternate 0.014-inch guidewires include the Choice PT and Journey (Boston Scientific, Natick, Mass.) or the Balance Middleweight universal guidewire (Abbott Laboratories). If these wires have not been able to traverse an occlusion, alternate 0.014-inch choices include the Victory (Boston Scientific) or the ASAHI MiracleBros 6 and Spartacore (Abbott Laboratories) guidewires. The guidewire should be advanced beyond the lesion to avoid losing access during the procedure, with wire position intermittently assessed to avoid injuring the distal vasculature. Heparin (100 units per kilogram of body weight) may be given directly after sheath placement and before lesion manipulation, with the activated clotting time maintained above 300 seconds (Fig. 49-1).

Balloon Angioplasty

A balloon catheter is advanced over the wire and placed across the lesion. The choice of balloon catheter depends on the characteristics of the lesion and the diameter of the adjacent nondiseased vessels, as well as the profile of the catheter tip and deflated balloon to ensure that the catheter is able to pass through the lumen of the stenosis. As an example, the Coyote (Boston Scientific) balloon catheter is a low-profile, 0.014-inch balloon that is available in monorail or over-the-wire platforms, diameters between 1.5 and 4 mm, and lengths up to 220 mm. Once the balloon is placed across the lesion, it is inflated to a pressure of 10 to 12 atm under direct fluoroscopic guidance and kept inflated for approximately 30 to 40 seconds. If a residual stenosis remains, the lesion can be reballooned at a higher pressure or with a larger balloon (Fig. 49-1).

Postangioplasty Imaging

The need for stent placement is based on degree of residual stenosis, amount of recoil of the vessel wall, and residual dissection or flap. If required, the shortest possible stent sufficient to treat the lesion stent is selected and oversized by 1 to 2 mm. Poststent completion angiograms should be performed to document full expansion of the stent and brisk flow across the treated lesion. Postprocedure clinical examination, including full lower extremity pulse examination, is performed before transfer of the patient to the recovery area.

TIBIAL ARTERY SUBINTIMAL ANGIOPLASTY AND STENTING

Subintimal angioplasty may be most suitable for chronic, moderate to severely calcified, long occlusions or a previously failed attempt at intraluminal angioplasty.[16]

Arterial Access

Patients are positioned, prepped, and accessed in the same manner as an intraluminal angioplasty. A 5-Fr angled catheter is introduced in an antegrade fashion, the patient is systemically heparinized, and a vasodilator, such as papaverine (30 mg) or nitroglycerin (200 mcg) is administered intraarterially before crossing the lesion.

Crossing the Lesion

The tip of a straight floppy wire is curved and advanced to the origin of the occlusion. The guidewire is then passed into the subintimal plane by deliberate, purposeful application of force. Resistance is overcome by advancing the catheter along with the guidewire. Alternatively, a directional catheter can be used to direct the guidewire into the subintimal plane (Fig. 49-2). Wire location within the subintimal plane is confirmed by a characteristic "looped appearance," with the diameter of the loop larger than the luminal diameter of the artery, along with a small hand injection of contrast.

Entry back to the true lumen occurs spontaneously with the looped guidewire in approximately 80% of the cases. If reentry does not occur spontaneously, a reentry device, such as the Outback catheter (Cordis Corp., Miami) can be used to reenter the true lumen. This catheter uses a constrained needle, which is oriented by markers to facilitate the delivery of the guidewire into the true lumen.

Balloon Angioplasty

After crossing the lesion and reentering the true lumen, an appropriately sized balloon is introduced and inflated to 10 to 12 atm for approximately 30 to 40 seconds throughout the length of the lesion.

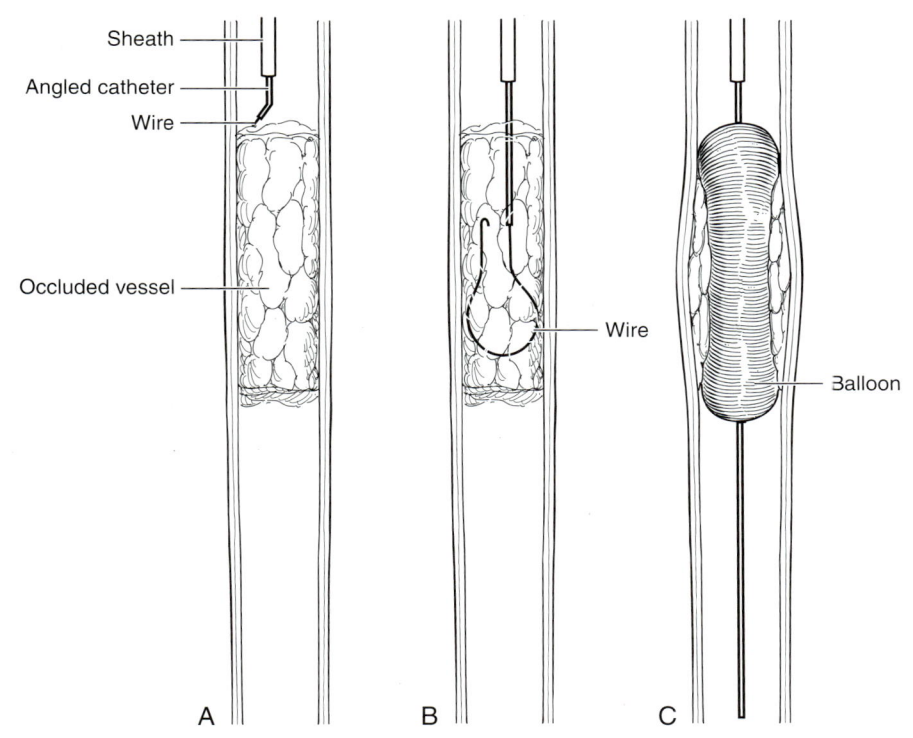

Figure 49-2. A, The wire dissection for subintimal angioplasty is initiated by advancing a hydrophilic 0.035-inch wire through a 5-Fr angled-tip catheter (e.g., Berenstein) into the subintimal plane immediately proximal to the occlusion. This requires a deliberate, purposeful motion to essentially "force" the wire into the appropriate plane. The catheter is subsequently advanced over the wire into the subintimal plane. **B,** The subintimal dissection is continued by allowing the wire to form a large loop within the subintimal plane. The wire and catheter combination is then advanced within the subintimal plane to separate the lesion from the deeper layers of the vessel wall. After the presumed distal endpoint is reached, the catheter is advanced and the wire is withdrawn to remove its loop. The wire is then advanced into the patent, distal vessels using the angled catheter to direct its orientation. The catheter is subsequently advanced over the wire, and its location within the distal vessels is confirmed with a puff of contrast. **C,** The subintimal plane is then dilated using the same technique and balloons as used for the intraluminal approach.

Postangioplasty Imaging

An angiogram is performed to evaluate the success of treatment. A decision to stent is based on the presence of residual stenosis or dissection (Fig. 49-3).

TIBIAL ARTERY LASER ANGIOPLASTY AND STENTING

Indications for laser angioplasty are similar to those considered for subintimal angioplasty, with careful case selection in patients with diabetes and renal failure. Laser-assisted angioplasty devices, such as the TurboElite laser ablation catheter (Spectranetics, Colorado Springs, Colo.), generally use a 6-Fr sheath for vessels between 3 and 3.5 mm in diameter. Otherwise, similar guidewire and catheter techniques are used to reestablish inline flow as with intraluminal angioplasty. One important consideration is the high rates of distal emboli generated from laser tissue ablation. In a single-center prospective registry of excimer laser ablative therapy, 67% of the patients had evidence of distal emboli, compared with 35% of the patients with angioplasty or stenting. However, clinically significant macrodebris was approximately 20% in both groups.[17]

Postoperative Care

- **Antiplatelet therapy.** Patients are loaded with 300 mg of clopidogrel in the recovery room and then begun on a daily dosage of 75 mg for 1 month. Concurrently, aspirin at a daily dosage of 325 mg is initiated in the recovery room if it is not part of the patient's current medication regimen. After 1 month the clopidogrel is stopped and daily aspirin (325 mg) continued indefinitely.

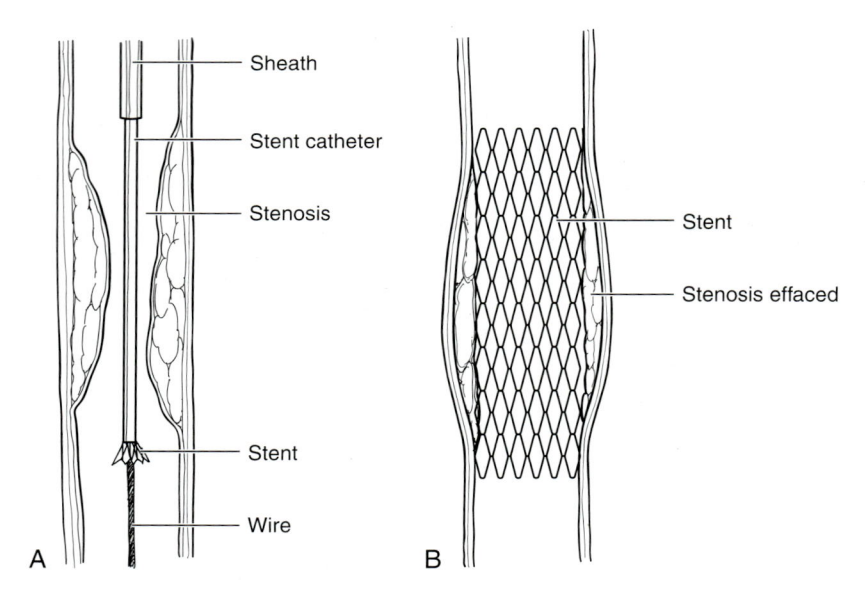

Figure 49-3. Placement of an intraluminal stent in an infrapopliteal vessel is illustrated. **A,** The stent delivery catheter is advanced through the long sheath beyond the lesion. The stent is positioned a few millimeters beyond the critical lesion. The stent is partially deployed until the ends begin to flare and is then positioned precisely before continuing the deployment. **B,** The stent is subsequently angioplastied with the appropriately sized balloon to complete the procedure. A completion arteriogram is used to confirm precise position of the stent across the lesion.

- **Postoperative surveillance.** Patients are evaluated at 1- and at 6-month intervals with serial ABIs and, if appropriate, by exercise treadmill testing. Repeat intervention is indicated for recurrent clinical symptoms of critical limb ischemia. Restenosis in the absence of clinical symptoms is not sufficient to compel for repeat intervention.

Complications

- **Morbidity.** The incidence of complications range from 5% to 26%.[18,19] Bleeding is the most common complication, with a frequency of 2% to 8%.
- **Arterial rupture.** The key step to successful endovascular management of rupture is to ensure that the guidewire traversing the ruptured artery remains in the true lumen distal to the rupture, as confirmed by angiography. Once the wire is known to cross the ruptured area, gentle inflation of an appropriately sized angioplasty balloon is adequate to prevent further extravasation. The addition of a bare metal stent may control hemorrhage when angioplasty alone is not sufficient. Coil embolization may be used if there is adequate collateral flow distally. Coils should be placed both distal and proximal to the site of rupture. Surgical revascularization or surgical repair may be necessary depending on the clinical situation, and the balloon can be used for temporary control during surgical dissection. Wire perforation of a small branch vessel with minimal extravasation may be treated by reversal of heparin, compression, and careful monitoring.
- **Arterial dissection.** An inadvertent arterial dissection is managed with the prime goal of reestablishing flow into the true lumen. Once a dissection is noted, it is important to ensure that the guidewire is in the true lumen by performing an angiogram. Although the true lumen can also be identified by intravascular ultrasound, this can be difficult given the small diameter of tibial arteries. Once wire placement in the true lumen is confirmed, the flap is stented.
- **Embolization or thrombosis.** An acute occlusion may be treated by crossing the lesion with either a 0.018- or a 0.014-inch weighted-tip wire or by entering the subintimal plane. If repeat angioplasty fails to open the lesion, an end-hole or flush catheter can be guided to the point of embolization or occlusion for direct intraarterial infusion of tissue plasminogen activator (tPA), with a 6-mg bolus followed by continuous infusion at 1 mg/hr until clinical improvement is noted. Risks of tPA include hemorrhagic stroke (1%) and major (5%) or minor (15%) hemorrhage.[20] If thrombolytic therapy does not produce the desired clinical improvement, open embolectomy should be considered.

- **Access site complications.** The access site should be assessed for hematoma, which may be associated with an underlying pseudoaneurysm or arteriovenous fistula or, in the event of acute ischemia, with thrombosis or local dissection at the site of access.

REFERENCES

1. Schwarten DE, Cutcliff WB: Arterial occlusive disease below the knee: Treatment with percutaneous trans-luminal angioplasty performed with low-profile catheters and steerable guide wires, *Radiology* 169:71-74, 1988.
2. Brown KT, Schoenberg NY, Moore ED, et al: Percutaneous trans-luminal angioplasty of infrapopliteal vessels: Preliminary-results and technical considerations, *Radiology* 169:75-78, 1988.
3. Bakal CW, Sprayregen S, Scheinbaum K, et al: Percutaneous transluminal angioplasty of the infrapopliteal arteries: Results in 53 patients, *Am J Roentgenol* 154:171-174, 1990.
4. Schwarten DE: Clinical and anatomical considerations for nonoperative therapy in tibial disease and the results of angioplasty, *Circulation* 83(Suppl):86-90. 1991.
5. Bolia A, Miles KA, Brennan J, et al: Percutaneous transluminal angioplasty of occlusions of the femoral and popliteal arteries by subintimal dissection, *Cardiovasc Intervent Radiol* 13:357-363, 1990.
6. Nydahl S, Hartshorne T, Bell PRF, et al: Subintimal angioplasty of infrapopliteal occlusions in critically ischaemic limbs, *Eur J Vasc Endovasc Surg* 14:212-216, 1997.
7. Cothern RM, Hayes GB, Kramer JR, et al: A multishield catheter with an optical shield for laser angiosurgery, *Lasers Life Sci* 1:1-12, 1986.
8. Bosiers M, Peeters P, Elst FV, et al: Excimer laser assisted angioplasty for critical limb ischemia: Results of the LACI Belgium study, *Eur J Vasc Endovasc Surg* 29:613-619, 2005.
9. Serino F, Cao Y, Renzi C, et al: Excimer laser ablation in the treatment of total chronic obstructions in critical limb ischaemia in diabetic patients. Sustained efficacy of plaque recanalisation in mid-term results, *Eur J Vasc Endovasc Surg* 39:234-238, 2010.
10. Feiring A, Wesolwski A, Lade S: Primary stent-supported angioplasty for treatment of below-knee critical limb ischemia and severe claudication: Early and one-year outcomes, *J Am Coll Cardiol* 44:2307-2314, 2004.
11. Rand T, Basile A, Cejna M, et al: PTA versus carbofilm-coated stents in infrapopliteal arteries: Pilot study, *Cardiovasc Intervent Radiol* 29:29-38, 2006.
12. Boisiers M, Kallakuri S, Deloose K, et al: Infragicular angioplasty and stenting in the management of critical limb ischaemia: One year outcome following the use of MULTI-LINK VISION stent, *EuroIntervention* 3:470-474, 2007.
13. Deloose K, Bosiers M, Peeters M: One year outcome after primary stenting of infrapopliteal lesions with the CHROMIS DEEP stent in the management of critical limb ischaemia, *EuroIntervention* 5:318-324, 2009.
14. Siablis D, Kraniotis P, Karnabatidis D, et al: Sirolimus-eluting versus bare stents for bailout after suboptimal infrapopliteal angioplasty for critical limb ischemia: 6-month angiographic results from a nonrandomized prospective single-center study, *J Endovasc Therapy* 12:685-695, 2005.
15. Norgren L, Hiatt WR, Dormandy JA, et al: Inter-society consensus for the management of peripheral arterial disease (TASC II), *J Vasc Surg* 45(Suppl S):S5-S67, 2007.
16. Bolia A, Sayars RD, Thompson MM, et al: Subintimal and intraluminal recanalization of occluded crural arteries by percutaneous balloon angioplasty, *Eur J Vasc Surg* 8:214-219, 1994.
17. Shammas NW, Coiner D, Shammas GA, et al: Distal embolic event protection using excimer laser ablation in peripheral vascular interventions: Results of the DEEP EMBOLI registry, *J Endovasc Ther* 16:197-202, 2009.
18. Matsi PJ, Manninen HI: Complications of lower-limb percutaneous transluminal angioplasty: A prospective analysis of 410 procedures on 295 consecutive patients, *Cardiovasc Intervent Radiol* 21:361-366, 1998.
19. Mousa A, Rhee J, Trocciola S, et al: Percutaneous endovascular treatment for chronic limb ischemia, *Ann Vasc Surg* 19:186-191, 2005.
20. Berridge DC, Makin GS, Hopkinson BR: Local low dose intraarterial thrombolytic therapy: The risk of stroke or major haemorrhage, *Br J Surg* 76:1230-1233, 1989.

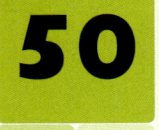

50 Endovascular Treatment of Popliteal Aneurysm

RAGHUVEER VALLABHANENI • LUIS A. SANCHEZ • PATRICK J. GERAGHTY

Historical Background

Although open surgical treatment remains the gold standard for treatment of popliteal artery aneurysm, endovascular repair has become a viable alternative. In 1994 Marin and colleagues described the first endovascular approach to exclusion of a popliteal artery aneurysm, using an expanded polytetrafluoroethylene (ePTFE) graft supported by two Palmaz stents.[1] Since that report, flexible, self-expanding endoprostheses, including the Wallgraft (Boston Scientific, Natick, Mass.) and the Viabahn endoprosthesis (W.L. Gore and Associates, Newark, Del.) have been introduced. These commercial devices have been adapted for endovascular popliteal aneurysm repair (EVPAR). To date, a multicenter, randomized trial of EVPAR has not been conducted, but multiple single-center series have documented acceptable primary and secondary patency rates in select patients with favorable anatomy.[2-6]

Indications

The primary goals of repairing popliteal artery aneurysms are the prevention of thromboembolic complications and limb loss. Complication rates of 15% to 25% at 1 year and 60% to 75% at 5 years have been reported for untreated popliteal artery aneuryms.[7,8] Thus in all ambulatory patients, elective repair of popliteal artery aneurysms greater than 2 cm in diameter, especially those with mural thrombus, should be undertaken to prevent embolization, thrombosis, and major amputation.[9,10]

Selection of open surgical treatment or EVPAR requires an individualized assessment of the patient. Suitable operative candidates with adequate saphenous vein should be offered surgical repair of popliteal artery aneurysm. Patients with symptomatic compression of the adjacent tibial nerve or popliteal vein should also undergo open surgical repair with aneurysm decompression and aneurysmorrhaphy, maneuvers best accomplished via the posterior approach. Finally, when thromboembolic complications require immediate revascularization, open surgical reconstruction with on-table adjunctive endovascular therapy offers the most expedient and anatomically flexible approach. However, a number of factors favor the choice of EVPAR, including patients with inadequate saphenous vein conduit or those with critical limb ischemia in the contralateral extremity who will require a venous conduit for tibial bypass. Likewise, the diagnosis of concomittant aortoiliac and popliteal aneurysms poses a challenge for frail patients. In those recovering from aortoiliac reconstruction, EVPAR permits timely popliteal artery aneurysm exclusion with minimal periprocedural morbidity. Patients undergoing endovascular repair should be able to tolerate lifelong antiplatelet therapy and potentially oral anticoagulation as well.

Several anatomic factors influence whether is EVPAR can be safely performed, including the diameters and lengths of the landing zones, the presence of mismatch between proximal and distal diameters of the landing zones, arterial angulation, and arterial runoff. Most experience has centered on use of the Viabahn endoprosthesis, which is available in 5- to 13-mm diameters. With appropriate oversizing, landing zone diameters may range from 4 to 12 mm, with at least 2 cm of nonaneurysmal artery proximal and distal to the popliteal aneurysm to affect a seal. Intravascular ultrasound (IVUS) may be used to verify the quality of the proposed seal zone. Excessive arterial angulation, which may occur at the junction of healthy and aneurysmal arterial segments, may predispose endografts to strut fracture and thrombosis. Tapered Viabahn endoprostheses are not commercially available. Therefore "pleating" or infolding of telescoped endografts to accomodate diameter mismatch may occur if the discrepancy between proximal and distal diameters is substantial. Partial or complete coverage of a patent tibial artery orifice must be avoided, and single-vessel tibial runoff should be present.

Preoperative Preparation

- **Preoperative imaging.** Although ultrasonography provides a cost-effective means of screening for popliteal artery aneurysms, computed tomography (CT) angiography with three-dimensional reconstruction is the imaging modality of choice for preoperative assessment and endovascular repair planning. CT angiography delineates the arterial wall, defining the extent of the aneurysm, permitting measurement of potential landing zones, and providing simultaneous screening for aortoiliac, femoral, and contralateral popliteal artery aneurysms.
- **Antiplatelet therapy.** Clopidogrel therapy is initiated before or immediately after endovascular repair to limit the risk of endograft thrombosis.[11]
- **Patient consent.** Patients should be counseled with regard to expected outcomes and that endograft use in EVPAR is not an FDA-approved indication for these devices.

Pitfalls and Danger Points

- Inadequate recognition of spatial constraints in selecting a suitable endograft
- Inaccurate intraprocedural identification of landing zones
- "Bowstringing" of the Viabahn delivery catheter

Endovascular Strategy

SELECTION OF AN ACCESS SITE

Although vascular surgeons are comfortable with retrograde femoral access from the contralateral groin, the larger introducer sheaths required for EVPAR may make the typical crossover technique cumbersome, if not impossible. Antegrade access of the ipsilateral common femoral artery or proximal superficial femoral artery is preferred via a percutaneous technique or by surgical exposure under local or regional anesthetic (Fig. 50-1).

SELECTION OF AN ENDOGRAFT

The Viabahn endoprosthesis, consisting of a flexible nitinol self-expanding stent with an inner lining of ePTFE, has been the stent graft of choice for EVPAR. The Viabahn is FDA approved for treatment of atherosclerotic occlusive disease of the iliac and superficial femoral arteries. Introducer sheaths of 7 to 12 Fr are required and the endograft diameter oversized by 1 to 2 mm. Oversizing the endograft by more than 15% should be avoided.

When it is necessary to use two or more endografts to achieve adequate exclusion of the popliteal artery aneurysm, there should be at least a 2-cm overlap between the grafts to avoid a type III endoleak. In addition, the diameters of the two devices should not differ by more than 2 mm. A larger difference may result in longitudinal

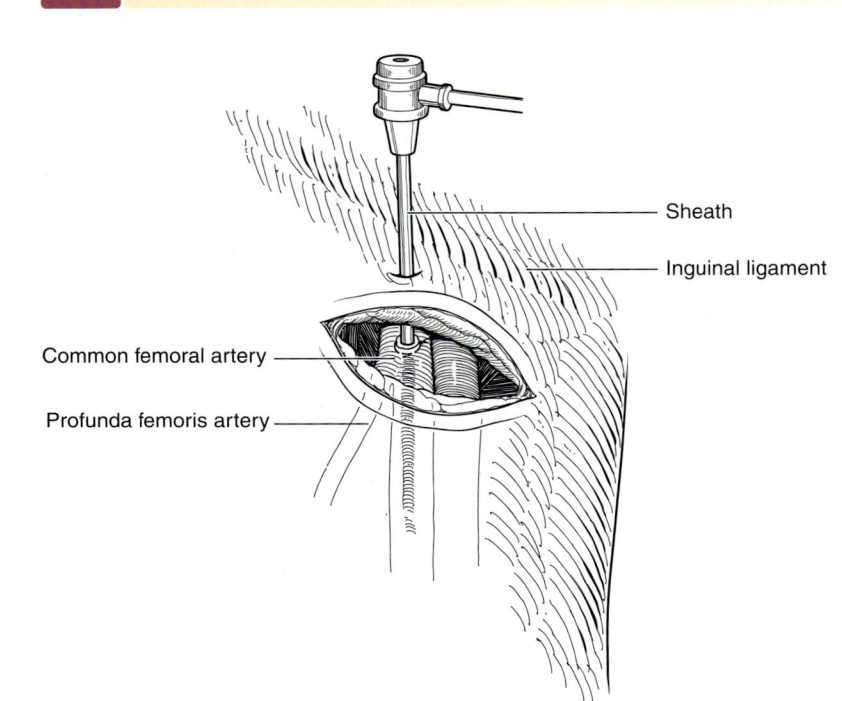

Figure 50-1. Antegrade puncture or a small cutdown on the common femoral artery should be used for delivery of the sheath. A small transverse incision is made below the inguinal ligament, and the distal common femoral artery is exposed. A mattressed, pledgeted polypropylene suture is placed on the anterior artery wall, followed by central needle puncture and wire introduction. An atraumatic 0.035-inch guidewire is inserted, and a 7-Fr sheath is placed. This can be upsized depending on the size of the endograft.

pleating of the larger endograft with luminal obstruction. When a popliteal artery aneurysm displays a large discrepancy between inflow and outflow vessel diameters, the telescoping of multiple endografts may lead to a stiff, noncompliant construct that is prone to mechanical kinking. In this setting open repair should be considered.

Endovascular Technique

ACCESS

Access is most commonly achieved using the antegrade approach, particularly when larger diameter endografts are required (Fig. 50-1 and Video 50-1). A small ipsilateral cutdown is used to expose the distal common femoral artery. A purse string polypropylene suture is placed on the anterior artery wall, followed by central needle puncture and wire introduction. In those patients with scarred common femoral arteries, surgical exposure of the proximal superficial femoral artery is a useful alternative. A 0.035-inch guidewire is inserted, a 7-Fr or larger sheath is placed, and systemic heparinization is instituted once access is obtained.

INTRAOPERATIVE IMAGING

Angiography of the extremity is performed before introduction of the device. Lateral views with the knee flexed may be used to determine the "hinge point" of the femoral-popliteal arterial segment. Documenting the location of maximum arterial flexion is salient if using multiple grafts, because there may be a higher likelihood of stent fracture if the stiffer overlap zone lies within this region. IVUS complements standard fluoroscopic imaging during EVPAR. The 0.018-inch compatible IVUS probe (Volcano Corp., Rancho Cordoba, Calif.) can be used to verify landing zone diameters and ensure these sites are free of mural thrombus.

A 0.018-inch guidewire, such as the 200-cm V-18 (Boston Scientific), is negotiated through the aneurysm and into a tibial outflow vessel under road map guidance. Use of a 0.018-inch guidewire facilitates atraumatic tibial vessel selection and subsequent IVUS examination. Although the Viabahn device permits the use of a stiffer 0.035-inch guidewire, its use is unnecessary if careful endograft deployment technique is used. The Viabahn endograft accommodates moderate vessel

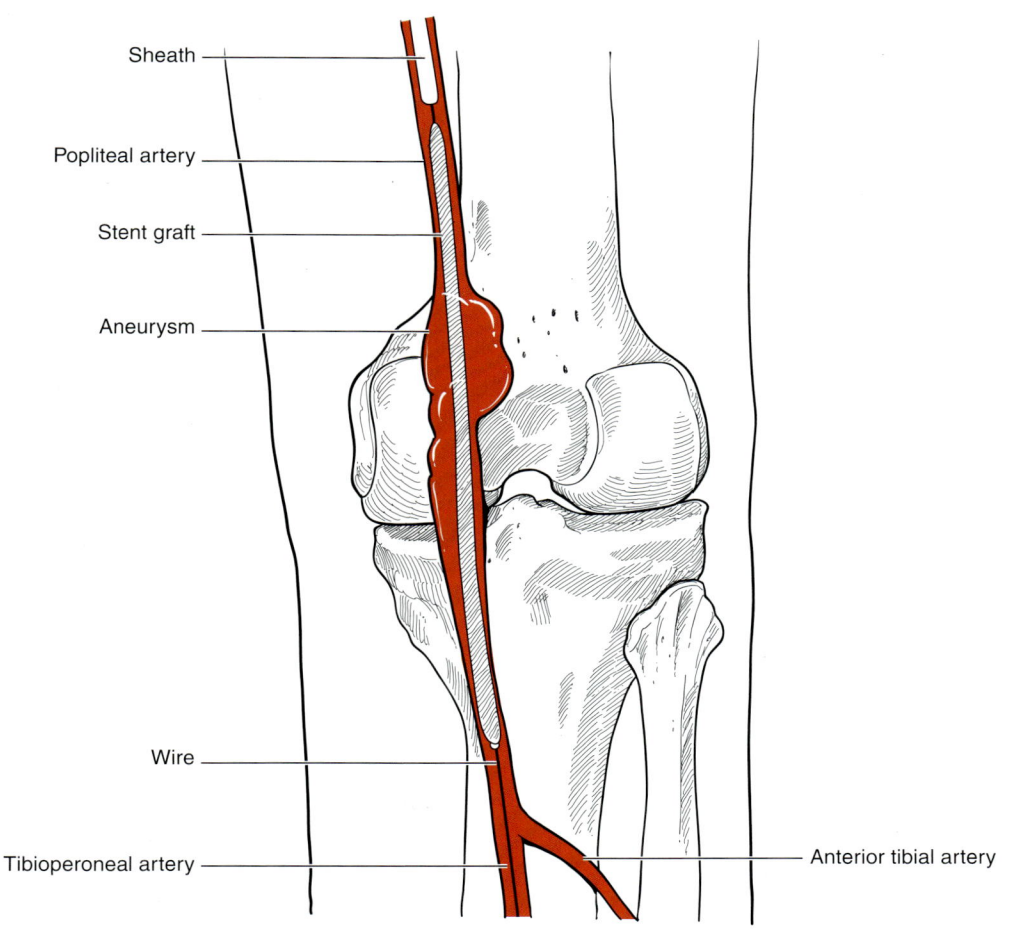

Figure 50-2. Proper positioning for stent-graft deployment. The sheath is placed above the proximal landing zone over the stiff 0.035-inch wire. A road mapping technique should be used for precise endograft deployment, and care should be taken to place the stent graft above the takeoff of the tibial and peroneal arteries.

angulation and arterial straightening through the use of stiffer guidewires is rarely required.

SHEATH PLACEMENT FOR PLANNED INTERVENTION

With the landing zone sites and diameters identified by angiography and confirmed by IVUS, the access sheath may be upsized to accommodate the diameter of the largest endograft to be deployed (Fig. 50-2). Road map imaging of the aneurysm is used to guide the sheath. The sheath can be advanced across the entire aneurysm if tortuous anatomy is thought to increase the risk of embolization with "bareback" advancement of the endograft delivery catheter.

ENDOGRAFT DEPLOYMENT

The Viabahn endoprosthesis deploys tip to hub, which facilitates accurate deployment of the distal end of the endograft. The graft should be inserted with the radiopaque markers in the proper position under angiographic visualization. The deployment suture lies along the lateral aspect of the endograft's constraining ePTFE jacket, and overly aggressive retraction of the deployment suture can bow the delivery catheter in a lateral direction. This "bowstringing" phenomenon can lead to retraction of the distal catheter tip, pulling the endograft back into the aneurysm sac at the moment of device expansion. A slow, steady pulling force on the deployment suture under continuous fluoroscopic visualization helps to avoid this complication.

After endograft deployment (Fig. 50-3), gentle balloon conformation of the landing zones and overlap regions is performed. At the proximal and distal landing zones, gentle hand inflations of a balloon equal in diameter to the endograft is performed.

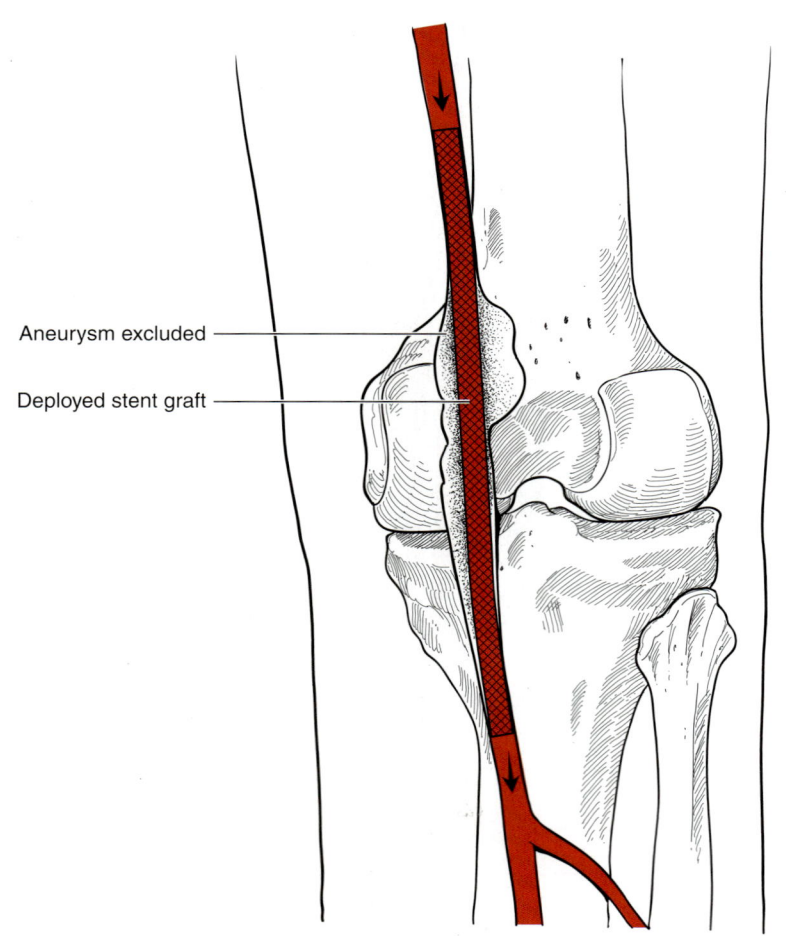

Figure 50-3. Deployed stent graft. The stent graft should have adequate seal above and below the aneurysm with at least single-vessel tibial runoff. A completion angiogram should be performed to ensure that there are no endoleaks and that embolization of mural thrombus has not occurred.

To avoid trauma to adjacent arterial segments, care is taken to keep the balloon shoulder within the endograft during inflations. At overlap zones, the balloon should be sized according to the smaller of the two endografts.

COMPLETION IMAGING STUDIES

Completion angiography is performed through the introducer sheath after removal of the endograft deployment catheter but before removal of the guidewire. Attention should be directed to the proximal and distal attachment sites to assess for the presence of a type I endoleak. If a proximal type I endoleak is noted, further proximal extension with an appropriately sized endograft may be necessary. A distal type I endoleak may be addressed with repeat balloon conformation of the landing zone or deployment of an additional endograft, provided tibial artery patency is not compromised. Images of the endograft with the knee in the flexed and extended positions can ensure that endograft patency is not compromised by normal range of motion. Distal outflow is assessed to confirm the absence of inadvertent periprocedural embolization.

Postoperative Care

- **Antiplatelet therapy.** Patients should be placed on lifelong aspirin after EVPAR. Although not supported by definitive data, the addition of clopidogrel may decrease the incidence of early graft thrombosis.[11]
- **Postoperative surveillance.** Evaluation should include history and physical examination, ankle-brachial indices, and duplex ultrasound to assess the diameter of the aneurysm sac and detect any endoleak at 1 month and annually thereafter.

Complications

- **Access site complications.** Access site complications are rare, particularly if sheath placement and arterial hemostasis are accomplished through a small surgical cutdown. Immediate postprocedural ambulation is possible and transient oral analgesics suffice for pain control.
- **Endoleak.** Type I and type III endoleaks may be noted at initial operation or at follow-up. These should be treated by endovascular methods if feasible, but surgical conversion may be necessary. Type II endoleaks may be observed in the absence of aneurysm sac growth. In the setting of a type II endoleak and aneurysm sac growth, percutaneous thrombin injection may be used to thrombose the sac.[3,12]
- **Thrombosis.** Most patients present with claudication after endograft thrombosis. The degree of ischemia dictates which salvage options are available with conversion to surgical bypass as an option. Thrombolytic therapy with endovascular salvage has been used to restore blood flow.[4,11,12]
- **Late outcomes.** Long-term primary patency after EVPAR has ranged from 70% to 83%, with secondary patency between 86% and 100%.[12,13] Limb loss after EVPAR is an uncommon event.

REFERENCES

1. Marin ML, Veith FJ, Panetta TF, et al: Transfemoral endoluminal stented graft repair of a popliteal artery aneurysm, *J Vasc Surg* 19:754-757, 1994.
2. Rosenthal D, Matsuura JH, Clark MD, et al: Popliteal artery aneurysms: Is endovascular reconstruction durable? *J Endovasc Ther* 7:394-398, 2000.
3. Curi MA, Geraghty PJ, Merino OA, et al: Mid-term outcomes of endovascular popliteal artery aneurysm repair, *J Vasc Surg* 45:505-510, 2007.
4. Mohan IV, Bray PJ, Harris JP, et al: Endovascular popliteal aneurysm repair: Are the results comparable to open surgery? *Eur J Vasc Endovasc Surg* 32:149-154, 2006.
5. Antonello M, Frigatti P, Battocchio P, et al: Open repair versus endovascular treatment for asymptomatic popliteal artery aneurysm: Results of a prospective randomized study, *J Vasc Surg* 42:185-193, 2005.
6. Gerasimidis T, Sfyroeras G, Papazoglou K, et al: Endovascular treatment of popliteal artery aneurysms, *Eur J Vasc Endovasc Surg* 26:506-511, 2003.
7. Dawson I, Sie R, van Baalen JM, et al: Asymptomatic popliteal aneurysm: Elective operation versus conservative follow-up, *Br J Surg* 81:1504-1507, 1994.
8. Whitehouse WM Jr, Wakefield TW, Graham LM, et al: Limb-threatening potential of arteriosclerotic popliteal artery aneurysms, *Surgery* 93:694-699, 1983.
9. Lowell RC, Gloviczki P, Hallett JW Jr, et al: Popliteal artery aneurysms: The risk of nonoperative management, *Ann Vasc Surg* 8:14-23, 1994.
10. Michaels JA, Galland RB: Management of asymptomatic popliteal aneurysms: The use of a Markov decision tree to determine the criteria for a conservative approach, *Eur J Vasc Surg* 7:136-143, 1993.
11. Tielliu IF, Verhoeven EL, Zeebregts CJ, et al: Endovascular treatment of popliteal artery aneurysms: Is the technique a valid alternative to open surgery? *J Cardiovasc Surg (Torino)* 48:275-279, 2007.
12. Antonello M, Frigatti P, Battocchio P, et al: Endovascular treatment of asymptomatic popliteal aneurysms: 8-year concurrent comparison with open repair, *J Cardiovasc Surg (Torino)* 48:267-274, 2007.
13. Jung E, Jim J, Rubin BG, et al: Long term outcome of endovascular popliteal artery aneurysm repair, *Ann Vasc Surg* 24:871-875, 2010.

51 Above- and Below-Knee Amputation

JOHN F. EIDT • VENKAT R. KALAPATAPU

Historical Background

The first recorded instance of amputations and prosthetic replacement appears in the Rig-Veda, written in Sanskrit between 3500 and 1800 BC.[1] The ancient Greek text, "On Joints," written in the latter half of the fifth century BC, recommends amputation for gangrene below the "boundaries of blackening" as soon as it is "fairly dead and lost its sensibility."[1,2] In the first century, Celsus described circumferential compression above the operative site, the technique of amputation through healthy tissue, and the ligation of vessels. Over the ensuing centuries, there was a return to the use of cautery to prevent hemorrhage with ligation reintroduced by Paré in the sixteenth century. The development of the Morel tourniquet in 1674 led to control of hemorrhage so that attention could be directed to the operative site. Because of a necessity for speed, amputation was initially performed in one cut, as a "classic circular cut," with detachment of skin, muscles, and bone at the same level. In 1718 Petit promoted a "two-stage circular cut" to reduce suture line tension, with initial transection the skin followed by the muscles and bone more proximally. During the seventeenth and early eighteenth centuries, Lowdham, Verduyn, and Langenbeck introduced the concept of a "flap amputation" with use of a soft-tissue flap to cover the bone without tension.[3]

Indications

The level of the amputation is selected based on the capacity for the surgical site to heal and the ambulatory potential of the patient. There is a substantially lower energy requirement for ambulation and commensurate greater likelihood to ambulate with a below-knee amputation. Thus even in the presence of marginal circulation, a below-knee amputation may be attempted. When the foot is severely infected, active cellulitis should be brought under control before performing the amputation. If necrosis and infection are severe, a guillotine amputation, 2 to 3 cm above the ankle, should be performed to remove the septic source. Several days later, a more definitive below-knee amputation is performed, with the area of the guillotine amputation carefully excluded from the operative field. Above-knee amputations are typically performed at the supracondylar level. Rarely, if the line of temperature demarcation is at the knee or higher, a midthigh or high-thigh amputation may be required.

Preoperative Preparation

- Evaluation of cardiac and pulmonary status is necessary to optimize perioperative course and rehabilitation.[4]
- Optimal nutritional status is essential for stump healing.
- Anesthesia may be general or regional based on preference and needs.
- Prophylactic antibiotics reduce perioperative wound infection rates.[5]

- Venous thromboembolism prophylaxis is mandatory.[6]
- Preoperative physiotherapy may help prevent flexion contracture.

Pitfalls and Danger Points

- Inappropriate stump length
- Stump trauma because of shear injury to the skin, subcutaneous tissue, and deep tissue
- Stump trauma because of pressure-induced necrosis from the underlying bony structure
- Stump trauma because of a tourniquet-type dressing
- Flexion contracture of the hip in above-knee amputations or the knee in below-knee amputations

Operative Strategy

The basis of selection of amputation level depends on the indication for the amputation, potential for rehabilitation after the amputation, and presence of an adequate blood supply as assessed by physical examination and vascular laboratory studies. Although not commonly performed, other studies that have been used to assess adequate perfusion include intradermal isotope blood flow measurement, skin perfusion pressure, skin fluorescence, and transcutaneous oxygen measurements. An above-knee amputation is often performed as a final level of amputation after a previous failed below-knee amputation but may be the initial amputation appropriate for patients who are unlikely to be ambulatory or those with severe ischemia or infection that precludes healing of a below-knee amputation.

Operative Technique for a Long Posterior Flap Below-Knee Amputation

SKIN INCISION

The most common technique for a below-knee amputation uses a long posterior flap.[7-9] The tibia should be divided 10 to 12 cm or approximately four fingerbreadths distal to the tibial tuberosity, but functional stumps may be achieved with as little as 5 cm of residual tibia (Fig. 51-1). The anterior skin incision extends two thirds of the circumference of the leg. A thicker posterior flap results in more prominent "dog ears" but may be better vascularized. The length of the posterior flap is approximately one third the circumference of the leg and should be gently curved to reduce dog ears. After venous exsanguination and application of the pneumatic thigh-high tourniquet, the skin and fascia are incised together beginning with the transverse component and then extending to complete the posterior flap. The anterior and lateral compartment muscles are divided.

DIVISION OF THE TIBIA AND FIBULA

The periosteum of the tibia is separated proximally for 2 cm and incised circumferentially, and the tibia is divided using a powered saw perpendicular to the long axis of the bone. The anterior lip of the tibia is beveled to eliminate sharp edges that may protrude through thin skin. The fibula is divided with a saw or bone cutter no more than 1 to 2 cm proximal to the tibia. Excessive resection of the fibula results in a conical stump that is difficult to fit with a suitable prosthesis.

CREATION OF A POSTERIOR MYOCUTANEOUS FLAP

The posterior flap is completed by dividing the residual posterior compartment musculature, the posterior tibial, flexor digitorum longus, and flexor hallucis longus muscles, at a plane just deep to the tibia and fibula with a long amputation knife. Major vascular bundles are suture ligated, and the tibial and peroneal nerves are sharply divided and allowed to retract to avoid formation of a neuroma. The tourniquet is released, and complete hemostasis is obtained. If necessary, the length and thickness of the posterior gastrocnemius-soleus flap may be tailored, but excessive attempts to eliminate dog ears should be avoided, because the stump will remodel with time. Some surgeons prefer to advance the posterior flap 3 to 4 cm proximal to the tibial osteotomy. If the posterior flap is too bulky to allow tension-free closure, the soleus muscle can be excised at the level of the tibial osteotomy, taking care to preserve the gastrocnemius muscle and fascia. The sural nerve is identified in the subcutaneous tissue in the middle

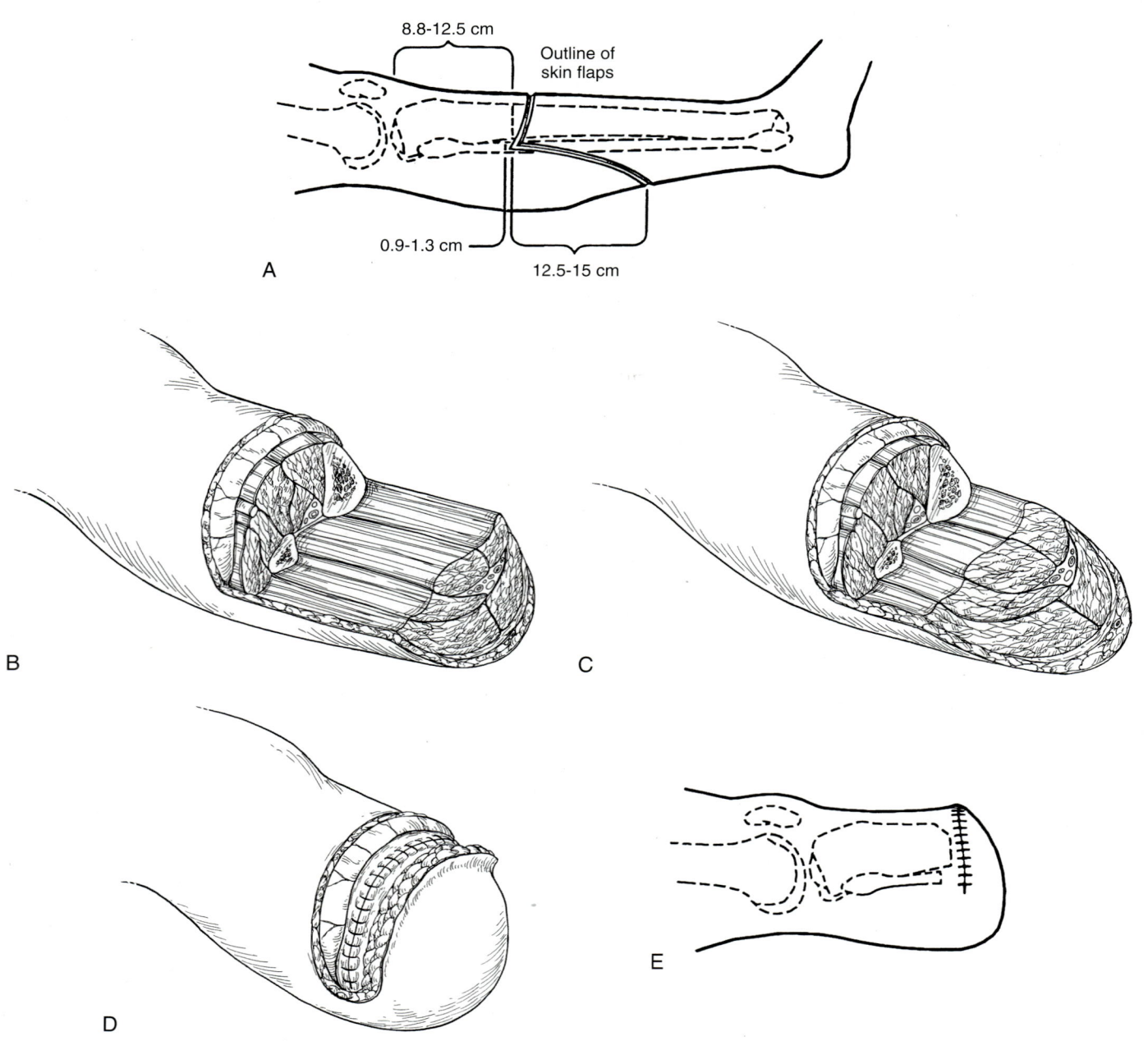

Figure 51-1. Incision and steps in the creation and closure of the posterior flap of a below-knee amputation. Note the transected tibia and fibula. **A,** The skin incision is usually placed approximately 10-12 cm distal to the tibial tuberosity. The length of the anterior transverse skin incision is approximately two-thirds of the circumference of the extremity at the site of amputation with the length of the posterior skin flap approximately one third the circumference of the extremity. **B,** The fibula is transected 1-2 cm proximal to the tibia. **C,** The soleus muscle, which derives its primary blood supply from the peroneal artery, may be resected to create a thinner posterior flap. The gastrocnemius muscle is usually supplied by arterial branches arising directly from the popliteal artery and is usually well vascularized. **D,** The fascia is closed with interrupted absorbable sutures. **E,** The posterior flap should be free of tension. It is unnecessary to remove "dog ears" at the ends of the incision because the stump will rapidly remodel in a short time. *(From Canale, ST: Campbell's operative orthopaedics, ed 10. St. Louis, 2003, Mosby, p 578, Fig. 11-2. Redrawn from Burgess EM, Zettl JH: Amputations below the knee. Artif Limbs 13:1, 1969.)*

of the posterior flap and divided 5 or 6 cm proximal to the skin edge to prevent neuroma formation.

WOUND CLOSURE

The wound is irrigated to remove bone dust. The deep fascia is approximated with interrupted absorbable sutures, taking care to cover the tibia without tension. The skin is closed with staples or monofilament suture. A bulky dressing is applied for protection, and a posterior splint is fashioned and used to prevent a flexion contracture of the knee.

Operative Technique for an Above-Knee Amputation

SKIN INCISION

A hemostatic tourniquet may be used if the femur has sufficient length. In most patients the femur can be divided at the junction between the middle and the distal thirds (Fig. 51-2). Almost any incision that results in sufficient soft-tissue coverage can be used. A transversely oriented fish mouth with equal anterior and posterior flaps is commonly used, but sagittal flaps are equally effective. Some surgeons prefer a simple, circular incision that is progressively deepened as the bone is approached. The superficial femoral artery and vein are divided and suture ligated.

DIVISION OF THE FEMUR

The femur is transected proximal to the skin incision. The edges of the transected femur are shaped with a rasp if desired. Bleeding from the bone marrow can be controlled with bone wax. The sciatic nerve is divided sharply under mild tension, ligated, and allowed to retract. The wound is irrigated. It is important to flex the patient's hip before wound closure, checking for tension on the muscle and skin. If there is tension, the femur should be further shortened.

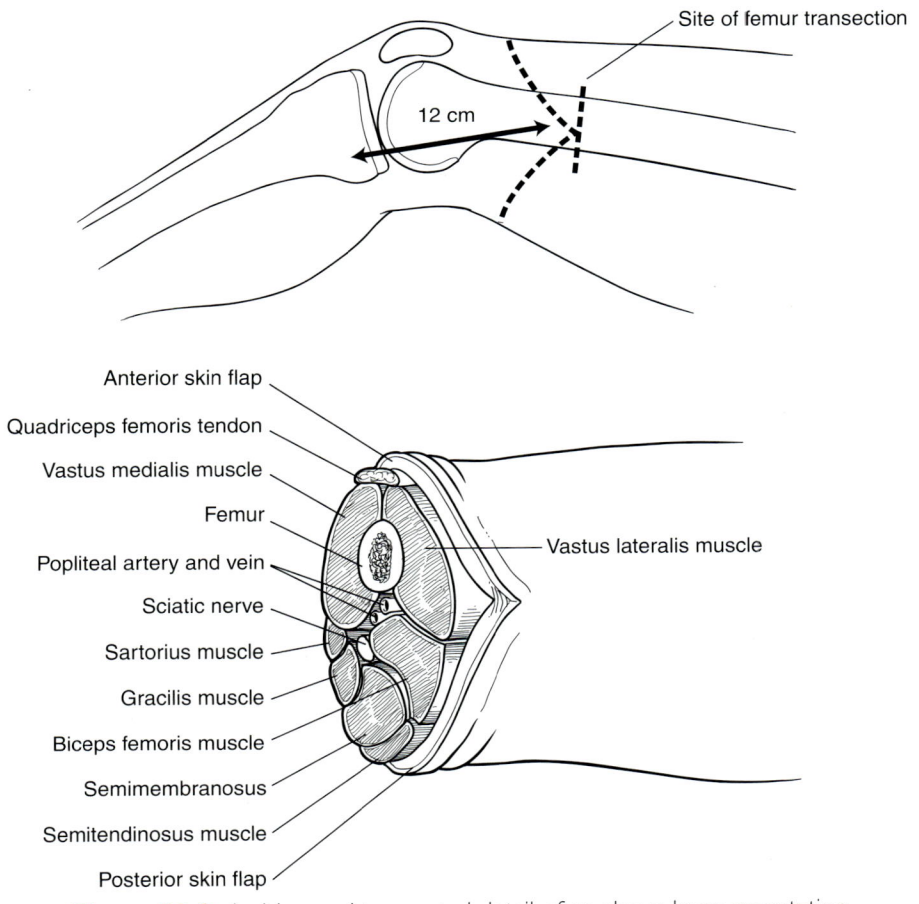

Figure 51-2. Incision and transected detail of an above-knee amputation.

WOUND CLOSURE

Some surgeons have recommended stabilization of the adductors by myopexy or myoplasty to avoid abduction and flexion of the proximal femur because of the unopposed action hip flexors. Myopexy is performed by sewing the muscles of the posterior and medial compartment to the periosteum anterolateral to the femur. Direct myoplasty of the adductor muscles involves securing the muscles by placement of nonabsorbable suture through drilled holes in the anterolateral femur. After either myoplasty or myopexy, the deep fascia is approximated with absorbable suture. The skin is closed using either staples or interrupted monofilament sutures. In elderly patients with diabetes and peripheral arterial disease, sutures or staples may be removed in approximately 4 to 6 weeks.

Postoperative Care

- **Supportive care.** Pain management and psychological support are critical to successful amputation surgery.
- **Incision site care.** A postoperative dressing protects the wound from contamination and trauma, allows easy access for wound examination, and minimizes edema without restricting arterial inflow. A soft dressing is appropriate for an above-knee amputation, but preventing fecal and urine wound contamination may be challenging. Care must be taken to avoid constrictive, circumferential dressings that impair blood flow. A simple and effective dressing consists of Vaseline gauze or nonadherent gauze on the suture line covered with a protective sheet of adhesive Ioban.
- **Prevention of knee contracture.** A rigid, removable, knee immobilizer with Velcro straps or posterior splint is used to prevent knee contracture after below-knee amputation. A foam cylinder can be cut to shape and inserted into the end of the knee immobilizer to provide additional protection to the stump. Care must be taken to avoid immobilizer pressure on the patella, which can result in skin necrosis and conversion to above-knee amputation.
- **Ambulation.** Immediate plaster dressings and early prosthetic ambulation are not recommended in patients with vascular insufficiency. Ambulation with weight bearing on the stump is progressively undertaken under the direction of a multidisciplinary rehabilitation team.
- **Edema.** After adequate wound healing, an elastic stump "shrinker" should be applied to reduce edema.

Complications

- **Hematoma.** Bleeding in the early postoperative period may result from inadequate hemostasis or from trauma to the stump. Significant hematoma should be evacuated to avoid creating a nidus for future infection.
- **Stump ischemia.** Ischemia of the amputation stump manifests coolness and pallor of the flap and continued pain. Necrosis of the skin and skin blisters are other indicators of ischemia. Stump ischemia occurs from either lack of adequate blood supply at the level of amputation or local pressure from a tourniquet-type postoperative dressing.
- **Wound infection.** Infection is more likely to occur in amputation stumps in which the indication for the procedure was infection. Other risk factors for infection include diabetes, malnutrition, malignancy, wound hematoma, and prior prosthetic grafts.[5,10] Perioperative antibiotics for skin infection and stump exploration for deeper infections should be performed as necessary. In cases of overwhelming sepsis in the foot, a transmalleolar "guillotine" amputation should precede a staged definitive transtibial amputation to minimize the likelihood of infection.

- **Knee contracture.** Inadequate early postoperative physical therapy may lead to knee contracture that impedes prosthetic rehabilitation.
- **Functional outcomes.** After transtibial amputation, approximately 20% to 30% of wounds fail to heal primarily. Of these, about 50% can be salvaged at the same level. Amputation at a higher level is necessary in 10% to 20%.[11,12] Complete healing of a transtibial amputation may be quite protracted; Nehler and colleagues reported that 100 days after the operation, only 55% were completely healed.[12] The energy required for ambulation with an above-knee amputation is approximately 50% higher than that needed after below-knee amputation. Fewer than 10% of elderly, vascular amputees ambulate effectively after transfemoral amputation.

REFERENCES

1. Duraiswami PK, Orth M, Tuli SM: 5000 years of Orthopaedics in India, *Clin Ortho* 75:269-280, 1971.
2. Vanderwerker EE Jr: A brief review of the history of amputations and prostheses, *ICIB* 15:15-16, 1976.
3. Sachs M, Bojunga J, Encke A: Historical evolution of limb amputation, *World J Surg* 23:1088-1093, 1999.
4. Aulivola B, Hile CN, Hamdan AD, et al: Major lower extremity amputation: Outcome of a modern series, *Arch Surg* 139:395-399, 2004.
5. Sadat U, Chaudhuri A, Hayes PD, et al: Five day antibiotic prophylaxis for major lower limb amputation reduces wound infection rates and the length of in-hospital stay, *Eur J Vasc Endovasc Surg* 35:75-78, 2007.
6. Burke B, Kumar R, Vickers V, et al: Deep vein thrombosis after lower limb amputation, *Am J Phys Med Rehabil* 79:145-149, 2000.
7. Allcock PA, Jain AS: Revisiting transtibial amputation with the long posterior flap, *Br J Surg* 88:683-686, 2001.
8. Burgess EM, Romano RL, Zettl JH, et al: Amputations of the leg for peripheral vascular insufficiency, *J Bone Joint Surg Am* 53:874-890, 1971.
9. Smith DG, Fergason JR: Transtibial amputations, *Clin Orthop Rel Res* 361:108-115, 1999.
10. Fisher DF Jr, Clagett GP, Fry RE: One-stage versus two-stage amputation for wet gangrene of the lower extremity: A randomized study, *J Vasc Surg* 8:428-433, 1988.
11. Dillingham TR, Pezzin LE, Shore AD: Reamputation, mortality, and health care costs among persons with dysvascular lower-limb amputations, *Arch Phys Med Rehabil* 86:480-486, 2005.
12. Nehler MR, Coll JR, Hiatt WR, et al: Functional outcome in a contemporary series of major lower extremity amputations, *J Vasc Surg* 38:7-14, 2003.

52 Amputations of the Forefoot

NICHOLAS J. BEVILACQUA • LEE C. ROGERS • GEORGE ANDROS

Historical Background

In 1946 McKittrick[1] described the use of the transmetatarsal amputation for the diabetic foot, along with specific indications including infection, ischemia, and neuropathic ulcerations of the toes and forefoot. He noted that forefoot amputation just proximal to the heads of the metatarsals, with primary closure, was practical only because of the introduction of penicillin for control of infection. The first transmetatarsal amputation was performed in 1944, and by 1946, 75 operations had been performed with preservation of ambulatory function. It was estimated that at least 10% to 15% of these patients would have undergone a major amputation before the use of this procedure.

Indications

Primary indications for a transmetatarsal amputation include gangrene of the digits, severe infection or abscess, chronic osteomyelitis, and nonhealing ulceration with prior digital amputation. Amputations of the hallux are most often indicated as a definitive procedure for an infected distal hallux ulcer complicated by osteomyelitis. If the infection spreads proximal to the metatarsophalengeal joint (MTPJ), a first ray resection is indicated.

Preoperative Preparation

- **Selection of an amputation level.** Evaluation of perfusion, residual infection, and nutritional status are determinants in operative planning and selecting the appropriate level for amputation.
- **Functional foot.** Assessment of the balance of forces in the foot while standing and ambulating is important to determine the ability to maintain a functional foot after healing.

Pitfalls and Danger Points

- Nonfunctional amputation because of muscle and tendon imbalances or inadequate preservation of the midfoot may predispose the patient to increased pressures, subsequent ulceration, and the need for a more proximal amputation.
- Excessive undermining of tissue, harsh handling of tissue, inadequate removal of nonviable or infected tissue, and poor hemostasis leading to hematoma may all contribute to necrosis of the incision.

Operative Strategy

SELECTION OF AN AMPUTATION LEVEL

Determining the level at which to amputate is not always obvious. In emergent situations appropriate debridement is essential, and the extent of infection initially dictates the level of debridement and amputation. Concerns of reconstruction and function should not discourage the surgeon from removing all infected tissue. After infection is controlled, it is important to determine the level of adequate tissue perfusion and tissue coverage of the defects. Physical examination augmented by noninvasive vascular studies, tests of tissue oxygenation or perfusion, and angiography help determine the need for vascular surgical intervention and the ultimate level of amputation healing.

The goals of a partial foot amputation are to first control infection and then perform the most distal, functional amputation. In the presence of an infection, the amputation is often performed in two stages. Certain lower-level, foot-sparing amputations are generally better tolerated and result in a more functional outcome than do higher-level amputations.

CHOICE OF ANESTHESIA

All forefoot amputations may be performed under local, regional, or general anesthesia.

Operative Technique

Proper surgical technique is paramount to reducing the risk of complications. Procedures are generally performed without a tourniquet to help determine tissue viability, because all necrotic tissue must be removed.[2] Skin incisions are made full thickness with minimal undermining. Medial and lateral incisions should be performed at the glabrous juncture between the dorsal and the plantar circulation. Dorsal and plantar incisions should be to bone, without undermining the soft tissue, to preserve arterial perfusion and thick soft-tissue coverage. Meticulous handling of the skin is essential, and a "no-touch" technique is used to prevent further injury. The area is irrigated, and deep tissue cultures are obtained using sterile, unused instrumentation as indicated.

TRANSMETATARSAL AMPUTATION

Incision

A fish-mouth incision is made proximal to all infected and nonviable tissue. The plantar skin incision extends farther distal to preserve a plantar soft-tissue flap so that the final suture line lies on the dorsal aspect of the stump (Fig. 52-1, *A*).

Transection of the Metatarsals

The metatarsals may be resected using a gigli or sagittal saw or using bone cutters. Resecting only about 20% of the metatarsal length results in maximal function, which is important to preserve the metatarsal parabola.[3] The metatarsal bone cuts are angled dorsal-distal to plantar-proximal, and the first and fifth metatarsals are beveled medially and laterally to reduce bony prominences. The first and fifth metatarsal bases are left intact to preserve the attachments of the tibialis anterior and peroneus brevis, respectively (Fig. 52-1, *B* and *C*).

Closure

The wound is irrigated, hemostasis is achieved, and the skin is approximated with interrupted nylon sutures. A bulky dressing is applied, and a posterior splint at 90 degrees may be considered to prevent an equinus contracture of the Achilles tendon.

DIGITAL OR METATARSAL RAY RESECTION

Incision

If the soft-tissue and bone infection is confined to the distal phalanx, a fish-mouth incision is planned preserving a plantar flap. If the infection involves the proximal phalanx or distal metatarsal, a racket-type incision with a plantar flap is made circumscribing the hallux and extending proximally along the medial glabrous junction.

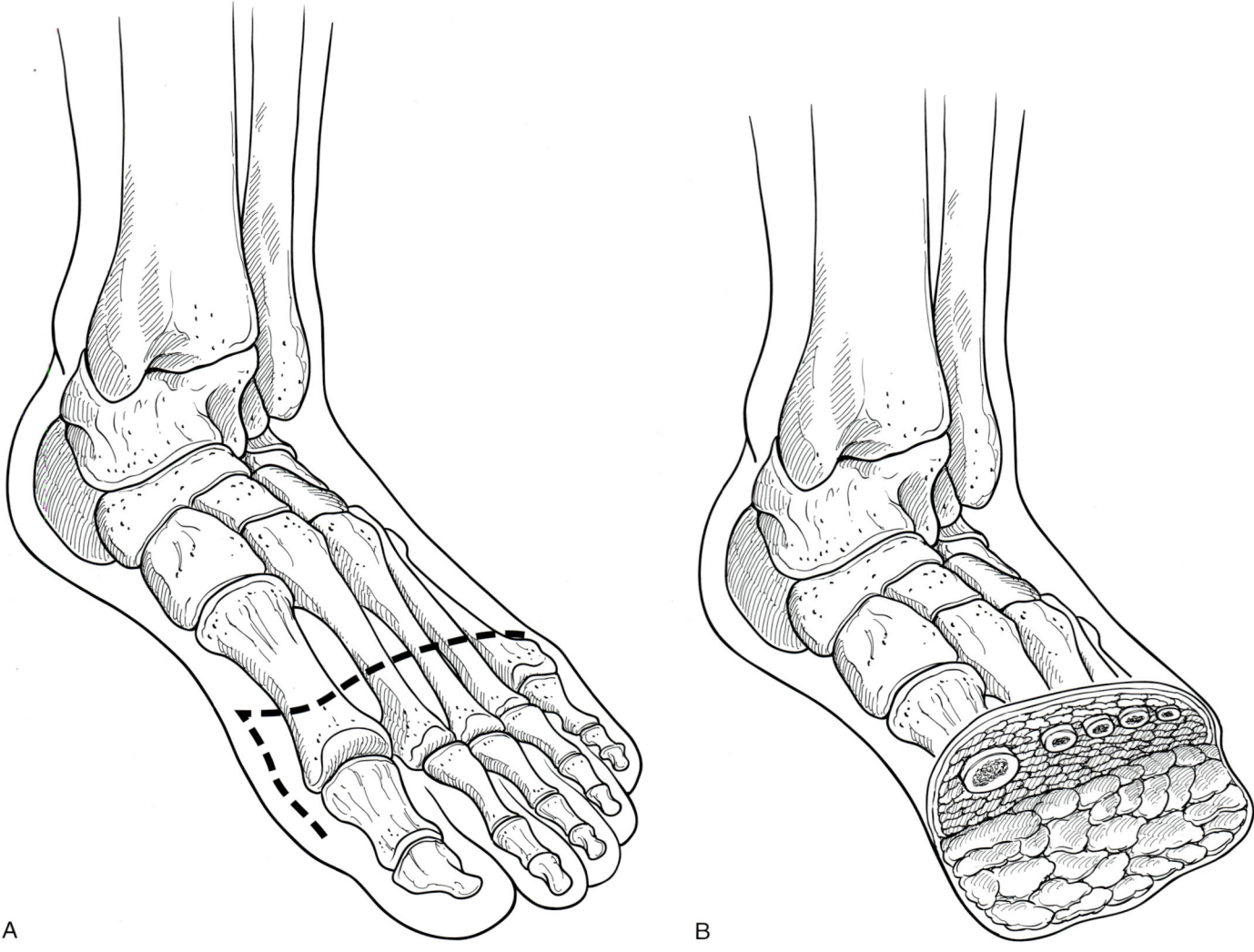

Figure 52-1. A, Appropriate incision for a transmetatarsal amputation. The incision is made proximal to all infected and necrotic tissue. **B,** The plantar skin incision is extended distal to preserve a plantar soft-tissue flap.

Transection of the Digit or Metatarsal

The hallux is disarticulated at the interphalangeal joint or MTPJ, depending on the extent of necrosis. This determines whether a digital or a metatarsal ray amputation will be performed. The resultant proximal phalanx or metatarsal bone is cut with a double-action bone cutter or sagittal saw until bleeding and normal marrow are noted. If possible, the base of the proximal phalanx is left intact to preserve the flexor mechanism and improve function. The metatarsal is cut using a sagittal saw and is ultimately angled from dorsal-distal to plantar-proximal and proximal-medial to distal-lateral to avoid resultant bone prominences (Fig. 52-2).

Central Metatarsal Ray Resection

Central metatarsal (toes 2-4) amputations often result in a deformed foot that is at risk for further breakdown.[4] Strauss and colleagues[5] described a forefoot narrowing technique later modified by Bernstein and Guerin[6] and then Bevilacqua and co-workers[4] using an external fixator for the management of cleft wounds resulting from resection of central metatarsal amputations to assist in wound closure after central ray resections (Fig. 52-3, *A* and *B*). Using fluoroscopy for guidance, the appropriately sized half-pins are percutaneously placed perpendicular into the central aspect of the distal shaft of the first and fifth metatarsals.[4] The fixator is then loosely secured approximately 2 cm above the dorsum of the foot to allow for postoperative

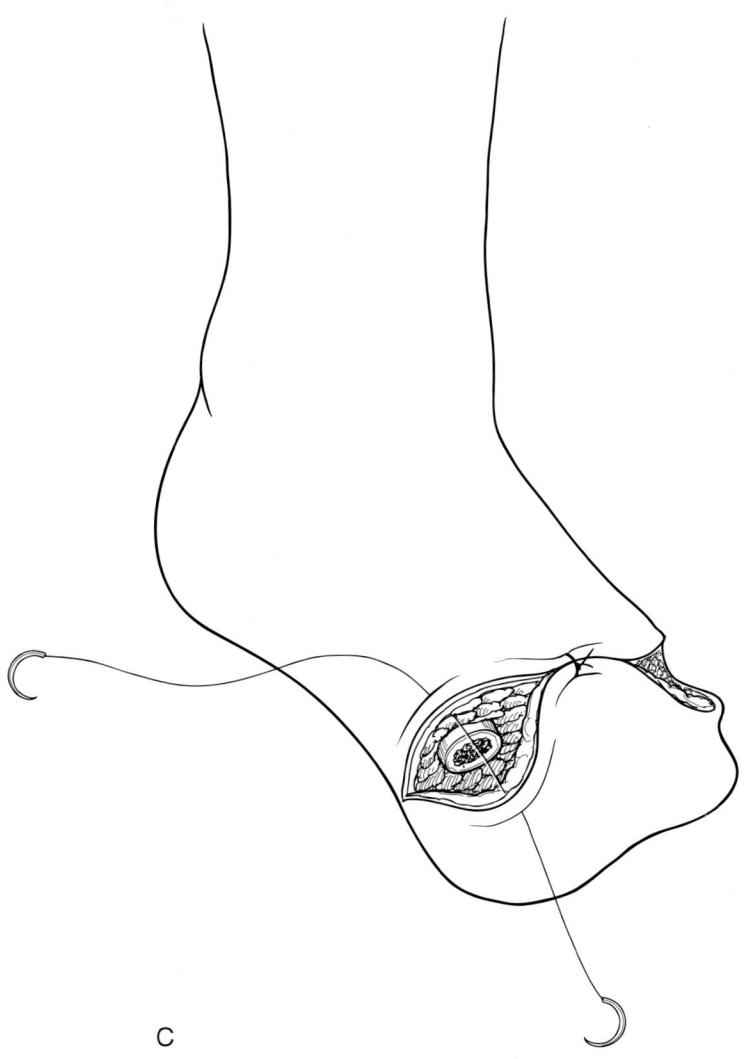

Figure 52-1, cont'd **C,** The skin incision is closed with minimal tension, and the final suture line should lie on the dorsal aspect of the stump.

swelling. The forefoot is manually compressed side to side until the plantar skin edges are apposed to facilitate primary wound closure, and the fixator is closed down to hold the position (Fig. 52-3, *C* and *D*).

Closure

The surgical site is irrigated, and hemostasis is achieved. Selective debridement of nonviable tissue is performed, and tendons within the flap are excised under traction. Soft tissue may have to be debulked to allow primary closure with minimal tension. The wound is closed, being careful to avoid dead space, and a closed suction drain may be used to reduce the risk of hematoma. Nonabsorbable sutures, skin staples, or a combination of the two can be used.

If there is concern with residual infection or if revascularization is necessary, the wound is left open until there are no signs and symptoms of infection before delayed primary closure. The wound may packed open, or a negative pressure wound therapy system may be used (see Fig. 52-2, *B*). A large, randomized, controlled trial has demonstrated that patients with diabetes and partial foot amputation have improved clinical outcomes when treated with negative pressure wound therapy.[7] The surgical site is dressed.

Metatarsal ray amputees are placed in a postoperative shoe or removable cast walker to eliminate a propulsive gait unless an external fixation device was placed. Patients should be non–weight bearing for 2 weeks and transitioned to partial weight bearing before removal of the external fixation device at 4 to 5 weeks in the

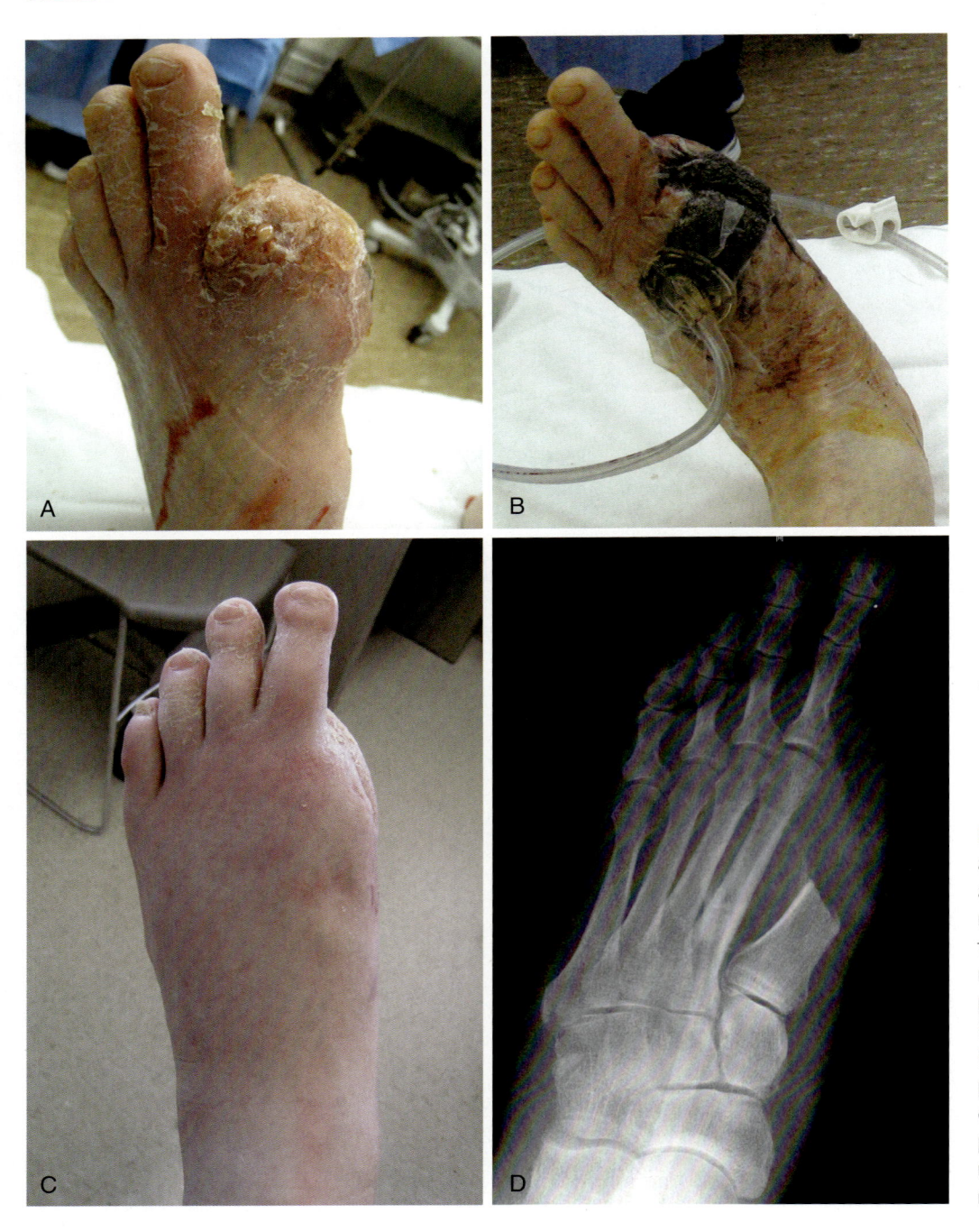

Figure 52-2. A, Ulceration and infection in a patient with a previous hallux amputation requiring a more proximal partial ray resection. **B,** First ray resection treated with negative pressure wound therapy. **C,** Healed first ray resection. **D,** Radiograph demonstrating a partial ray resection. The bone cut is angled from dorsal-distal to plantar-proximal and proximal-medial to distal-lateral to avoid resultant bone prominences.

office. Patients with a digital amputation may ambulate postoperatively and are instructed to keep the surgical site clean and dry.

If there is an equinus contracture of the Achilles tendon, consideration must be given to performing a tendo-Achilles lengthening or other soft-tissue balancing procedures at the time of initial surgery.

Postoperative Care

- In diabetic patients, sutures or skin staples are removed in 4 to 6 weeks and patients are transferred to extra-depth orthotic shoes.
- Long-term follow-up focuses on accommodating the residual foot and addressing accompanying deformities, often with a multidisciplinary team approach. Partial foot amputation often predispose the patient with diabetes to increased foot pressure and the development of a foot deformity, further placing the patient at risk for skin breakdown and subsequent amputation.[8]

AMPUTATIONS OF THE FOREFOOT 615

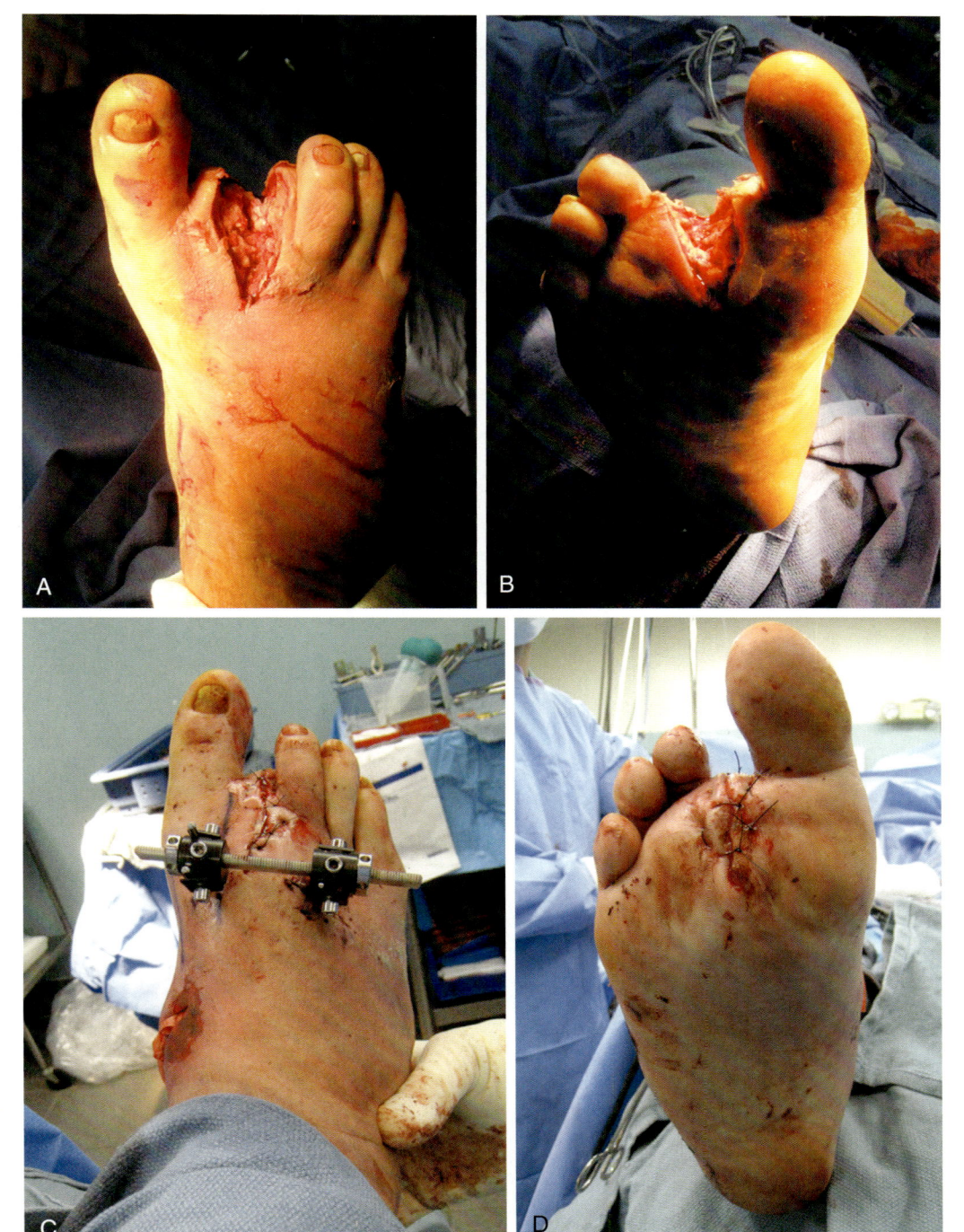

Figure 52-3. **A,** Infected bone and soft tissue resulting in a second ray resection. Full thickness skin incisions are made along the margins of the affected digit extending proximal and converging dorsal and plantar. **B,** The plantar incision extends farther proximal to incorporate the ulcer, and the digit and ulcer are removed. **C,** External fixator (minirail) is applied to the dorsum of the foot. **D,** Forefoot narrowing allows the plantar incision to be closed with minimal tension.

Complications

- **Infection.** Infection in the residual stump or amputation site can occur and should be treated aggressively to avoid further amputation.
- **Nonfunctional amputations.** Failure to address muscle and tendon imbalances predisposes the patient to increased pressure, resulting in skin breakdown and distal stump failure.

REFERENCES

1. McKittrick LS: Recent advances in the care of the surgical complications of diabetes mellitus, *N Engl J Med* 235:929-932, 1946.
2. Attinger CE, Bulan E, Blume PA: Surgical debridement: The key to successful wound healing and reconstruction, *Clin Podiatr Med Surg* 17:599-630, 2000.
3. Wallace GF, Stapleton JJ: Transmetatarsal amputations, *Clin Podiatr Med Surg* 22:365-384, 2005.

4. Bevilacqua NJ, Rogers LC, DellaCorte MP, et al: The narrowed forefoot at 1 year: An advanced approach for wound closure after central ray amputations, *Clin Podiatr Med Surg* 25:127-133, 2008.
5. Strauss MB, Bryant BJ, Hart JD: Forefoot narrowing with external fixation for problem cleft wounds, *Foot Ankle Int* 23:433-439, 2002.
6. Bernstein B, Guerin L: The use of mini external fixation in central forefoot amputations, *J Foot Ankle Surg* 44:307-310, 2005.
7. Armstrong DG, Lavery LA: Negative pressure wound after partial diabetic foot amputation: A multicentre, randomised controlled trial, *Lancet* 366:1704-1710, 2005.
8. Armstrong DG, Lavery LA, Harkless LB, et al: Amputation and reamputation of the diabetic foot, *J Amer Podiatr Med Assn* 87:255-259, 1997.

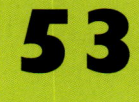

53 Upper and Lower Extremity Fasciotomy

TODD E. RASMUSSEN • JOSEPH M. WHITE

Historical Background

Fasciotomy is designed to prevent nerve injury and myonecrosis resulting from compartment syndrome characterized by elevated pressure within a fixed extremity compartment. Compartment syndrome is most often observed after reperfusion of an acutely ischemic extremity or among patients who present after severe limb trauma with associated soft-tissue and orthopedic injuries leading to elevated compartment pressures, compromised venous and arterial circulation, and direct barotrauma. In 1881 Volkmann[1] was the first to describe acute limb compartment syndrome when he noted the development of contracture as a common sequela after application of tight bandages to an extremity. The first reported treatment of compartment syndrome was described by Petersen[2] in 1888, and in 1926 Jepsen[3] was the first to demonstrate an experimental model of ischemic contracture. In 1975 Whitesides and colleagues[4] reported the development of a needle manometer to measure tissue compartment pressures as an adjunctive tool for determining the need for fasciotomy.

Indications

Fasciotomy may be performed either prophylactically in an extremity at high risk for compartment syndrome or therapeutically in the presence of an established compartment syndrome. For example, a prophylactic fasciotomy can be performed at the time of a severe crush injury or immediately after restoration of blood flow to a severely ischemic extremity. Prophylactic fasciotomy is most often performed after restoration of blood flow to an extremity that has been ischemic for 3 or more hours,[5] in the presence of concomitant major venous injury, after repair of vascular injury with associated soft-tissue or nerve injury,[6] following reduction and fixation of long bone fractures with severe crush injury, in the setting of an electrical injury, or when the mechanism of injury places a patient at high risk but serial clinical examination cannot be performed because of brain injury, the need for mechanical ventilation, or evacuation to another facility.[7]

A therapeutic fasciotomy is performed after the diagnosis of compartment syndrome is established by clinical findings or through direct measurement of compartment pressures. The clinical diagnosis of compartment syndrome may be noted in the presence of pain out of proportion to examination, paresthesias, pallor, paralysis, and poikilothermia. However, the most reliable indicator is pain, which is commonly aggravated on passive stretch of the affected muscle groups. In the lower extremity, the anterior compartment if often the first compartment to be affected. An early indicator of compartment syndrome is pain on palpation of the anterior compartment, as well as anterior compartment pain elicited on passive dorsiflexion of the ankle. Decreased sensation on the dorsum of the foot over the first web space is also consistent with compartment syndrome because of injury to the deep peroneal nerve, which courses within the anterior compartment. Paresthesias are a relatively late and ominous finding. Palpable pulses may be present in the setting of a compartment syndrome. Compartment pressures greater than 30 mm Hg or greater than 20 mm Hg below diastolic blood pressure are suggestive of compartment syndrome. Nonetheless, normal pressures in the presence of a consistent clinical examination does not reliably exclude compartment syndrome, and fasciotomy should be performed.

Preoperative Preparation

- **History and physical examination.** Acute ischemia often occurs as a result of an embolism or thrombosis in patients with multiple existing comorbidities, such as diabetes, renal insufficiency, and heart disease. A thorough history of existing medication, including oral anticoagulants, should be obtained.
- **Resuscitation.** Fluid resuscitation and alkalinization of the urine with intravenous bicarbonate should be initiated to reduce the risk of myoglobinemia-induced renal dysfunction. Patients with extremity trauma may also present with coagulopathy related to shock, anemia, or hypothermia, which should be corrected.[7,8]

Pitfalls and Danger Points

- Inadequate release extremity compartments
- Iatrogenic injury to extremity nerves and blood vessels
- Failure to implement postoperative surveillance

Operative Strategy

UNRECOGNIZED COMPARTMENT SYNDROME

The time during which nerve and muscle are exposed to elevated compartment pressures correlates with tissue damage and is eventually irreversible. A high index of suspicion or anticipation for the development of compartment syndrome should be maintained with a low threshold to perform fasciotomy. Patterns of injury prone to the development of elevated compartment pressures include venous injury, restoration of perfusion after prolonged ischemia (>3 hours), crush or soft-tissue injury, and large volume resuscitation, all of which increase extremity edema in the postinjury period.[5,9,10]

FAILURE TO RELEASE EXTREMITY COMPARTMENTS

Familiarity with limb anatomy is necessary to ensure all compartments have been adequately opened. The deep posterior and anterior compartments of the lower leg are commonly missed, potentially resulting in neurovascular compromise. The deep posterior compartment contains the posterior tibial, flexor digitorum, and flexor hallucis longus muscles, as well as the posterior tibial nerve and artery, which control plantar flexion of foot. The compartment is bound by the posterior tibia, fibula, and interosseous membrane in the proximal two thirds of the leg.

IATROGENIC INJURY

The common peroneal nerve becomes subcutaneous behind the head of the fibula, before penetrating the posterior intermuscular septum, and becomes closely opposed to the periosteum of the proximal fibula, after which it divides into superficial and deep peroneal nerves. Thus the common peroneal nerve is at risk for injury at the superior extent of the lateral fasciotomy incision, which can lead to weakness in ankle dorsiflexion or foot drop. Injury to the posterior tibial artery can occur at the inferior extent of the medial incision as the artery becomes superficial. Injury to the saphenous vein, when conducting the medial incision, can lead to bothersome bleeding in the postoperative period if unrecognized.

In the upper extremity, injury to the median nerve and its branches is most common. The anterior interosseous and palmar cutaneous branches in the arm and the recurrent branch in the hand can be injured as the volar compartment and carpal tunnel are opened. Injury to the median nerve may lead to weak pronation of the forearm, flexion, and radial deviation of wrist, as well as weakness of intrinsic hand muscles, thenar atrophy, and inability to oppose or flex the thumb. Numbness of the radial palm, thumb, index finger, middle finger, and radial aspect of the ring finger may be noted. The median nerve enters the forearm between the two heads of pronator teres, passes superficial to the flexor digitorum profundus and beneath the flexor digitorum superficialis, and runs between and deep to the flexor carpi radialis and palmaris longus into the carpal tunnel.

INADEQUATE POSTOPERATIVE SURVEILLANCE

Frequent repeat examinations of the extremity are required regardless of whether a fasciotomy has been performed. If a fasciotomy has not been performed, inspection is necessary to monitor for signs of compartment syndrome. Otherwise, the extremity should be examined after fasciotomy to assess for adequacy of perfusion, decompression, and signs of reperfusion injury. Second-look procedures are necessary to assess tissue viability, with debridement as indicated.[9,11]

Operative Technique

LOWER LEG FASCIOTOMY

The lower leg is composed of four compartments that are termed anterior, lateral, superficial posterior, and deep posterior (Fig. 53-1). The deep posterior and the anterior compartments contain the most vital neurovascular structures and are therefore the most important to release during fasciotomy. Although minimally invasive or single-incision fasciotomies have been described, the most reliable technique uses generous medial and lateral incisions.

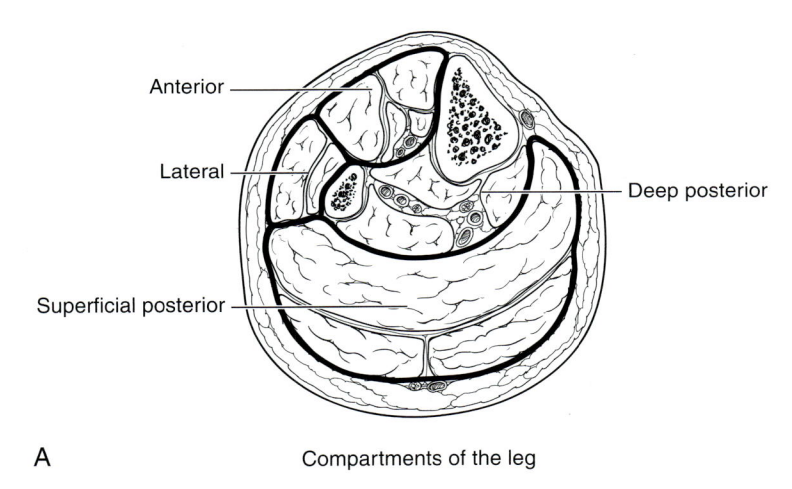

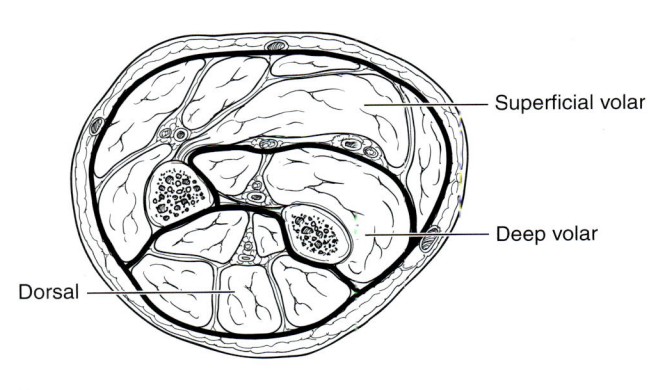

Figure 53-1. Cross-sectional anatomic representation of the leg and forearm illustrating the four compartments of the leg (**A**) and the three compartments of the arm (**B**).

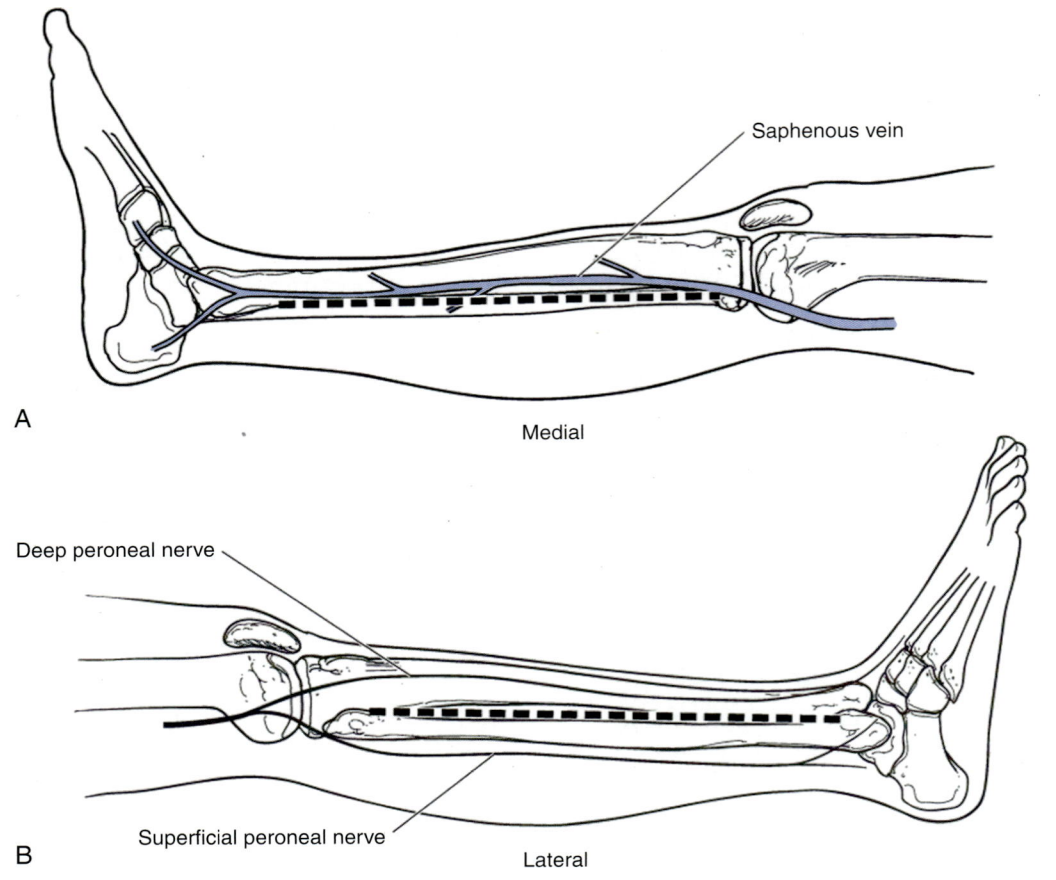

Figure 53-2. Lower extremity medial fasciotomy (**A**) and lateral fasciotomy (**B**) incision sites. For the medial fasciotomy, the saphenous vein lies nearly parallel to the skin incision and the posterior tibial artery lies in a superficial position at the distal extent of this fascial incision. For the lateral fasciotomy, the peroneal nerve is located at the superior extent of the lateral incision and fascial opening behind the head of the fibula.

Anterior Compartment

The anterior and lateral compartments of the lower leg are approached through the same lateral, longitudinal skin incision parallel to the tibia and positioned approximately 6 to 8 cm lateral to the anterior edge of the tibia (Fig. 53-2). The incision extends a distance that is one half to three quarters the distance from the lateral tibial tuberosity to the lateral malleolus. Through this skin incision, the anterior compartment is opened via a longitudinal incision of the fascia 2 cm lateral to the anterior edge of the tibia (Fig. 53-3). It is important during this step to visualize and firmly palpate the tibia under the superior or medial skin flap to verify that the anterior, not the lateral, compartment is released. The skin must be opened for an adequate length to ensure it is not hampering a full compartment release.

Lateral Compartment

The intermuscular septum between the anterior and the lateral compartments must be identified after opening of the anterior compartment (see Fig. 53-1), either by making a transverse incision in the anterior fascia or by dissecting around the anterior compartment muscles circumferentially to expose the anteromedial aspect of the lateral compartment. The lateral compartment is opened via a longitudinal incision 1 cm posterior to the intermuscular septum (Fig. 53-4). Protection of the common peroneal nerve, which lies behind the head of the fibula, is important at the superior extent of the incision while decompressing the anterior and lateral compartments.

Superficial and Deep Posterior Compartments

The superficial and deep posterior compartments of the lower leg are approached through the same medial skin incision 2 to 3 cm posterior to the medial border of the tibia (see Fig. 53-2). Like the lateral leg incision, it should be at least one half to three quarters the distance from the medial tibial tuberosity to the medial malleolus. A longitudinal opening in the fascia is created 2 to 3 cm posterior to

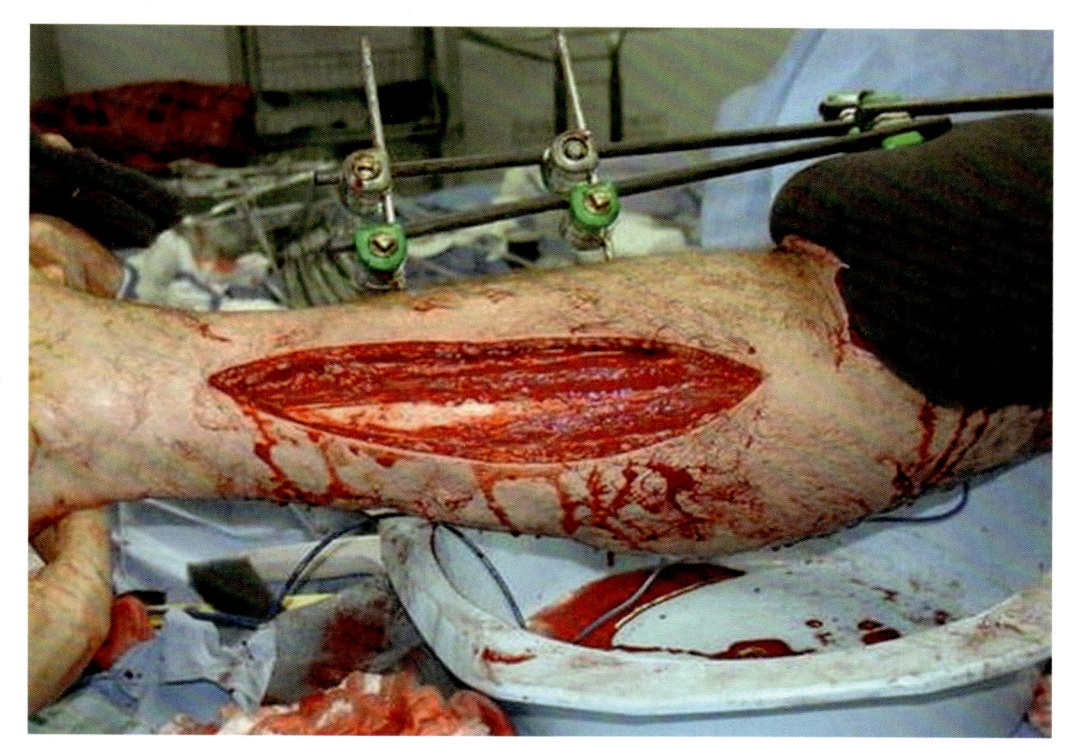

Figure 53-3. Lower extremity lateral fasciotomy incision of the leg through which the anterior compartment is opened longitudinally 2 cm posterior to the lateral edge of the tibia. The intermuscular septum dividing the anterior and the lateral compartments is identified, allowing the opening of the lateral compartment. The right (black knee cover) is proximal, and the left side is distal.

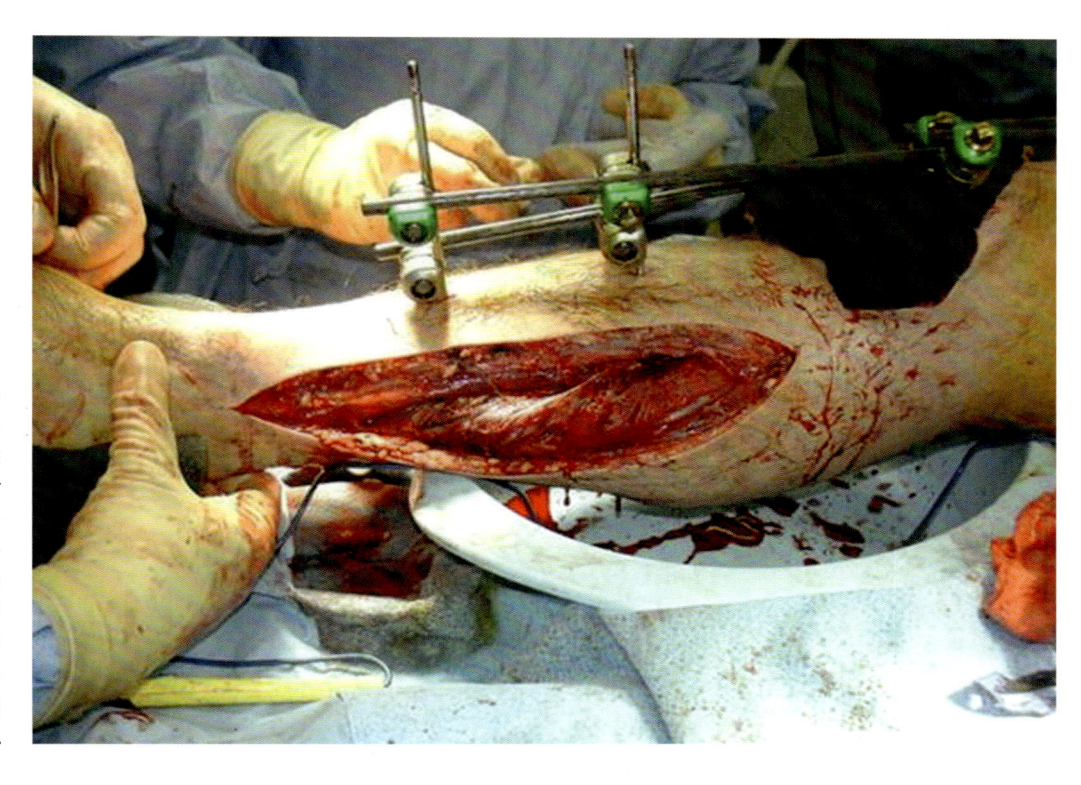

Figure 53-4. Lower extremity medial fasciotomy incision of the leg through which the superficial and deep posterior compartments are opened longitudinally. The initial compartment to be entered through the medial incision is the superficial posterior compartment, which contains no significant neurovascular structures. The right side is proximal, and the left side is distal.

the posteromedial border of the tibia, opening the superficial posterior compartment (Fig. 53-5). Opening this plane does not release the deep compartment.

Decompression of the deep posterior compartment requires detaching the soleus from the posterior edge of the tibia and the underlying interosseous membrane. This maneuver can be facilitated by elevating the upper skin flap and palpating the tibia at its confluence with the soleus fibers (Fig. 53-6). The soleus is separated from the tibia and the interosseous membrane in this location using electrocautery over a right-angled clamp. The deep posterior compartment is then opened nearly the length of the skin incision by carefully incising the interosseous fascial membrane, taking care not to injure the distal posterior tibial artery as it becomes more superficial in the lower leg.

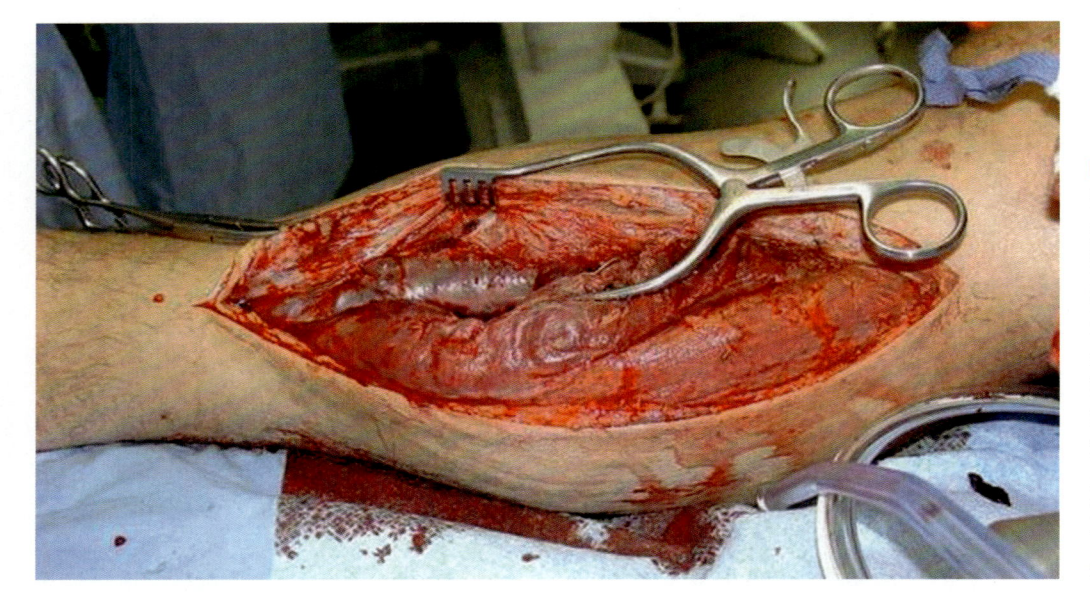

Figure 53-5. Lower extremity superficial posterior compartment fasciotomy. The initial incision is the same as the medial incision, after which a longitudinal opening in the fascia is created 2 to 3 cm posterior to the posteromedial border of the tibia. This opens the superficial posterior compartment, exposing the gastrocnemius and soleus muscles. The right side is proximal, and the left side is distal.

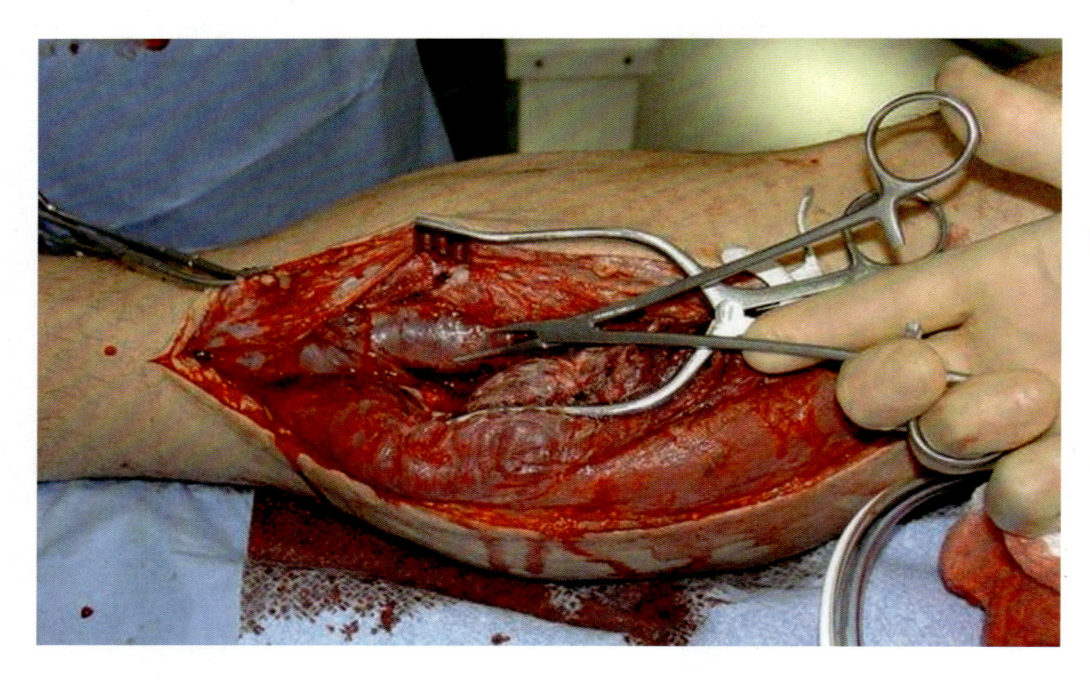

Figure 53-6. Lower extremity deep posterior compartment fasciotomy. After the superficial posterior compartment has been exposed, decompression of the deep compartment is achieved by separating the soleus from the posterior edge of the medial tibia using electrocautery over a clamp and opening the interosseous fascial membrane. The right side is proximal, and the left side is distal.

THIGH FASCIOTOMY

Anterolateral Extensor Compartment of the Thigh

An anterolateral, longitudinal incision is made along the iliotibial tract, which extends from the intertrochanteric space to lateral condyle of the femur. The vastus lateralis muscle is opened with another longitudinal incision and bluntly reflected off the intermuscular septum, releasing the anterior compartment of the thigh. Manual elevation of the anterior leaf of the fascia facilitates decompression of the remaining muscles of the quadriceps femoris group.

Posterolateral Flexor Compartment of the Thigh

The vastus lateralis is freed from its posterior attachments and retracted superomedially. The intermuscular septum, positioned lateral to the posterior flexor compartment, is then incised longitudinally to decompress the biceps femoris muscles of the posterior compartment of the thigh.

Medial Adductor Compartment of the Thigh

An anteromedial, longitudinal incision is created over the adductor-pectineus-gracilis muscle groups. Care must be taken not to injure the great saphenous vein.

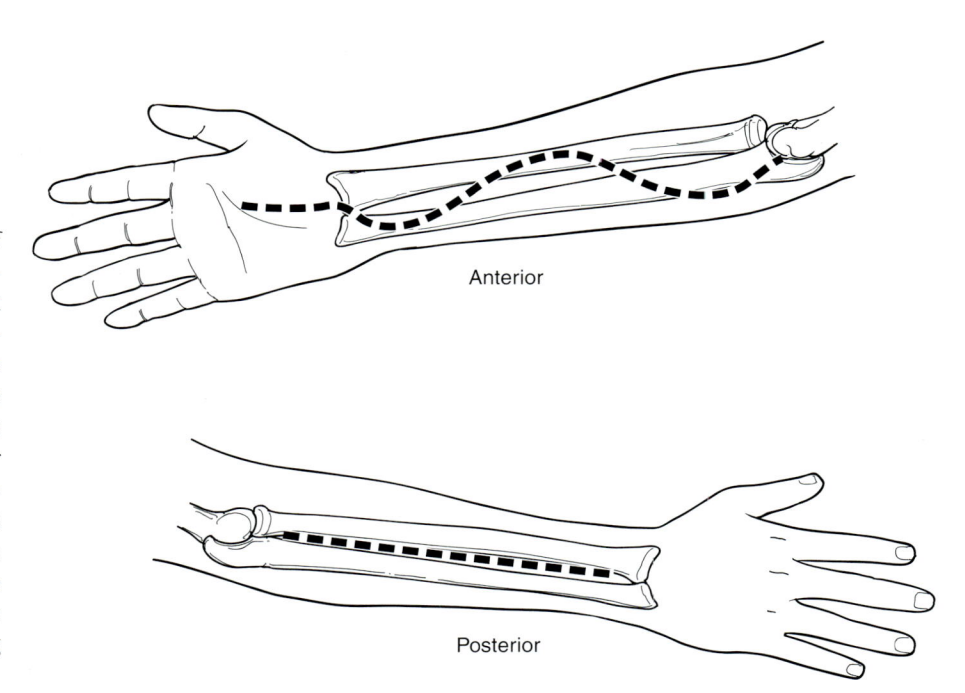

Figure 53-7. Volar fasciotomy incision of the forearm beginning at the medial epicondyle and extending across the wrist and transverse carpal ligament of the carpal tunnel onto the palmar surface of the hand. The skin and fascial incisions at the distal portion of the forearm and across the carpal tunnel are kept to the ulnar side, thereby avoiding injury to the anterior interosseous and palmar cutaneous branches of the median nerve in the arm and the recurrent branch in the hand. The dorsal fasciotomy is performed through an incision in the posterior forearm, releasing the extensor muscle compartment.

A longitudinal incision of the fascia is performed, completing the release of the medial adductor compartment.

UPPER EXTREMITY

Flexor (Superficial and Deep) and Mobile Wad Compartments of the Arm

To release the superficial volar compartment of the forearm (see Fig. 53-1), a curvilinear skin incision should be started on the ulnar aspect of the arm anterior to the medial epicondyle and proximal to the anticubital fossa (Fig. 53-7). At this location the medial antebrachial cutaneous nerve can be identified and protected near the medial epicondyle. To create a curvilinear fasciocutaneous release, the incision should be initially directed distal and radially toward the brachioradialis to open the mobile wad or lateral compartment. The mobile wad can be decompressed by elevating the medial fascial flap resulting from the fasciotomy of the superficial flexor compartment.

In the proximal one third of the forearm, the incision should be transitioned back toward the ulna and the radial aspect of the flexor carpi ulnaris tendon in the distal one third of the forearm (Fig. 53-7). Maintaining the incision and fascial opening to the ulnar side at the midforearm and distal forearm lessens the likelihood of injury to the median nerve and its branches in the arm and hand. Finally, the incision should be continued in a transverse orientation along the wrist and at the midpoint, vertically extending onto the palm crossing the carpal tunnel. Although controversial, release of the transverse carpal ligament at the carpal tunnel is generally considered necessary to fully decompress the volar compartment and median nerve. This is especially true in the setting of electrical injury.

To open the deep compartment of the arm, the space between the flexor carpi ulnaris and the flexor digitorum superficialis muscles must be identified, and the ulnar nerve and artery, which can be visualized in the deep flexor compartment, must be manually separated. A longitudinal fasciotomy of the deep compartment is performed by retracting the vessel and nerve laterally.

Extensor Compartment of the Arm

A longitudinal incision is created from the lateral epicondyle of the humerus and is extended to the distal one third of the posterior forearm. Extensor fasciotomy is performed between the extensor carpi radialis brevis and the extensor digitorum communis muscles, avoiding injury to the posterior cutaneous nerves.

Postoperative Care

- Negative pressure wound therapy with reticulated open cell foam (Vacuum Assisted Closure, Kinetic Concepts, San Antonio, Tex.) can be used to cover fasciotomy wounds. This adjunct removes fluid from the wound, decreases edema, and assists with delayed primary closure or skin grafting.[12,13] However, saline dressings can also be used.
- Patients undergoing fasciotomy require careful monitoring for 24 to 48 hours to assess for myoglobinemia and hyperkalemia that may accompany reperfusion or crush injury.[14]
- Repeat detailed examination of the extremity is required to confirm continued neurovascular integrity and viability of skeletal muscle.
- Bulky soft splinting and elevation of the upper extremity can assist in pain control but should not impair serial neurovascular examination.
- There should be a low threshold for operative evaluation of the extremity in the first 24 to 48 hours depending on the extent of injury or ischemia to evaluate muscle viability and perform debridement when necessary. Fasciotomy closure can also be initiated at this time or subsequently depending on the tissue viability and edema of the wound.[11,12]

Complications

- Myonecrosis and nerve deficit may be secondary to incomplete compartmental release.
- Systemic ischemia reperfusion or postcrush injury sequelae include lactic acidosis, hyperkalemia, myoglobinemia, and renal dysfunction.[14]
- Sepsis may occur as a result of unrecognized myonecrosis.
- The risk of wound infection is increased in the presence of chronic limb ischemia in elderly patients with medical comorbidities, such as diabetes.
- Wound complications are rare when appropriate surgical principles are combined with delayed primary closure or skin grafting.

REFERENCES

1. Volkmann R: Die ischämischen muskellähmungen und kontracturen. Centralblatt für Chirurgie, Leipzig, 8:801–803, 1881.
2. Rorabeck CH: The treatment of compartment syndromes of the leg, *J Bone Joint Surg Br* 66:93-97, 1984.
3. Jepson PN: Ischaemic contracture: Experimental study, *Ann Surg* 84:785-795, 1926.
4. Whitesides TE, Haney TC, Morimoto K, et al: Tissue pressure measurements as a determinant for need of fasciotomy, *Clin Ortho Rel Res* 113:43-51, 1975.
5. Gifford SM, Eliason JL, Clouse WD, et al: Early versus delayed restoration of flow with temporary vascular shunt reduces circulating markers of injury in a porcine model, *J Trauma* 67:259-265, 2009.
6. Fox CJ, Gillespie DL, O'Donnell SD, et al: Contemporary management of wartime vascular trauma, *J Vasc Surg* 41:638-644, 2005.
7. Rasmussen TE, Clouse WD, Jenkins DH, et al: Echelons of care and the management of wartime vascular injury: A report from the 332nd EMDG/Air Force Theater Hospital, Balad Air Base, Iraq. *Perspect Vasc Surg Endovasc Ther* 18:91-99, 2006.
8. Clouse WD, Rasmussen TE, Peck MA, et al: In-theater management of vascular injury: 2 years of the Balad Vascular Registry, *J Am Coll Surg* 204:625-632, 2007.
9. Woodward EB, Clouse WD, Eliason JL, et al: Penetrating femoropopliteal injury during modern warfare: Experience of the Balad Vascular Registry, *J Vasc Surg* 47:1259-1264, 2008.
10. Clouse WD, Rasmussen TE, Perlstein J, et al: Upper extremity vascular injury: A current in-theater wartime report from Operation Iraqi Freedom, *Ann Vasc Surg* 20:429-434, 2006.
11. Peck MA, Clouse WD, Cox MW, et al: The complete management of extremity vascular injury in a local population: A wartime report from the 332nd Expeditionary Medical Group/Air Force Theater Hospital, Balad Air Base, Iraq. *J Vasc Surg* 45:1197-1204, 2007.
12. Leininger BE, Rasmussen TE, Smith DL, et al: Experience with wound VAC and delayed primary closure of contaminated soft tissue injuries in Iraq, *J Trauma* 61:1207-1211, 2006.

13. Yang CC, Chang DS, Webb LX: Vacuum-assisted closure for fasciotomy wounds following compartment syndrome of the leg, *J Surg Orthop Adv* 15:19-23, 2006.
14. Collard CD, Gelman S: Pathophysiology, clinical manifestations, and prevention of ischemia-reperfusion injury, *Anesthesiology* 94:1133-1138, 2001.

Section II

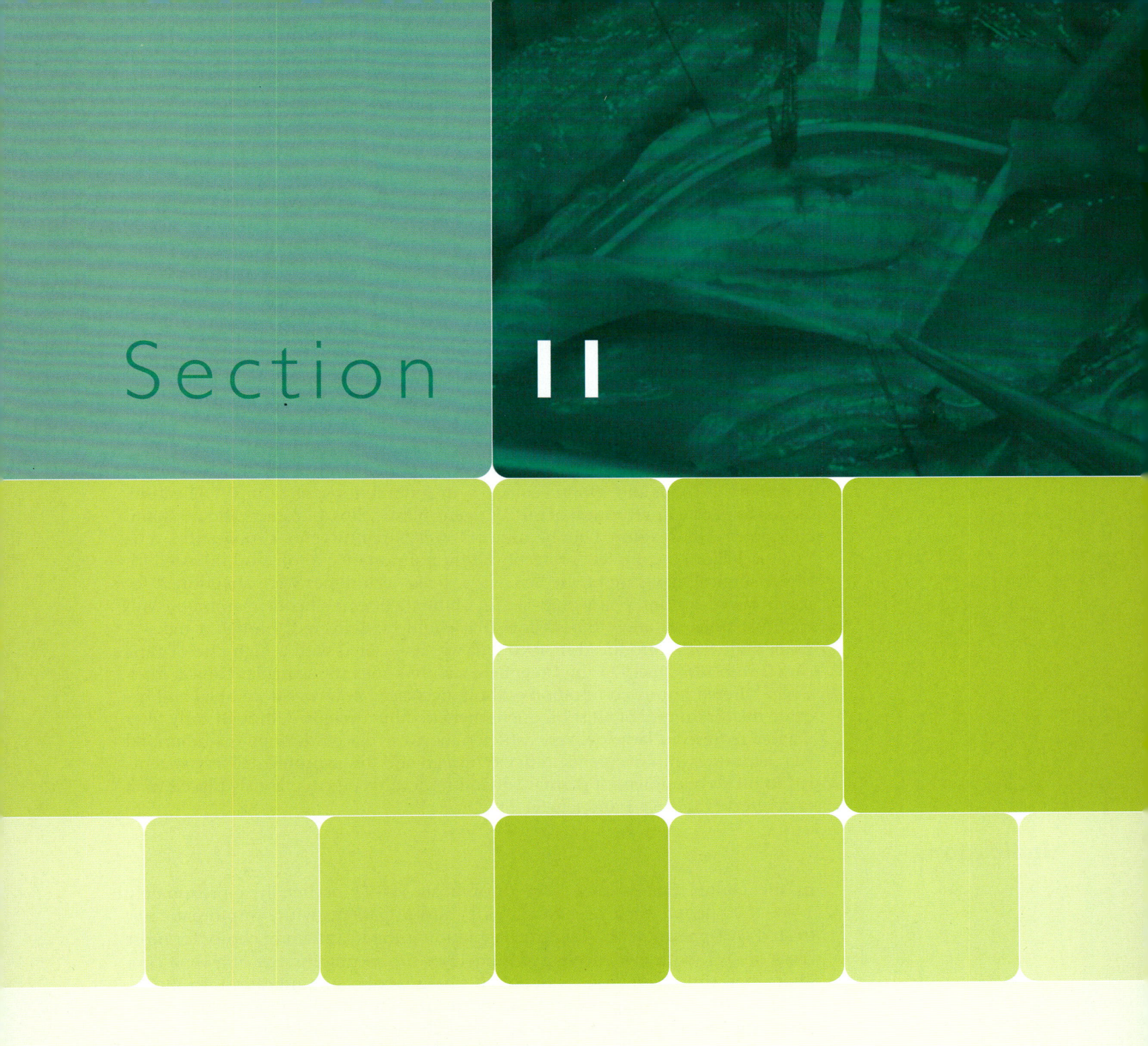

VENOUS DISEASE

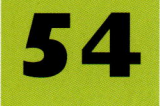

54 Placement of Vena Cava Filter

BRENTON E. QUINNEY • MARC A. PASSMAN

Historical Background

Vena cava interruption for prevention of pulmonary embolism (PE) was introduced in the 1950s and 1960s. Femoral vein and inferior vena cava (IVC) ligation, as well as partial interruption of the IVC using plastic clips, plication, and mechanical staplers, were explored but because of lower extremity venous congestion, vena cava occlusion, incomplete protection from pulmonary emboli, and the need for direct surgical exposure of the vena cava, these techniques were abandoned for less invasive options. The Mobin-Uddin umbrella filter, a silicone membrane with multiple holes to allow blood flow that could be delivered through a transvenous route, was introduced in 1967 but was associated with a high rate of vena cava thrombosis. In 1973 the Greenfield stainless-steel intravascular conical filter, which offered improved filtration without decreased flow, was developed and became the forerunner of all subsequent metallic filter designs. Although early filter devices required a large delivery catheter and were placed through open femoral vein exposure, improvements in device design and lower-profile delivery systems led to the development of permanent and retrievable percutaneously placed vena cava filters (Table 54-1 and Fig. 54-1).

Indications

In the United States, deep vein thrombosis (DVT) occurs in approximately 1 per 1000 people each year. Nearly one third of patients with symptomatic untreated DVT present with PE.[1] Anticoagulation is the treatment of choice for most cases of DVT, with evidence-based guidelines supporting the use of a vena cava filter when anticoagulation is not possible because of contraindications to anticoagulation or hemorrhagic complications, recurrent PE despite therapeutic anticoagulation, or an inability to achieve therapeutic anticoagulation.[2]

Expanded indications have been based on clinical factors that place a patient at high risk for both PE and bleeding, prohibiting use of prophylactic anticoagulation.[3] Likewise, relative indications for filter placement include poor compliance with anticoagulation, free-floating iliocaval thrombus, renal cell carcinoma with extension into the renal vein and vena cava, thrombolysis or thromboembolectomy of the iliofemoral veins or IVC, and risk of recurrent PE with preexisting pulmonary hypertension or limited cardiopulmonary reserve. Filter placement may also be considered after DVT in patients with cancer, burns, and pregnancy or for prophylaxis in multitrauma patients, including those with severe closed head injury (Glasgow Coma Scale score < 8), spinal cord injury, complex pelvic or multiple long-bone fractures, intraabdominal injury, pelvic or retroperitoneal hematoma, and ocular trauma. Contraindications to vena cava filter placement include chronic occlusion or significant compression of the vena cava or agenesis of the vena cava. The latter occurs when the right subcardinal vein fails to connect with the hepatic sinusoids during fetal development, which leads to infrahepatic interruption of the IVC segment with azygos continuation.

TABLE 54-1 Comparison of Current U.S. FDA–Approved Vena Cava Filters

Filter Device	Company	Material	Design	Access	Delivery Catheter Diameter (Fr)	Maximum Caval Diameter (mm)	Maximum Deployed Length (mm)	FDA-Approved Use
ALN optional filter	ALN	Stainless steel	Conical	Femoral/jugular/brachial	7	28	55	Optional
Option	Rex Medical Angiotech	Nitinol	Conical	Femoral/jugular	5	30	55	Optional
Eclipse	Bard Peripheral Vascular	Nitinol	Bilevel, conical	Femoral/jugular	Femoral 7 Jugular 10	28	47	Optional
G2 X filter	Bard Peripheral Vascular	Nitinol	Bilevel, conical	Femoral/jugular	Femoral 7 Jugular 10	28	47	Optional
G2 filter	Bard Peripheral Vascular	Nitinol	Bilevel, conical	Femoral/jugular	Femoral 7 Jugular 10	28	44	Optional
Simon Nitinol filter	Bard Peripheral Vascular	Nitinol	Bilevel, conical	Femoral/jugular/brachial	7	28	38	Permanent
Meridian	Bard Peripheral Vascular	Nitinol	Bilevel, conical	Femoral/jugular	Femoral 8 Jugular 10	28	47	Permanent or optional
Denali	Bard Peripheral Vascular	Nitinol	Bilevel, conical	Femoral/jugular		8.4	28	Permanent or optional
Vena Tech LP filter	B. Braun/Vena Tech	Phynox	Conical	Femoral/jugular	7	28	43	Permanent
Vena Tech LGM filter	B. Braun/Vena Tech	Phynox	Conical	Femoral/jugular	10	28	38	Permanent
Stainless-steel Greenfield	Boston Scientific	Stainless steel	Conical	Femoral/jugular	12	28	50	Permanent
Titanium Greenfield	Boston Scientific	Titanium	Conical	Femoral/jugular	12	28	50	Permanent
Bird's Nest	Cook Medical	Stainless steel	Variable	Femoral/jugular	12	40	80	Permanent
Celect	Cook Medical	Conichrome	Conical	Femoral/jugular	Femoral 8.5 Jugular 7	30	48	Optional
Günther Tulip	Cook Medical	Conichrome	Conical	Femoral/jugular	Femoral 8.5 Jugular 7	30	50	Optional
TrapEase	Cordis Corp.	Nitinol	Double basket	Femoral/jugular/brachial	6	30	50	Permanent
OPTEASE	Cordis Corp.	Nitinol	Double basket	Femoral/jugular/brachial	6	30	54	Optional
Crux Vena Cava Filter System	Crux Biomedical Inc.	Nitinol	Helical	Femoral/jugular	9	17-28	Depends on vena cava diameter	Permanent or optional
SafeFlo	Rafael Medical Technologies	Nitinol	Double-ring anchor with spiral filter element	Femoral/jugular	6	27	60	Permanent

Adapted from Endovascular Today. Welcome to the 2013 Buyer's Guide. *Endovasc Today* 2012;11:114. Available at http://bmctoday.net/evtoday/buyersguide/2013/chart.asp?id=vena_cava_filters. (Accessed October 9, 2013.)

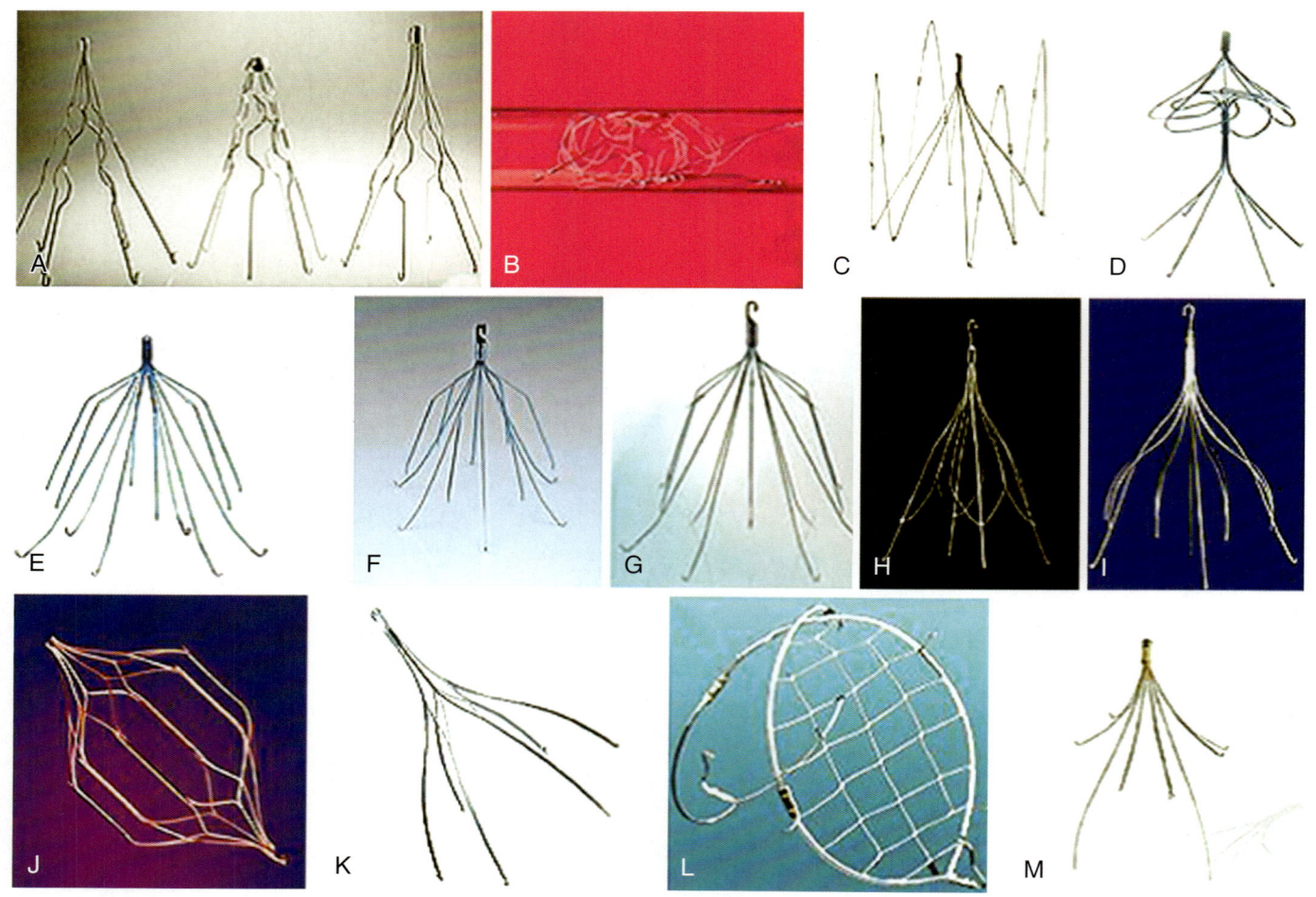

Figure 54-1. Structural design features of FDA-approved filters. **A**, From left to right, Boston Scientific titanium Greenfield filter, original stainless steel Greenfield filter, and low-profile stainless steel Greenfield filter; **B**, Cook Medical Gianturco-Roehm Bird's Nest filter; **C**, Vena Tech LP filter; **D**, Bard Peripheral Vascular/Simon Nitinol filter; **E**, Bard Peripheral Vascular Recovery G-2 filter; **F**, Bard Peripheral Vascular Eclipse filter; **G**, Bard Peripheral Vascular Meridian filter; **H**, Cook Medical Günther Tulip filter; **I**, Cook Celect filter; **J**, Cordis Corporation OPTEASE filter; **K**, Argon Medical Devices Option filter; **L**, Crux Biomedical Vena Cava Filter; **M**, ALN International Inc Optional filter. *(Photos courtesy respective manufacturers.)*

Preoperative Preparation

- A review of the indications for filter placement and hemorrhagic risk should be conducted prior to filter placement. Based on the clinical scenario, either a permanent or a retrievable filter should be selected.
- Central venous catheters that may be present at the proposed site of access or across the intended location for filter deployment should be removed.
- Coagulopathy or other hematologic issues should be assessed. Discontinuation of anticoagulation before the procedure should be considered based on clinical indication and hemorrhagic risk profile.
- Preprocedure review of duplex ultrasound or available computed tomography (CT) images should be performed to identify anatomic vena cava variants or other venous anomalies that could potentially alter the treatment plan. During filter placement, selective venography may also help to identify venous anomalies. In this regard accessory renal veins, retroaortic, and circumferential left renal vein anomalies (5%-7%) are the most common anatomic variation but do not affect filter position. Transposition of the vena cava to the left side with drainage into the left renal vein is rare (0.2%-0.5%) but necessitates accurate anatomic definition and could require a suprarenal filter. Duplication of the vena cava is also rare (0.2%-0.3%), with the right-sided IVC draining the right iliac vein and right renal vein, whereas the left-sided IVC drains the left iliac veins and joins the left renal vein where it crosses over into the right-sided vena cava. Undiagnosed duplication of the IVC may leave the duplicated vena cava

unprotected against PE and would require either separate filters in each vena cava or a suprarenal filter, above the junction of the left renal vein and the right-sided vena cava. Agenesis of the vena cava is extremely rare, but when present, filter insertion should be avoided, although filter placement into an enlarged azygous segment has been described.[4]

- A preprocedure duplex ultrasound should be obtained to evaluate the presence of venous thrombosis at the intended percutaneous access site or extending into iliofemoral or vena cava. Jugular venous access may be needed if femoral vein access is not possible. Additional imaging should be performed just before positioning and deployment of a filter to assess whether there is thrombus in the vena cava. The presence of thrombus in the infrarenal IVC may necessitate suprarenal filter placement.
- Ultrasound-guided percutaneous access is recommended to allow direct visualization of the access vein and real-time image guidance for the needle stick, as well as to avoid concomitant arterial injury.
- The diameter of the IVC, including major and minor axes, should be measured either from venography, transabdominal duplex ultrasound, intravascular ultrasound (IVUS), or a preprocedure CT scan to assist in appropriate filter selection. Vena cava diameter measurements can vary depending on intravascular fluid status and respiratory variation. Vena cava geometry can also range from circular to elliptical.[5] Both major and minor axes should be measured.
- Accurate identification of both renal and common iliac veins is important before filter deployment. The tip of the filter should be positioned below the lowest renal vein after adequate clearance of the filter base from the iliac vein confluence.
- An algorithm incorporating clinical indications, filter type, and preferred endovascular technique can be used to guide treatment (Fig. 54-2).[6]

Pitfalls and Danger Points

- **Vena cava anatomy.** Before filter placement it is best to define the vena cava diameter, the location of the iliac vein confluence and renal veins, as well as the presence of vena cava and renal vein anomalies or thrombus in the vena cava.
- **Access site thrombosis.** Ultrasonography-guided access can evaluate whether there is thrombus at the access site before puncture and also help to avoid concomitant arterial injury.
- **Limitations of imaging.** Although the third lumbar vertebral body has been used as a landmark for filter deployment, bony lumbar vertebral anatomy alone is not adequate for proper filter placement as the renal veins and the iliac vein confluence may be found at this level in 5% to 10% of patients.[7] Whether venography, transabdominal duplex ultrasound, or IVUS is used for placement, understanding the limitations of each modality is critical for accurate filter placement.
- **Filter deployment problems.** Filter tilt, crossing of filter legs, entrapment of the filter device inside the filter delivery catheter, filter migration, and vena cava penetration can occur during filter deployment. A thorough understanding of catheter-based techniques, imaging, and specific filter delivery systems is required.

Endovascular Strategy

SELECTION OF A PERMANENT OR RETRIEVABLE FILTER

Permanent filters are designed to provide lifelong filtration, with features that allow maximal fixation to the vena cava intimal surface and promote tissue ingrowth. Optional or retrievable filters are similar to permanent filters but have additional features that limit tissue ingrowth to allow removal at a later interval. If removal is not indicated or desired, these filters can function as permanent filters (Fig. 54-3).[7] Current indications for filter retrieval include patients for whom the

VENOUS DISEASE

VTE Risk Assessment

Standard Indications
- Recurrent PE despite full anticoagulation
- Proximal DVT and contraindications to full anticoagulation
- Proximal DVT and major bleeding while on full anticoagulation
- Progression of iliofemoral clot despite anticoagulation

Relative Indications
- High-risk bleeding: severe closed head injury (GCS < 8), spinal cord injury, complex pelvic fractures, multiple long-bone fractures, critical illness

AND

- Increased DVT risk: intracranial hemorrhage, solid intraabdominal organ injury, pelvic or retroperitoneal hematoma, ocular injury, medical problems (cirrhosis, ESRD, medication, coagulation)

Filter Type

Permanent Filter
- Extended anticipated risk of DVT based on injury

Optional/Retrievable Filter
- Definable end-point for retrieval

Bedside Imaging
Transabdominal US
IVUS

Bedside imaging inadequate

Standard Imaging
Venography

Bedside Placement
- Critically ill (ICU)
- Injury type and severity
- Transportation risk

Endosuite Placement
- Non-critically ill
- Venous anomalies
- Jugular access needed (bilateral leg DVT)
- IVC thrombosis
- Transportation risk acceptable

Figure 54-2. Clinical decision algorithm for vena cava filter placement options. *DVT*, Deep vein thrombosis; *ESRD*, end-stage renal disease; *GCS*, Glasgow Coma Scale; *ICU*, intensive care unit; *IVC*, inferior vena cava; *IVUS*, intravascular ultrasound; *PE*, pulmonary embolism; *US*, ultrasound; *VTE*, venous thromboembolism. *(Adapted from Killingsworth CD, Taylor SM, Patterson MA, et al: Prospective implementation of an algorithm for bedside intravascular ultrasound-guided filter placement in critically ill patients,* J Vasc Surg *51:1215-1221, 2010.)*

Filter Retrieval Should Be Considered If:
Retrievable filter type
Placement < 6 months
VTE prophylaxis indication at time of placement
Prior DVT/PE resolved
Risk of VTE currently low
Risk of bleeding low—anticoagulation possible
Ambulatory—functional status improved

Filter Retrieval Should Not Be Considered If:
Permanent filter type
Placement > 6 months
DVT/PE indication at time of placement
Risk of VTE remains high
Bleeding risk high—anticoagulation contraindicated
Non-ambulatory—immobile—functional status impaired
Spinal cord paraplegia

Venous ultrasound → (+) DVT → Leave filter as permanent

(−) DVT → Filter retrieval

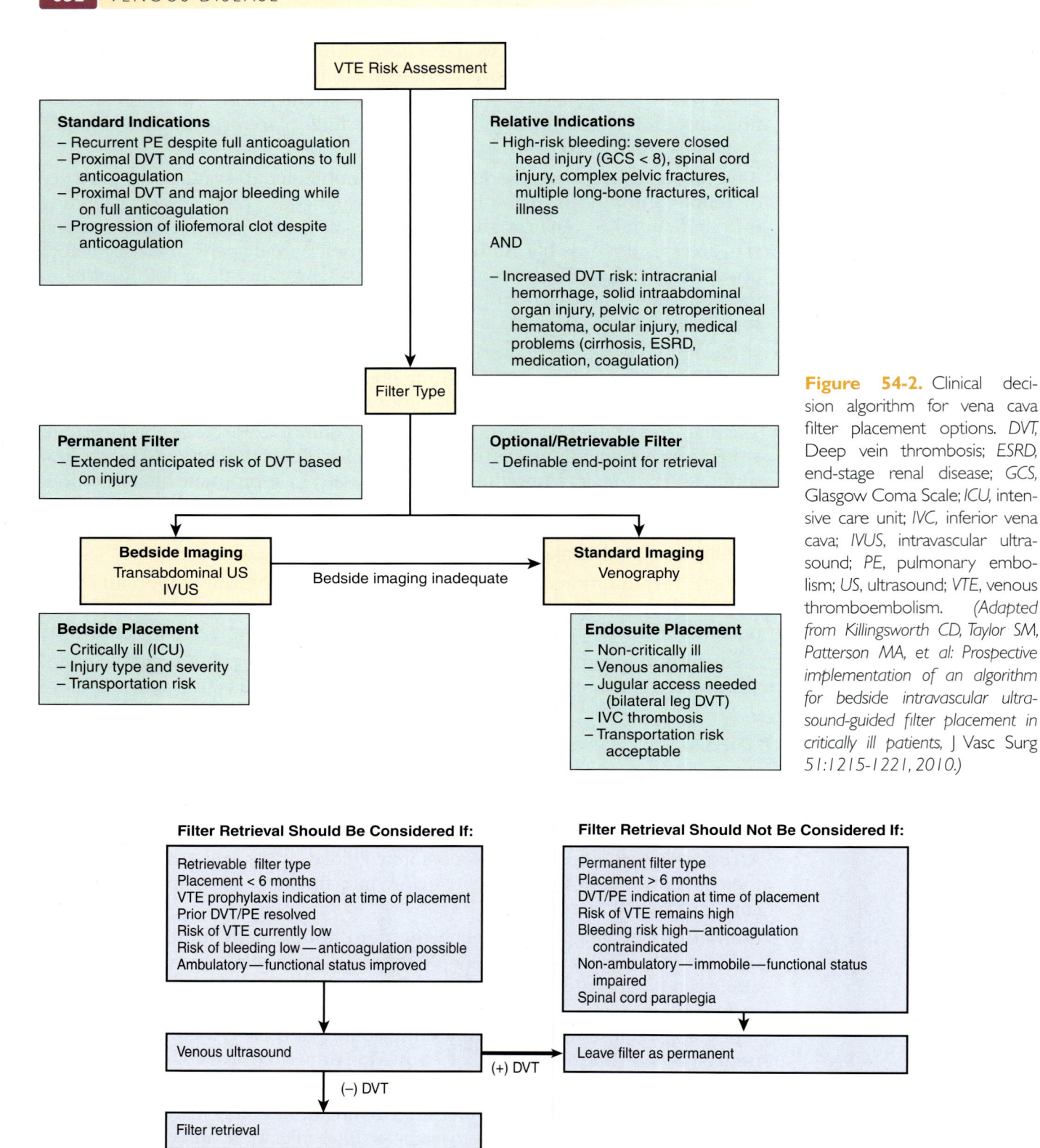

Figure 54-3. Clinical decision algorithm for filter retrieval. *DVT*, Deep vein thrombosis; *PE*, pulmonary embolism; *VTE*, venous thromboembolism.

duration of risk for PE may be limited, particularly in young multitrauma or perinatal patients, as well as morbidly obese patients undergoing bariatric or orthopedic procedures.

CONTRAST VENOGRAPHY AND ULTRASOUND IMAGING

Venography, with subsequent determination of the lowest renal vein and iliac vein confluence, assures appropriate filter position. In some instances further selective branch venography is required to delineate the anatomy if venous landmarks cannot be identified. Renal vein catheterization and imaging across the iliac confluence can aid in demonstrating aberrant anatomy, especially a duplicated caval system. A change of intended preoperative filter location may occur in up to 11% to 30% of patients after venography.[8-10]

In immobilized or critically ill patients, bedside filter placement using transabdominal or IVUS may be preferred. Transabdominal ultrasound-guided filter placement is technically feasible in 86% to 88% of patients, with success rates of 98% when visualization is adequate.[11] IVUS, which is not limited by body habitus, offers technical success rates of 96% to 99%.[12-14]

AVOIDING INADVERTENT SUPRARENAL FILTER PLACEMENT

The ideal position for filter placement is in the infrarenal IVC with the tip just caudal to the lowest renal vein (Fig. 54-4, A). Intended suprarenal filter placement may be required in the case of IVC thrombus, a malpositioned infrarenal filter, duplicate IVC, ovarian vein thrombosis, or a pregnant patient. Avoiding inadvertent suprarenal placement is important to prevent thrombus from extending into the renal veins after filter deployment. Renal veins should be identified on an initial nonselective venogram with provocative maneuvers, such as breath holding and valsalva. Additional selective branch venography may be required if the renal vein or iliac vein confluence anatomy cannot be defined. Additional imaging with IVUS can be used if venographic imaging is inadequate. Vena cava diameters exceeding 28 mm are too large for most filter designs and may require either a bird's nest filter or the placement of filter devices into both common iliac veins.

SPECIAL CONSIDERATIONS FOR THE PREGNANT PATIENT

Indications for filter placement in the pregnant patient include DVT with contraindication to anticoagulation. A suprarenal filter is preferred because of compression of the infrarenal portion of the IVC by the gravid uterus. Jugular access should be considered, and limiting radiation exposure through use of IVUS is advantageous. Contrast venography or IVUS imaging is required to confirm the level of the renal veins and the hepatic vein confluence as distal and proximal landmarks, respectively (Fig. 54-4, B). The suprarenal vena cava is usually larger than the IVC, and measurements should confirm a diameter less than 28 mm. The filter leg attachment point should be just above the most cephalad renal vein, to avoid deployment into a renal vein and filter tilt, but below the hepatic vein confluence, to avoid potential hepatic vein thrombosis. This usually positions the filter between the T11 and the L1 vertebral bodies.

Endovascular Technique

PERCUTANEOUS FILTER PLACEMENT WITH VENOGRAPHY

Percutaneous access may be obtained at the femoral, jugular, or antecubital veins. When obtaining access through the jugular vein, fluoroscopic guidance may be necessary to avoid the right atrium and guide the wire into the IVC.

Initial contrast venography is performed through the catheter or sheath to identify anatomy and confirm absence of thrombus. A marker or calibrated catheter is positioned at the confluence of the IVC and iliac veins, and a power injection of 20 mL/sec of contrast for 2 seconds should confirm normal vena cava and iliac vein relationships. The marker catheter facilitates accurate diameter measurements of the IVC. Depending on the specific filter device used, deployment sequence may vary, and understanding of the sheath and delivery catheter interactions is essential for each filter type.

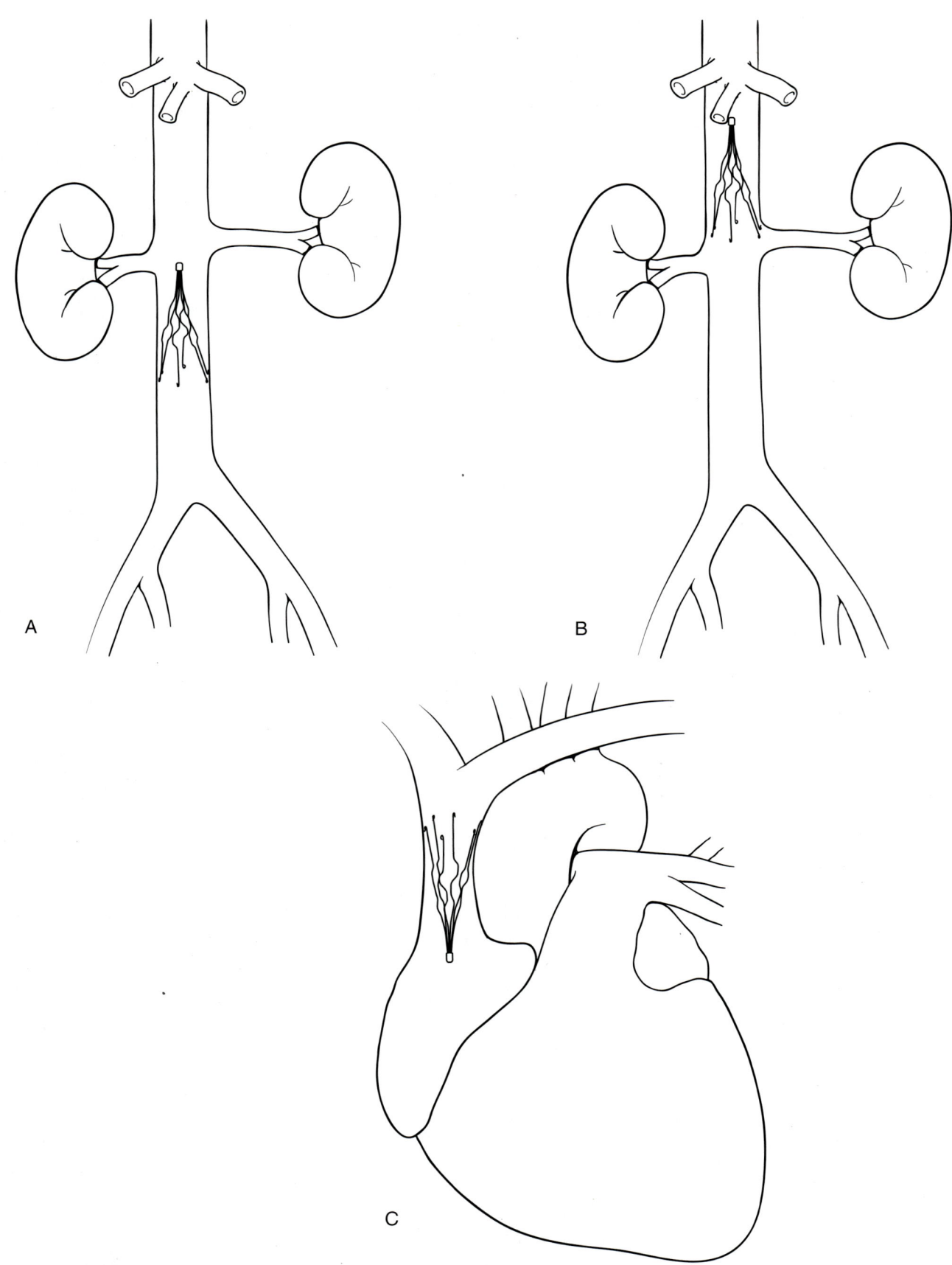

Figure 54-4. A, The infrarenal vena cava filter is positioned with the filter base above the iliac vein confluence and the filter tip at the lowest renal artery. **B,** A suprarenal vena cava filter is positioned with its base above the highest renal vein and the filter tip below the level of the hepatic veins. **C,** A superior vena cava filter is positioned with the filter base just beyond the confluence of the innominate veins and the tip proximal to the right atrium.

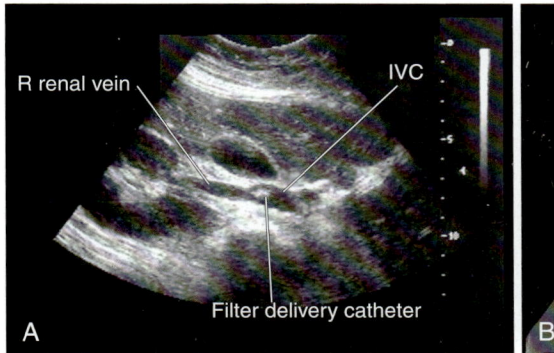

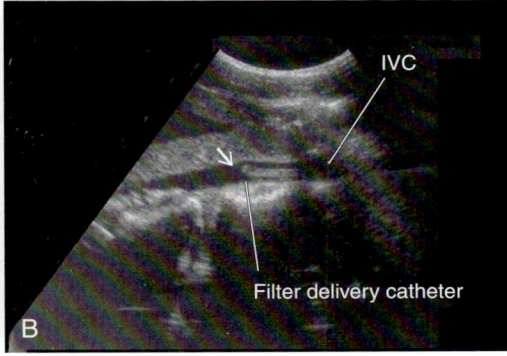

Figure 54-5. Transabdominal duplex ultrasound guidance for inferior vena cava (IVC) filter placement with visualization of the tip of the filter delivery catheter at the junction of the right renal vein and IVC in the transverse (**A**) and longitudinal (**B**) planes. *(From Passman MA, Dattilo JB, Guzman RJ, et al: Bedside placement of inferior vena cava filters by using transabdominal duplex ultrasonography and intravascular ultrasound imaging, J Vasc Surg 42:1027-1032, 2005, Fig. 2.)*

PERCUTANEOUS FILTER PLACEMENT WITH BEDSIDE TRANSABDOMINAL OR INTRAVASCULAR ULTRASOUND

For immobilized, critically ill, or intubated patients, bedside transabdominal or IVUS-guided filter placement avoids potential transportation risk. Thorough understanding of the filter delivery and imaging system is necessary before applying these advanced bedside techniques. Effectiveness of filter device visualization with transabdominal duplex ultrasound depends on profile and echogenicity of the filter system. Feasibility of filter placement with IVUS guidance with either a single- or a dual-access technique depends on sheath profile and delivery catheter interactions. Gaining initial experience is best achieved by filter placement in the endovascular suite under ultrasound guidance and real-time venographic confirmation.

FILTER PLACEMENT WITH TRANSABDOMINAL DUPLEX ULTRASOUND

Transabdominal duplex-directed filter placement requires adequate imaging of the IVC and renal veins in both the longitudinal and the transverse axis (Fig. 54-5).[14] In the transverse cross-sectional view, both renal veins should be visualized. In the longitudinal plane, the right renal vein is usually lowest and the crossing right renal artery behind the IVC can serve as an indirect marker for renal vein level.

Once percutaneous access is obtained, a guidewire is advanced into the IVC under duplex ultrasound visualization. An introducer sheath is inserted into the vena cava just beyond the renal vein level. Transverse imaging of the IVC at the level of the right renal vein is obtained, and the filter delivery catheter is advanced within the sheath to this level. The guidewire is removed, and the filter delivery catheter is slowly pulled back to allow more precise localization of the tip of the filter below the renal veins. Confirmation of position can occur by moving the filter delivery catheter in and out of view in the IVC at the renal vein level. The longitudinal view shows the filter delivery catheter in proper alignment with the vena cava and the filter deployed under direct visualization (Fig. 54-6).

Proper filter deployment is confirmed by transabdominal duplex ultrasound in both the longitudinal and the transverse planes, and an abdominal radiograph is obtained to confirm the position and full expansion of the filter.

FILTER PLACEMENT WITH INTRAVASCULAR ULTRASOUND

Intravascular Ultrasound System and Filter Choice

IVUS-guided filter placement can be accomplished using a single or dual venous access technique, which depends on the relationship between IVUS probe size and filter catheter or sheath size.[15-17] Lower-megahertz probes limited to 8-Fr or larger sheaths are required to adequately image vena cava dimensions. For the

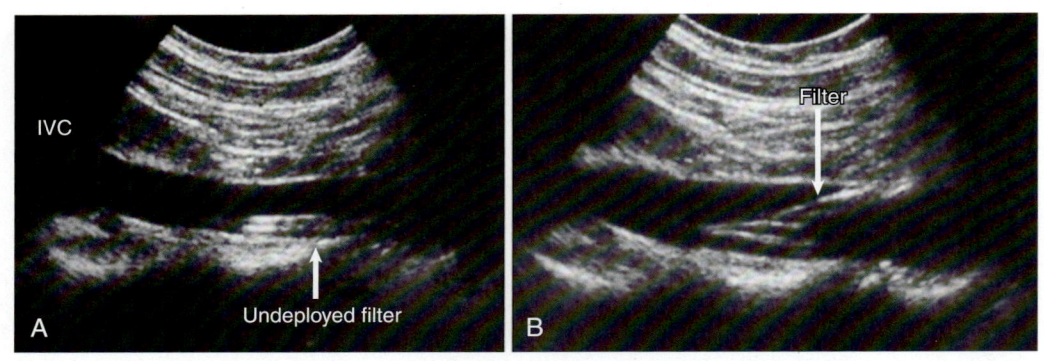

Figure 54-6. Transabdominal duplex ultrasound-guided inferior vena cava (IVC) filter placement before and after deployment. (**A,** *From Passman MA. Vena cava interruption. In: Cronenwett JL, Johnston KW, editors. Rutherford's vascular surgery, ed 7. Philadelphia, 2010, Saunders, p 827, Fig. 52-8.* **B,** *From Passman MA, Dattilo JB, Guzman RJ, et al: Bedside placement of inferior vena cava filters by using transabdominal duplex ultrasonography and intravascular ultrasound imaging,* J Vasc Surg *42:1027-1032, 2005, Fig. 3.*)

Volcano s5 or s5i system (Volcano Corp., San Diego), the company's Visions PV8.2F (8 Fr/8.3 MHz) IVUS probe is preferred over its Eagle Eye Gold (5 Fr/20 MHz) probe. In the case of Boston Scientific (Natick, Mass.) systems, the cart version of the iLab ultrasound system with Sonicath Ultra-9 (9 Fr/9 MHz) or the Atlantis PV peripheral imaging catheter (8 Fr/15 MHz) is preferred for imaging the entire vena cava and surrounding landmarks. Although IVUS probes are available that fit through smaller sheath sizes, the higher megahertz levels of these probes is inadequate to visualize the entire diameter and branch anatomy of the vena cava. Thus the IVUS-guided, single-puncture technique can only be used if the filter delivery sheath exceeds 8 Fr.

Preprocedural Imaging

After adequate local anesthesia, percutaneous femoral venous access is obtained. The IVUS probe is inserted into the sheath over the guidewire and directed into the IVC to the level of the right atrium of the heart. Using a pullback technique, the venous anatomic landmarks are sequentially identified, including the right atrium, hepatic veins, renal veins, and confluence of the iliac veins (Fig. 54-7). If the location of the iliac vein confluence is unclear, additional contralateral femoral venous access is obtained for passage of a second guidewire, allowing precise identification of the iliac confluence at the level where this second contralateral wire is visualized in the IVC. The IVUS probe is directed just below the level of the lowest renal vein, and IVC diameter measurements are made before proceeding with IVC filter deployment. The IVUS probe is then withdrawn to the iliac confluence to confirm the measured distance between the renal and iliac veins. The IVUS probe is subsequently removed with attention to the distance from the end of the IVUS probe to a finger held on the probe where it exits the sheath. This finger pinch mark helps to estimate the length of the filter delivery catheter from femoral access level to the renal vein.

Single Venous Access Technique

A single venous access technique can be used if the filter delivery kit sheath exceeds 8 Fr. Sheath exchange is performed over the guidewire, and the sheath is advanced to the predetermined level of the renal veins. The IVUS probe is used to precisely direct the end of the sheath to the level of the lowest renal vein. In this regard IVUS is guiding sheath positioning, which, because of the measured length of the different filter delivery systems, indirectly guides the intended filter position. For filter systems with predetermined marks, such as Günther Tulip and Celect filters (Cook Medical, Bloomington, Ind.), the filter delivery catheter is advanced to the mark, aligning the tip of the filter with the end of the sheath. Then the sheath is withdrawn to the second mark in a "pin-pull" fashion to allow deployment of the filter at the infrarenal level. For filter systems without

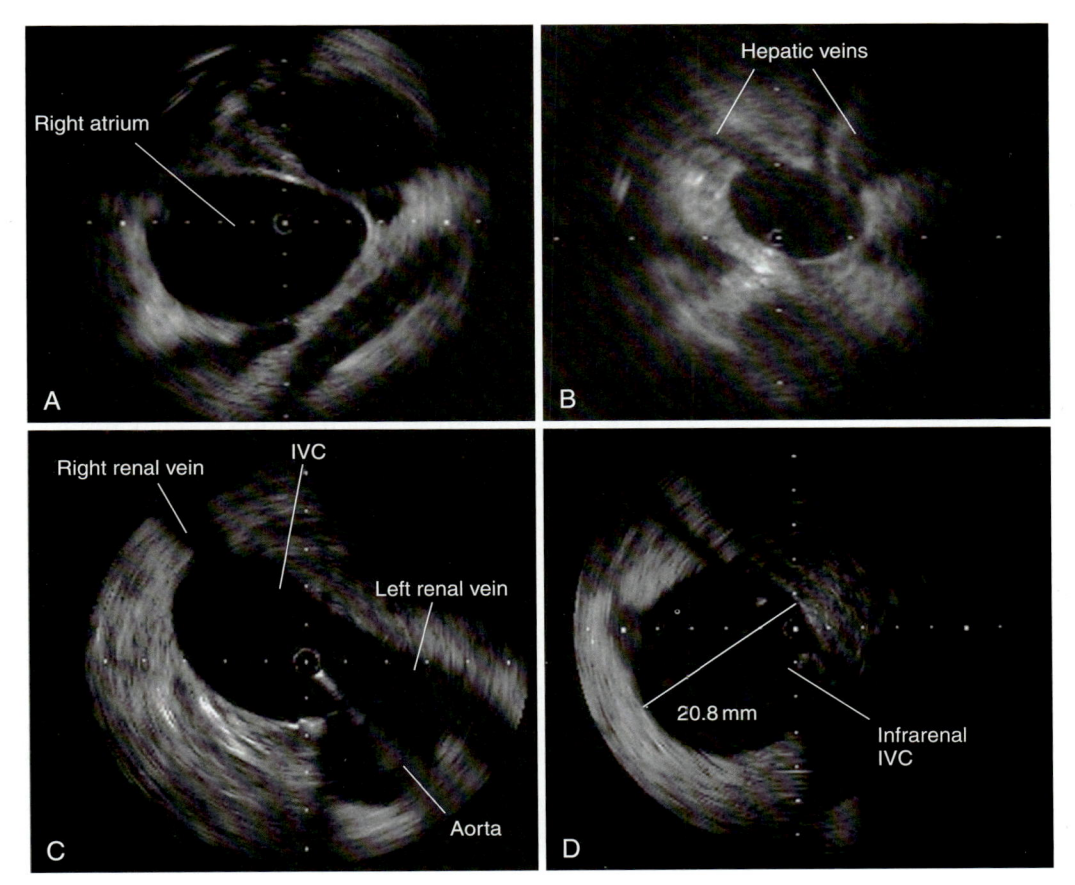

Figure 54-7. Intravascular ultrasound imaging of the inferior vena cava (IVC) identifying venous landmarks at the right atrium (**A**), hepatic veins (**B**), renal veins (**C**), and infrarenal IVC above the iliac vein confluence (**D**). *(From Passman MA, Dattilo JB, Guzman RJ, et al: Bedside placement of inferior vena cava filters by using transabdominal duplex ultrasonography and intravascular ultrasound imaging,* J Vasc Surg *42:1027-1032, 2005, Fig. 4.)*

predetermined marks, such as the Greenfield filter (Boston Scientific), the sheath is first pulled back over the intravascular probe for a distance equivalent to the length that the filter delivery catheter extends beyond the sheath. For the Greenfield filter, this distance is approximately 7 cm. Thus when the filter delivery catheter is loaded into the sheath, the tip of the filter will precisely align with the lowest renal vein upon deployment.

Dual Venous Access Technique

If filter placement is not feasible with the single-puncture technique or if a lower-profile filter system (<8 Fr) is used, a dual venous access technique is required. The IVUS probe is left at a position just below the renal veins. Separate percutaneous access is obtained preferably in the contralateral femoral vein, which allows confirmation of the iliac confluence and avoids double large sheaths in the same femoral vein. If contralateral venous thrombosis is present, the ipsilateral femoral vein adjacent to the IVUS can be used, but potential for access site thrombosis is increased. With real-time IVUS imaging, the filter delivery catheter is directed to the level of the renal veins through the additional femoral access. Once position of the filter delivery catheter tip is confirmed, the IVUS probe is pulled back and the filter is deployed. An abdominal radiograph confirms alignment and position of the filter.

PERCUTANEOUS SUPERIOR VENA CAVA FILTER PLACEMENT

Upper extremity DVT is becoming more common with the increasing use of central venous lines, pacemakers, and implantable defibrillators, with an estimated risk of PE approaching 9% in some series.[18] Standard treatment involves anticoagulation, but with contraindications or complications arising from anticoagulation, superior vena cava (SVC) filter placement may be a consideration.

Filters that are specifically designed for the SVC do not exist, and adaptation of an IVC filter and techniques is required. A conical filter with a filter leg hook attachment is most appropriately placed at the confluence of the innominate veins. Filter length should be considered to prevent protrusion into the right atrium. Filter placement in a SVC with a diameter greater than 28 mm is not recommended.

After access is achieved, a venogram is obtained to identify the innominate vein and SVC confluence and unexpected anatomic venous anomalies. Duplication of the SVC occurs in 0.1% to 0.3%. The presence of occlusion, stenosis, or thrombus in the SVC precludes filter placement. Percutaneous jugular, subclavian, or femoral venous access can be used for deployment of a filter in the SVC. However, correct orientation of the filter requires use of a jugular filter kit from the femoral position or a femoral filter set deployed from the jugular or subclavian position. The filter is deployed so that leg hooks attach at the confluence of the innominate veins and the tip extends into the SVC (see Fig. 54-4, C). A chest radiograph is obtained to confirm filter position.

RETRIEVAL OF A VENA CAVA FILTER

Optimal timing for filter retrieval remains poorly defined, with some case reports noting successful late retrieval but a higher failure rate. Until further data are available, optimal retrieval likely falls within a few months of placement but in general should occur at the earliest possible time when either anticoagulation can be restarted or venous thromboembolic risk has diminished, assuming the risk of PE or contraindication to anticoagulation no longer exists.

Before retrieval, the filter should be evaluated radiologically to detect potential technical problems that would prohibit removal. Removal is contraindicated if venography or duplex ultrasound demonstrates thrombus in the filter or if an abdominal radiograph suggests filter migration, severe tilt, fracture, or other mechanical failure.

Different filter types have different mechanisms for retrieval, but all require recapture of a caudal or cranial hook or attachment apex. Once the filter is engaged, the snared filter is retracted into an appropriately sized sheath. The filter legs should release from the vena cava wall with ease. If resistance is met or difficulty is encountered, retrieval should be aborted. A completion venogram should be obtained to confirm absence of extravasation or other evidence of vena cava injury.

Postoperative Care

- **Access site.** Initial postoperative care dictates removal of the sheath from the accessed vein and manual pressure over the puncture site for approximately 15 minutes. A pressure dressing is applied for a few hours, and then the access site is reinspected. Swelling, hematoma, or bruit would indicate the need for a groin ultrasound to rule out a pseudoaneurysm or arteriovenous fistula.
- **Postprocedural imaging.** An abdominal radiograph is obtained after filter placement to document the position of the filter. The tip should reside between the L1 and the L2 vertebral bodies, but bony vertebral level can vary in relation to renal vein position. Filter tilt should be less than 15 degrees. Tilt greater than 15 degrees suggests filter malpositioning in the iliac vein or migration of the filter tip into a renal or gonadal vein.

Complications

- Reported technical success rates for a properly positioned filter range between 98% and 100%. Early complications involve access site hematoma, ecchymosis, arteriovenous fistulae, or maldeployment of the filter. Late complications include vena cava thrombosis, pulmonary embolus, access site thrombosis, migration, tilt, and leg penetration through the wall of the vena cava.[19,20] Although most filters types are roughly equivalent in prevention of PE, there is some variation in complication rates among devices.[21-25]

- **Vena cava thrombosis (6%-30%).** Filter design and shape may have some impact on propensity for vena cava thrombosis. Conical filter designs seem to have less flow impedance compared with nonconical designs. In a conical design, filling of the filter with thrombus occurs centrally while blood flows peripherally, which may help to maintain vena cava patency.
- **Venous access site thrombosis (2%-28%).** Factors contributing to access site thrombosis may include larger filter delivery catheter and sheath size, multiple venous access attempts, extended postprocedure puncture site pressure, and clotting tendency.
- **Filter malpositioning and misplacement (1%-10%).** Filter tilt exceeding 15 degrees may decrease filtration efficiency and lead to pulmonary emboli or vena cava occlusion.[26] Inadvertent misplacement of the filter in the suprarenal vena cava can lead to renal vein thrombosis, and deployment in the iliac vein can contribute to iliofemoral venous thrombosis.
- **Filter leg or hook penetration (9%-24%).** Filter leg or hook penetration through the vena cava wall is fairly common and is usually asymptomatic. Filter design features such as recurved hooks, thickened J hooks, and longitudinal filter struts have decreased but not eliminated the risk of penetration. Occasional erosion into the aorta, duodenum, small bowel, colon, ureter, and adjacent vertebral body has been described and, if associated with pseudoaneurysm or infection, may necessitate operative filter removal.
- **Filter migration (2%-5%).** Filters can migrate to a more distal vena cava segment or to the heart and can be associated with severe cardiopulmonary compromise and death. Migration is usually the result of inappropriate sizing, deployment over a thrombus with inadequate attachment to the wall of the vena cava, or dislodgement when catheters or guidewires becoming entangled within the filter struts.
- **Filter fracture (<1%).** Filters made from nitinol tend to be more prone to material fatigue and fracture, with an attendant risk of migration.
- **Guidewire entrapment (<1%).** Entrapment of guidewires, central venous catheters, or other intravascular devices has been reported.
- **PE and death.** Nonfatal PE (2%-5%), fatal PE (0.7%), and deaths linked to filter insertion (0.12%) are rare.

REFERENCES

1. Office of the Surgeon General and National Heart, Lung, and Blood Institute, editor: The surgeon general's call to action to prevent deep vein thrombosis and pulmonary embolism. U.S. Department of Health and Human Services 2008. Available at http://www.surgeongeneral.gov/topics/deepvein. (Accessed April 28, 2010.)
2. Kearon C, Kahn SR, Agnelli G, et al: Antithrombotic therapy for venous thromboembolic disease: American College of Chest Physicians evidence-based clinical practice guidelines, *Chest* 133:454S-545S, 2008.
3. Rogers FB, Cipolle MD, Velmahos G, et al: Practice management guidelines for the prevention of venous thromboembolism in trauma patients: The EAST Practice Management Guidelines Work Group, *J Trauma* 53:142-164, 2002.
4. Tanju S, Dusunceli E, Sancak T: Placement of an inferior vena cava filter in a patient with azygos continuation complicated by pulmonary embolism, *Cardiovasc Intervent Radiol* 29:681-684, 2006.
5. Murphy EH, Arko FR, Trimmer CK, et al: Volume associated dynamic geometry and spatial orientation of the inferior vena cava, *J Vasc Surg* 50:835-842, 2009.
6. Killingsworth CD, Taylor SM, Patterson MA, et al: Prospective implementation of an algorithm for bedside intravascular ultrasound-guided filter placement in critically ill patients, *J Vasc Surg* 51:1215-1221, 2010.
7. Danetz JS, McLafferty RB, Ayerdi J et al: Selective venography versus nonselective venography before vena cava filter placement: Evidence for more, not less. *J Vasc Surg* 38:928-934, 2003.
8. Hicks ME, Malden ES, Vesely TM, et al: Prospective anatomic study of the inferior vena cava and renal veins: Comparison of selective renal venography with cavography and relevance in filter placement, *J Vasc Interv Radiol* 6:721-729, 1995.

9. Martin KD, Kempczinski RF, Fowl RJ: Are routine inferior vena cavograms necessary before Greenfield filter placement? *Surgery* 106:647-650, 1989.
10. Mejia EA, Saroyan RM, Balkin PW, et al: Analysis of inferior venacavography before Greenfield filter placement, *Ann Vasc Surg* 3:232-235, 1989.
11. Conners M, Becker S, Guzman R, et al: Duplex scan-directed placement of inferior vena cava filters: A five year institutional experience, *J Vasc Surg* 35:286-291, 2002.
12. Garrett J, Passman MA, Guzman RJ, et al: Expanding options for bedside placement of inferior vena cava filters with intravascular ultrasound when trans-abdominal duplex ultrasound imaging is inadequate, *Ann Vasc Surg* 18:329-334, 2004.
13. Oppat WF, Chiou AC, Matsumura JS: Intravascular ultrasound-guided vena cava filter placement, *J Endovasc Surg* 6:285-287, 1999.
14. Passman MA, Dattilo JB, Guzman RJ, et al: Bedside placement of inferior vena cava filters by using transabdominal duplex ultrasonography and intravascular ultrasound imaging, *J Vasc Surg* 42:1027-1032, 2005.
15. Jacobs DL, Motaganahalli RL, Peterson BG: Bedside vena cava filter placement with intravascular ultrasound: A simple, accurate, single venous access method, *J Vasc Surg* 46:1284-1286, 2007.
16. Wellons ED, Rosenthal D, Shuler FW, et al: Real-time intravascular ultrasound-guided placement of a removable inferior vena cava filter, *J Trauma* 57:20-25, 2004.
17. Rosenthal D, Wellons ED, Levitt AB, et al: Role of prophylactic temporary inferior vena cava filters placed at the ICU: Bedside under intravascular ultrasound guidance in patients with multiple trauma, *J Vasc Surg* 40:958-964, 2004.
18. Munoz FJ, Mismetti P, Poggio R, et al: Clinical outcome of patients with upper-extremity deep vein thrombosis: Results from the RIETE Registry, *Chest* 133:143-148, 2008.
19. Ballew KA, Philbrick JT, Becker DM: Vena cava filter devices, *Clin Chest Med* 16:295-305, 1995.
20. Ray CE Jr, Kaufman JA: Complications of inferior vena cava filters, *Abdom Imaging* 21:368-374, 1996.
21. Becker DM, Philbrick JT, Selby JB, et al: Inferior vena cava filters: Indications, safety, effectiveness, *Arch Intern Med* 152:1985-1992, 1992.
22. Greenfield LJ, Rutherford RB: Participants in the Vena Caval Filter Consensus Conference. Recommended reporting standards for vena caval filter placement and patient followup, *J Vasc Surg* 30:573-579, 1999.
23. Streiff MB: Vena caval filters: A comprehensive review, *Blood* 95:3669-3677, 2000.
24. Young T, Tang H, Aukes J, et al: Vena caval filters for the prevention of pulmonary embolism, *Cochrane Database of Systematic Reviews* 2007, 4:CD006212; DOI:10.1002/14651858.CD006212.pub3.
25. Hann CL, Streiff MB: The role of vena caval filters in the management of venous thromboembolism, *Blood Reviews* 19:179-202, 2005.
26. Kinney TB, Rose SC, Weingarten KE, et al: IVC filter tilt and asymmetry: Comparison of the over-the-wire stainless-steel and titanium Greenfield IVC filters, *J Vasc Interv Radiol* 8:1029-1037, 1997.

55 Surgical Reconstruction for Superior Vena Cava Syndrome

PETER GLOVICZKI • MANJU KALRA

Historical Background

In 1757 Hunter[1] was the first to describe a patient with compression of the superior vena cava (SVC) by a large syphilitic aortic aneurysm leading to thrombosis. In 1954 Schechter[2] reported a series of 400 patients with SVC syndrome of which 75% were due to malignant neoplasm, predominantly primary lung tumors.

Initial descriptions of surgical reconstruction of the SVC using polytetrafluoroethylene (PTFE), Dacron, or autologous conduits were published in the 1970s.[3-5] Gladstone and colleagues[6] were the first to report venous decompression using a segment of autogenous femoral vein, and Doty[7,8] reported successful long-term treatment of SVC syndrome with autogenous spiral vein grafts in 1982.

Indications

Surgical treatment is considered for symptomatic patients with benign disease if endovascular treatment is not appropriate because of the extent of venous occlusion or if attempted endovascular treatment is unsuccessful or subsequently fails. Surgical reconstruction in the presence of malignant disease is indicated when curative tumor resection is possible.

Although tuberculosis and syphilitic mediastinitis or aortitis were frequently noted causes of SVC syndrome in the 19th century, lung cancer with metastatic mediastinal lymphadenopathy and primary mediastinal malignancies are now the most common etiologies of SVC syndrome.[9] The most frequent primary mediastinal malignancies causing SVC syndrome include mediastinal lymphoma, medullary or follicular carcinoma of the thyroid, thymoma, teratoma, angiosarcoma, and synovial cell carcinoma. Non–small cell lung cancer is responsible for half of all SVC syndromes, whereas small cell lung cancer, lymphoma, metastatic cancer, germ cell tumors, and thymoma cause the remainder. Although mediastinal fibrosis, most frequently caused by histoplasmosis, was the most frequent cause of benign SVC syndrome in earlier studies, thrombosis because of central lines and pacemaker wires is now the most frequent cause of benign SVC syndrome.[10,11] SVC syndrome occurs with an estimated prevalence ranging from 1:40,000 to 1:250 people after pacemaker insertion after a mean interval of approximately 48 months.[12] The risk of SVC syndrome is also increased in patients with previous radiation to the mediastinum and in those with thrombophilia.

Preoperative Preparation

- **Signs and symptoms.** Upper body venous congestion is suggested by the presence of swelling, bluish discoloration of the skin, and dilated veins of the head,

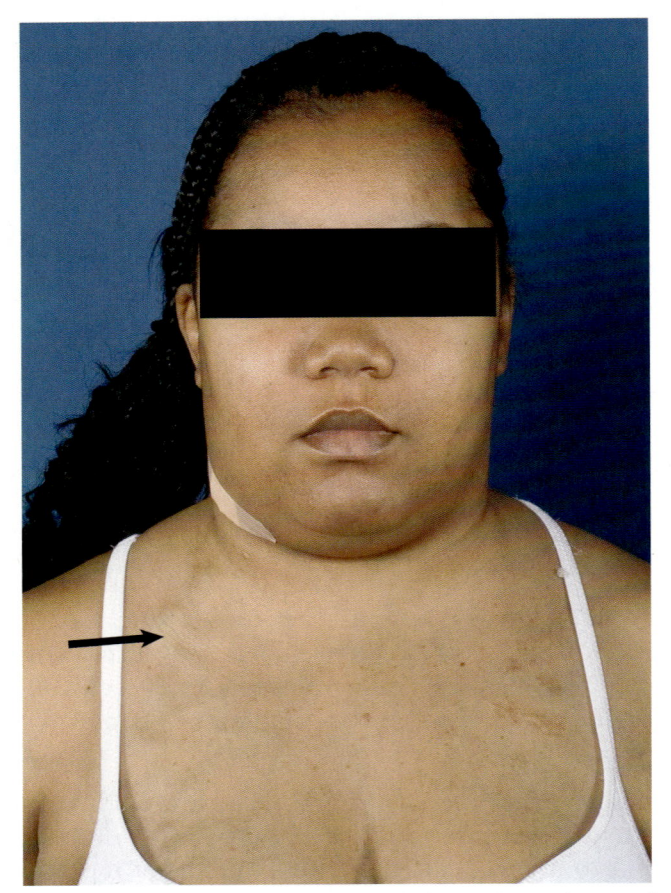

Figure 55-1. Physical signs of SVC syndrome. Arrow indicates large chest wall venous collaterals.

neck, upper chest, and less frequently, upper extremities (Fig. 55-1). Complaints include a sense of fullness in the head, headaches, and visual symptoms, which worsen when bending over, as well as dyspnea and dizziness. Sleeping on several pillows because of orthopnea when lying flat is common.[10] Signs and symptoms of malignancy, such as weight loss, lethargy, fever, night sweats, and palpable lymph nodes, in addition to hemoptysis, hoarseness, or dysphagia, may be present.

- **Imaging studies.** Preoperative chest radiography, computed tomography (CT) or magnetic resonance angiography is recommended to evaluate for the presence of benign or malignant disease, as well as to assess the extent of SVC occlusion, to determine the presence of venous collaterals, and to classify the severity of SVC syndrome.[10] Duplex scanning of jugular veins may be helpful for endovascular treatment planning. If the SVC is not adequately visualized by CT (Fig. 55-2) or magnetic resonance imaging, conventional venography should be performed.

- **Nonoperative measures.** A measure of symptomatic relief may be obtained by using pillows to keep the head elevated when sleeping and by avoiding bending over or constrictive garments.

- **Acute SVC syndrome.** Management of acute SVC syndrome includes anticoagulation with administration diuretics to decrease, at least temporarily, edema of the head and neck. Catheter-directed thrombolysis with or without stenting may be considered, followed by intravenous unfractionated or subcutaneous low-molecular-weight heparin and warfarin to prevent recurrence.

- **SVC syndrome secondary to malignancy.** Chemotherapy, radiation therapy, or a combination of both may be used based on tumor histology for patients who have SVC syndrome because of mediastinal malignancy. The tumor shrinks and symptoms resolve in 80% of patients, with the remaining patients considered for endovascular treatment.

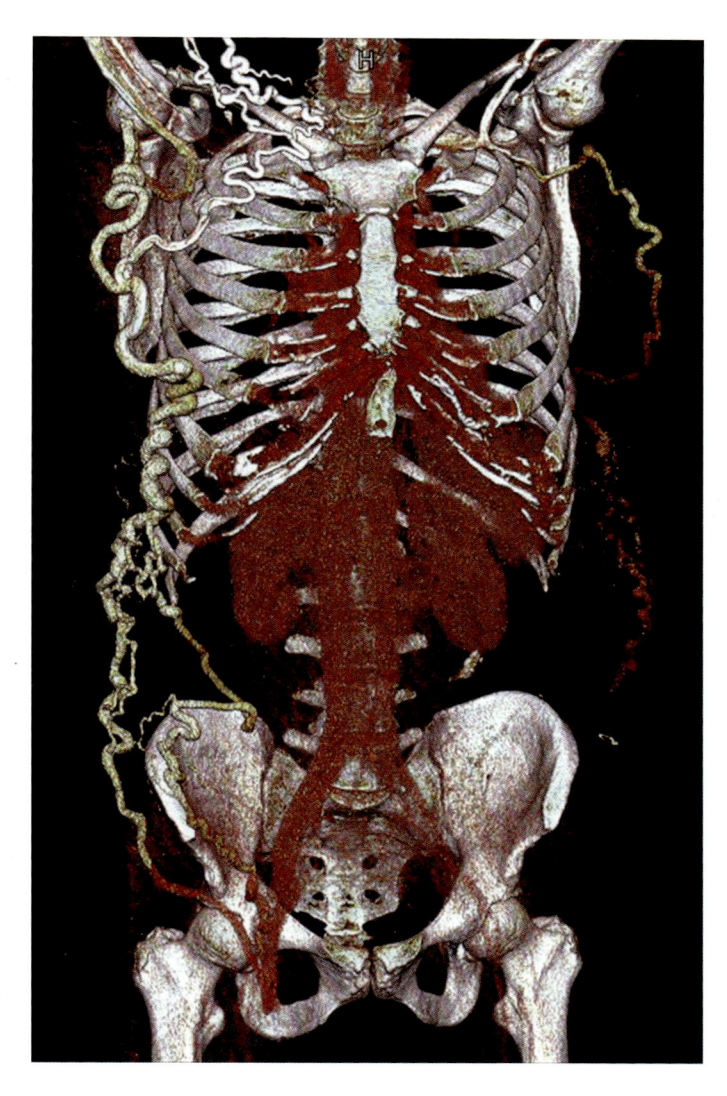

Figure 55-2. CT angiogram of a patient with SVC syndrome. Axillary and chest wall venous collaterals are present as a consequence of extensive central venous occlusion.

Pitfalls and Danger Points

- **Bleeding complications.** Bleeding can be excessive during the course of incising skin and subcutaneous tissue, as well as median sternotomy, because of extensive venous collaterals and elevated venous pressure.
- **Graft thrombosis.** Patency grafts in the venous system are inferior because of low venous pressure, especially in patients with a network of collateral circulation, and poor inflow because of extensive venous occlusion. The frequent presence of thrombophilia may also contribute to graft failure, as well as delayed graft stenosis because of intimal hyperplasia or external compression.

Operative Strategy

AVOIDING INTRAOPERATIVE BLEEDING

Preoperative oral anticoagulation must be stopped at least 5 days before open surgical reconstruction. If bridging with subcutaneous low-molecular-weight heparin is needed, the last dose should be given at least 12 hours before surgical incision. Careful planning, thorough hemostasis, and rapid autotransfusion of blood products are helpful to decrease bleeding and correct blood loss. Finally, collaboration with thoracic or cardiac surgeons may be required in the presence of mediastinal malignancy, in redo median sternotomy, or in placement of the central venous anastomosis at the right atrium, as well as if a concomitant cardiac procedure is required.

TABLE 55-1 Surgical Repair for Superior Vena Cava Syndrome

Type of Repair	No. Patients	%
Autologous vein graft	28	67
Spiral saphenous vein	22	52
Straight grafts	19	43
Bifurcated grafts	2	5
Straight graft + innominate vein reimplantation	1	2
Femoral vein	6	14
Iliocaval allograft	1	2
Externally supported PTFE graft	13	31
Total	42	100

From Rizvi AZ, Kalra M, Bjarnason H, et al: Benign superior vena cava syndrome: Stenting is now the first line of treatment, *J Vasc Surg* 47:372-380, 2008.

AVOIDING PULMONARY EMBOLISM

Careful flushing of the graft to remove thrombus or air before reestablishing venous circulation is mandatory so as to avoid inadvertent pulmonary embolism.

SELECTION OF A VASCULAR CONDUIT

Externally supported PTFE grafts that are 10 to 14 mm are excellent conduits as short grafts for replacement of the SVC or the innominate vein (Table 55-1). A 12-mm externally supported PTFE graft can be used for bypass from the internal jugular vein to SVC or right atrium, although patency is reduced unless there exists a pressure gradient greater than 10 mm Hg. PTFE grafts below 8 mm in diameter have decreased long-term patency. An externally supported PTFE graft is preferred for all patients with malignancy, because recurrent tumor may compress and occlude a vein graft.

A spiral saphenous vein graft is preferred if a saphenous vein of appropriate dimension is available.[8,10,11,13-15] The femoral vein has been successfully used for SVC replacement, although residual limb swelling has been noted in some patients with thrombophilia.[10] Bovine pericardium can also be fashioned as a conduit, and fresh or cryopreserved allografts may be used for venous reconstruction. The great saphenous vein is too small to be used as a conduit.

SELECTION OF VENOUS INFLOW AND OUTFLOW SITES

The right innominate vein is the preferred inflow site, followed by the left innominate vein and the right and then the left internal jugular vein. Grafts that do not cross the midline reportedly have somewhat greater long-term patency.[16] Outflow sites are either the right atrial appendage or the SVC. The latter option is used in those patients who present with an innominate vein occlusion or a short segment occlusion of the SVC in proximity to the innominate veins.

CHOICE OF UNILATERAL OR BILATERAL VENOUS RECONSTRUCTION

Collateral venous circulation in the head and neck is usually sufficient to preclude the need for bilateral reconstruction. However, sole reconstruction of a left brachiocephalic vein results in a significant rate of occlusion. Thus reconstruction of a right brachiocephalic vein or bilateral brachiocephalic vein reconstruction is recommended; in the latter case, separate reconstruction of veins is preferred to use of a Y graft.[16]

Operative Technique

CHOICE OF ANESTHESIA

The operation is performed under general anesthesia with endotracheal intubation and mechanical ventilation.

POSITION AND INCISION

The neck, chest, abdomen, groins, and lower limbs are prepped and draped in a sterile fashion. The legs are prepped to the midcalf level, and the knees are bent in a frog-leg position for access to the saphenous vein. Draping is performed so that the neck up to the jaw is exposed, allowing a neck incision, if needed, to expose the internal jugular veins. A midline skin incision is made on the sternum, two fingerbreadths distal to the suprasternal or jugular notch for better cosmetic appearance. The incision is carried down to the sternum, and hemostasis is required to control bleeding from large venous collaterals of the chest wall. A full sternotomy is performed with an oscillating saw. Partial sternotomy or a "trapdoor" incision can be made for isolated innominate vein reconstruction if the cranial portion of the SVC or the contralateral innominate vein is patent.

DISSECTION OF THE INNOMINATE VEINS AND THE SUPERIOR VENA CAVA

The first structure in the upper anterior mediastinum is the thymus. It frequently must be divided or a portion must be excised between ligatures to expose the left innominate vein, which is an upper midline structure. The left innominate vein is frequently thrombosed in the presence of SVC syndrome, and the dissection is carried to the left, laterally under the sternum to expose an area that is patent, and close to the confluence of the left jugular and subclavian veins. If both innominate veins are thrombosed, then an oblique neck incision is made along the anterior border of the medial head of the sternocleidomastoid muscle to expose the internal jugular vein. On the left, injury to the thoracic duct should be avoided.

To expose the SVC, the pericardium is opened in the midline. In most patients with benign disease because of fibrosing mediastinitis, the right atrial appendage is selected for outflow and no attempt is made to dissect the sclerosed and fibrosed SVC. Biopsies, if needed, can be taken from the mediastinal tissues.

PREPARATION OF A SPIRAL VEIN GRAFT

To prepare the spiral saphenous vein graft, the saphenous vein is harvested from the groin to the knee. Side branches are ligated or oversewn with 6-0 or 7-0 polypropylene sutures and distended with a diluted papaverine-saline solution. The vein is opened longitudinally, valves are excised, and the vein is wrapped around a 32- or 36-Fr chest tube, depending on the size of the vein needed, with the endothelial surface facing the chest tube (Fig. 55-3, *A* and *B*). The opposing edges of the vein are sutured together with 6-0 polypropylene to form a conduit, interrupting the suture line at every three-quarter turn to prevent purse stringing and narrowing of the graft. Alternatively, nonpenetrating metal vascular clips may be used. However, the clips may not always hold firmly, and placement of additional interrupted sutures may be needed. The length of saphenous vein needed to produce a spiral vein graft of the required length can be calculated as

$$l = [(R)(L)]/r$$

where r and l represent the radius and length, respectively, of the saphenous vein and R and L represent the radius and length, respectively, of the spiral graft.[17] For example, a 40-cm-long saphenous vein graft with a mean radius of 3 mm affords an 8-cm-long spiral vein graft with a radius of 15 mm.

PERFORMING THE ANASTOMOSES

The central anastomosis should be performed initially to the right atrial appendage, followed by the peripheral anastomosis to the inflow site. The atrial anastomosis, in the presence of cardiac motion, is easier to perform if the vein graft is freely mobile. The patient is fully heparinized (100 units per kilogram

646   VENOUS DISEASE

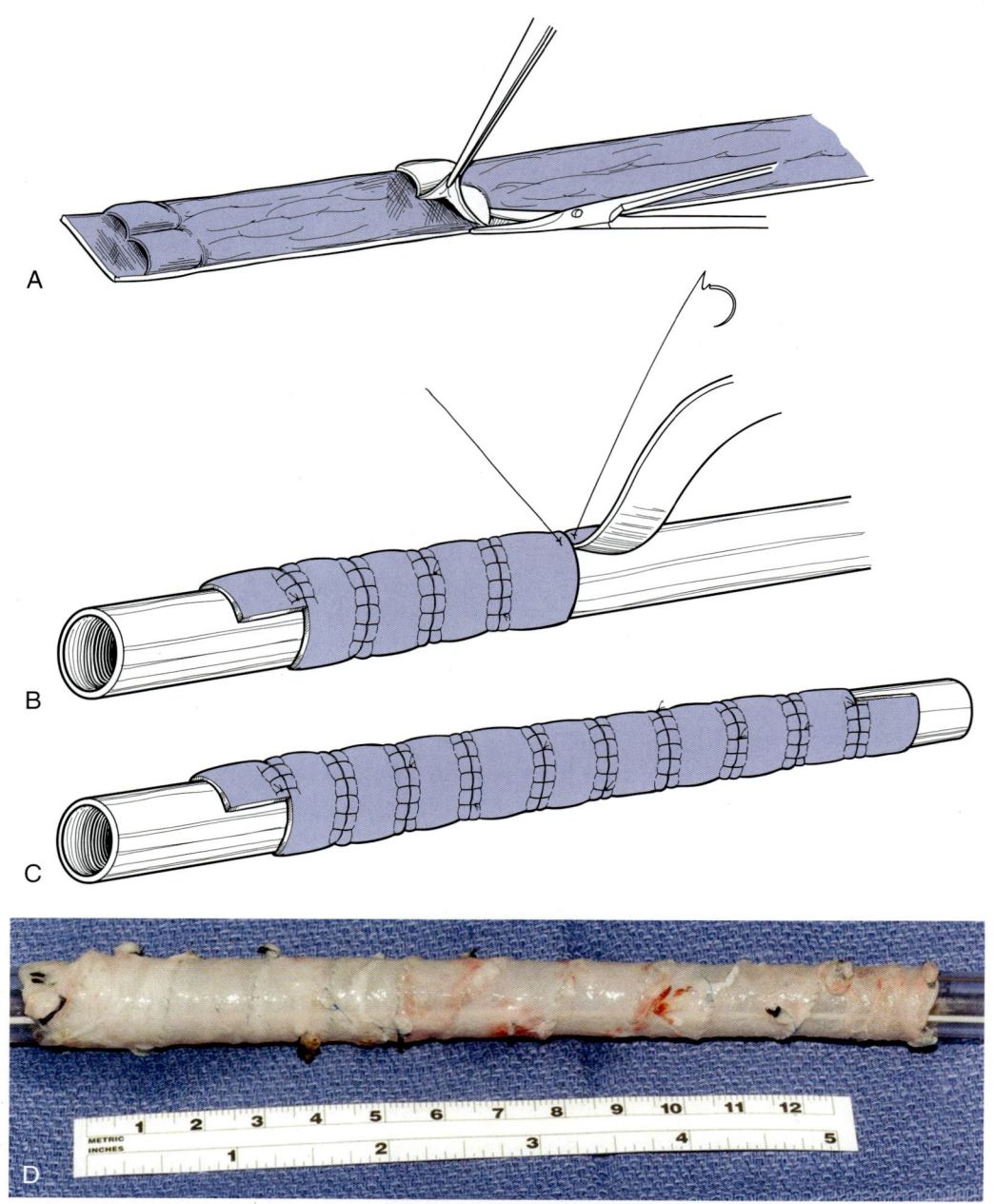

Figure 55-3. A, The great saphenous vein is opened longitudinally, and all valves are excised to prepare a spiral vein graft. **B**, The vein is wrapped around a chest tube, with the endothelial surface facing the chest tube and the opposing edges of the vein are sutured together to form the conduit. Interrupting the suture line at every three-quarter turn is necessary to prevent purse stringing and narrowing of the graft. **C** and **D**, Completed spiral vein graft. The length of saphenous vein needed to produce a spiral vein graft of the required length can be calculated according to an equation proposed by Chiu and colleagues.[17]

of body weight), and a Satinsky clamp is placed on the atrial appendage (Fig. 55-4, *A*). The edge of the appendage is opened longitudinally over a length of about 2 cm using a No. 11 scalpel blade or fine scissors. The trabecular muscles in the appendage are excised with fine scissors to optimize inflow to the heart. An oblique end-to-end anastomosis is then performed between the spiral vein graft or a 12-mm PTFE graft and the atrial appendage using 5-0 polypropylene (see Fig. 55-4, *B*). The graft is filled with heparinized saline before the clamp is removed from the atrial appendage to avoid air embolism. Soft bulldogs are placed on the graft a few centimeters proximal to the anastomosis. An end-to-end or end-to-side anastomosis is then performed to the innominate or internal jugular vein using 5-0 polypropylene. Before reestablishment of flow, blood and air are flushed out of the graft to avoid embolism (Fig. 55-5, and see Fig. 55-4, *C*).

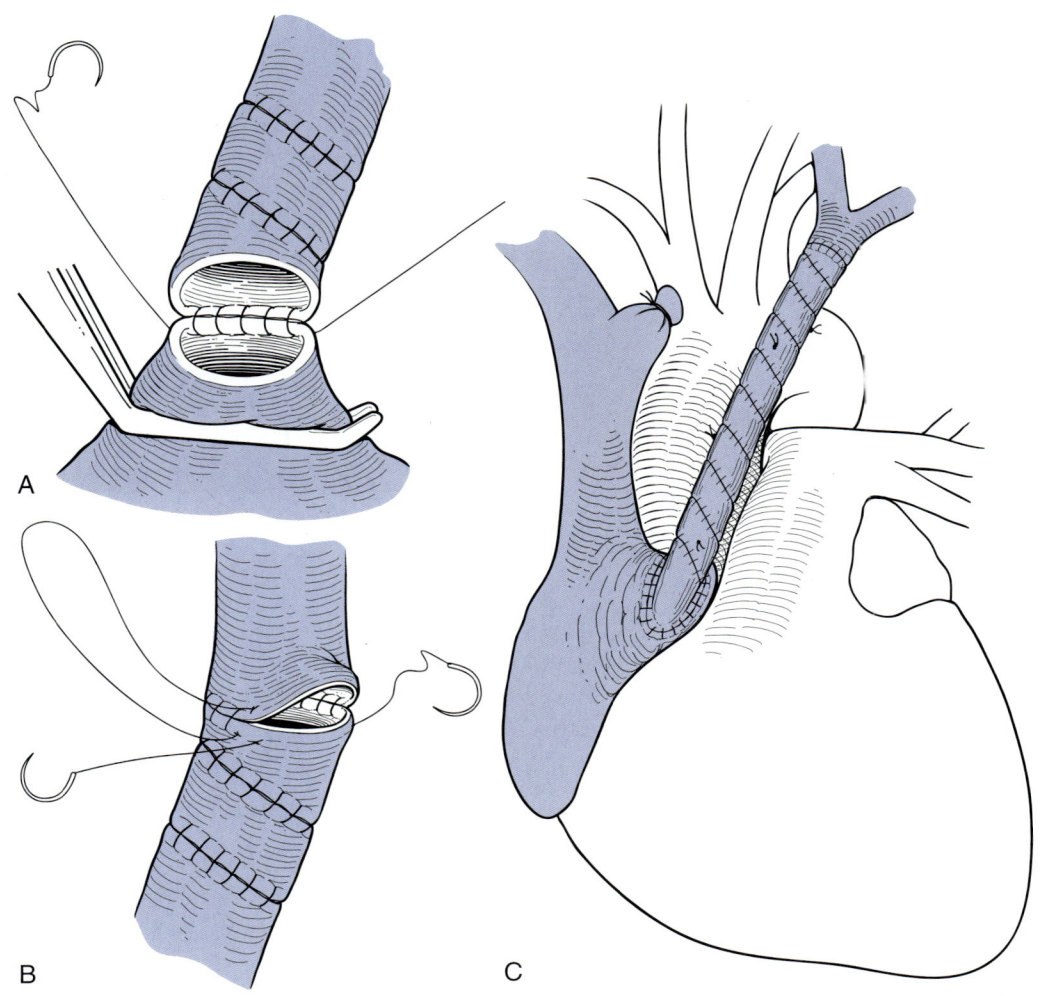

SURGICAL RECONSTRUCTION FOR SUPERIOR VENA CAVA SYNDROME | 647

Figure 55-4. **A**, A spiral saphenous vein bypass between the left innominate vein and the right atrial appendage requires performance of an initial anastomosis to the right atrial appendage. A Satinsky clamp is placed on the atrial appendage, which is opened longitudinally over 2 cm, followed by excision of the trabecular muscular network and construction of an end-to-side anastomosis. **B**, An end-to-end anastomosis is then performed to the innominate vein. **C**, Blood and air are flushed out of the graft to avoid embolism before reestablishment of flow.

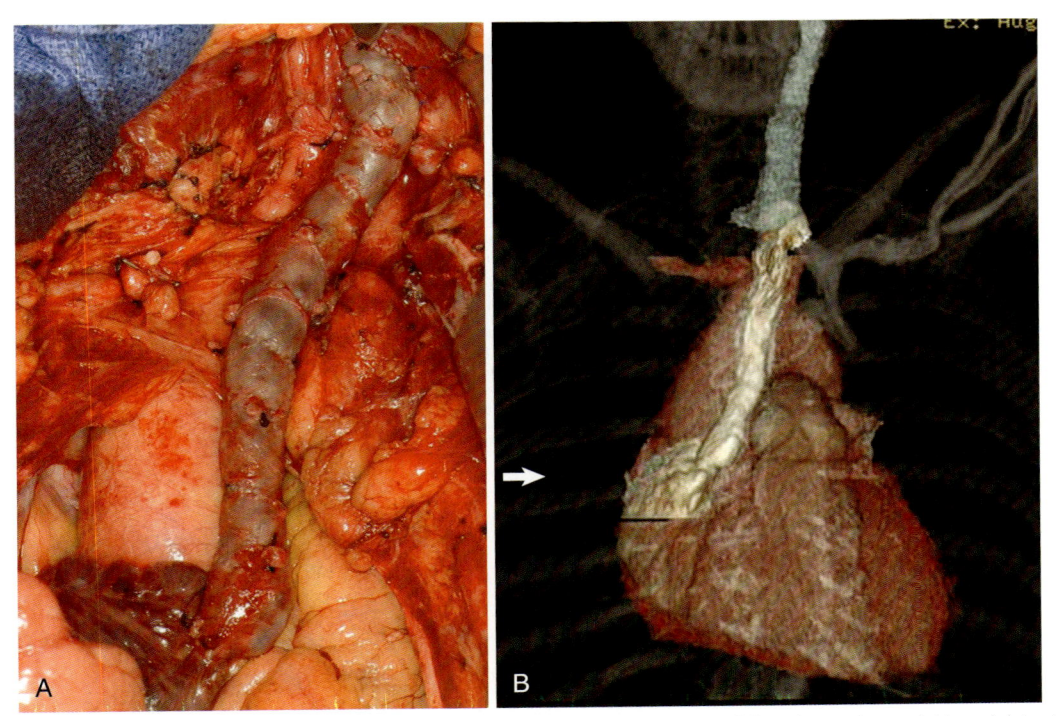

Figure 55-5. **A**, Completed spiral saphenous vein graft between the left internal jugular vein and the right atrial appendage. **B**, Postoperative CT angiogram demonstrating graft patency. Arrow indicates anastomosis of the graft with the atrial appendage.

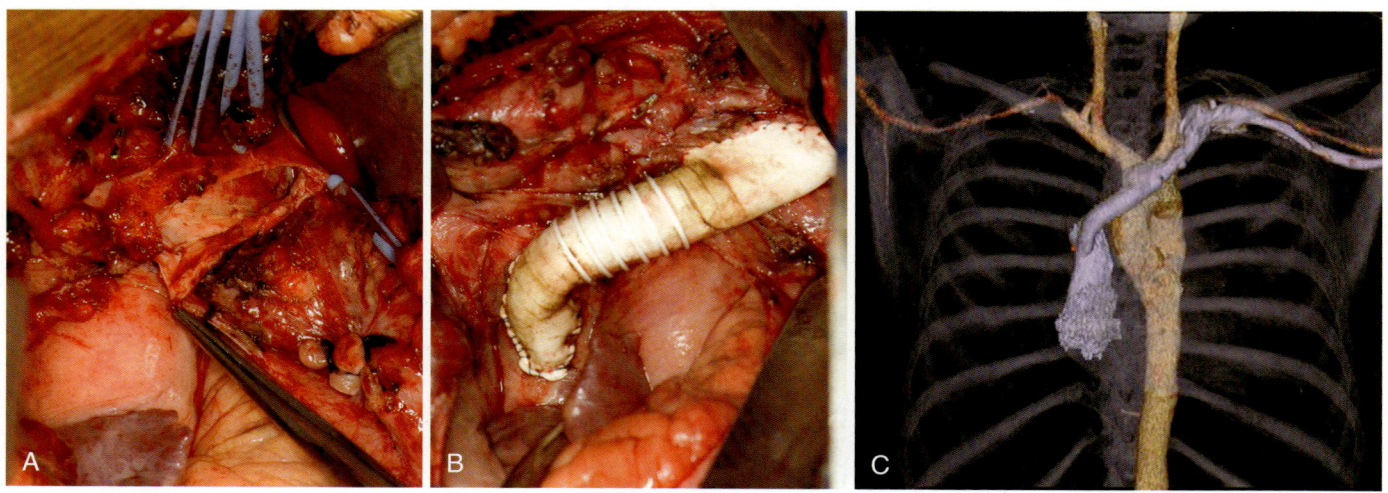

Figure 55-6. A, Left innominate vein after the recanalized thrombus has been excised and the vein is prepared for anastomosis. **B,** Completed PTFE graft between the left innominate vein and the SVC. **C,** Postoperative CT angiogram demonstrating graft patency.

In patients who require a short innominate vein–SVC graft using a PTFE or a spiral vein graft, the proximal anastomosis is usually completed initially followed by the distal anastomosis. This technique permits brief removal of the clamp once the proximal anastomosis is completed to fully distend the graft to avoid kinking and to determine appropriate graft length (Fig. 55-6, A and B).

CLOSURE OF THE MEDIAN STERNOTOMY

Heparin is partially reversed by intravenous administration of 30 mg of protamine sulfate and adequate hemostasis achieved. The pericardium is loosely approximated with 4-0 polypropylene sutures to avoid graft compression. If required, thymus, regional lymph nodes, or portions of the strap muscles can be resected to avoid graft compression. If the sternum compresses the graft, especially if the graft originates in the neck, a small portion of the posterior sternal wall can be carefully removed. A mediastinal drain is placed, avoiding graft compression. If the chest cavity was entered, chest tubes are placed. The sternum is closed using wire sutures, followed by closure of the subcutaneous tissue and skin.

Postoperative Care

- **Anticoagulation.** Low-dose unfractionated heparin is administered intravenously 24 hours after surgery at 500 unit/hr, with full anticoagulation within 72 to 96 hours. Patients should be discharged on an oral anticoagulation regimen. Patients with a femoral vein or spiral vein graft are maintained on warfarin for 3 months, whereas those who have a PTFE graft, as well as those with an underlying thrombophilia, require lifelong anticoagulation.
- **Imaging.** All patients should undergo CT angiography within 1 year. Earlier and more frequent imaging is recommended for symptomatic patients. Endovascular therapy with stenting can prolong graft patency if a stenosis is observed on imaging studies.

Complications

- **Mortality and pulmonary embolism.** Among 42 surgical reconstructions for benign disease, mortality was not observed, and only one patient had a nonfatal pulmonary embolism (Table 55-2). Patients who undergo SVC reconstruction in conjunction with resection of a malignant tumor have a reported 1-year mortality rate of up to 30%.[18]
- **Deep venous thrombosis.** Duplex imaging may be required to exclude deep venous thrombosis if significant leg swelling occurs after femoral vein harvest.

TABLE 55-2 Thirty-Day Complications After Surgical Reconstruction for Superior Vena Cava Syndrome

Complication	No. Patients (n = 42)
Mediastinal hematoma requiring evacuation	1
Pericardial effusion requiring drainage	1
Deep venous thrombosis	2
Pulmonary embolus	1
Prolonged mechanical ventilation	2
Tracheostomy, prolonged mechanical ventilation, pleural effusion requiring drainage, pneumonia	1
Total	8

From Rizvi AZ, Kalra M, Bjarnason H, et al: Benign superior vena cava syndrome: Stenting is now the first line of treatment, *J Vasc Surg* 47:372-380, 2008.

- **Pericardial effusion or mediastinal hematoma.** Given the need for early anticoagulation, there should be a high index of suspicion in the presence of clinical signs suggestive of pericardiac tamponade. For example, Beck's triad is characterized by hypotension, jugular venous distention, and muffled heart sound because of decreased stroke volume, impaired venous return, and fluid within the pericardial sac, respectively.
- **Graft patency.** Secondary 5-year patency of 86% has been reported for spiral vein grafts, and 90% patency noted after a mean follow-up of 23 months for large-diameter externally supported PTFE grafts.[1C,19]

REFERENCES

1. Hunter W: The history of an aneurysm of the aorta with some remarks on aneurysms in general, *Med Obs Inq (Lond)* 1:323-357, 1757.
2. Schechter MM: Superior vena cava syndrome, *Amer J Med Sci* 227:46-56, 1954.
3. Gomes MN, Hufnagel CA: Superior vena cava obstruction, *Ann Thorac Surg* 20:344-359, 1975.
4. Scherck JP, Kerstein MD, Stansel HC: The current status of vena caval replacement, *Surgery* 76:209-233, 1974.
5. Avasthi RB, Moghissi K: Malignant obstruction of the superior vena cava and its palliation, *J Thorac Cardiov Surg* 74:244-248, 1977.
6. Gladstone DJ, Pillai R, Paneth M, et al: Relief of superior vena caval syndrome with autologous femoral vein used as a bypass graft, *J Thorac Cardiov Surg* 89:750-752, 1985.
7. Doty DB: Bypass of superior vena cava: Six years' experience with spiral vein graft for obstruction of superior vena cava due to benign and malignant disease, *J Thorac Cardiov Surg* 83:326-338, 1982.
8. Doty JR, Flores JH, Doty DB: Superior vena cava obstruction: Bypass using spiral vein graft, *Ann Thorac Surg* 67:1111-1116, 1999.
9. Rice TW, Rodriguez RM, Light RW: The superior vena cava syndrome: Clinical characteristics and evolving etiology, *Medicine* 85:37-42, 2006.
10. Rizvi AZ, Kalra M, Bjarnason H, et al: Benign superior vena cava syndrome: Stenting is now the first line of treatment, *J Vasc Surg* 47:372-380, 2008.
11. Kalra M, Gloviczki P, Andrews JC, et al: Open surgical and endovascular treatment of superior vena cava syndrome caused by nonmalignant disease, *J Vasc Surg* 38:215-223, 2003.
12. Riley RF, Petersen SE, Ferguson JD, et al: Managing superior vena cava syndrome as a complication of pacemaker implantation: A pooled analysis of clinical practice, *Pacing Clin Electrophysiol* 33:420-425, 2010.
13. Doty JR, Flores JH, Doty DB: Superior vena cava obstruction: Bypass using spiral vein graft, *Ann Thorac Surg* 67:1111-1116, 1999.
14. Gloviczki P, Pairolero PC, Cherry KJ, et al: Reconstruction of the vena cava and of its primary tributaries: A preliminary report, *J Vasc Surg* 11:373-381, 1990.
15. Gloviczki P, Pairolero PC, Toomey BJ, et al: Reconstruction of large veins for nonmalignant venous occlusive disease, *J Vasc Surg* 16:750-761, 1992.
16. Shintani Y, Ohta M, Minami M, et al: Long-term graft patency after replacement of the brachiocephalic veins combined with resection of mediastinal tumors, *J Thorac Cardiov Surg* 129:809-812, 2005.
17. Chiu CJ, Terzis J, MacRae ML: Replacement of superior vena cava with the spiral composite vein graft. A versatile technique, *Ann Thorac Surg* 17:555-560, 1974.
18. Magnan PE, Thomas P, Giudicelli R, et al: Surgical reconstruction of the superior vena cava, *Cardiovasc Surg* 2:598-604, 1994.
19. Dartevelle PG, Chapelier AR, Pastorino U, et al: Long-term follow-up after prosthetic replacement of the superior vena cava combined with resection of mediastinal-pulmonary malignant tumors, *J Thorac Cardiov Surg* 102:259-265, 1991.

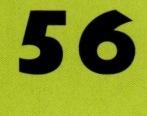

56 Surgical Reconstruction of the Inferior Vena Cava and Iliofemoral Venous System

THOMAS C. BOWER

Historical Background

The first direct venous reconstruction using a saphenous vein graft for "postphlebitic stasis" was reported in 1954 by Warren and Thayer.[1] In the late 1950s and 1960s venous reconstructions for benign occlusions using a cross-pubic venous bypass were introduced by Palma and Esperon[2] in Uruguay and later popularized in the United States by Dale.[3] Although Perl[4] first described the entity of venous leiomyosarcoma in 1971, descriptions of surgical resection for primary and secondary malignancies of the iliocaval venous system have been largely limited to series reported since 1993.[5-21]

Indications

BENIGN ILEOFEMORAL VENOUS OCCLUSION

Surgical reconstruction of the inferior vena cava (IVC) and iliac veins for benign disease has been relegated to symptomatic patients with long-segment iliac vein or vena cava occlusions who either are not candidates for stenting or have failed attempts at percutaneous recanalization.[22] The most common cause of benign occlusions is deep venous thrombosis because of May-Thurner syndrome, iatrogenic or blunt trauma, radiation, or external compression from retroperitoneal fibrosis, tumors, or large iliac or abdominal aortic inflammatory aneurysms. Congenital causes of venous obstruction include membranous obstruction of the suprahepatic IVC in either the absence or the presence of hepatic vein occlusion, as in Budd-Chiari syndrome, or hypoplasia of the iliofemoral veins, as observed in Klippel-Trenaunay syndrome.[22,23]

MALIGNANT ILIOFEMORAL VENOUS OCCLUSION

Select patients with primary or secondary malignancies of the iliac veins or IVC may be offered operation (Box 56-1). Candidates include patients without metastatic disease and good cardiopulmonary function who are able to perform daily activities with minimal limitation.[5,8,11,21] Patients with renal cell cancer tumor thrombus extending to the right heart who have limited pulmonary metastases may also benefit from tumor thrombectomy and postoperative chemotherapy.

Preoperative Preparation

- **Duplex ultrasonography and venous plethysmography.** Venous duplex ultrasonography, in combination with lower extremity air plethysmography, can be used to determine the site of venous occlusion and assess inflow from the common and deep femoral veins; determine the severity of valve incompetence, which is present in about two thirds of patients; and provide a measure of calf muscle pump function.[22] In addition, exercise testing by conducting 10 ankle

> **Box 56-1** **TUMORS OF THE INFERIOR VENA CAVA**
>
> *Primary*
> - Leiomyosarcoma
>
> *Secondary*
> - Retroperitoneal soft-tissue tumors
>   - Liposarcoma
>   - Leiomyosarcoma
>   - Malignant fibrous histiocytoma
> - Hepatic tumors
>   - Cholangiocarcinoma
>   - Hepatocellular carcinoma
>   - Metastatic (e.g., colorectal)
> - Pancreaticoduodenal cancers
> - Osteosarcoma, osteochondroma, or chordomas involving the lumbar spine or sacrum
>
> *Secondary Tumors With Caval Thrombus*
> - Renal cell carcinoma
> - Pheochromocytoma
> - Adrenocortical carcinoma
> - Sarcomas of uterine origin
>   - Leiomyomatosis
>   - Endometrial stromal cell
> - Germ cell tumors
>   - Embryonal
>   - Teratocarcinoma

dorsiflexions or 20 isometric calf muscle contractions should mimic symptoms and produce a twofold increase in lower extremity ambulatory venous pressure.

- **Three-dimensional computed tomography (CT) or magnetic resonance imaging (MRI).** CT and MRI can be used to exclude abdominal or pelvic pathology and with appropriate venous phase imaging to define iliofemoral and vena caval obstruction, as well as collateral veins and the proximity of tumor, if present, to adjacent organs (Figs. 56-1 and 56-2).

- **Transesophageal echocardiography (TEE).** TEE may be helpful to determine the proximity of an intracaval tumor thrombus to the hepatic veins or right heart.[21]

- **Ascending and descending venography.** Conventional venography via femoral vein access can define venous anatomy, as well as determine whether a stenosis is hemodynamically significant by the presence of a 3 to 5 mm Hg pressure gradient. Normal pressures, however, may be observed at rest because of large collaterals. Intravascular ultrasound is a helpful adjunct in identifying lesions that may otherwise be difficult to identify by conventional, CT, or magnetic resonance venography.[22]

- **Duplex mapping of the saphenous vein.** A donor saphenous vein of at least 5 mm in diameter is preferred for a cross-pubic femoral vein bypass (Palma procedure).

- **Cardiopulmonary function.** Cardiopulmonary function is assessed with dobutamine stress echocardiography or perfusion studies of the heart.

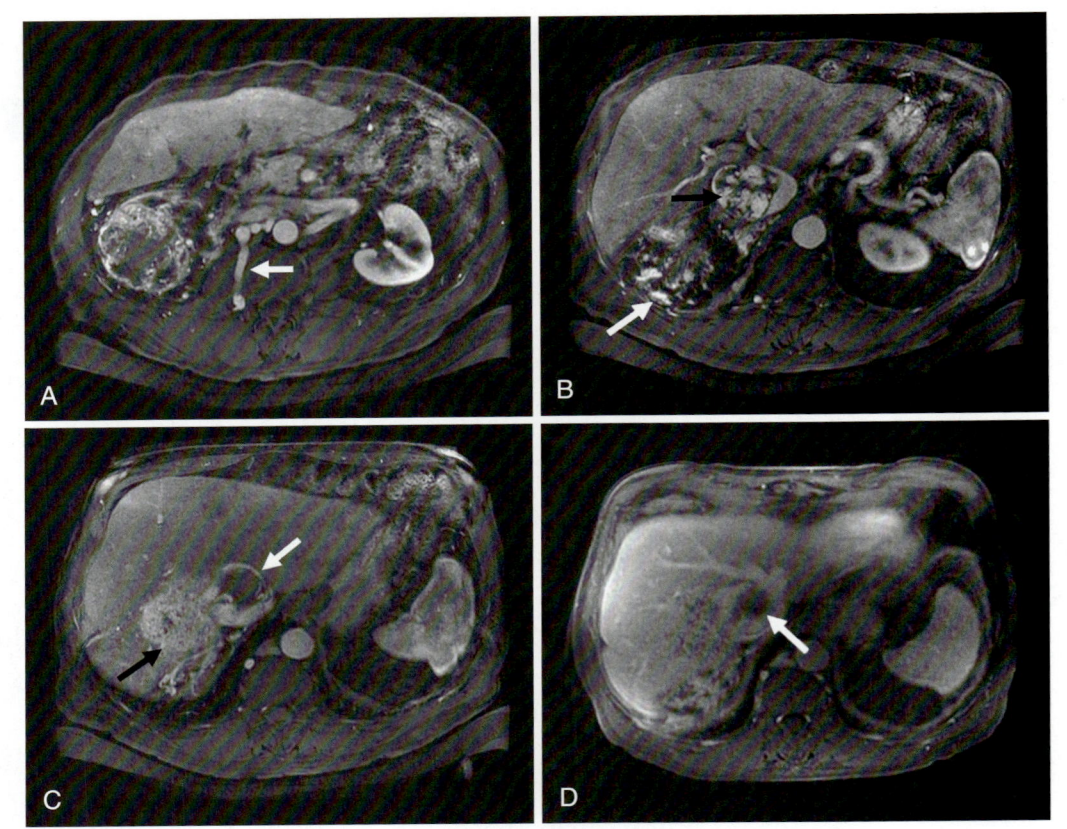

Figure 56-1. Axial CT images in a caudal to cephalad direction of large vascular renal cell cancer, right liver lobe hepatic metastasis, and intracaval tumor thrombus extending to the hepatic vein–caval confluence. **A**, A dilated lumbar vein *(white arrow)* is a consistent finding with suprarenal inferior vena cava (IVC) obstruction and may be a source of significant backbleeding during removal of caval thrombus. A highly vascular renal cell carcinoma is adjacent to the vein. **B**, The top of the renal cell cancer *(white arrow)* and beginning of the hepatic metastasis *(black arrow)* causing compression of the IVC. **C**, The hepatic metastasis is highly vascular *(black arrow)*, with tumor thrombus within the retrohepatic IVC *(white arrow)*. **D**, The tumor thrombus extends to the junction of the IVC and right hepatic vein *(white arrow)*. (From Bower TC. Venous tumors. In: Cronenwett JL, Johnston KW, editors: Rutherford's vascular surgery, ed 7. Philadelphia, 2010, Saunders, pp 983-995, Fig. 63-6.)

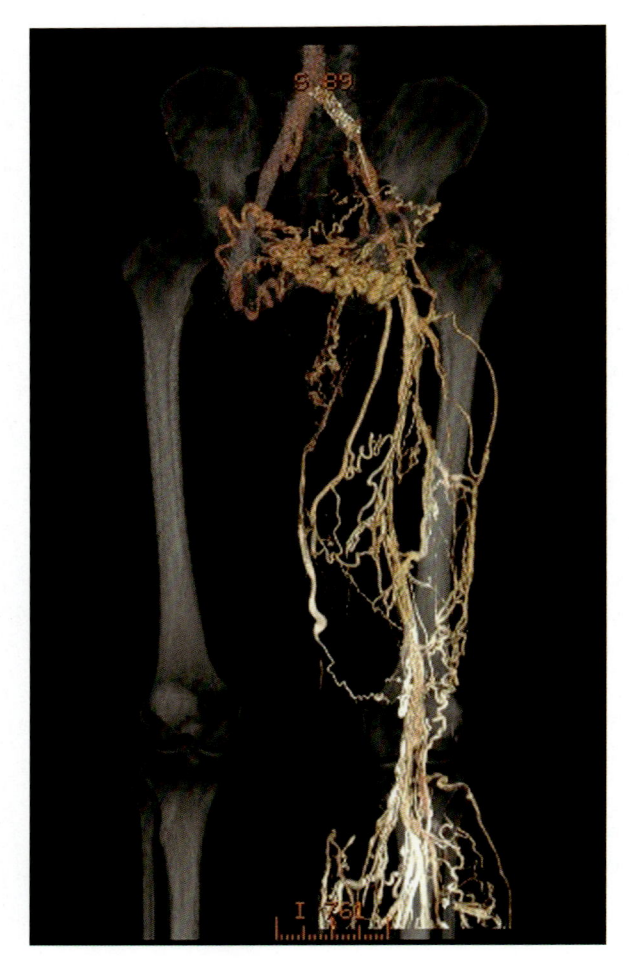

Figure 56-2. Three-dimensional CT venogram confirming occluded left iliac stent with large suprapubic venous collaterals. (From Gloviczki P, Oderich GS: Open surgical reconstructions for non-malignant occlusion of the inferior vena cava and iliofemoral veins. In: Gloviczki P, editor: Handbook of venous disorders: Guidelines of the American Venous Forum. London, 2009, Hodder Arnold, pp 514-522.)

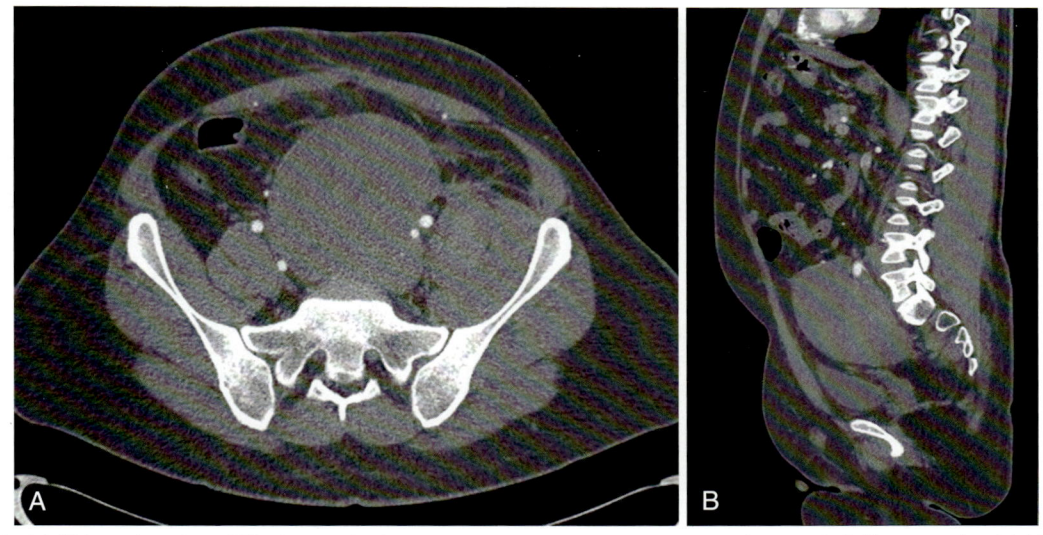

Figure 56-3. Axial (**A**) and sagittal (**B**) views of a large pelvic sarcoma partially encasing the left iliac arteries, highlighted with contrast. Venous phase images are not shown, but veins were encased by tumor. The tumor was large and immobile, and endovascular occlusion of distal internal iliac artery and vein branches was performed. *(From Bower TC: Primary and secondary tumors of the inferior vena cava and iliac veins. In: Gloviczki P, editor: Handbook of venous disorders: Guidelines of the American Venous Forum. London, 2009, Hodder Arnold, pp 574-582.)*

- **Pulmonary function.** Pulmonary function studies and arterial blood gases are performed in those patients with moderate to severe chronic obstructive lung disease.
- **Preoperative embolization of the renal artery.** In patients with a large renal cell cancer, renal artery embolization 24 hours before operation may shrink the tumor.[21,24] Preoperative embolization of internal iliac artery and venous branches may be helpful in patients with large immobile tumors of the sacrum and pelvis to minimize blood loss during resection (Fig. 56-3).

Pitfalls and Danger Points

- **Early failure of a cross-femoral venous bypass.** A cross-femoral venous bypass may occlude because of small saphenous vein (<4 mm), poor inflow related to obstruction or venous incompetence in the femoral-popliteal and deep femoral systems, inadequate cross-pubic tunnel, kinking at the donor saphenofemoral junction, or lack of an arteriovenous fistula when a prosthetic bypass is used.
- **Selection of cross-femoral bypass conduit.** An 8- to 10-mm-diameter expanded polytetrafluoroethylene (ePTFE) bypass should be used when the donor saphenous vein is of small caliber, diseased, or absent.
- **Common femoral vein as an inflow source.** If there are thrombophlebitic changes in the common femoral vein, an endovenectomy should be considered. This consists of excising the dense synechiae and endoluminal fibrous tissue with placement of a vein patch (Fig. 56-4, *A*).
- **Cross-femoral pubic tunnel.** The suprapubic tunnel should admit two fingers throughout its course.
- **Kinking of a cross-femoral venous bypass.** If the saphenous vein kinks at the donor saphenofemoral junction, it should be disconnected from the femoral vein with a 2-mm cuff, rotated 180 degrees, and reanastomosed to the femoral vein.[22]
- **Arteriovenous fistula.** The addition of an arteriovenous fistula is important if a prosthetic bypass is used. A 4-mm-diameter branch of saphenous vein or ePTFE graft between the superficial femoral artery and the hood of the donor venous anastomosis is preferred (see Fig. 56-4, *B*).[22] A larger-diameter arteriovenous fistula increases the pressure within the venous system and should be avoided.
- **Internal iliac or lumbar vein bleeding.** Ineffectual ligation of short, broad-based internal iliac or lumbar vein branches may lead to hemorrhage. Ligation of only

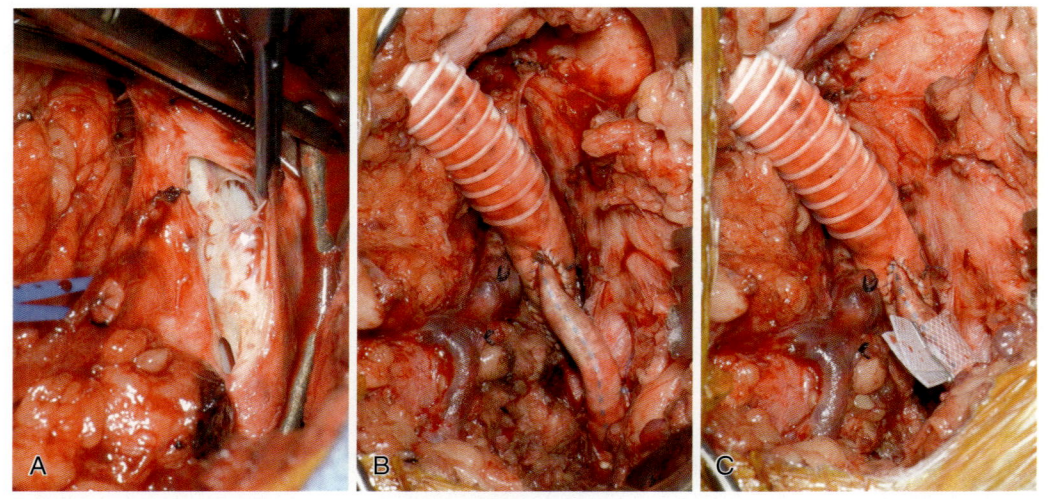

Figure 56-4. **A,** A partially recanalized femoral vein is identified after venotomy. Endovenectomy i performed to remove the organized thrombus and improve inflow into a femoral-femoral crossover venous polytetrafluoroethylene (PTFE) bypass. **B,** An arteriovenous fistula is placed between the superficial femoral artery and the hood of the cross-femoral PTFE graft. **C,** A small Silastic sheath is placed around the fistula and marked with metal clips to facilitate identification at reoperation to close the fistula. *(Courtesy Mayo Foundation for Medical Education and Research.)*

the internal iliac vein trunk in the course of sacral resection or hemipelvectomy increases blood loss when the bone is transected. As many branches of the internal iliac vein as are possible should be ligated and divided to minimize blood loss. To avoid distention of internal iliac vein branches, it is best to initially isolate but not ligate the main trunk or trunks of the internal iliac vein, after which the branches are ligated. Dilated lumbar veins at the renal vein–IVC confluence are a source of significant bleeding when extracting intracaval thrombus (Fig. 56-1, *C*).

- **Thromboembolism.** Malposition of the upper (cephalad) caval clamp during removal of the intracaval tumor thrombus may inadvertently fracture the thrombus and result in pulmonary embolism. Early renal artery ligation to promote tumor thrombus retraction and the use of intraoperative transesophageal echocardiography to be certain that the suprahepatic IVC is free of tumor thrombus may help avoid this problem. Some patients with intracaval tumor thrombus also have occlusive or partially occlusive bland thrombus in the infrarenal cava (Fig. 56-5). If there is concern about maintaining IVC patency, the infrarenal thrombus must be removed in its entirety. Otherwise, a caval filter should be placed.[14]

- **Air embolism.** Retrograde and prograde flushing of the iliocaval prosthesis should be performed with the patient in a head-down position and the lungs inflated to a pressure of 30 cm of water to avoid inadvertent air embolism. The graft can also be filled with heparinized saline, and punctures of the graft with a 25-Ga needle can be used to remove air before restoration of blood flow.

- **Iliocaval graft thrombosis and stenosis.** Early thrombosis of a large-diameter iliac or caval graft is uncommon. Failure occurs if there is purse stringing of the suture line, causing stenosis, redundancy or compression of the graft, or inadequate inflow. Anastomotic stenosis is avoided by beveling the graft, triangulating the suture lines, and when tying the suture, incorporating at least 2 mm of "growth factor" (air knot).

- **Selection of an iliocaval conduit.** Autogenous vein grafts in the abdomen are prone to compression; therefore the use of ePTFE grafts is preferred for iliocaval replacements, with preservation of as many graft rings as feasible, even in the region of the beveled anastomosis.[5,8,21]

- **Avoiding graft torsion at the hepatic veins.** When the retrohepatic IVC requires replacement, the tendency is to cut the graft too long. This is avoided by measuring the length of the graft needed with the lungs maximally inflated and then deflated before cutting the graft to length. In addition, the graft is cut with the

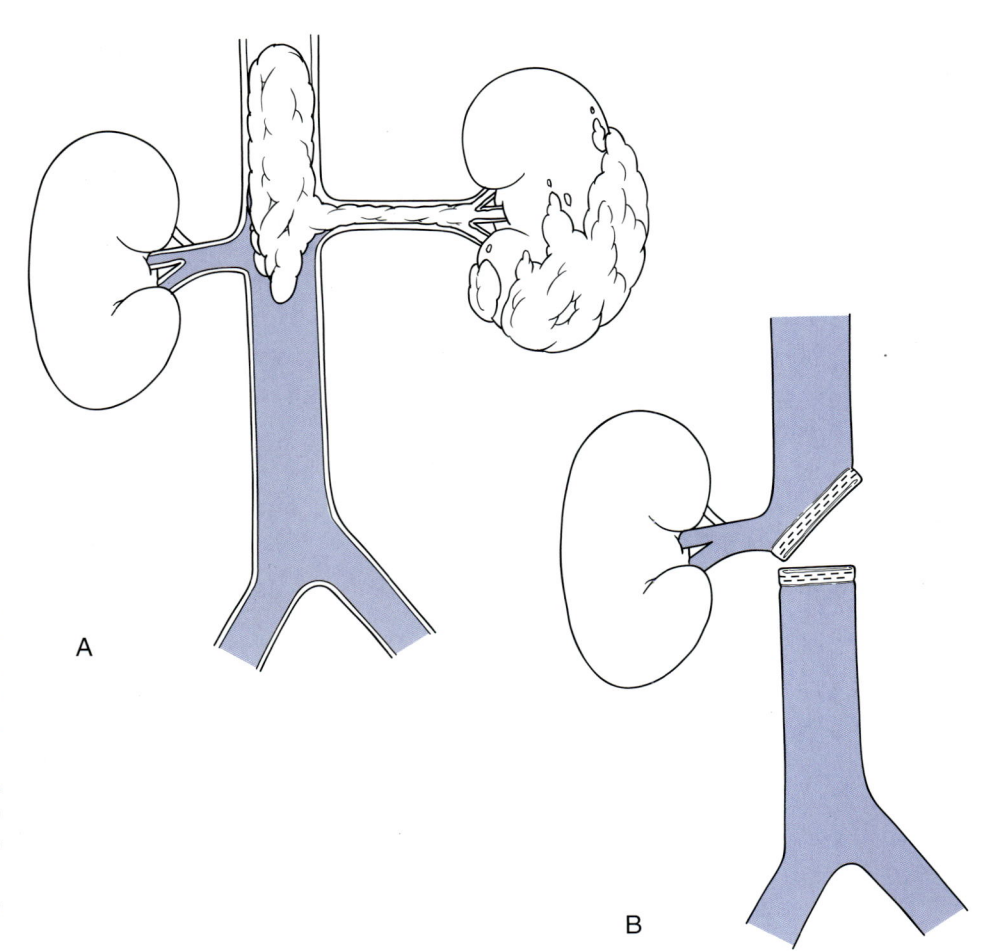

Figure 56-5. A, Schematic of a renal cell carcinoma and tumor thrombus extending from the renal vein into the suprarenal and infrarenal vena cava with associated chronic occlusive bland thrombus. **B**, Once the tumor thrombus is removed, the IVC is obliquely transected and either oversewn or stapled to avoid a cul-de-sac. *(Adapted from illustrations created by David Factor, Mayo Foundation. Courtesy Mayo Foundation for Medical Education and Research.)*

liver or the liver remnant rotated to its normal position to avoid torsion at the hepatic veins. If the upper graft anastomosis is at the level of the hepatic veins, the suprahepatic clamp is best secured in a supradiaphragmatic extrapericardial position so that the vein cuff does not slip through the clamp (Fig. 56-6). Manipulation of stiff grafts can be difficult, so a parachute suture technique may be helpful.

- **Necessity for venovenous bypass.** It is important to test clamp the suprahepatic IVC before resection to be certain that appropriate hemodynamics can be maintained with volume loading. If it cannot, venovenous bypass is needed.
- **Liver ischemia.** Liver ischemia should be less than 30 minutes when total vascular isolation of the liver is used, regardless of whether concomitant major hepatic resection is undertaken. Perfusion techniques should be considered if an ischemic period of greater than 60 minutes is anticipated. If hepatic resection is needed, ischemic preconditioning of the liver may be of benefit to those patients with large cancers polycystic liver disease, preexisting liver dysfunction, or those undergoing reoperation.[8,11,21] Nonetheless, the presence of intrinsic hepatic dysfunction may be a relative contraindication to any procedure necessitating liver ischemia because tolerance to ischemia is reduced.
- **Graft infection.** Although the risk of prosthetic graft infection is low, it can be further minimized by wrapping the graft with omentum or with bovine pericardium.[5,8,11] A spiral or panel femoral vein graft or cryopreserved homograft provides an alternative option in the presence of enteric contamination.

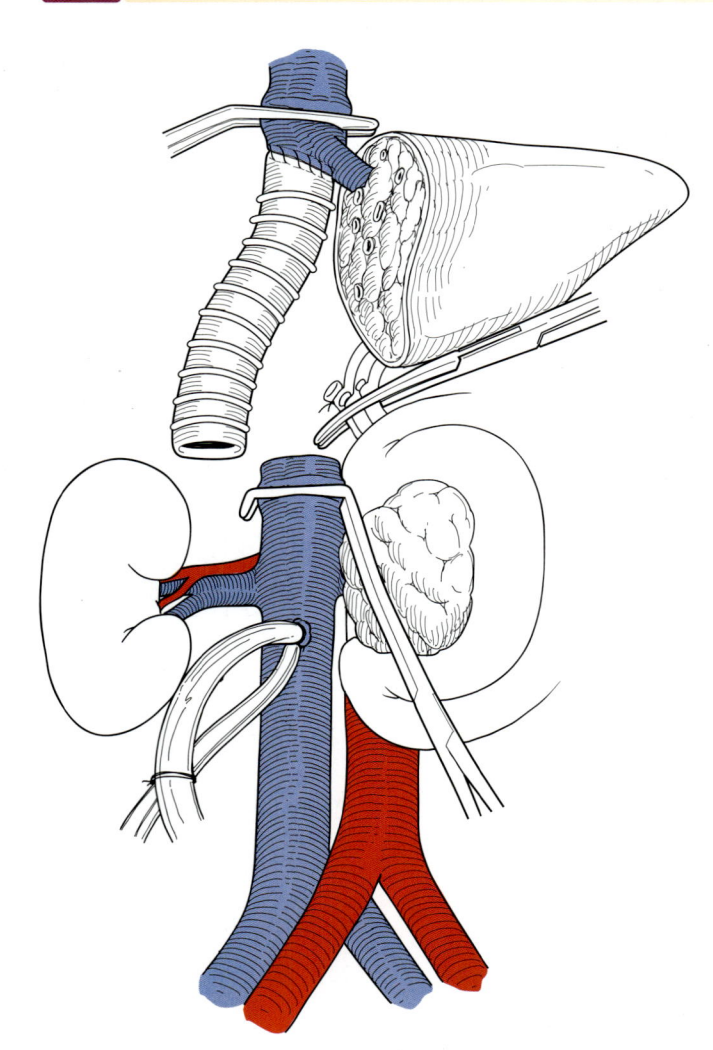

Figure 56-6. Reconstruction of the retrohepatic inferior vena cava (IVC) often requires total vascular isolation of the liver. The sequence of clamping begins with the infrahepatic IVC, followed by inflow occlusion across the portal triad, and then placement of the suprahepatic caval clamp. Individual dissection of the hepatic artery and the portal vein is not required and use a soft vascular clamp on the portal triad will minimize the risk of injury to its structures. The upper caval anastomosis is performed first. If systolic blood pressure cannot be maintained at or above 100 mm Hg upon suprahepatic IVC clamping, venovenous bypass is instituted with a cannula placed in the infrarenal IVC and tubing to a large-bore catheter in the jugular vein. *(Adapted from illustrations created by David Factor, Mayo Foundation. Courtesy Mayo Foundation for Medical Education and Research.)*

Operative Strategy

ANATOMY

Resection of the iliac veins or the IVC can lead to bleeding from the internal iliac vein and its branches, the iliolumbar or middle sacral veins, or the lumbar veins. The internal iliac vein receives extrapelvic and pelvic tributaries, which correspond to the branches of the internal iliac artery. The internal iliac vein may be a single trunk or composed of several medial and lateral trunks that may be short and broad. The iliolumbar veins, which may be short and broad, drain directly into the common iliac veins, and the medial sacral vein empties near the confluence of the left common iliac vein and IVC. The lumbar veins are either single or paired, dilate in response to proximal IVC occlusion, and drain through collateral pathways, which include the paravertebral and ascending lumbar veins (Fig. 56-1, *C*). The latter lies between the psoas major muscle and the roots of the transverse process of the lumbar vertebrae. The paravertebral collaterals drain into the azygos or hemiazygos systems and through the second lumbar or lumborenal vein, which is a tributary of the left renal vein.

CHOICE OF INCISION

Midline incisions are used for iliocaval bypass for benign conditions, replacing the infrarenal IVC in patients with primary or secondary malignancies, and mobilizing the major arteries and veins during lumbar spine, pelvic, and sacral resections. Many patients with sacral resection require a rectus abdominis musculocutaneous flap to close the defect, obviating a retroperitoneal approach. Midline or extended subcostal incisions are used for resection of renal cell cancers with level I to III tumor thrombus and malignancies involving the suprarenal IVC including the retrohepatic segment. As defined by a Mayo Clinic classification system for renal cell

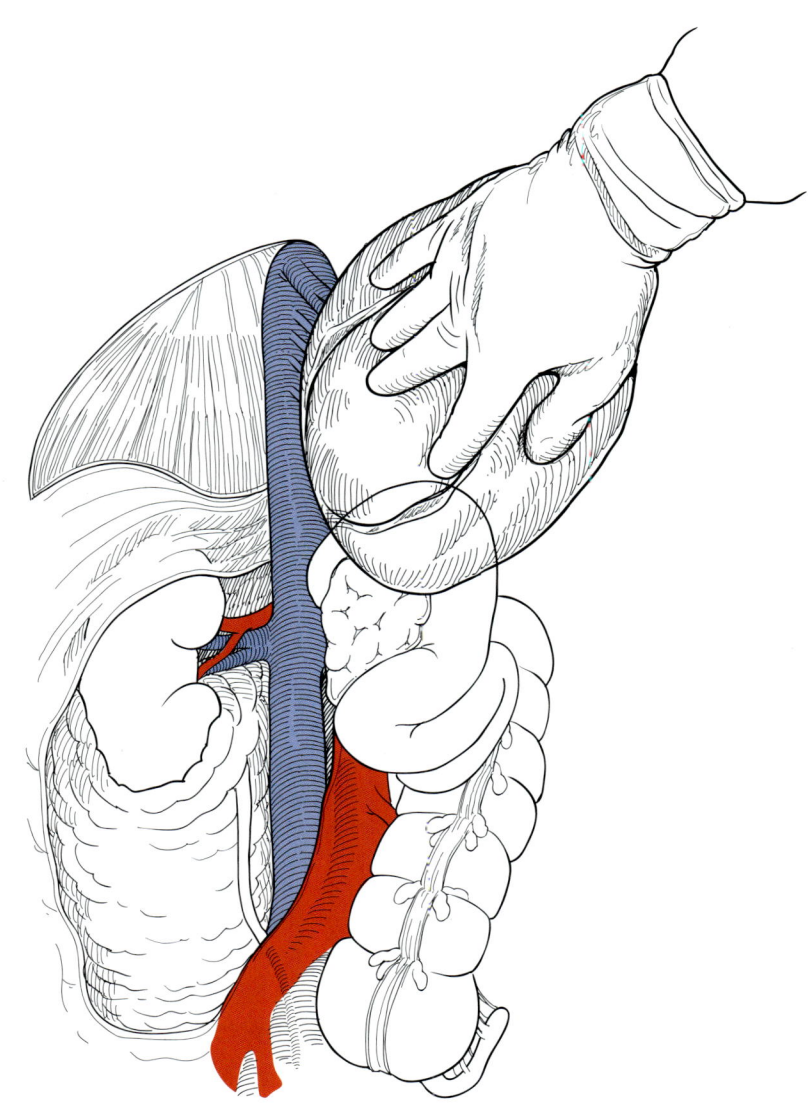

Figure 56-7. The retrohepatic IVC can be approached through a bilateral subcostal or a right thoracoabdominal incision, using a medial visceral rotation with division of the falciform and right triangular ligaments of the liver. While dividing the triangular ligament, care should be taken not to injure the paired large diaphragmatic veins that enter the vena cava at the diaphragm. Control of individual hepatic veins is not needed and best avoided even in those cases where suprahepatic control of the vena cava is required. *(Adapted from illustrations created by David Factor, Mayo Foundation. Courtesy Mayo Foundation for Medical Education and Research.)*

carcinoma, a level 1 tumor thrombus is located either at the entry of renal vein or within the IVC less than 2 cm from the confluence of renal vein and IVC. A level II tumor thrombus extends within the IVC greater than 2 cm above the confluence of renal vein and IVC, but below the hepatic veins. A level III tumor thrombus involves the intrahepatic IVC. A level IV tumor thrombus extends above diaphragm or into the right atrium. Bilateral subcostal or midline incisions can be extended with a median sternotomy should the patient require concomitant cardiopulmonary bypass to remove intracardiac tumor thrombus (Fig. 56-7). Patients with large primary or secondary hepatic malignancies involving the retrohepatic IVC can be approached through a right thoracoabdominal incision via the eighth or ninth interspace. With this incision, part of the diaphragm is radially incised to facilitate exposure.

RESECTION OF THE SUPRARENAL INFERIOR VENA CAVA IN CONJUNCTION WITH MAJOR LIVER RESECTION

Intraabdominal regional metastases should be excluded, and intraoperative ultrasound should be used to define the intrahepatic vascular anatomy, the presence of multicentric disease within the liver, and the relationship between the tumor and the afferent and efferent vasculature. Total vascular isolation of the liver is needed to minimize blood loss while sewing the upper caval anastomosis. In situ or ex situ perfusion techniques may be needed if liver ischemia time approaches 60 minutes or if reconstruction of the hepatic veins, portal vein, and IVC is required.[9-13,21] Ex situ liver perfusion carries a risk of liver failure, requiring salvage orthotopic liver transplant.[11]

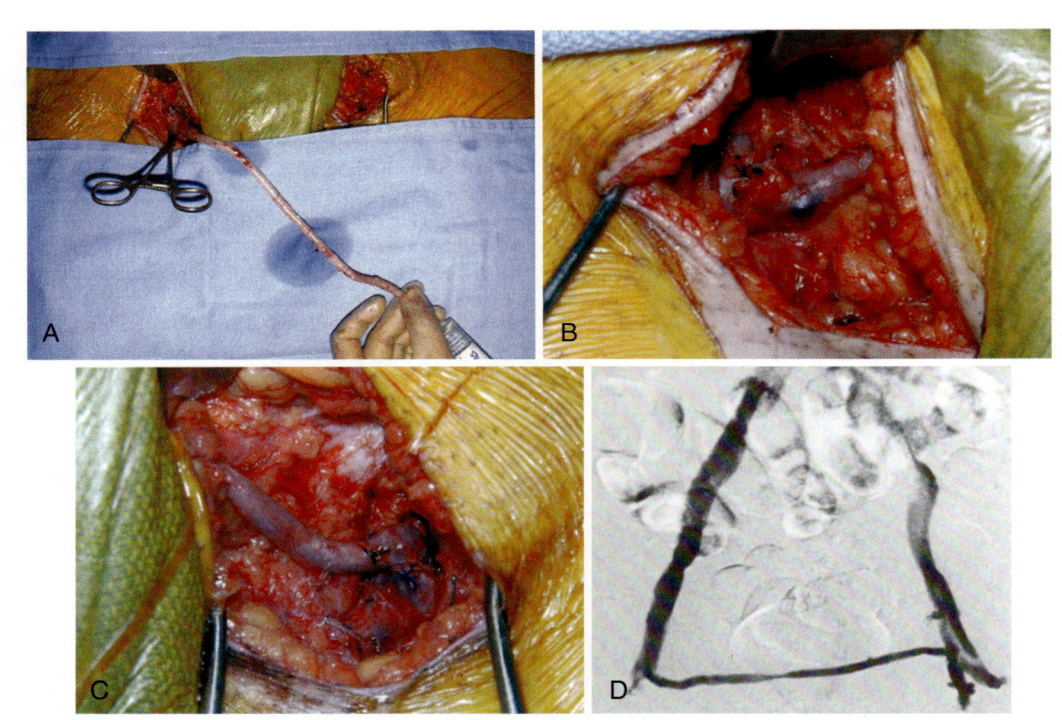

Figure 56-8. A, Preparation of the right great saphenous vein before suprapubic saphenous vein transposition (Palma procedure). Bilateral groin incisions were performed to expose the left common femoral vein and the right saphenofemoral junction. The right saphenous vein is harvested through short incisions in the thigh, and a clamp is placed to occlude the saphenous vein and part of the common femoral vein. The vein is distended with heparin solution before being tunneled to the left side for anastomosis with the femoral vein. **B,** The right saphenofemoral junction after tunneling the vein to the left side in the suprapubic space. There should be no kinks in the saphenous vein. **C,** Anastomosis of the saphenous vein to the left common femoral vein. **D,** Postoperative venography confirms a patent saphenous vein graft. *(Courtesy Mayo Foundation for Medical Education and Research.)*

Operative Technique

FEMORAL-FEMORAL VENOUS BYPASS

Patients with unilateral iliac vein obstruction not amenable to endovascular procedures are candidates for a femoral-femoral bypass with saphenous vein transposition (Fig. 56-8). An ePTFE graft of 8 to 10 mm in diameter with an arteriovenous fistula is suitable if the saphenous vein is absent or of poor quality.[22,23,25]

Patency is improved if the saphenous vein graft is at least 5 mm in diameter and the pressure difference between the two femoral veins is greater than 3 to 5 mm Hg. If the saphenous vein is less than 5 mm and the pressure gradient is less than 3 mm Hg, an arteriovenous fistula should be added to enhance vein graft patency.[22]

ILIOCAVAL VENOUS BYPASS

An iliocaval bypass is best performed using an ePTFE graft with end-to-side proximal and distal anastomoses. The diameter of the graft is based on the size of the inflow iliac or femoral vein and of the IVC at the outflow anastomosis. In general 12- to 16-mm-diameter grafts are preferred. A long femorocaval or iliocaval bypass should be supplemented with an arteriovenous fistula. In addition, a polypropylene catheter should be threaded through a small vein branch and placed near the proximal anastomosis of the graft at the femoral or iliac vein level so that heparin can be administered directly through the graft during the early postoperative period (Fig. 56-9).[22,23,25] To avoid graft compression the, inguinal ligament should be released when performing a femorocaval bypass. If a cavoatrial bypass is performed, the graft can be passed along side the native IVC behind the right or the left lobe of the liver through the diaphragm.

A silicone elastomer (Silastic) sheath or a small piece of thin-walled polytetrafluoroethylene (PTFE), with a polypropylene suture around it, can be placed around the

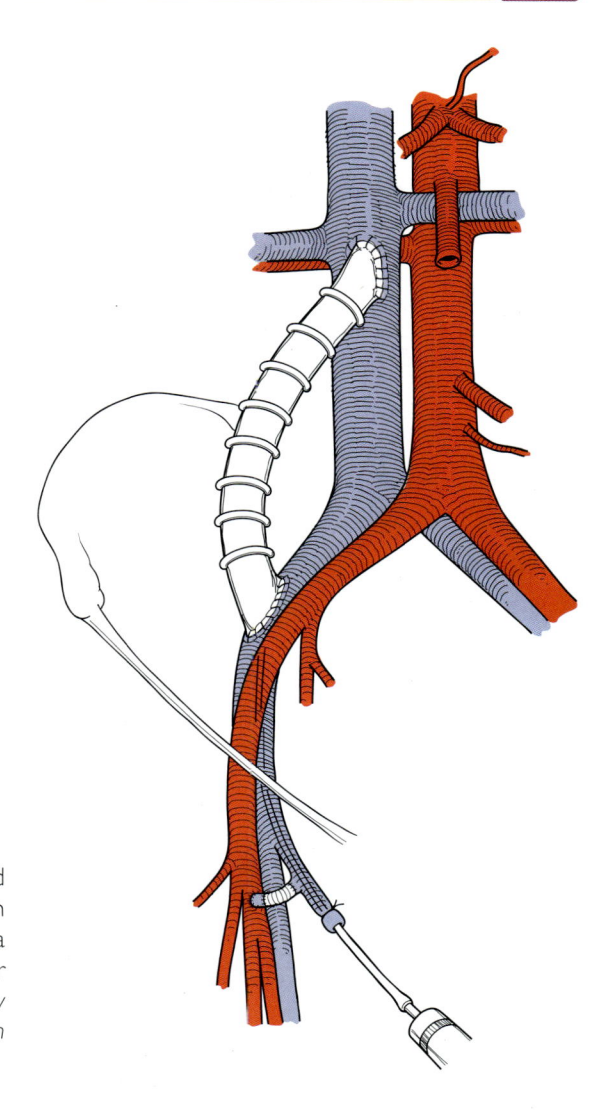

Figure 56-9. A right iliac vein–inferior vena cava externally supported expanded polytetrafluoroethylene graft. An arteriovenous fistula has been constructed between the right femoral artery and the saphenous vein, and a 20-Ga catheter has been placed through a tributary of the saphenous vein for perioperative administration of heparin. *(Adapted from illustrations created by David Factor, Mayo Foundation. Courtesy Mayo Foundation for Medical Education and Research.)*

arteriovenous fistula to facilitate operative ligation of the fistula at a later date (see Fig. 56-4, C).[22] Alternatively, the fistula can be closed with an endovascular coil or plug.[25]

RECONSTRUCTION OF THE INFERIOR VENA CAVA

The infrarenal IVC can be resected and not replaced if it is chronically occluded and adjacent collateral veins are not disrupted during the course of resection.[7] However, the pararenal IVC should be replaced because of the risk of postoperative renal failure and severe lower extremity edema.[6,8,11,16]

Patch closure is preferred to interposition graft replacement of the iliac veins or vena cava and can be used for reconstruction of up to one half to two thirds of the vein circumference.[21] A formula has been developed to determine patch width and length and to avoid underestimating the requisite diameter of the bovine pericardial patch and buckling or kinking at the cranial and caudal portions of the patch (Fig. 56-10).

An interposition graft should be used if more than two thirds of the vein circumference is involved by tumor, preferably an externally supported ePTFE prosthesis. Graft diameters may range between 16 and 20 mm for replacement of the IVC and between 10 and 14 mm for reconstruction of the external and common iliac veins. However, others have advocated using a graft size smaller than the IVC, between 12 and 16 mm, to reduce the risk of thrombosis by promoting higher shear rates through the IVC graft segment. Graft rings should be preserved close to the level of the anastomosis. Proximal and distal venous control may also require mobilization of the lower aorta and the iliac arteries. Resection of the pararenal IVC necessitates salvage of the remnant renal vein by reimplantation or use of a

660 VENOUS DISEASE

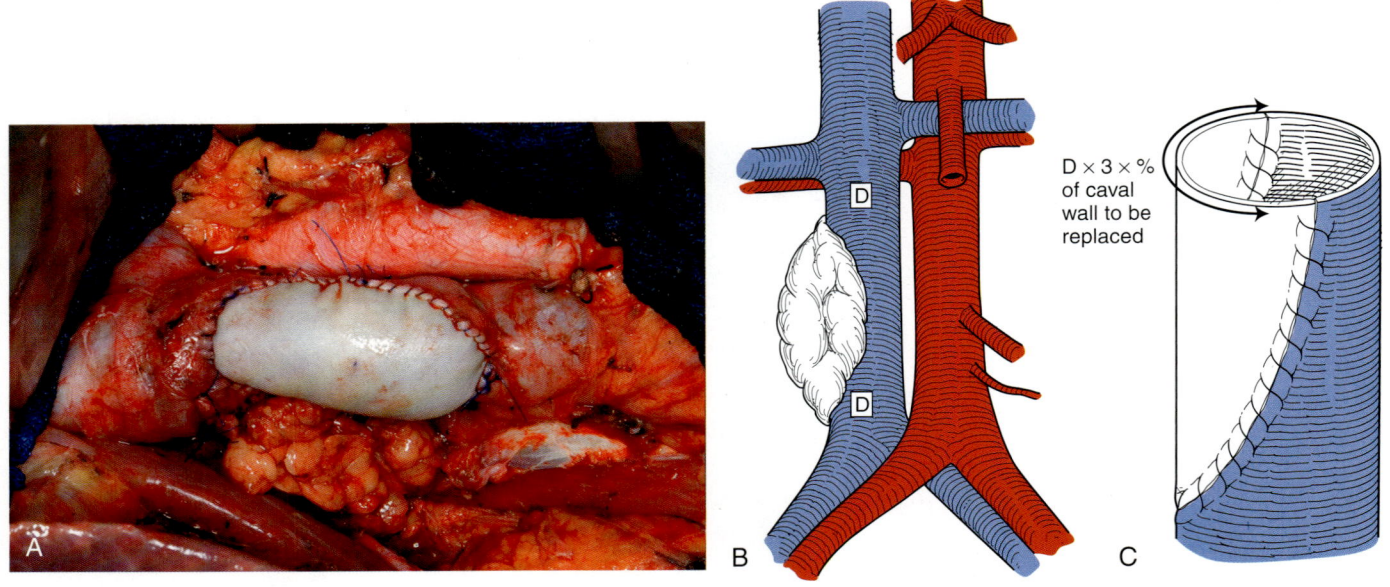

Figure 56-10. **A**, As much as one half to two thirds of the vena cava wall can be resected and replaced with a patch. Bovine pericardium is preferred for the patch. **B and C**, The estimated diameter of the patch can be determined by the formula, $D \times 3 \times \%$, where D is the diameter of the vena cava and % represents the percentage of the vena cava to be replaced. *(Adapted from illustrations created by David Factor, Mayo Foundation. Courtesy Mayo Foundation for Medical Education and Research.)*

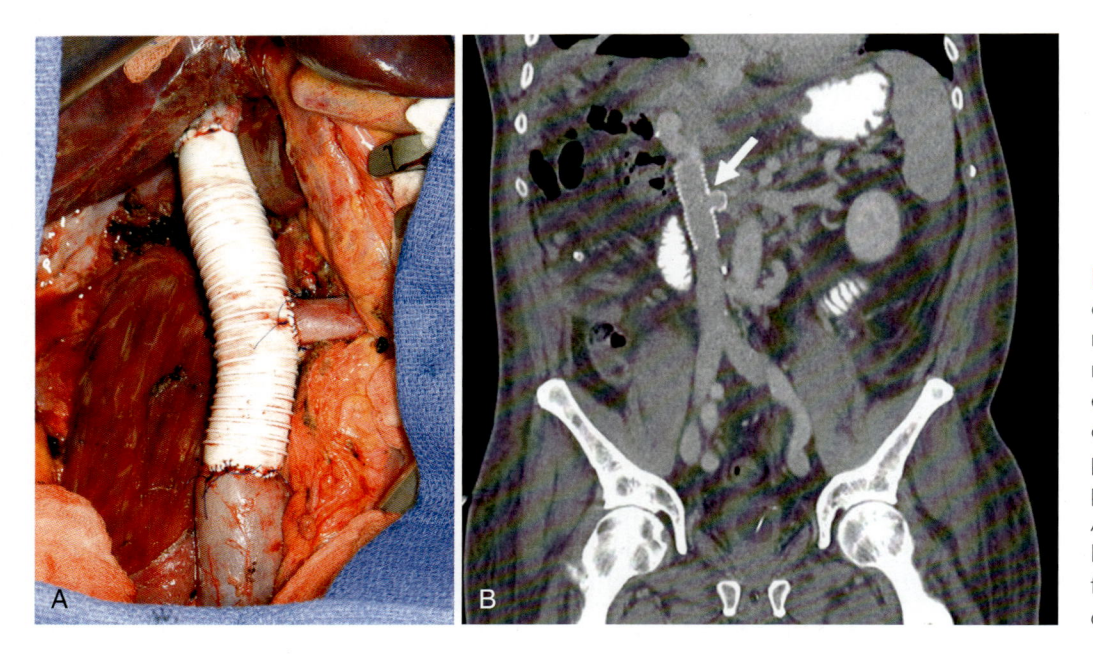

Figure 56-11. Resection of the pararenal vena cava requires salvage of the remnant renal vein. This can be achieved either by reimplantation (**A**) or by a separate ePTFE interposition graft, as shown in the postoperative CT image (**B**). A button is cut out of the PTFE graft to ensure blood flow from the renal vein is not compromised.

10- to 14-mm interposition graft with a circular button cut out of the caval graft to avoid compromise at the anastomotic site (Fig. 56-11).[21] When reconstructing the perirenal IVC, the cephalad anastomoses is performed first, allowing early restoration of outflow from the kidneys. Routine reimplantation of the left renal vein should be considered because the adequacy of collateral drainage may be difficult to assess after radical tumor resection. If both renal veins are to be reimplanted, the right renal vein is reimplanted first because of the lack of collateral drainage. Control of the right renal artery can prevent organ congestion. A continuous suture line is appropriate because preserved rings at the graft opening will prevent purse-stringing.

In controlling the suprarenal IVC, control of each renal vein is required. In particular, ligation of the right adrenal vein is recommended as a tear of this branch during retraction can lead to significant hemorrhage. Likewise, ligation of the hepatic vein draining the caudate lobe may be necessary to provide additional exposure of the IVC.

Special techniques are needed when the retrohepatic IVC requires replacement with concomitant major liver resection or when tumor thrombus is adherent to the caval wall.[5,8,11,12,18,21] The latter can be anticipated if tumor thrombus distends the IVC to 40 mm or more, if tumor thrombus is located at level III or IV, or if the renal vein orifice is dilated more than 14 mm on preoperative imaging.[21,26] Test clamping of the suprahepatic IVC should be performed to determine whether systolic blood pressure can be maintained at or above 100 mm Hg. If test clamping is not tolerated, venovenous bypass is required. This is achieved using a Bio-Medicus pump (Eden Prairie, Minn.), with placement of a right-angle cannula into the infrarenal IVC at the gonadal vein junction and extracorporeal return of venous blood into a large-bore jugular vein catheter (≥ 8 Fr).[21]

Total vascular isolation of the liver by inflow occlusion of the portal triad is used when the upper (cephalad) caval anastomosis is near the hepatic veins (see Fig. 56-6). This provides a bloodless field except in a rare patient who has a replaced right or left hepatic artery or lumbar veins in the retrohepatic cava. To facilitate correct positioning of the ends of graft and vena cava at the anastomosis, two double armed, 3-0 polypropylene sutures can be initially placed at the 4- and 8-o'clock positions. The back wall can then be run in continuous fashion followed by the anterior wall. The rings of the graft should be preserved up to the level of the anastomosis. Once the upper caval anastomosis is completed, inflow occlusion of the portal triad is released to wash out acid metabolites from the liver. Backbleeding is conducted in a head-down position, and the lungs are inflated to 30 cm of water by Valsalva maneuver. The graft is filled with heparanized saline and clamped distal to the caval anastomosis before the suprahepatic clamp is released.[8,11,21] Because the graft is thick walled, two aortic or coarctation clamps may be needed to avoid troublesome venous backbleeding through the graft while the lower (caudal) caval anastomosis is performed. To avoid graft redundancy, the length of the graft should be cut after maximal inflation and deflation of the lungs. Systemic heparinization is used selectively in patients with a history of deep vein thrombosis or partial caval thrombosis. Low-dose intravenous heparin (1000-3000 units) is administered for both iliac and IVC graft replacement. The dose of heparin is adjusted based on the weight of the patient, the amount of blood loss preceding the venous reconstruction, and the anticipated liver ischemia time. Alternatively, in the absence of a history of deep vein thrombosis, partial thrombosis of the IVC, or need for arterial reconstruction, heparinized saline (10 U/mL) alone can be used during the procedure.[27] Although intermittent pneumatic compression boots should be used throughout the procedure, this device should be turned off while performing the caval anastomoses.

If total liver isolation is used after the retrohepatic anastomosis is completed, the infradiaphragmatic clamp should be transiently released during a Valsalva maneuver. The portal triad clamp is then temporarily released, allowing back bleeding through the graft. The graft is then controlled, followed by release of the infradiaphragmatic clamp. The portal triad clamp is then released and the liver is allowed to reperfuse and is returned to its normal anatomic position.

A few points warrant comment for mobilization of the iliac arteries and veins during resection of pelvic and sacral tumors. For patients undergoing sacral resection, the anterior stage of the operation is done first. If the proximal extent of resection is to the L5 vertebral body, the lower IVC and aorta require mobilization. Mobilization of the common and external iliac arteries improves exposure of the veins. Control of the common and external iliac veins is done before attempting dissection of the internal iliac artery and vein branches. Blood loss during transection of the bone is reduced if branches of the internal iliac artery and vein are ligated to the superior, inferior, and lateral margins of resection. In select cases of high sacral resection, the posterior division branches of the internal iliac artery, such as the superior gluteal, should be preserved. The internal iliac artery branches are ligated and divided first, followed by the branches of the internal iliac veins. The main trunk of the internal iliac vein should be controlled but not ligated, whereas venous branches are isolated and ligated to avoid distention of the vein branches. Short, broad-based internal iliac vein branches require suture ligature for control. Care is required in mobilizing the posterior walls of the proximal common iliac veins and IVC, because short, broad, lateral and middle sacral veins often tether the larger veins to the periosteum and are easily torn, especially in irradiated or reoperative fields. A thick Silastic mesh is placed anterior to the sacrum but posterior to the vessels to protect against vascular injury when osteotomies are performed during the posterior stage of the operation. Omentum is used to wrap IVC grafts and to cover iliac vein grafts. Bovine pericardium is used in the absence of omentum.

Postoperative Care

- **Anticoagulation.** Heparin is administered through a small polyethylene catheter inserted near the inflow (caudal) venous anastomosis at 500 and 800 unit/hr after placement of a cross-pubic, iliocaval, or femorocaval graft. The dose is slowly increased, normally within 48 hours after operation, until the activated partial thromboplastin time is twice normal. The catheter is then removed and heparin is continued through a peripheral line.[22] Subcutaneous heparin the night of or morning after surgery may be a better alternative for patients whose surgery was conducted for resection of a pelvic or sacral tumor. Warfarin is begun with a goal of achieving an international normalized ratio of between 2 and 3 and is continued for at least 3 months in those with autogenous bypass and indefinitely in those with a prosthetic bypass or if thrombus of 20% or more of the lumen is noted in follow-up imaging.[21]
- **Intermittent pneumatic compression.** A lower extremity compression device is applied to the extremities, and the legs are kept elevated, with early ambulation encouraged. Patients are fitted with 30 to 40 mm Hg elastic compression stockings before discharge.
- **Management of an arteriovenous fistula.** If a fistula is created, it is left open for at least 6 months after operation but may be kept open longer for those with prosthetic iliocaval or femoral-caval bypasses that are longer than 10 cm.[22]
- **Vena cava filter.** Placement of a retrievable caval filter may be required after resection of a sacral or pelvic tumor resections.
- **Serial liver function tests (LFTs).** LFTs are monitored after combined major hepatic resection and retrohepatic IVC replacement. LFTs peak within the first 3 days after operation and then gradually return to baseline unless the liver ischemia time exceeded 30 to 40 minutes. In these cases LFTs may remain abnormal for as long as 7 days. Persistent elevation of the LFTs should prompt imaging of the hepatic artery, the IVC, and the hepatic and portal veins.[8,11,21]
- **Postoperative imaging.** Surveillance imaging with duplex ultrasound or CT imaging should be performed at 1, 6, and 12 months after surgery and annually thereafter.

Complications

- **Deep venous thrombosis.** The risk of lower extremity deep venous thrombosis is highest after resection of sacral and pelvic malignancies.
- **Lower extremity edema**
- **Graft thrombosis**
- **Graft infection**
- **Renal failure**
- **Coagulopathy**

REFERENCES

1. Warren R, Thayer TR: Transplantation of the saphenous vein for postphlebitic stasis, *Surgery* 35:867-878, 1954.
2. Palma EC, Esperon R: Vein transplants and grafts in the surgical treatment of postphlebitic syndrome, *J Cardiov Surg* 1:94-107, 1960.
3. Dale WA: Peripheral venous reconstructions. In Dale WA, editor: *Management of vascular surgical problems*, New York, 1985, McGraw-Hill, pp 493-521.
4. Perl L: Ein fall von sarkom der vena cava inferior, *Virchows Arch* 53:378-383, 1971.
5. Bower TC, Nagorney DM, Toomey BJ, et al: Vena cava replacement for malignant disease: Is there a role? *Ann Vasc Surg* 7:51-62, 1993.
6. Huguet C, Ferri M, Gavellia A: Resection of the suprarenal inferior vena cava: The role of prosthetic replacement, *Arch Surg* 130:793-797, 1995.
7. Beck SD, Lalka SG: Long-term results after inferior vena caval resection during retroperitoneal lymphadenectomy for metastatic germ cell cancer, *J Vasc Surg* 28:808-814, 1998.
8. Bower TC, Nagorney DM, Cherry KJ Jr, et al: Replacement of the inferior vena cava for malignancy: An update, *J Vasc Surg* 31:270-281, 2000.
9. Oldehafer KJ, Lang H, Schlitt HJ, et al: Long-term experience after ex situ liver surgery, *Surgery* 127:520-527, 2000.
10. Lodge JPA, Ammori BJ, Prasad KR, et al: Ex vivo and in situ resection of inferior vena cava with hepatectomy for colorectal metastases, *Ann Surg* 231:471-479, 2000.
11. Sarmiento JM, Bower TC, Cherry KJ, et al: Is combined partial hepatectomy with segmental resection of the inferior vena cava justified for malignancy? *Arch Surg* 138:624-630, 2003.
12. Arii S, Teramoto K, Kawamura T, et al: Significance of hepatic resection combined with inferior vena cava resection and its reconstruction with expanded polytetrafluoroethylene for treatment of liver tumors, *J Am Coll Surg* 239:712-721, 2004.
13. Hemming AW, Reed AI, Langham MR, et al: Combined resection of the liver and inferior vena cava for hepatic malignancy, *Ann Surg* 239:712-721, 2004.
14. Blute ML, Leibovich BC, Lohse CM, et al: The Mayo Clinic experience with surgical management, complications and outcome for patients with renal cell carcinoma and venous tumor thrombus, *BJU Int* 94:33-41, 2004.
15. Leibovich BC, Cheville JC, Lohse C, et al: A scoring algorithm to predict survival for patients with metastatic clear cell renal cell carcinoma: A stratification tool for prospective clinical trials, *J Urol* 174:1759-1763, 2005.
16. Yoshidome H, Takeuchi D, Ito H, et al: Should the inferior vena cava be reconstructed after resection for malignant tumors? *Am J Surg* 189:419-424, 2005.
17. Kieffer E, Alaoui M, Piette JC, et al: Leiomyosarcoma of the inferior vena cava: Experience in 22 cases, *Ann Surg* 244:289-295, 2006.
18. Cicnacio G, Livingstone AS, Soloway M: Surgical management of renal cell carcinoma with tumor thrombus in the renal and inferior vena cava: The University of Miami experience in using liver transplantation techniques, *Europ Urol* 51:988-995, 2007.
19. Haferkamp A, Bastian PJ, Jakobi H, et al: Renal cell carcinoma with tumor thrombus extension into the vena cava: Prospective long-term follow-up, *J Urol* 177:1703-1708, 2007.
20. Illuminati G, Calio FG, D'Urso A, et al: Prosthetic replacement of the infrahepatic inferior vena cava for leiomyosarcoma, *Arch Surg* 141:919-924, 2008.
21. Bower TC: Venous tumors. In Cronenwett JL, Johnston KW, editors: *Rutherford's vascular surgery*, ed 7, Philadelphia, 2010, Saunders, pp 983-995.
22. Gloviczki P, Oderich GS: Open surgical reconstructions for non-malignant occlusion of the inferior vena cava and iliofemoral veins. In Gloviczki P, editor: *Handbook of venous disorders: Guidelines of the American Venous Forum*, London, 2009, Hodder Arnold, pp 514-522.
23. Jost CJ, Gloviczki P, Cherry KJ, et al: Surgical reconstructions of iliofemoral veins and the inferior vena cava for nonmalignant occlusive disease, *J Vasc Surg* 33:320-328, 2001.
24. Nesbitt JC, Soltero ER, Dinney CPN, et al: Surgical management of renal cell carcinoma with inferior vena cava tumor thrombus, *Ann Thorac Surg* 63:1592-1600, 1997.
25. Garg N, Gloviczki P, Karimi KM, et al: Factors affecting outcome of open and hybrid reconstructions for nonmalignant obstruction of iliofemoral veins and inferior vena cava, *J Vasc Surg* 53:383-393, 2011.
26. Zini L, Destrieux-Garnier L, Leroy X, et al: Renal vein ostium wall invasion of renal cell carcinoma with inferior vena cava tumor thrombus. Prediction by renal and vena caval vein diameters and prognostic significance, *J Urol* 179:450-454, 2008.
27. Quinones-Baldrich WJ, Farley S: Techniques for inferior vena cava resection and reconstruction for retroperitoneal tumor excision, *J Vasc Surg Venous and Lym Dis* 1:84-89, 2013.

57 Transjugular Intrahepatic Portosystemic Shunt Procedure

EUGENE HAGIWARA • DARREN B. SCHNEIDER

Historical Background

In 1969 Rosch and colleagues[1] reported the first transjugular portal venography and portacaval shunt placement in a canine model. At that time, they foresaw the potential therapeutic benefits of transjugular intrahepatic portosystemic shunt (TIPS) placement and recognized the importance of selecting the appropriate stent material for optimal shunting. In 1982 Colapinto and co-workers[2] performed the first TIPS in a 54-year-old man with cirrhosis and bleeding esophageal varices. In 1988 the first successful TIPS performed with a bare metal stent was reported by Rössle and associates[3] at the University of Freiburg. However, in-stent stenosis and occlusion complicated a large number of early TIPS procedures. In the past decade the development of expanded polytetrafluoroethylene (ePTFE)–covered stents has led to improved patency rates and decreased clinical relapse rates.

Preoperative Preparation

- **Predicting survival after a TIPS procedure.** The Child-Pugh score and model for end-stage liver disease (MELD) score predict survival after a TIPS procedure. The Child-Pugh score includes serum albumin, bilirubin, and prothrombin time, as well as degree of hepatic encephalopathy and ascites. Using these five variables, a score between 1 and 15 is determined, and patients are categorized as class A, B, or C, with C indicative of the most severe level of hepatic dysfunction. The MELD score is calculated using an empirically derived formula based on serum creatinine, bilirubin, and international normalized ratio (INR) levels.

- **Management of upper gastrointestinal (UGI) bleeding.** UGI bleeding from variceal hemorrhage is initially managed by endoscopy and medical treatment, which successfully control bleeding in 80% to 90% of cases.[4] In both acute and recurrent variceal hemorrhage, endoscopy is required before the TIPS procedure for diagnosis, localization of bleeding site, and possible treatment. Placement of a Sengstaken-Blakemore tube in the acute setting may temporarily tamponade UGI bleeding. Early intubation should be considered to prevent aspiration. Packed red blood cell transfusion and fluid resuscitation may be required for hemodynamic stabilization, and fresh frozen plasma or platelets may be needed to correct coagulopathy.

- **Management of ascites.** TIPS may be considered for patients with ascites that is refractory to treatment by sodium restriction and diuretic therapy. Paracentesis may be performed prior to a TIPS procedure in those patients with large or tense ascites.

- **Cardiovascular evaluation.** Suspicion of right heart failure or pulmonary hypertension should prompt cardiology evaluation as both are relative contraindications to TIPS placement. In all patients, arterial blood pressure monitoring is recommended during the TIPS procedure.

- **Management of hepatic encephalopathy.** TIPS may lead to or exacerbate hepatic encephalopathy. Use of nonabsorbable disaccharides or antibiotics has not reduced this risk.
- **Duplex ultrasound examination.** Before the TIPS procedure, portal and hepatic venous systems should be evaluated by duplex ultrasound.
- **Prophylactic antibiotics.** Cephalosporin or, in the presence of a penicillin allergy, vancomycin is administered before the TIPS procedure.

Pitfalls and Danger Points

- **Intraperitoneal hemorrhage and injury to perihepatic structures.** Potential injury may occur to the gallbladder, kidney, bowel, pericardium, and abdominal wall. Avoiding these complications requires the intrahepatic portal vein to be accessed at least 2 cm from the left-right bifurcation while minimizing puncture of the liver capsule.
- **Correct selection and identification of the target hepatic vein**
- **Visualization and access of the target portal vein**
- **Selection of adequate shunt diameter and length**
- **Avoiding an acutely angulated shunt**

Endovascular Strategy

AVOIDING INTRAPERITONEAL HEMORRHAGE AND INJURY TO PERIHEPATIC STRUCTURES

Localizing the Catheter Tip in the Right Hepatic Vein

TIPS can be constructed from any large hepatic vein, but the right or middle hepatic vein is preferred. Most important, however, is recognizing which vein has been selectively catheterized. The ostium of the right hepatic vein lies more lateral to the middle hepatic vein and tends to course in a more lateral, often posterolateral direction, approximately in the coronal plane. Oblique projections during fluoroscopic imaging, as well as attention to the direction of the TIPS access needle hub, aid in this distinction with contrast injection further differentiating the right from the middle hepatic vein. In 85% of patients the middle hepatic vein and left hepatic vein originate from a shared ostium. The marginal right vein, a small tributary that courses within the superior right lobe and parallels the right hemidiaphragm, joins the right hepatic vein within a few centimeters of the inferior vena cava (IVC) and is not visualized in a middle hepatic venogram.

Mapping the Portal Venous System

Balloon occlusion wedged carbon dioxide (CO_2) venography helps map the portal venous system and aids in targeting and cannulation (Fig. 57-1). In some cases, however, hepatic vein collateral vessels may shunt away the injected CO_2 and thus prevent successful portal venography. It should be noted that iodinated contrast should not be used for wedged portal venography, because it does not easily cross the hepatic sinusoids and may lead to parenchymal staining. Wedged CO_2 venograms may be repeated in multiple projections to provide a mental map of the three-dimensional relationship between the hepatic vein and the portal vein. If wedged portal venography cannot be successfully performed, portal system access can still be established with "blind" passes toward the expected anatomic location of the right portal vein. Reviewing available cross-sectional imaging before the procedure is recommended.

Accessing the Portal Vein

Establishing access into the targeted portal vein is the crucial step in the TIPS procedure. The needle should be advanced in a single motion from the selected hepatic vein toward the portal vein, with a firm movement, only after careful consideration of the direction and approximate distance to the targeted vessel. It

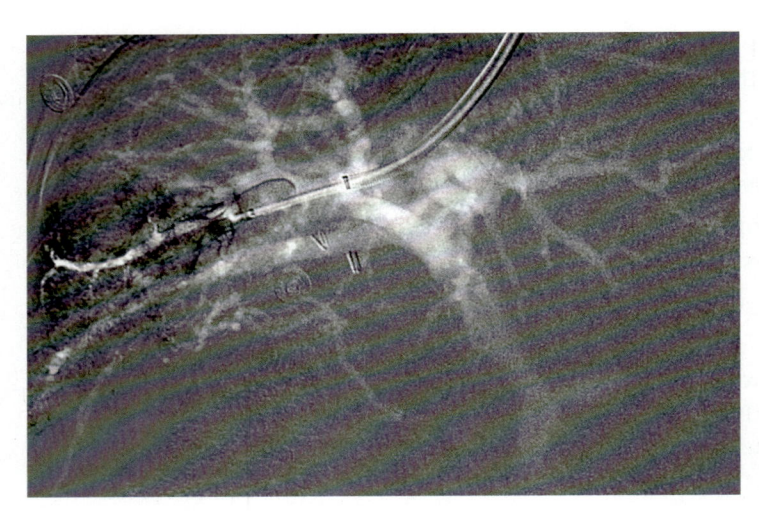

Figure 57-1. Wedged CO_2 hepatic venogram. CO_2 is injected through an occlusive balloon-tip catheter in the right hepatic vein, opacifying the portal system.

should be remembered that the consistency, as well as the size and morphology of the liver, is altered depending on the severity of cirrhosis.

AVOIDING DETERIORATION OF LIVER FUNCTION AND HEPATIC ENCEPHALOPATHY

Portosystemic Gradient Measurements

Measurement of baseline and the post-TIPS portosystemic gradient is necessary for determining the most appropriate size of the shunt, as well as for subsequent monitoring of stent function. Pressure measurements should be made at consistent, reproducible locations.

Target Portosystemic Gradient

The portosystemic gradient after TIPS should be no more than 12 mm Hg when performed for variceal hemorrhage and no more than 8 mm Hg for refractory ascites. Higher portosystemic gradients (e.g., 50% of baseline) have been advocated by some to minimize hepatic encephalopathy, but this must be balanced against the risk of clinical recurrence.[5]

AVOIDING TRANSJUGULAR INTRAHEPATIC PORTOSYSTEMIC SHUNT IN-STENT STENOSIS

Ideal Parenchymal Tract

The TIPS stent should follow either a straight or a gentle C-curve configuration. Acute angulation along the tract increases the risk of turbulence and shunt thrombosis. A TIPS tract from the right hepatic vein to the central right portal vein generally provides the straightest path. Access to or from different vessels or access of the portal system more peripherally increases the likelihood of angulation.

Selecting and Deploying the Appropriate Stent

The TIPS stent should extend from the portal vein to the junction of the hepatic vein and IVC. Simultaneous opacification of the portal-parenchymal junction and hepatic vein–IVC junction by injection through a marker pigtail catheter in the portal system and the TIPS introducer sheath in the hepatic vein allows accurate measurement of this distance. Depending on the curvature of the tract, it may be necessary to add 1 to 2 cm to the measured tract length. Outflow stenosis occurs if the covered stent is deployed short of the hepatic vein junction with the IVC.

Endovascular Technique

CHOICE OF ANESTHESIA

TIPS can be performed under conscious sedation, but general anesthesia may be preferred, because the procedure can be long and uncomfortable and requires careful physiologic monitoring and, in many cases, early intubation.[6]

PATIENT POSITIONING AND VENOUS ACCESS

The patient is placed in the supine position, and a limited ultrasound examination of the right internal jugular vein (IJV) is performed to confirm patency. The right IJV is the preferred route of access, because it provides a straight course to the IVC and favorable angulation to the hepatic veins. If access cannot be achieved through the right IJV, the right external jugular vein, left IJV, or right subclavian vein may also be used, though such access increases the difficulty of the procedure.

The right neck is prepped and draped in a standard sterile fashion. The right IJV access site should be slightly more superior relative to the clavicle than the typical site used for central line placement, because this allows better manipulation of stiff, large sheaths and introducers and facilitates manual compression for hemostasis. After local anesthesia is achieved with subcutaneous lidocaine, a small dermatotomy is made with a No. 11 blade and the right IJV is punctured with a 21-Ga needle under ultrasound guidance. Using modified Seldinger technique, after serial dilation, a 10-Fr TIPS introducer sheath is advanced into the right IJV over a 0.035-inch wire, across the right atrium, and into the intrahepatic IVC. The importance of serial dilation, using 8-, 10-, and possibly 11-Fr dilators cannot be overstated, because atraumatic introduction of the TIPS sheath with an angled obturator can be difficult.

SELECTIVE HEPATIC VENOGRAPHY

Once the sheath tip is placed within the IVC, the internal obturator is removed over the wire. The 0.035-inch wire should be kept in place with the tip in the infrarenal IVC to serve as a safety wire in maintaining IVC access. The right, or less preferably the middle or left, hepatic vein is then selectively catheterized. This can be accomplished with an angled-tip 4- or 5-Fr angiographic catheter and 0.035-inch angled-tip hydrophilic guidewire. The angiographic catheter and wire are advanced through the sheath alongside the safety wire into the IVC. The sheath is then retracted into the right atrium just superior to the IVC–right atrial junction, leaving the angiographic catheter and guidewire, as well as the safety wire, in place within the IVC.

Cannulation of the right hepatic vein can be performed by orienting the angled catheter tip laterally while slowly retracting the catheter until it falls into the hepatic vein. Once the selected hepatic vein is cannulated, the catheter is advanced into the hepatic vein. Oblique projections help to confirm selective catheterization of the laterally or posterolaterally oriented right hepatic vein. A selective hepatic venogram confirms both position of the catheter and adequate vessel size.

PORTOSYSTEMIC PRESSURE GRADIENT MEASUREMENT

Once the catheter is positioned peripherally within the main trunk of the right or other selected hepatic vein, the guidewire is exchanged for a stiffer 0.035-inch Amplatz wire. The catheter is then exchanged over the stiff wire for a 5-Fr occlusion balloon catheter (Boston Scientific, Natick, Mass.). The occlusion balloon should be positioned centrally, within 5 cm of the hepatic vein–IVC junction, to obtain more accurate pressure readings and to avoid vessel injury. The stiff wire can then be removed, and pressure measurements can be made through the occlusion balloon catheter, first without balloon inflation for measurement of the free hepatic vein pressure and then with balloon inflation to measure the wedged hepatic vein pressure. Adequate wedging can be verified by injecting a small amount of contrast through the balloon catheter and visualizing complete vessel occlusion with stasis of the injected contrast. The portosystemic pressure gradient is the difference between the wedged and the free hepatic vein pressure.

MAPPING THE PORTAL SYSTEM

A wedged CO_2 hepatic venogram is then performed, which requires digital subtraction angiography with image acquisition at 4 to 9 frame/sec (see Fig. 57-1). Approximately 40 mL of CO_2 is injected at a steady rate through the occlusion balloon catheter with the occlusion balloon inflated. Forceful injection can lead to hepatic laceration. Despite correct technique, the wedged CO_2 hepatic venogram may fail to opacify the portal venous system. This may be because of large collateral vessels among the hepatic veins or spontaneous portosystemic shunts. Although portal vein thrombosis is also possible, this cause should have been excluded by an initial ultrasound examination. Regardless, establishing portal vein access can be, and often is, accomplished without the benefit of fluoroscopic portal system road mapping. In conventional anatomy, the right and left portal veins both lie inferior to the central hepatic veins. In the anterior-posterior direction, the right portal vein lies between the right and the middle hepatic veins, whereas the left portal vein lies between the middle and the left hepatic veins. Thus when creating the preferred right hepatic vein–to–right portal vein tract, the needle should be advanced from the central right hepatic vein in an inferior and anterior direction.

ACCESSING THE PORTAL VEIN

A stiff wire, such as a Rosen or Amplatz wire, is advanced through the occlusion balloon catheter, and both are advanced peripherally in the hepatic vein for increased purchase. The 10-Fr TIPS introducer sheath is then advanced over the balloon catheter and stiff wire into the central hepatic vein. Timing the gradual advancement of the 10-Fr sheath with the patient's respiration is often helpful to avoid buckling.

With the tip of the 10-Fr sheath secure within the hepatic vein, the balloon catheter is removed. The TIPS puncture needle with its outer catheter is advanced over the stiff wire through the 10-Fr sheath. The stiff wire is removed, with slight forward pressure continuously applied to the sheath and needle to prevent retraction out of the hepatic vein. For a TIPS procedure from right hepatic vein to right portal vein, the needle is directed anteriorly and advanced in a single motion toward the anticipated location of the right portal vein. Depending on the particular TIPS kit used, the needle or the outer catheter is slowly retracted while gently aspirating with a contrast-filled syringe attached to the hub. For example, with the Rosch-Uchida access kit (Cook Medical, Bloomington, Ind.), the needle is first removed and the outer catheter is slowly retracted. When using the Colapinto needle (Cook Medical), the needle is slowly retracted.

Blood return within the syringe indicates access of the portal venous, hepatic venous, or hepatic arterial system. Once blood return is seen, a small amount of contrast is injected, revealing which of these systems has been accessed. Needle passes are repeated in this manner until the portal venous system is accessed. Once accessed, a 0.035-inch angled-tip hydrophilic guidewire is advanced through the access needle or catheter into the portal venous branch and directed through the main portal vein into the splenic vein. The outer catheter in both the Rosch-Uchida kit and the Colapinto system is advanced over the wire through the main portal vein into the splenic vein. The hydrophilic wire is exchanged for a stiffer wire, and the TIPS needle is exchanged for a 5-Fr calibrated pigtail catheter. The pigtail catheter is positioned within the splenic vein. Portal venous pressure is measured through the pigtail catheter. This is followed by a power-injected portal venogram, typically using 20-mL intravenous contrast at a rate of 10 mL/sec and a pressure of 800 to 1000 psi (Fig. 57-2). A portal venogram at the confluence of the splenic vein and superior mesenteric vein usually demonstrates multiple collateral vessels. Finally, a small amount of contrast is injected through the pigtail catheter while simultaneously injecting through the 10-Fr sheath. This allows measurement of the length of the TIPS tract from the portal-parenchymal junction to the hepatic vein–IVC junction for selection an appropriate covered stent.

CREATING THE PARENCHYMAL TRACT

Once the portal venogram has been performed and the length of the parenchymal tract has been measured, the pigtail catheter is exchanged over a stiff wire for an

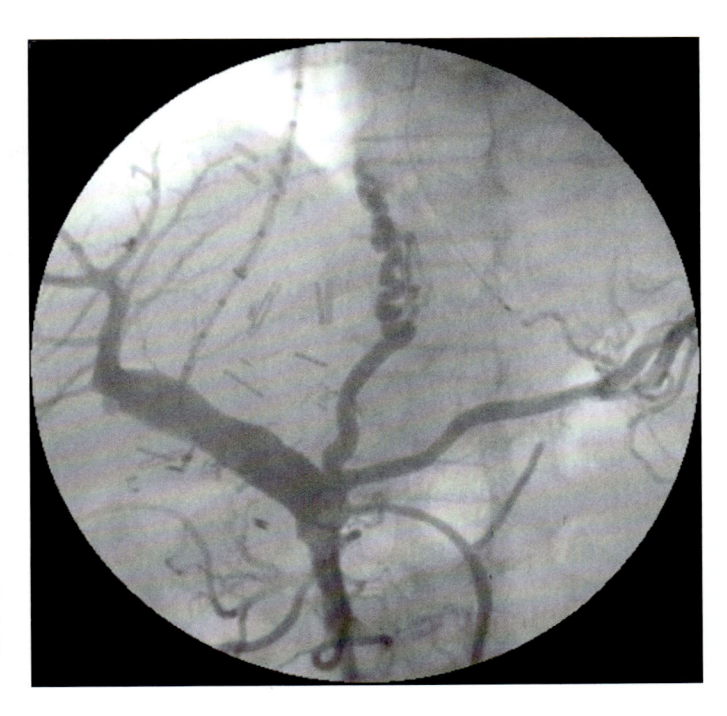

Figure 57-2. Transjugular portal venogram. A marker pigtail flush catheter is positioned in the main portal vein. Hepatofugal flow is demonstrated with opacification of gastroesophageal varices.

8-mm-diameter angioplasty balloon catheter. Balloon inflation is performed to dilate the parenchymal tract from the portal vein to the hepatic vein. The 10-Fr sheath is then advanced through the parenchymal tract into the portal vein.

DEPLOYMENT OF THE TRANSJUGULAR INTRAHEPATIC PORTOSYSTEMIC SHUNT STENT

The Viatorr endoprosthesis (W.L. Gore & Associates, Newark, Del.) is a self-expanding nitinol stent partially covered with ePTFE, designed for deployment along the parenchymal tract, with an additional 2-cm uncovered end, designed for deployment in the portal vein. The stent is loaded into the 10-Fr TIPS sheath and advanced to the sheath tip in the portal vein. The bare portion of the stent is not constrained by the rip cord and expands when unsheathed. Once the stent is in the appropriate position, the sheath is withdrawn, allowing the bare portion to expand. The sheath and stent are then gently retracted as a unit to fit the stent graft snugly into the parenchymal tract. The radiopaque marker that delineates the uncovered-covered seam is at the portal vein entry site. The sheath is then fully withdrawn, and the deployment rip cord is pulled to release the endoprosthesis, followed by balloon dilation with an 8-mm angioplasty balloon catheter.

COMPLETION PORTOSYSTEMIC GRADIENT MEASUREMENT AND PORTOGRAPHY

Venous pressures are measured through the TIPS sheath in the hepatic vein–IVC junction, as well as through a pigtail catheter in the portal system, with target gradients of no more than 12 mm Hg for variceal hemorrhage and no more than 8 mm Hg for ascites. However, these values are not universally agreed upon, and preventing hepatic encephalopathy is thought to require a gradient of at least 10 mm Hg. If the calculated portosystemic gradient exceeds the desired levels, balloon dilation of the TIPS stent can be performed.

A completion portogram is performed through a pigtail flush catheter in the portal system and should demonstrate good flow through the shunt, with minimal or no variceal opacification (Fig. 57-3). If the post-TIPS portogram demonstrates persistent opacification of large gastroesophageal varices or other portosystemic shunts, such as a splenorenal shunt, selective venography and transcatheter embolization should be performed.

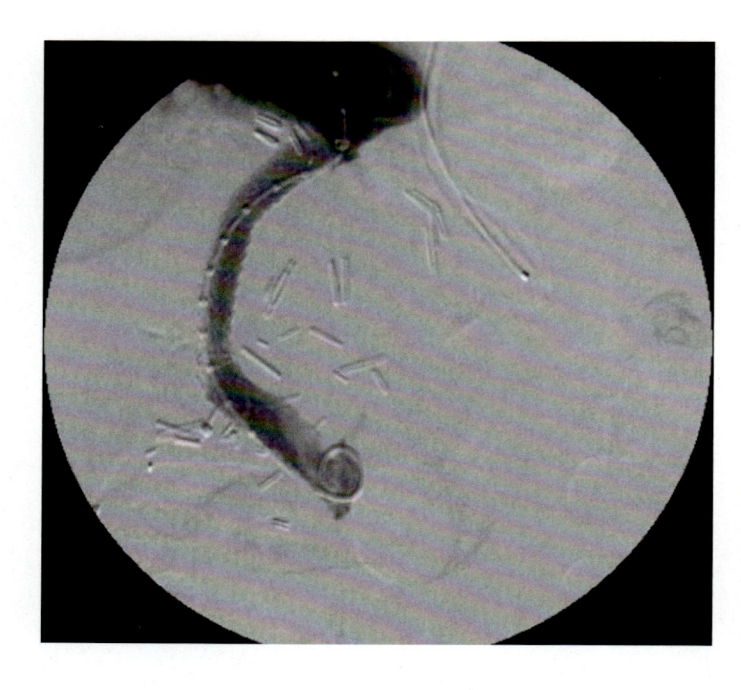

Figure 57-3. TIPS portal venogram. A marker pigtail flush catheter is positioned in the main portal vein. There is hepatopetal flow in the main portal vein with flow through the newly created TIPS and no evidence of opacification of gastroesophageal varices. The superior end of the stent extends to the hepatic vein–IVC junction.

Postoperative Care

- **Cardiovascular monitoring.** Patients should be transferred to the intensive care unit after TIPS placement. Right atrial pressure may be elevated with the newly diverted portal venous blood and in turn increase cardiac output.
- **Hematologic monitoring.** Monitoring is required for other potential complications, including intraperitoneal hemorrhage, hematobilia, and gastrointestinal bleeding. Given the risk of hemorrhage, serial blood counts should be followed and coagulopathy should be corrected.
- **Neurologic monitoring.** Patients should also be assessed for exacerbation of hepatic encephalopathy.
- **Renal function monitoring.** Serum creatinine levels should be monitored, because renal failure resulting from contrast nephropathy is a potential complication.
- **Shunt patency.** Duplex ultrasound examination should be performed within 2 weeks to confirm shunt patency.

Complications

- **Outcomes.** The technical success rate of TIPS is reported to be greater than 90%, with a low procedural mortality rate of 0.5% to 3% and a 30-day mortality of 3% to 42%.[7] The risk of significant intraperitoneal hemorrhage in elective cases is 1% to 2%. However, mortality from this complication increases to 27% to 50% when TIPS is performed emergently for acute variceal hemorrhage.[4]
- **Hemorrhage.** Intraabdominal bleeding and massive hematobilia may occur because of arterial injury during the TIPS procedure. If intraperitoneal or retroperitoneal hemorrhage is suspected, contrast-enhanced computed tomography imaging should be performed. Hematobilia may also be evaluated by upper endoscopy. Transcatheter angiography and embolization may be necessary to control bleeding.
- **Hepatic encephalopathy.** Worsening liver function and hepatic encephalopathy are the most important complications after TIPS, and both result from shunting of blood away from the liver. New or worsened hepatic encephalopathy occurs in 5% to 47% of patients, which can be controlled in the majority by medical therapy that includes lactulose and nonabsorbable antibiotic administration, but 3% to 7% of cases prove refractory and require TIPS revision or

other invasive treatment.[7-9] Options include liver transplantation, TIPS occlusion, and TIPS reduction using covered and bare stents.

- **Persistent or recurrent variceal bleeding.** In the acute setting, TIPS placement has a 89% to 100% success rate in controlling variceal hemorrhage, with a rebleeding rate of only 15%.[5] Failure to control bleeding indicates that the portosystemic gradient was not sufficiently reduced. In the early postprocedure setting, embolization of large varices, TIPS revision, or a new TIPS may be considered.
- **In-stent stenosis.** Shunt dysfunction because of TIPS in-stent stenosis is the cause of recurrent symptoms in most patients, including late rebleeding. Stents covered with ePTFE have dramatically improved 1-year primary and secondary patency rates to 76% to 84% and 98% to 100%, respectively, and have decreased the need for reintervention.[8] Repeat angioplasty or additional stent placement may be required.
- **Reaccumulation of ascites.** In patients with refractory ascites, a clinical response to TIPS is observed in 70% to 75% of patients. In those who do not respond, TIPS revision may be considered. Other options include continued aggressive medical therapy, serial paracenteses, and liver transplantation.
- **Portal vein thrombosis.** In the acute setting, portal vein thrombosis can be treated by mechanical thrombolysis. The risk of hemorrhage far outweighs the potential benefit of pharmacologic thrombolysis. In late occlusion, an uncovered stent can be extended along the TIPS stent to the level of the patent, non-thrombosed portal, splenic, or superior mesenteric vein.
- **TIPS stent infection.** The estimated incidence of a shunt infection is less than 2%. If infection of the stent graft is suspected, long-term antibiotics and/or liver transplantation may be required.[10]

REFERENCES

1. Rosch J, Hanafee W, Snow H: Transjugular portal venography and radiologic portacaval shunt: An experimental study, *Radiology* 92:1112-1114, 1969.
2. Colapinto R, Stronell R, Birch S, et al: Creation of an intrahepatic portosystemic shunt with a Grüntzig balloon catheter, *Can Med Assoc J* 126:267-268, 1982.
3. Rössle M, Richter GM, Nöldge G, et al: New non-operative treatment for variceal haemorrhage, *Lancet* 334:153, 1989.
4. Bouza E, Munoz P, Rodriguez C, et al: Endotipsitis: An emergic prosthetic-related infection in patients with portal hypertension, *Diagn Microbiol Infect Dis* 49:77-82, 2004.
5. Riggio O, Ridola L, Lucidi C, et al: Emerging issues in the use of transjugular intrahepatic portostystemic shunt (TIPS) for management of portal hypertension: Time to update the guidelines? *Dig Liver Dis* 42:462-467, 2009.
6. Kalva S, Salazar G, Walker G: Transjugular intrahepatic portosystemic shunt for acute variceal hemorrhage, *Tech Vasc Interv Radiol* 12:92-101, 2009.
7. Maleux G, Verslype C, Heye S, et al: Endovascular shunt reduction in the management of transjugular portosystemic shunt-induced hepatic encephalopathy: Preliminary experience with reduction stents and stent-grafts, *Am J Radiol* 188:659-664, 2007.
8. Rossle M, Grandt D: TIPS: An update, *Best Pract Res Clin Gastroenterol* 18:99-123, 2004.
9. Owen A, Stanley A, Vijayananthan A, et al: The transjugular intrahepatic portosystemic shunt (TIPS), *Clin Radiol* 62:664-674, 2009.
10. Kurmis TP: Transjugular intrahepatic portosystemic shunt: An analysis of outcomes, *ANZ J Surg* 79:745-749, 2009.

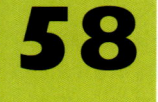

58 Endovascular Treatment of Iliofemoral and Femoral-Popliteal Deep Vein Thrombosis

ERIN H. MURPHY • MIHAIELA ILVES • FRANK R. ARKO III

Historical Background

Anticoagulation has long been considered the gold standard for treatment of lower extremity deep vein thrombosis (DVT). This therapy is effective at preventing DVT extension, pulmonary embolism, and DVT-related death. However, because anticoagulation does not dissolve thrombus, clot resolution is slow, relying on the intrinsic thrombolytic pathways. Although this is sufficient for isolated calf DVT, prolonged venous obstruction can lead to pronounced long-term morbidity in those with more proximal iliofemoral DVT.[1,2] Five-year follow-up of patients with iliofemoral DVT treated with anticoagulation alone demonstrates that up to 95% develop venous hypertension, 90% display venous reflux, 15% exhibit venous claudication, and another 15% develop venous ulceration.[2] Poor quality of life has been substantiated by further study.[2,3]

Early clot removal with surgical venous thrombectomy for iliofemoral DVT was first reported by Fogarty and colleagues in 1966.[4] Venous thrombectomy was demonstrated to improve long-term patency and substantially reduced the occurrence of postthrombotic symptoms and morbidity.[4,5] Nonetheless, this technique was highly invasive, which prevented widespread acceptance and implementation.

Systemic thrombolysis was assessed as an alternative to venous thrombectomy, with improvement in patient outcomes and venous patency correlating directly with the degree of lysis. Complete lysis, however, was only achievable in up to 50% of patients with nonocclusive thrombus and 10% of patients with occlusive thrombus. Clinical applicability of this strategy was further limited by unacceptably high rates of bleeding complications.[6] Thus for nearly a decade, strategies of early thrombus removal were abandoned, because the immediate risks of the procedure outweighed the significant long-term morbidity of iliofemoral DVT.

In 1994 Semba and Dake[7] were the first to demonstrate the effectiveness of catheter-directed thrombolysis using urokinase in the treatment of 21 patients with ileofemoral DVT. Complete lysis was achieved in 18 patients (72%) and partial lysis in 5 patients (20%). There were no major complications or clinically detectable PE. At 3 months, 12 limbs were studied with Doppler ultrasonography and veins were patent in 92%. Subsequent advancements in endovascular techniques have demonstrated the ability to achieve more effective clot removal while limiting systemic thrombolytic drug exposure and bleeding risks. In 2001 Kasirajan and colleagues[8] demonstrated the potential value of percutaneous mechanical thrombectomy to

ENDOVASCULAR TREATMENT OF ILIOFEMORAL AND FEMORAL-POPLITEAL DEEP VEIN THROMBOSIS

achieve symptomatic relief and clot removal in ileofemoral DVT using a rheolytic AngioJet catheter (Medrad, Inc., Warrendale, Pa.). In 2006 Lin[9] demonstrated that additional infusion of a thrombolytic agent via the AngioJet catheter increased the effectiveness of percutaneous mechanical thrombectomy in a technique referred to as power pulse spray mode. With limited risk and significant improvements in long-term clinical outcomes and venous patency, endovascular interventions should be considered for all healthy patients with proximal lower extremity DVT, good functional status, and reasonable life expectancy.

Preoperative Preparation

- **Preoperative imaging.** Because isolated calf DVT is best managed with anticoagulation, thrombus within the iliofemoral system should be documented before the decision to intervene. Although venography remains the gold standard for both the diagnosis and the assessment of DVT, this test is invasive and is reserved as a confirmatory study during intervention (Fig. 58-1). Alternatively, preoperative imaging with lower extremity duplex ultrasonography is noninvasive, convenient, and cost effective for the diagnosis of DVT (Fig. 58-2). Duplex imaging has a sensitivity and a specificity of 95% and 97%, respectively, for diagnosing proximal lower extremity DVT. Ultrasonographic evidence of

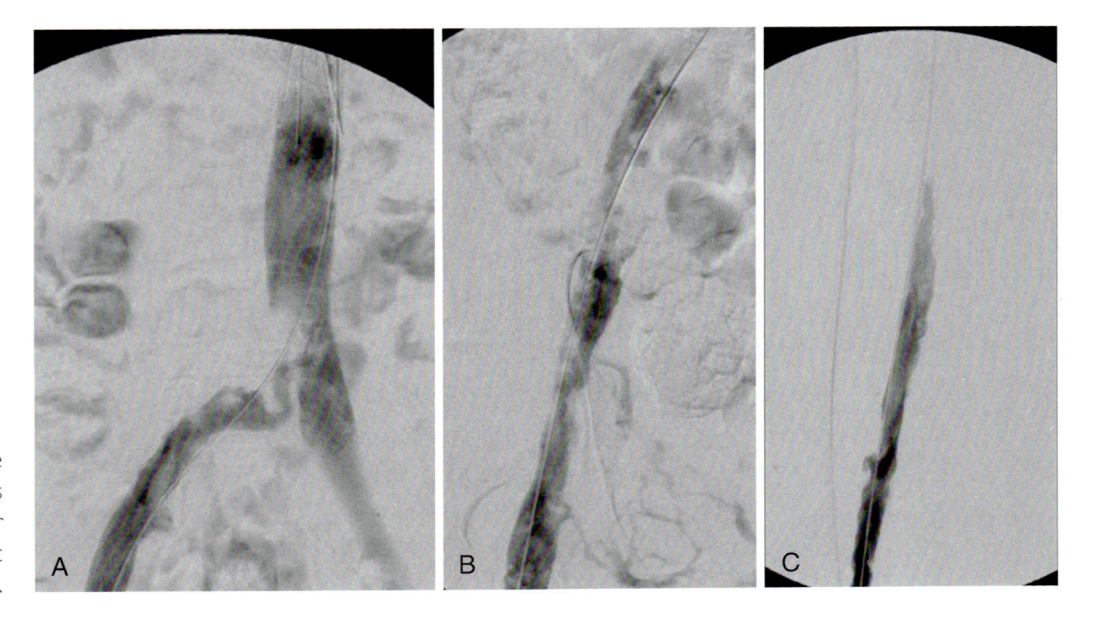

Figure 58-1. Intraoperative venography demonstrates thrombus within the inferior vena cava (**A**), common iliac vein (**B**), and femoral vein (**C**).

Figure 58-2. Ultrasound confirms thrombosis of the right common femoral vein in a woman with acute onset of right thigh pain. **A,** Before compression of the femoral vein with the ultrasound probe, an echogenic filling defect is noted within the lumen of the vein. **B,** Noncompressibility of the femoral vein confirms the diagnosis of DVT. *A,* Common femoral artery; *V,* common femoral vein.

DVT includes noncompressible or partially compressible venous segments with continuous venous flow patterns that lack normally phasic flow variation.[10]

- **Thrombophilia evaluation.** Evaluation for inherited thrombophilia is indicated for patients who present under 50 years of age with an unprovoked DVT, a family history of thromboembolism, unusual thrombus location, or with a recurrent DVT. Screening should include evaluation for protein C or S deficiency, antithrombin deficiency, factor V Leiden, protein C resistance, prothrombin gene mutation 20210A, hyperhomocysteinemia, and antiphospholipid antibody syndrome. Diagnosis of a thrombophilic disorder should prompt referral to a hematologist for long-term anticoagulation. A history of oral contraceptive use and malignancy should be sought, and evaluation for occult cancer should be considered.
- **Anticoagulation.** Therapeutic anticoagulation with unfractionated heparin or low-molecular-weight heparin should be administered preoperatively once the diagnosis is established and blood is drawn for evaluation of an inherited thrombophilia. Full anticoagulation should continue throughout the procedure and for at least 6 months thereafter. Longer periods of anticoagulation may be necessary for treatment of an underlying thrombophilia.

Pitfalls and Danger Points

- **Hemorrhagic complications.** Bleeding complications have been substantially reduced with the introduction of catheter-directed endovascular therapy for thrombolysis. The use of thrombolytics enhances the success of intervention, but if the risk is deemed too high, percutaneous mechanical thrombolysis (PMT) may be performed with saline infusate alone.
- **Recurrent DVT.** Treatment of recalcitrant thrombus and stenting of underlying lesions may reduce the risk of recurrent DVT.

Operative Strategy

TIMING OF INTERVENTION

Endovascular thrombolysis and thrombectomy procedures are ideally suited for early intervention. Patients can expect complete or near-complete clot and symptom resolution and preservation of venous valvular function if treated when symptoms have been present for less than 14 days.

Efficacy of DVT intervention decreases significantly as time from initial presentation increases. Several difficulties are encountered when attempting to treat chronic DVT. First, organized thrombus is often difficult to lyse even with aggressive treatment. Patients with chronic DVT and postthrombotic symptoms have also often developed venosclerosis, or diffuse venous scarring. In addition, damage to venous valves is likely irreversible after 14 to 30 days.

Nonetheless, venous recanalization and subsequent clinical improvement have been documented in patients with subacute and chronic DVT. In a series of 287 patients from the North American Venous Registry, complete lysis was achieved with catheter-directed thrombolysis (CDT) in 34% and 19% of patients with acute and chronic DVT, respectively. Significant partial lysis of greater than 50% was achievable in 64% and 47% of acute and chronic DVT patients, respectively. Better results have been obtained with the use of PMT alone or in combination with overnight CDT. Rao and associates reported that 17 patients (89%) with more than 14 days of symptoms underwent successful lysis and clinical symptom resolution. The two failures were in patients who were not considered candidates for adjunctive CDT after PMT.[11] Ultrasound-accelerated thrombolysis led to partial lysis in 96% of acute DVT (<14 days), 100% of subacute DVT (15-28 days), and 78% of chronic (>28 days) and acute-on-chronic DVT cases.[12]

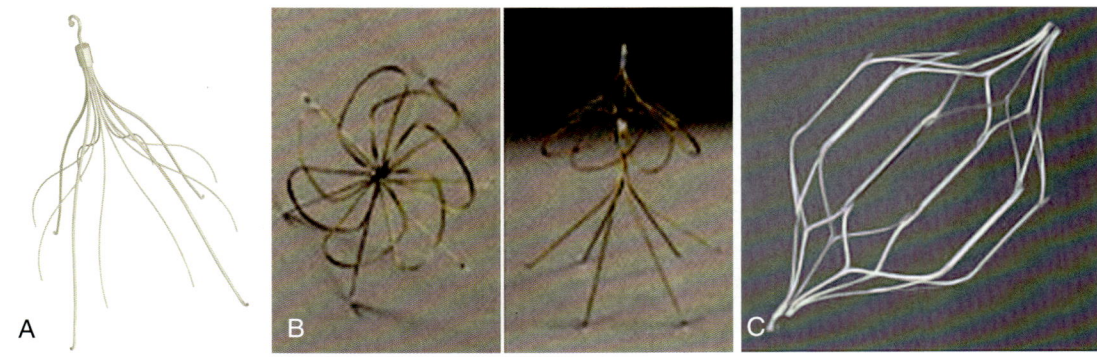

ENDOVASCULAR TREATMENT OF ILIOFEMORAL AND FEMORAL-POPLITEAL DEEP VEIN THROMBOSIS

Figure 58-3. Examples of temporary inferior vena cava filters. **A**, Gürther tulip. **B**, Simon Nitinol. **C**, OptEase/TrapEase. *(A, Courtesy Cook Medical, Bloomington, Ind.; B, Courtesy Bard Medical, Covington, Ga.; C, Courtesy Cordis, Bridgewater, N.J.)*

Patients with subacute and chronic DVT may be candidates for treatment with pharmacomechanical thrombectomy and catheter directed thrombolysis if debilitating symptoms are present in otherwise healthy, functional patients, who have a reasonable life expectancy.

ACCESS AND CROSSING THE LESION

Access is achieved in the vein distal to the occluded segment. An ipsilateral femoral puncture may be sufficient for isolated iliac and femoral DVT. More extensive DVT, particularly involving the femoral-popliteal segments, is best accessed from the ipsilateral popliteal vein. It is essential to use ultrasound guidance to confirm venous entry, because blood return may not be obtained upon venous puncture secondary to occlusion of venous flow. Use of a micropuncture technique is recommended to minimize bleeding complications in an anticoagulated patient who will be further exposed to a thrombolytic agent. A venogram should be obtained and the lesion crossed with a 0.035-inch guidewire before any intervention is initiated.

INFERIOR VENA CAVA FILTERS

Retrievable filters may be considered to prevent pulmonary embolization as the clot is disrupted (Fig. 58-3). Approximately 30% to 40% of patients have thrombus in filters retrieved after intervention.[13,14] The true incidence of symptomatic emboli is unknown but appears to be low.[15]

If a filter is used, it should be placed prior to intervention below the renal veins via a delivery route that is free of thrombus; most often from the contralateral femoral vein or right internal jugular vein. The filter can be retrieved at the end of the procedure or later if thrombus remains or a contraindication to anticoagulation exists.

Operative Technique

CATHETER-DIRECTED THROMBOLYSIS

Technique

A small multisidehole infusion catheter, such as a 4 or 5 Fr Uni-Fuse catheter (Angiodynamics, Latham, N.Y.) is advanced directly into the venous thrombus and secured at the most distal end of the thrombus load. The 4 Fr Uni-Fuse catheter is available in 90 and 135 cm lengths with infusion slit patterns of 5, 10, and 20 cm. The 5 Fr Uni-Fuse catheter is available in 45, 90, and 135 cm lengths with infusion slit patterns between 5 and 50 cm. Both catheters are compatible with a 0.035-inch guidewire. A thrombolytic agent is slowly administered while the patient is monitored in the intensive care unit (ICU). Blood sampling should be performed at 6-hour intervals to monitor hematocrit, platelet count, fibrinogen levels, and aPTT. Although debated, halting thrombolysis should be considered if fibrinogen levels fall below 150 mg/dL. The external portion of the catheter should be rolled into a coil that is secured under a transparent barrier film that should be monitored for hematoma formation. Repeat venography and assessment of clot lysis is performed at least once every 24 hours until complete lysis is achieved.

Thrombolytic Agents

Tissue plasminogen activator (tPA, Activase, Genentech, South San Francisco) or recombinant tissue plasminogen activator (r-tPA, Retavase, PDL BioPharma, Fremont, Calif.), or tenecteplase (TNK, Genentech) are commonly used thrombolytic agents and no significant differences have been observed with regard to success rate or major complications. Recommended doses for continuous catheter-directed thrombolytic infusion include tPA 0.5 to 1.0 mg/hour, r-tPA 0.25 to 0.75 U/hour, and TNK 0.25 to 0.5 mg/hour. Concomitant heparin is delivered at 500 U/hour.

Outcomes

Successful clot lysis has been reported in 60% to 90% in patients with proximal DVT.[16-18] Improvements in long-term venous patency and prevention of postthrombotic syndrome correlate with the degree of thrombolysis.

Advantages

CDT allows lytic infusion at the location of venous thrombosis, thus maximizing effect and limiting overall drug dosages and systemic lytic exposure.

Disadvantages

The ICU stay during drug infusion may range from 36 to 72 hours. Expensive drug costs can be attributed to the large amount of lytics used during lysis. Significant bleeding complications are not eliminated, with insertion site bleeding as high as 45%, transfusion requirements in up to 22% of patients, and intracranial bleeding in up to 33% of patients.[19]

ULTRASOUND-ACCELERATED THROMBOLYSIS: EKOSONIC ENDOVASCULAR SYSTEM

Mechanism

The EkoSonic endovascular system uses low-power, high-frequency (2 MHz) ultrasound, in combination with catheter-directed thrombolysis, to achieve clot lysis. Ultrasound waves create microstreams through the thrombus, allowing greater permeability and distribution of lytics.

Device

The EkoSonic device consists of an infusion and aspiration catheter, an ultrasound core wire, and a drive unit (Fig. 58-4). Catheters are available in treatment lengths of 6 to 50 cm, which accommodate the 0.035-inch ultrasound wire and normal saline infusate used for central cooling during use. Three infusion channels containing microinfusion pores for drug delivery are arranged in a triangular distribution around the central lumen. Thermocouples monitor changes in temperature and flow patterns. The ultrasound core wire has transducers (2.2 MHz) located at 1-cm intervals. When the drive unit is activated, ultrasound waves are delivered to the core wire and transmitted through the catheter, penetrating thrombus and allowing lytic dispersion.

Technique

The catheter is positioned so that the treatment zone extends through the length of the thrombosed venous segment. The guidewire is exchanged for the ultrasound core wire. Three separate drug infusion lumens are primed with unfractionated heparin. The control unit is activated delivering ultrasound energy via the core wire while the thrombolytic agent of choice is administered. Normal saline

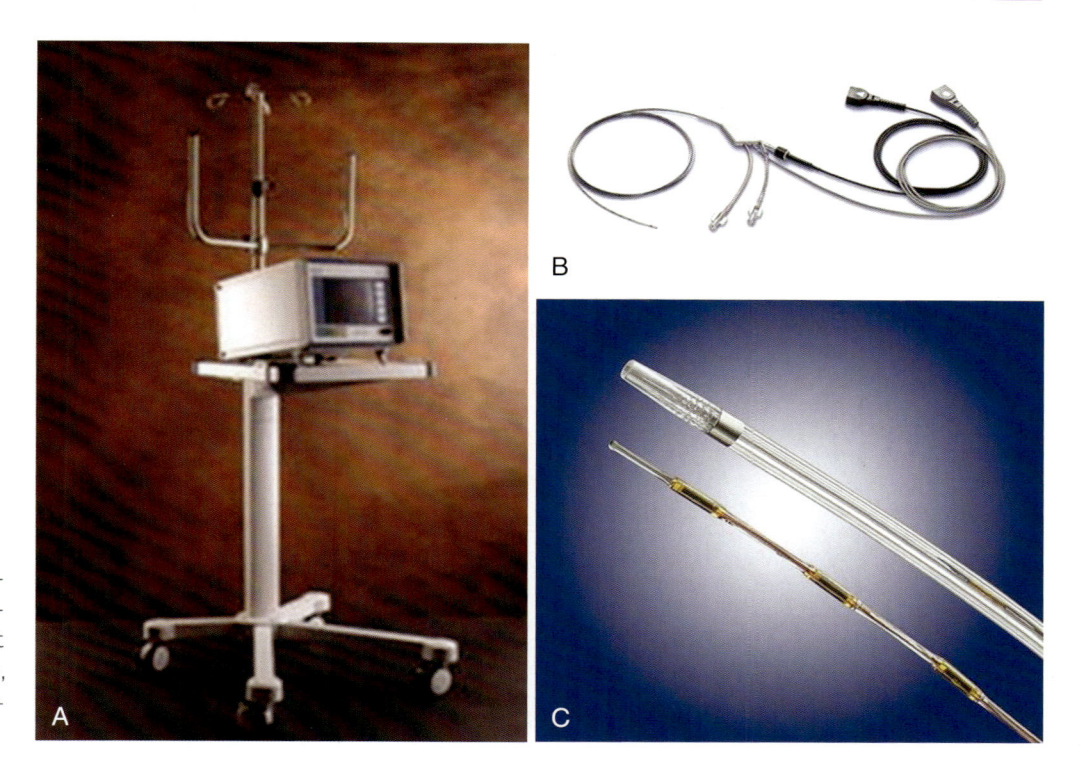

Figure 58-4. EkoSonic endovascular system. Three components include the control unit (**A**), drug delivery catheter (**B**), and ultrasound core (**C**). *(Courtesy Ekos, Bothell, Wash.)*

is infused continuously through the central lumen during the procedure to dissipate heat produced during the process. The power of the ultrasound energy is adjusted automatically as flow is restored in the venous segment. The procedure is continued until complete lysis is achieved.

Outcomes

Ultrasound-mediated increase in thrombus permeability leads to a 44% reduction in the diameter of fibrin strands and a 65% increase in the number of fibrin strands exposed to the thrombolytic agent.[20] Thrombus uptake of recombinant tissue plasminogen activator during ultrasound-accelerated thrombolysis increases by 48%, 84%, and 89% at 1, 2, and 4 hours, respectively.[21] Greater than 90% clot lysis was demonstrated in 70% and partial thrombus resolution achieved in 91% of patients.[12]

Advantages

Lower median lytic infusion times of 22 hours and a low incidence of bleeding complications (3.8%) have been noted.[12] These lead to decrease in overall ICU stay and lower perioperative risk compared with standard CDT.

Disadvantages

ICU stay is still required during drug infusion, and bleeding complications have not been eliminated. Total drug costs remain high compared with PMT.

RHEOLYTIC THROMBECTOMY: ANGIOJET POWER PULSE SPRAY TECHNIQUE

Mechanism

High-velocity infusion jets create a localized low-pressure zone in accordance with Bernoulli's principle at the catheter tip, macerating thrombus and redirecting flow and debris into outflow channels behind the catheter tip for aspiration and removal.

Device

The AngioJet catheter system is composed of a single-use catheter, a single-use pump set, and a drive unit. The drive unit is capable of generating 10,000 psi of pulsatile infusion flow, which is released from the catheter in retrograde-directed, high-velocity

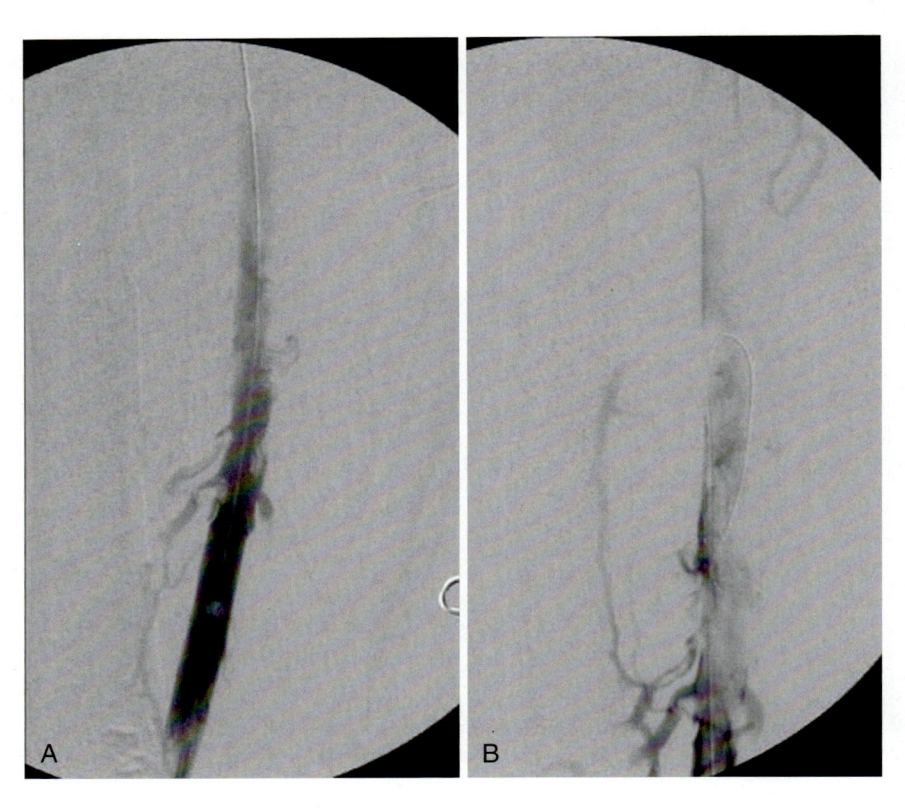

Figure 58-5. Residual thrombus after AngioJet pulse spray therapy is noted on venography (**A** and **B**) in a patient with DVT of the left iliac, femoral, and popliteal veins.

saline jets. The catheter, which is available in working lengths of 60, 100, and 120 cm, contains a central lumen for the infusate and a larger lumen encompassing the central channel, the guidewire, and aspirate from the thrombus. Thrombolytics may be added to the infusate to improve the degree of achievable thrombolysis.

Technique

The AngioJet catheter is advanced over a 0.035-inch guidewire through the thrombus load. With the aspiration port clamped, the infusate is released into the thrombosed venous segment during a slow pullback of the catheter, effectively lacing the clot with thrombolytic drug. After 10 minutes, the aspiration function of the catheter is turned on. The catheter is then slowly advanced through the thrombosed segment a second time, removing macerated thrombus through the aspiration ports as the catheter is advanced. This process may be repeated if there is remaining thrombus burden at the end of the first pass (Fig. 58-5).

Outcomes

Modest results, with 59% of patients achieving at least 50% lysis, have been reported without the addition of lytics to the infusate during use of the AngioJet system.[22] However, superior results are clearly obtained with the use of thrombolytics. In this setting at least partial resolution can be expected in all patients, and complete resolution has been demonstrated in more than 60% of patients.[23] Venous patency may be restored in 90% of patients and venous valvular function may be maintained in 88% of patients over a 6-month follow-up period.[24]

Advantages

The AngioJet device may be used without the addition of thrombolytics in patients with absolute contraindications to anticoagulation, although outcomes are suboptimal. However, even with the use of a thrombolytic agent, systemic exposure is limited, with a relatively low risk of hemorrhagic complication.

Disadvantages

Bradyarrythmias ranging from bradycardia to complete asystole can occur during rheolytic thrombectomy. The mechanism is unknown but may be related to stretching of receptors in the vein wall.[25] Anesthesia should be forewarned about the possibility of intraprocedural arrhythmias before starting the thrombectomy. Rare cases of pancreatitis have also been reported and attributed to hemolysis that occurs with rheolytic thrombectomy.[26]

TRELLIS-8 PERIPHERAL INFUSION SYSTEM

Mechanism

Lytic infusion is limited between two isolation balloons inflated proximal and distal to the thrombosed venous segment, while a dispersion wire oscillates in the treated segment to increase thrombus permeability. The Trellis-8 device (Covidien, Mansfield, Mass.) allows high local drug concentration while limiting systemic lytic exposure.

Device

The Trellis-8 device consists of a single-use catheter, a dispersion wire, and an integral drive unit. The catheter contains proximal and distal occlusion balloons and has a central lumen to accommodate both the dispersion wire and the infusate. Catheters are available in lengths of 80 or 120 cm, with varied distances between occlusion balloons, allowing treatment of 10-, 15-, or 30-cm venous segments.

Technique

The catheter is positioned across the thrombosed segment. With proximal and distal balloons inflated, 5 to 10 mg of lytic is infused within the thrombus. After 10 minutes, the dispersion wire, which is attached to the integral drive unit, is inserted into the catheter. The drive unit creates catheter oscillation at 500 to 3500 rpm, causing dispersion of lytics within the thrombus load and mechanical clot disruption. The dispersion wire may be advanced farther and retracted once a minute during the treatment interval to further assure mixing of the lytics within the thrombus. After 5 to 15 minutes, the distal balloon is deflated and the catheter is aspirated via a side port to remove macerated thrombus and a substantial portion of the remaining lytics. During aspiration the proximal balloon is left inflated to prevent thrombus embolization. After aspiration, with both balloons deflated, the system may be removed or advanced into adjacent thrombosed segments, repeating the procedure until the thrombus load is resolved (Fig. 58-6).

Outcomes

The Trellis-8 has been demonstrated to achieve more effective clot lysis than CDT, with 93% of patients achieving at least 50% lysis, compared with only 79% of patients for CDT. There were no bleeding complications, as compared to an 8.5% incidence of bleeding in patients undergoing CDT.[27] Additional studies have confirmed up to 96% grade II or III lysis and 100% venous patency at 30 days.[28] Clot resolution has been observed in 80% of patients in a single setting, with 88% venous patency at 6-month follow-up.[24] Although slightly less effective clot lysis has been noted compared with the AngioJet system (72% vs. 88%), clinical outcomes are similar with both devices (Figs. 58-7 and 58-8).

Advantages

Hemorrhagic complications are rare because systemic lytic exposure is limited. Lower overall cost can be achieved because of lower drug dosages, shorter hospital stays, and a decreased or eliminated ICU stay.[24,27,28]

Disadvantages

Even though thrombolytic exposure is minimized, the Trellis-8 technique is probably not suitable for patients with an absolute contraindication to thrombolysis.

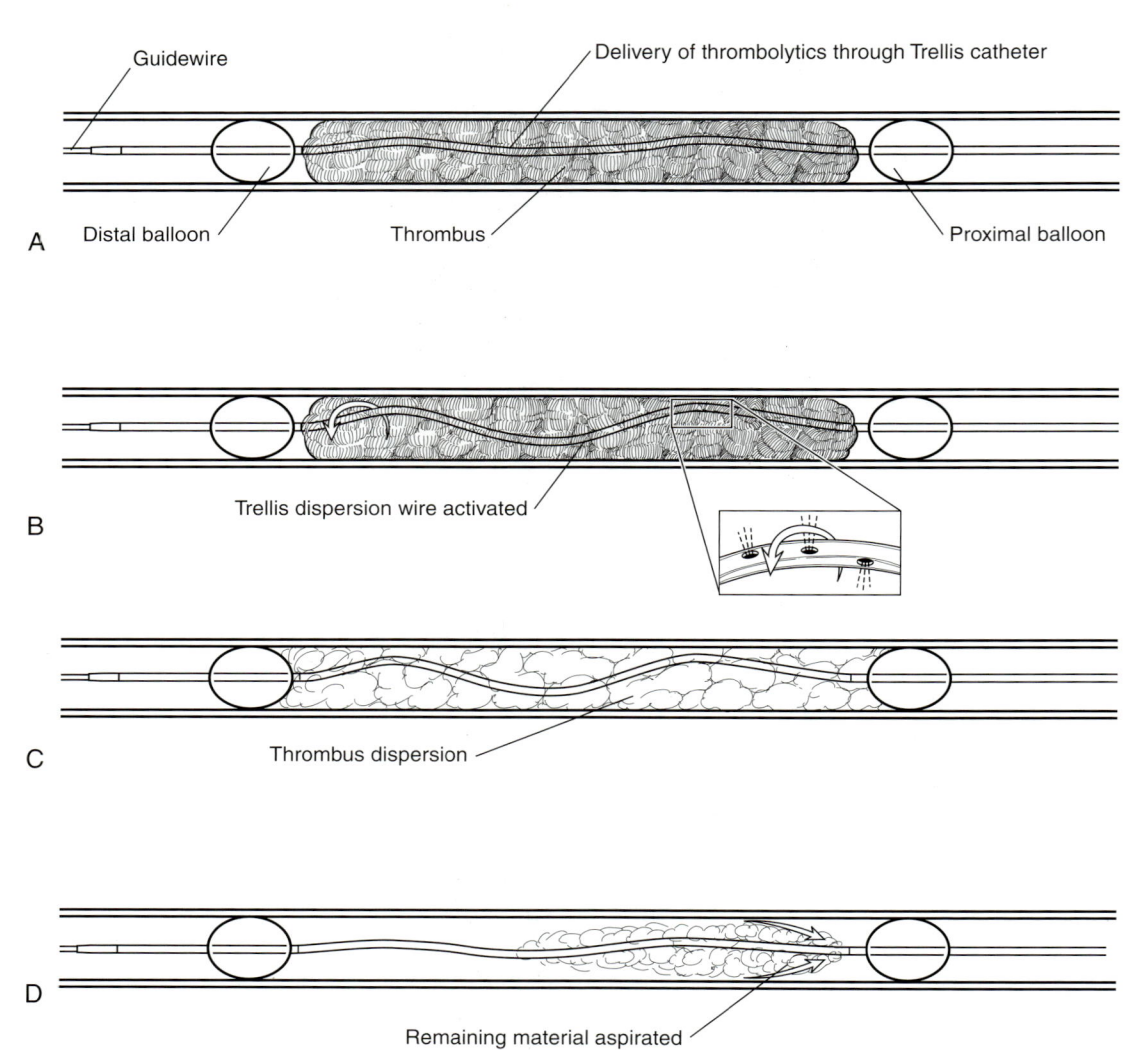

Figure 58-6. Thrombolytic treatment for DVT using the Trellis-8 peripheral infusion system. **A**, After percutaneous access, the Trellis catheter is advanced through the clot. The distal and proximal occluding balloons are inflated, after which delivery of the thrombolytic agent is initiated. **B**, The Trellis dispersion wire is activated using a motorized drive unit. **C** and **D**, Residual thrombus debris after clot dispersion is aspirated through the Trellis catheter.

Adjunctive Treatment

RECALCITRANT THROMBUS

Outcomes are directly correlated with the degree of thrombolysis achieved. If more than 30% of the lumen is occupied by thrombus as noted by completion venography or intravascular ultrasound, further treatment is warranted.

Multiple options exist for treatment of the remaining thrombus. A second PMT device can be used with a lower dose of thrombolytic. Alternatively, overnight CDT therapy may be used after clot debulking with PMT. This significantly reduces the time required for effective CDT and the associated bleeding risk.[11,23,24]

ILIAC VEIN STENOSIS

Most patients with iliofemoral DVT have an underlying venous stenosis. May-Thurner syndrome is the most common anomaly noted, with a venous stenosis occurring secondary to compression of the left common iliac vein against the fifth lumbar vertebrae by the overlying right common iliac artery (Fig. 58-9). This condition predisposes to left iliofemoral DVT, particularly among women.[29] Early thrombus removal without treatment of the underlying stenosis can lead to recurrent DVT.[30] This anatomic variant requires venous angioplasty and stenting with 100% symptom resolution, preservation of valve function, and prevention of postthrombotic syndrome.[30]

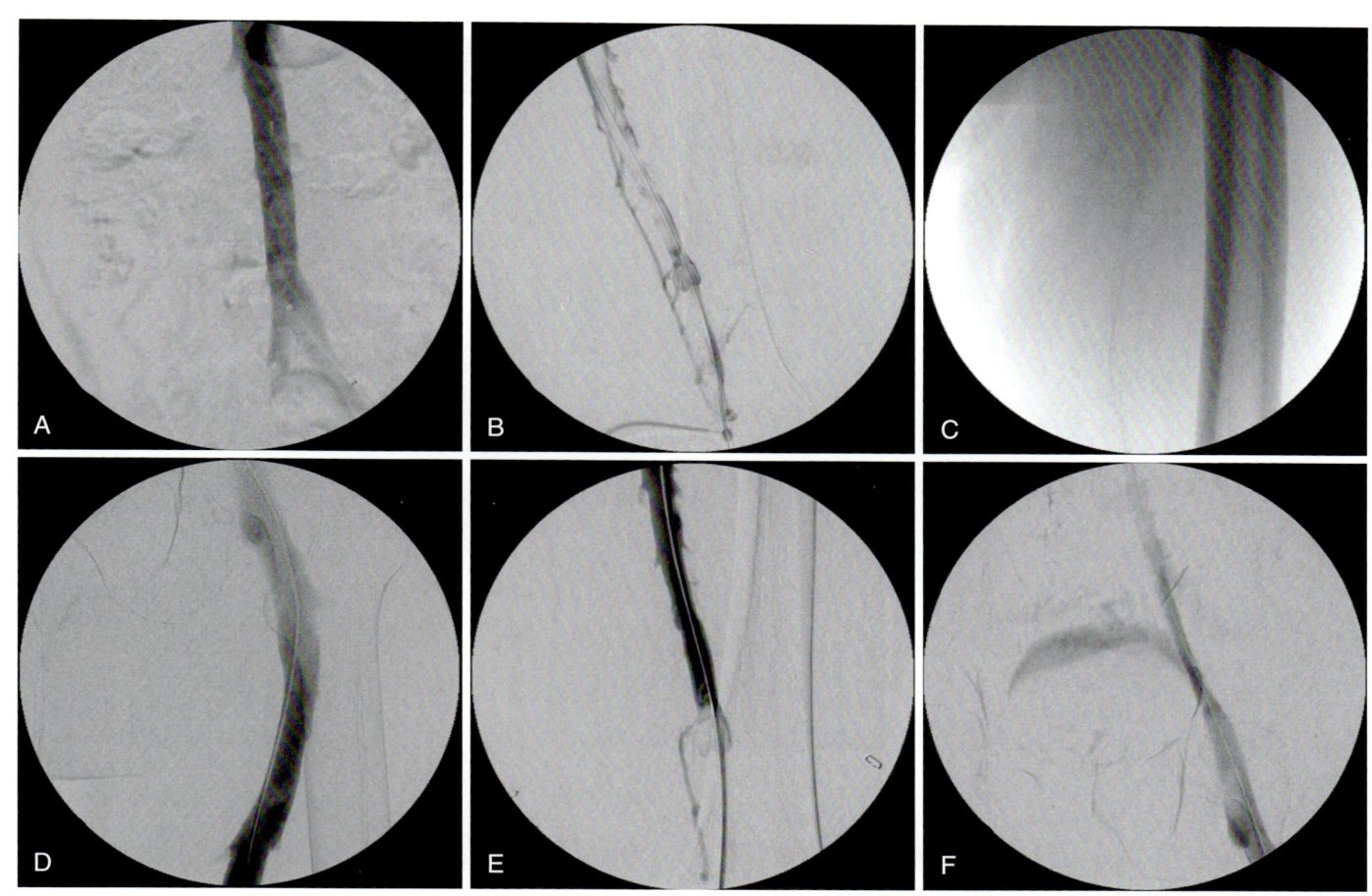

ENDOVASCULAR TREATMENT OF ILIOFEMORAL AND FEMORAL-POPLITEAL DEEP VEIN THROMBOSIS   681

Figure 58-7. Clot lysis of a symptomatic DVT in the left lower extremity using the Trellis-8 peripheral infusion system. **A**, An inferior vena cava filter is placed from an access site in the right femoral vein. **B**, Venography confirms thrombosis of the femoral vein. **C**, The Trellis catheter is positioned across the thrombus, with visualization of the sine wave of the Trellis wire. **D** and **E**, The femoral vein is cleared of thrombus after mechanical thrombectomy, and no residual thrombus noted in the common femoral vein (**F**).

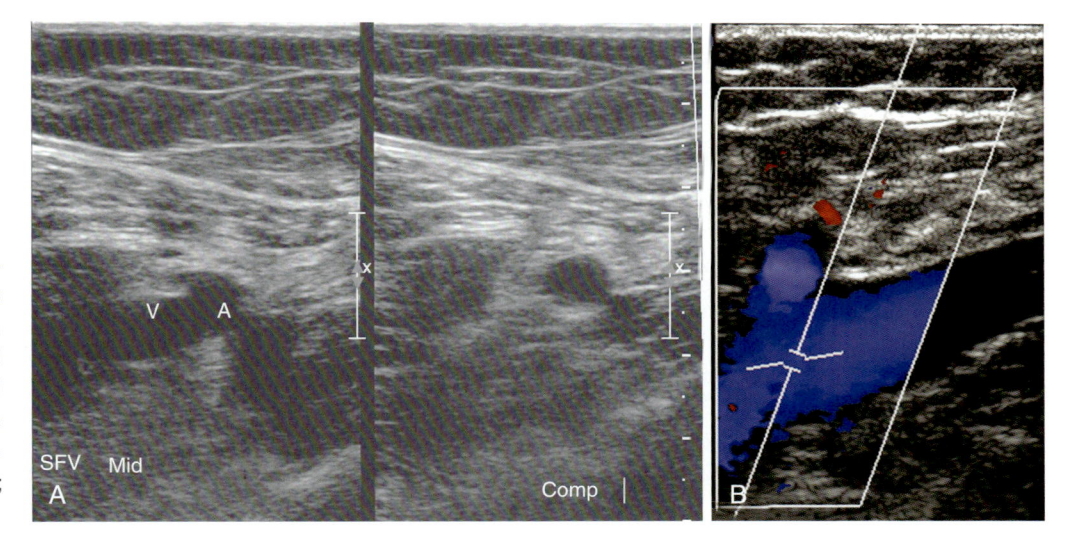

Figure 58-8. Ultrasound confirms the absence of thrombus within the midfemoral vein with B-mode ultrasound (**A**) and color flow duplex ultrasound (**B**) after treatment with the Trellis-8 peripheral infusion system. *A*, Superficial femoral artery; *V*, femoral vein.

Postoperative Care

- **Anticoagulation.** Patients should be anticoagulated with unfractionated heparin or low-molecular-weight heparin and transitioned to oral warfarin for 6 months. Lifelong aspirin (81 mg/day) should be considered in all patients with venous stents. Hematology consultation is recommended for patients with recurrent DVT or hypercoagulable disorders, because longer duration or higher levels of anticoagulation may be required.

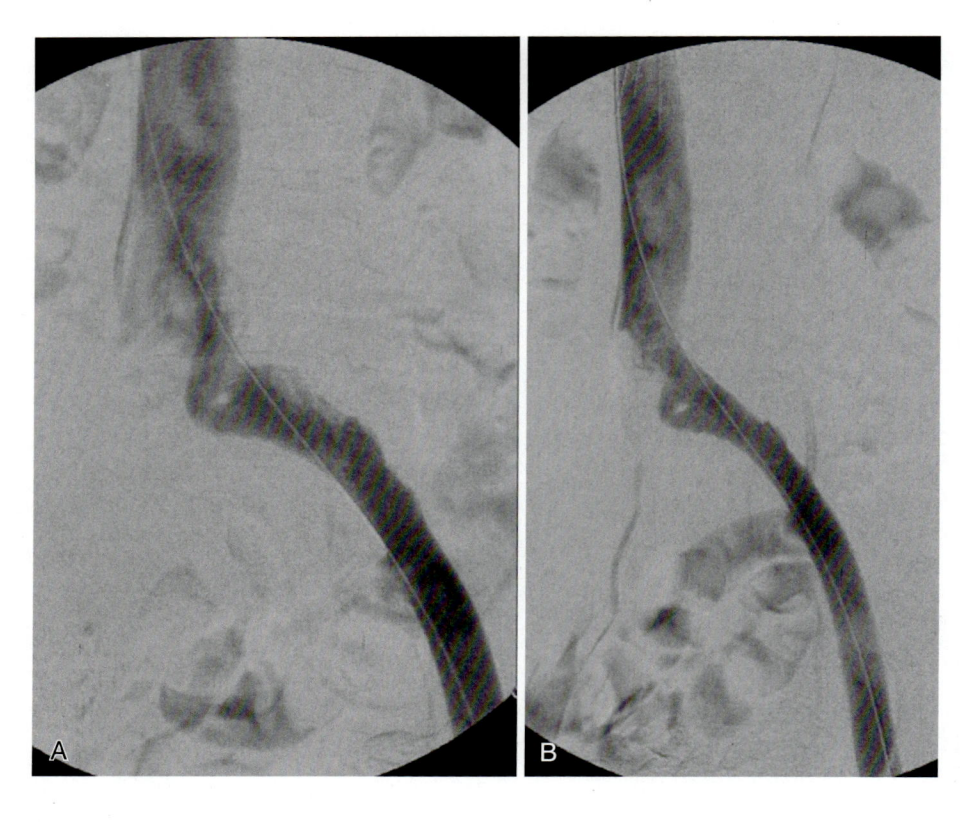

Figure 58-9. A, Imaging of the left iliac vein after treatment of an iliofemoral DVT secondary to May-Thurner syndrome with the Trellis-8 catheter system. **B,** Completion venography after angioplasty and stenting of the left iliac vein.

- **Surveillance imaging.** Patients should be followed with duplex ultrasonography at 1 month, 6 months, and yearly thereafter. Repeat venography and intervention should be considered for patients with recurrent DVT, with thorough evaluation for untreated venous stenosis.

Complications

- Bleeding
- Stroke
- Recurrent venous thrombosis

REFERENCES

1. Akesson H, Brudin L, Dahlstom JA, et al: Venous function assessed during a 5 year period after ilio-femoral venous thrombosis treated with anticoagulation, *Eur J Vasc Surg* 4:43-48, 1990.
2. O'Donnell TF Jr, Browse NL, Burnand KG, et al: The socioeconomic effects of an iliofemoral venous thrombosis, *J Surg Res* 22:483-488, 1977.
3. Delis KT, Bountouroglou D, Mansfield AO: Venous claudication in iliofemoral thrombosis: Long-term effects on venous hemodynamics, clinical status, and quality of life, *Ann Surg* 239:118-126, 2004.
4. Fogarty TJ, Dennis D, Krippaehne WW: Surgical management of iliofemoral venous thrombosis, *Am J Surg* 112:211-217, 1966.
5. Plate G, Eklof B, Norgren L, et al: Venous thrombectomy for iliofemoral vein thrombosis: 10 year results of a prospective randomized study, *Eur J Vasc Endovasc Surg* 14:367-374, 1997.
6. Comerota AJ, Aldridge SA: Thrombolytic therapy for acute deep vein thrombosis, *Semin Vasc Surg* 5:76-84, 1992.
7. Semba CP, Dake MD: Iliofemoral deep venous thrombosis: Aggressive therapy with catheter-directed thrombolysis, *Radiology* 191:487-494, 1994.
8. Kasirajan K, Gray B, Ouriel K: Percutaneous AngioJet thrombectomy in the management of extensive deep venous thrombosis, *J Vasc Interv Radiol* 12:179-185, 2001.
9. Lin PH, Zhou W, Dardik A, et al: Catheter-direct thrombolysis versus pharmacomechanical thrombectomy for treatment of symptomatic lower extremity deep venous thrombosis, *Am J Surg* 192:782-788, 2006.
10. Kraaijenhagen RA, Lensing AW, Wallace JW, et al: Diagnostic management of venous thromboembolism, *Baillieres Clin Haematol* 11:541-586, 1998.

11. Rao A, Konig G, Leers S, et al: Pharmacomechanical thrombectomy for iliofemoral deep venous thrombosis: An alternative in patients with contraindications to thrombolysis, *J Vasc Surg* 50:1092-1098, 2000.
12. Parikh S, Motarjeme A, McNamara T, et al: Ultrasound-accelerated thrombolysis for the treatment of deep vein thrombosis: Initial clinical experience, *J Vasc Interv Radiol* 19:521-528, 2008.
13. Trerotola SO, McLennan G, Eclavea AC, et al: Mechanical thrombolysis of venous thrombosis in an animal model with use of temporary caval filtration, *J Vasc Interv Radiol* 12:1075-1085, 2001.
14. Thery C, Bauchart J, Lesenne M, et al: Predictive factors of effectiveness of streptokinase in deep venous thrombosis, *Am J Cardiol* 69:117-122, 1992.
15. Herrera S, Comerota AJ: Embolization during treatment of deep venous thrombosis: Incidence, importance, and prevention, *Tech Vasc Interv Radiol* 14:58-64, 2011.
16. Comerota AJ, Throm RC, Mathias SD, et al: Catheter-directed thrombolysis for iliofemoral deep venous thrombosis improves health-related quality of life, *J Vasc Surg* 32:130-137, 2000.
17. Mewissen MW, Seabrook GR, Meissner MH, et al: Catheter-directed thrombolysis for lower extremity deep venous thrombosis: Report of a national multicenter registry, *Radiology* 211:39-49, 1999.
18. AbuRahma AF, Pekins SE, Wulu JT, et al: Iliofemoral deep vein thrombosis: Conventional therapy versus lysis and percutaneous transluminal angioplasty and stenting, *Ann Surg* 233:752-760, 2001.
19. Ouiel K, Grey B, Clair DG, et al: Complications associated with the use of urokinase and recombinant tissue plasminogen activator for catheter directed peripheral arterial and venous thrombolysis, *J Vasc Interven Radiol* 11:295-298, 2000.
20. Braaten JV, Goss RA, Francis CW: Ultrasound reversibly disaggregates fibrin fibers, *Thromb Haemost* 78:1063-1068, 1997.
21. Francis CW, Blinc A, Lee S, et al: Ultrasound accelerates transport of recombinant tissue plasminogen activator into clots, *Ultrasound Med Biol* 21, 1995. 419424.
22. Kasirajan K, Grey B, Ouriel K: Percutaneous AngioJet thrombectomy in the management of extensive deep venous thrombosis, *J Vasc Interv Radiol* 12:179-185, 2001.
23. Bush RL, Lin PH, Bates JT, et al: Pharmacomechanical thrombectomy for treatment of symptomatic lower extremity deep venous thrombosis: Safety and feasibility study, *J Vasc Surg* 40:965-970, 2004.
24. Arko Fr Davis CM, Murphy EH, et al: Aggressive percutaneous mechanical thrombosis: Early clinical results, *Arch Surg* 142:513-518, 2007.
25. Zhu DW: The potential mechanisms of bradyarrhythmias associated with AngioJet thrombectomy, *J Invasive Cardiol* 20(8 Suppl A):2A-4A, 2008.
26. Piercy KT, Ayerdi J, Geary RL, et al: Acute pancreatitis: A complication associated with rheolytic mechanical thrombectomy of deep venous thrombosis, *J Vasc Surg* 44:1110-1113, 2006.
27. Hillman DE, Pharm D, Razavi MK: Clinical and economic evaluation of the Trellis-8 infusion catheter for deep vein thrombosis, *J Vasc Interv Radiol* 19:377-383, 2008.
28. O'Sullivan GJ, Lohan DG, Gough N, et al: Pharmacomechanical thrombectomy of acute deep vein thrombosis with the Trellis-8 isolated thrombolysis catheter, *J Vasc Interv Radiol* 715-724, 2007.
29. May R, Thurner J: The cause of predominately sinistral occurance of thrombosis of the pelvic veins, *Angiology* 8:419-427, 1957.
30. O'Sullivan GJ, Semba CP, Bittner CA, et al: Endovascular management of iliac vein compression (May-Thurner) syndrome, *J Vasc Interv Radiol* 11:823-836, 2000.

59 Varicose Vein Stripping and Ambulatory Phlebectomy

HARRY MA • MARK D. IAFRATI

Historical Background

By the 1890s Trendelenburg[1] not only had developed the compression test to evaluate saphenous vein reflux but also had performed great saphenous vein ligations using a transverse upper thigh incision, thus establishing the foundation for surgical treatment of varicose veins. In 1916 Homans[2] described ligation of the saphenofemoral junction as it is commonly practiced today. A major advancement was contributed by Mayo,[3] who postulated additional benefit by removing the saphenous vein. Although quite effective at eliminating great saphenous vein reflux, this extensive surgical approach resulted in long operative times and significant wound complications. The introduction of an intraluminal stripping technique by Babcock[4] reduced the invasiveness of vein stripping, which has persisted with few refinements for most of the last century. Development of noninvasive venous testing in the 1980s improved the ability to target appropriate veins for intervention. Although sclerotherapy and endovenous ablation occupy preeminent roles in the contemporary management of superficial venous disease, open surgical approaches remain relevant when applied appropriately and executed expertly.

Indications

Chronic venous insufficiency may lead to debilitating pain, swelling, skin changes, and ulcerations. Conservative treatment including gradient compression remains important, but surgical correction of superficial venous reflux has proved superior to compression alone for a number of indications in a large prospective randomized trial (Box 59-1).[5]

Because of the less invasive nature of endovenous ablation, the use of open surgical approaches to varicose vein surgery has declined in recent years. However, there remain situations in which open venous surgery has advantages and is indicated. Specifically, endovenous ablation is contraindicated in the following situations:

1. The target vein, such as the great saphenous vein, small saphenous vein, or accessory saphenous vein, adheres closely to the skin.
2. It is not possible to create a 1-cm zone between the catheter and the skin, with tumescent anesthesia increasing the risk of thermal injury to the skin.
3. The endovenous ablation catheter or sheath cannot be passed through a tortuous great saphenous vein or a great saphenous vein in which synechia have formed because of chronic thrombophlebitis. In this situation it is often possible to pass a more rigid vein stripper or the more flexible Codman stripper. If these instruments cannot be passed, then ligation and phlebectomy may be appropriate.
4. Segments of the saphenous vein are extremely dilated or aneurysmal, with diameters greater than 2.5 cm. They may not ablate effectively and may be prone to thrombotic complications.

> **Box 59-1** | **INDICATIONS FOR VARICOSE VEIN SURGERY**
>
> - Symptomatic varicose veins or venous insufficiency
>   - Pain and tenderness associated with varicosities
>   - Heavy sensation in the extremity after prolonged standing
>   - Edema
> - Complications related directly to varicose veins
>   - Lipodermatosclerosis
>   - Venous ulceration
>   - Superficial thrombophlebitis
>   - External hemorrhage
> - Cosmetic appearance

5. Acute thrombosis in the target vein buffers the thermal effect and reduces the effectiveness of the endovenous ablation procedure. In addition, crossing the thrombus with an endovenous ablation catheter without proximal ligation risks embolization.
6. In certain settings, the cost of endovenous ablation may represent an economic barrier to its use.

Preoperative Preparation

- **History.** The first step in preparing for venous surgery is to obtain a history, including symptoms, complications related to the varicose veins, history of deep vein thromboses, prior venous interventions, and recurrent thrombotic episodes or varicose veins. It is also important to assess for concomitant peripheral arterial disease and associated medical comorbidities.
- **Physical examination.** Examination of the axial venous system from groin to ankles should be performed with the patient standing, noting edema, telangiectasias, varicose veins, skin discoloration, and evidence of ulcerations. Palpation of the lower extremities should focus on the compliance of the subcutaneous tissue and the turgidity of the veins.
- **Duplex ultrasound.** A detailed ultrasound assessment of the axial venous system focused on identifying areas of reflux in the superficial, deep, and perforating veins and areas of obstruction or postthrombotic changes provides a road map of the functional venous anatomy of the leg. To plan the appropriate procedure, it is crucial to understand the anatomy of the great saphenous vein. The great saphenous vein runs from the medial malleolus cephalad to the anteromedial surface of the calf. Around the knee, the great saphenous vein continues in a more superficial plane. As it courses farther cephalad, it enters the superficial fascia and most commonly remains between the deep and the superficial fascia. The great saphenous vein may be "duplicated" such that two veins run the length of the thigh, both within the fascial envelope. Particularly relevant is the "S-type" anatomy, where the great saphenous vein is only a partially duplicated, the dominant vein remains above the fascia, and the intrafascial vein is atretic. Preoperative knowledge of which variation is present is important to ensure that all refluxing segments or accessory veins are treated.
- **Evaluation.** Detailed evaluation of the popliteal fossa is also important given the highly variable location of the saphenopopliteal junction and local venous anatomy. Accurately assessing the relationship between the small saphenous vein and the gastrocnemius veins, intersaphenous vein, and other tributaries increases the success of small saphenous vein ligation and stripping. Approximately one third of small saphenous vein terminate in the popliteal vein above the knee, whereas a low termination occurs in approximately 10% of patients.[6-8] Likewise, determining

whether the gastrocnemius vein is incompetent is important, because it must be ligated with the small saphenous vein to prevent persistent reflux and recurrence. Duplex ultrasound has become the standard of care in evaluating venous insufficiency. However, the presence of venous outflow obstruction is better assessed by computed tomography, intravascular ultrasound, or venography.

- **Preoperative marking.** Before surgery, the patient should be marked in the standing position with an indelible marker. Such markings are crucial in cases of ambulatory phlebectomy, because visualization of the varicose veins may be impossible when the patient is supine. Areas of vein clusters should be marked for removal by phlebectomy, and only segments of either the great saphenous vein or the small saphenous vein with venous reflux should be marked for vein stripping. Duplex-guided marking of the saphenofemoral or saphenopopliteal junctions also allows precise placement of incisions.

Pitfalls and Danger Points

- **Varicose vein recurrence.** The most common reason for recurrent varicose veins is a missed refluxing great saphenous vein segment.[9] Overdissection of the groin region can also result in neovascularization at the saphenofemoral junction.[10] Finally, inadequate preoperative evaluation may fail to identify segments contributing to venous reflux, such as the small saphenous vein with posterior calf varices.
- **Nerve injury with ligation and stripping.** Injury to the saphenous nerve, which accompanies the great saphenous vein behind the medial border of the tibia, may lead to a sensory deficit to the medial aspect of the lower leg and foot. Injury to the sural nerve, which lies close to the small saphenous vein, may lead to a sensory deficit to the lateral lower leg and foot. Several motor nerves are also at risk for injury, including the tibial nerve, the common peroneal nerve, and occasionally a low-lying sciatic nerve, all of which course through or arise within the popliteal fossa and may be near the saphenopopliteal junction.
- **Arterial or venous injury.** Ligation of the common femoral vein may occur if it is mistaken for the saphenous vein. Ligation and stripping of the posterior tibial artery has been reported when it is mistaken for the saphenous vein at the ankle.
- **Great saphenous vein stump.** Ligation and division of the great saphenous vein that leaves a substantial blind stump may lead to thrombus formation with risk of pulmonary embolus.
- **Hematoma, extensive ecchymosis, and pain**

Operative Strategy

GENERAL CONSIDERATIONS

The technical goal of most venous surgery is elimination of axial reflux because of incompetent valves in the great saphenous vein and small saphenous vein, varicose vein clusters, and incompetent perforators. The best way to ensure that these goals are achieved is to perform a complete preoperative ultrasound assessment before the procedure. In addition, several intraoperative strategies can be used to avoid the major pitfalls of varicose vein surgery.

PREVENTING RECURRENCE

Preoperative markings with duplex ultrasound of the saphenofemoral or saphenopopliteal junction are helpful for proper placement of incisions. This reduces both incision size and unnecessary subcutaneous dissection, potentially reducing neovascularization and recurrent varicose vein formation.[11] Ligation of incompetent accessory saphenous veins also reduces recurrence. Ligation of the great saphenous vein alone without vein stripping is associated with a higher recurrence rate.[11,12] However, stripping of competent portions of the great saphenous vein can result in removal of important venous collateral pathways that may exacerbate the presence and development of varicose veins (Fig. 59-1). Inadequate attention to the small saphenous vein and posterior calf varicosities is another cause of recurrence. In a recent survey nearly 90% of surgeons carried out preoperative duplex imaging, but only 50% marked the saphenopopliteal junction and even fewer explored this region, thus limiting treatment of gastrocnemius veins or other incompetent veins that could serve as a source of persistent reflux.[13] Awareness of small saphenous vein anatomy, careful preoperative marking, and gentle retraction and dissection can increase the success and reduce the morbidity of small saphenous vein ligation.

AVOIDING NERVE INJURY

The saphenous nerve is prone to injury during great saphenous vein stripping, especially if the vein is stripped to the ankle.[14] Stripping the vein in a caudal direction, from the top down, diminishes this risk.[15] When exposing the small saphenous vein in the popliteal fossa, it is possible to injury either the sural or the tibial nerves by aggressive retraction or dissection.

AVOIDING ARTERIAL OR VENOUS INJURY

Failure to clearly define the saphenofemoral or saphenopopliteal junctions has resulted in injury to the femoral or the popliteal vein and artery.[16] Passage of the vein stripper in a caudal direction can reduce accidental removal of the femoral vein and confirms the lack of competent valves.

HEMATOMA, ECCHYMOSIS, AND PAIN

Minimizing skin incisions and subcutaneous dissection through the use of preoperative marking limits unnecessary soft-tissue trauma, whereas leg elevation during stripping and vein avulsion reduces venous bleeding and postoperative ecchymosis. Use of a proximal tourniquet with Esmarch bandage drainage of

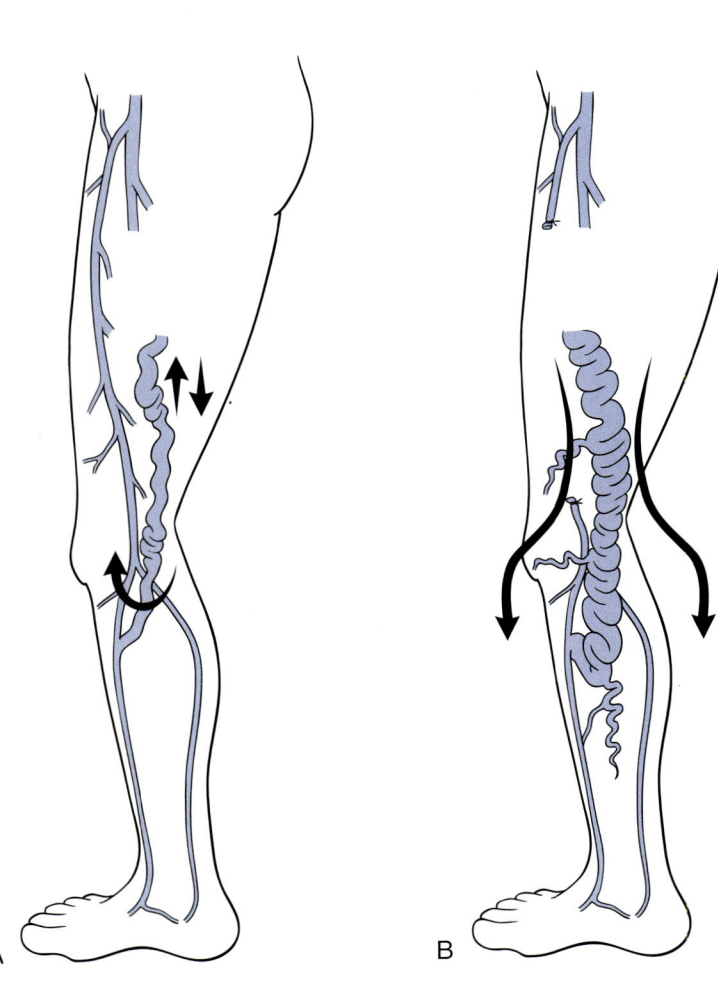

Figure 59-1. Collateral varicosities may worsen because of outflow resistance. **A**, A competent great saphenous vein serves as runoff for a collateral varicose vein, with arrows indicating the direction of blood flow. **B**, Without the great saphenous vein serving as a runoff vessel, worsening of collateral varicose veins may be observed.

the limb is rarely necessary but may be a potential helpful adjunct for patients with massive varices, such as those associated with Klippel-Trenaunay syndrome. Because the great saphenous vein resides within a fascial envelope, the use of tumescent anesthesia, supplemented with epinephrine, reduces bleeding from both direct compression and vasoconstriction. When tumescent anesthesia is not used, a piece of lidocaine- and epinephrine-soaked gauze can be attached to the vein stripper. As the vein is removed, the gauze is left in place temporarily to provide compression of avulsed tributary veins, absorb blood, and deliver epinephrine and anesthesia to the traumatized area. The gauze is then removed before wound closure.

Operative Technique

If it is determined that a patient is best served with open varicose vein surgery, then some combination of ligation, axial stripping, and ambulatory phlebectomy is used to remove the relevant venous segments.

ANESTHESIA

The surgical procedure can be performed under general, regional, or local anesthesia in an operating room or in an office procedure room that is appropriately equipped and staffed. Tumescent anesthesia is generally preferred either alone or in combination with other modalities.

GREAT SAPHENOUS VEIN LIGATION AND STRIPPING

For the best cosmetic results and the most reliable access to the saphenofemoral junction, the great saphenous vein should be approached through an oblique incision, typically 1 cm above and parallel to the groin crease. The incision is guided by preoperative duplex ultrasound marking. Otherwise, the incision should start over the palpable femoral artery and extend medially to ensure visualization of the saphenofemoral junction and its tributaries. Dissection through the subcutaneous tissue proceeds in a cephalad-caudal axis to limit injury to lymphatics. Once the main trunk of the great saphenous vein is identified, a small self-retaining retractor is helpful, so the plane over the saphenous vein can be extended toward the saphenofemoral junction with minimal dissection. Each of the tributaries to the great saphenous vein should be identified. Failure to clearly define the saphenofemoral junction can result in injury to the femoral vein or artery.[10,12] Because of the anatomic variations in the number and position of the saphenofemoral venous tributaries, the dissection should be 2 cm above and below the confluence to ensure that no additional tributaries enter the femoral vein directly. Careful isolation and ligation of both lateral and medial accessory saphenous veins should be performed. Once the saphenofemoral junction has been clearly identified, suture ligation of the great saphenous vein is performed close to the femoral vein, taking care not to narrow the femoral vein or leave a long great saphenous vein stump that might serve as nidus for a thrombus and potential embolus.

After ligation and division of the great saphenous vein the vein stripper is passed down the great saphenous vein which should proceed with relative ease to the level of the knee, consistent with a system of incompetent valves. It is not necessary to remove the great saphenous vein below the knee unless it is incompetent and dilated. This approach results in less postoperative pain, ecchymosis, or risk of nerve injury.

Once the stripping device has reached an appropriate level, a small transverse counter incision is made over the palpable distal end of the vein stripper. The saphenous vein is identified within the subcutaneous tissue, divided, and ligated distally before stripping the vein. Using a top-down method of introducing the stripping device ensures that false entry into the common femoral vein is avoided.

To avulse the vein with the endoluminal stripping device, the vein must be affixed to the stripper head at the cephalad portion of the vein at the level of the groin incision. This can be accomplished with a suture ligature, fixing the vein around the stripper device just below the head of the stripper. A long trailing suture is also placed on the stripper head to facilitate the extraction of the vein from the groin incision once the vein has been fully avulsed or as a means to pull a lidocaine with epinephrine-soaked gauze sponge into the subcutaneous track. In selecting the size of the head, a larger head improves the ability to avulse the tributary segments and recover a greater portion of the vein but does so at the cost of more trauma and increased bruising. The vein is stripped in a downward direction, from head to toes, which results in both improved tributary avulsion and reduced saphenous nerve injury.[17] The great saphenous vein may be drawn back up and out through the groin incision by pulling the attached trailing suture (Fig. 59-2, A).

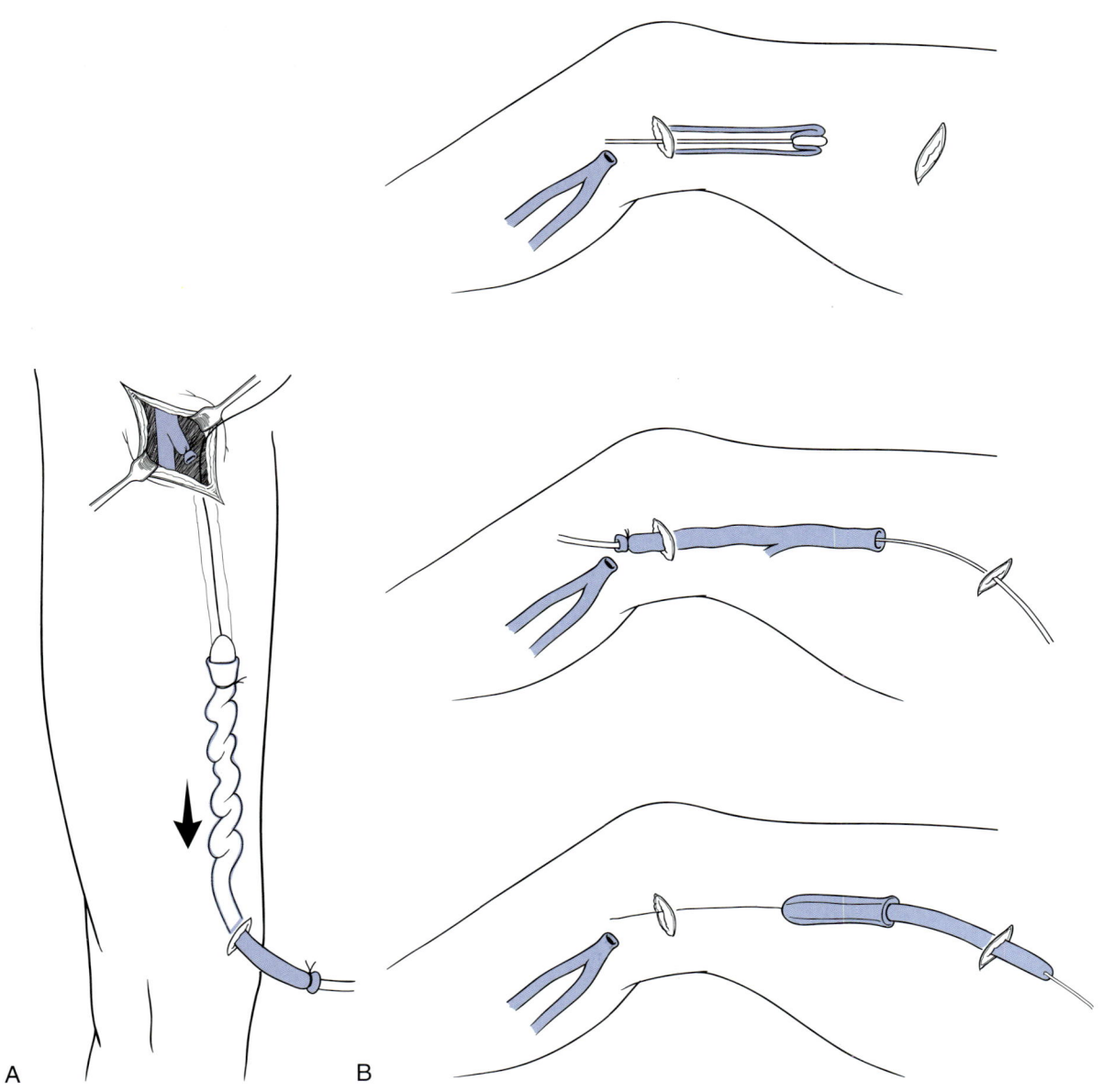

Figure 59-2. Alternative methods of vein stripping. **A,** The intraluminal stripper is passed top down from the groin incision, and the vein is fixed proximally by a ligature. A lidocaine-epinephrine soaked gauze sponge can be pulled into the vein track by a trailing suture. **B,** The perforate invaginate method with the vein inverted into itself and removed through the distal above-knee incision *(upper)*. Although uncommon, if the vein is torn during the stripping process, then removal of the residual segment can be accomplished by attaching the distal segment of vein to the intraluminal stripper and reversing the invagination by applying traction in cephalad direction *(middle)*, with the remaining venous segment removed via the groin incision *(lower)*.

Continued

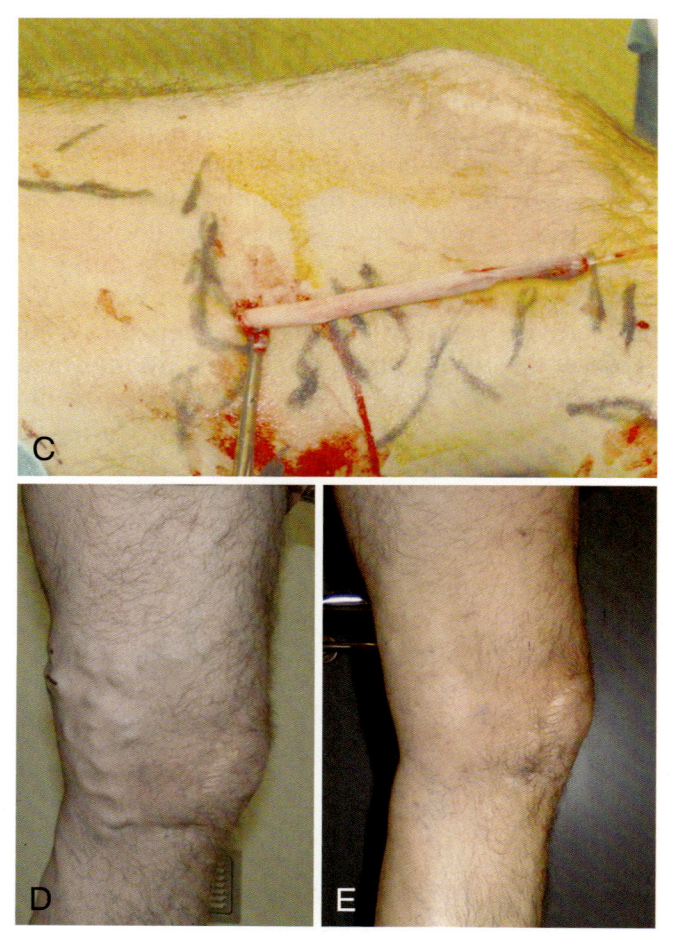

Figure 59-2, cont'd C, Stripping and avulsion of the great saphenous vein by passing an intraluminal stripper top down from the groin incision to an incision above the knee. **D**, Varicosities of the great saphenous vein before vein stripping, which are effectively eliminated by stripping (**E**).

Many alternative approaches to this technique have been described. One common alternative is to invaginate the great saphenous vein into itself as it is being stripped. The initial steps are identical to the conventional method. However, after passing the stripper device through the great saphenous vein, the vein is ligated to the stripper device without attaching the stripper head to the device. As distal traction is applied, the vein is then inverted into itself and removed through the distal incision (Fig. 59-2, B). Flexible or rigid strippers may be used with this technique. The advantage to this method is that diameter of the tunnel created by removal of the vein is minimized, reducing trauma to the soft tissues and nerves. In addition, the vein tends not to bunch up and is easily extracted from the smaller caudal incision. Because the great saphenous vein is prone to tearing at the sites of tributary confluence, it should be examined after removal to determine whether complete stripping of the target segment was achieved. If the vein tears, resulting in incomplete stripping, the torn segment is removed distally, and the stripping is repeated in the opposite direction to remove remaining portions of the great saphenous vein (Fig. 59-2, B). The groin incision is closed in layers with absorbable suture, and the skin is closed with an absorbable subcuticular suture. A single absorbable subcuticular suture may be required to close the small counter incision above the knee. A compressive dressing is placed, with padding over the area where the vein was stripped to minimize hematoma and bruising.

SMALL SAPHENOUS VEIN LIGATION

The patient is placed prone on a padded operating table with the affected limb flexed slightly at the knee. Preoperative duplex ultrasound marking facilitates

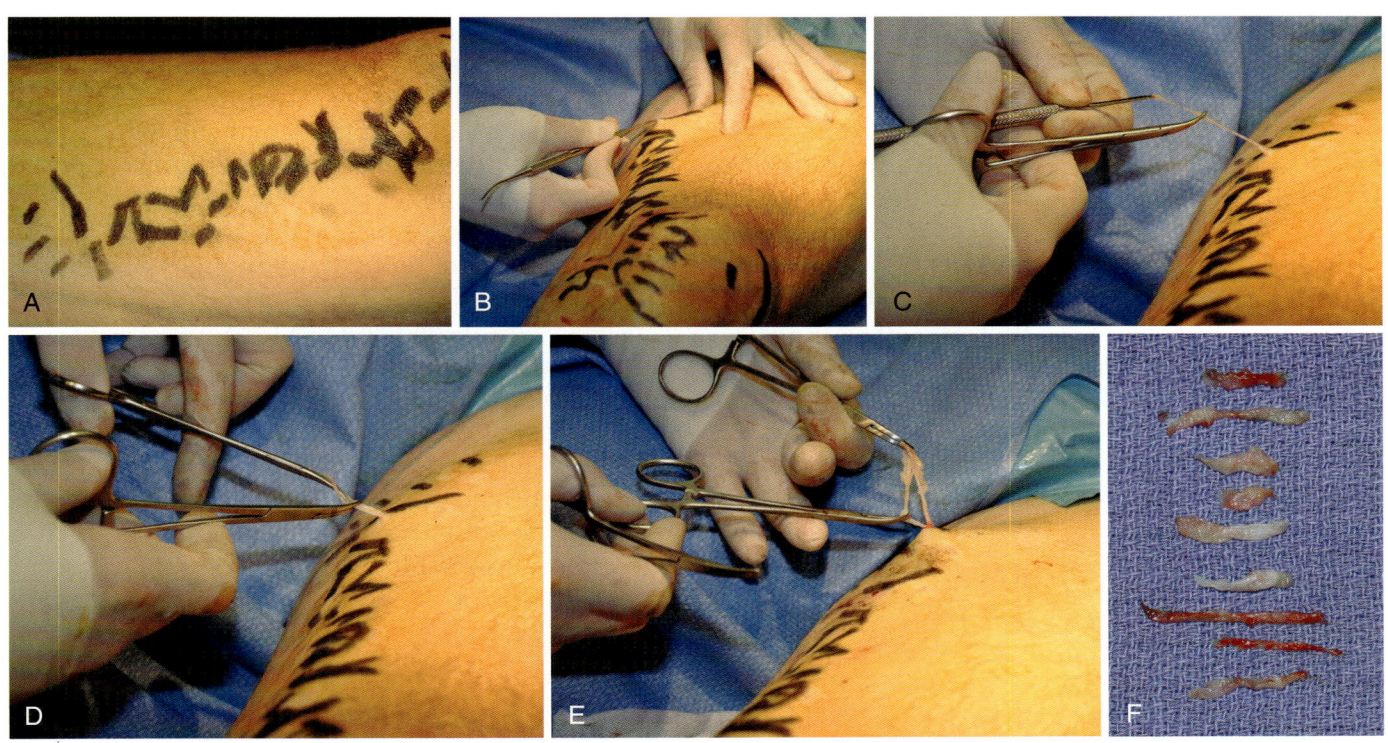

Figure 59-3. Ambulatory phlebectomy. **A**, Before the initiation of the procedure and with the patient standing, all varicose veins are marked on the skin using an indelible marker. **B**, Stab incisions, 2 mm in length, are placed over the site of previously marked varicose veins and are typically oriented longitudinally—except in the groin, knee, and ankle, where a transverse orientation aligns with the lines of Langer. **C** and **D**, A vein hook is used to initially pull the vein out through the incision. Retrieval of the vein can be assisted by use of a curved snap. **E**, The vein can be divided and avulsed proximally and distally by direct traction with or without rolling the vein onto the clamp. **F**, Typical lengths of avulsed varicose veins.

placement of a small transverse incision just distal from the saphenopopliteal junction. The incision may need to be increased for larger legs. The superficial fascia is opened transversely, the small saphenous vein is identified, and the perivascular tissue is carefully dissected to avoid injury to the sural nerve. Gentle retraction of the surrounding tissue avoids traction injury to the tibial nerve. Once isolated, the small saphenous vein is divided distally between clamps and ligated. Using light retraction on the transected vein, the dissection is carried cephalad to the saphenopopliteal junction. If the gastrocnemius or intersaphenous veins share a common trunk or are incompetent, they should be ligated and divided. The small saphenous vein is then ligated and divided at the saphenopopliteal junction, allowing excision of this 5-cm cephalad portion of the small saphenous vein. The popliteal fossa is closed in layers, with particular attention given to approximating the fascia to prevent a popliteal fossa hernia. The skin is closed with a running 5-0 subcuticular suture.

STAB OR AMBULATORY PHLEBECTOMY

After removing the source of axial reflux by ligation and stripping of the great saphenous vein, small saphenous vein, or both, the remaining superficial varicosities, if left uninterrupted, will drain via alternate pathways and may remain both symptomatic and cosmetically displeasing. Use of 2-mm "stab incisions" to effectively isolate and eliminate these tributary varices produces excellent results.[18,19] Preoperative markings are essential, because these veins cannot be visualized when the patient is supine (Fig. 59-3). In excess of 20 phlebectomies are commonly required to adequately address varices.

The technique of ambulatory phlebectomy or stab avulsion is straightforward. When done in isolation, it is well suited to local anesthesia either with a superficial subdermal infiltration around the vessel of interest or with larger volume tumescent techniques. Ambulatory phlebectomy is best performed on a horizontal plane, and because many patients are treated under a local anesthetic, it is often possible to have the patient assist in positioning the extremity during the procedure to maximize exposure. Skin incisions of 2 mm in length are made with a No. 11 blade and are typically oriented longitudinally; exceptions are incisions where a transverse orientation aligns with the lines of Langer in the groin, knee, and ankle. Small dermal varicosities are grasped or hooked and avulsed proximally and distally. Larger veins are grasped and brought up through the incision, cleared of fat, doubly clamped, and divided (Fig. 59-3). By applying inline traction, several centimeters of varicose vein can be teased out from each end. The vein is rolled onto the hemostat, which prevents the vein from avulsing prematurely. The varicose segments should be removed in their entirety, and if the vein breaks during the process, it may be reobtained through a new incision. There is no need to ligate the veins; avulsion alone is adequate, unless there is a perforating vein within the varicose cluster. At the end of the procedure, skin incisions are closed by approximating skin edges with adhesive Steri-strips. Rarely, larger incisions can be closed with an interrupted absorbable subcuticular suture.

Postoperative Care

- **Bandaging the extremity.** When the procedure is complete, the patient is dressed in compressive bandages. This bandaging, along with intraoperative measures including tumescent anesthesia, decreases postoperative ecchymosis and hematoma formation, which in turn reduces pain. The primary dressing is usually removed on the second postoperative day, after which a compression garment is worn.
- **Ambulation.** Upon discharge, ambulation is encouraged, but patients are advised to avoid long walks, prolonged standing, or vigorous exercise for 1 to 2 weeks.

Postoperative Complications

- **Recurrence.** The most common complication of venous surgery is recurrent varices, which may vary widely, occurring in 20% to 80% of patients over a follow-up period of 5 to 20 years.[20] The recurrent varices after surgery group demonstrated that in a series of 199 lower extremities with recurrent varicose veins, 47% were found to have reflux present at the saphenofemoral because of neovascularization or inappropriate ligation.[9] Recurrence in the popliteal region commonly results from the inadequate ligation noted in 29% to 47% of patients.[21,22] Venous outflow obstruction is implicated in about 10% to 15% of patients.
- **Nerve injury.** The incidence of saphenous nerve injury has been documented in up to 39% of patients, where the great saphenous vein is stripped to the ankle. Stripping the great saphenous vein to the knee reduced this incidence to 7% of patients.[23] Clinical experience suggests that paresthesia improves over time. Chronic pain and the development of saphenous neuritis are quite rare. The sural nerve is prone to injury when the small saphenous vein is ligated.
- **Arterial or venous injury.** Injury to the femoral artery or vein is rare.[24] Partial stripping of the common femoral vein can occur by passing the stripper through a large perforator vein. By passing the stripper using the top-down method, this complication can be reduced. When an arterial injury occurs during vein stripping, diagnosis is often delayed, and the outcome is poor, with up to one third of cases requiring an amputation.[24]

REFERENCES

1. Trendelenburg F: Uber die unterbindung der vena faphena magna bei unterschendelzaricen, *Berl Klin Chir* 7:195, 1890.
2. Homans J: The operative treatment of varicose veins and ulcers, based upon a classification of these lesions, *Surg Gynecol Obstet* 22:143-159, 1916.

3. Mayo C: The surgical treatment of varicose veins, *Saint Paul Med J* 6:695, 1904.
4. Babcock W: A new operation for the extirpation of varicose veins of the legs, *NY Med J* 86:153, 1907.
5. Gohel MS, Barwell JR, Taylor M, et al: Long-term results of compression therapy alone versus compression plus surgery in chronic venous ulceration (ESCHAR): Randomised controlled trial, *BMJ* 335:83, 2007.
6. Labropoulos N, Giannoukas AD, Delis K, et al: The impact of isolated lesser saphenous vein system incompetence on clinical signs and symptoms of chronic venous disease, *J Vasc Surg* 32:954-960, 2000.
7. Hobbs JT: Preoperative venography to ensure accurate sapheno-popliteal vein ligation, *Br Med J* 280:1578-1579, 1980.
8. Kosinski C: Observations on the superficial venous system of the lower extremity, *J Anat* 60:131-142, 1926.
9. Perrin MR, Labropoulos N, Leon LR Jr: Presentation of the patient with recurrent varices after surgery (REVAS), *J Vasc Surg* 43:327-334, 2006.
10. Fischer R, Chandler JG, De Maeseneer MG, et al: The unresolved problem of recurrent saphenofemoral reflux, *J Am Coll Surg* 195:80-94, 2002.
11. Lofgren KA: Management of varicose veins: Mayo Clinic experience. In Bergan JJ, Yao JST, editors: *Venous problems*, Chicago, 1978, Yearbook, pp 71-83.
12. Rivlin S: The surgical cure of primary varicose veins, *Br J Surg* 62:913-917, 1975.
13. Winterborn RJ, Campbell WB, Heather BP, et al: The management of short saphenous varicose veins: A survey of the members of the vascular surgical society of Great Britain and Ireland, *Eur J Vasc Endovasc Surg* 28:400-403, 2004.
14. Munn SR, Morton JB, Macbeth WA, et al: To strip or not to strip the long saphenous vein? A varicose veins trial, *Br J Surg* 68:426-428, 1981.
15. Jacobsen BH, Wallin L: Proximal or distal extraction of the internal saphenous vein? *Vasa* 4:240-242, 1975.
16. Eger M, Golcman L, Torok G, et al: Inadvertent arterial stripping in the lower limb: Problems of management, *Surgery* 73:23-27, 1973.
17. Negus D: Should the incompetent saphenous vein be stripped to the ankle? *Phlebology* 1:33-36, 1986.
18. Barwell JR, Davies CE, Deacon J, et al: Comparison of surgery and compression with compression alone in chronic venous ulceration (ESCHAR study): Randomised controlled trial, *Lancet* 363:1854-1859, 2004.
19. Michaels JA, Brazier JE, Campbell WB, et al: Randomized clinical trial comparing surgery with conservative treatment for uncomplicated varicose veins, *Br J Surg* 93:175-181, 2006.
20. Perrin MR, Guex JJ, Ruckley CV, et al: Recurrent varices after surgery (REVAS), a consensus document: REVAS group, *Cardiovasc Surg* 8:233-245, 2000.
21. Rashid HI, Ajeel A, Tyrrell MR: Persistent popliteal fossa reflux following saphenopopliteal disconnection, *Br J Surg* 89:748-751, 2002.
22. Labropoulos N, Touloupakis E, Giannoukas AD, et al: Recurrent varicose veins: Investigation of the pattern and extent of reflux with color flow duplex scanning, *Surgery* 119:406-409, 1996.
23. Holme JB, Skajaa K, Holme K: Incidence of lesions of the saphenous nerve after partial or complete stripping of the long saphenous vein, *Acta Chir Scand* 156:145-148, 1990.
24. Rudstrom H, Bjorck M, Bergqvist D: Iatrogenic vascular injuries in varicose vein surgery: A systematic review, *World J Surg* 31:228-233, 2007.

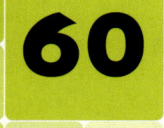

60 Endovenous Thermal Ablation of Saphenous and Perforating Veins

JULIANNE STOUGHTON

Historical Background

Venous valve anatomy was first described in the 1500s, but with the exception of compression wraps, treatment for chronic venous disease (CVD) was not considered until several centuries later. Trendelenburg[1] described saphenous vein ligation in 1891 as a treatment of varicose veins, but it was soon recognized to be associated with a high recurrence rate. Ligation and stripping of the entire saphenous vein became a mainstay of therapy in the twentieth century, but this method was later modified to selective stripping of the upper portion of the great saphenous vein to reduce of the risk of neuralgia observed with vein stripping below the knee.

Sclerotherapy, or chemical ablation of the saphenous vein, was described over the past 2 centuries, but the safety profile of ablative chemical agents was not considered acceptable until the 1960s. The application of ultrasound guidance proved to be a useful adjunct, but the success rates of chemical ablation remained suboptimal with a high risk of recanalization. In the late 1990s endovenous thermal ablation was first described using radiofrequency (RF) energy,[2] and soon thereafter endovenous laser[3] treatment was developed.

Indications

The types and stages of CVDs have been defined by a classification system composed of four components: clinical stage (1-6), etiology (primary, secondary, or congenital), anatomy (deep, superficial, or perforator system), and pathophysiology (reflux, obstruction, or both), known by the acronym CEAP (Fig. 60-1).[4] Another scoring system that has gained popularity is the venous clinical severity score,[5] which assigns a score to various clinical attributes, such as pain, varicose veins, edema, skin changes, use of compression, and ulceration. Such scoring systems can be helpful in evaluating outcomes and disease progression.

Varicose veins may be associated with distinct pattern of clinical findings, categorized into six clinical stages (C1-C6) in the CEAP classification system. Early symptoms (C1) are mild and include aching, tiredness, heaviness, or throbbing while upright without overt varicosities. Conservative measures such as support hose at 20 to 30 or 30 to 40 mm Hg of external compression often alleviate early symptoms. As the degree of venous hypertension increases, enlarging varicosities can cause local discomfort. Pain, cramping, or restless leg symptoms at night, as well as itching, can be associated with venous disease. Numbness or sharp or radiating pain are not usually attributable to venous insufficiency. Varicose veins (C2) are often associated with one or multiple sources of reflux and may be symptomatic, progressive, or of cosmetic concern. Although edema (C3) may result from CVD, other causes, including lymphedema, lipedema, medication effects,

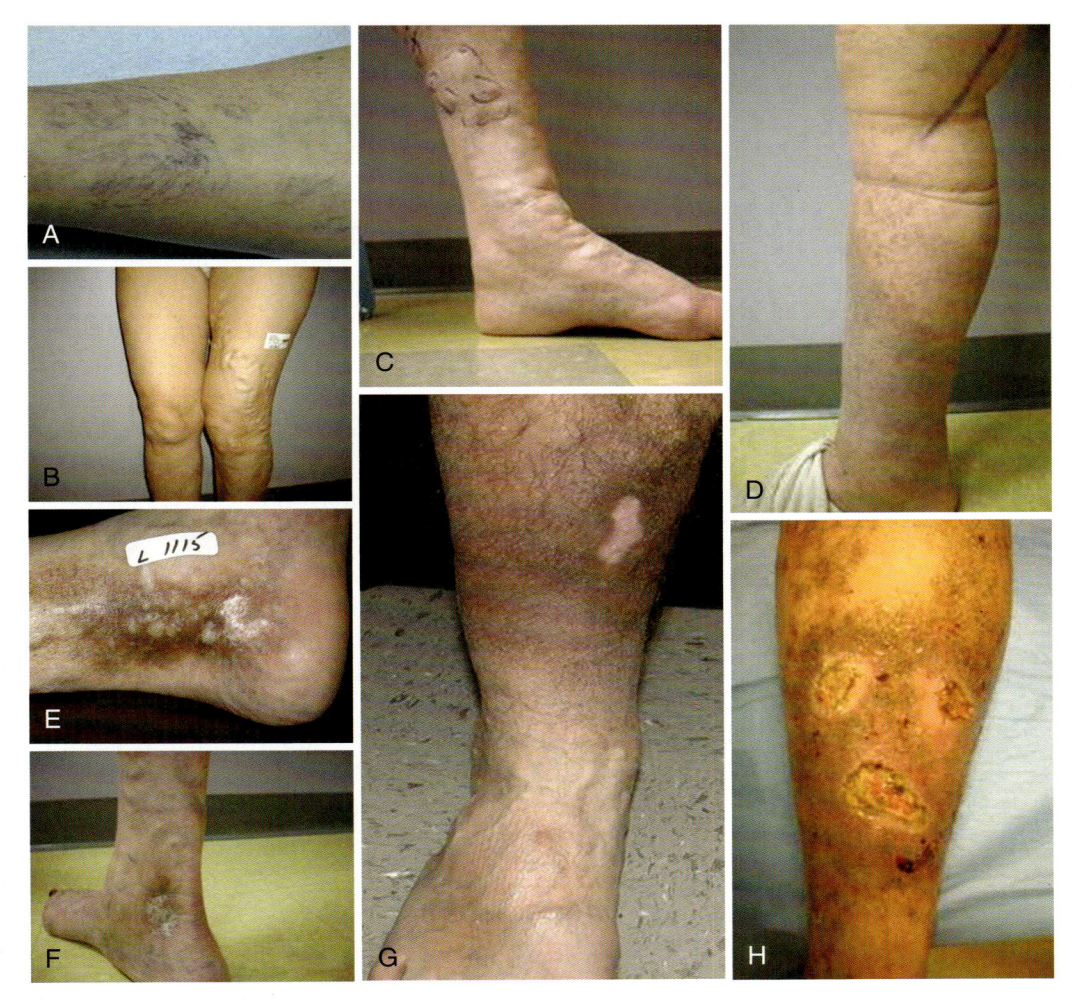

Figure 60-1. The classification of venous disease using CEAP system. **A**, Stage C1: Telangiectasia and reticular veins. **B**, Stage C2: Varicosities. **C**, Stage C3: Edema. Stage C4: Skin changes, including eczema and pigmentation (**D**) or lipodermatosclerosis and atrophie blanche (**E**). Stage C5: Preulcerative (**F**) or healed (**G**) ulcer. **H**, Stage C6: Active ulceration.

pulmonary, cardiac, renal, hepatic, endocrine, or sleep apnea, should be excluded. Venous stasis skin changes (C4) in the gaiter distribution, including pigmentation, eczema, lipodermatosclerosis, inflammation, and ulceration, are associated with multiple sources of reflux with or without obstruction. Skin changes are an indication for treatment of superficial venous reflux, if present. Skin ulceration (C5-C6) requires compression and local wound care, which should precede treatment of CVD. Surgical stripping of the great saphenous vein has decreased ulcer recurrence, but multiple sources of reflux, including superficial, perforator veins, and deep venous reflux, may be present.[6]

Treatment should always begin with conservative measures, including compression therapy, exercise, weight loss, and intermittent elevation. Continued signs or symptoms of progressive venous insufficiency consistent with CEAP C2 to C6 venous disease are indications for endovenous or surgical treatment. A history of superficial vein thrombosis (SVT) does not preclude endovenous treatment. Both thermal and chemical ablation techniques can be used to treat recanalized refluxing veins after SVT.

Absolute contraindications to endovenous thermal ablation of saphenous and perforating veins include an inability to ambulate, the presence of arteriovenous malformation or uncompensated deep venous obstruction with poorly developed collaterals, pregnancy, and allergic reaction local anesthetic. Relative contraindications include the presence of superficial veins that lie within 1 cm of the skin, because a risk of skin burn exists. This can be prevented by injecting tumescent anesthesia to increase the depth of the vein to greater than 1 cm from the skin. If the vein is immediately subdermal, alternatives to thermal ablation should be considered given the risk of a phlebitic reaction, prolonged pain, and skin changes with retraction or pigmentation. Likewise, tortuous veins may increase the difficulty of advancing the catheter. Aneurysmal vein segments or larger vein diameters (>25 mm), as well as short refluxing vein segments (<3 cm long) and veins with small diameters (<3 mm) may be best treated with other approaches.

Preoperative Preparation

- **Ultrasound evaluation.** Duplex evaluation of the superficial venous system should be performed in the upright position (Fig. 60-2). All major leg veins should be evaluated in B mode for compressibility, wall thickness, and the presence of internal echoes. Axial veins should be described with regard to diameters, depths, length within the fascia, degree of tortuosity, and communications with perforators or other enlarged tributaries. Perforators are assessed for diameter at the fascia level, location, and the presence of reflux with the patient seated and dangling the leg. Augmentation of venous flow with distal compression cuffs or manual squeeze of the calf are used with color flow Doppler waveform analysis of each refluxing vein.
- **Preoperative vein assessment.** The target vein is mapped by ultrasound and marked, and diameters and depths are measured. Major tributaries; large refluxing perforators; tortuous, partially occluded, and aneurysmal segments; and refluxing duplicate veins should be noted using a marker pen. Entry sites are selected where the vein is superficial, but ablation is halted proximal to the entry point to prevent skin burn or phlebitis. Preprocedure photographs are helpful for documentation (Fig. 60-3).
- **Assessment of thrombotic risk.** Evaluation of personal or family history of thrombosis should be conducted, and those at increased risk of thrombosis should be assessed for an inherited thrombophilia.[7] Endovenous ablation can be performed while on warfarin, and low-molecular-weight heparin can be administered perioperatively to those patients at increased risk.[8]
- **Medications and compression.** An oral benzodiazepine and an antibiotic are prescribed 1 and 2 hours before the procedure, respectively. If indicated, low-molecular-weight heparin is also administered 1 to 2 hours before the procedure. A 30 to 40 mm Hg thigh-high stocking with an open toe and a waist attachment should be available and applied immediately after the procedure.

Pitfalls and Danger Points

- Bruising and hematoma
- Superficial phlebitis
- Deep vein thrombosis
- Thrombus extension to deep vein junction
- Thermal skin injury
- Paresthesia
- Recanalization
- Neovascularization

Endovascular Strategy

DEEP AND PERFORATING VEINS

The perforator veins connect the superficial and deep venous system and have unidirectional valves. A clinically significant source of reflux may be present if the valves are incompetent and the perforator is greater than 3.5 mm in diameter. However, perforator incompetence may resolve after treatment of superficial venous insufficiency alone.[9]

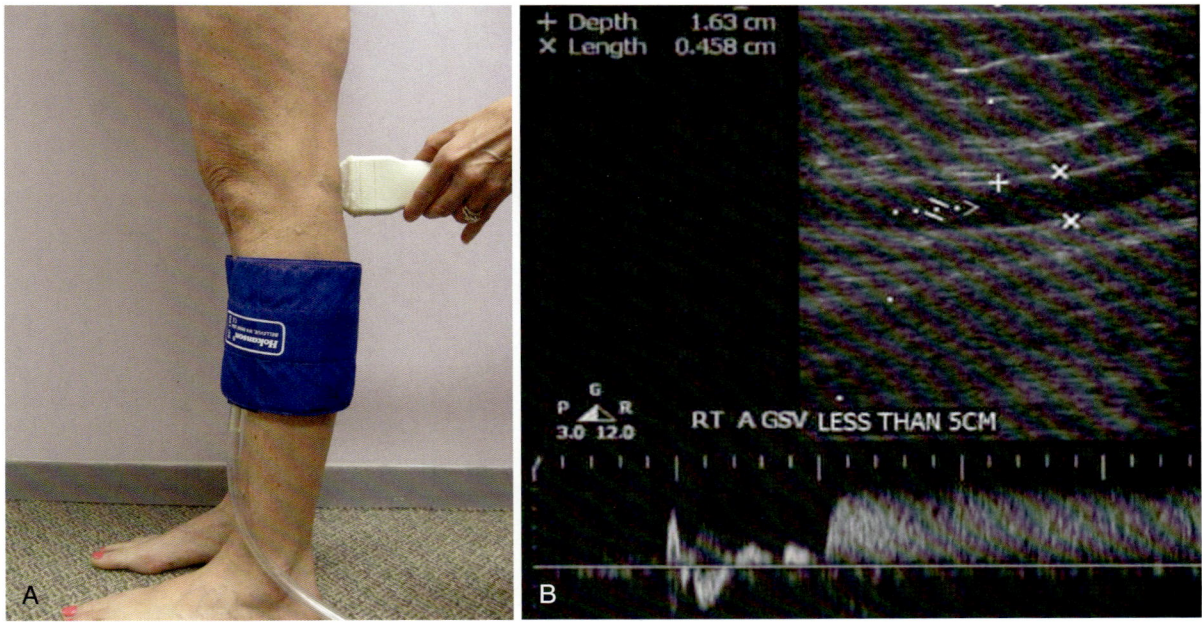

Figure 60-2. Duplex ultrasound examination of venous reflux. **A**, Patient is in the standing position, and reflux is induced with rapid cuff inflation. **B**, Flow is measured proximally over the veins using Doppler waveform analysis. After cuff deflation, reversal of flow for more than 0.5 seconds is consistent with reflux within the vein segment.

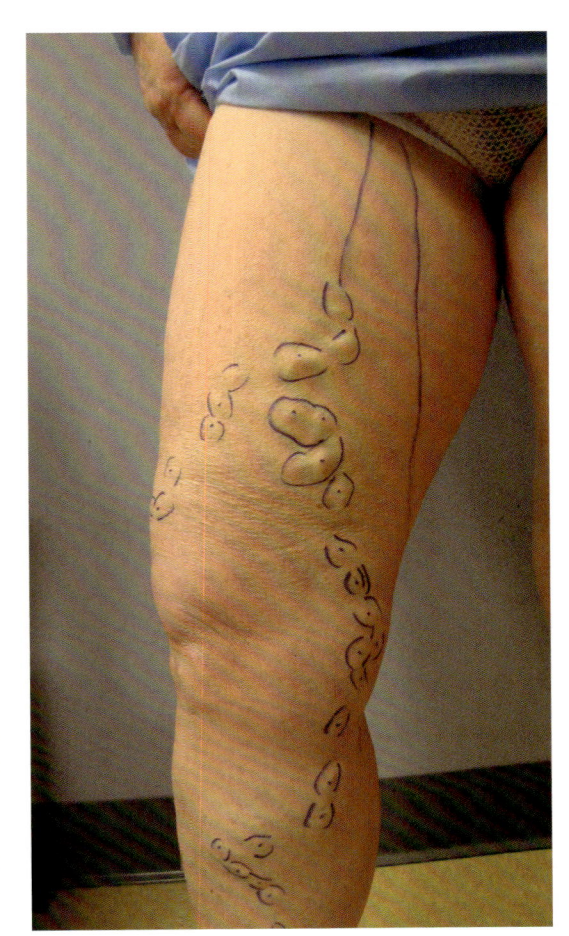

Figure 60-3. Preoperative marking of the varicose veins. Before the endovenous thermal ablation, the refluxing vein segments should be carefully mapped by ultrasound and marked percutaneously. Diameters, depths, aneurysmal segments, and partially occluded or tortuous segments should be indicated, as well as communication with tributaries or perforating veins. This information is used to plan the treatment of each segment of the target vein to use the minimal effective amount of energy and decrease the risk of complication.

GREAT SAPHENOUS VEINS

The great saphenous vein begins anterior to the medial malleolus of the ankle, travels up the medial thigh, and terminates at the saphenofemoral junction (SFJ) at or below the inguinal ligament and medial to the femoral artery (Fig. 60-4). Anterior and posterior accessory saphenous veins may be present and may be a source of concurrent or recurrent varicosities after treatment of the great saphenous vein.

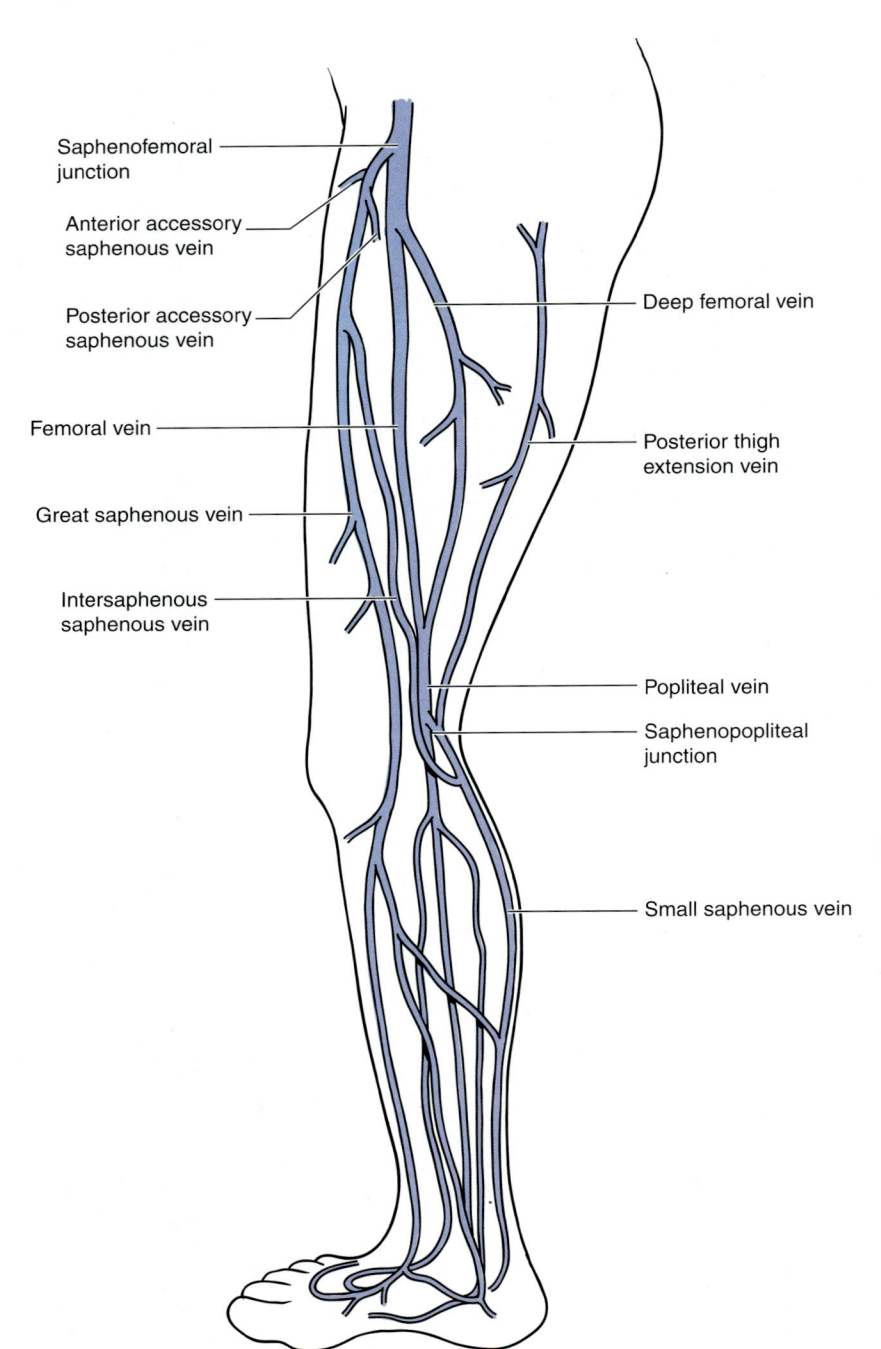

Figure 60-4. Lower extremity venous anatomy. The great saphenous vein travels up the medial aspect of the leg from the ankle to the saphenofemoral junction (SPJ). Major tributaries or accessory saphenous veins are variable at the junction and can include the anterior accessory great saphenous vein and the posterior accessory great saphenous vein. The small saphenous vein starts at the lateral ankle and travels up the posterior calf. It can extend above the popliteal fossa into the posterior thigh vein or can communicate medially with the great saphenous vein as the intersaphenous vein. The SPJ is usually at or above the popliteal fossa, where the vein enters the deep popliteal vein. The anatomy of this junction is highly variable, and connections from the muscular veins in the popliteal fossa must be preserved when performing ablation of the small saphenous vein.

SMALL SAPHENOUS VEINS

The small saphenous vein begins at the lateral aspect of the foot, continues over the Achilles tendon, and runs up the posterior calf to the saphenopopliteal junction (SPJ) within 10 cm of the popliteal fossa (Fig. 60-4). The anatomy of the small saphenous vein is highly variable and commonly duplicate. A cranial or posterior thigh extension can continue from the small saphenous vein up the posterior thigh, emptying into the femoral vein. The intersaphenous vein, previously known as the "vein of Giacomini," can communicate from the small saphenous vein in the popliteal fossa to the medial thigh great saphenous vein. Refluxing perforators are found in the popliteal fossa, often lateral and superior to the SPJ, which must be carefully distinguished from small saphenous vein reflux. Gastrocnemius and soleus veins are deep to the muscular fascia but can be mistaken for the small saphenous vein by inexperienced ultrasound technicians. The saphenous veins are identified outside the muscular fascia and beneath the saphenous fascia. The administration of tumescent anesthesia is facilitated by injecting into this saphenous compartment.

SUPERFICIAL TRIBUTARIES

Tributaries or varicosities consist of an interconnecting network of subcutaneous veins communicating with the main saphenous trunks and are best treated with phlebectomy. Significantly, ultrasound can be used to evaluate whether tributaries are associated with refluxing axial veins or enlarged incompetent perforators that require treatment.

PROXIMAL PELVIC VEINS

Medial labial and thigh varicosities may be associated with pelvic venous insufficiency and abdominal wall and suprapubic varicosities related to a proximal source of obstruction. Varicosities in these areas should not be treated without assessment of proximal iliac and vena cava anatomy.

SMALLER VEINS

Reticular veins are flat, blue, and less than 3 mm in diameter, whereas spider veins are more superficial, present as red or purple dermal veins, and are less than 1 mm in diameter. These veins are not suitable for endovenous thermal ablation but are amenable to cosmetic sclerotherapy. A flare or confluence of spider veins at the medial ankle and foot (corona phlebectatica) may indicate deep or perforator vein insufficiency.

Endovascular Technique

POSITION

The patient is placed in the supine position for great saphenous vein or accessory great saphenous vein ablation after circumferential sterile preparation of the leg. Although a staged approach for treatment of great saphenous vein and small saphenous vein is preferred if concomitant small saphenous vein ablation is planned, the posterior midcalf may be accessed in the externally rotated frog-leg position. Alternatively, the patient may be placed in the lateral decubitus or prone position if the small saphenous vein is technically too difficult to access from the front. If ablations of only the small saphenous vein or the posterior thigh extension of the small saphenous vein are planned, the patient can be placed in the prone position.

ACCESS

The ultrasound probe is covered by a sterile sleeve, and the vein is accessed at the distal aspect of the target vein. The insertion site should be chosen that is distal from most major refluxing tributaries and at a point where the vein is easily accessible. Most clinicians avoid thermal ablation of the great saphenous vein below-knee segment or the distal small saphenous vein segment below the bifurcation of the gastrocnemius muscle because of an increased risk of paresthesia or skin injury. A reverse Trendelenburg position can facilitate venopuncture, and the patient should be kept warm and calm to avoid venospasm. Tourniquets have been used to help dilate the veins, and the use of topical nitroglycerin ointment (Nitropaste) before venopuncture has been described.[10] Imaging of the target vein is performed in the longitudinal or transverse view, a small skin wheel is raised using local anesthesia, and the vein is entered using a micropuncture needle. After the needle is used to tent the vein wall, the needle is rapidly advanced into the vein (Fig. 60-5). Blood return is confirmed, and a 0.018-inch micropuncture wire is inserted and advanced into the vein. If the treatment of duplicate veins is considered, access should be obtained for all veins before injection of tumescent anesthesia. If there is a partially occluded segment or an impassable tortuous segment of vein, a second access site can be obtained cephalad to the obstruction.

CATHETER PLACEMENT

Radiofrequency Catheter

The RF catheter is flushed, the end is capped, and the catheter is advanced into the vein to the SFJ via a 7- or 11-cm-long, 7-Fr sheath using ultrasound guidance (Fig. 60-6). Prior to catheter insertion, the length of catheter to be inserted in the

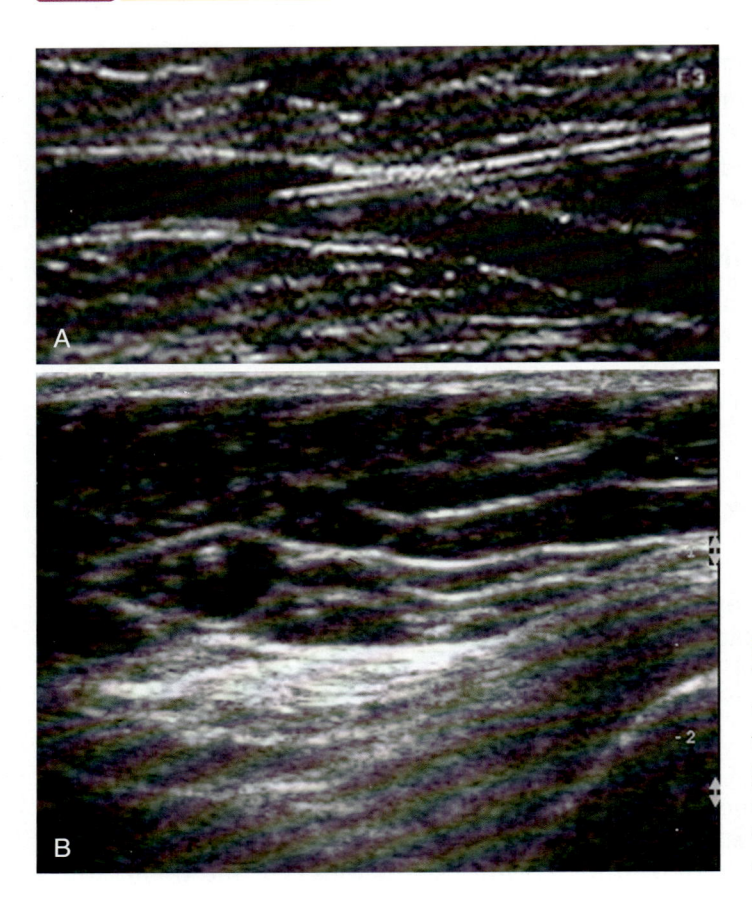

Figure 60-5. Access of the vein using ultrasound guidance. The vein is imaged in either the longitudinal (**A**) or the transverse (**B**) direction, advancing the ultrasound the needle up to the wall of the vein. The tenting of the vein wall helps ensure proximity. The needle is then rapidly advanced into the vein lumen. Transverse images are most accurate to determine whether the needle is intraluminal, although longitudinal images can be helpful to assess needle depth and direction.

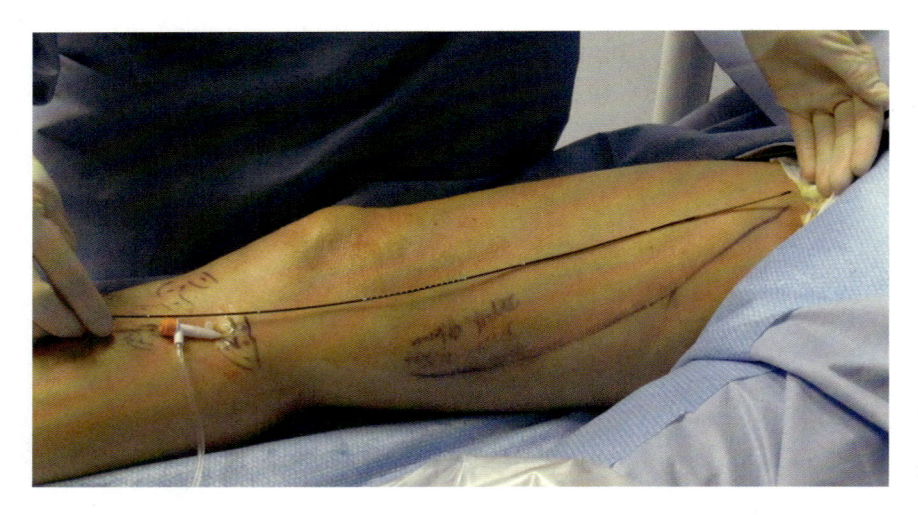

Figure 60-6. The RF segmental catheter. The RF catheter heats a 7-cm segment of vein over 20 seconds at 120°C. The catheter is marked in 6.5-cm increments to avoid skipping areas of thermal ablation within the vein. Care should be taken not to withdraw the heating element too close to the entry site to prevent skin burn.

vein should be estimated and the approximate length of catheter that will remain outside the vein noted. A 0.025-inch Glidewire can be advanced through the catheter lumen to assist passage through tortuous segments. The wire is removed, and the catheter is flushed and recapped.

Endovenous Laser

A full-length sheath is used through which the laser fiber is advanced. Care should be taken not to advance the laser fiber alone, as this may result in perforating the vein wall. The 4- or 5-Fr sheath is positioned over a 0.035-inch J-tipped guidewire, and the tip of the sheath is positioned just below the junction. The fiber is advanced to the end of the sheath, and the sheath is retracted 2 cm, leaving the tip of the fiber exposed. Radial-type fibers can be advanced alone through a shorter sheath. The position of the laser tip should be confirmed by ultrasound and by visualizing the light beam through the skin.

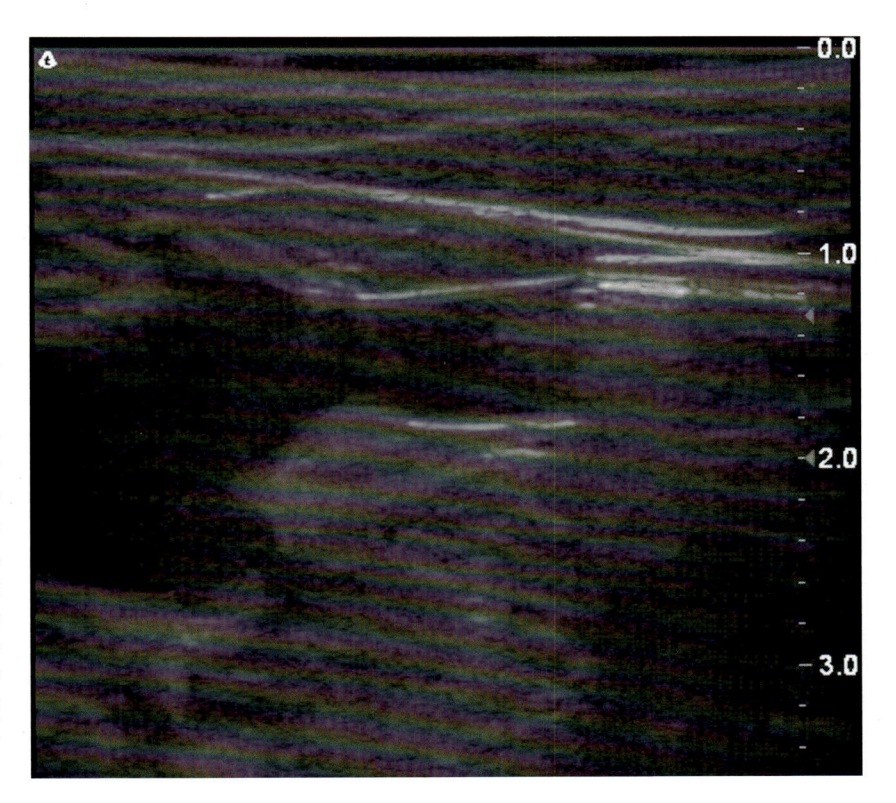

Figure 60-7. Ideal placement of catheter related to the junctions between the superficial and deep venous system. Ultrasound guidance is used to evaluate the catheter tip position before delivering energy to the vein wall. A safe distance is generally 2 cm from the catheter tip to the saphenofemoral or saphenopopliteal junction, ensuring preservation of the superficial epigastric vein in the groin or the gastrocnemius and soleus veins in the popliteal fossa. The positioning of the catheter tip in the small saphenous vein is ideally at the area where the vein is still superficial and is just beginning to descend through the muscular fascia toward the popliteal vein.

Confirmation of Catheter Tip Position

For both types of thermal ablation, tip position must be reconfirmed immediately before treatment. The catheter tip in the great saphenous vein should be 2 cm from the SFJ and below the superficial epigastric vein, if present (Fig. 60-7). In the small saphenous vein system the tip should be positioned farther from the SPJ, usually caudal to the point where the vein begins to dive deeper toward the SPJ. In addition, care should be taken to stay distal from the junction of the gastrocnemius and soleus veins to the small saphenous vein to preserve the muscular venous drainage. If a refluxing posterior thigh vein extension is present, the catheter tip should be positioned in the superficial portion of the vein before it begins to dive into the muscle to join the femoral vein.

Tumescent Anesthesia

Tumescent anesthesia consists of a mixture of large volumes of saline with a small amount of local anesthetic, epinephrine, and bicarbonate and provides adequate local anesthesia, as well as an excellent heat sink during thermal ablation. Epinephrine creates venospasm, and injection of the anesthetic around the vein helps to create better wall contact with the catheter. Tumescent anesthesia is injected into the saphenous fascial sheath around axial veins, and subcutaneous injections are performed for subdermal varicosities. Hand injection is possible, but the use of a roller pump allows larger volumes to be injected under higher pressure. A small skin wheal of anesthetic is delivered every 5 to 10 cm along the veins with a small 30-Ga needle, followed by deeper injection using a 20-Ga spinal needle. Approximately 10 mL of tumescent anesthesia per cm of vein to be treated should be injected to optimize contact between the heating element and the vein wall. After confirmation of final tip position, infiltration over and beyond the SFJ or SPJ should be performed. Ultrasound visualization when injecting helps avoid injection outside of the saphenous sheath or within the lumen of the vein. Every attempt is made to surround the vein with the tumescent solution, and an additional volume is injected adjacent to the catheter tip to avoid proximal propagation of heat. Additional anesthesia should be injected if patients report sensation during the ablation (Fig. 60-8). Adequate tumescent anesthesia is necessary to avoid thermal skin injury and minimizes the risk of postprocedure paresthesia.

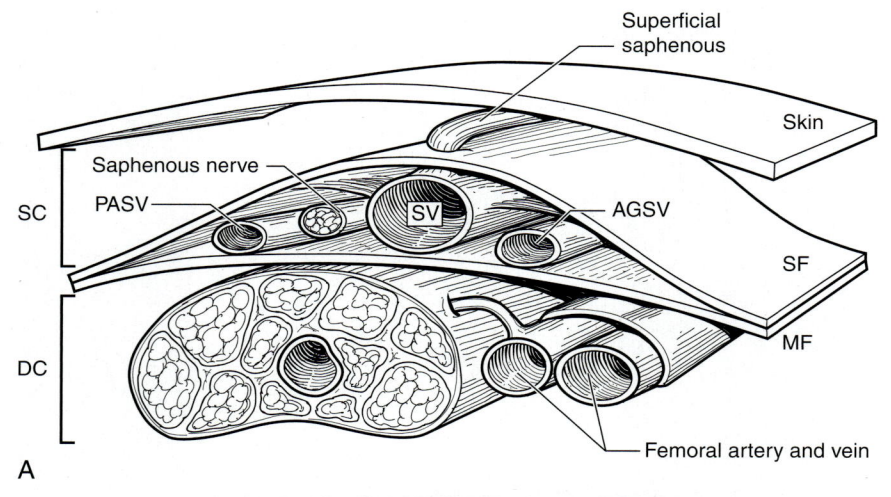

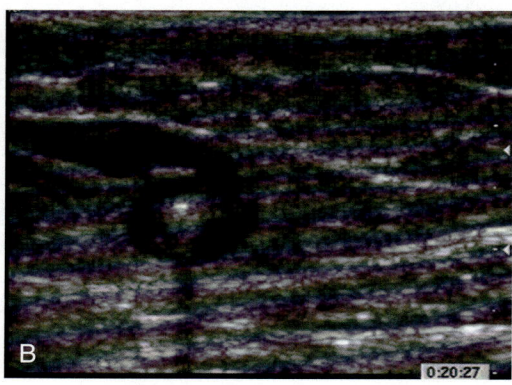

Figure 60-8. Placement of tumescent anesthesia in the saphenous sheath. **A**, Cross-sectional anatomy of the saphenous sheath and related structures. **B**, Transverse ultrasound views of the saphenous vein above the muscular fascia, below the saphenous fascia, and within the saphenous sheath. Tumescent anesthesia is injected into this sheath to provide anesthesia for ablation, to externally compress the vein around the catheter, and to minimize the risk of thermal injury to the skin. *AGSV*, Anterior accessory great saphenous vein; *DC*, deep compartment; *MF*, muscular fascia; *PASV*, posterior accessory saphenous vein; *SC*, superficial compartment; *SF*, saphenous fascia; *SV*, saphenous vein.

TREATMENT OF AXIAL VEINS

Tumescent anesthesia creates venospasm and mechanically compresses the vein. In addition, the patient should be placed in the Trendelenburg position to empty the veins, and surface pressure should be applied to improve wall contact. Impedance values can be followed while using RF ablation, which can signify the need for further compression.

Radiofrequency Energy

The RF catheter is designed with a 7-cm-long coil, which achieves 120° C (248° F) and treats the vein over this length in 20-second cycles. The RF generator (VNUS Medical, San Jose, Calif.) is preprogrammed for the appropriate temperature, and the RF cycles are controlled by the operator via a button on the catheter. The number of treatment cycles, the treatment time, and the length of the treated vein should be recorded. Initially a double cycle is performed just below the SFJ, followed by sequential single cycles throughout the remainder of the vein. Double cycles may be advantageous, particularly in large-diameter or aneurysmal veins, as well as for previously treated or phlebitic veins. The RF catheter is marked in 6.5-cm segments to have a small overlap zone between treatment lengths. The catheter is "indexed" by keeping it in place and sliding the sheath back to the first visible mark on the catheter. The catheter is then withdrawn at 6.5-cm intervals by following the markings on the catheter related to the sheath. While administering RF energy, the catheter is visualized by ultrasound, care should be taken not to withdraw the coil into the sheath, and pressure is applied along the length of the coil. During each treatment cycle, the power will typically begin at 40 watts and drop to below 20 watts within 10 seconds if compression is appropriate and the vein segment properly exsanguinated. If the set temperature is not reached within 5 seconds or the power level is maintained above 20 watts there may be flow within the vein that is cooling the treatment segment. RF energy delivery should cease and the effectiveness of exsanguination and proper tip position confirmed.

RF treatment should not be performed adjacent to the entry site in the skin. Skin burn at the entry site can be difficult to heal and is preventable. Most catheters are marked with a triple line, which indicates that the coil is getting close to the skin and should not be withdrawn farther. If the line is close, the catheter can be slightly readvanced to complete the treatment of the distal vein segment.

If treating multiple veins, the catheter can be flushed and reused to treat each vein. The coil should not be reused if there are defects or breaks. Thrombus, which rarely accumulates on the catheter, can be gently wiped away. If chemical ablation is planned at a certain site, injection through the catheter lumen is possible under ultrasound guidance.

Although the view is obscured after the injection of tumescent anesthesia, confirmation of occlusion, as well as patency of the common femoral vein is performed by ultrasound and compression of the deep system before completion. Both the catheter and the cord are disposable and should not be resterilized.

Endovenous Laser Ablation

The 600-micron laser fiber tips are available in bare-tip, coated-tip, and radial-tip designs and are positioned within a long sheath, with 1 to 2 cm exposed. The tip position should be confirmed both by ultrasound and by visualization of the aiming beam through the skin in a darkened room. After confirming tip position with the patient in Trendelenburg position, laser safety measures are instituted. Although the fiber-optic laser is positioned inside the patient, the laser energy, which is focused at the tip, could be released elsewhere through a fiber break. Wavelength-specific safety goggles, signs, and trained staff are required.

Laser energy is delivered to the vein wall by selective photothermolysis. Specific wavelengths of laser energy are targeted to absorb either hemoglobin or water within the vein. The energy delivered is measures in joules (joules = watts × seconds). Optimal energy delivery is considered to be between 60 to 100 J per linear centimeter of vein, defined as linear endovenous energy density (LEED). Generally, the proximal aspect of the vein is treated with at least 100 J/cm, and then a slightly lower LEED is delivered to the distal aspect of the vein if the diameter is not enlarged. Higher energies (>120 J/cm) can be used if needed for previously treated, recanalized phlebitic veins and larger-diameter or aneurysmal vein segments. Each laser has an optimal setting for wattage, and the pullback can be adjusted to deliver the appropriate joules to each vein segment. The principle of using the least energy possible should be followed, especially in smaller or more superficial vein segments, to reduce complication risk.

Various wavelength lasers are available (810, 940, 980, 1064, 1320, and 1470 nm), but the wavelength is not as important as the technique. After endovenous laser ablation, occlusion should be confirmed and compression of the deep system should be performed to assess the common femoral vein. For treatment of multiple veins, the dilator, sheath, and fiber may be reused; however, the tip can deteriorate or accumulate a large amount of coagulum, which may alter energy delivery.

TREATMENT OF PERFORATOR VEINS

Percutaneous access using ultrasound guidance is easily obtained, and veins can be treated even in areas of severely compromised skin. These procedures are easily performed using local anesthesia, with minimal risk of complication. Treatment of perforator veins adjacent to arterial perforators should be avoided. Laser delivery should be halted immediately if the patient has the perception of heat, and further tumescent anesthetic should be administered. Care is taken to avoid heating too close to the skin to prevent skin burn. Careful visualization of the tip is essential, keeping the tip of the fiber at least 2 cm away from the deep veins and more than 1 cm from the skin.

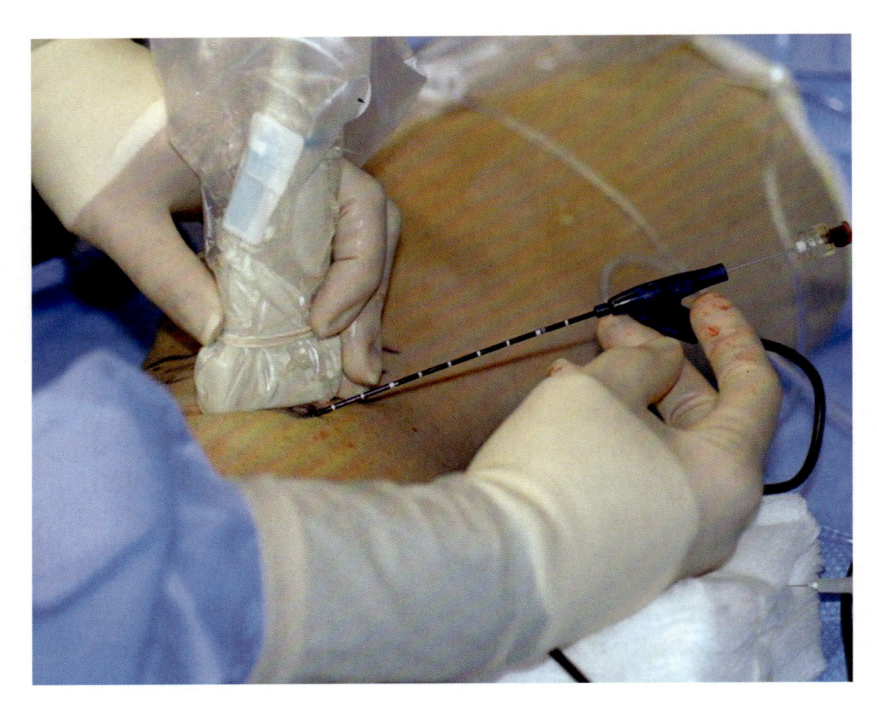

Figure 60-9. Positioning of a thermal ablation catheter in an incompetent perforating vein. The RF stylet catheter is tilted to treat the perforator vein in four quadrants for 1 minute each. While treating the vein, gentle pressure is applied externally with the ultrasound probe and the impedance levels are followed. RF must be stopped if the patient perceives sensation of heat so that additional tumescent anesthetic can be administered.

The steps in thermal ablation of perforator veins are similar to those for the saphenous vein. Ultrasound guidance is essential, percutaneous access into the suprafascial or perifascial perforator is performed, local anesthetic is injected, the vein is treated, and pressure is applied after removal of the device.

Endovenous Laser Ablation

Ultrasound-guided micropuncture is used to access the suprafascial or perifascial perforator. A 4-Fr sheath is inserted over the micropuncture wire, the laser fiber is advanced into the sheath, and the sheath is withdrawn to expose the fiber tip. Tumescent anesthesia is injected using ultrasound guidance around the tip, just under the fascia, and around the subcutaneous portion of the vein. Tip position is confirmed, the patient is placed in Trendelenburg position, and the laser is used to treat the perforator while withdrawing the catheter into the tributary.

Radiofrequency Ablation

A stylet catheter is available for RF ablation, which can be advanced over a 0.018-inch wire. The catheter has a sharp cutting tip, which must be advanced cautiously to prevent shearing of the wire. After advancing the catheter tip into the vein, the stylet is pulled back and the blunt-tipped portion of the catheter is advanced over the wire to optimally position the tip. Feedback from the RF generator can help confirm an intravascular position, because the impedance values should be less than 400 ohms if the tip is within the vein. After careful positioning of the tip at the perifascial region, the course of the catheter is infiltrated with local anesthetic, the tip position is reconfirmed with ultrasound and impedance feedback, the patient is placed in Trendelenburg position, and pressure is applied with the ultrasound probe over the treatment area (Fig. 60-9). The RF generator is initiated at the preset 85°C (185°F), and the RF stylet catheter is gently tilted to treat in four quadrants for 1 minute in each direction. If the perforator vein is sufficiently long, the catheter is withdrawn 0.5 to 1 cm and the procedure is repeated.

Postoperative Care

- **Dressings.** Steri-strips and Tegaderm dressings are used to cover the microincisions and entry sites. Absorbent dressings are applied under the compression where phlebectomy was performed to absorb excess tumescent anesthesia. In addition, both adequate compression and careful technique can minimize bruising and hematoma formation.

- **Compression therapy.** Compression does not improve the closure rate, but it does improve patient comfort during the first 2 weeks after the procedure. A thigh-high garment with a waist attachment applying 30 to 40 mm Hg of external compression is applied immediately after the ablation and is worn continuously for at least 24 hours. Eccentric compression in which pads are applied along the treated vein under the compression decreases the incidence of postoperative pain and bruising.[11] Compression is continued for 1 to 3 weeks, until tenderness has diminished over the treated vein segment. Routine knee-high compression is recommended thereafter.

- **Pain management.** Application of ice is encouraged for local discomfort for 48 hours. Acetaminophen or ibuprofen is prescribed for pain. If a phlebitic reaction occurs, a nonsteroidal antiinflammatory agent may be helpful. A delayed form of "pulling" discomfort often occurs at 1 to 2 weeks after ablation. This can be treated with gentle stretching, continued compression, and a nonsteroidal antiinflammatory agent.

- **Activity.** Patients are encouraged to ambulate frequently, and routine activities are resumed immediately after the procedure. Intermittent elevation every few hours is recommended for patients in the first 24 to 48 hours and as needed throughout the first week. Routine activity is encouraged, but high-impact activities and weight lifting should be avoided in the 1 to 2 weeks after the ablation to avoid swelling, bruising, and discomfort. The importance of continued exercise and weight management should be emphasized.

- **Clinical and duplex follow-up evaluation.** Ultrasound is used to evaluate ablation of the treated vein and to exclude deep vein thrombosis. Although consensus does not exist as to the optimal time for this study, it is often performed 24 to 72 hours after the procedure. When examination is performed early within the first week, thrombus extension to the SFJ, common femoral vein, SPJ, and popliteal vein ranges between 0.3% and 1%. In centers that assess patients after the first week, almost no incidence of thrombus extension is observed.[12] Ultrasound and clinical examination should be performed at 6 to 12 months to determine whether recanalization or recurrent varicose veins are present.

Complications

- **Bruising and discomfort.** Discomfort and bruising are usually present in the first 1 to 2 days. Pulling pain may be present after the first week. Inner thigh or abductor stretching is recommended for patient comfort.

- **Numbness and paresthesias.** The incidence of numbness and paresthesias ranges between 0.2% and 14%, which may be minimized by copious injection of tumescent anesthesia within the saphenous sheath. The saphenous nerve adjacent to the great saphenous vein below midcalf and the sural nerve adjacent to the small saphenous vein in the midcalf to distal calf are at increased risk.

- **Skin burns.** These can be avoided by using sufficient tumescent anesthesia, and assuring that the catheter is greater than 1 cm from the skin.

- **Pigmentation.** Persistent pigmentation can occur if treating subdermal veins.

- **Deep vein thrombosis.** The risk of deep vein thrombosis is less than 1%, although one small study reported an incidence of 7.7% (3/39) with extension into the common femoral vein.[13] Endovenous heat-induced thrombosis describes extension of thrombus to the SFJ or into the common femoral vein (Fig. 60-10). If the thrombus extends into the common femoral vein, serial ultrasound with or without short-term anticoagulation should be instituted.[14]

- **Superficial phlebitis.** The risk of superficial phlebitis is reduced when enlarged tributaries are removed with concomitant phlebectomy.

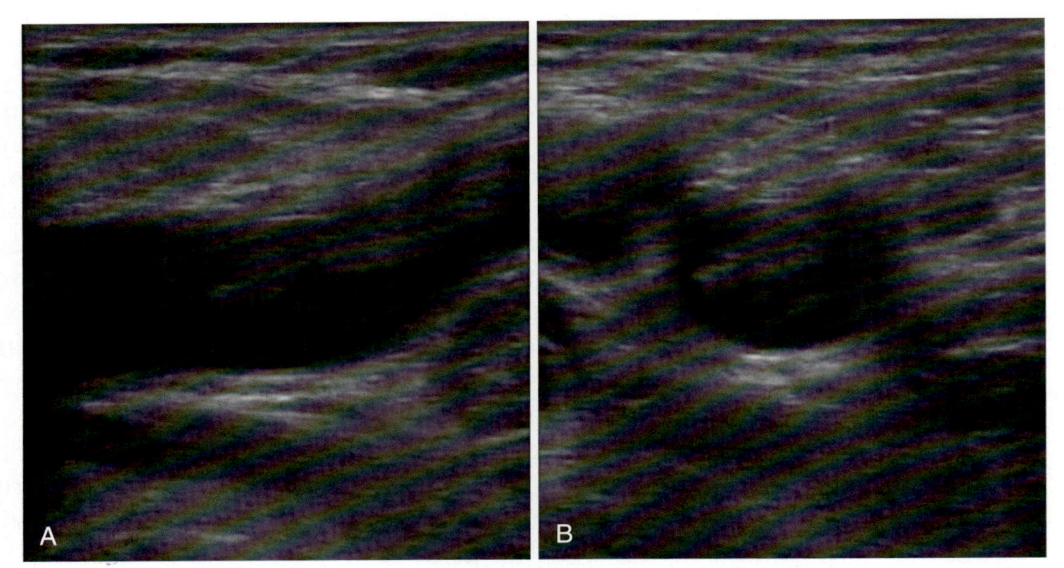

Figure 60-10. Endovenous heat-induced thrombosis within the common femoral vein. **A,** Longitudinal view of the saphenofemoral junction (cephalad to the left) with thrombus. **B,** Transverse view of the common femoral vein with thrombus at the saphenofemoral junction. This process is usually visualized within the first week after ablation. If the thrombus extends close to the superficial-deep vein junction but not into the femoral vein, conservative management and repeat ultrasound are appropriate. If the hyperechoic thrombus extends into the deep vein, the patient should be treated with short-term anticoagulation until the clot resolves.

- **Neovascularization.** Neovascularization is more likely after surgical ligation and stripping and less commonly after ablation.[15]
- **Arteriovenous fistula.** An arteriovenous fistula is rare and is attributed to thermal injury or needle trauma.[16]
- **Failure to close.** Primary, primary-assisted, and secondary occlusion rates are similar for RF and laser ablation. Failures more frequently occur in larger or recanalized veins. Segmental patency may occur in veins adjacent to an incompetent perforator or a large refluxing tributary. If the patient becomes symptomatic, a short patent segment can be treated with chemical ablation. Most clinical failures become apparent within 6 months after the procedure. Recanalization is often a consequence of a refluxing tributary or perforating vein, which requires additional treatment.

REFERENCES

1. Trendelenburg F: Uber die unterbindung der vena saphena magna bie unterschenkel varicen, *Beitr Z Clin Chir* 7:195, 1891.
2. Weiss RA, Weiss MA: Controlled radiofrequency endovenous occlusion using a unique radio-frequency catheter under duplex guidance to eliminate saphenous varicose vein reflux: A 2 year follow up, *Dermatol Surg* 28:38-42, 2002.
3. Navarro L, Min RJ, Bone C: Endovenous laser: A new minimally invasive method of treatment of varicose veins. Preliminary observations using an 810 nm diode laser, *Dermatol Surg* 27:117-122, 2001.
4. Kistner RL, Eklof B, Masuda EM: Diagnosis of chronic venous disease of the lower extremities: The CEAP classification, *Mayo Clin Proc* 71:338-345, 1996.
5. Rutherford RB, Padberg FT Jr, Comerota AJ, et al: Venous severity scoring: An adjunct to venous outcome assessment, *J Vasc Surg* 31:1307-1312, 2000.
6. Barwell JR, Davies CE, Deacon J, et al: Comparison of surgery and compression with compression alone in chronic venous ulceration (ESCHAR study): Randomized controlled trial, *Lancet* 363:1854-1859, 2004.
7. Caprini J: Risk assessment as a guide for the prevention of the many faces of venous thromboembolism, *Am J Surg* 199:S3-S10, 2010.
8. Theivacumar NS, Gough MJ: Influence of warfarin on the success of endovenous laser ablation (EVLA) of the great saphenous vein (GSV), *Eur J Vasc Endovasc Surg* 38:506-510, 2009.
9. Parks T, Lamka C, Nordestgaard A: Changes in perforating vein reflux after saphenous vein ablation, *J Vasc Ultrasound* 32:141-144, 2008.

10. Morrison N: VNUS Closure of the saphenous vein. In Bergan J, editor: *The vein book*, ed 1., Burlington, Mass, 2007, Academic Press, pp 283-298.
11. Lugli M, Cogo A, Guerzoni S, et al: Effects of eccentric compression by a crossed-tape technique after endovenous laser ablation of the great saphenous vein: A randomized study, *Phlebology* 24:151-156, 2009.
12. Mozes G, Kalra M, Carmo M, et al: Extension of saphenous thrombus into the femoral vein: A potential complication of new endovenous ablation techniques, *J Vasc Surg* 41:130-135, 2005.
13. Hingorani AP, Ascher E, Markevich N, et al: Deep vein thrombosis after radiofrequency ablation of the greater saphenous vein: A word of caution, *J Vasc Surg* 40:500-504, 2004.
14. Kabnick L, Ombrellino M, Agis H, et al: Endovenous heat induced thrombosis (EHIT) at the superficial-deep venous junction: A new post-treatment clinical entity, classification and patient treatment strategies, American Venous Forum 18th Annual Meeting, February 23, 2006, Miami.
15. Lurie F, Creton D, Eklof B, et al: Prospective randomised study of endovenous radiofrequency obliteration (closure) versus ligation and vein stripping (EVOLVeS): Two-year follow-up, *Eur J Vasc Endovasc Surg* 29:67-73, 2005.
16. Timperman PE: Arteriovenous fistula after endovenous laser treatment of the short saphenous vein, *J Vasc Interv Radiol* 15:625-627, 2004.

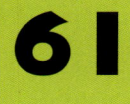

61 Surgical Treatment of Lower Extremity Deep and Perforator Vein Incompetence

ALESSANDRA PUGGIONI

Historical Background

In 1968 Kistner[1] was the first to describe direct surgical repair of incompetent deep venous valves. Indirect valve repair was first popularized in the early 1980s after report of the axillary vein transfer technique, which was followed by Gloviczki and colleagues'[2] description of angioscope-assisted external repair of venous valves in 1991. Surgical interruption of incompetent perforating veins to mitigate the effects of venous hypertension and promote venous ulcer healing was first described by Linton[3] in 1938. Relatively high wound complication rates limited this approach, and as a minimally invasive alternative, subfascial endoscopic perforator surgery (SEPS) was first described in 1985 by Hauer[4] in Germany and was subsequently popularized in the United States by Gloviczki and associates.[5]

Indications

DEEP VENOUS VALVE SURGERY

Indications for deep vein valve surgery include venous valve reflux in the presence of intractable, advanced symptoms of lower extremity chronic venous insufficiency (CEAP classes C4-C6), or the presence of significant pain that interferes with quality of life. Typically, intervention follows long-standing compressive therapy and the correction of iliac or iliofemoral venous outflow obstruction, and superficial or perforator vein reflux. Lower extremity axial reflux is present that extends from groin to calf, along with an incompetent deep venous valve, which is amenable to direct surgical repair, or a postthrombotic vein segment that is suitable for indirect repair or replacement.

SUBFASCIAL ENDOSCOPIC PERFORATOR SURGERY

The role of perforating vein surgery in treating symptoms of venous insufficiency remains controversial. Chronic venous insufficiency (CEAP C4-C6) with a medially located leg ulcer in association with perforator vein reflux of greater than 3.5 seconds on duplex scan are usually present. Appropriate candidates for intervention are those patients with low operative risk and acceptable ambulatory status without significant peripheral arterial occlusive disease, calf pump failure, morbid obesity, or a hypercoagulable state.

Preoperative Preparation

DEEP VENOUS VALVE SURGERY

- Preoperative diagnostic workup should include lower extremity arterial and venous duplex studies.
- Ascending and descending venography is performed to identify the sites of reflux and obstruction. When proximal venous obstruction is suspected in the iliac system, intravascular ultrasound should be performed, because it is often superior to conventional venography at diagnosing venous stenoses.
- Duplex imaging of the axillary veins can be performed to evaluate its suitability as a donor segment for lower extremity valve transplantation.
- Assessment for underlying thrombophilia is indicated to guide postoperative anticoagulation.
- A sequential compression device is applied at the time of anesthesia to decrease the risk of deep vein thrombosis (DVT) and postoperative edema.

SUBFASCIAL ENDOSCOPIC PERFORATOR SURGERY

- Duplex imaging is performed preoperatively to identify the number, location, and size of incompetent perforators and to evaluate the superficial and deep venous systems.
- The day before surgery perforators are marked on the skin with a semipermanent marker.
- Preoperative and postoperative strain gauge or air plethysmography may be used as a physiologic tool to evaluate the impact of treatment on the degree of valve incompetence, calf muscle pump function, outflow obstruction, and related hemodynamic changes.
- Prophylactic low-molecular-weight heparin may be considered during the perioperative period, especially in patients with a prior history of DVT.

Pitfalls and Danger Points

DEEP VENOUS VALVE SURGERY

- **Deep vein thrombosis.** The risk of DVT in deep vein valve surgery is less than 5%, but may involve the site of repair, the distal venous system, or the opposite unoperated limb.[6] Sequential pneumatic boots, heparin prophylaxis, and perioperative anticoagulation may help diminish the risk of DVT. Lower extremities should be elevated in the postoperative period until the patient is ambulatory to decrease venous stasis and edema.
- **Hematoma.** Meticulous hemostasis is required and a drain left at the operative site, particularly, if postoperative anticoagulation will be instituted.
- **Incompetent reconstructed valve.** The construction of a neovalve or vein valve transfer can be considered if direct repair is unsuccessful.

SUBFASCIAL ENDOSCOPIC PERFORATOR SURGERY

- **Missed perforators.** Failure to identify incompetent perforators that may be located in the intermuscular septum, paratibial, or retromalleolar region may contribute to delayed ulcer healing or a recurrent ulcer. The medial insertion of the soleus muscle may need to be exposed to visualize proximal paratibial perforators. Retromalleolar, lower posterior tibial perforators cannot be reached by current endoscopes and, if incompetent, may need to be interrupted by an open technique.
- **Nerve injury.** Damage to the saphenous nerve, which runs along the saphenous vein below the knee, can cause dysesthesia and a loss of sensation along the

medial aspect of the lower leg. In addition, the tibial nerve runs posterior to the medial malleolus into the foot and is also at risk of injury. Tibial injury may present as dysesthesia and weakness of the foot and toes.

- **Infection.** The risk of a surgical site infection is increased in the presence of an open ulcer, even if remote from the surgical incision. The procedure should be deferred in the presence of active cellulitis and prophylactic antibiotics considered routine.
- **Deep vein thrombosis**
- **Hematoma**

Operative Strategy

DEEP VENOUS VALVE SURGERY

Direct valve repair is used more often for patients who present with primary valvular incompetence, whereas deep vein valve reconstruction, such as vein valve transfer, is most often performed for those with postthrombotic syndrome.

Proximal Venous Obstruction

Patients who present with an incompetent deep venous valve and a concomitant iliocaval venous stenosis should first undergo treatment of the obstruction, typically by venous stenting. Relief of pain and edema may be achieved in a substantial number of patients even in the presence of persistent deep valvular incompetence.

Selection of Valve Site for Repair

Femoral vein, profunda femoral vein, popliteal vein, and posterior tibial vein valves are all amenable to repair. Repair of a single incompetent valve, most commonly the proximal femoral vein valve, is sufficient in most cases of primary venous insufficiency, whereas for those patients with postthrombotic syndrome, if present, an incompetent profunda femoral vein valve should be repaired as well.[7,8]

Avoiding Early Deep Vein Thrombosis at the Site of Valve Surgery

Surgical manipulation should be minimized to preserve normal vein morphology and limit endothelial damage. Closure of a venotomy should be performed with everting sutures to avoid creation of a thrombogenic nidus. External valvuloplasty carries risk of stenosis because of improper placement of sutures with a stenosis that exceeds 20% dictating the potential need for vein valve transfer.

Anticoagulation

Intravenous heparin is administered should vein clamping be required. Low-molecular-weight heparin should be continued postoperatively and then converted to warfarin. Duration of anticoagulation is patient specific but usually continues for a minimum of 2 to 4 months.

Avoiding an Incompetent Venous Valve Repair

Once a valve repair has been completed and the venotomy closed, intraoperative assessment of valve competence should be conducted. In the strip test, the distal inflow vein segment is temporarily occluded and blood is milked across the valve by sliding a finger upward against the wall. Blood is then forced back against the valve. If the vein below the valve remains collapsed, then the valve is competent; if incompetent, refilling of the emptied distal vein segment will be observed. An intraoperative duplex study of the repaired valve or reconstructed vein segment can also be performed. Surgical correction of an incompetent repair should be performed and, if unsuccessful, axillary vein valve transfer considered.

SUBFASCIAL ENDOSCOPIC PERFORATOR SURGERY

SEPS can be performed in the presence of an open but not an infected ulcer; however, patients with extensive skin changes and circumferential leg ulcers should not undergo SEPS. If there are signs of cellulitis or erysipelas, pain, erythema, and purulent discharge, antibiotics and local treatment should be initiated before surgery. Small upper calf incisions should be placed remote from the ulcer or affected skin. Proper wound cleaning before the procedure and coverage of the extremity with a transparent, occlusive dressing will help minimize intraoperative bacterial contamination and surgical wound infection.

Operative Technique

DEEP VENOUS VALVE SURGERY

General or spinal anesthesia can be used for deep venous valve surgery. The patient is positioned supine with the thigh slightly externally rotated. The common femoral vein, femoral vein, great saphenous vein, and profunda femoral vein can be exposed through a groin incision; dissecting through the sartorius muscle fascia helps expose the profunda femoral vein. The popliteal vein can be exposed by a supragenicular, an infragenicular, or a posterior approach. Target veins and their branches are isolated by blunt dissection for several centimeters. Although the attachment lines of primary incompetent valves are readily identifiable on inspection, postthrombotic veins are often surrounded by thickened, fibrous periadvential tissue, which will need to be sharply dissected to expose the segment to be treated. Absent or incomplete valve leaflet attachment lines predict a nonrepairable, destroyed valve that is not suitable for direct repair.

VALVULAR REPAIR TECHNIQUES

Internal Valvuloplasty

Most primary incompetent valves and some valves affected by postthrombotic changes are amenable to direct valvuloplasty. In the classic Kistner procedure, a longitudinal venotomy is performed between the valve cusps 1 to 1.5 cm below the valve attachment lines with extension using a Potts scissors through the anterior commissural apex.[1] Plicating 7-0 polypropylene double-needled sutures are used to suture the valve edges together with the posterior commissural apex. All sutures are tied with knots outside the vein (Fig. 61-1). Plication shortens the valve cusps to eliminate valve leaflet redundancy. For the divided anterior commissure, separate sutures are needed for each half before closing the venotomy. This kind of repair requires a precise initial venotomy. Otherwise, entering the vein may result in damage to the valve.

As an alternative approach, a 1.5-cm supravalvular transverse incision can be performed 2.5 cm above the commissural apex.[9] The valve cusps are sutured together at their free edges, starting from the more central portion of the vein toward the commissures to shorten about 20% of the leaflet length. A transverse venotomy can be converted into a T venotomy by extending the venotomy toward but not across the valve annulus, which increases exposure.[10] Another incision is the "trapdoor" incision in which two partial transverse incisions are connected by a vertical incision through the anterior commissure.[11] The choice of technique is dictated by surgeon preference with similar results reported for all approaches.

External Valvuloplasty

Valve leaflet attachment lines are brought together by placing external, partial-thickness, plicating sutures to decrease vein diameter in the absence of a venotomy.[12] Interrupted sutures are initially placed at the commissural apex and then caudally placed over one fifth of the attachment line to narrow the commissural angle and decrease the vein diameter. Usually four to seven stitches are necessary at each commissural side until competence is noted by the strip test. A variation of this technique is limited anterior plication, in which only the anterior commissure is addressed by external valvuloplasty.

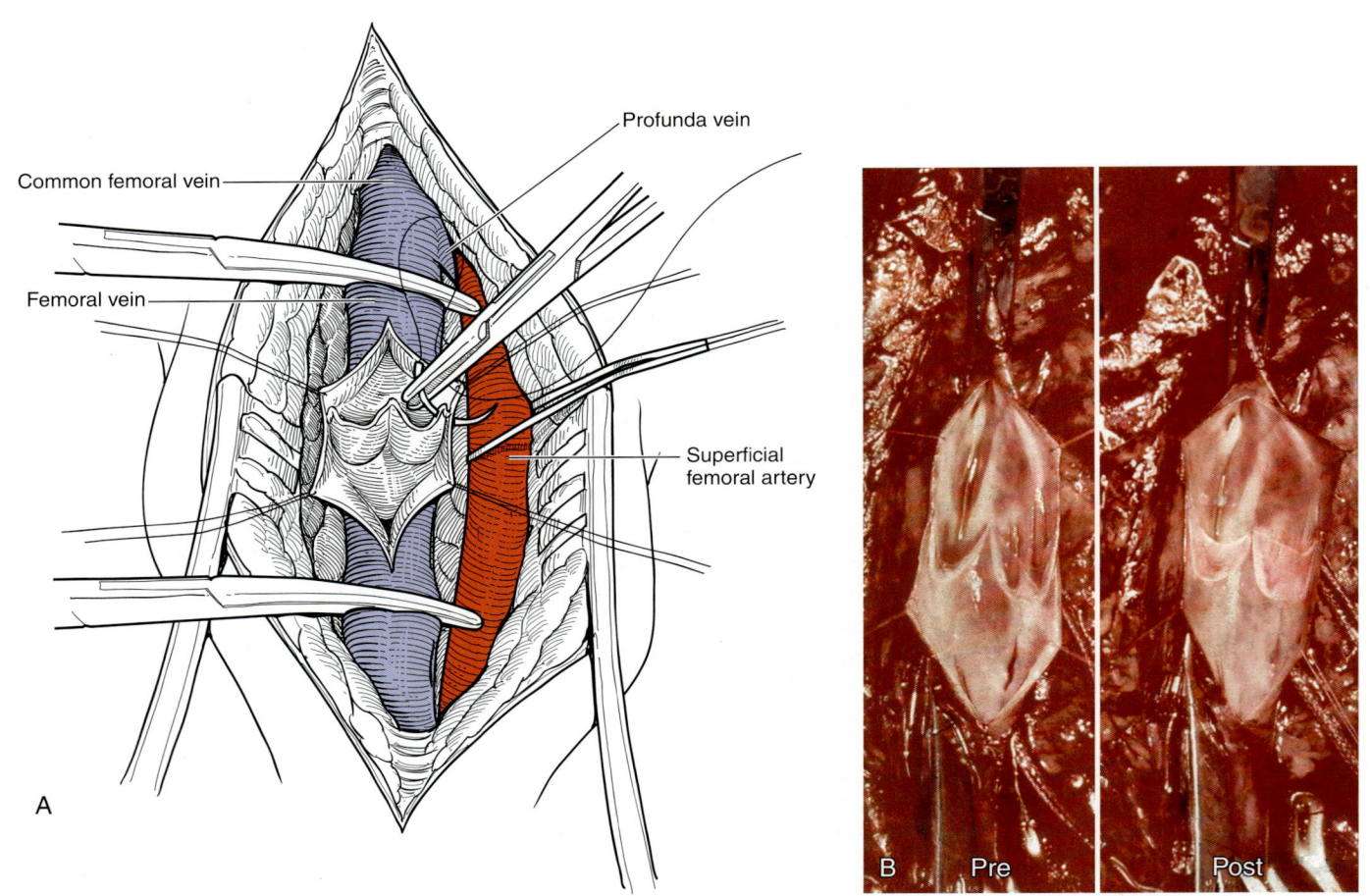

Figure 61-1. Kistner internal valvuloplasty. **A**, A longitudinal venotomy through the anterior commissure optimally exposes the valvular apparatus. Femoral vein internal valve repair is performed by applying multiple plicating sutures at each commissure through the valve cusps and the vein wall. **B**, Valve before and after repair. Sutures placed at each commissure tighten the angle and shorten the valve cusp. (**B**, *From Kistner RL: Surgical repair of a venous valve*, Straub Clin Proc 34:41-43, 1968.)

Angioscope-Assisted Valvuloplasty

An angioscope is used to identify valve attachment lines while external suturing is performed.[2] The vein is surgically exposed, and the scope is inserted through a great saphenous vein tributary or a venotomy proximal to the valve. If needed, a purse string may be placed around the scope entry site, because continuous irrigation with heparinized saline is required for optimal visualization. Suturing takes place from outside to inside the lumen and across each commissure encompassing the redundant free edges of the valve.

Transcommissural Valvuloplasty

Sutures are externally placed in a blind fashion without a venotomy. The first sutures lie at the commissural apex and are kept shallow. The lower sutures are deepened farther into the vein to encompass the cusp edges, like in angioscopic-assisted valvuloplasty. This closes the valve attachment angle and tightens the valve cusps.

External Banding Valvuloplasty

Some veins are incompetent because their diameter exceeds valve leaflet length, and a reduction in diameter may restore competence by allowing the cusps to meet. A 2- to 3-cm-long sleeve of polytetrafluoroethylene or polyester is wrapped around the valve, tightened to the desired diameter until competence is achieved, sutured longitudinally, and then secured to the adventitia.[13] This technique can be used to reinforce other valvuloplasties if the vein appears to be particularly dilated.

Autologous Neovalve Construction

Postthrombotic valves have been reconstructed without implantation of foreign material. Valves can be created de novo in the shape of semilunar cusps made by trimming the adventitia and part of the media of the great saphenous vein or one of its tributaries.[6] The nonintimal surface is then sewn in place and directed toward the lumen to decrease the risk of thrombosis. Alternatively, the great saphenous vein or a tributary of a deep vein is obliquely transected near its origin, and its stump is invaginated to be secured with a stitch to the opposite wall of the deep vein and thus create a pseudoneovalve.[14] The fibrous tissues of postthrombotic veins have also been used to create de novo, in situ neovalves, with the femoral vein used for most repairs.[15] In brief, the femoral vein is exposed and the valve reconstruction site is determined based on preoperative and intraoperative assessment. The venotomy can be longitudinal, T-shaped, or transverse. Dissection of the valve flap is initiated after endovenectomy using an ophthalmic scalpel or microsurgical scissors to lift a flap of intimal tissue. The depth of the valve is determined empirically so that the flap is sufficiently wide to occlude the lumen. Either a bicuspid or monocuspid valve can be created depending on the circumferential distribution of thrombotic thickening. The free edge of the flap near the attachment of neocommissure to the vein wall is secured in a semi-open position by applying 7-0 polypropylene sutures to fix it to the vein wall. The venotomy is closed, the vessel opened, and the flap assessed.

Vein Segment Transposition

In the presence of a great saphenous vein or profunda femoral vein segment with a competent valve, the incompetent common femoral vein can be divided distal from the incompetent valve and anastomosed end-to-end or end-to-side to the adjacent valve-bearing vein.[16] The profunda femoral vein is preferred because of the higher likelihood of late incompetence of the proximal valve of the great saphenous vein.

After performing a standard groin incision, the common femoral vein and its tributaries are dissected over a 10-cm length. Venous clamps are applied, and the femoral vein is transected at its confluence with the common femoral vein. The distal stump of the femoral vein is anastomosed to the anterior surface of the profunda femoral vein; alternatively, an end-to-end anastomosis is performed between the femoral vein and the first profunda femoral vein branch. An incompetent profunda femoral vein can be sewn to a competent great saphenous vein in similar fashion.

Vein Valve Transplantation

A vein segment containing one or more competent valves, characteristically the axillary or brachial vein, is interposed within an femoral vein or popliteal vein segment whose valves are destroyed or unrepairable by conventional valvuloplasty techniques.[6,8] A two-team approach significantly reduces operative time. The recipient vein is initially exposed (Fig. 61-2, A), followed by exposure of the donor vein. With the contralateral arm abducted and externally rotated, an 8- to 10-cm-long longitudinal incision is performed in the axilla parallel to the neurovascular bundle. The axillary vein is exposed, its branches are dissected and ligated, and the anterior wall is marked longitudinally with a marking pen to help prevent torsion at the time of transposition. Before harvesting the axillary vein, valve competence should be confirmed by duplex imaging or a strip test. Up to 40% of axillary vein valves may be incompetent but amenable to transcommissural or internal valvuloplasty. However, identifying a more proximal or distal segment containing a competent valve or harvesting the ipsilateral axillary vein is preferred.

Systemic heparin is administered, and 3 cm of the recipient vein is removed between clamps, which is usually half the length of the donor vein to be implanted. Intraluminal synechiae and masses within the recipient vein should be removed.

A 6- to 8-cm segment of axillary vein with competent valves is anastomosed to the recipient vein, proximal side first, with interrupted 7-0 polypropylene sutures, taking care not to entrap the valvular elements in the anastomosis (Fig. 61-2, *B*). Excess kinking or tension on the transposed segment should be avoided, and after completion of the distal anastomosis, a strip test is performed to confirm valve competence. A polyester or polytetrafluoroethylene sleeve can be wrapped around the transplanted segment to prevent future dilation of the vein segment.

Artificial Valve Implantation

When incompetent deep valves are unrepairable, implantation of an artificial venous valve may provide an alternative option in the future. Experimental studies

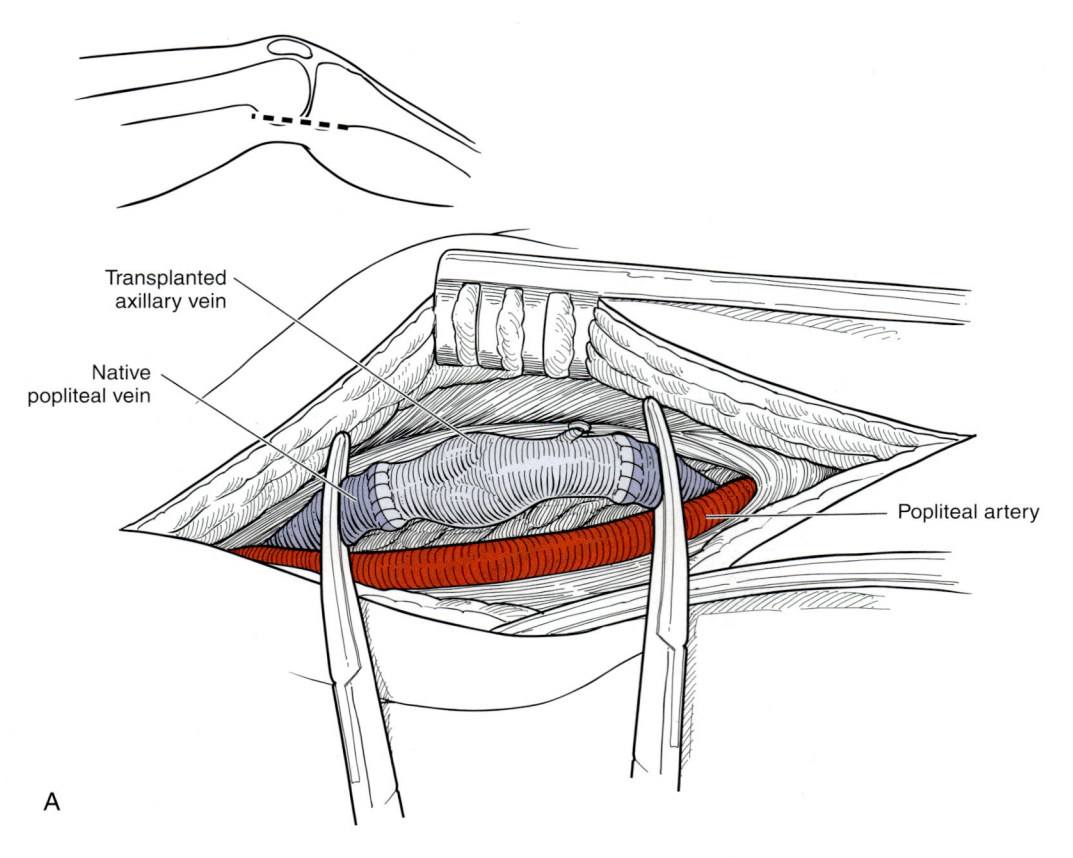

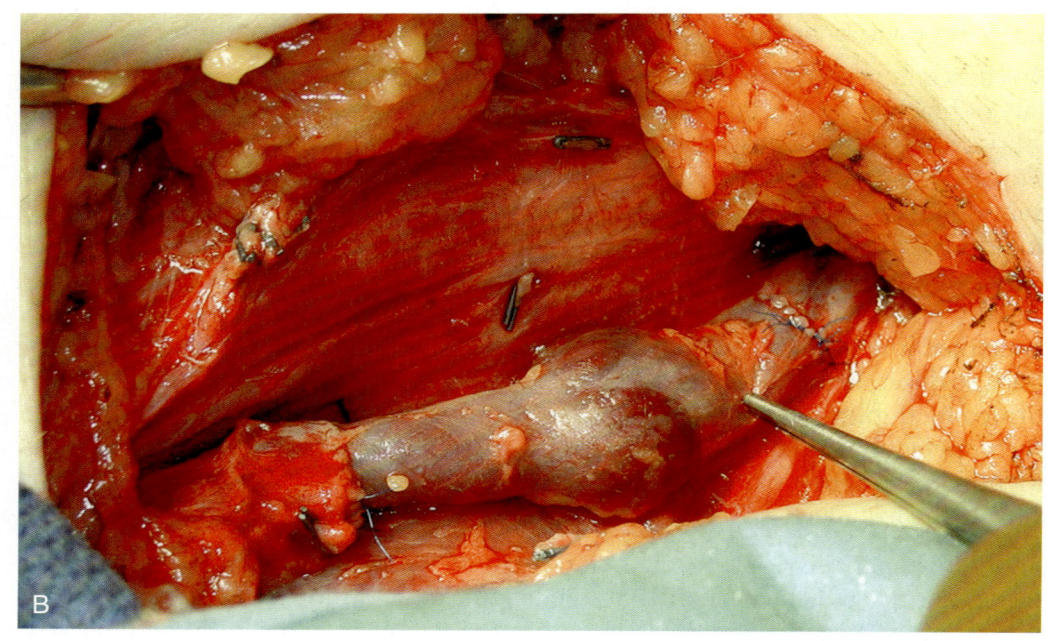

Figure 61-2. Axillary vein transfer. **A**, The above-the-knee popliteal vein has been exposed through a medial incision, and a segment of vein has been removed. A portion of axillary vein has been harvested and anastomosed as an interposition graft to the recipient popliteal vein. Correct orientation of the valve should be maintained to facilitate distal to proximal venous flow. **B**, Axillary vein transfer to the femoral vein. The transplanted axillary vein bears a competent valve whose attachment lines are visible through the thin wall, as opposed to the recipient vein, which has thickened, scarred walls. The patient's foot is located to the right and head to the left of the photograph. (**B**, *Courtesy Peter Neglen, MD, SP Vascular Center, Limassol, Cyprus.*)

with cryopreserved femoral vein and glutheraldehyde-preserved bovine vein have failed in early or midterm clinical follow-up.[17] Xenograft bicuspid valves produced by mounting decellularized small intestine submucosa on a stent have been reported, but clinical efficacy has yet to be demonstrated.[18]

Closure

Venous branches are tied individually to avoid hematoma. Heparin should not be reversed and placement of a drain considered since postoperative anticoagulation is anticipated.

SUBFASCIAL ENDOSCOPIC PERFORATOR SURGERY

Choice of Anesthesia

General or spinal anesthesia is required, especially when concomitant procedures are planned. SEPS under tumescent anesthesia alone has been reported.

Incision

The equipment required for SEPS can be adapted from that typically used for laparoscopic general surgery (Box 61-1). The patient is placed in the supine position, and the limb is elevated and exsanguinated with an Esmarch bandage. A thigh tourniquet is inflated to 300 mm Hg, and the limb rested on a leg holder (Fig. 61-3). The two-port technique uses one port for the camera and a separate

Box 61-1	SUBFASCIAL ENDOSCOPIC PERFORATOR SURGERY EQUIPMENT

- Esmarch bandage
- Thigh pneumatic tourniquet
- Dissection balloon
- Laparoscopic ports (10 and 5 mm)
- Camera with light source and video monitor
- CO_2 insufflator
- Laparoscopic scissors
- Laparoscopic harmonic scalpel, electrocautery, or clip applier

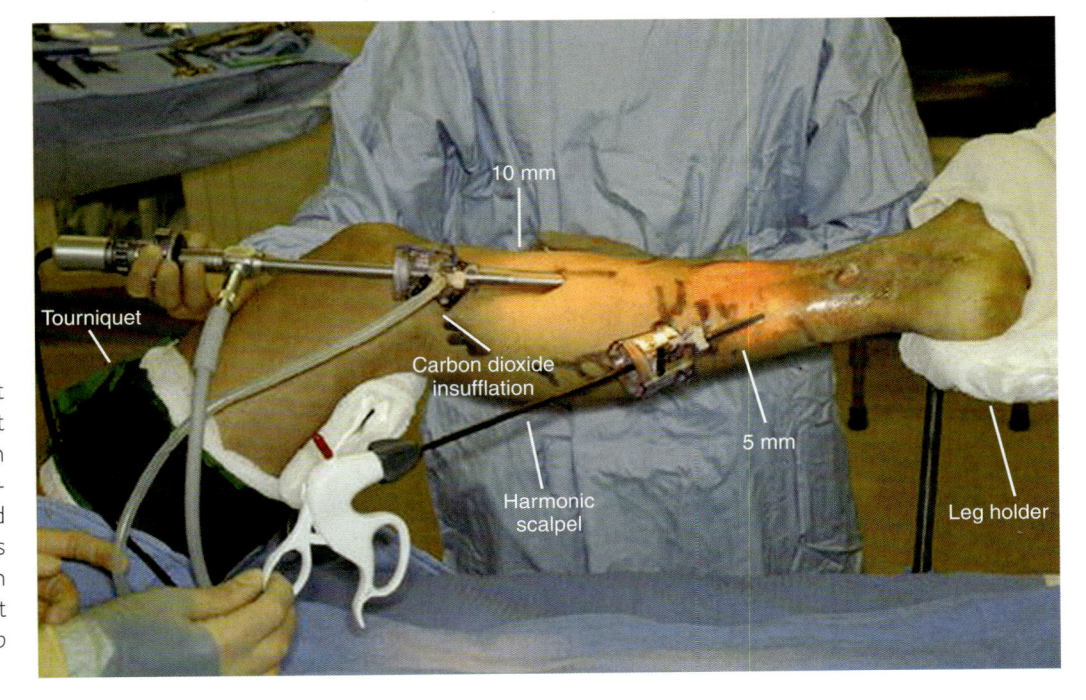

Figure 61-3. SEPS two-port technique with a 10-mm port for the camera and a 5-mm port for a harmonic scalpel. Carbon dioxide insufflation is used to visualize the perforator veins in the subfascial space; a thigh tourniquet and leg holder assist with hemostasis. *(Courtesy Mayo Foundation, Rochester, Minn.)*

port for instrumentation. A vertical 10-mm incision is placed in the medial aspect of the calf 10 cm distal from the tibial tuberosity, the fascia is identified by blunt dissection, grasped with mosquito clamps, and incised longitudinally. A large opening should be avoided to minimize gas leakage and poor visualization.

Port Insertion

A 10-mm endoscopic port is placed through the incision, and a space-maker balloon inserted and then inflated to widen the subfascial space (Fig. 61-4). The distal 5-mm port is placed halfway between the first port and the ankle, approximately 10 to 12 cm away from each. Carbon dioxide is insufflated into the subfascial space, and pressure is maintained at 30 mm Hg.

Exploration of the Subfascial Space

The loose connective tissue between the calf muscles and the superficial fascia is sharply divided, and the subfascial space is explored from the medial border of the tibia to the posterior midline, between the ankle and the 10-mm port. A thorough knowledge of the anatomy of medial leg perforating veins and their relationships to the deep fascia is essential (Fig. 61-5). Perforators are identified between the fascia of the posterior superficial compartment and the posterior tibial veins. Important medial perforators include the lower and upper posterior tibial perforators, as well as the proximal paratibial perforating veins (Fig. 61-6). The upper posterior tibial and the lowest proximal paratibial perforators are also accessible from the subfascial space. All perforators encountered are divided with a harmonic scalpel, with an electrocautery, or between clips (Fig. 61-7).

Paratibial Fasciotomy

A paratibial fasciotomy is made by sharply incising the fascia of the deep posterior compartment close to the tibia to avoid injury to the posterior tibial vessels and nerve. The posterior tibial perforators are identified behind the paratibial fascia or the intermuscular septum, which also has to be incised. The medial insertion of the soleus muscle on the tibia may need to be exposed to visualize proximal paratibial perforators. Proximal perforating veins can also be divided by rotating the ports cephalad and continuing the dissection to the level of the knee.

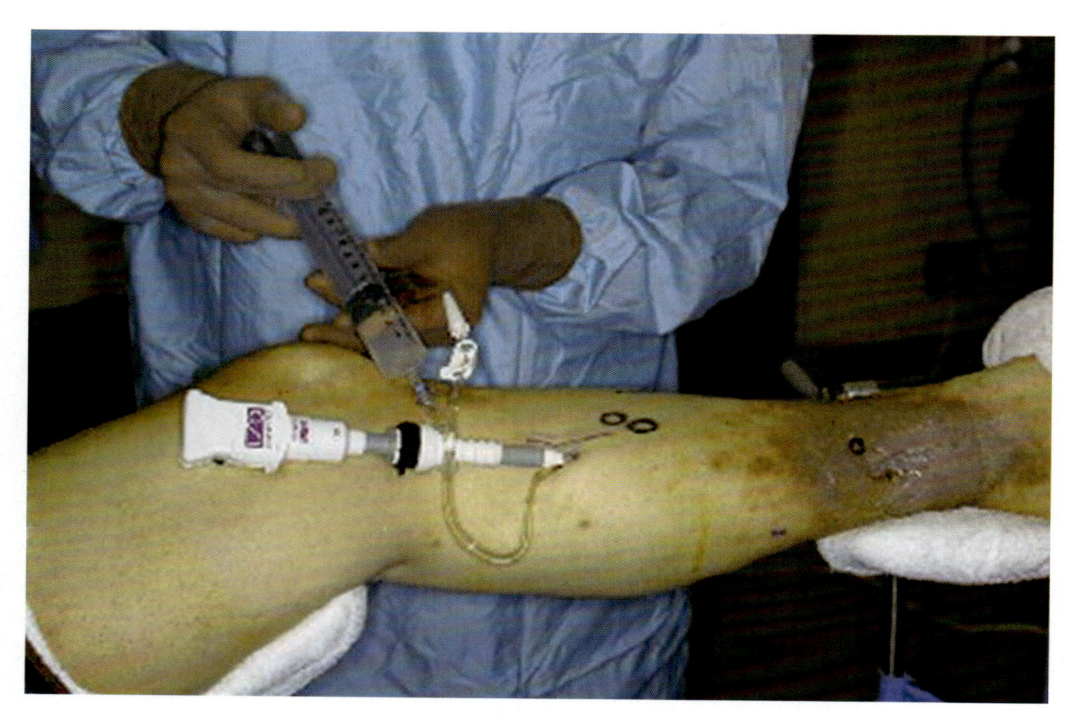

Figure 61-4. Endoscopic port insertion during SEPS procedure. The proximal port is inserted in the medial calf, 10 cm from the tibial tuberosity. The space-maker balloon is then inserted and inflated to widen the subfascial space. *(Courtesy Mayo Foundation, Rochester, Minn.)*

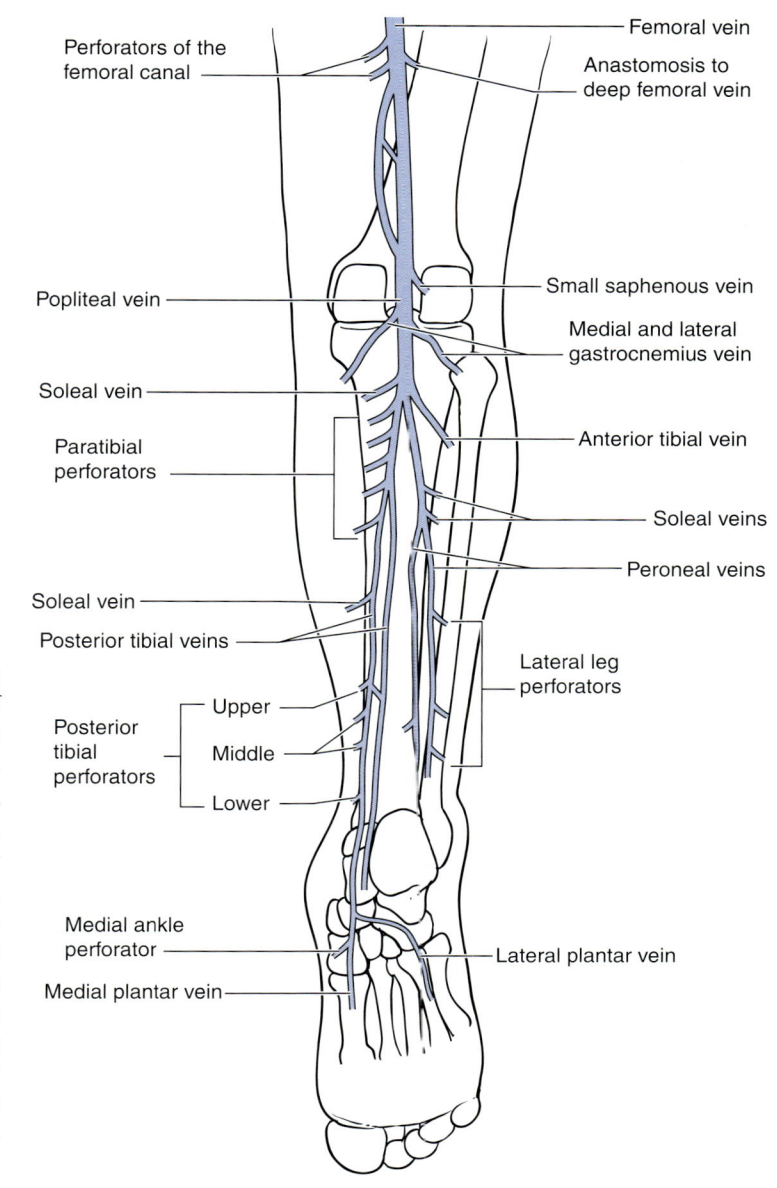

SURGICAL TREATMENT OF LOWER EXTREMITY DEEP AND PERFORATOR VEIN INCOMPETENCE

Figure 61-5. Anatomy of the perforating veins of the leg. The lower extremity consists of four main groups of perforating veins: foot, medial calf, lateral calf, and thigh perforators. The direct medial calf or posterior tibial perforators, which cross the superficial posterior compartment, contribute to venous ulcer formation when incompetent. Cockett I perforators, now referred to as lower posterior tibial perforators, are located behind the medial malleolus, whereas middle and upper posterior tibial perforators, formerly Cockett II and III perforators, respectively, are located more proximally in the calf, approximately 7 to 9 and 10 to 12 cm from the medial malleolus, respectively, and about 1 inch medial to the tibia. These perforators connect the posterior arch vein to the posterior tibial veins. Paratibial direct perforators are located closer to the tibia and 18 to 22 cm from the medial malleolus. *(Redrawn from art provided by Mayo Foundation, Rochester, Minn.)*

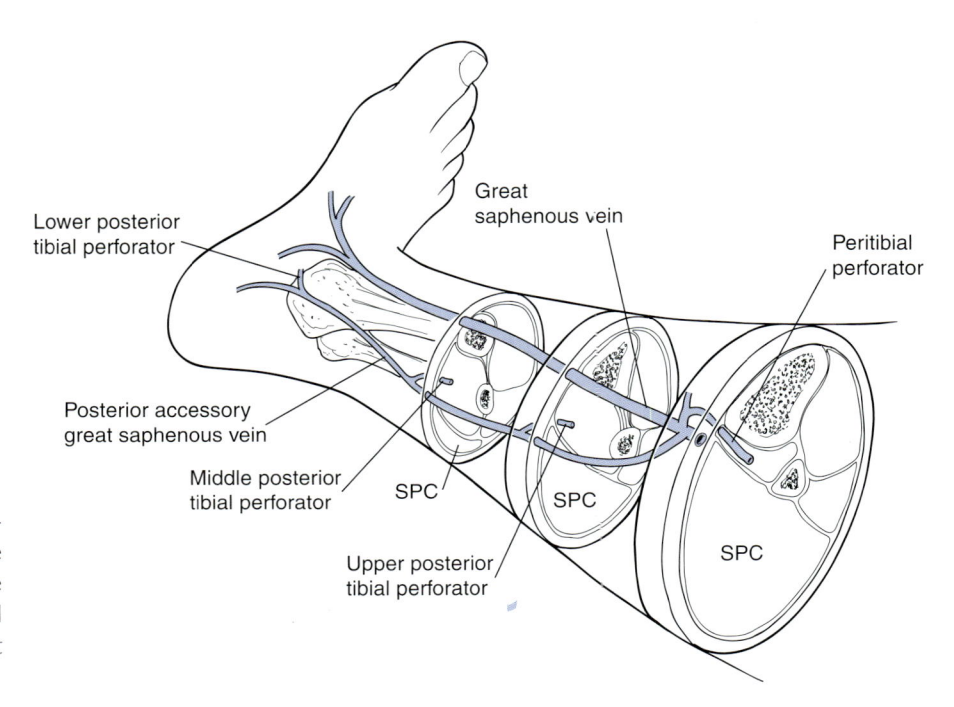

Figure 61-6. Proximal paratibial perforators. These perforating veins connect the great saphenous vein and its tributaries to the tibial vein or popliteal vein. *SPC,* Superficial posterior compartment. *(Redrawn from art provided by Mayo Foundation, Rochester, Minn.)*

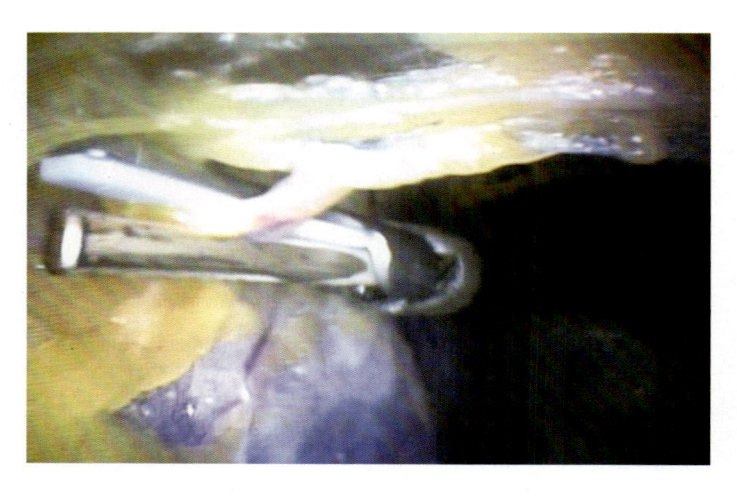

Figure 61-7. Perforator vein interruption. A perforating vein encountered in the subfascial space is dissected and divided with a harmonic scalpel.

Distal Ankle Perforators

Access to retromalleolar, lower posterior tibial perforator endoscopically is usually not possible through a paratibial fasciotomy, and if the perforator is incompetent, a separate incision may be required to gain direct exposure.

Closure

After completion of the endoscopic portion of the procedure, the instruments and ports are removed, CO_2 is manually expressed from the limb, and the tourniquet is deflated. To relieve postoperative pain, 20 mL of 0.5% bupivacaine solution is instilled into the subfascial space. Port sites are closed in two layers, and the limb is wrapped with an elastic bandage.

Concomitant Procedures

Endovenous ablation or high ligation and stripping of the great saphenous vein or small saphenous vein, if incompetent, are performed, along with stab avulsions, at the end of the SEPS procedure.

Postoperative Care

DEEP VENOUS VALVE SURGERY

- Gradual increase in activity is allowed the day after surgery, but leg elevation and sequential compression devices should be continued until the patient is fully ambulatory.
- Intravenous heparin or subcutaneous low-molecular-weight heparin should be converted to warfarin in the postoperative period.
- Prophylactic antibiotics, such as cefazolin, should be administered within 1 hour before surgical incision and discontinued within 24 hours from the end of surgery.
- A postoperative duplex scan of both lower extremities is performed before discharge to confirm patency of the valve repair and to exclude early DVT.
- Most patients are able to return to work within 2 to 3 weeks. However, those patients whose usual activity requires prolonged standing or heavy lifting should wait up to 6 weeks before returning to work.
- Postoperative arm swelling after axillary or brachial vein harvest can be prevented by arm elevation and through the use of an elastic compression bandage. An upper extremity sling may also be worn for the first 48 to 72 hours.

SUBFASCIAL ENDOSCOPIC PERFORATOR SURGERY

- Leg elevation at 30 degrees and an elastic compression bandage should be maintained postoperatively. Ambulation is permitted after an initial 3-hour period.

- SEPS is an outpatient procedure, and patients are discharged the same day or after overnight observation.
- Patients may return to work in 10 to 14 days and are advised to wear elastic compression stockings providing 30 to 40 mm Hg of external pressure.

Complications

DEEP VENOUS VALVE SURGERY

- **Deep vein thrombosis.** Incidence of early thrombosis is 2% to 10%, higher in secondary cases but often does not involve the reconstructed valve.[19] Pulmonary embolism is rare (<1%).
- **Hematoma.** Hematoma occurs in about 2% to 16% of cases, as a consequence of perioperative anticoagulation.[20] Evacuation is recommended to avoid vein compression and thrombosis of the reconstructed valve.
- **Wound complications.** The incidence of wound complications, including infection, seroma, and lymphatic leak, is 2% to 4%.[20]
- **Late recurrence.** Valve competence after repair has been reported to range between 50% and 70% at 10 years, depending on the type of repair and indication.[20] Internal valvuloplasty offers the best long-term results, and the success rate of primary valvuloplasty exceeds valve transposition (73% vs. 43%).[21] Reoperative valve reconstruction because of failure of initial valve repair may be quite difficult.[6] In these cases, selecting a more distal valve for repair or performing a valve transposition may be a wiser option.

SUBFASCIAL ENDOSCOPIC PERFORATOR SURGERY

- **Ulcer nonhealing and recurrence.** After SEPS, with or without superficial venous ablation, ulcers heal in about 88% of limbs and the recurrence rate is 13% at 21 months.[22] Risk factors for failure of ulcer healing or a recurrent ulcer include missed, new, or recurrent incompetent perforators, postthrombotic syndrome, deep vein obstruction, or an ulcer greater than 2 cm in size. An intact intermuscular septum or deep posterior fascia that hides incompetent middle posterior tibial perforators may lead to treatment failure. Redo-SEPS can be performed; however, the rate of postoperative complications such as hematoma or cellulitis increases.
- **Hematoma.** Significant intraoperative bleeding is rare, especially if the tourniquet is properly inflated. Nonetheless, an accidental injury to a tibial vessel or venous branch may result in postoperative subfascial or wound hematomas, which occur in 9% or 5% of cases, respectively.[23]
- **Nerve injury.** Saphenous, sural, and tibial nerve injury causing neuralgia, neuropraxia, or both may occur at a rate of between 0% and 9%. Long-lasting hypoesthesia and paresthesia of the medial ankle, plantar surface of the foot, or both may occur in up to 4% of patients.[24]
- **Infection.** Wound infection occurs in up to 6% of patients. The risk can be reduced by providing appropriate perioperative care of open ulcers and avoiding contamination during surgery.
- **Deep vein thrombosis.** DVT occurs in less than 1% of cases.

REFERENCES

1. Kistner RL: Surgical repair of a venous valve, *Straub Clin Proc* 34:41-43, 1968.
2. Gloviczki P, Merrell SW, Bower TC: Femoral vein valve repair under direct vision without venotomy: A modified technique with use of angioscopy, *J Vasc Surg* 14:645-648, 1991.
3. Linton RR: The operative treatment of varicose veins and ulcers, based upon a classification of these lesions, *Ann Surg* 107:582-593, 1938.
4. Hauer G: Endoscopic subfascial discussion of perforating veins: Preliminary report, *Vasa* 14:59-61, 1985.

5. Gloviczki P, Cambria RA, Rhee RY, et al: Surgical technique and preliminary results of endoscopic subfascial division of perforating veins, *J Vasc Surg* 23:517-523, 1996.
6. Raju S, Hardy J: Technical options in venous valve reconstruction, *Am J Surg* 173:301-307, 1997.
7. Raju S, Fredericks RK, Neglen PN, et al: Durability of venous valve reconstruction techniques for "primary" and postthrombotic reflux, *J Vasc Surg* 23:357-366, 1996.
8. Eriksson I, Almgren B: Influence of the profunda femoris vein on venous hemodynamics of the limb: Experience from thirty-one deep vein valve reconstructions, *J Vasc Surg* 4:390-395, 1986.
9. Raju S, Fredericks R: Valve reconstruction procedures for nonobstructive venous insufficiency: Rationale, techniques, and results in 107 procedures with two- to eight-year follow-up, *J Vasc Surg* 7:301-310, 1988.
10. Sottiurai VS: Technique in direct venous valvuloplasty, *J Vasc Surg* 8:646-648, 1998.
11. Tripathi R, Ktenidis KD: Trapdoor internal valvuloplasty: A new technique for primary deep vein valvular incompetence, *Eur J Vasc Endovasc Surg* 22:86-89, 2001.
12. Kistner RL: Surgical technique of external valve repair, *Straub Found Proc* 55:15-16, 1990.
13. Jessup G, Lane RJ: Repair of incompetent valves: A new technique, *J Vasc Surg* 8:569-575, 1988.
14. Plagnol P, Ciostek P, Grimaud JP, et al: Technique de reconstruction valvulaire autogene dans le syndrome de reflux post-phlebitique, *Ann Chir Vasc* 13, 1999. 399-342.
15. Maleti O, Lugli M: Neovalve construction in postthrombotic syndrome, *J Vasc Surg* 43:794-799, 2006.
16. Ferris EB, Kistner RL: Femoral vein reconstruction in the management of chronic venous insufficiency: A 14-year experience, *Arch Surg* 117:1571-1579, 1982.
17. Dalsing MC, Raju S, Wakefield TW, et al: A multicenter, phase I evaluation of cryopreserved venous valve allografts for the treatment of chronic venous insufficiency, *J Vasc Surg* 30:854-866, 1999.
18. Pavcnik D, Uchida B, Kaufman J, et al: Percutaneous management of chronic deep venous reflux: Review of experimental work and early clinical experience with bioprosthetic valve, *Vasc Med* 13:75-84, 2008.
19. Cheatle TR, Perrin M: Venous valve repair: Early results in fifty-two cases, *J Vasc Surg* 19:404-413, 1994.
20. Masuda EM, Kistner RL: Long term results of venous valve reconstruction: A four- to twenty-one year follow-up, *J Vasc Surg* 19:391-403, 1994.
21. Tripathi R, Sieunarine K, Abbas M, et al: Deep venous valve reconstruction for non-healing leg ulcers: Techniques and results, *ANZ J Surg* 74:34-39, 2004.
22. Gloviczki P, Bergan JJ, Rhodes JM, et al: Midterm results of endoscopic perforator vein interruption for chronic venous insufficiency: Lessons learned from the North American subfascial endoscopic perforator surgery registry. North American Study Group, *J Vasc Surg* 29:489-502, 1999.
23. Kulbaski M, Salam A, Castor S, et al: Subfascial hemorrhage after endoscopic perforator vein ligation. Control with balloon tamponade, *Surg Endosc* 12:990-991, 1998.
24. Ciostek P, Myrcha P, Noszcyk W: Ten years experience with subfascial endoscopic perforator vein surgery, *Ann Vasc Surgery* 16:480-487, 2002.

62 Sclerotherapy

ERIC MOWATT-LARSSEN • CYNTHIA SHORTELL

Historical Background

Sclerotherapy is the chemical ablation of abnormal veins. The modern goal of therapy is an irreversible fibrotic occlusion, followed by reabsorption of the target vessel. Sclerotherapy is an old technique revolutionized by recent technological advances. Elsholz performed the first known endovenous treatment when he used a chicken bone needle and pigeon bladder syringe in 1665 to treat venous ulcers. Pravaz invented the syringe in 1831, and Rynd invented the hypodermic needle in 1845. Sclerotherapy's popularity has increased and decreased sporadically over the last 200 years. A randomized, controlled trial in the 1970s showed sclerotherapy to be less durable than surgery.[1] Sclerotherapy was then revolutionized by the advent of foamed sclerosants and ultrasound guidance, which have greatly improved efficacy and decreased risk. Foaming detergent sclerosants improved sclerosant potency and allowed sclerosant visualization by ultrasound. Ultrasound guidance allowed better anatomic visualization, greater hemodynamic understanding, more precise foam targeting and delivery, and monitoring for unwanted foam passage into deep veins. With these advances, sclerotherapy has now become an appropriate treatment for any type or size of vein.

The development of sclerotherapy has been limited by the range in techniques. This practice variation has produced inconsistent results that make generalizations about the procedure difficult. In the last few years, however, variations in technique have begun to be evaluated and the resulting knowledge has improved overall results. There have been two European consensus meetings on foam sclerotherapy, in 2003 and 2006, which arrived at a consensus opinion from a panel of those experienced in sclerotherapy.[2]

Preoperative Preparation

- **History and physical examination.** Symptoms and signs of chronic vein disease include varicose veins, telangiectasias, extremity pain or swelling worsened with standing and improved by elevation, and skin changes around the ankle area.
- **Duplex ultrasound.** The duplex ultrasound examination permits determination of venous anatomy and hemodynamics. Superficial, perforator, and deep venous systems are examined for obstruction or reflux. Venous reflux is retrograde blood flow of over 0.5 seconds.
- **Magnetic resonance angiography.** Patients with evidence of a vascular malformation, such as lesions present since birth, or abnormal anatomy or blood flow on ultrasound, should have further testing, usually magnetic resonance angiography, to determine whether the malformation is high flow or low flow. Such malformations should be treated by a multidisciplinary team, often containing experts in phlebology, vascular surgery, plastic surgery, dermatology, and orthopedic surgery. Low-flow venous malformations can often be treated successfully by foam sclerotherapy.

- **Sequence of treatment of chronic venous disease.** Abnormal veins are usually treated beginning with the superficial system, followed by the perforator veins and finally the deep system. Superficial vein therapies have good efficacy and minimal side effects. Perforator vein treatments are technically efficacious but of uncertain patient benefit in many cases. Deep vein treatments carry a higher risk, have more variable success rates, and are usually treated only in patients with particularly severe symptoms and only at a specialized center.

- **Sequence of treatment of superficial venous disease.** Superficial veins are usually treated in the following order when symptomatic reflux is present: saphenous veins, tributary veins, and localized veins. Sclerotherapy can be used to treat almost any abnormal vein. It is most effective for veins less than 6 to 7 mm in diameter, but is still effective with excellent technique at almost any vein diameter.[3] Endovenous thermal ablation and surgical ligation and stripping are performed more often than sclerotherapy in the United States for symptomatic incompetent saphenous veins. Ambulatory phlebectomy is an alternative for tributary veins or localized varicosities, especially at larger vein diameters. Surface laser therapy can be used for telangiectasias and reticular varicosities, but sclerotherapy is considered first-line therapy for these veins on the lower extremity.

- **Preoperative patient counseling.** In a recent randomized, controlled trial, polidocanol microfoam proved noninferior to surgical treatment for saphenous vein reflux.[4] In a recent metaanalysis, ultrasound-determined pooled saphenous ablation rates at 3 years were 77% for sclerotherapy, 78% for stripping, 84% for radiofrequency ablation, and 94% for laser ablation.[5] Sclerofoam injection improved ulcer healing rates in patients with severe chronic venous insufficiency in one study.[6] Sclerotherapy success rates around 80% have been reported for tributary veins, perforator veins, and recurrent varicose veins after surgery.[7] Sclerotherapy produces minimal procedural and postprocedural pain. It is easier to perform than most alternative strategies. However, even with recently improved techniques, the need for repeat treatment is high. Therefore it is important to inform patients that retreatment may be required.

Pitfalls and Danger Points

- **Deep vein thrombosis (DVT) and thrombophilia.** Active DVT or obstruction is a contraindication to sclerotherapy, because abnormal superficial flow is often required to bypass the obstruction. Risks and benefits in patients with increased risk of DVT, such as patients with thrombophilia, cancer, or limited mobility, should be carefully weighed. Screening for thrombophilia should be considered in patients with prior unprovoked or multiple episodes of thrombosis. Prophylactic anticoagulation should be considered for these more complicated patients if treatment is necessary. A typical prophylactic regimen is enoxaparin 40 mg subcutaneous just before sclerotherapy and then daily thereafter for 7 days.

- **Symptomatic patent foramen ovale.** Foam sclerotherapy should be avoided in patients with symptomatic patent foramen ovale, because these patients may be at increased risk of neurologic complications because of passage of foam through a right to left shunt. Symptoms associated with patent foramen ovale include stroke or transient ischemic attack of undefined etiology and migraine or migrainelike headaches. Patients with other known but asymptomatic right to left shunts may have a greater risk of neurologic complications. Sclerofoam injection may precipitate a migraine headache, and patients with this history should be warned of the risk.

- **Allergic reaction.** Allergy to a sclerosant may necessitate avoiding the agent. Having multiple allergies is a relative contraindication to sclerotherapy.

Anaphylaxis after sclerotherapy is a rare complication, but physicians should be equipped for and prepared to manage such an emergency.

- **Pregnancy.** The safety of sclerotherapy during pregnancy has not been established. In addition, varicosities appearing during pregnancy often decrease in size or resolve spontaneously. Treatment is usually delayed until around 3 months postpartum if possible.
- **Arterial insufficiency.** Sclerotherapy is less successful in patients in whom external compression is difficult to apply, such as patients with arterial insufficiency or severe obesity.

Endovascular Strategy

SEQUENCE OF TREATMENT OF SUPERFICIAL VEINS

Veins are first treated at the proximal source of reflux and then closed distally until ablation is complete. This strategy allows the interruption of proximal sources of pressure, which plays a major role in the pathophysiology of chronic venous disease. Abnormal proximal vein pressure because of reflux is relayed distally through the venous system in refluxing veins when the patient's extremity is below heart level because of the increased blood volume and the weight of the blood column from gravity. Ambulatory venous hypertension, the inability to reduce venous pressure through calf muscle contraction and venous valve closure, is the major cause of symptoms of chronic venous disease.[8]

SELECTION OF A SCLEROSANT SOLUTION

Sodium tetradecyl sulfate (STS) is the most frequently used sclerosant in the United States because of good efficacy, low risk of side effects, and its approval by the U.S. Food and Drug Administration as a liquid sclerosant. Polidocanol is another detergent sclerosant used often in Europe. By using varying concentrations and foaming techniques, STS can be used in almost any type of vein. Liquid sclerosant is most often used to correct reticular varicosities and telangiectasias, whereas foam is most often used for all sizes of varicose veins. Table 62-1 is a general guideline for recommended STS concentrations. Emerging evidence, however, indicates that higher sclerosant concentrations may not always be more effective than lower concentrations, as had been previously assumed.[9]

Other sclerosants are also used, such as glycerin and hypertonic saline. Glycerin is effective for telangiectasias and has a lower side effect rate than that of STS. Glycerin can be used after dilution with lidocaine to 50% concentration. For example, glycerin at a 72% concentration and a dose of 2.0 mL can be mixed with lidocaine at a 1% concentration and dose of 1.0 mL. The lidocaine reduces injection pain. Hypertonic saline carries more side effects than STS or glycerin but is useful is patients with allergy to other sclerosants. It can be used at a 23.4% concentration or diluted as far down as 11.7%.

TABLE 62-1 Sodium Tetradecyl Sulfate Concentration Guidelines

Vein	Concentration (%), Technique
Great saphenous vein	3.0, foam
Small or accessory saphenous veins	1.0, foam
Tributary vein	1.0, foam
Perforator vein	1.0, foam
Localized 7- to 10-mm diameter	0.5-1.0, foam
Localized 3- to 7-mm diameter	0.25-0.50, foam
Reticular varicosity	0.25, liquid
Telangiectasia	0.25, liquid or glycerin

Endovascular Technique

POSITIONING

Patient positioning is an important variable, especially with the use of sclerofoam. A reverse Trendelenburg position facilitates venous access by increasing vein diameter. In patients whose varicose veins and reticular varicosities collapse with extremity elevation, veins can be accessed in a dependent position with a 27-Ga butterfly needle with normal saline and then taped in place. Subsequent extremity elevation decreases vein diameter, making sclerotherapy more effective and less risky. Tumescent anesthesia can also potentially be used to decrease vein diameter. In principle elevating the treated extremity to 45 degrees may limit passage of bubbles into the pulmonary and cardiac circulations.

FOAMING THE SCLEROSANT SOLUTION

The Tessari method[10] is most often used to foam the detergent sclerosants such as STS. Video 62-1 shows this technique. One syringe of 1.0 mL of liquid sclerosant is connected by a three-way stopcock valve to a syringe with 4.0 mL of air. The stopcock valve is turned 30 to 45 degrees from flat to make the foamed bubbles as small as possible but still allow mixing of the two syringes. The syringes are mixed vigorously back and forth at least 20 times. Current consensus recommendations are to limit total volume injected per site to 2 to 4 mL and per session to 10 mL of foam. Sclerofoam bubble size and stability (how long the bubbles remain small) may be key variables in decreasing systemic symptoms, as discussed elsewhere. With the preceding technique (4:1 air-to-STS volume), the foam should be used within 60 to 90 seconds. Other techniques that may decrease bubble size, increase foam stability, or both include the use of carbon dioxide or CO_2-O_2 mixtures, low silicone content syringes, larger-bore needles, filters, or variation in the gas-to-liquid volume ratio.[11]

INJECTION OF THE TARGET VEIN

A 27-Ga butterfly needle can be used with a syringe for treatment of localized varicose veins and reticular varicosities. The appearance of blood in the butterfly tubing indicates successful cannulation. The sclerosant is then injected into the target vein and the vessel blanches, showing the replacement of blood with sclerosant. The injection is halted immediately when the target vein is filled, with injection volume per site usually less than 0.5 mL (Video 62-2).

For telangiectasias the target vessel can be injected with a syringe, 30-Ga needle, and STS that is a 0.25% concentration liquid. The target vessel should blanch immediately. The injection is halted if any bleb appears. When treating smaller vessels, magnification is highly recommended. Keeping the needle flat to the skin surface and aiming superficially also helps.

For larger veins or veins near deep junctions, ultrasound guidance can be used to guide needle and catheter placement into the target vein and to monitor for foam migration into deep veins. In general, the catheter should be placed more than 10 cm from a major deep-superficial junction, such as the saphenofemoral junction. After ultrasound-guided venous access, the patient can be placed in the Trendelenburg position. The sclerofoam is then mixed and injected into the target vein under ultrasound guidance. The foam is easily visible on ultrasound as hyperdense bubbles displacing hypodense blood, as shown in Figure 62-1.

Postoperative Care

- **Elevation.** After sclerofoam injection, patients are kept with the treated extremity elevated another 5 to 10 minutes to allow the foam to liquefy as much as possible and prevent early proximal foam movement. If asymptomatic, compression can be applied and the patient can be allowed to walk.

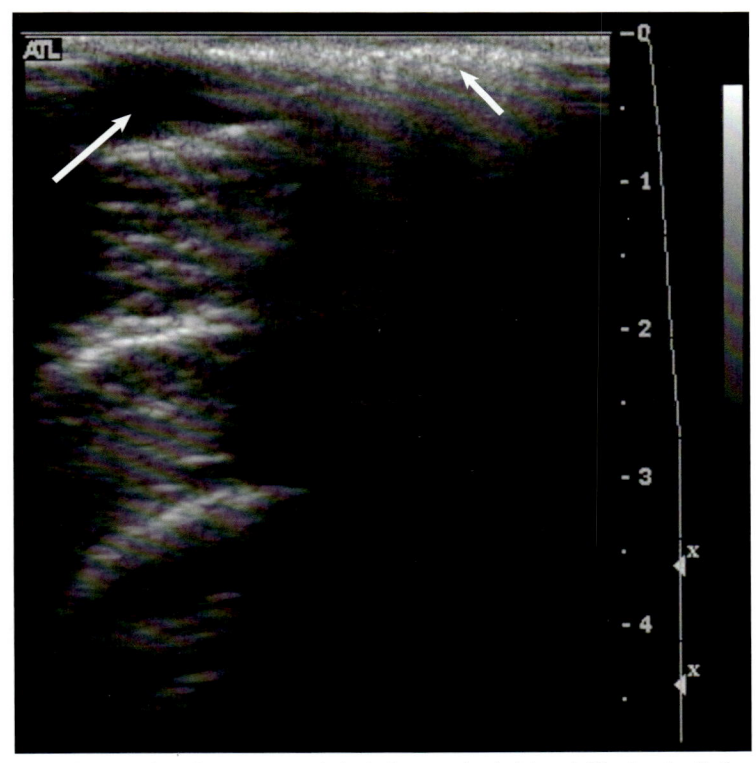

Figure 62-1. Duplex ultrasound picture showing a normal dark, hypoechoic blood-filled vein *(left arrow)* and a white, hyperechoic foam-filled vein *(right arrow).*

- **Compression.** Postsclerotherapy compression improves efficacy and theoretically reduces the risk of DVT. Some research shows a benefit to postsclerotherapy compression for as long as 6 weeks, but this result must be balanced with likelihood of patient compliance. Use of a 20 to 30 mm Hg knee- or thigh-high compression hose that covers the treated area is recommended day and night for 1 week. Large varicosities are compressed with a localized compression dressing of cotton gauze and self-adherent elastic wrap during the initial 48 hours after treatment to reduce the risk of trapped blood.
- **Management of intravascular hematoma.** Trapped blood, which is also referred to as a "thrombus" or "intravascular hematoma," manifests as a hard, tender vein in an area treated recently with sclerotherapy. It should be drained after around 2 to 3 weeks with a large-caliber, 18-Ga needle and pressure to decrease pain and reduce the risk of hyperpigmentation, as discussed later.

Complications

- **Thrombotic complications.** The risk of DVT is low, well under 1% for most veins,[12] but may be higher in large-diameter veins. Postsclerotherapy ultrasound is usually unnecessary unless treating a higher-risk patient (e.g., less mobile) or a higher-risk vein (e.g., larger diameter or near a major junction). Treatment for DVT includes anticoagulation, ultrasound surveillance for clot improvement and resolution, and compression stocking. Superficial thrombophlebitis can usually be treated with microphlebectomy, compression, or both. One study showed an increased risk of DVT in veins greater than 5 mm in diameter and for total sclerofoam volumes greater than 10 mL. STS foam at a 2.0% to 2.5% concentration had an increased risk compared with lower or higher concentrations.[13]
- **Gas embolization.** Rare neurologic and pulmonary symptoms are believed to result from passage of gas bubbles into the systemic circulation.[14] Gas emboli from sclerofoam frequently pass into the right ventricle, as detected by

transthoracic echocardiography. These emboli can then pass into the cerebral circulation via the left ventricle if a right to left shunt is present because of a patent foramen ovale or pulmonary arteriovenous malformation. Sclerofoam has been associated with rare episodes of cerebrovascular accident, transient ischemic attack, visual disturbances similar to a migraine aura, and migraine headaches. Systemic bubbles in the pulmonary circulation may produce chest tightness or dry cough. Injecting very small bubbles and using carbon dioxide–predominant gas mixtures may reduce systemic symptoms. Other technique modifications that are thought to reduce risk include limiting the total foam volume below 10 mL, elevating the extremity to 45 degrees, keeping the patient immobile for 5 to 10 minutes after injection to allow the foam to liquefy, and occluding the saphenofemoral junction with direct pressure. The sclerosant has probably been "scrubbed off" and replaced with serum by the time it reaches a distant systemic target. Thus potential damage is attributable to the gas bubble, which may occlude smaller arterial side vessels.[15]

- **Allergic reaction.** Treatment of an allergic reaction depends on severity but may include oxygen, intravenous fluids, epinephrine, antihistamines, and corticosteroids.

- **Arterial or arteriolar occlusion.** Ultrasound needle guidance of veins not visible on the skin surface should prevent arterial or arteriolar occlusion, which may lead to tissue necrosis. High-risk areas include the groin, popliteal fossa, and ankle. Skin necrosis can result from sclerosant extravasation at higher concentrations, causing direct injury or inadvertent injection into skin arterioles. Routine wound care produces acceptable results.

- **Hyperpigmentation.** A brown discoloration at injected sites caused by hemosiderin deposition may occur in 20% of injection sessions. Drainage of trapped blood may reduce the risk of hyperpigmentation. Most hyperpigmentation resolves spontaneously within 1 year, with surface laser or intense pulsed light therapy considered in those instances in which hyperpigmentation does not resolve. Topical bleaching agents are also sometimes used.

- **Matting.** The development of tiny red vessels around the site of an injected vein may be a result of neovascularization. Matting occurs in 15% to 20% of sessions and usually resolves within 1 year. Sclerotherapy or surface laser treatment can be considered for persistent matting.

- **Recurrence.** Abnormal veins may recur at injected sites or at new sites, but recurrence rates may be reduced by excellent technique.

REFERENCES

1. Hobbs JT: Surgery and sclerotherapy in the treatment of varicose veins, *Arch Surg* 190:793-796, 1974.
2. Breu FX, Guggenbichler S, Wollmann JC: Second European Consensus Meeting on Foam Sclerotherapy 2006, *Vasa S* 71:3-29, 2008.
3. Myers KA, Jolley D, Clough A, et al: Outcome of ultrasound-guided sclerotherapy for varicose veins: Medium-term results assessed by ultrasound surveillance, *Eur J Vasc Endovasc Surg* 33:116-121, 2006.
4. Wright D, Gobin JP, Bradbury AW, et al: Varisolve polidocanol microfoam compared with surgery or sclerotherapy in the management of varicose veins in the presence of trunk vein incompetence: European randomized controlled trial, *Phlebology* 21:180-190, 2006.
5. Van den Bos R, Arends L, Kochaert M, et al: Endovenous therapies of lower extremity varicosities: A meta-analysis, *J Vasc Surg* 49:230-239, 2009.
6. Pascarella L, Bergan JJ, Menkenas LV: Severe chronic venous insufficiency treated by foamed sclerosant, *Ann Vasc Surg* 20:83-91, 2006.
7. Mowatt-Larssen E: Management of secondary varicosities, *Semin Vasc Surg* 23:107-112, 2010.
8. Bergan JJ, Scmid-Schonbein GW, Coleridge Smith PD, et al: Mechanisms of disease: Chronic venous disease, *N Engl J Med* 355:488-498, 2006.
9. Hamel-Desnos C, Ouvry P, Benigni JP, et al: Comparison of 1% and 3% polidocanol foam in ultrasound guided sclerotherapy of the great saphenous vein: A randomized, double-blind trial with 2 year-follow-up. "The 3/1 Study," *Eur J Vasc Endovasc Surg* 34:723-729, 2007.

10. Tessari L, Cavezzi A, Frullini A: Preliminary experience with a new sclerosing foam in the treatment of varicose veins, *Dermatol Surg* 27:58-60, 2001.
11. Myers KA, Roberts S: Evaluation of published reports of foam sclerotherapy: What do we know conclusively? *Phlebology* 24:275-280, 2009.
12. Guex JJ, Allaert FA, Gillet JL, et al: Immediate and midterm complications of sclerotherapy: Report of a prospective multicenter registry of 12,173 sclerotherapy sessions, *Dermatol Surg* 31:123-128, 2005.
13. Myers KA, Jolley D: Factors affecting the risk of deep venous occlusion after ultrasound-guided sclerotherapy for varicose veins, *Eur J Vasc Endovasc Surg* 36:602-605, 2008.
14. Morrison N, Neuhardt DL: Foam sclerotherapy: Cardiac and cerebral monitoring, *Phlebology* 24:252-259, 2009.
15. Guex JJ: Complications and side-effects of foam sclerotherapy, *Phlebology* 24:270-274, 2009.

Section 12

ARTERIOVENOUS ACCESS FOR HEMODIALYSIS

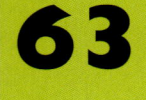

63 Radial Artery–Cephalic Vein and Brachial Artery–Cephalic Vein Arteriovenous Fistula

MATTHEW J. DOUGHERTY • DANIEL J. HAYES, JR. • KEITH D. CALLIGARO

Historical Background

Although Kolff and colleagues[1] reported the development of a hemodialysis machine for renal replacement therapy in 1944, maintenance hemodialysis did not become a reality for another 2 decades because of a lack of reliable vascular access.[2] Simple venipuncture was initially employed,[3] but peripheral veins would not support the flow rates necessary for dialysis.[2] The Scribner-Quinton shunt was the earliest solution proposed and consisted of a cannulated artery and vein connected by an external Teflon tube. At the time of dialysis the Teflon tube could be disconnected so that the artery and vein extensions could be connected directly to the hemodialysis system. The Scribner-Quinton shunt was prone to infection, thrombosis, and dislodgement, and as an exteriorized shunt, it provoked patient apprehension.[2]

The ability to achieve reliable arteriovenous access was solved in 1966 when Cimino and Brescia, two nephrologists at the Bronx Veterans Affairs Hospital's chronic dialysis unit, reported the successful dialysis of 13 patients by repeated venipuncture of arteriovenous fistulas constructed between the radial artery and the cephalic vein by Appel.[4] They theorized that a surgically created arteriovenous fistula would provide durable venous access with reliable flow rates without high-output heart failure or hand ischemia.

Unfortunately, many patients lack a cephalic vein suitable for creation of an arteriovenous fistula at the wrist, because repeated venipunctures often render the forearm cephalic vein unusable. Alternative fistula constructions, including the anastomosis of the cephalic vein to the brachial artery at the elbow, have since been described. Although a number of options for hemodialysis access, including large-bore central catheters, ports, and synthetic bridge grafts, are in wide use, the radiocephalic or Cimino arteriovenous fistula and the brachiocephalic arteriovenous fistula remain the preferred options for access.

Indications

As outlined in Kidney Disease Outcomes Quality Initiative (KDOQI), every patient with chronic kidney disease (CKD) should have a functioning arteriovenous fistula ready for use when dialysis is initiated.[5] Most surgeons and nephrologists prefer to wait a minimum of 6 weeks between the creation of a fistula and its use. This interval allows time for fistula maturation, which Saad succinctly defines as "a general term used to refer to multiple processes that occur from the time of surgical fistula construction until the time the arteriovenous fistula becomes a functional hemodialysis access. The desired end result of the maturation process is a high-flow, large-caliber, superficial vessel with robust wall structure suitable for reliable repeated dialysis needle access."[6]

Most nephrologists refer patients to a surgeon when they anticipate a need for dialysis within 1 year to allow time for preoperative planning, scheduling of the procedure, maturation of the fistula, and necessary revisions to the fistula. Typically, a patient will likely require dialysis within 1 year when serum creatinine is 4 mg/dL or greater and creatinine clearance is less than 25 mL/min.[7] The initiation of maintenance hemodialysis is driven by multiple factors, including uremic symptoms, hyperkalemia, and fluid overload.

Preoperative Preparation

- **History.** A successful arteriovenous fistula requires an artery with adequate "inflow" and a vein of adequate size and "outflow." Thus the history and physical should be directed toward identifying a suitable vein, as well as arterial or venous lesions that might limit flow. Arteriovenous fistulas are preferentially placed in the nondominant extremity if the upper extremity vessels are equally suitable. Given the advanced age and increased comorbidities of patients with chronic renal disease, a history of central venous catheters or cardiac devices with transvenous wires, such as pacemakers or defibrillators, is not uncommon. Patients with a history of such devices are at increased risk for central venous stenoses that may compromise outflow, especially when the subclavian vein has been used. Finally, the patient must be asked whether there is prior history of arm trauma or surgery, including prior attempts at hemodialysis access that might compromise flow or complicate the dissection.

- **Physical examination.** On physical examination, both radial and brachial pulses are assessed and blood pressure is measured in both arms. Allen's test can identify the rare patient whose palmar arch depends on radial artery flow, although this does not preclude its use for access. Visual inspection of the neck and chest often reveals evidence of pacemakers, defibrillators, scarring, or venous collaterals consistent with a history of central venous devices. Similarly, examination of the arms can reveal scars from previous injuries or surgical procedures.

- **Duplex ultrasound.** Visual inspection and palpation of the cephalic vein is often sufficient. However, many patients, especially those who are obese, may have a cephalic vein of suitable caliber that cannot be seen or palpated. Furthermore, even a cephalic vein of adequate size on physical examination may be compromised proximally. Therefore duplex ultrasound "vein mapping" should be used to accurately assess the diameter of the arm veins before surgery.[5,7-9] Preoperative duplex ultrasound can also reveal a central venous stenosis or occlusion. A cephalic vein measuring at least 3 mm in diameter without tourniquet placement and less than 1 cm deep by duplex ultrasound usually matures to a usable fistula. Noninvasive arterial studies are used selectively for patients in which there is the suspicion of arterial occlusive disease.

- **Assessment of comorbidities.** Preoperative medical clearance may occasionally be indicated, because patients presenting for access frequently have significant comorbidities. Fortunately, the creation of a fistula is a relatively minor procedure that can usually be completed under local anesthesia. Electrolytes should be routinely assessed before the procedure.

Pitfalls and Danger Points

- **Failure of the cephalic vein to mature.** A cephalic vein with an insufficient diameter or without the ability to dilate may fail to mature. The vein should measure a minimum of 3.5 mm and preferably 4 mm to interrogation with a coronary dilator.

- **Anastomotic tension.** Inadequate dissection of a sufficient length of distal cephalic vein will limit the ability of the vein to reach the artery without tension.
- **Vein kinking.** Proximal "skeletonization" of the cephalic vein is necessary to avoid kinking in the subcutaneous space.
- **Vein twisting.** Failure to maintain proper orientation of the cephalic vein causes twisting and stenosis.
- **Inadequate arterial inflow.** Poor choice of inflow vessel due to size or because of the presence of a stenosis or occlusion of the proximal inflow vessel may lead to steal or access occlusion.
- **Nerve or vessel injury.** Injury to the nerve or vessel may occur because of traction or through use of electrocautery.

Operative Strategy

SELECTION OF A FISTULA SITE

If a suitable cephalic vein is found at the wrist, the first choice is to perform a radiocephalic fistula, because it is the simplest fistula to construct and preserves more proximal veins as future access sites.[5,9] If vein size at the wrist is borderline in size, the vein can be explored through a small incision and an attempt made to pass a dilator. If the vein accommodates a 3.5-mm dilator, the incision is extended and the fistula is created. A brachiocephalic fistula at the elbow is performed if a radiocephalic fistula does not prove feasible.[5,9] The presence of an internal jugular venous catheter in a patient already receiving dialysis is not a contraindication to access placement when suitable veins are found in the ipsilateral arm.

ALTERNATIVES IN THE ABSENCE OF SUITABLE CEPHALIC VEIN

For patients without adequate cephalic vein, the best alternatives are either a basilic vein transposition or a synthetic arteriovenous graft, which are described in subsequent chapters. The basilic vein transposition requires a significantly larger incision and dissection, whereas a synthetic bridge graft is associated with higher rates of infection and thrombosis.[5,9]

ANESTHESIA

In the operating room, light sedation or anxiolytics are administered, along with local anesthesia.

OPERATIVE FIELD

The entire arm, including the hand, is prepared circumferentially up to the shoulder and chest to allow easy mobilization of the operative site during the procedure. The entire hand is prepared to allow evaluation of hand perfusion at the conclusion of the case and prevent contamination from sudden and unexpected patient movement. Care must be taken to allow adequate exposure up into the axilla when the patient has consented for possible basilic vein transposition. Magnifying surgical loupes are routinely used.

HEPARINIZATION

Regional rather than systemic heparinization is preferred.

Operative Technique

RADIOCEPHALIC (CIMINO) ARTERIOVENOUS FISTULA

Incisions

Although separate incisions for the radial artery and cephalic vein exposures are described, a single, oblique incision extending from the cephalic vein distally to

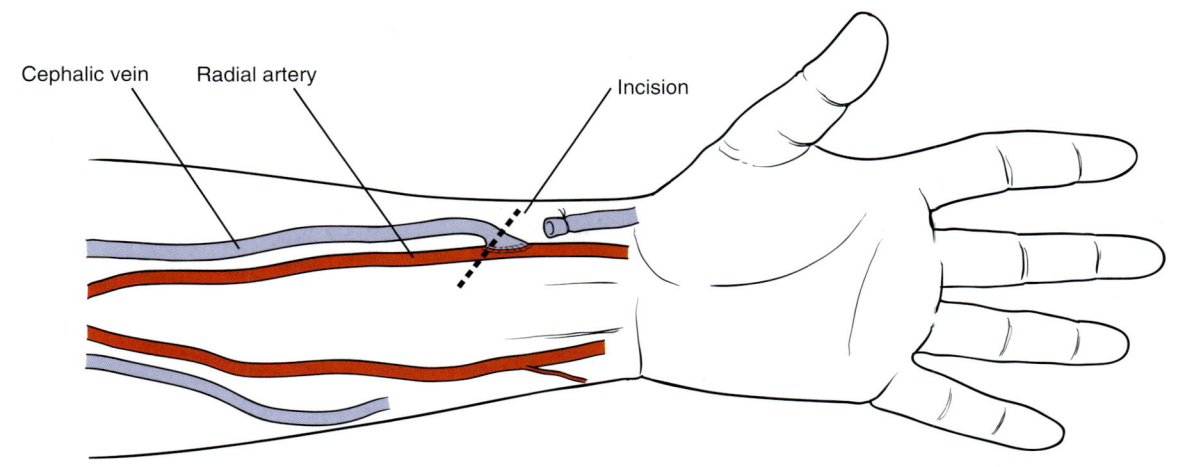

Figure 63-1. The proper orientation of the wrist incision to optimize exposure to the cephalic vein distally for ligation and the radial artery proximally for anastomosis.

the radial artery pulse proximally is preferred (Fig. 63-1). This orientation facilitates mobilization of the vein to the artery. When the cephalic vein is appreciable only with duplex ultrasound, it can be initially identified through a smaller incision that is then extended to the radial pulse.

Operative Exposure of the Cephalic Vein

The cephalic vein is dissected free from surrounding tissue proximally and distally. "Cat paw" retractors are useful for raising the skin flaps to expose the vein, and Lincoln or fine Metzenbaum scissors are preferred for the delicate dissection. Once a length of cephalic vein long enough to reach the radial artery without tension is exposed, the vein is divided as far distally as possible, and the distal stump is ligated with a silk suture. The proximal end of the vein is flushed with heparinized saline to ensure low resistance in the outflow and to dilate the vein. The vein's diameter and potential for dilation can be confirmed by passing serial dilators, beginning with 3.0 mm probe, followed by a 3.5 mm and 4 mm dilator. The proximal vein is flushed with heparin and clamped.

Operative Exposure of the Radial Artery

Once the vein is prepared, the radial artery is exposed after injecting 1% lidocaine (Xylocaine) under the volar fascia. The fasciotomy is extended transversely to eliminate constriction by fascial bands. The median nerve is carefully avoided. The artery is controlled proximally and distally either with vessel loops or fine-angled bulldog clamps. A longitudinal arteriotomy is made on the anterior volar wall of the artery, slightly toward the vein, using a No. 11 scalpel. The arteriotomy is then extended to a total length of 6 to 7 mm using fine iris or Potts scissors. The artery is then flushed proximally and distally with heparinized saline. If the artery is especially small or in spasm, a dilute papaverine solution is infused. This maneuver can be quite painful to the awake patient.

Arteriovenous Anastomosis

The end of the transected cephalic vein is brought over to the arteriotomy to determine the proper orientation and necessary length of vein. Excess vein is transected to prevent kinking from too much laxity. The end of the vein is then spatulated by inserting one blade of the Potts or iris scissors into the lumen and incising one wall. The spatulation must match the arteriotomy both in size and in orientation such that the heel of the vein aligns with the proximal end of the arteriotomy when the vein lies in a neutral, untwisted orientation.

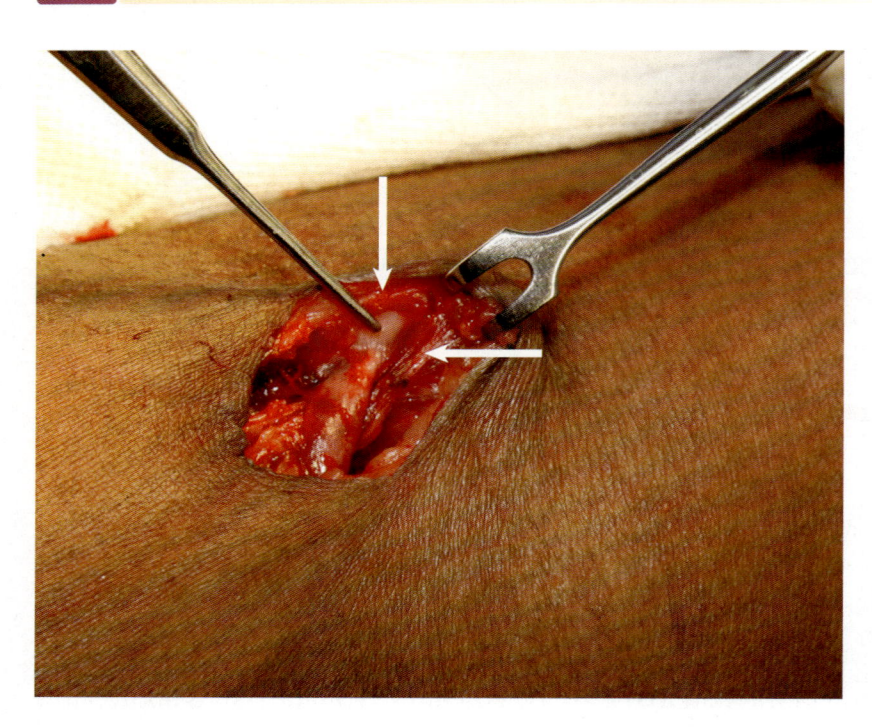

Figure 63-2. Example of tissue bands (*arrows*) around the proximal vein that can lead to stenosis and kinking. Careful dissection of these bands often converts a pulse to a thrill.

The end-to-side anastomosis is then performed using one double-armed 6-0 or 7-0 monofilament suture. The anastomosis begins at the heel, and the back wall is completed first. If the artery is small or spastic, gentle dilatation with a 3-mm Bakes dilator is performed just before completion of the anastomosis. The vein clamp or loop is then released, followed by release of the distal and then the proximal arterial clamps.

Confirmation of Flow and Closure

Once the anastomosis and wound are hemostatic, the cephalic vein is palpated to confirm the presence of a thrill, which confirms continuous, low-resistance outflow. A weak thrill suggests poor inflow, possibly because of arterial spasm, obstruction, or hypotension, whereas a strong pulse in the absence of a thrill suggests outflow obstruction. Inspection of the vein under the proximal skin flap often reveals tissue bands that narrow or kink the now-engorged vein (Fig. 63-2). Careful dissection of these bands to free the vein frequently changes a pulse to a thrill. The wound is then closed in two layers with 3-0 and 4-0 absorbable suture, and the incision is covered with a surgical glue or sealant without the use of other strips or bandages.

BRACHIOCEPHALIC ARTERIOVENOUS FISTULAS

Incision

For brachiocephalic arteriovenous fistulas, a transverse incision is made 1 to 2 cm or approximately one fingerbreadth distal to the elbow crease extending from the cephalic vein to the brachial artery pulse (Fig. 63-3). A small incision can be used to confirm the presence of a suitable cephalic vein before extending the incision toward the artery.

Operative Exposure of the Cephalic Vein

The cephalic vein is exposed and prepared in a manner similar to that described earlier. However, the venous anatomy at the elbow frequently provides additional options for the anastomosis. If there is an adequate median antecubital or basilic vein, it can frequently be transected and anastomosed to the brachial artery without interrupting the cephalic vein. If the cephalic vein caliber is adequate in the forearm, this vein can be used to construct what is effectively a side-to-side anastomosis. Valves in the distal cephalic vein are then gently ruptured by retrograde passage of Bakes dilators to increase the total length of vein usable for dialysis

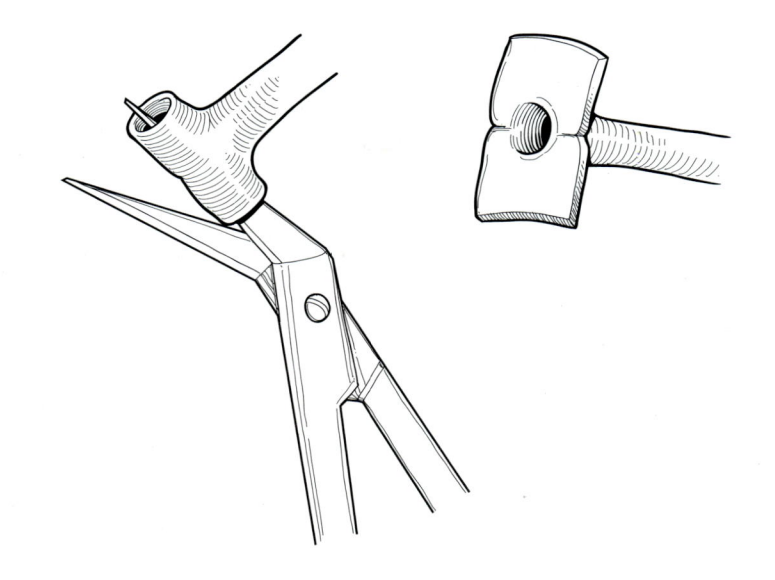

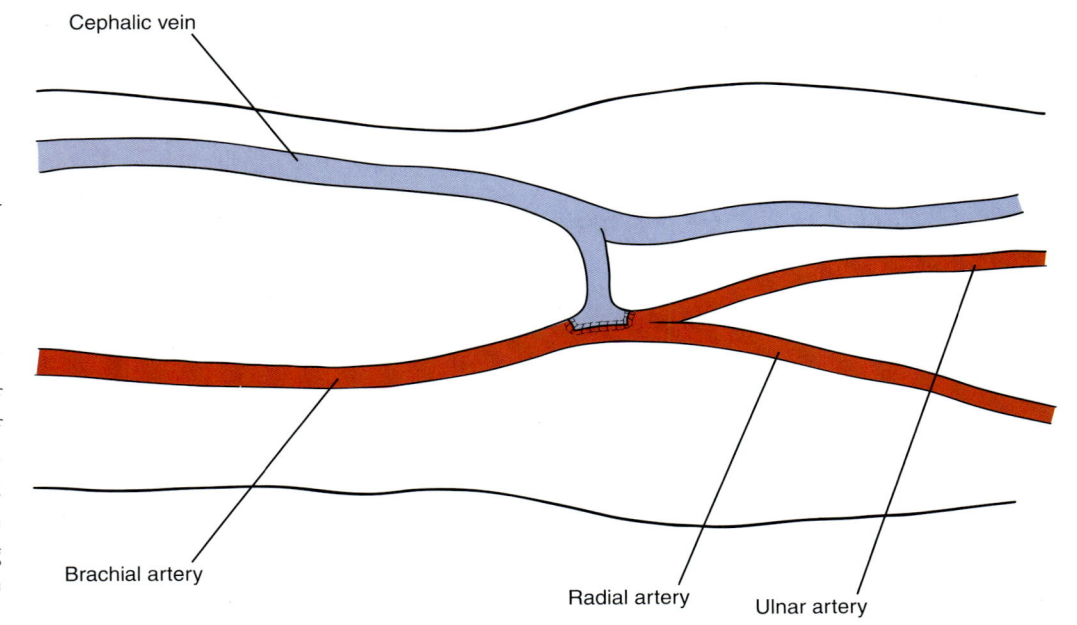

Figure 63-3. Anastomosis of the median antecubital vein to the brachial artery, combined with lysis of the valves in the distal cephalic vein, increases the length of cephalic vein available for dialysis access. If the distal cephalic vein is of inadequate size or quality, the antecubital or basilic vein is used to create a natural patch for anastomosis by opening the confluence of the vein junction longitudinally.

access. If the distal cephalic vein is of inadequate size or quality, the antecubital or basilic vein may be used to create a natural patch for the anastomosis. The confluence of the vein junction is opened longitudinally, providing a larger venous cuff for anastomosis.

Operative Exposure of the Brachial Artery

The brachial artery lies beneath the flexor retinaculum of the brachioradialis muscle. Local anesthetic is injected under this layer before incising it to provide effective anesthesia to this space. The brachial venae comitantes must be carefully dissected free of the artery to avoid bothersome bleeding. If the brachial bifurcation can be exposed, the radial and ulnar arteries are separately controlled with vessel loops to improve length of brachial artery exposure. The ulnar artery tends to be dominant and is the more medial vessel. The brachial artery bifurcation is occasionally above the elbow crease. In this situation, the larger of the radial or ulnar artery should be chosen for the anastomosis. The anastomosis is constructed with 6-0 or 7-0 monofilament suture in a technique identical to that used for the radiocephalic fistula (Fig. 63-4).

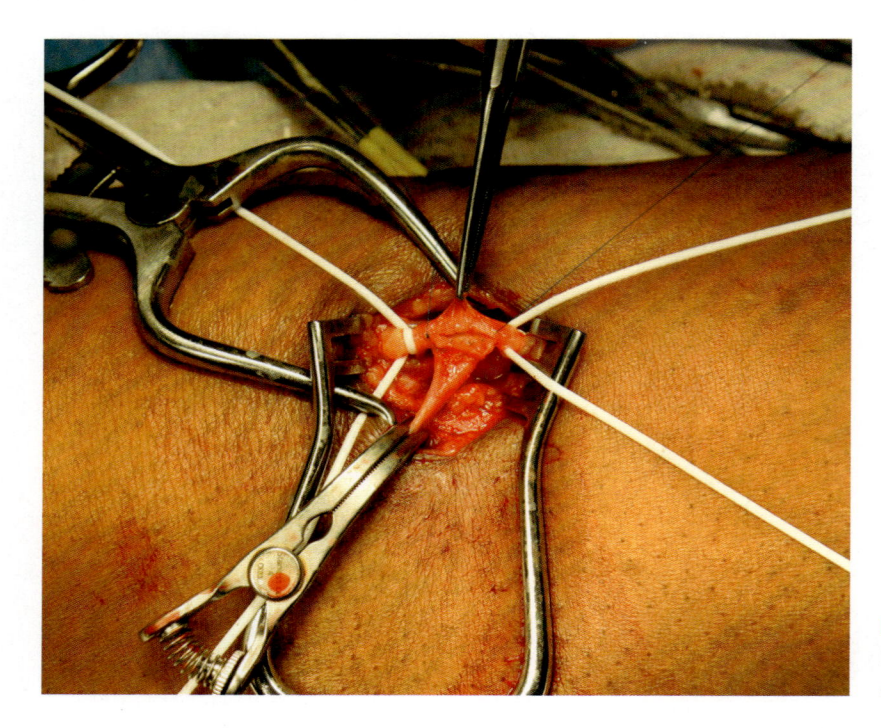

Figure 63-4. Exposure and vessel control for a brachiocephalic arteriovenous fistula. The back wall of the anastomosis has been completed.

Postoperative Care

- **Discharge instructions.** After surgery, the patient is discharged with instructions to keep the incision dry for 24 hours. No elastic compression or other wound care is necessary. Patients are instructed to expect mild swelling and hand coolness but cautioned to call if significant hand pain, numbness, or weakness is noted.
- **Follow-up care.** Patients are evaluated in 1 to 2 weeks and thereafter followed by their nephrologist, who generally determines when the fistula can be accessed. Hand exercises, such as the use of a squeeze ball, do not impact maturation of the fistula, because increased skeletal muscle arterial flow does not significantly increase flow within the maturing fistula.

Complications

- **Failure of fistula maturation because of small vein caliber.** The most frequent complication after the creation of an arteriovenous fistula with a cephalic vein is failure of the fistula to mature, which occurs more commonly with radiocephalic arteriovenous fistulas. Some of these failures stem from the use of a vein of small caliber. However, an initial attempt to use a marginally adequate vein to create a more distal autogenous fistula is reasonable. Patients should be made aware that a fistula may not mature.
- **Failure of fistula maturation because of diversion of flow or stenosis.** Diversion of flow away from the main cephalic vein through side tributaries can hinder maturation. Stenosis of the vein from prior venipuncture or postoperative neointimal hyperplasia can also limit flow and maturation. A fistula that has not matured within 12 weeks should be evaluated by duplex ultrasound, which can be used to identify diverting vessels or a stenosis. Diverting venous side branches can be treated by ligation or coil embolization, and a stenosis treated by surgical revision or balloon angioplasty. Miller and associates[10] have reported the technique of balloon-assisted maturation in which nonmaturing veins without discrete stenoses were dilated serially with long balloons of increasing diameter.

- **Difficult access of fistulas in obese patients.** Puncture of the vein for dialysis may prove difficult in obese patients or in those with deeper superficial veins, which is more common for brachiocephalic arteriovenous fistulas. If the vein is more than 1.5 cm deep in the subcutaneous space, it is unlikely to be reliably accessed and superficialization of the vein is recommended. Surgical revision should be delayed until the vein has arterialized, generally 3 months or more after the initial procedure. At that time, three 2-cm transverse incisions are created, perpendicular to the axis of the vein and approximately 3 cm apart from each other above the elbow crease. Although a longitudinal incision is simpler, it is more prone to dehiscence and vessel exposure, and the scarring along the length of the fistula can make needle access more difficult. The vein is skeletonized along its entire length, lysing subcutaneous fat to the immediate subdermal level. The tissue is then reapproximated with absorbable suture beneath the vein, which now lies just deep to the dermis.

- **Arm edema.** Significant or disabling arm edema may occur after the creation of an arteriovenous fistula, which usually indicates an occult central venous stenosis. These lesions are diagnosed by venography, with angioplasty, as needed. For patients not yet on dialysis in whom contrast exposure might precipitate the need for acute dialysis, compression therapy may be used initially and intervention delayed. It is rare for a central vein lesion to cause occlusion of an autogenous access.

- **Arterial steal syndrome.** A difficult complication of upper extremity access surgery is arterial steal syndrome. Although Cimino and Brescia were correct in their assumption that most patients with a surgical arteriovenous fistula adequately perfuse the ipsilateral hand, steal symptoms occur in up to 5% to 10% of patients, with more proximal arteriovenous anastomoses being more prone to this complication. It is significantly more common in diabetic patients and patients with collagen vascular disease, likely a reflection of the higher rates of distal arterial occlusive disease in these patients. Symptoms range from mild coolness, numbness, pain, or weakness in the hand that may occur only during dialysis, months after access placement, to constant and severe pain, numbness, and paralysis that may develop immediately after access construction. In severe cases, urgent treatment, usually ligation, is necessary to avoid permanent disability in the hand. For milder cases, further observation is warranted. The most convincing physical finding is that of relief of symptoms and signs of ischemia with fistula compression. When steal is suspected, in addition to physical examination, pulse volume recordings (PVRs) should be obtained in the fingers of the ipsilateral hand with and without fistula compression and compared with finger PVRs measured from the contralateral hand. All patients with arteriovenous fistula have diminished plethysmographic waveforms, but with clinically significant ischemia, digital waveforms are usually flat. If steal is responsible, there should be substantial augmentation of PVRs with fistula compression. If this is not observed, a structural occlusive arterial lesion proximal to or distal from the arteriovenous fistula should be considered. When steal syndrome is confirmed, mild cases can be observed and frequently improve. When the symptoms are significant or ischemia is critical, management must balance the desire to preserve the access against the need for adequate hand perfusion. Ligation of the fistula is the simplest option, but this should be reserved for only the most severe and acute circumstances. There is little reason to anticipate that a contralateral or more proximal hemoaccess procedure is less prone to this complication. A definitive method for managing the competing concerns of access preservation and hand perfusion is distal revascularization interval ligation (DRIL) procedure. Most patients with steal syndrome can be initially treated by "banding" the outflow vein. Monitoring digital Doppler signals, the surgical team serially applies medium-sized metallic clips to create a tapered stenosis about 1.5 cm in length near the arterial anastomosis. The degree of narrowing is balanced by Doppler interrogation, aiming for a good monophasic digital flow signal while preserving brisk diastolic flow through the fistula. Once satisfied with this balance, the clips are secured with mattress sutures. Many discount the usefulness of banding because of the difficulty and imprecise nature of determining how much the venous lumen should be decreased to reduce flow enough to treat the steal but not so much that the fistula thromboses. However, given the lesser morbidity of banding versus the DRIL procedure, in which the patient's native artery is ligated and distal perfusion becomes dependent on a bypass graft, the risk of requiring a secondary procedure or losing the fistula may be acceptable.

- **Neuropathic pain.** Steal must be differentiated from neuropathy, which is not uncommon, particularly in diabetic patients. Median nerve neuropathy usually follows its dermatome, and may be secondary to carpal tunnel compression from increased limb perfusion, or from surgical manipulation or hematoma at the surgical site abutting the median nerve. Patients with diabetic neuropathy are predisposed to a more variable and often severe "acute monomelic neuropathy," the pathophysiology of which is suggested to be microvascular ischemia within peripheral nerves.

- **Fistula thrombosis.** Although native fistulas have a higher patency rate than synthetic arteriovenous grafts, thrombosis can occur. Salvage can be more difficult than for grafts because of variable luminal diameter, inflammation, and clot adherence. Therefore endovascular techniques, such as pharmacomechanical thrombolysis and angioplasty, are preferred. Success at reopening a thrombosed arteriovenous fistula is higher when it has matured.

REFERENCES

1. Kolff WJ, Berk HTJ, ter Welle M, et al: The artificial kidney: A dialyser with a great area, *Acta Med Scand* 117:121-134, 1944.
2. Cimino JE, Brescia MJ: The early development of the arteriovenous fistula, *ASAIO J* 40:923-927, 1994.
3. Cimino JE, Brescia MJ, Aboody R: Simple venipuncture for hemodialysis, *N Engl J Med* 267:608-609, 1962.
4. Brescia MJ, Cimino JE, Appel K, et al: Chronic hemodialysis using venipuncture and a surgically created arteriovenous fistula, *N Engl J Med* 275:1089-1092, 2006.
5. National Kidney Foundation. KDOQI: 2006 vascular access guidelines, *Am J Kidney Dis* 48:S177-S322, 2006.
6. Saad TF: Management of the immature autologous arteriovenous hemodialysis fistula, *Vascular* 18:316-324, 2010.
7. National Kidney Foundation: NKF-DOQI clinical practice guidelines for vascular access, *Am J Kidney Dis* 37:S137-S181, 2001.
8. Silva MB, Hobson RW, Pappas PJ, et al: A strategy for increasing use of autogenous hemodialysis access procedures: Impact of preoperative noninvasive evaluation, *J Vasc Surg* 27:302-308, 1998.
9. Sidawy AN, Spergel LM, Besarab A, et al: The Society for Vascular Surgery clinical practice guidelines for the surgical placement and maintenance of arteriovenous hemodialysis access, *J Vasc Surg* 48:2S-25S, 2008.
10. Miller GA, Goel N, Khariton A, et al: Aggressive approach to salvage non-maturing arteriovenous fistulae: A retrospective study with follow-up, *J Vasc Access* 10:183-191, 2009.

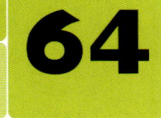

64 Forearm Loop Graft and Brachial Artery–Axillary Vein Interposition Graft

SHAWN M. GAGE • DAVID A. PETERSON • JEFFREY H. LAWSON

Historical Background

Kolff's development of hemodialysis in the 1930s led to a series of advances in the care of patients with end-stage renal disease (ESRD). Although native arteriovenous fistulas and homografts were initial cannulation options for dialysis access, the availability of prosthetic grafts in the 1970s afforded a number of new access sites.[1] Nonetheless, this new type of access generated a new set of complications and expenditures to the health care system, with economic costs of ESRD in the United States at more than $26 billion in 2006.[2]

Indications

The National Kidney Foundation's Kidney Disease Outcomes Quality Initiative guidelines promote initial fistula formation in the nondominant extremity.[3] The "fistula first" initiative would suggest creating autogenous access on the dominant upper extremity once native fistula options have been exhausted on the nondominant side. However, a common practice is to remain on the ipsilateral nondominant limb and proceed with a forearm loop or upper arm brachial artery–to–axillary vein arteriovenous graft (AVG).

Preoperative Preparation

- **History and physical examination.** The decision to implant a forearm loop or brachial-axillary AVG depends on the existing arterial and venous anatomy. A thorough past medical history and a physical examination of the extremities and sites of previous vascular access should be obtained to preserve the greatest number of sites for future access (Fig. 64-1). A strong palpable pulse is required to provide adequate inflow, and a weak pulse may indicate a proximal defect of the artery or heavily calcified vessels, neither of which allows ample flow to support hemodialysis and both of which may predispose the patient to arterial steal syndrome.
- **Venous imaging.** Determining target vein patency and the quality of venous outflow is essential to careful planning (Fig. 64-2). Venous duplex mapping is limited to determining the adequacy of venous outflow in the antebrachium, antecubital fossa, and axilla, but venography is required to effectively evaluate the central veins, if it is deemed clinically necessary because of a history of prior interventions. Magnetic resonance venography is an alternative to conventional venography, but images are less dynamic and patients with severe renal dysfunction are at risk of nephrogenic systemic fibrosis.[4,5] However, recent advances in imaging and contrast technology allow for the use of Feraheme as a contrasting agent, which can safely be used in ESRD patients.
- **Preoperative dialysis.** Patients taking hemodialysis require dialysis the day before or the morning of surgery.

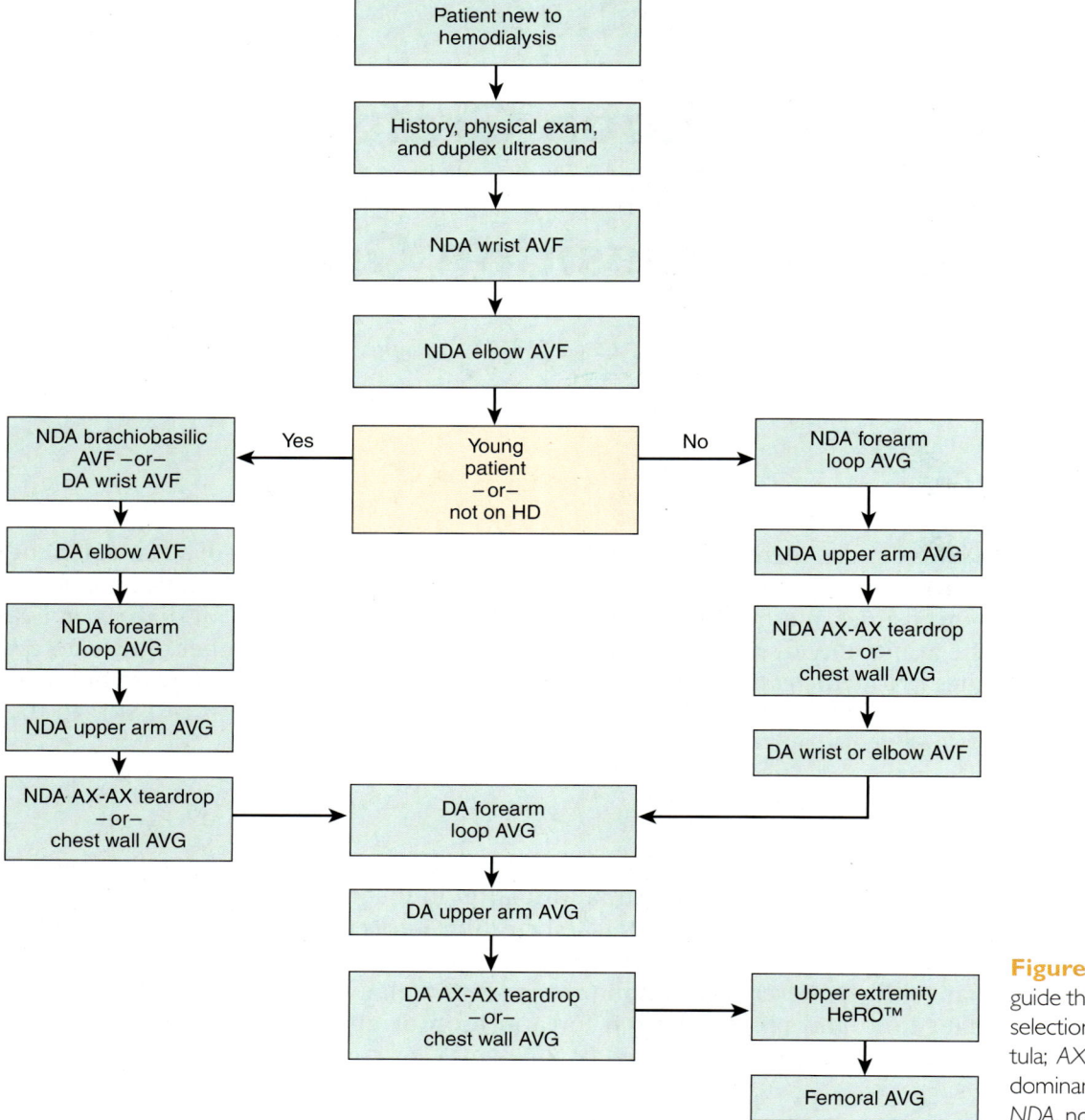

Figure 64-1. An algorithm to guide the sequence of access site selection. *AVF,* Arteriovenous fistula; *AX-AX,* axillary-axillary *DA,* dominant arm; *HD,* hemodialysis; *NDA,* nondominant arm.

Pitfalls and Danger Points

- **Selection of adequate inflow and outflow sites.** Inflow arteries must be relatively soft and amenable to clamping. Outflow veins should be greater than 3 mm in diameter and free from prior traumatic injury, thrombus, scar, or occlusion.
- **Arterial and nerve injury.** Distraction performed too forcefully on neurovascular structures can lead to injury, including arterial dissection or neuropraxia.
- **Graft tunneling.** Tunneling the graft too deeply can lead to difficulties in accessing the graft. Care must also be taken to prevent conduit twisting or kinking, which may occur when tunneling too tight of a loop for a forearm graft. When placing a brachial-axillary AVG, the preference is to position the graft posterior to the median nerve to avoid kinking, which can occur if the graft is draped anteriorly over the nerve.
- **Anastomosis.** The anastomosis must be constructed at an appropriate angle and beveled to avoid kinking of the hood. Likewise, excessive tension can lead to tenting of the back wall of the artery at the anastomosis.
- **Central venous stenosis.** A long-standing tunneled dialysis catheter may increase the risk of a central venous stenosis. Likewise, this catheter may need

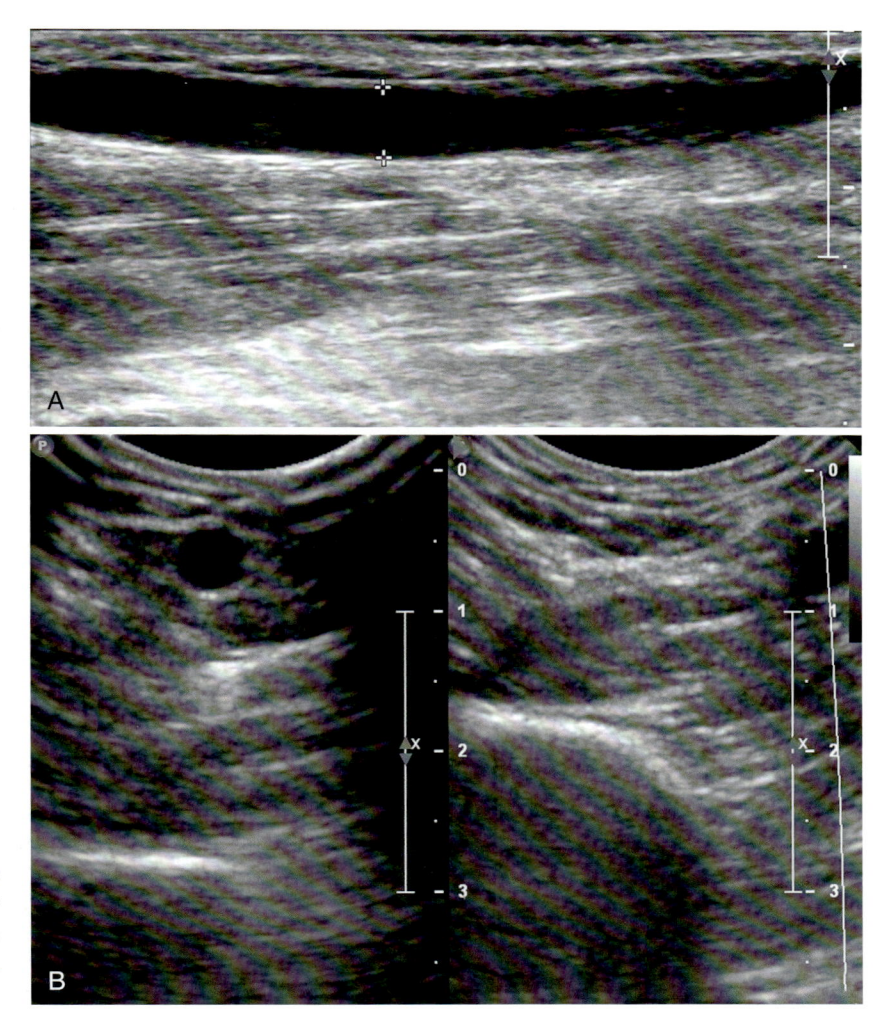

Figure 64-2. B-mode ultrasound is used to visualize the cephalic vein in the longitudinal view (**A**) and the basilic vein in the transverse view (**B**) with compression *(right)* and without compression *(left).*

to be relocated before the placement of the access graft to minimize the risk of postoperative arm edema.

Operative Strategy

SELECTION OF AN ARTERIOVENOUS GRAFT

Once native fistula possibilities in the nondominant extremity have been exhausted, placement of a forearm AVG may be considered. A brachial-axillary AVG is a more proximal option usually reserved after failure of a forearm graft without the possibility for endovascular or surgical revision. Additional options include axillary artery–to–axillary vein grafts, chest wall grafts, or the hemodialysis reliable outflow (HeRO, Hemosphere, Eden Prairie, Minn.) "graft catheter" device.

SELECTION OF SITES FOR VENOUS OUTFLOW AND ARTERIAL INFLOW

Potential venous outflow options for a forearm loop AVG include the median antebrachial, median cubital, basilic, cephalic, and brachial veins, but their utilization limits future use for fistula creation. Options for arterial inflow include the brachial, proximal ulnar, and radial arteries. A palpable brachial pulse or use of the proximal radial or ulnar artery decreases the incidence of steal syndrome.[6]

Potential venous outflow options for a brachial-axillary arteriovenous graft include the proximal brachial or basilic veins or the distal axillary vein. As in the loop graft, options for arterial inflow include the brachial, proximal radial, and ulnar arteries. If these arteries are too small, then an axillary-axillary teardrop AVG should be considered (see Fig. 64-1).

Operative Technique

FOREARM LOOP GRAFT

Incision

A forearm graft requires control of the brachial artery and antecubital veins through a transverse incision approximately 2 cm distal from the antecubital fossa. The vessels are dissected free from the surrounding tissue and encircled with vessel loops for control. In some cases it may be necessary to use the most proximal aspect of the radial or ulnar artery for inflow. Similarly, options for venous outflow can vary considerably. Common choices include the brachial, median antebrachial, median cubital, cephalic, and basilic veins. A minimal touch technique is used to dissect the vein with silicone elastomer (Silastic) vessel loops used for gentle distraction and manipulation of the vein.

Tunneling of the Graft

A tunneling device is used to place the graft in the subdermal space, thus facilitating cannulation, and a counterincision in the distal forearm is required for tunneling. The tunneler is passed from the counterincision in the distal forearm to the antecubital incision, and as the graft is pulled back through the tunnel, avoidance of twisting or kinking of the conduit must be maintained (Fig. 64-3). The tunneling device is then passed from the antecubital incision to the counterincision to pull the graft back through and complete the loop.

Anastomoses

Intravenous heparin is administered at 50 mg per kilogram of body weight after the vessels have been dissected and once tunneling is complete. It may be preferable to sew the venous anastomosis first to reduce the amount of needle-hole bleeding that can occur if the arterial side is sewn first. Vascular clamps are applied and a 1-cm longitudinal venotomy is created, followed by an anastomosis using a running 6-0 polypropylene. Once the anastomosis is complete, clamps are released and the conduit is flushed with heparinized saline. Vascular clamps are then applied to the artery, a 1-cm longitudinal arteriotomy is made, and a running 6-0 polypropylene is used to fashion an end-to-side anastomosis. In the case of biologic grafts, such as Procol or Artegraft, the arterial anastomosis should be performed first and the conduit should be distended under pressure to avoid redundant regions and allow full graft elongation.

Confirmation of Flow and Closure

After completion, a thrill should be apparent and Doppler should confirm robust flow at the venous anastomosis, as well as radial and ulnar signals. A signal is not immediately appreciated over a newly implanted expanded polytetrafluoroethylene graft, because the presence of air within the graft wall attenuates the ultrasound signal. Within a week enough serum has saturated the graft for detection of flow by Doppler examination. Reversing systemic heparinization is rarely required. Incisions are closed with a deep layer of absorbable suture and a superficial layer of absorbable monofilament suture. Sterile dressings are applied, and the patient is discharged after a period of observation.

BRACHIAL-AXILLARY ARTERIOVENOUS GRAFT

Incision

A brachial artery–to–axillary vein graft requires exposure of the axillary vein through a longitudinal incision, with care taken to avoid injury to the axillary artery and median nerve, which lie adjacent to the vein. The vein should be greater than 4 mm in diameter. The brachial artery is then exposed proximal to the antecubital fossa through a longitudinal incision, and a subdermal tunnel is

FOREARM LOOP GRAFT AND BRACHIAL ARTERY–AXILLARY VEIN INTERPOSITION GRAFT | 743

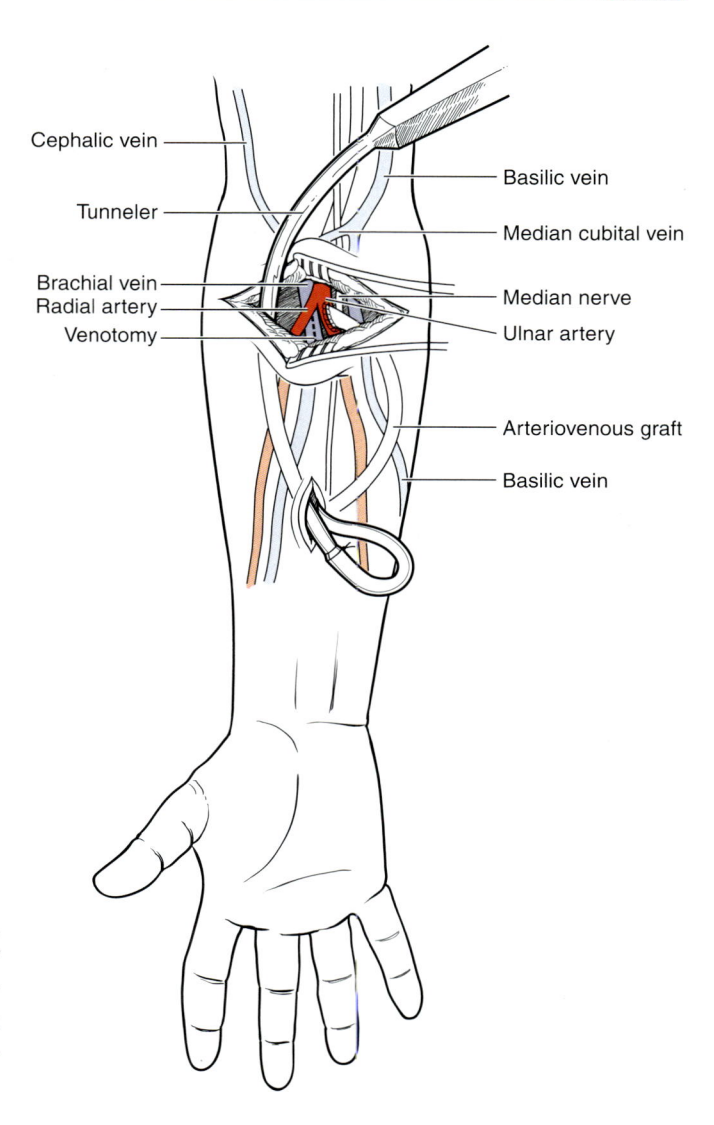

Figure 64-3. A right-sided forearm loop graft in which the arterial anastomosis has been created at the proximal aspect of the ulnar artery. The graft has been tunneled from the primary operative site to the counterincision and is now being pulled back toward the antebrachial vein confluence with the aid of the tunneling device.

created posterolaterally with a curved tunneling device to form an elongated C configuration.

Anastomoses

Intravenous heparin is administered, vascular clamps are applied, and a 1-cm longitudinal venotomy is created, followed by creation of an end-to-side anastomosis with running 6-0 polypropylene (Fig. 64-4). Once the venous anastomosis is complete, clamps are released and the conduit is flushed with a heparinized saline solution. Vascular clamps are then applied to the artery, a 1-cm longitudinal arteriotomy is made, and an end-to-side anastomosis is created with running 6-0 polypropylene. Flow is restored, and Doppler is used to confirm distal arterial flow and venous outflow. Incisions are closed in two layers, and sterile dressings are applied.

Postoperative Care

- **Discharge examination.** Most patients receiving grafts are observed for signs of complications until the morning after surgery, but some are comfortable with discharge on the day of surgery after several hours of postoperative monitoring. In both cases the surgical team must ensure that the postoperative neurovascular examination is unchanged. The hand must be warm and well perfused with a capillary refill time of 2 seconds or less. A palpable radial or ulnar pulse may be diminished to a biphasic or triphasic Doppler signal with significant augmentation upon graft occlusion.

744 ARTERIOVENOUS ACCESS FOR HEMODIALYSIS

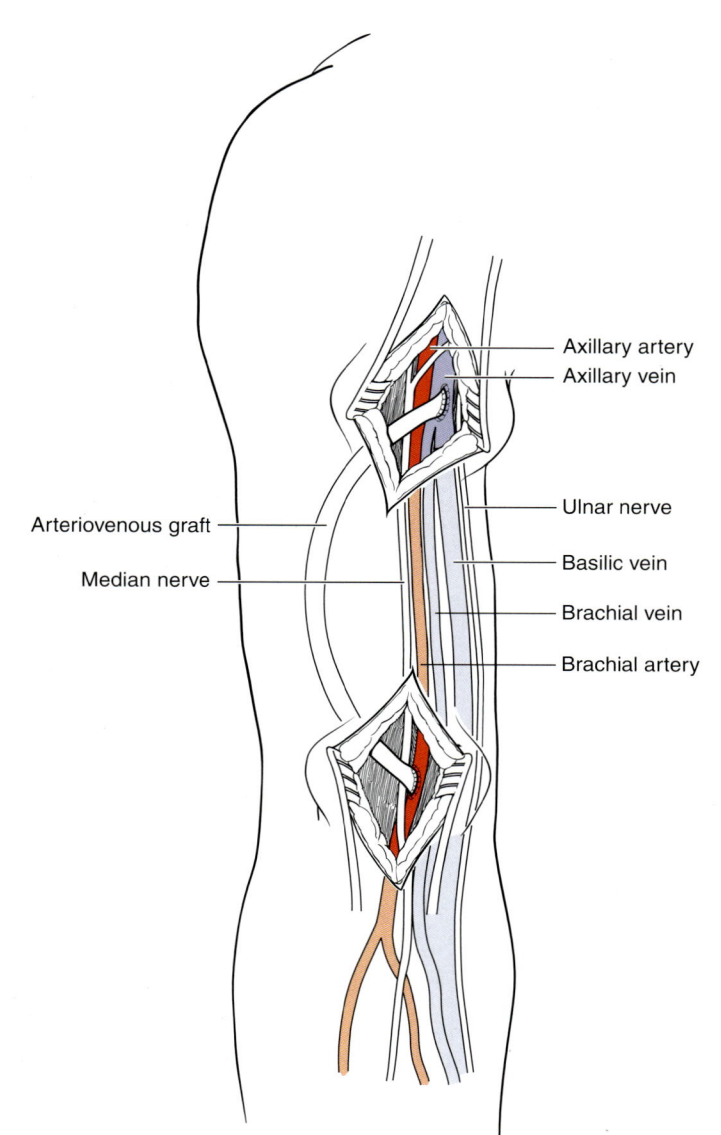

Figure 64-4. A right-sided upper arm brachial artery–to–axillary vein interposition graft. A gradual arch configuration increases the length of the cannulation segment.

- **Postoperative follow-up.** Subcuticular skin closure is preferred to avoid the return of the patient for removal of staples 10 to 14 days after surgery. Otherwise, 4-week follow up is sufficient, by which time a weak thrill, as well as a bruit, should be present over the graft. Early graft failure within 2 weeks after surgery mandates surgical exploration for correction of a presumed technical failure. Waiting at least 4 weeks after surgery before initiating graft cannulation is recommended to reduce the risk of early perigraft hematoma, especially for those patients who require anticoagulation or have a bleeding disorder.

- **Communication with the nephrologist and dialysis center.** Communication with the referring nephrologist regarding the type of access and special considerations is important. It is essential that the technologists and charge nurse at the patient's dialysis center comprehend the type and location of access, as well as the direction of flow. Once the access is deemed appropriate for cannulation, it is good practice to trace the outline of the graft and indicate the direction of flow to facilitate safe and effective cannulation practices.

Complications

- **Infection.** Infections often result from a breach of aseptic technique and frequent cannulation of nonautogenous grafts. Erythema in the immediate postoperative period, confined to the incision, can often be managed with antibiotics and expectant wound care. Traumatic cannulation can lead to the development of an overlying eschar or ulcer with a risk of hemorrhage. Thus surgical revision and exclusion of the affected segment are essential. Endovascular stent-graft exclusion of a graft defect is minimally invasive; however, bacteremia or sepsis could ensue if concomitant infection exists.[7] In such cases segmental graft replacement or even total graft excision is recommended.

- **Hematoma.** Postoperative hematoma of significant size can lead to pain, graft compression, and thrombosis. Furthermore, if the hematoma expands within the brachial sheath, the median or ulnar nerve is at risk of injury, which requires expeditious evacuation of the hematoma.

- **Neuropathic pain.** Neuropathic pain can occur after AVG placement and can be attributed to one of three causes: direct nerve trauma, steal syndrome, or ischemic monomelic neuropathy. Neuropraxia can be induced secondary to retractor placement or vigorous nerve manipulation. Reassurance that neuropraxia is self-limited should be provided. However, ongoing neuropathy may require treatment with neuroleptic medications and neurologic consultation. If a motor deficit is apparent, physical or occupational therapy may be necessary.

- **Steal syndrome.** Steal syndrome occurs most commonly when the brachial artery is used for inflow, and the incidence can be reduced if the proximal radial or ulnar artery is an appropriate site for inflow.[8] Coolness in the fingers, tingling, numbness, and mild discomfort in the hand occur in 10% of patients.[9] Moderate to severe pain or decreased motor function mandates prompt evaluation, and if steal syndrome is suspected, urgent treatment is required to avoid permanent neurovascular compromise. Clinically significant steal syndrome is usually present within the first 12 hours after surgery. Banding, ligation, and distal revascularization with interval ligation are options for management of steal syndrome (see Chapter 68). Access surgery carries a risk of ischemic insult to the hand. This issue typically manifests as a mild to moderate noncritical ischemia of the hand or digits. Clinical ischemia can arise from a number of causes, including arterial dissection, thromboembolic events, and steal syndromes. Arterial dissection occurs from vigorous artery manipulation or back wall injuries during the creation of an anastomosis. Thromboembolic events are more likely to occur if the procedure was performed without systemic anticoagulation or with a prolonged period of clamping.

- **Monomelic neuropathy.** Distinguishing between steal syndrome and ischemic monomelic neuropathy can be confusing. Steal syndrome occurs because of the reversal of distal blood flow, which manifests as pain and paresthesias in the hand or digits but may lead to digit or limb loss. Ischemic monomelic neuropathy causes pain and paresthesias, but vascular findings are less pronounced and rarely result in digit or limb loss. It has been attributed to axonal loss and manifests as multiple distal mononeuropathies.[10]

- **Arm edema.** Edema can be quite common. If localized to the graft, it is usually attributed to graft tunneling and resolves within a few weeks. Edema because of venous hypertension often resolves over a short period, but an undiagnosed venous outflow lesion may cause persistent painful edema, which requires intervention (Fig. 64-5).

- **Venous outflow obstruction.** Late venous outflow obstruction is characterized by elevated venous pressure, flow abnormalities while on hemodialysis, excessive bleeding at decannulation, or graft thrombosis.[11,12] A variety of techniques, including surgical revision or endovascular intervention, have been suggested for treatment of outflow lesions.[13]

- **Graft thrombosis.** Management of graft thrombosis that occurs less than 4 weeks postoperatively is likely related to a technical issue and should be assessed in the operating room.

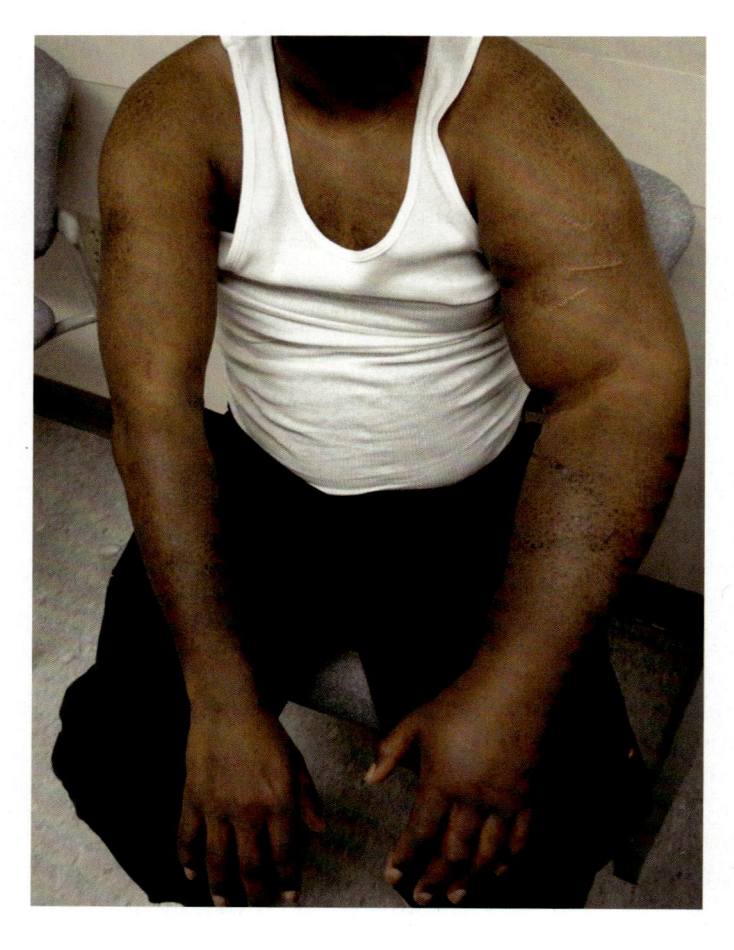

Figure 64-5. Severe upper extremity edema because of a central venous stenosis after the implantation of an upper arm arteriovenous graft.

REFERENCES

1. Baker LD Jr, Johnson JM, Goldfarb D: Expanded polytetrafluoroethylene (PTFE) subcutaneous arteriovenous conduit: An improved vascular access for chronic hemodialysis, *Trans Am Soc Artif Intern Organs* 22:382-387, 1976.
2. U.S. Renal Data System: USRDS 2008 annual data report: Atlas of chronic kidney disease and end-stage renal disease in the United States, Bethesda, Md., 2008, National Institutes of Health, National Institute of Diabetes and Digestive and Kidney Diseases.
3. National Kidney Foundation: Kidney Disease Outcomes Quality Initiative (KDOQI) clinical practice guidelines and clinical practice recommendations for diabetes and chronic kidney disease, *Am J K Dis* S12-S154, 2007.
4. Swaminathan S, Ahmed I, McCarthy JT, et al: Nephrogenic fibrosing dermopathy and high-dose erythropoietin therapy, *Ann Intern Med* 145:234-235, 2006.
5. Grobner T: Gadolinium: A specific trigger for the development of nephrogenic fibrosing dermopathy and nephrogenic systemic fibrosis? *Nephrol Dial Transplant* 21:1104-1108, 2006.
6. Rivers SP, Scher LA, Veith FJ: Correction of steal syndrome secondary to hemodialysis access fistulas: A simplified quantitative technique, *Surgery* 112:593, 1992.
7. Kim CY, Guevara CJ, Engstrom BI, et al: Analysis of infection risk following covered stent exclusion of pseudoaneurysms in prosthetic arteriovenous hemodialysis access grafts, *J Vasc Interv Radiol* 23:69-74, 2012.
8. White GH, Wilson SE: Patient assessment and planning for vascular access surgery. In Wilson SE, editor: *Vascular access: Principles and practice*, ed 5, Philadelphia, 2010, Lippincott Williams & Wilkins, pp 7-12.
9. Morsy A, Kulbaski M, Chen C, et al: Incidence and characteristics of patients with hand ischemia after a hemodialysis access procedure, *J Surg Res* 74:8-10, 1998.
10. Wilbourn AJ, Furlan AJ, Hulley W, et al: Ischemic monomelic neuropathy, *Neurology* 33:447-451, 1983.
11. Tordoir JH, Van Der Sande FM, De Haan MW: Current topics on vascular access for hemodialysis, *Minerva Urol Nefrol* 56:223-235, 2004.
12. Roy-Chaudhury P, Sukhatme VP, Cheung AK: Hemodialysis vascular access dysfunction: A cellular and molecular viewpoint, *J Am Soc Nephrol* 17:1112-1127, 2006.
13. Haskal ZJ, Trerotola S, Dolmatch B, et al: Stent graft versus balloon angioplasty for failing dialysis access grafts, *N Engl J Med* 362:494-503, 2010.

65 Basilic and Femoral Vein Transposition

WAYNE S. GRADMAN • SIDNEY GLAZER

Historical Background

In 1976 Dagher and colleagues[1] reported a series of 23 upper arm basilic vein transpositions for hemodialysis. The procedure did not achieve widespread acceptance until after the first National Kidney Foundation's Kidney Disease Outcomes Quality Initiative (KDOQI) guidelines were published in 1997.[2] The first large series of femoral vein transpositions was published by Gradman and associates in 2001.[3] The procedures are analogous but differ in their indications, magnitude, technique, and complications.

Basilic Vein Transposition

Indications

An upper arm basilic vein transposition should be considered whenever a forearm fistula fails or is not feasible. Preference should be given to either a brachiocephalic fistula or a basilic vein transposition, depending on vein size.

Preoperative Preparation

- **Preserving veins.** Antecubital venipuncture should be discouraged and the jugular vein should be used used whenever possible for intravenous lines or pacemaker wires to preserve axial vein integrity.
- **Preoperative imaging.** Duplex ultrasound with a proximal tourniquet can be used to determine the size of the basilic and cephalic veins and identify common anatomic variations.[4] Duplex ultrasound is best conducted when the patient is hydrated, in a warm environment, and free of anxiety. Veins should be marked and sized on a nondialysis day to limit venoconstriction associated with volume shifts. Patients with long-standing ipsilateral central venous catheters, pacemakers, or previous dialysis catheters should have an imaging study to rule out central venous occlusive disease.

Pitfalls and Danger Points

- **Venous variations.** The basilic vein occasionally joins the brachial vein in the midarm, rather than in the axilla. Antecubital vein variations are common. The median cubital vein, which extends from the midantecubital fossa to join the basilic vein, may be diseased, atretic, or nonexistent.
- **Nerve injury.** The medial antebrachial cutaneous nerve of the forearm, a sensory nerve originating directly from the medial cord of the brachial plexus, crosses directly in front of the basilic vein at or just central to the entry of the median cubital vein. Dividing this nerve can lead to medial forearm anesthesia. The median nerve lies medial to the brachial artery at the level of the elbow and must be protected from injury during dissection and retraction.
- **Steal syndrome**

Operative Strategy

ONE- OR TWO-STAGE PROCEDURE

Surgeons may choose to construct a basilic vein transposition in one or two stages. The single-stage procedure is cost effective but results in a higher frequency of primary failures.[5] The two-stage procedure is most beneficial when the upper arm veins are of borderline size (2.5-3.5 mm; Fig. 65-1). A one-stage basilic vein transposition usually matures if the basilic vein is larger than 3.5 mm, but a two-stage basilic vein transposition should be constructed if the vein is between 2.5 and 3.5 mm. If the basilic vein is smaller than 2.5 mm, failure is common.

Harvest of the Basilic Vein

Whether done in one or two stages, the basilic vein must be transected distally and care must be taken to avoid injury to the medial antebrachial cutaneous nerve, which crosses anterior to the basilic vein at or just before the entry of the median cubital vein (Fig. 65-2, A). Surgeons often encounter a stout large branch between the basilic and the brachial veins in the midarm. They should ligate or, if necessary, suture this branch carefully to avoid narrowing the lumen of the basilic vein. The basilic vein also occasionally joins the brachial vein in the midarm. Experience shows that if extra length is needed, the brachial vein may be harvested in continuity to the axilla without resulting in disabling postoperative arm edema. The brachial vein may be the dominant arm vein and can be used when no other autogenous vein is available. However, it is more fragile and has more branches than the basilic vein. The basilic vein should be freed to the proximal arm, marked to maintain orientation and tunneled over the anterior arm before anastomosis of the vein onto the brachial artery. Mere elevation of the vein makes for awkward cannulation and uncomfortable dialysis (Fig. 65-2, B).[5] The basilic vein can also be harvested endoscopically or via a "keyhole" technique.[6,7] The benefit of decreased incisional pain has not been established.

STEAL SYNDROME

Steal syndrome occurs less frequently with a basilic vein transposition (<4%) than with a prosthetic bridge graft. Upper arm fistulas may be originated from the proximal radial artery to reduce the incidence of steal syndrome.[8]

Operative Technique

Preoperative duplex vessel mapping is essential and may be assisted by placing a tourniquet on the proximal arm with gentle massage of the venous column centrally to distend the vein. Prophylactic antibiotics should be administered. Supraclavicular brachial plexus block can be used for anesthesia, along with 0.5% to 1.0% lidocaine to infiltrate the line of incision. Additional lidocaine can be administered into the fascial compartment. General anesthesia may be an alternative. The harvest incision extends the full length of the upper arm to the axilla. Exposure of the vein may begin anywhere along its length, but the venous anatomy is most reliably defined either in the axilla or at the median cubital vein. The basilic vein distal from its junction with the median cubital vein is occasionally harvested to gain additional length.

TWO-STAGE PROCEDURE

First Stage

An incision is made over the median cubital vein, which is dissected for a short distance. The adjacent brachial artery is exposed, a 4- to 5-mm-long arteriotomy is made, and an end-to-side, vein-to-artery anastomosis is created with 6-0 or 7-0 polypropylene.

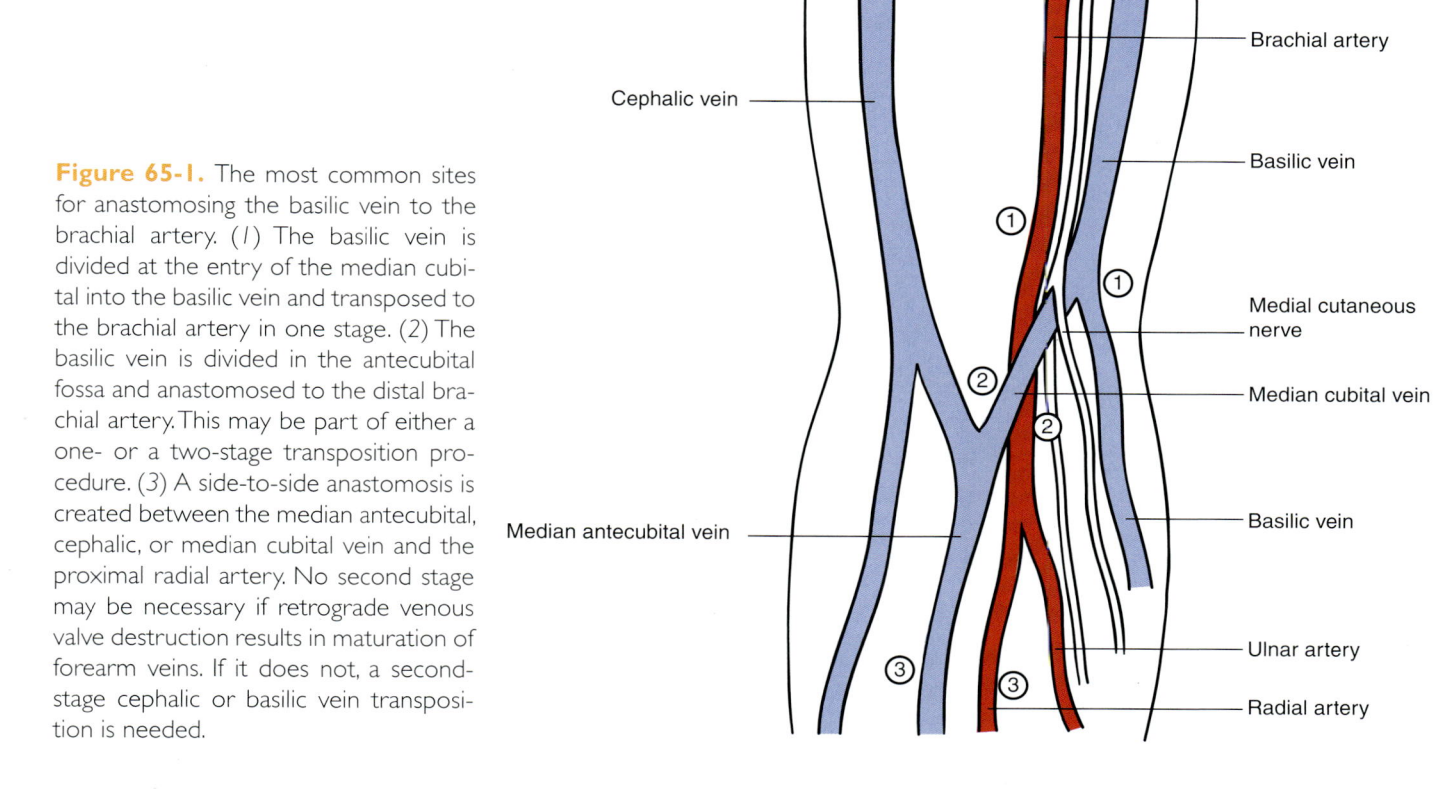

Figure 65-1. The most common sites for anastomosing the basilic vein to the brachial artery. (1) The basilic vein is divided at the entry of the median cubital into the basilic vein and transposed to the brachial artery in one stage. (2) The basilic vein is divided in the antecubital fossa and anastomosed to the distal brachial artery. This may be part of either a one- or a two-stage transposition procedure. (3) A side-to-side anastomosis is created between the median antecubital, cephalic, or median cubital vein and the proximal radial artery. No second stage may be necessary if retrograde venous valve destruction results in maturation of forearm veins. If it does not, a second-stage cephalic or basilic vein transposition is needed.

Figure 65-2. A, The left basilic arm vein is exposed from the elbow to the axilla and marked for orientation before transection and tunneling. The medial antebrachial cutaneous nerve of the forearm, which crosses the basilic vein in the distal arm, should not be divided. Simple elevation of the vein, in contrast to transposition, results in medial forearm anesthesia and makes for uncomfortable and awkward cannulation for hemodialysis. **B,** The basilic vein has been tunneled anteriorly and anastomosed to the distal brachial artery. Twists and kinks must be avoided.

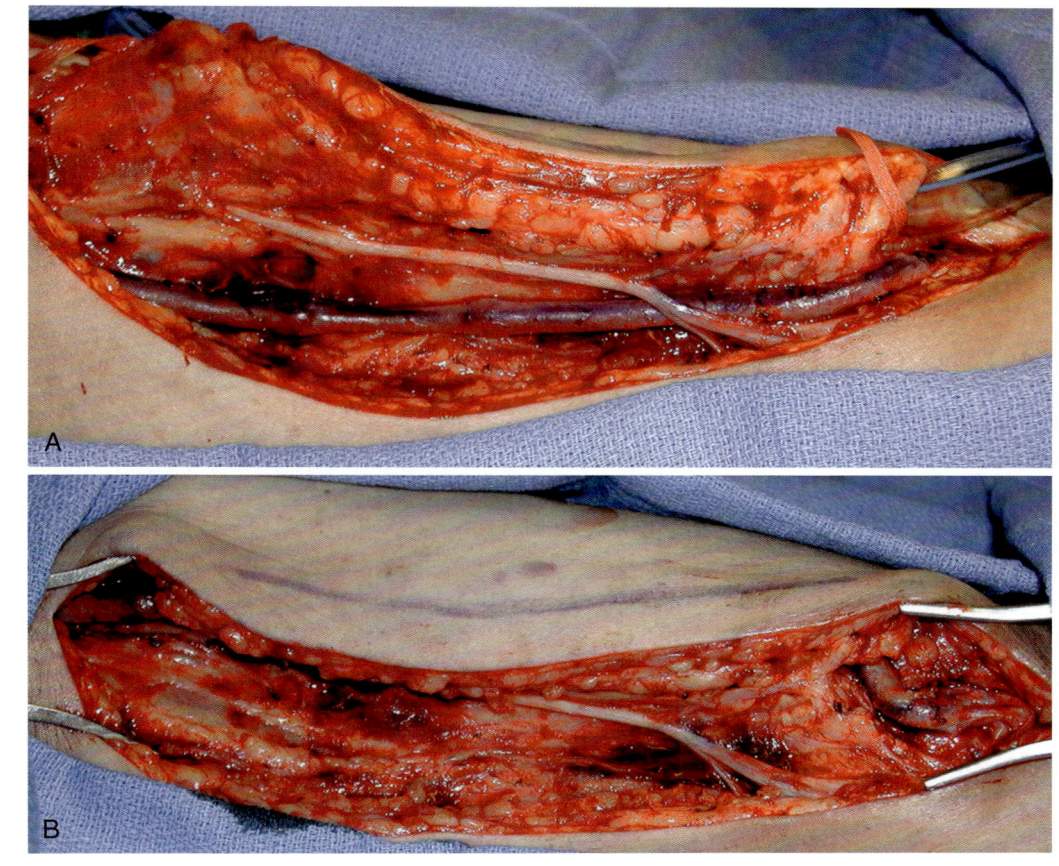

Second Stage

After 4 weeks, ultrasound confirms that the basilic vein is suitable, as indicated by slight thickening and enlargement of the vein. At the second stage, the basilic vein is exposed to the axilla. A tunnel is created about 2 to 3 cm anterior to the basilic vein with a sheathed tunneler. The basilic vein is marked along its anterior surface, transected distally, gently dilated with heparinized saline, and drawn through the tunnel, with care taken to avoid rotation or kinking. The transposed basilic vein is reanastomosed to the distal vein. Subcutaneous tissue is reapproximated with a running 3-0 absorbable suture. A drain is usually unnecessary. Skin is closed with 5-0 subcuticular suture, and a sterile adhesive dressing is applied.

Superficialization of the Fistula

An additional popular variation involves performing an initial end-to-side basilic vein to brachial artery anastomosis. After a 4- to 6-week maturation period, the basilic vein is exposed, branches are divided and ligated, and the vein is superficialized by approximating the subcutaneous tissue below the vein. The fistula can be accessed after healing of the skin incision.

Use of the Radial Artery

Variations at the second stage include creating an anastomosis to the brachial artery at a more proximal site or transecting the vein close to the original arteriovenous anastomosis. Jennings[8] has described a variation in which the radial artery is exposed in the proximal forearm and a side-to-side anastomosis is created to the adjacent median antebrachial, median cubital, or cephalic vein. Before creating the anastomosis, the valves in the distal vein are disrupted with a valvulotome to allow both antegrade and retrograde flow. The upper arm cephalic vein, cubital veins, and forearm veins may dilate and mature sufficiently for dialysis. If not, the upper arm cephalic or basilic vein can be transposed.

SINGLE-STAGE PROCEDURE

Most basilic veins are 4 mm in diameter or greater, and a one-stage procedure is usually possible if the vein is of sufficient size and free of intimal disease. The vein is exposed to the axilla, and a tunnel is created 2 to 3 cm anterior to the main harvest incision. The vein is marked on its anterior surface, transected distally at the level of the median cubital vein, and drawn through the tunnel, avoiding vein rotation or kinking. The vein is anastomosed end to side to the brachial artery. In most patients the brachial artery is exposed through the main incision about 2 to 3 cm proximal to the basilic vein transection. In the obese patient a second incision may be necessary to expose the artery.

An important variation of this procedure is to begin the basilic vein harvest starting at the confluence of basilic and median cubital veins. The advantage of transecting the basilic vein at this more proximal site is that the vein is usually 4 mm or larger and is unaffected by previous venipuncture, catheters, or revision of forearm prosthetic grafts. The obvious drawback is that there is less basilic vein for the transposition, but this has not proved detrimental in practice. If the basilic vein ends in the midarm, the surgeon needs to harvest the brachial vein in the upper arm to achieve adequate length. Subcutaneous tissue is reapproximated with a running 3-0 absorbable suture. A drain is usually unnecessary. Skin is closed with 5-0 subcuticular suture, and a sterile adhesive dressing is applied.

Postoperative Care

- **Follow-up care.** The patient should be evaluated 2 to 4 weeks postoperatively to assess vein enlargement and flow.

Complications

- **Thrombosis and maturation.** Major complications are thrombosis and failure of the fistula to mature. Ultrasound can be used to assess vein size, depth, areas of stenosis, and blood flow.[4] Fistulas with robust flow experience an increase in vein diameter of 1 to 2 mm in the early postoperative period.
- **Wound breakdown.** Wound complications are uncommon but can be encountered in the obese patient.
- **Steal syndrome.** Steal symptoms such as mild numbness or coolness often resolve spontaneously.[9] If severe, angiography is mandatory, and angioplasty of inflow or outflow arterial lesions may relieve the steal. The basilic vein may dilate considerably over time. If excess fistula flow is identified, then reducing flow can be achieved by tapering the proximal vein or interposing a short segment of vein or tapered polytetrafluoroethylene (PTFE). Alternatively, if there is redundant vein, the fistula can be extended to the proximal radial artery if the ulnar artery is patent or a distal revascularization interval ligation (DRIL) procedure can be performed (see Chapter 67).
- **Fistula thrombosis.** Success in constructing a functional basilic vein transposition varies widely. Two-year secondary patency rates of 85% have been achieved.[10] Early thrombosis before initiation of dialysis suggests a technical error or poor-quality vein. Immediate thrombectomy and correction of any technical problem may occasionally result in useful access. Late thrombosis usually results from intimal hyperplasia or vein degradation because of repeated use. Pharmacomechanical thrombolysis can be used to determine whether salvage is feasible.

Femoral Vein Transposition

Indications

KDOQI guidelines recommend exhausting upper extremity access before constructing one in the lower extremities. Nonetheless, it is preferable to proceed to a lower extremity access whenever it becomes necessary either to surgically salvage an upper extremity access by repairing a subclavian, innominate, or superior vena cava obstruction or to bypass to the internal jugular vein. Reoperation on the jugular vein can be formidable, and the vein should remain available for future temporary catheter access. For most individuals a femoral vein transposition should be considered for the first lower extremity access. Femoral vein transposition is not recommended for frail, elderly individuals with a life expectancy of less than 2 years. Patients with appreciable arterial occlusive disease should also be excluded, unless angioplasty can restore pedal pulses and the ankle brachial index exceeds 0.85. In patients with good popliteal pulses but absent pedal pulses, a loop composite PTFE–femoral vein may provide all the benefits and avoid the ischemic complications of a nonlooped femoral vein access. Postoperative edema is well tolerated even if the great saphenous vein has been harvested and seldom exceeds a 2-cm increase in leg circumference.

Preoperative Preparation

- **Catheter-based dialysis.** Prolonged use of femoral vein catheters for temporary vascular access while waiting for an upper extremity access to mature is strongly discouraged. This tactic greatly reduces the usefulness of the extremity for either femoral vein or prosthetic access grafts. If an iliac vein stenosis is suspected, a stent may be placed.
- **Preoperative imaging.** Patients should undergo duplex ultrasonography to ensure that the femoral vein is at least 5 mm in diameter and to exclude deep vein thrombosis, a duplicated femoral vein, or the presence of a dominant

profunda femoris vein. Iliac venography is advisable if the patient has had a long-standing ipsilateral femoral catheter.
- **Patient communication.** Patients should be advised to expect some degree of postoperative pain and initial difficulty ambulating.

Pitfalls and Danger Points

- Steal syndrome
- Compartment syndrome
- Excessive flow
- Edema
- Wound complications
- Nerve damage
- Venous anomalies and previous thrombophlebitis

Operative Strategy

STEAL SYNDROME

The increased incidence of steal and compartment syndromes after femoral vein transposition derives from a combination of high flow through the fistula, increased distal venous pressure, and prevalence of obstructive and calcific arterial disease. If arterial insufficiency is present, angiography with angioplasty of iliac, femoral, or popliteal disease may allow an otherwise unqualified individual to undergo the procedure. Postoperative ischemic complications can be reduced by tapering the femoral vein to 4 to 5 mm before anastomosis to the femoral artery. If pedal pulses are not palpable after completion of the femoral vein transposition, the systolic arterial pressure should be measured in the distal popliteal artery. If the systolic pressure in the popliteal artery is not at least 60% of systolic blood pressure in the arm, then additional flow-reducing measures should be considered.

AVOIDING WOUND COMPLICATIONS

Wound complications include infection, full-thickness skin necrosis of the posterior flap, and lymphocutaneous fistulas, which are more common in the obese patient, diabetics, and individuals who have had multiple previous surgeries. The incision for harvesting the femoral vein should be placed directly over the arterial pulse to avoid ischemic skin flaps. Division of femoral artery branches while harvesting the femoral vein should be avoided to assure optimal perfusion of the thigh.

Operative Technique

INCISION

A Bair Hugger (Arizant Healthcare, Eden Prairie, Minn.) conserves upper body heat. At the end of a long procedure, palpating a pedal pulse in a cold, vasoconstricted patient may be difficult. General anesthesia with arterial blood pressure monitoring is recommended. Prophylactic antibiotics are administered. The incision begins at the level of the inguinal crease directly over the femoral pulse, where the artery is easiest to identify, and is extended distally. The common femoral artery is not exposed unless a loop composite fistula with PTFE is planned.

EXPOSURE OF THE FEMORAL VEIN

Although the femoral vein is always deep to the artery along its entire course in the thigh, it is usually easier to expose the vein lateral to the artery throughout its length. The femoral artery pulse is used to guide the incision's distal extension.

Division of arterial branches while dissecting the vein and dividing its tributaries should be avoided. Each tributary is ligated adjacent to the femoral vein; hemoclips or ligatures are applied distally. Transected lymphatic vessels should also be clipped.

EXPOSURE OF THE DISTAL FEMORAL AND POPLITEAL VEIN

As the incision is extended, the overlying sartorius muscle is encountered, which is mobilized as needed to expose the vein. The thick fascia distal from the sartorius may make it difficult to feel the arterial pulse in the distal half of the thigh. A few centimeters distal from the lateral border of the sartorius muscle is the adductor tendon, which can be divided, taking care not to injure the saphenous or other adjacent nerves. The popliteal vein is dissected beyond the divided adductor tendon until it dives deep into the popliteal fossa. Sufficient popliteal vein is harvested to bring the vein to the surface and back to the artery for anastomosis. In the obese patient, the vein is harvested as far distal as possible with a supragenicular incision. The distal popliteal vein is transected and ligated with a 2-0 ligature.

MOBILIZATION OF THE PROXIMAL FEMORAL VEIN

The femoral vein is now dissected back to its confluence with the profunda femoris vein, which at this point is as large as the femoral vein and dives directly posterior from the bifurcation. The bifurcation is at least 1 cm distal from the arterial bifurcation, which need not be exposed. The profunda vein should not be confused with the lateral circumflex vein, which is often divided when exposing the profunda femoral artery. The venous tributaries of the distal common femoral vein are routinely divided to allow complete mobilization of the femoral vein.

TRANSPOSITION PROCEDURE

To conserve length, the femoral vein is transposed lateral to the femoral artery before tunneling (Fig. 65-3). Some believe that lateral positioning may induce stenosis of the femoral vein at its junction with the common femoral vein and therefore have advocated curving the femoral vein medially around the artery to begin anterior thigh tunneling. Two counter incisions are made to help pass the femoral vein back to the distal femoral artery. Freely incise fascia at either end of the tunnel to allow the vein to lie unconstricted and without kinks. The distance between the incisions is typically 12 to 15 cm, which is the cannulated segment of the fistula. This length may not seem adequate, given the effort to mobilize almost the entire length of the thigh vein, but it is more than adequate if nurses are encouraged to move the needle sites or use the buttonhole technique. The tunnel is created 2 to 3 cm lateral to the main incision, and a 32-Fr chest tube may be used to enlarge the tunnel. Wound problems and skin necrosis usually involve the medial flap.

ARTERIOVENOUS ANASTOMOSIS

Options for anticoagulation include intravenous heparin administration at 2000 units without protamine reversal or full anticoagulation at 100 units per kilogram of body weight with protamine reversal. The vein is typically anastomosed on the superficial femoral artery halfway between the sartorius muscle and the divided adductor tendon. Veins larger than 5 mm in diameter should be tapered to reduce the incidence of steal (Fig. 65-3).[9] A wedge of the vein is excised, usually one third of its diameter, and the vein is then sutured so as to taper it. The resultant diameter of the vein is reduced about 50%, which reduces its cross-sectional area by 75%. The superficial femoral artery is often calcified or has markedly thickened intima, and an arterial clamp is used to control flow. The anastomosis is performed with continuous 5-0 polypropylene. Fistula and pedal flows are checked with continuous-wave Doppler after completing the anastomosis.

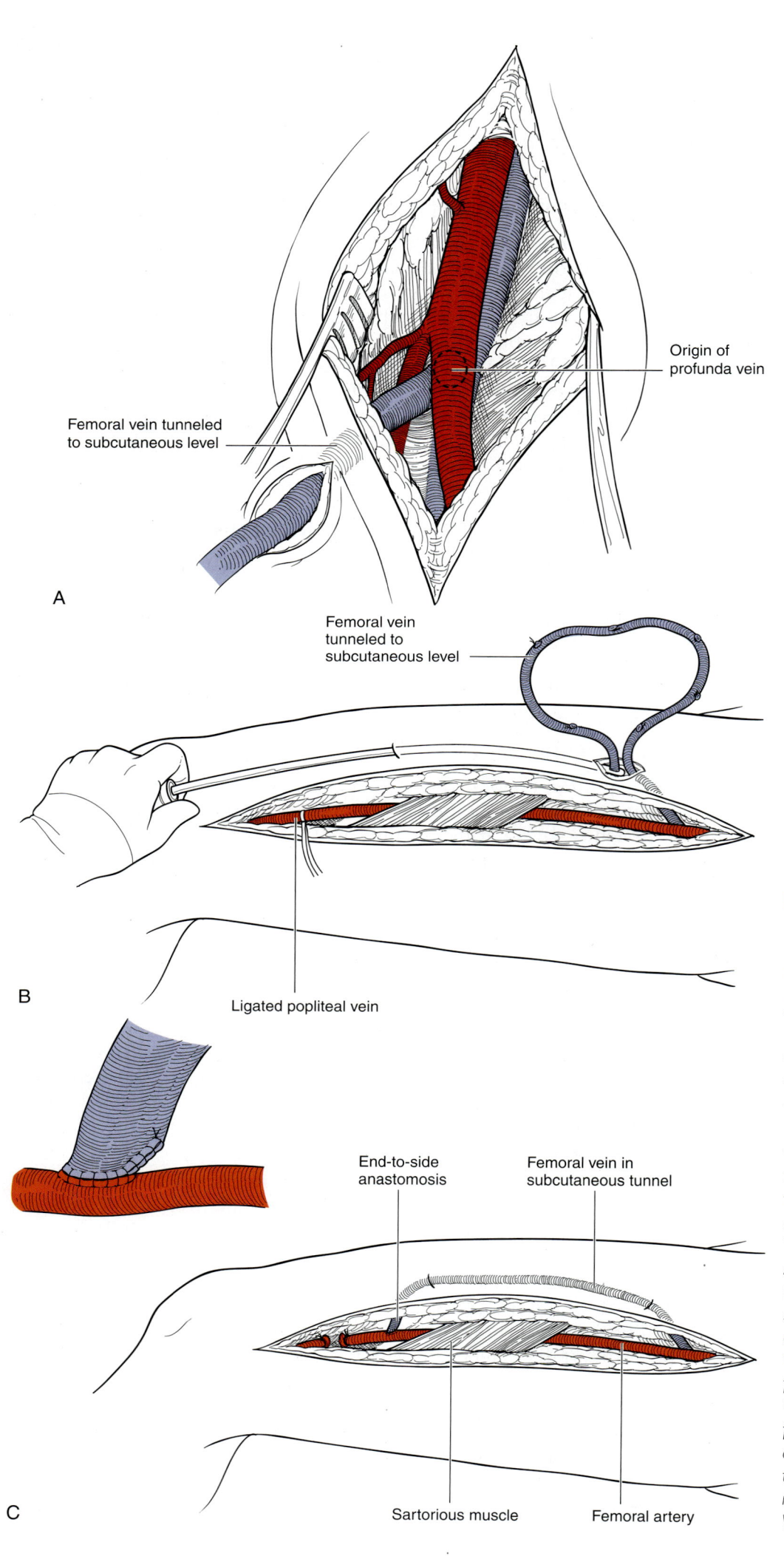

Figure 65-3. A, The mobilized femoral vein is passed deep to the femoral artery and brought through a separate small skin incision in preparation for tunneling. **B**, The femoral vein is tunneled distally with the help of a second small distal skin incision. **C**, Completed femoral vein transposition. The inset shows how the femoral vein is tapered to a 4.5- to 5.0-mm diameter before implantation on the distal femoral artery. (**A-C**, Redrawn from Gradman WS, Cohen W, Haji-Aghaii M: Arteriovenous fistula construction in the thigh with transposed superficial femoral vein: Our initial experience. *J Vasc Surg* 33:970-971, 2001; **B**, inset, Redrawn from Gradman WS, Laub J, Cohen W: Femoral vein transposition for arteriovenous hemodialysis access: Improved patient selection and intraoperative measures reduce postoperative ischemia. *J Vasc Surg* 41:280, 2005.)

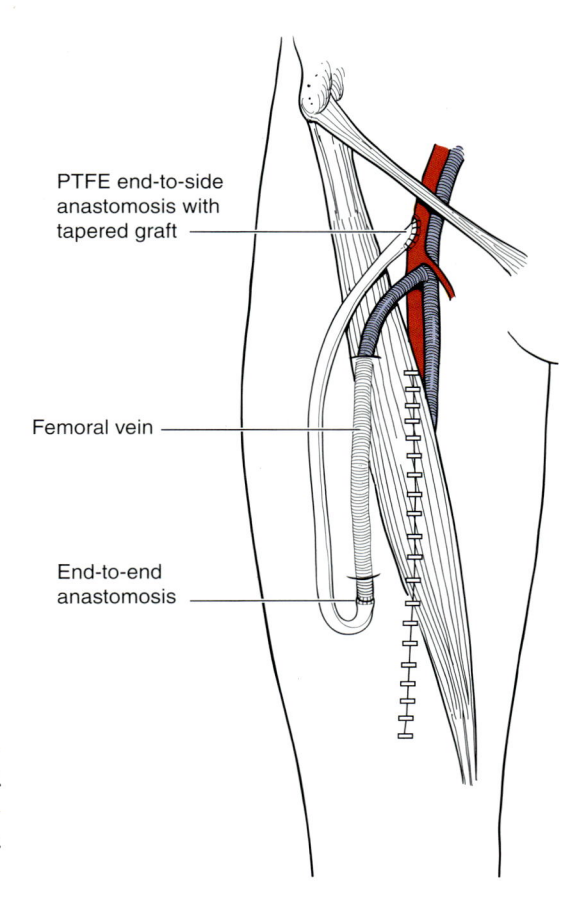

Figure 65-4. Loop composite PTFE-transposed femoral vein fistula. A 4- to 7-mm, tapered PTFE graft reduces fistula flow and helps prevent a steal. (Redrawn from Gradman WS, Cohen W, Haji-Aghaii M: Arteriovenous fistula construction in the thigh with transposed superficial femoral vein: Our initial experience. J Vasc Surg 33:971, 2001.)

LOOP COMPOSITE POLYTETRAFLUORETHYLENE–FEMORAL VEIN ARTERIOVENOUS ACCESS

In the presence of a patient at risk for steal syndrome, loop composite PTFE–femoral vein access can be constructed with a 4- to 7-mm, tapered PTFE graft (Fig. 65-4). The typical patient may have a palpable popliteal but not pedal pulses. The proximal end of the graft should be tapered to about 5 mm before implanting the PTFE graft on the common femoral artery. A third counter incision is made between the 5- and 7-o'clock positions in the loop access to avoid a kink. The 7-mm end is usually a good fit with the vein. The PTFE limb does not need to be buried as previously reported. Nonetheless, both dialysis needles should be placed into the femoral vein to avoid cannulating the PTFE. The advantage of keeping the PTFE near the skin surface is that if the vein later degenerates, the PTFE graft can be extended to the common femoral vein and the original PTFE arteriovenous conduit used exclusively until the new interposed segment matures. This approach is especially useful for patients with extremely limited sites for temporary access. Intimal hyperplasia in a composite graft typically occurs initially at the junction of the PTFE and the femoral vein, a site that is surgically accessible if angioplasty is necessary.

A prophylactic closed medial and lateral calf fasciotomy may be advisable and adds little morbidity to the procedure. A drain is not routinely used. The main incision is closed with 2-0 or 3-0 absorbable subcutaneous suture and 5-0 absorbable subcuticular skin suture. Bupivacaine without epinephrine may be injected into the wound for postoperative pain control.

Postoperative Care

- **Compartment syndrome.** In the first 24 to 48 hours observe closely for a compartment syndrome, especially the anterior compartment. If the compartment is firm and tender and the patient cannot dorsiflex the foot, proceed to fasciotomy at the bedside under local anesthesia even if a palpable dorsalis pedis pulse is present. An open fasciotomy is preferable to a closed fasciotomy. The incisions may be closed after swelling resolves.

- **Anticoagulation.** Patients do not need routine anticoagulation after femoral vein transposition. Transient postoperative edema and calf pain may lead to venous ultrasound studies commonly showing thrombus in the midpopliteal and distal popliteal veins, but the benefit of anticoagulation in this setting has not been established.
- **Ambulation.** Patients have trouble walking in the immediate postoperative period, so it is beneficial to keep them in the hospital a few days for pain control and physical therapy.
- **Initiation of dialysis.** In patients without another site for temporary catheter placement, the access can be used as soon as 2 to 3 days if 17-gauge needles are used. This is preferable to placing a temporary dual lumen catheter in the ipsilateral femoral vein. If possible, wait for 2 months before using the access, but after 3 to 4 weeks, 17-gauge needles can be used for access.

Complications

- **Patency rates.** It is challenging to reoperate in the vicinity of the artery-vein anastomosis after the original surgery.[11] If an inflow problem develops at the arterial anastomosis that is uncorrectable with angioplasty, it is easier to convert the fistula to a loop composite PTFE–femoral vein rather than revising the original anastomosis.
- **Steal syndrome.** Steal syndrome may appear early or late, but prompt diagnosis and treatment are important to prevent limb damage. Early fasciotomy, especially of the anterior compartment, can provide time for proper strategic evaluation of the steal. Angiography with angioplasty is highly desirable if time permits. Of the many options available for treatment of a steal, proximalization with a 4- to 7-mm PTFE graft, as described earlier, is probably the easiest and is consistently effective. As a second option, a 6- or 7-mm PTFE femoral-popliteal bypass from the common femoral artery can be constructed to the proximal popliteal artery. The typical patient has no pedal flow after tapering the vein. It is not necessary to ligate the interval femoral artery, as performed in the DRIL procedure. Wound and technical problems may ensue upon reexploration of the femoral artery–femoral vein anastomosis to taper the anastomosis or in creating a femoropopliteal bypass with or without interval ligation.
- **Lymphatic disruption.** Small lymphocutaneous fistulas may occasionally be closed with skin sutures one month after the incision has healed. Larger collections of lymph fluid may respond to repeated aspiration but in many cases need to be explored.
- **Late thrombosis.** Pharmacomechanical thrombectomy with percutaneous angioplasty is more successful with a femoral vein access than in the upper extremity. If a loop composite access occludes, the stenosis is often noted at the vein-PTFE graft junction. In this instance, and surgical patch angioplasty is more durable than percutaneous angioplasty.
- **Wound problems.** Wound complications are common, especially in the obese patient with a history of prior lower extremity surgery. A patch of full-thickness necrosis may develop in the medial thigh flap and, if uninfected, may be observed rather than debrided. Even full-thickness necrosis usually heals by secondary intention. Wound infections will respond to antibiotics and drainage.

REFERENCES

1. Dagher F, Gelber R, Ramos E, et al: The use of basilic vein and brachial artery as an A-V fistula for long term hemodialysis, *J Surg Res* 20:373-376, 1976.
2. National Kidney Foundation: K/DOQI clinical practice guidelines for vascular access, *Am J Kidney Dis* 30:S150-S191, 1997.
3. Gradman WS, Cohen W, Haji-Aghaii M: Arteriovenous fistula construction in the thigh with transposed superficial femoral vein: Our initial experience, *J Vasc Surg* 33:968-975, 2001.
4. Wiese P, Nonnast-Daniel B: Colour Doppler ultrasound in dialysis access, *Nephrol Dial Transplant* 19:1956-1963, 2004.
5. Hossny A: Brachiobasilic arteriovenous fistula: Different surgical techniques and their effects on fistula patency and dialysis-related complication, *J Vasc Surg* 37:821-826, 2003.
6. Martinez BD, LeSar CJ, Fogarty TJ, et al: Transposition of the basilic vein for arteriovenous fistula: An endoscopic approach, *J Am Coll Surg* 192:233-236, 2001.
7. Hill BB, Chan AK, Faruqi RM, et al: Keyhole technique for autologous brachiobasilic transposition arteriovenous fistula, *J Vasc Surg* 42:945-950, 2005.
8. Jennings WC: Creating arteriovenous fistulas in 132 consecutive patients, *Arch Surg* 141:27-32, 2006.
9. Gradman WS: Prevention and treatment of hemodialysis access-related steal: A new classification. In Henry M, editor: *Vascular access for hemodialysis*, Chicago, 2008, W.L. Gore and Associates, pp 155-160.
10. Chemla ES, Morsey MA: Is basilic vein transposition a real alternative to an arteriovenous bypass graft? A prospective study, *Sem Dial* 21:352-356, 2008.
11. Gradman WS, Laub J, Cohen W: Femoral vein transposition for arteriovenous hemodialysis access: Improved patient selection and intraoperative measures reduce postoperative ischemia, *J Vasc Surg* 41:279-284, 2005.

66 Unconventional Venous Access Procedures for Chronic Hemodialysis

DAVID L. CULL

Historical Background

Despite the success of the Brescia-Cimino type subcutaneous arteriovenous fistula in 1962, the absence of suitable forearm vessels in many patients led to the evaluation of alternative conduits. In 1969 May and colleagues[1] described the creation of a forearm arteriovenous fistula using autogenous saphenous vein. This was soon followed by the evaluation of nonautogenous conduits, including the bovine carotid heterograft, as described by Chivitz and associates[2] in 1972, and microporous expanded polytetrafluoroethylene (PTFE), which was first reported by Baker and co-workers[3] in 1975. PTFE grafts, as either loop or straight arteriovenous conduits, was applied both in the upper and lower extremity in these early reports. In the decades that followed, patients presenting with limited vascular access options in the upper extremity continued to challenge surgeons with increasing frequency. Thus the use of unconventional sites and means of achieving vascular access for hemodialysis continued to be explored. Use of the anterior chest wall axillary artery and vein for arteriovenous access was reported by Ono and colleagues[4] in 1995, and the transposition of the brachial vein in the upper extremity and saphenous vein in the lower extremity for henodialysis access described in 1998.[5,6] Katzman and associates[7] described their initial experience with the hybrid HERO graft-catheter vascular access device in 2009.

Indications

Although algorithms have been developed to define a general "order of preference" for access placement in the upper extremity, a similar algorithm for patients who require more complex access placement is problematic given the lack of evidence-based reports. It is possible, however, to provide recommendations for specific clinical situations in which a particular complex access procedure would be most helpful and in which it should be avoided. These recommendations are outlined in Table 66-1.

Preoperative Preparation

- **History.** A complete history that specifies the presumed cause for prior vascular access failures requires a thorough review of operative notes, as well as consultation with treating nephrologists and dialysis nurses.
- **Preoperative imaging.** Noninvasive vascular testing may not provide sufficient anatomic information for patients who have had multiple access procedures. Accordingly, contrast angiography may be required to identify arterial and venous pathology that may influence outcome.

TABLE 66-1 Considerations for Major Complex Access Procedures

Access Procedure	Indications	Ideal Clinical Situations	Relative Contraindications
Femoral or saphenous vein transposition	Patent femoral or saphenous vein Femoral or saphenous vein > 3 mm in diameter Patent, noncalcific femoral artery	Pediatric or young healthy patients Thrombophilia with no other autogenous access option Patients at high risk for infection (poor hygiene, immunosuppressed, multiple previous access infections)	Significant obesity of the thigh Patients who are medically fragile Access sites for temporary catheter placement not readily available Patients at high risk for access-related limb ischemia
Brachial vein transposition	Brachial vein > 2.5 mm in diameter	Pediatric or young healthy patient Patients at high risk for infection (poor hygiene, immunosuppressed, multiple previous access infections)	Patients who are candidates for autogenous radial-cephalic, brachial-cephalic, or brachial-basilic access Significant obesity of the upper arm
Prosthetic midthigh or proximal loop femoral-femoral access	Patent femoral or common femoral vein Patent, noncalcific superficial femoral artery (midthigh access), common femoral artery	Patients who are elderly or have significant medical comorbidities	Patients at high risk for infection (poor hygiene, immunosuppressed, multiple previous access infections) Patients who are morbidly obese
Prosthetic chest wall access	Patent axillary or subclavian artery and vein Patient central vein	Patients who are morbidly obese	Patients who are reasonable candidates for an autogenous or prosthetic thigh access procedure
Transthoracic cuffed dialysis catheter	Patent superior vena cava (long stump preferable) Access to the superior vena cava via the femoral vein for pigtail catheter placement	Patients who have limited life expectancy (<6 months) Patients for whom all alternative access procedures have been used	Patients who are candidates for an alternative complex access procedure Patients who are candidates for cuffed dialysis catheter placement via the internal jugular or subclavian vein Patients with severe cardiac or pulmonary disease
HERO device	Patent central veins Brachial artery anatomy suitable for arteriovenous access placement	Patients whose only option for chronic hemodialysis access is a tunneled cuffed dialysis catheter	Patients who are candidates for an alternative complex access procedure

- **Preoperative preparation.** The patient's medical condition should be optimized before surgery, including fluid status, which may require coordination with the treating nephrologist and the patient's dialysis schedule. In addition, healing of all open wounds and resolution of coexistent infection, as well as stabilization of significant comorbid conditions that may increase anesthetic risk, should be undertaken before surgery. Preoperative vascular and neurologic status of the extremity should be documented.
- **Prevention of surgical site infection.** Appropriate prophylactic antibiotics should be administered, and an antimicrobial adhesive film barrier should be applied over the operative field.

Pitfalls and Danger Points

- Relevant vascular anatomy should be delineated.
- Factors contributing to prior access failures, including undetected thrombophilia, should be identified. Strategies to prolong patency may include adjusting medications and the patient's dry weight to minimize the risk of hypotension during or after hemodialysis. In addition, initiating anticoagulation therapy immediately after thrombectomy or access placement may be appropriate.
- All access options must be considered to formulate a long-term vascular access strategy.

Operative Strategy

OPTIONS FOR TEMPORARY DIALYSIS ACCESS

Planning for the potential need for future access should begin long before surgical intervention is necessary. Strategic considerations should also include options for temporary access. If options for a temporary dialysis catheter are limited, an "early stick" vascular graft may be of value. If possible, catheters located at or near the region where new access is planned should be removed several days before the operative procedure.

ASSESSMENT OF REMAINING OPTIONS FOR UPPER EXTREMITY ACCESS

The complication rate of vascular access in the lower extremity, chest wall, and other so-called exotic access sites is higher than in the upper extremity, and management of these problems can be challenging. Therefore one should ensure that alternative options in the upper extremity no longer exist. For example, a venogram may reveal paired brachial veins or an open cephalic vein in the deltopectoral groove, either of which could provide adequate venous outflow. Occasionally upper extremity arterial and venous anatomy is adequate, but an ipsilateral central venous stenosis or occlusion seemingly precludes vascular access. Although long-term durability of central vein angioplasty is modest, with primary patency rates of about 40% at 6 months, repeat angioplasty with or without stenting does extend secondary patency rates.[8] Thus treatment of a central vein stenosis with a percutaneous intervention followed by placement of an upper extremity arteriovenous access site should be considered before proceeding to the thigh or chest wall. For patients who are obese, standard basilic, brachial, or femoral transpositions through a separate subcutaneous tunnel may be impractical because vein length will not be sufficient. However, a transposition may be possible if the vein is elevated into the incision.[9]

THE PEDIATRIC PATIENT

For small children, peritoneal dialysis may be advisable. If necessary, hemodialysis via percutaneously or surgically placed catheters can be achieved, but infectious complications are common. Ideally, pediatric patients should receive an autogenous vascular access placed distally in the extremity. Microsurgical techniques, including the use of microsurgical instruments, interrupted sutures, and adequate magnification, greatly facilitate pediatric vascular access placement. To minimize vessel dissection and vasospasm, the use of a sterile tourniquet may be helpful.

BRACHIAL VEIN TRANSPOSITION

Brachial vein transposition should be considered if vein diameter exceeds 2.5 mm on preoperative vein mapping and if a brachial-cephalic fistula or basilic vein transposition is precluded. Brachial vein transposition should be performed as a two-stage procedure, whereby the arteriovenous anastomosis is created first and is followed 6 weeks later by vein transposition. A one-stage procedure may be considered if the preoperative brachial vein diameter exceeds 4 mm. Obese patients with significant upper arm adipose tissue are not ideal candidates for brachial vein transposition because the vein length may be too short to transpose superficially.

SAPHENOUS VEIN TRANSPOSITION

Use of skip incisions or endoscopic techniques to harvest the saphenous vein may decrease the risk of wound complications. Because the great saphenous vein does not readily dilate after creation of a fistula, only veins greater than 3 mm in diameter should be used. Cannulation of the access must be delayed at least 6 weeks postoperatively to avoid puncture site bleeding and hematoma. The procedure may not be practical for patients who are morbidly obese, because cannulation may require the patient to lie supine and to retract the pannus to expose the access site.

PROSTHETIC LOWER EXTREMITY VASCULAR ACCESS

Sites used for prosthetic arteriovenous access in the lower extremity are the femoral artery to great saphenous or femoral vein loop access, and the midthigh, midsuperficial femoral artery to femoral vein loop access. Prosthetic access in the lower extremity is preferred once options in the upper extremity have been exhausted because of simplicity and accessibility of femoral vessels, with patency rates that are comparable if not superior to upper extremity procedures. In addition, graft infection and an anastomotic stenosis are easier to manage than if the access site is in the chest wall, and both hands are free to self-cannulate or to perform other activities during dialysis. By basing the arterial and venous anastomoses in the midthigh superficial femoral artery and femoral vein, node-bearing tissue and panniculus in the groin are avoided. As a result, prosthetic midthigh loop access appears to carry a lower infection rate compared with prosthetic procedures in the groin. The prosthetic midthigh loop access also preserves proximal femoral vessels for future access placement. Preoperative duplex ultrasonography should be performed to verify patency of both artery and vein, as well as to determine the degree of calcification in the arterial wall.

PROSTHETIC CHEST WALL VASCULAR ACCESS

The most common sites and graft configurations for prosthetic arteriovenous access placement on the chest wall are axillary artery to ipsilateral axillary vein loop access and axillary artery to contralateral axillary vein straight or necklace access. An advantage of the looped graft configuration over the axillary-axillary straight or necklace access is that the contralateral axillary vessels are preserved as a site for future access placement. It is important that central venous patency be confirmed before surgery. If the proximal axillary, subclavian, or brachiocephalic vein has recently undergone angioplasty or stenting, an alternative site for arteriovenous access should be chosen, because recurrent stenosis after central venous intervention is common and influences patency. If there is a significant difference in blood pressure between the arms, the axillary artery on the side with the highest pressure is the preferred donor vessel. A preoperative contrast arteriogram or computed tomography angiogram should be considered. Access-related ischemia has not been reported, even when chest wall access was performed using vessels ipsilateral to an arm in patients with a prior history of steal syndrome. Chest wall prosthetic access may be associated with a lower risk of infection or wound complications than a lower extremity prosthetic arteriovenous access graft in a morbidly obese patient. A major disadvantage of chest wall access is that proximal control of the axillary vessels can be challenging if the graft becomes infected and excision required.

TRANSTHORACIC CUFFED DIALYSIS CATHETER PLACEMENT

The procedure using a transthoracic cuffed dialysis catheter should be considered only after conventional central venous catheter placement is precluded by internal jugular and subclavian vein thrombosis. Severe cardiopulmonary disease is a relative contraindication to transthoracic cuffed dialysis catheter placement. The risk of bleeding is increased in patients with a short superior vena cava stump that requires cannulation of the vessel through the pericardial sac.

HEMODIALYSIS RELIABLE OUTFLOW VASCULAR ACCESS DEVICE PLACEMENT

Blood cultures should be obtained before Hemodialysis Reliable Outflow (HERO) device placement (Hemosphere, Minneapolis) and if present, bacteremia should be treated with appropriate antibiotics. If the silicone catheter component of the HERO device is inserted over a wire after removal of a tunneled dialysis catheter, the catheter tip should be cultured. Antibiotics should be considered if the culture is positive. Placement of the HERO device through a previously infected field should be avoided. If a tunneled dialysis catheter is present, the catheter should be removed as soon as the HERO device is ready for cannulation in 2 to 3 weeks and the tip should be cultured.

Operative Technique

BRACHIAL VEIN TRANSPOSITION

There are important differences between brachial and basilic vein transpositions. Transposition of the brachial vein is technically more challenging because of its short length, greater depth, and numerous venous tributaries. Furthermore, although use of basilic vein transposition is well established, the role of brachial vein transposition is poorly defined. The largest experience consists of 58 brachial vein transpositions, most of which were completed in two stages. Primary and secondary patency rates were 52% and 92% at 12 months, respectively.[10]

Anesthesia and Patient Positioning

Initial creation of an arteriovenous anastomosis is performed under local anesthesia. In the second stage, local sedation can be used in select cases of mobilization and transposition of the vein; however, a regional interscalene block or general anesthesia is preferred. For both stages, the patient is positioned at the table edge with the upper extremity abducted to 90 degrees and centered on an arm board.

Stage 1: Creation of the Arteriovenous Anastomosis

A longitudinal incision over the brachial pulse in the antecubital fossa exposes both the brachial artery and the brachial vein. Where multiple veins are present, the largest is used for the arteriovenous anastomosis. The vein is ligated distally and divided. The proximal vein is gently dilated hydrostatically with heparinized saline. Use of the most proximal radial artery, rather than the brachial artery, may reduce the risk of steal syndrome. An end-to-side vein to artery anastomosis is performed using a running 6-0 polypropylene suture (Fig. 66-1).

Stage 2: Mobilization and Transposition of the Arterialized Vein

The second stage is performed 4 to 6 weeks later to allow the vein wall to arterialize and facilitate its mobilization. A longitudinal incision is made over the course of the brachial artery and vein in the upper arm. This incision is extended proximally several centimeters at a time, while sequentially exposing the anterior surface of the vein from the antecubital fossa to the axilla. Mobilization of the

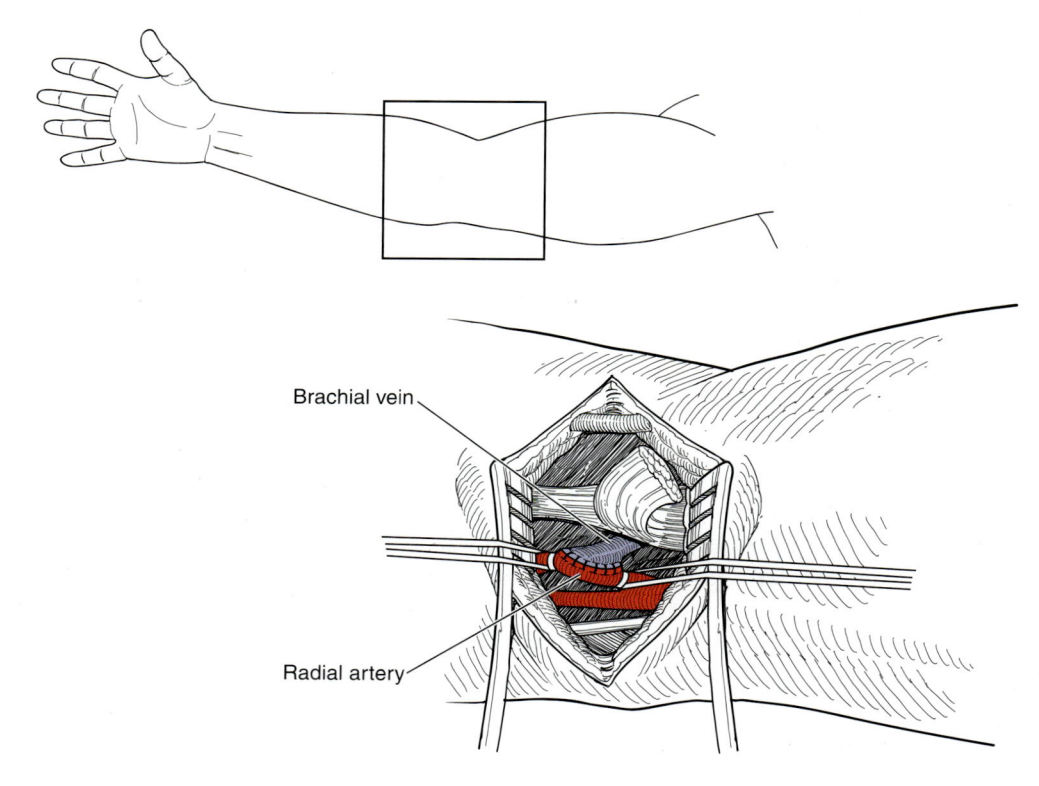

Figure 66-1. Brachial vein transposition, stage 1. The brachial artery and vein are exposed near the antecubital fossa. If multiple brachial veins are present, the largest should be selected for anastomosis to either the brachial or the radial artery.

vein can be challenging and requires patience. The medial antebrachial cutaneous and median nerves are adjacent to the vein and must be protected from injury. Because the vein can be adherent to the adjacent brachial artery, it can be easily torn during mobilization (Fig. 66-2). Venous tributaries are individually ligated with 4-0 silk sutures, and short, broad tributaries are oversewn with 7-0 polypropylene. The anterior surface of the vein is marked to prevent twisting during transposition.

A number of techniques for transposing the vein have been described. If the length of mobilized vein is adequate, it may be passed through a separate subcutaneous tunnel using a tunneling device, previously placed lateral to the upper arm incision from antecubital fossa to axilla. The vein is divided near the arteriovenous anastomosis, passed through the subcutaneous tunnel, taking care to prevent twisting or kinking, and an end-to-side anastomosis of the vein is performed using 6-0 polypropylene (Fig. 66-3, *A*). If the vein is too short to be transposed through a separate subcutaneous tunnel, it can be elevated by closing the subcutaneous tissue beneath it with interrupted 3-0 absorbable suture. The skin is closed over the fistula with running 4-0 absorbable suture (Fig. 66-3, *B*). Alternatively, a subcutaneous flap, about 3 mm below the skin incision, can be created for the placement of the vein away from the overlying incision. The arteriovenous access can be cannulated once the skin incision has completely healed, usually 3 weeks after the second-stage procedure. If the fistula is located directly beneath the skin incision, dialysis personnel are instructed to cannulate the fistula through the overlying scar.

SAPHENOUS VEIN TRANSPOSITION

Outcomes after saphenous vein transposition are limited to small case series. Early failure has been reported in about 25% of cases, with secondary patency of 80% at 1 year.[11-13]

Anesthesia and Patient Positioning

Saphenous vein transposition is performed under general or regional anesthesia. With the patient in a supine position, a roll is used to externally rotate the knee and thigh to expose the greater saphenous vein.

Exposure and Mobilization of the Saphenous Vein

The proximal superficial femoral artery and saphenofemoral junction are approached through a single longitudinal groin incision over the femoral pulse. The saphenous vein is exposed using skip incisions from groin to knee. Tributaries of the vein are divided and ligated with 4-0 silk, and the vein is mobilized from the saphenofemoral junction to the knee. Alternatively, using endoscopic vein harvest equipment, the saphenous vein can be mobilized through a single small incision.

Figure 66-2. Brachial vein transposition, stage 2. The brachial vein in the upper arm is exposed and mobilized. The medial antebrachial cutaneous and median nerves should be protected from injury. Small venous tributaries are ligated with silk suture. Short, broad venous tributaries are oversewn with 7-0 polypropylene suture.

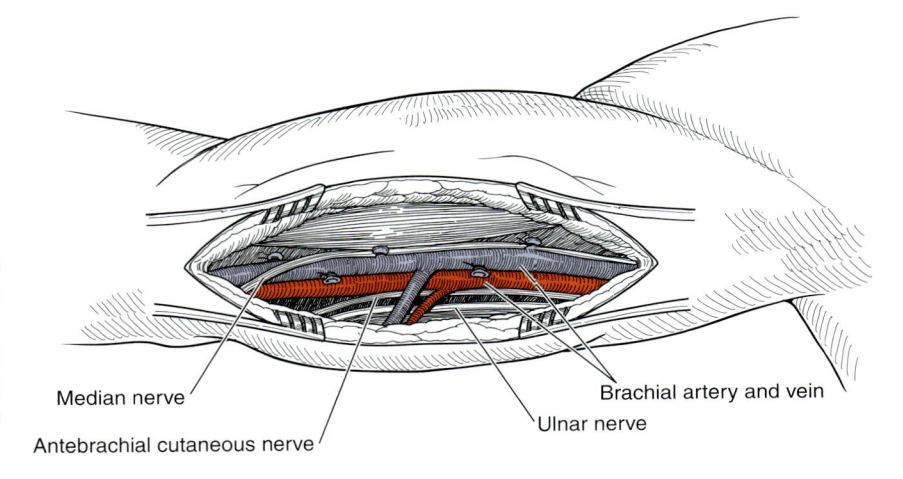

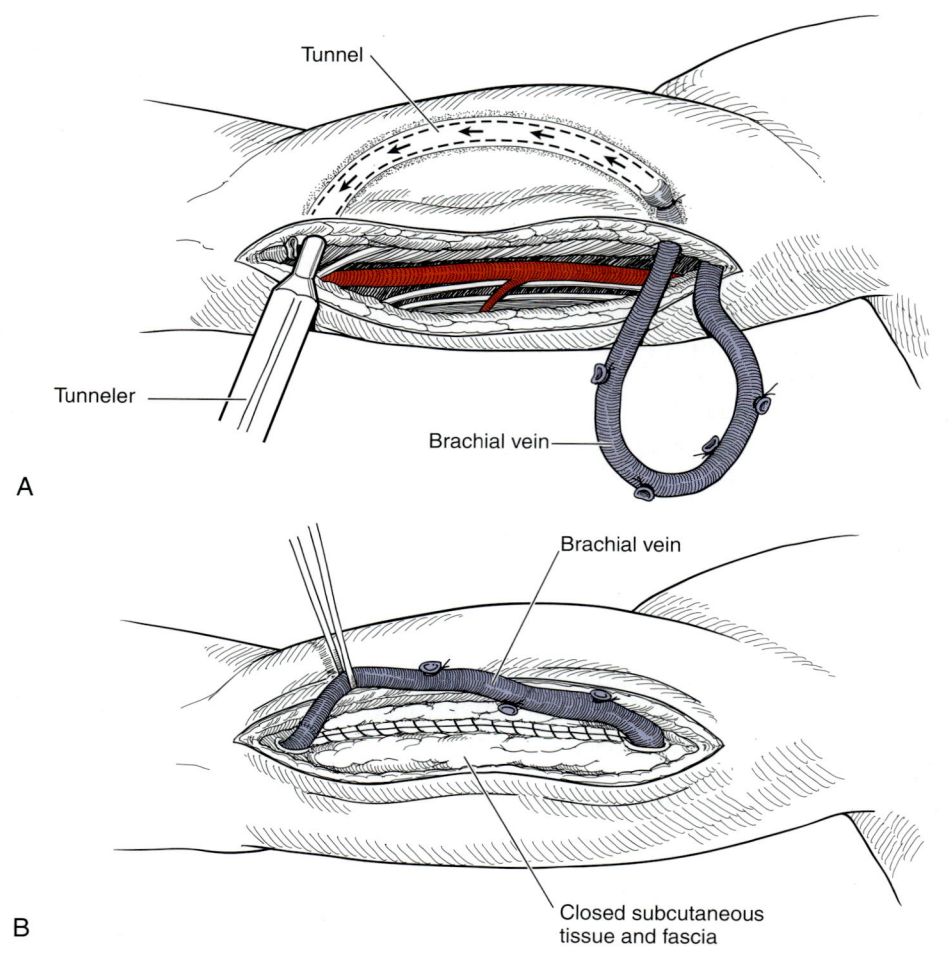

Figure 66-3. Brachial vein transposition: Tunneling techniques. **A,** The preferred transposition technique is to bring the fistula through a subcutaneous tunnel over the ventral aspect of the upper arm. To accomplish this, the fistula is divided near the arteriovenous anastomosis. Using a tunneling device, the vein is passed through a subcutaneous tunnel lateral to the upper arm incision and reanastomosed to the proximal end of the fistula. **B,** If the fistula is too short to be transposed through a separate subcutaneous tunnel, it can be simply elevated by closing the fascia and subcutaneous tissue of the wound beneath it with 3-0 absorbable suture. The skin is closed over the fistula with a running 4-0 absorbable suture. Postoperatively, dialysis personnel are instructed to cannulate the fistula directly through the overlying scar.

Tunneling the Vein and Constructing the Arteriovenous Anastomosis

The saphenous vein is ligated and transected distally at the knee, with the saphenofemoral junction left intact. The proximal superficial femoral artery is then exposed. Using a tunneling device, a subcutaneous tunnel is created below the dermis along the anterior aspect of the thigh through two separate skin incisions. The saphenous vein is brought through the tunnel in a loop configuration and anastomosed end-to-side to the proximal superficial femoral artery with a running 6-0 polypropylene suture. The anastomosis can be performed to the common femoral artery if the proximal superficial femoral artery is occluded or has significant atherosclerotic occlusive disease. Alternatively, if the superficial femoral artery is normal, the saphenous vein can be tunneled lateral to the medial thigh incision and anastomosed to the distal superficial femoral artery (Fig. 66-4). Likewise, the femoral vein can be mobilized and transposed to create an arteriovenous fistula (Video 66-1).

PROSTHETIC LOWER EXTREMITY VASCULAR ACCESS

Prosthetic arteriovenous access in the lower extremity is associated with secondary patency rates between 68% and 85% at 1 year and 54% and 82% at 2 years. The infection rate for thigh access ranges from 16% to 41% and limb ischemia in 3% of cases.[14-16] Prosthetic loop access originating from the superficial femoral artery and femoral vein in the midthigh have been associated with a risk of infection in one of five patients, which compares favorably with the risk of infection for common femoral arteriovenous grafts.[17,18]

Anesthesia and Patient Positioning

Prosthetic vascular access procedures in the thigh are usually performed with general or regional anesthesia. The patient is placed in the supine position.

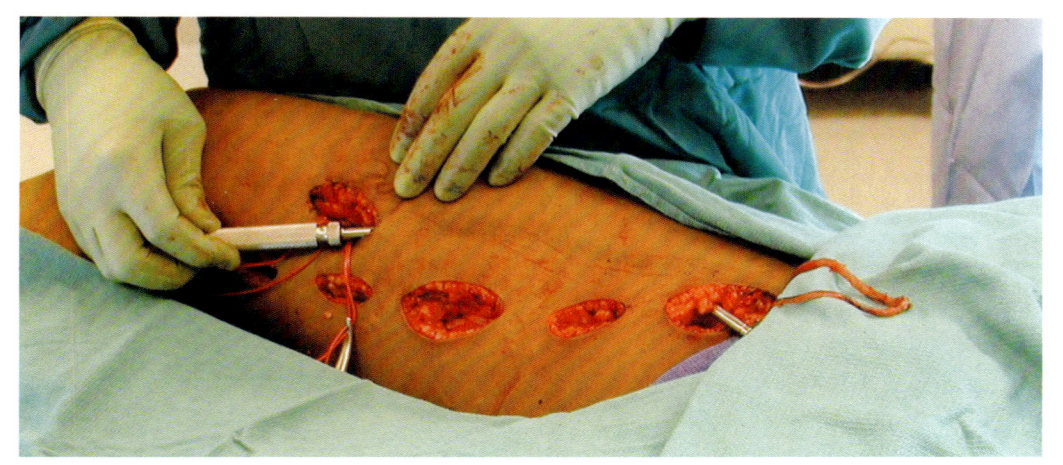

Figure 66-4. Saphenous vein transposition. The saphenous vein is exposed and mobilized from the saphenofemoral junction to the knee using skip incisions. The distal superficial femoral artery is exposed proximal to the adductor hiatus through a separate incision. The vein is transected distally and brought through a subcutaneous tunnel over the anterior thigh to the artery. The photograph shows the vein attached to a tunneling device before passing it through the subcutaneous tunnel. Alternatively, if the superficial femoral artery is diseased, the saphenous vein can be tunneled in a loop configuration over the anterior thigh and anastomosed to the common femoral artery.

Exposure and Technique for Proximal Prosthetic Thigh Access

The femoral artery and great saphenous vein are exposed through a single longitudinal groin incision over the femoral pulse. The proximal superficial femoral artery and great saphenous vein near the saphenofemoral junction are mobilized for a distance of 3 to 4 cm. The superficial femoral artery is the preferred site for arterial inflow, because graft complications, such as arterial steal or graft infection are more easily treated than for grafts using the common femoral artery. However, the common femoral artery should be chosen if occlusive disease is present in the superficial femoral artery. The preferred site for the venous anastomosis is the saphenous vein. Alternatively, the femoral or common femoral vein can be used, as dictated by venous anatomy. A counterincision is necessary to place the graft in the loop configuration. A wide loop is created to obviate graft kinking. Usually the arterial limb is oriented laterally and the venous limb is oriented medially. Although some prefer an 8-mm polytetrafluoroethylene (PTFE) graft for thigh arteriovenous access, a 6-mm graft minimizes the risk of steal syndrome (Fig. 66-5). The graft should not be cannulated for 4 to 6 weeks after placement. If an option for temporary access is not available, an early-stick prosthesis may be considered.

Exposure and Technique for Midthigh Prosthetic Access

Exposure of the superficial femoral artery and femoral vein is gained via an incision along the medial border of the sartorius muscle in the midthigh. The muscle is then retracted laterally to expose the femoral vessels (Fig. 66-6, A). The superficial femoral artery and femoral vein are mobilized and encircled with vessel loops. The prosthetic graft is tunneled subcutaneously over the anterolateral thigh. This location facilitates graft cannulation without the patient having to externally rotate the leg. In most cases the venous limb of the graft is located medially and the arterial limb is located laterally. When the superficial femoral artery lies beneath the lateral edge of the sartorius muscle, the muscle border is mobilized and the arterial limb is tunneled lateral to it (Fig. 66-6, B).

PROSTHETIC CHEST WALL VASCULAR ACCESS

In 1996 McCann reported outcomes for 26 patients with prosthetic chest wall access. A straight graft configuration from the axillary artery to the contralateral axillary or internal jugular vein was used. Secondary patency was 60% at 2 years.[19] Two small series have also reported use of a prosthetic axillary-axillary loop access using the ipsilateral axillary artery and vein. Secondary patency at 2 years ranged

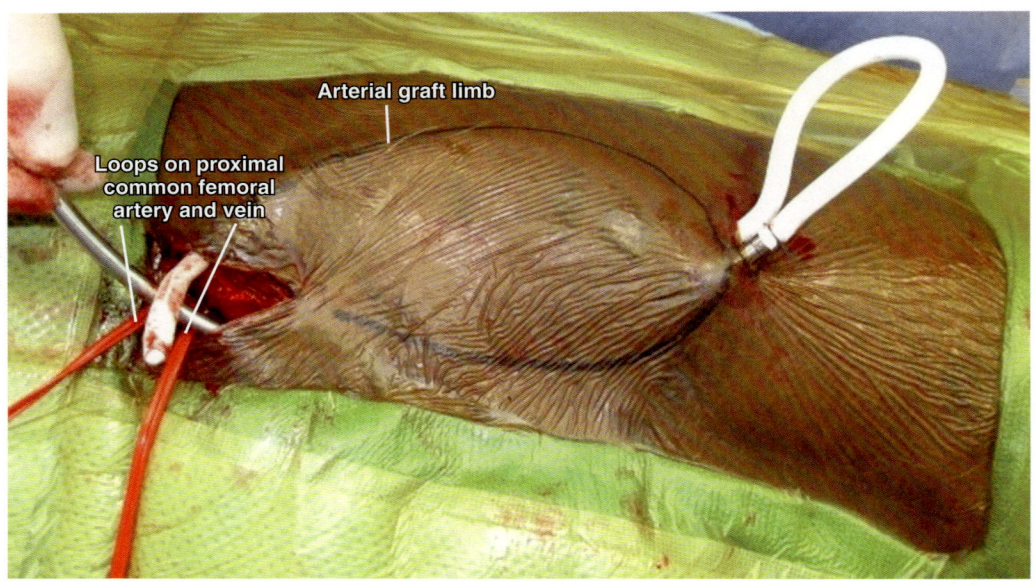

Figure 66-5. Prosthetic proximal thigh loop access. A single longitudinal groin incision is used to expose the femoral vessels. The proximal superficial femoral artery and great saphenous vein near the saphenofemoral junction are the preferred sites for the arteriovenous anastomoses. In this case there is extensive scarring of those vessels because of previous arteriovenous access procedures in the groin; therefore the proximal common femoral artery and vein were used for the anastomoses. A counterincision is used to pass a 6-mm graft in a loop configuration over the anterior thigh. A wide loop is created to prevent the graft from kinking. Generally, the arterial limb is oriented laterally and the venous limb is oriented medially on the thigh.

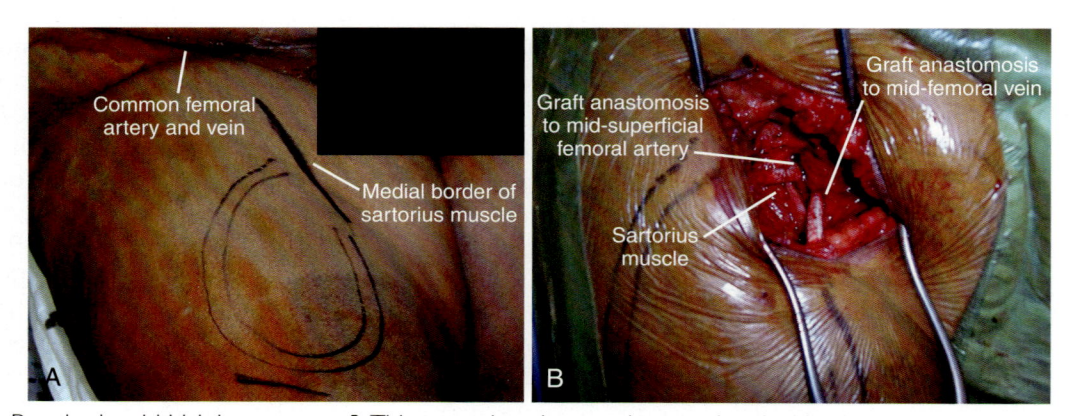

Figure 66-6. Prosthetic midthigh loop access. **A,** This access location may be associated with a lower infection rate, because it avoids the node-bearing tissue and the panniculus that overlies the common femoral artery and vein. It also preserves the proximal femoral vessels for future access placement. **B,** An incision is made along the medial border of the sartorius muscle in the midthigh. This muscle is retracted laterally to expose the superficial femoral artery and femoral vein. When the superficial femoral artery lies beneath the lateral border of the sartorius muscle, the lateral edge of the muscle is mobilized and the arterial limb is tunneled lateral to it.

between 37% and 80%.[20] Infection rates for prosthetic chest wall access range from 4% to 15%. Infection and patency rates do not appear to differ between obese and nonobese patients.[19-21]

Anesthesia and Patient Positioning

The procedure is performed using general anesthesia, with the patient placed supine and the arm extended 90 degrees on an arm board.

Technique for Prosthetic Axillary-Axillary Loop Arteriovenous Access

An incision is made one fingerbreadth below the clavicle from the sternoclavicular joint to the coracoid process. The pectoralis major muscle fibers are split. The clavipectoral fascia is divided, and the exposed axillary vein is mobilized for a distance of 5 to 6 cm. It may be necessary to ligate and divide several venous tributaries, as well as part of the pectoralis minor muscle. A fascial layer beneath

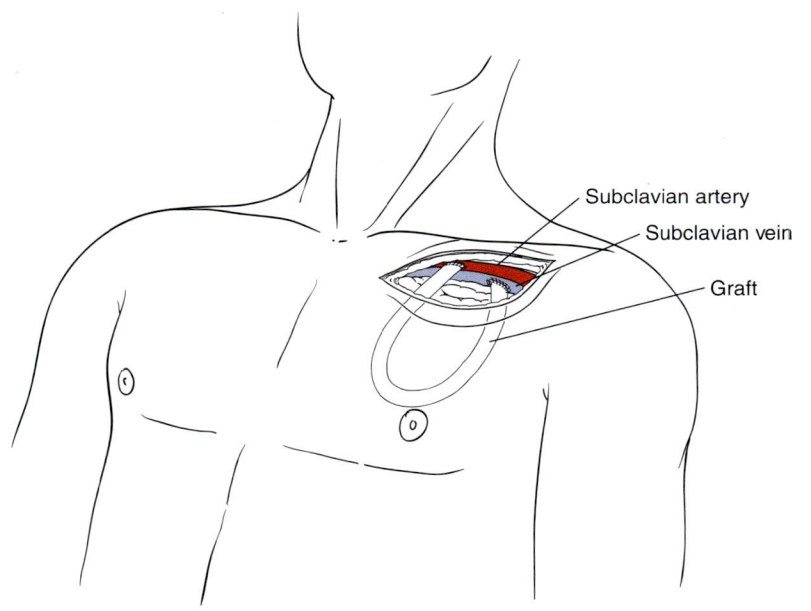

Figure 66-7. Prosthetic axillary-axillary loop access. An incision is made one fingerbreadth below the clavicle from the sternoclavicular joint to the coracoid process. The pectoralis major muscle fibers are split, and the clavipectoral fascia is incised to expose and mobilize the axillary vein. The fascial layer beneath the axillary vein is divided to expose the axillary artery. A 6-mm PTFE graft is tunneled in a looped configuration on the chest wall. The venous limb of the graft is positioned laterally on the chest and is oriented centrally and parallel to the axillary vein. This positioning facilitates percutaneous endovascular intervention of the graft should it thrombose because of the development of a venous outflow stenosis. End-to-side anastomoses are performed between the graft and the artery and vein. (From Kendall TW, Cull DL, Carsten CG, et al: The prosthetic axillo-axillary loop access: Indications, technique, and outcomes, J Vasc Surg 48:389-393, 2008.)

the axillary vein separates the vein from the axillary artery. The axillary artery is often not readily palpable until this fascial layer has been divided and the artery is then mobilized for 3 to 4 cm. Branches of the axillary artery, such as the supreme thoracic artery, may need to be ligated and divided. A counterincision placed cephalad to the breast areola is used to tunnel a 6-mm PTFE graft in a loop configuration on the chest wall. Before tunneling, the patient is tilted into a reverse Trendelenburg position to place the breast in a dependent location. This maneuver allows more accurate confirmation of graft length and is particularly useful in females with pendulous breasts.

The venous limb of the graft is positioned laterally on the chest. The venous end of the graft is oriented nearly parallel to the axillary vein and is directed centrally. This arrangement facilitates percutaneous endovascular intervention of the graft should it clot as a result venous outflow stenosis. The arterial end of the graft is placed perpendicular to the axillary artery. The graft is sewn end-to-side to the axillary artery and vein. The access can be cannulated 2 to 3 weeks postoperatively (Fig. 66-7).

Technique for Prosthetic Axillary-Axillary Straight (Necklace) Access

The patient is placed supine with both upper extremities extended 90 degrees on arm boards. The axillary artery and contralateral axillary vein are exposed, as described earlier. The graft is tunneled subcutaneously across the upper chest over the sternum and anastomosed end to side to the artery and contralateral vein.

COMPLEX CATHETER-BASED VASCULAR ACCESS

Tunneled dialysis catheters are used as a bridge until maturation of an autogenous or prosthetic vascular access or when all other options for vascular access have been exhausted. Compared with other access procedures, tunneled dialysis catheters provide less effective dialysis and are attended by a higher risk of infection, thus leading to increased morbidity, mortality, and hospitalization. The most

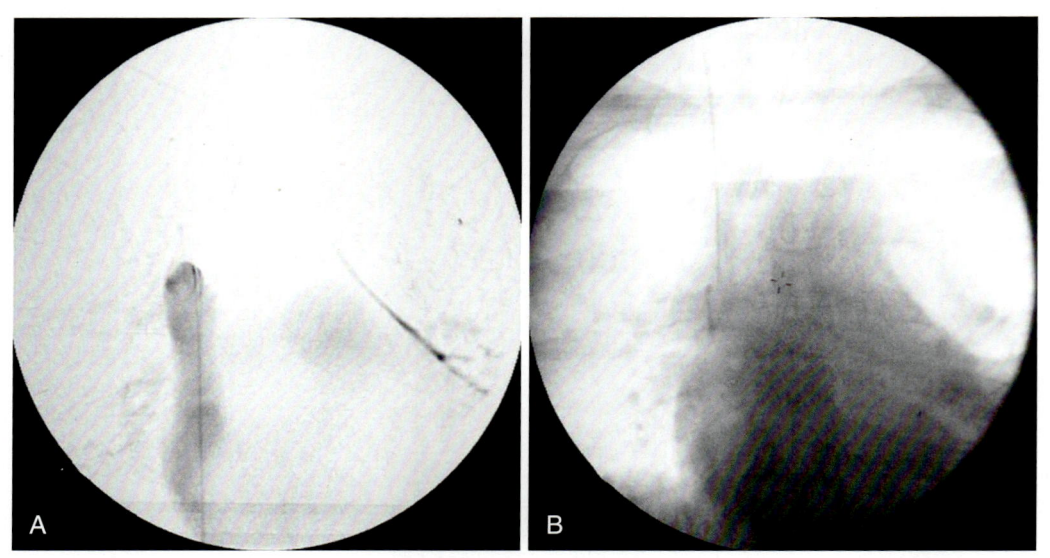

Figure 66-8. Transthoracic cuffed dialysis catheter placement. Via access from the femoral vein, a pigtail catheter is placed in the stump of the superior vena cava. An 18-Ga, 2.75-inch introducer needle is inserted into the skin at a point immediately cephalad to the head of the right clavicle. Using the anteroposterior (**A**) and lateral (**B**) fluoroscopic views of the pigtail catheter as guides to its location, the needle is advanced toward the superior vena cava. *(From Wellons ED, Matsuura J, Lai KM, et al: Transthoracic cuffed hemodialysis catheters: A method for difficult hemodialysis access, J Vasc Surg 42:286-289, 2005.)*

common veins chosen for tunneled dialysis catheter placement are the internal jugular and subclavian veins. However, these vessels may be stenosed or occluded in patients who have had multiple upper extremity vascular access procedures or central venous catheters. Alternative sites for tunneled dialysis catheter include transfemoral, translumbar, and transhepatic placement. Unfortunately, these are associated with a high incidence of infection, catheter malfunction, and dislodgement. A transthoracic tunneled cuffed dialysis catheter and the HERO vascular access device are two options in selected patients.

Transthoracic Cuffed Dialysis Catheter Placement

The transthoracic placement of a tunneled dialysis catheter involves percutaneously cannulating the superior vena cava directly from the neck. Wellons and colleagues have reported a 10% early complication rate, including pneumothorax and hemothorax, in a series of 22 patients.[22]

Superior vena cava imaging and cannulation are performed in an angiography suite or in the operating room using standard fluoroscopic equipment with the patient in a supine position. A pigtail catheter is placed in the superior vena cava via access from the femoral vein. Anteroposterior and lateral venograms of the superior vena cava are obtained to define anatomy and to determine the length of the superior vena cava stump. The pigtail catheter is positioned at the end of the superior vena cava stump. The right supraclavicular area is anesthetized with a local agent. An 18-Ga, 2.75-inch introducer needle is inserted into the skin at a point immediately cephalad to the head of the right clavicle. Using the anteroposterior and lateral fluoroscopic views of the pigtail catheter as guides to its location, the needle is advanced toward the superior vena cava (Fig. 66-8). In obese patients a 3.5-inch spinal needle may be required to reach the superior vena cava. Once the superior vena cava has been entered, a hydrophilic wire is inserted and passed into the inferior vena cava. To aid passage of the wire, it may be necessary to insert a snare from the groin to pull the wire into the inferior vena cava. After successful wire placement, a 5-Fr sheath is placed, and an exchange catheter is used to change the hydrophilic wire to a superstiff wire and thus allow tracking of large dilators into the superior vena cava. Once a tract to the superior vena cava has been dilated, a cuffed dialysis catheter is inserted.

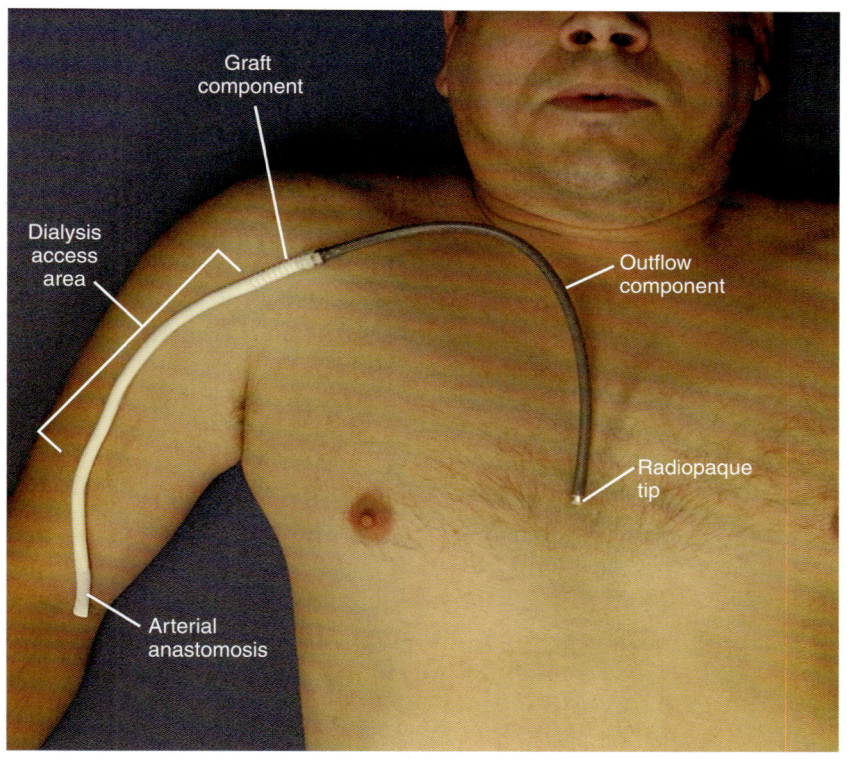

Figure 66-9. HERO vascular access device placement. The silicone catheter component of the HERO device is placed into the central veins using a similar technique to that of placing a cuffed dialysis catheter, with the exception that to facilitate passage of the catheter, it may be necessary to dilate the tract with an over-the-wire angioplasty balloon. A tunneling device is used to pass the silicone catheter from the neck incision to the counterincision at the deltopectoral groove. An end-to-side anastomosis between the graft component and the distal brachial artery is performed, and the graft is tunneled retrograde to the incision at the deltopectoral groove. Silicone catheter and graft components are connected using the titanium connector. *(From Katzman HE, McLafferty RB, Ross JR, et al: Initial experience and outcome of a new hemodialysis access device for catheter-dependent patients, J Vasc Surg 50:600-607, 2009.)*

Hemodialysis Reliable Outflow Vascular Access Device Placement

The HERO device may be used as an alternative to a tunneled dialysis catheter and consists of a standard PTFE graft implanted subcutaneously in the upper arm and anastomosed to the brachial artery. A 19-Fr silicone catheter is then percutaneously placed into the right atrium. The two components are joined through a titanium connector via a counterincision in the deltopectoral groove. The graft component is used for dialysis access (Fig. 66-9).

A multicenter study has reported bacteremia rates (0.70/1000 days) that were lower than rates in a metaanalysis of tunneled dialysis catheters (2.3/1000 days). The secondary patency for the HERO device is 72% at 8 months, with an average of 2.5 interventions each year to maintain patency.[7]

Anesthesia and Patient Positioning

The HERO device can be implanted with local anesthesia and sedation or under general anesthesia. The patient is placed in the supine position, and the upper extremity is extended 90 degrees on an arm board. The head is turned away from the side through which the HERO device is to be implanted.

Placement of the Graft Component

An incision is made over the brachial pulse in the distal upper arm. The brachial artery is dissected free from adjacent tissues. A counterincision for connecting the graft and catheter components is then made in the deltopectoral groove. Using a tunneling device, the graft component of the HERO device is brought through a subcutaneous tunnel from the exposed brachial artery into the counterincision.

Placement of the Silicone Catheter Component

If the silicone catheter of the HERO device is passed through the tract of an existing tunneled dialysis catheter in the internal jugular vein, a cutdown should be made in the neck over the tunneled catheter. The tunneled dialysis catheter is transected, and a stiff guidewire is inserted through the distal end of the catheter under fluoroscopic guidance. Both sections of the transected dialysis catheter are removed from the field. To enable passage of the introducer sheath and silicone catheter through the established tract, it is necessary to dilate the tract. A dilator and introducer sheath are inserted over the guidewire. The dilator and guidewire are removed, and the silicone catheter is inserted down the sheath. Fluoroscopy is used to ensure correct positioning of the catheter tip in the right atrium. A tunneling device is used to pass the silicone catheter from the neck incision to the counterincision in the deltopectoral groove.

Constructing the Arterial Anastomosis and Connecting the Components

After systemic heparin has been administered, an end-to-side anastomosis between the graft and the distal brachial artery is performed. Clamps are released briefly to flush air and thrombus from the graft. The graft and catheter are trimmed to the appropriate length at the incision in the deltopectoral groove and are connected using the titanium connector. Clamps are removed, and flow is established through the graft. A thrill should be palpable over the graft component of the access.

Postoperative Care

- **Postoperative course.** Patients are observed overnight for bleeding and steal syndrome.
- **Communication with the dialysis center.** Close communication with the dialysis center is essential, including operative drawings and illustrations on the patient's skin that are used to indicate access location and direction of blood flow.
- **Follow-up evaluation.** Patients should be seen within 2 weeks to assess patency, soft-tissue edema, and healing incision, and to remove sutures. If the thrill is weak, a pulsatile mass is noted, or significant limb edema is present, a fistulagram should be obtained.
- **Timing for access cannulation.** PTFE grafts should not be cannulated until 2 or 3 weeks after placement. Polyurethane early-stick grafts can be cannulated immediately if necessary. An autogenous access should not be cannulated earlier than 6 weeks after creation.

Complications

- **Complications.** Thrombosis, infection, and steal syndrome are the most common complications of unconventional vascular access procedures.
- **Salvage of the failing access graft.** Unconventional vascular access is often placed in patients who have limited access options, and a fallback strategy should be developed if the access fails. In addition, every effort should be made to preserve a functioning unconventional vascular access rather than to relegate the patient to a cuffed dialysis catheter. For example, rather than excising the entire access graft for treatment of a localized infection, salvage can be attempted by partial graft excision and bypass.[23]

REFERENCES

1. Chinitz JL, Tokoyama T, Bower R, Swartz C: Self-sealing prosthesis for arteriovenous fistula in man, *Trans Am Soc Artif Intern Organs* 18:452-457, 1972.
2. May J, Tiller D, Johnson J, Stewart J, Sheil AGR: Saphenous vein arteriovenous fistula in regular dialysis treatment, *N Engl J Med* 280:770, 1969.

3. Baker LD Jr, Johnson JM, Goldfarb D: Expanded polytetrafluoroethylene (PTFE) subcutaneous arteriovenous conduit: An improved vascular access for chronic hemodialysis, *Trans Am Soc Artif Intern Organs* 22:382-387, 1976.
4. Ono K, Muto Y, Yano K, Yukizane T: Anterior chest wall axillary artery to contralateral axillary vein graft for vascular access in hemodialysis, *Artif Organs* 19:1233-1236, 1995.
5. Salgado OJ, Teran NA, Garcia R, et al: Subcutaneous transposition of arterialized upper arm veins for hemodialysis angioaccess: Optimal alternative to grafts, *Vasc Surg* 32:81-85, 1998.
6. Gorski TF, Nguyen HQ, Gorski YC, et al: Lower-extremity saphenous vein transposition arteriovenous fistula: An alternative for hemodialysis access in AIDS patients, *Am Surgeon* 64:338-340, 1998.
7. Katzman HE, McLafferty RB, Ross JR, et al: Initial experience and outcome of a new hemodialysis access device for catheter-dependent patients, *J Vasc Surg* 50:600-607, 2009.
8. Quinn SF, Schuman ES, Demlow TA, et al: Percutaneous transluminal angioplasty versus endovascular stent placement in the treatment of venous stenoses in patients undergoing hemodialysis: Intermediate results, *J Vasc Interv Radiol* 6:851-855, 1995.
9. Bronder CM, Cull DL, Kuper SG, et al: The fistula elevation procedure: Experience with 295 consecutive cases over a seven year period, *J Am Coll Surg* 206:1076-1081, 2008.
10. Jennings WC, Sideman MJ, Taubman KE, et al: Brachial vein transposition arteriovenous fistulas for hemodialysis access, *J Vasc Surg* 50:1121-1126, 2009.
11. Pierre-Paul D, Williams S, Lee T, et al: Saphenous vein loop to femoral artery arteriovenous fistula: A practical alternative, *Ann Vasc Surg* 18:223-227, 2004.
12. Gorski TF, Nguyen HQ, Gorski YC, et al: Lower-extremity saphenous vein transposition arteriovenous fistula: An alternative for hemodialysis access in AIDS patients, *Am Surg* 64:338-340, 1998.
13. Illig KA, Orloff M, Lyden SP, et al: Transposed saphenous vein arteriovenous fistula revisited: New technology for an old idea, *Cardiovasc Surg* 10:212-215, 2002.
14. Cull JD, Cull DL, Taylor SM, et al: Prosthetic thigh arteriovenous access: Outcome with SVS/AAVS reporting standards, *J Vasc Surg* 39:381-386, 2004.
15. Bhandari S, Wilkinson A, Sellars L: Saphenous vein forearm grafts and Goretex thigh grafts as alternative forms of vascular access, *Clin Nephrol* 44:325-328, 1995.
16. Khadra MH, Dwyer AJ, Thompson JF: Advantages of polytetrafluoroethylene arteriovenous loops in the thigh for hemodialysis access, *Am J Surg* 173:280-233, 1997.
17. Flarup S, Hadimeri H: Arteriovenous PTFE dialysis access in the lower extremity: A new approach, *Ann Vasc Surg* 17:581-584, 2003.
18. Scott JD, Cull DL, Kalbaugh CA, et al: The mid-thigh loop arteriovenous graft: Patient selection, technique, and results, *Am Surg* 72:825-828, 2006.
19. McCann RL: Axillary grafts for difficult hemodialysis access, *J Vasc Surg* 24:457-462, 1996.
20. Kendall TW, Cull DL, Carsten CG, et al: The prosthetic axillo-axillary loop access: Indications, technique, and outcomes, *J Vasc Surg* 48:389-393, 2008.
21. Jean-Baptiste E, Hassen-Khodja R, Haudebourg P, et al: Axillary loop grafts for hemodialysis access: Midterm results from a single-center study, *J Vasc Surg* 47:138-143, 2008.
22. Wellons ED, Matsuura J, Lai KM, et al: Transthoracic cuffed hemodialysis catheters: A method for difficult hemodialysis access, *J Vasc Surg* 42:286-289, 2005.
23. Schwab DP, Taylor SM, Cull DL, et al: Isolated arteriovenous dialysis access graft segment infection: The results of segmental bypass and partial graft excision, *Ann Vasc Surg* 14:63-66, 2000.

67 Distal Revascularization Interval Ligation Procedure

LINDA M. HARRIS • HASAN H. DOSLUOGLU

Historical Background

The steal phenomenon was first described in 1969 by Storey and associates after creation of a Brescia-Cimino-Appel autogenous access.[1] Steal can be a potentially limb-threatening event and must be promptly evaluated and treated if clinically significant. The goals for treating steal syndrome are twofold: restoration of antegrade flow sufficient to maintain distal perfusion and maintenance of the access for dialysis. Steal is seen more commonly after graft placement rather than after autogenous access creation, and typically occurs soon after access creation, but has been reported months to years later in up to 25% of cases.[2,3] The incidence of clinically significant steal may range from 1% for an autogenous arteriovenous (AV) fistula placed in the distal forearm to as high as 9% for prosthetic grafts.[4-8] The brachial artery is the most frequently involved inflow vessel in cases of steal syndrome. High-flow–induced steal syndrome in the absence of a proximal stenosis and with normal outflow vessels requires a reduction in fistula blood flow to eliminate steal symptoms. Options for intervention include access ligation, banding, relocation of the arterial anastomosis to a more proximal artery, revision using distal inflow (RUDI),[9] and the distal revascularization interval ligation (DRIL) procedure.[3,10] DRIL has been recommended as the standard of care by a number of surgeons, because it maintains arteriovenous access while maintaining distal limb perfusion.[11]

The DRIL procedure was first described in 1988 by Schanzer and co-workers and subsequently popularized by Berman and colleagues.[2,12] Since that time, several groups have confirmed its success.[7,13] Reported long-term results have been excellent. Schanzer described 14 patients, all of whom had an access originating from the brachial artery and 13 of whom had complete recovery of function, including healing of gangrenous lesions after a DRIL procedure.[3] One-year patency was 81.7% and all bypass grafts remained open. Berman described 21 patients with limb salvage and graft patency of 100% and 94%, respectively, and coined the term DRIL.[2] Knox and co-workers published a series of 55 patients. Ninety percent had substantial or complete resolution of ischemia, and 15 of 20 patients had completely healed digital lesions. Access patency was 83% at 1 year, and 80% of DRIL bypass grafts were patent at 4 years.[13]

Indications

If steal syndrome is suspected, urgent vascular evaluation is necessary. A grading system has been developed as a measure of the degree of steal syndrome and to guide intervention. Intervention may be necessary for grade 2 steal (intermittent ischemia during dialysis) but is mandatory for grade 3 steal (ischemic rest pain or tissue loss) (Fig. 67-1). Many patients experience mild transient symptoms, which resolve within a few weeks. These patients should be closely monitored, because worsening symptoms may rapidly progress, leading to a permanent disability. Between one half and two thirds of the patients who develop steal do so within

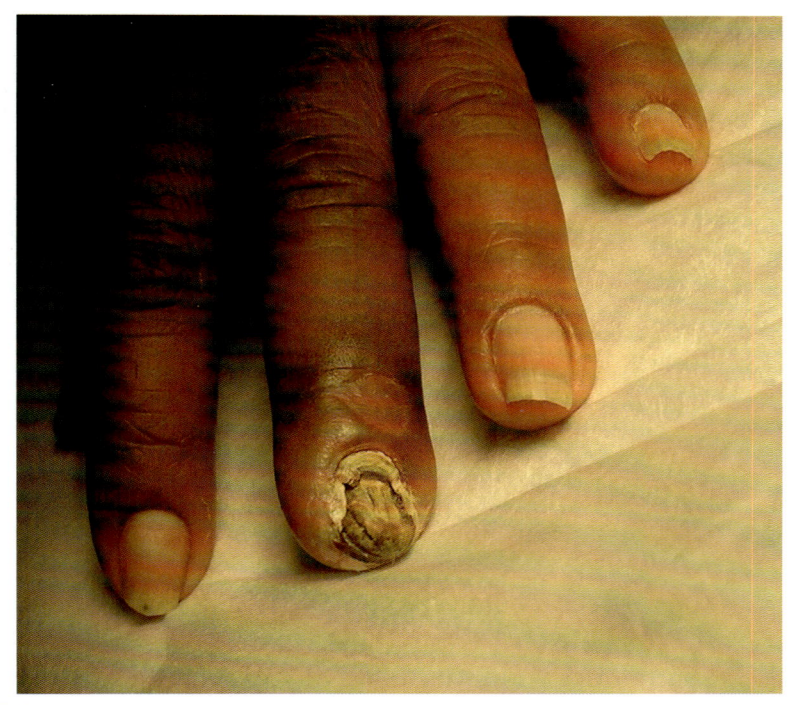

Figure 67-1. Digital gangrene in a patient with a brachiocephalic AV fistula and steal syndrome.

the first 30 days.[2,3] Rest pain or motor impairment immediately after surgery requires immediate reoperation.[14-17] Symptoms such as progressive numbness or pain, pallor, diminished sensation, ischemic ulcers, progressive dry gangrene, and muscle atrophy all demand intervention.[6] Early symptoms are accompanied by gradual tissue loss; however, if ignored, rapid progression leads to necrosis and gangrene of the digits. It is important to differentiate hand ischemia from carpal tunnel syndrome and tissue acidosis, and edema from venous hypertension and monomelic ischemic neuropathy.[15] Symptoms of steal syndrome are frequently exacerbated during dialysis. Although simpler options exist for the treatment of steal syndrome, including banding or ligation, the DRIL procedure maintains access and provides a means to revascularize the hand. Avoidance of dissecting at the site of the previous AV anastomosis is an additional benefit of the DRIL procedure.

Preoperative Preparation

- **Physical examination.** To determine the optimum method of treatment, it is important to identify the etiology of the problem and the flow state of the fistula. Absence of a palpable pulse distal to the arterial anastomosis in the absence of clinical symptoms is not an indication for intervention. However, in symptomatic patients, absence of a pulse, which is corrected by manual compression of the access, is diagnostic for steal syndrome.
- **Digital pulse oximetry.** Tissue oxygen saturation using pulse oximetry is low in the presence of steal and increases with compression of the access to greater than 90%.
- **Duplex ultrasound.** Duplex ultrasound can be used to evaluate distal flow, along with photoplethysmography tracings of digital flow with and without access compression. Duplex venous mapping of the great saphenous vein is recommended to ensure an adequate conduit for the DRIL procedure. If the saphenous vein is inadequate, mapping alternate veins should be undertaken.
- **Angiography.** Preoperative angiography may be used to identify the presence of a proximal arterial lesion, confirm the adequacy of the distal arterial vasculature, and identify a distal target vessel for revascularization. An arterial stenosis

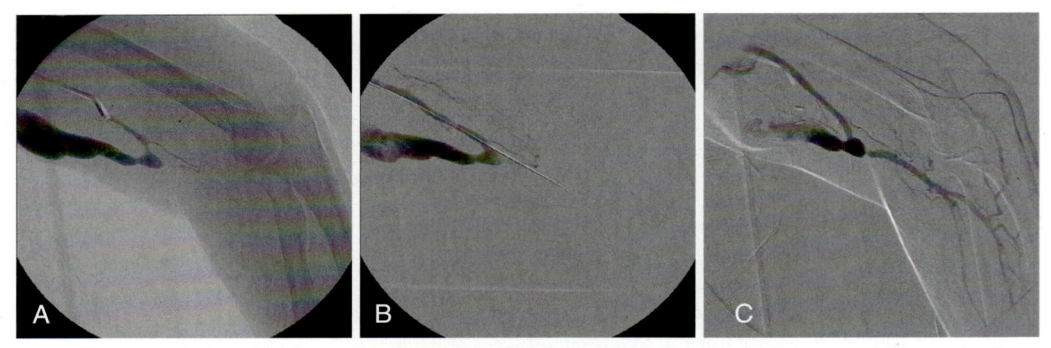

Figure 67-2. **A**, Angiogram of a brachial artery demonstrating flow through the fistula but without distal arterial flow. **B**, An angiogram of the brachial artery with passage of a wire into the radial artery. **C**, Angiography with manual compression of the fistula results in flow into distal vessels.

proximal to the anastomosis, such as a subclavian stenosis, may be treated by angioplasty or stenting[12] (Fig. 67-2, *A-C*).
- **Preprocedural dialysis.** Patients should undergo routine dialysis either the day before or the morning of surgery to optimize electrolytes and fluid status.
- **Antibiotics.** Prophylactic antibiotics are recommended.

Pitfalls and Danger Points

- **Complexity of the intervention.** Compared with banding, ligation, proximalization, or relocation of the anastomosis distally (RUDI), DRIL is a more complex procedure, with limb blood flow dependent on a newly created bypass graft rather than the native arterial system.
- **Inadvertent access of the bypass graft.** If the bypass is not clearly identified, it may be inadvertently accessed for dialysis, leading to further ischemia, aneurysmal degeneration, or graft occlusion.
- **Failure to ligate the brachial artery.** Failure to ligate the brachial artery proximal to the distal anastomosis may lead to persistent steal syndrome from retrograde flow. However, more recent data suggests that the ligation portion of the procedure only contributes about 10% of the flow, and could possibly be avoided in some patients.
- **Location of the proximal DRIL anastomosis.** Placement of the proximal anastomosis too close to the AV anastomosis may lead to failure of the DRIL procedure because of inadequate arterial inflow.

Operative Strategy

TIMING OF THE DRIL PROCEDURE

DRIL should be undertaken urgently once ischemic steal syndrome has been confirmed. Delay may lead to tissue loss or amputation of a digit or a limb. The DRIL procedure affords the best augmentation of flow to the hand of all available revascularization procedures.[7,18]

TYPE OF CONDUIT

Initial descriptions required use of a venous conduit for the bypass, whereas recent reports have shown good success with prosthetic grafts.[2,3]

Operative Technique

CHOICE OF ANESTHESIA

The DRIL procedure is typically performed with general anesthesia, although a regional block may be used.

DISTAL REVASCULARIZATION INTERVAL LIGATION PROCEDURE 775

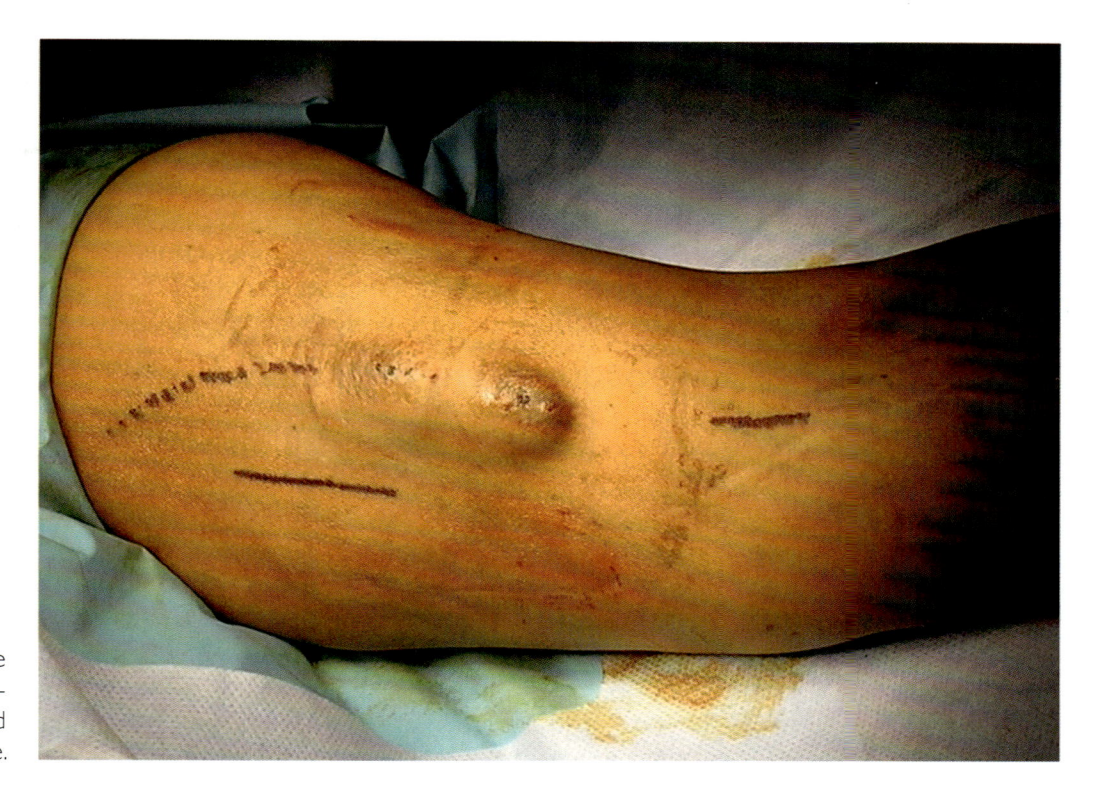

Figure 67-3. Preoperative marking of the autogenous arteriovenous fistula and planned incisions for the DRIL procedure.

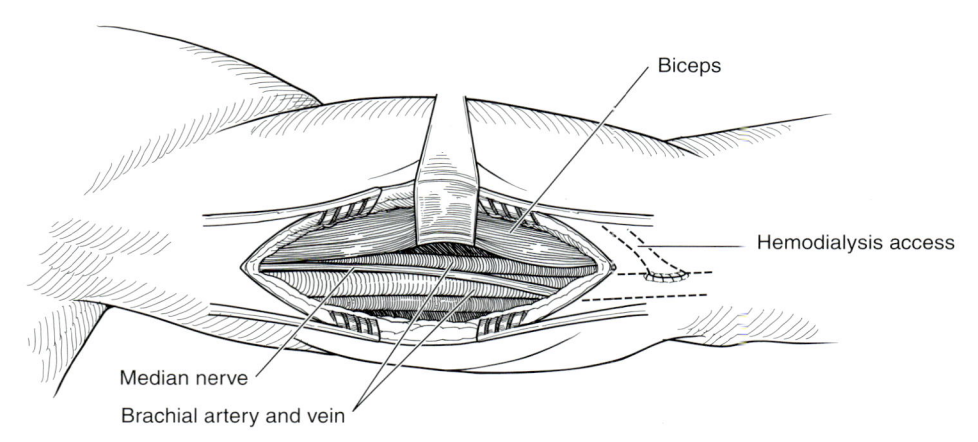

Figure 67-4. Brachial artery in the upper arm at the site of proximal anastomosis for distal revascularization interval ligation.

INCISION

Most frequently, the fistula or graft involves the brachial artery. When using a venous conduit, this is typically harvested from the great saphenous vein in the thigh to allow adequate size and length. Alternately, upper extremity veins, cadaveric veins, or prosthetics can be used. The arm is initially prepped and draped on an arm board in an extended, supinated position. The entire arm to the wrist should be prepped to allow evaluation of the radial and ulnar arteries at the completion of the procedure and to allow adequate proximal arterial access. The hand may also be prepped into the field to allow oxygen saturation monitoring of the digits before and after completion of the DRIL procedure. Marking the path of the arteriovenous conduit is recommended so as to avoid injury to the fistula from the incision or tunneling (Fig. 67-3). The proximal incision is made in the upper arm along the sulcus, separating the biceps and the triceps muscles, above the level of the existing arterial anastomosis.

DISSECTION OF THE INFLOW VESSEL

The brachial aponeurosis is opened, and the biceps muscle is retracted laterally to facilitate vision of the neurovascular bundle. The neurovascular sheath is opened (Fig. 67-4). Care should be taken not to injure the median nerve, which crosses the artery in the midarm, and the nearby median cutaneous nerve. The paired brachial veins are identified but are not dissected entirely free from the artery. The artery is dissected free from the surrounding veins proximally and distally to allow placement of vessel loops. Leaving the midsection of the artery adherent to the surrounding veins facilitates splaying of the artery once it is opened. The inflow vessel should be disease free and at least 5 to 7 cm above the arterial anastomosis of the fistula or access graft. This avoids the pressure sink, an area of reduced pressure in the artery just proximal to the autogenous access.[2,3,19] This region exists because the large capacitance of the venous outflow causes the pressure to fall, approximating central venous pressure within 1 cm of the anastomosis.

EXPOSURE OF THE DISTAL VESSEL

The distal longitudinal incision is made in the forearm, below the arterial anastomosis of the fistula or AV graft. The target vessel is often the distal brachial, proximal ulnar, or proximal radial artery, depending on the level of the bifurcation and the dominance of the vessels (Fig. 67-5). The brachial artery typically terminates about 2 cm below the elbow, where it divides into the radial and ulnar arteries. The common interosseous artery usually arises from the ulnar artery, although variants may be seen. The cubital vein may or may not need to be mobilized to allow access to the underlying artery, depending on whether this has been used in the prior access. To access the radial artery, the brachioradialis muscle is retracted laterally, and the artery is visible just beneath the muscle (Fig. 67-6). The proximal ulnar artery can be approached via retraction of the pronator muscle inferomedially. The distal anastomosis should be constructed to the dominant distal outflow vessel, chosen based on the preoperative angiogram. Once the chosen vessel is dissected from the surrounding tissues, vessel loops are again used for hemostatic control. The artery proximal to the planned distal DRIL anastomosis is dissected free, which will be ligated after completion of the bypass.

CONDUIT

The saphenous vein is harvested for sufficient length to complete the bypass. The vein is gently dilated using heparinized saline to test for leaks before creation of the proximal anastomosis. Alternate veins, such as the basilic vein, can be used but are usually avoided to allow future AV access. Alternatively, a prosthetic conduit of polytetrafluoroethylene may be used.

TUNNELING

A tunnel is created between the two incisions. This is typically placed medially and deeper on the arm to avoid confusion with the fistula, which continues to be accessed by the hemodialysis nursing staff. If a prosthetic is used, it is placed through the tunnel at this time. When a vein is used, it is recommended to complete the proximal anastomosis, check again for the integrity of all branch ligatures, and then pass the vein through the tunnel to avoid twists or kinks.

ARTERIOTOMY AND BYPASS

Patients are not typically given heparin before clamping of the brachial artery; rather, they are treated with locally injected heparinized saline into the artery proximally and distally, without systemic anticoagulation. Alternatively, systemic heparin can be given at 100 units per kilogram of body weight. A longitudinal arteriotomy is created in the proximal artery. The anastomosis is completed end to side with 6-0 polypropylene running sutures. The clamps or vessel loops are then released, with a vascular clamp placed distally on the vein graft (Fig. 67-7). The vein is then marked with a pen longitudinally to enable identification of twisting when brought through the tunnel. A tube-type tunneler is preferred when tunneling a venous conduit to decrease the risk of traction on side branch ligatures and branch avulsion. Once the graft has been brought through the tunnel, the clamp is temporarily released to confirm adequate inflow.

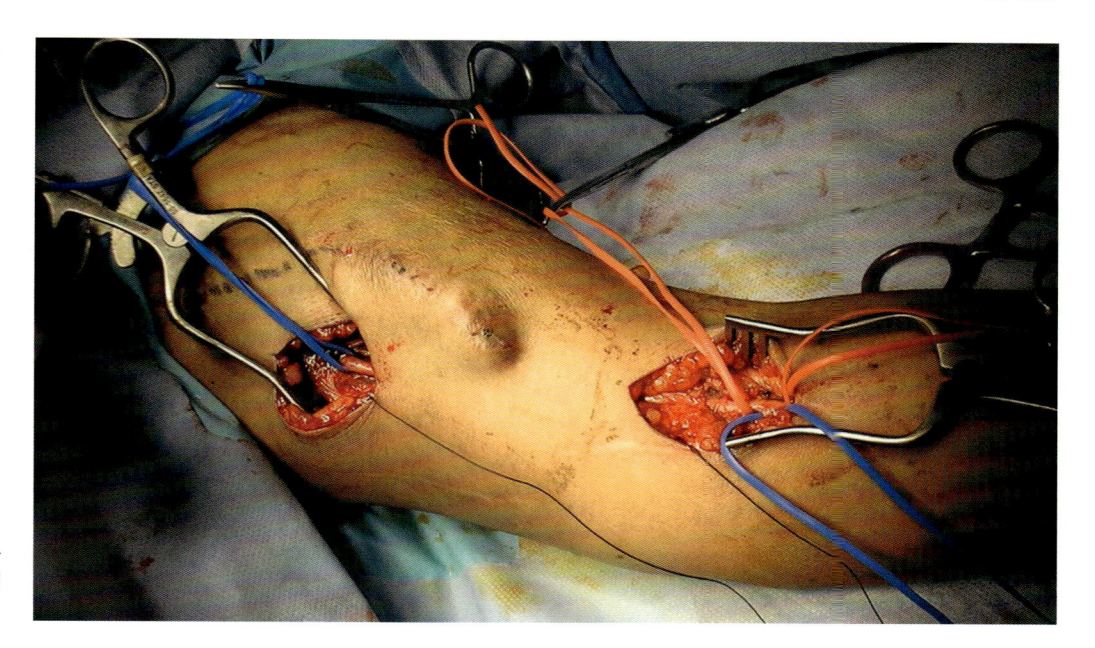

DISTAL REVASCULARIZATION INTERVAL LIGATION PROCEDURE 777

Figure 67-5. Exposed brachial artery and proximal radial artery.

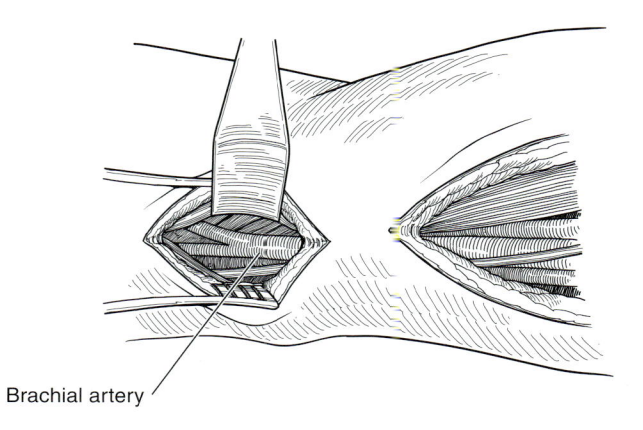

Figure 67-6. The brachial artery bifurcates into the radial and ulnar arteries.

Brachial artery

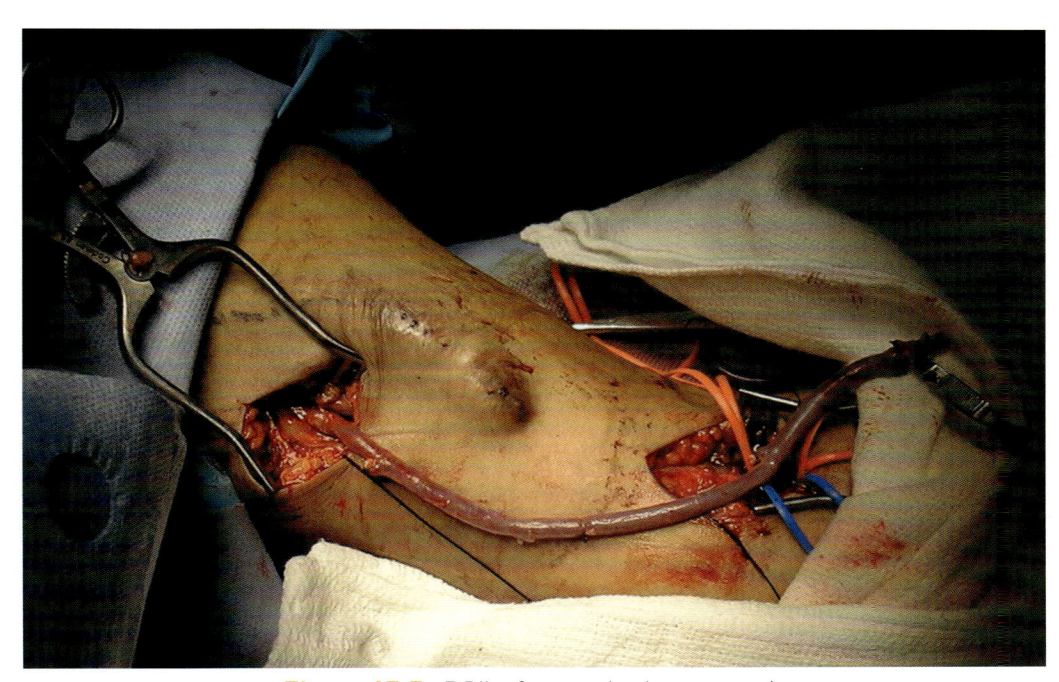

Figure 67-7. DRIL after proximal anastomosis.

778 ARTERIOVENOUS ACCESS FOR HEMODIALYSIS

Attention is then turned to the distal target artery. The artery is controlled with vessel loops or fine vascular clamps. To decrease risk of complications, internal occluders may also be used to prevent suturing of the back wall in the smaller distal vessel. An end-to-side anastomosis is created between the vein graft and the distal brachial artery or the ulnar or radial artery. This functionally is converted to an end-to-end anastomosis with the ligation of the proximal artery (Fig. 67-8). An end-to-end anastomosis can be created if this is technically easier. Before completion, all segments are backbled to remove air from the conduits and to confirm patency.

LIGATION OF THE ARTERY

If arteriotomy and bypass are successful, the artery proximal to the distal DRIL anastomosis is ligated with a 2-0 silk ligature, and the vessel loop or clamp is removed.

CLOSURE

Incisions are closed in at least two layers, with a subcutaneous and a subcuticular closure. The skin should be clearly marked to identify the location of the bypass graft and to distinguish it from the access vessel or graft, which can be used without interruption (Fig. 67-9).

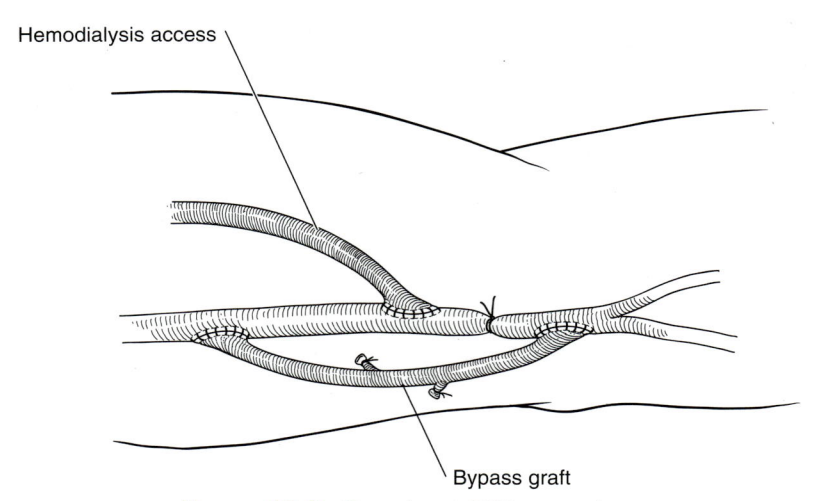

Figure 67-8. Completed DRIL procedure.

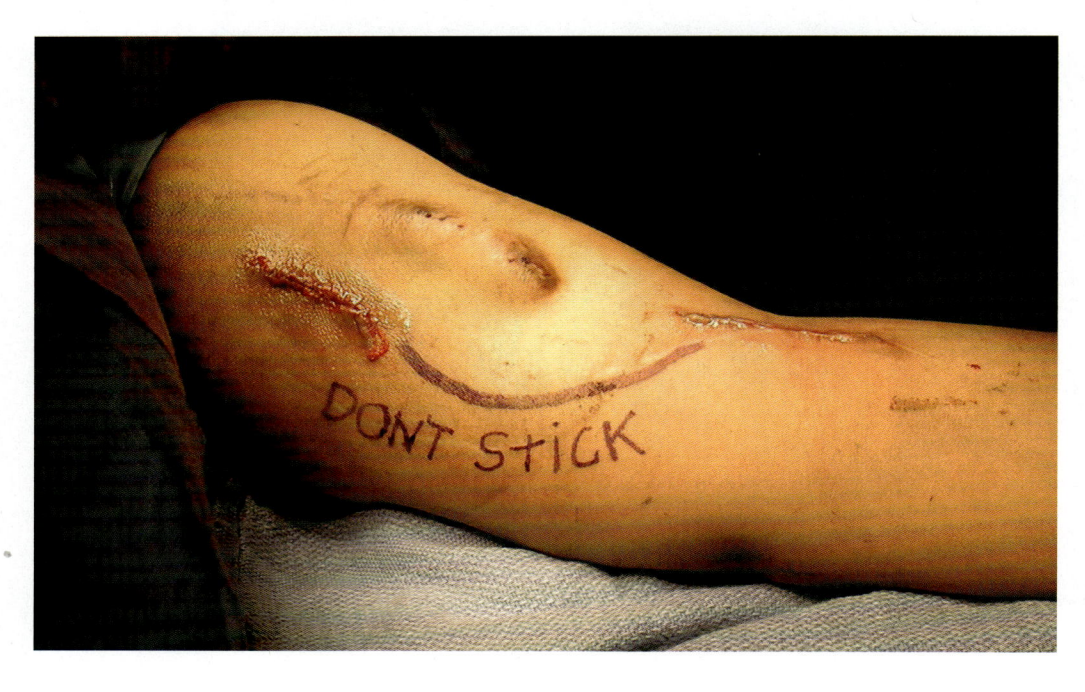

Figure 67-9. Arm after DRIL, marked for the dialysis unit.

Postoperative Care

- **Discharge evaluation and instructions.** The access is evaluated for the presence of a thrill, and the distal radial and ulnar arteries are evaluated for the presence of a palpable pulse before discharge from the hospital. Patients are discharged home the same day, and dry gauze dressings or Dermabond applied. It is important to have the access site for the fistula or graft uncovered to enable continued dialysis. The incisions should be kept dry for at least 2 days to decrease risk of wound infection. Use of the extremity is not restricted.
- **Follow-up evaluation.** The initial office visit is conducted 2 weeks postoperatively. If the patient has tissue loss, this may be treated expectantly, if an ulcer or dry gangrene. More extensive tissue loss may require amputation.

Complications

- **Local wound complications or infection.** Wound complications are uncommon, especially when venous conduits are used.
- **Failure to achieve symptom resolution.** A small percentage of patients fail to heal digital lesions despite a successful DRIL procedure. Partial digit or digit amputation is not uncommon for patients with advanced tissue loss.
- **Patency.** Long-term patency of the DRIL bypass has been reported to range from 67% to 100%, with access preservation ranging from 68% to 100%. With thrombosis of the DRIL bypass, some patients have no recurrent symptoms and do not require reintervention, whereas others may require a secondary DRIL procedure. Overall patient survival in this population is compromised with reports of 33% life expectancy at 5 years in one study[20] and 61% at 16 months in another.[21]

REFERENCES

1. Storey BG, George CR, Stewart JH, et al: Embolic and ischemic complications after anastomosis of radial artery to cephalic vein, *Surgery* 66:325-327, 1969.
2. Berman SS, Gentile AT, Glickman MH, et al: Distal revascularization-interval ligation for limb salvage and maintenance of dialysis access in ischemic steal syndrome, *J Vasc Surg* 26:393-404, 1997.
3. Schanzer H, Skadany M, Haimov M: Treatment of angioaccess-induced ischemia by revascularization, *J Vasc Surg* 16:861-866, 1992.
4. Lewis P, Wolfe JHN: Lymphatic fistula and perigraft seroma, *Br J Surg* 80:410-411, 1993.
5. Schanzer H: Overview of complications and management after vascular access creation. In Gray RJ, editor: *Dialysis access*, Philadelphia, 2002, Lippincott Williams & Wilkins, pp 93-97.
6. Miles AM: Upper limb ischemia after vascular access surgery: Differential diagnosis and management, *Semin Dial* 13:312-315, 2000.
7. Tordoir JH, Dammers R, van der Sande FM: Upper extremity ischemia and hemodialysis vascular access, *Eur J Vasc Endovasc Surg* 27:1-5, 2004.
8. Morsy AH, Kulbaski M, Chen C, et al: Incidence and characteristics of patients with hand ischemia after a hemodialysis access procedure, *J Surg Res* 74:8-10, 1998.
9. Mwipatayi BP, Bowles T, Balakrishnan S, et al: Ischemic steal syndrome: A case series and review of current management, *Curr Surg* 63:130-135, 2006.
10. Sessa C, Pecher M, Maurizi-Balsan J, et al: Critical hand ischemia after angioaccess surgery: Diagnosis and treatment, *Ann Vasc Surg* 14:583-593, 2000.
11. Odland MD, Kelly PH, Ney AL, et al: Management of dialysis-associated steal syndrome complicating upper extremity arteriovenous fistulas: Use of intraoperative digital photoplethysmography, *Surgery* 199;110:664-669.
12. Schanzer H, Schwartz M, Harrington E, et al: Treatment of ischemia due to "steal" by arteriovenous fistula with distal artery ligation and revascularization, *J Vasc Surg* 7:770-773, 1988.
13. Knox RC, Berman SS, Hughes JD, et al: Distal revascularization-interval ligation: A durable and effective treatment for ischemic steal syndrome after hemodialysis, *J Vasc Surg* 36:250-256, 2002.
14. Lazarides MK, Staamos DN, Panagopoulos GN, et al: Indications for surgical treatment of angioaccess-induced arterial "steal", *J Am Coll Surg* 187:422-426, 1998.
15. Pirzada NA, Morgenlander JC: Peripheral neuropathy in patients with chronic renal failure: A treatable source of discomfort and disability, *Postgrad Med* 102:249-261, 1997.

16. Wilbourn AJ, Furlan AJ, Hulley W, et al: Ischemic monomelic neuropathy, *Neurology* 33:447-451, 1983.
17. Hye RJ, Wolf YG: Ischemic monomelic neuropathy: An under-recognized complication of hemodialysis access, *Ann Vasc Surg* 8:578-582, 1994.
18. Gradman W, Pozrikidis C: Analysis of options for mitigating hemodialysis access-related ischemic steal phenomena, *Ann Vasc Surg* 18:59-65, 2004.
19. Wixon CL, Hughes JD, Mills JL: Understanding strategies for the treatment of ischemic steal syndrome after hemodialysis access, *J Am Coll Surg* 191:301-310, 2000.
20. Huber T, Brown M, Seeger J, et al: Midterm outcome after the distal revascularization and interval ligation (DRIL) procedure, *J Vasc Surg* 48:926-933, 2008.
21. Sessa C, Riehl G, Porcu P, et al: Treatment of hand ischemia following angio-access surgery using the distal revascularization interval-ligation technique with preservation of vascular access: Description of an 18-case series, *Ann Vasc Surg* 18:685-694, 2004.

68 Surgical and Endovascular Intervention for Arteriovenous Graft Thrombosis

GEORGE H. MEIER

Historical Background

As of 2007, 527,000 patients received treatment for end-stage renal disease in the United States.[1] During this same year, approximately 1500 access interventions were performed per 1000 patients. With the exception of dialysis itself, the most commonly performed procedures on patients with end-stage renal disease are open or endovascular interventions directed at maintenance of arteriovenous access.

The modern era of hemodialysis began with the availability of reusable silicone elastomer (Silastic) external shunts between the artery and the vein, pioneered by Hegstrom and colleagues in 1960.[2] For the first time repetitive arteriovenous access was available for maintenance hemodialysis in patients with renal failure. Although these shunts were cumbersome, prone to infection, and unsightly, they provided a simple means of allowing repetitive vascular access for dialysis of patients with renal failure.

In the mid-1960s Cimino and Brescia described the creation of a native arteriovenous fistula for chronic vascular access.[3,4] In this technique needle cannulation of an enlarged segment of autogenous vein allowed repetitive hemodialysis access. The self-contained nature of this access allowed patients to function normally when not receiving hemodialysis. With the increased durability achieved by the Brescia-Cimino fistula, however, surgical strategies for effective access maintenance and for the treatment of access complications, including fistula degeneration, false aneurysm formation, and thrombosis, became imperative. In the 1990s percutaneous interventions were applied with increasing frequency for arteriovenous access maintenance. Although less invasive, the limited durability led to a dramatic increase in vascular access interventions.

Surgical Intervention for Arteriovenous Access Thrombosis

Traditional management of arteriovenous graft thrombosis combined open surgical thrombectomy with surgical revision of the underlying cause of graft failure, often without the aid of direct intraoperative imaging techniques. However, the introduction of intraoperative venography has provided a means to define the cause of access failure as a routine component of the intervention.

Preoperative Preparation

- **Operative preparation.** Many patients will present with an arteriovenous access thrombosis at a regularly scheduled hemodialysis session and often have recently eaten. Patients should be instructed to cease all oral intake.

- **Temporary dialysis.** Preoperative discussion should include the possibility of placing a temporary hemodialysis catheter. Significant hyperkalemia or fluid overload warrants placement of a catheter for acute dialysis.
- **Prophylactic antibiotics.** Administration of a preoperative intravenous antibiotic active against *Staphylococcus* species is routine, particularly in the presence of synthetic graft material. In addition, topical rifampin can be applied to exposed graft material during the procedure to minimize secondary biofilm infections.

Pitfalls and Danger Points

- **Incomplete thrombectomy.** Residual thrombus may compromise the durability of the access graft, if complete visualization is not afforded by intraoperative contrast venography.
- **Incomplete treatment.** Anastomotic and other occult stenoses in the central venous system, as well as lesions in the graft and the arterial inflow, may be missed without thorough contrast imaging.

Operative Strategy

Treatment of arteriovenous access thrombosis that occurs 30 days or longer after the initial procedure has been traditionally approached by empirical operative revision of a stenotic venous anastomosis resulting from intimal hyperplasia, which remains the most common cause of access failure (Fig. 68-1).[5-14] In the absence of intraoperative imaging, revision of the distal anastomosis or distal portion of the access is often performed after open thrombectomy, where the presence of a pulse in the graft suggests a more distal obstruction or stenosis.[15,16] Without contrast venography, physical examination becomes critical to the success of the procedure (Fig. 68-2).[17-20] Normal venous segments of an arteriovenous fistula typically do not thrombose.

A segment of the synthetic arteriovenous graft distant from the previous skin incision chosen as the site to expose the prosthesis for planned thrombectomy. This segment is incorporated into the subsequent surgical plan for graft revision. By selecting a segment of graft underlying healthy skin, the risk of wound complications can be minimized. If intraoperative examination identifies the underlying cause of thrombosis, revision can be performed simultaneously with thrombectomy. Patch angioplasty or an interposition jump graft is often necessary to treat an underlying outflow stenosis. A limited dose of systemic intravenous heparin may be used, along with the administration of regional heparin using a heparin flush solution through the graft. Systemic doses of heparin range from 20 to 50 units per kilogram of body weight as an intravenous bolus, about one half the typical heparin dose used in patients without end-stage renal disease. Heparin flush solutions vary from 4 to 20 unit/mL, averaging about 10 unit/mL.

Operative Technique

ANESTHESIA AND INCISION

Graft thrombectomy and revision can often be performed under local anesthesia with intravenous sedation. The additional use of bupivacaine infiltration anesthesia can provide improved postoperative pain control. Typically, bupivacaine is used at a dose of 20 to 30 mL of 0.5% solution without epinephrine to a maximum dose of about 2 mg per kilogram of body weight. Systemic antibiotics should be given preoperatively. The use of a plastic antimicrobial skin barrier may also be helpful to prevent contact between skin and graft material. Generally, some form of barrier should be used to avoid skin flora contaminating the graft material. An incision is made over or near the distal anastomosis

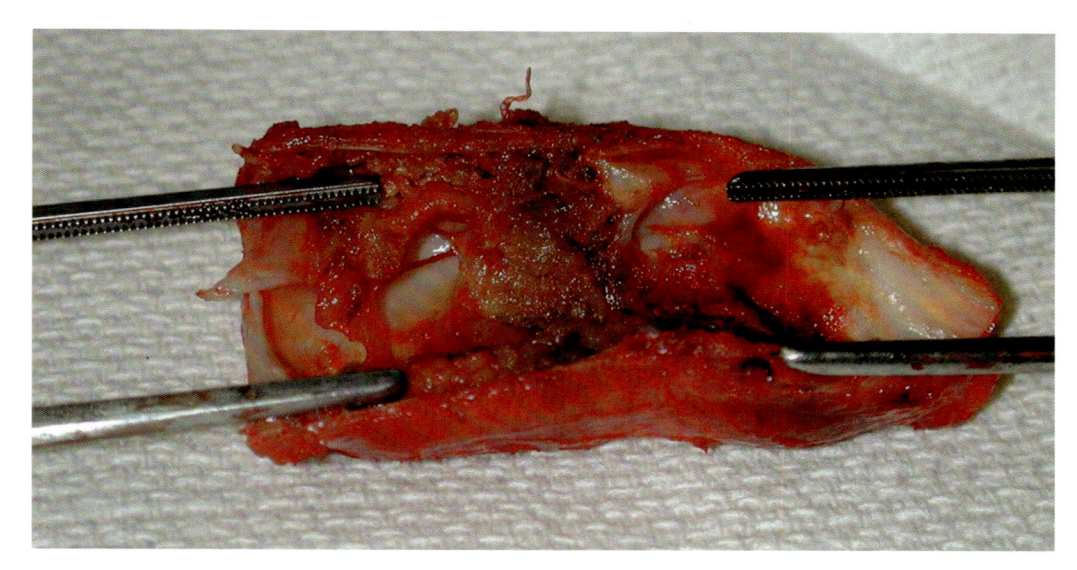

Figure 68-1. Resected anastomosis from an arteriovenous graft demonstrating intimal hyperplasia between the graft on the left and the native vein on the right.

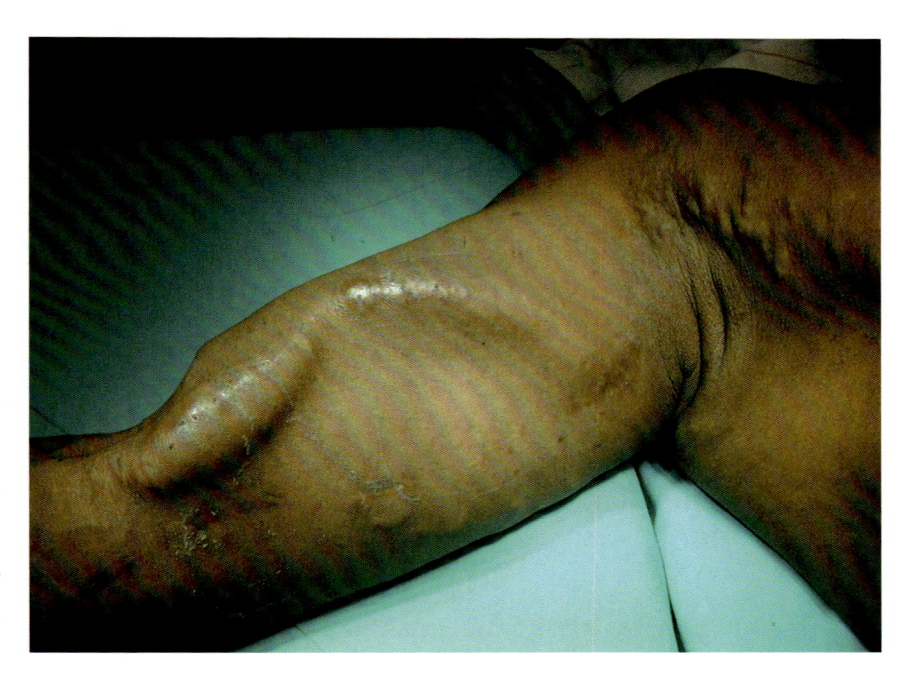

Figure 68-2. Physical examination is an important component of access assessment. This upper arm graft demonstrates access site aneurysmal degeneration. The presence of proximal collateral veins suggests an associated central venous obstruction.

of the arteriovenous graft in a segment of healthy skin. In many cases this may incorporate the prior incision, but extension of the incision proximally or distally may be required to fully expose the involved segment. A sigmoid-shaped incision is useful near areas of flexion at the antecubital fossa.

THROMBECTOMY

Mechanical thrombectomy is performed using a Fogarty embolectomy catheter. Typically, venous thrombectomy is performed first by passing the catheter distally and slowly withdrawing the venous thrombus. Resistance to catheter withdrawal is often sensed if a stenosis is encountered. Most normal outflow veins can accommodate a fully inflated 4-Fr balloon catheter. If surgical revision of venous outflow is planned, this should be performed before completing the arterial thrombectomy. Otherwise, if a cause for graft thrombosis is not apparent, then arterial thrombectomy should be undertaken. Arterial thrombectomy is performed segmentally to remove the more liquid thrombus in the body of the graft, before withdrawal of the fibrous cap often found at the arterial end of the prosthesis. This minimizes the risk of embolization of the arterial cap retrograde into the arterial tree. Residual debris is removed by repetitive flushing once pulsatile inflow is achieved.

REVISION OF THE DISTAL VENOUS ANASTOMOSIS

Revision of the distal venous anastomosis most often consists of either patch angioplasty (Fig. 68-3) or extension interposition grafting (Fig. 68-4). Although there is no consensus as to the best approach, patching is applied for short areas of stenosis and avoids loss of outflow vein. Interposition grafting is reserved for a longer-segment stenosis. Once the graft is free of thrombus and flow reestablished, a careful physical examination in the operating room should be performed. The graft should have an easily palpable pulse and thrill. Pulsatility in the absence of a thrill suggests significant residual outflow stenosis, and careful intraoperative imaging from the arterial anastomosis to the central veins is warranted.

CLOSURE

Antibiotic irrigation of all incisions should be performed, with some advocating routine application of a topical rifampin solution to exposed grafts for a more prolonged antibiotic effect and improved efficacy against *Staphylococcus* species, including *Staphylococcus epidermis*. Typically, the solution consists of 600 mg of rifampin in about 20 mL of saline. Rifampin has a high degree of topical adsorption onto prosthetic materials and tissues, and the antimicrobial effect is a local one, limited to about 2 weeks. Rifampin is renally excreted, often resulting in orange coloration of the urine if residual excretory renal function exists. Wound closure is performed with an absorbable subcuticular suture.

Endovascular Intervention for Arteriovenous Graft Thrombosis

Endovascular techniques for treatment of arteriovenous graft complications are evolving as newer devices and approaches become available.[21-28] In the process routine use of intraoperative imaging has led to improved visualization of the entire arteriovenous access, including the arterial inflow and central venous system (Fig. 68-5).

Preoperative Preparation

- **Operative preparation.** Most endovascular procedures can be performed under local anesthesia with conscious sedation. This mandates that the patient avoid oral intake for at least 6 hours before any planned procedure. Pretreatment with steroids is required if the patient relays a history of dye allergy.

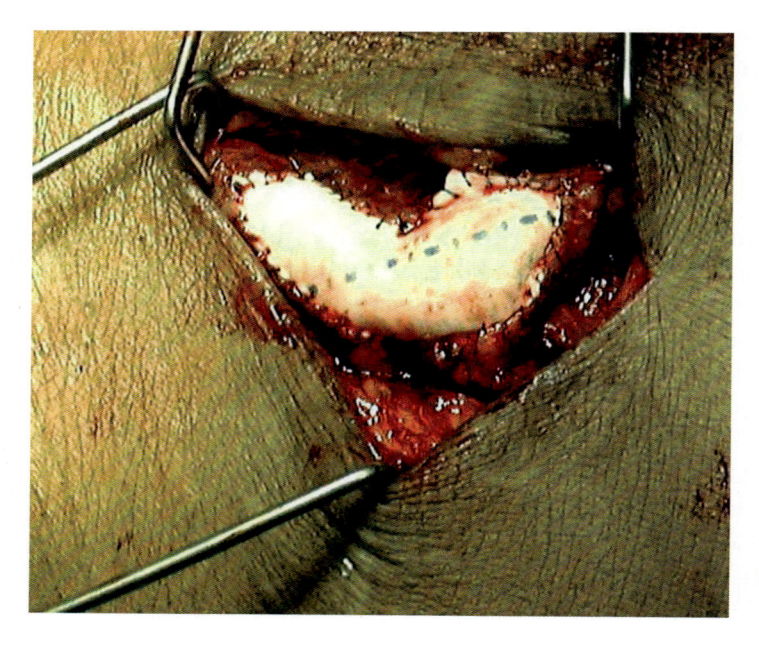

Figure 68-3. Surgical patch angioplasty of the venous anastomosis of a stenotic arteriovenous graft.

SURGICAL AND ENDOVASCULAR INTERVENTION FOR ARTERIOVENOUS GRAFT THROMBOSIS   785

- **Antibiotic prophylaxis.** A preoperative intravenous antibiotic active against *Staphylococcus* species should be administered. When the use of graft material is planned, an antibiotic effective against methicillin-resistant *Staphylococcus aureus*, such as vancomycin, should be selected. Otherwise, cefazolin is an acceptable choice.

Pitfalls and Danger Points

- **Incomplete thrombectomy.** Incomplete thrombectomy remains a concern for endovascular techniques but can be avoided by intraoperative imaging.
- **Clot embolization.** Endovascular treatment is associated with some embolization of clot to the pulmonary circulation. Although this does not appear to be clinically significant, this possibility should be considered if hemodynamic instability is noted during treatment.

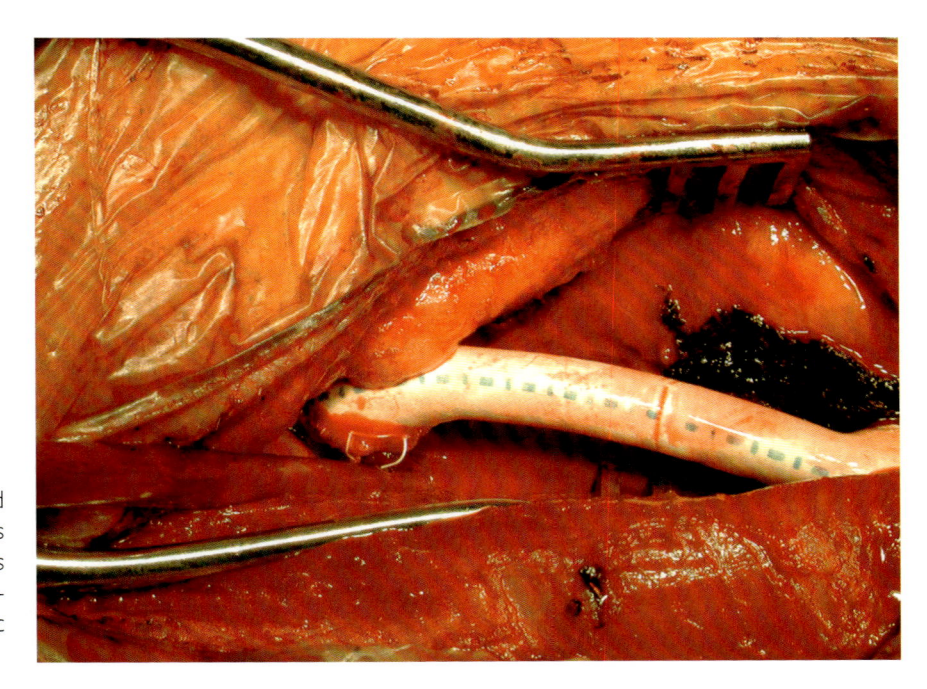

Figure 68-4. An interposition graft is used to bypass a venous anastomotic stenosis because of intimal hyperplasia. However, this type of revision results in loss of the intervening vein segment if a recurrent anastomotic stenosis occurs.

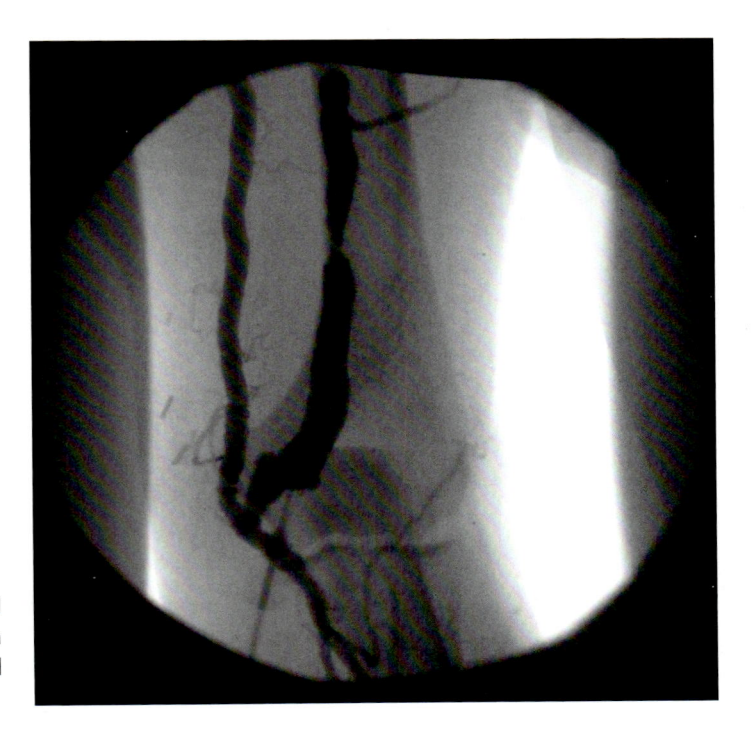

Figure 68-5. An angiogram is obtained to assess the proximal anastomosis of an arteriovenous fistula. Complete visualization of the access from the arterial inflow to the central veins should be performed before intervention of any type.

Operative Strategy

SHEATH PLACEMENT

Two sheaths are used for the procedure. The main treatment sheath originates near the arterial end and is directed toward the venous outflow. In some situations this single sheath may be sufficient. The secondary sheath is placed near the venous outflow and is directed toward the arterial end. This is used to assist in removal of the arterial cap or to treat flow-limiting lesions at the arterial inflow site (Fig. 68-6).

USE OF COVERED STENTS

A pseudoaneurysm in the conduit can be excluded by placement of a covered stent, but this approach does not treat the mass effect of the pseudoaneurysm. In some instances the thrombus remodels with a reduction in size of the subcutaneous mass.

Operative Technique

"LYSE-AND-GO" TECHNIQUE

Conscious sedation, either moderate or monitored, along with local anesthesia, is needed for most interventions. The lyse-and-go technique involves thrombolysis by direct injection of tissue plasminogen activator (tPA) into the access conduit in a preintervention holding area. Typically, a needle or catheter is introduced a few centimeters from the arterial anastomosis and pointed toward the venous anastomosis. In most cases a plastic 20-Ga catheter used for intravenous access is selected. An access sheath can be used, but must be changed to a treatment sheath during the operative procedure. The patient is given 3000 units of intravenous heparin, followed by slow injection within the conduit over a period of several minutes of 2 mg of tPA mixed in a total volume of 10 to 20 mL. Gentle compression is initially applied to the arterial end to encourage infiltration through the venous clot. Distal compression over the venous end is then used to infiltrate the lytic agent to the arterial anastomosis. This injection should proceed slowly and cautiously to avoid embolization of the arterial cap into the arterial circulation.

Using the lyse-and-go technique, the patient is taken to the operating room or angiography suite as soon as the tPA injection is complete. The "lyse-and-wait" technique relies on restoration of patency in the arteriovenous access graft before transfer to the interventional suite. However, if the access is not patent at the time of patient arrival, additional maneuvers can be performed percutaneously to restore patency.

REMOVAL OF RESIDUAL CLOT

Mechanical devices are often necessary to allow restoration of patency and remove residual clot. The needle or catheter used initially for injection of tPA is exchanged for a sheath, usually a short, bright tip, 7-Fr sheath (5.5 cm). An 8 mm by 8 cm high-pressure angioplasty balloon catheter is then introduced over a wire through the sheath, and balloon angioplasty of the venous outflow is often performed blindly. In many cases, patency is restored by this maneuver. Imaging can then be performed to evaluate for the presence of residual clot. If better visualization of the arterial end of the access is needed, then the balloon can be gently inflated distally and dye can be refluxed to the arterial end. In a significant proportion of cases, a second sheath will need to be placed from the distal end of the access graft toward the arterial anastomosis; typically a second short, bright tip, 7-Fr sheath. Dye can be injected close to the arterial anastomosis, and if the arterial cap remains, a 4-Fr Fogarty embolectomy catheter can be used to pull the arterial cap into the venous outflow (Fig. 68-7). Additional thrombolysis may be needed. Alternatively, a mechanical thrombectomy device such as the Teratola or Possis AngioJet can be used

SURGICAL AND ENDOVASCULAR INTERVENTION FOR ARTERIOVENOUS GRAFT THROMBOSIS 787

Figure 68-6. A, A patient presented with low flow of unknown etiology in a dialysis access graft. The arm was supinated at 90 degrees. **B**, "Crossed" sheaths were placed in the arteriovenous graft to allow access to arterial and venous anastomoses.

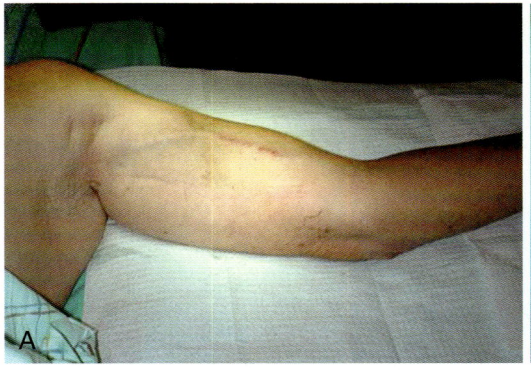

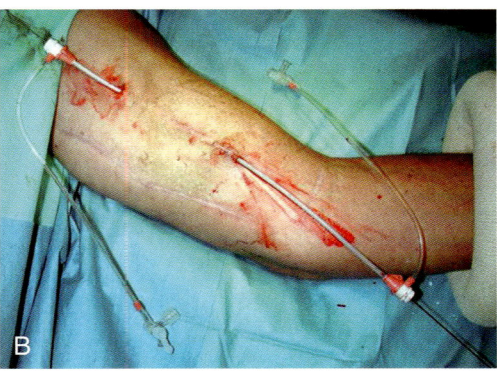

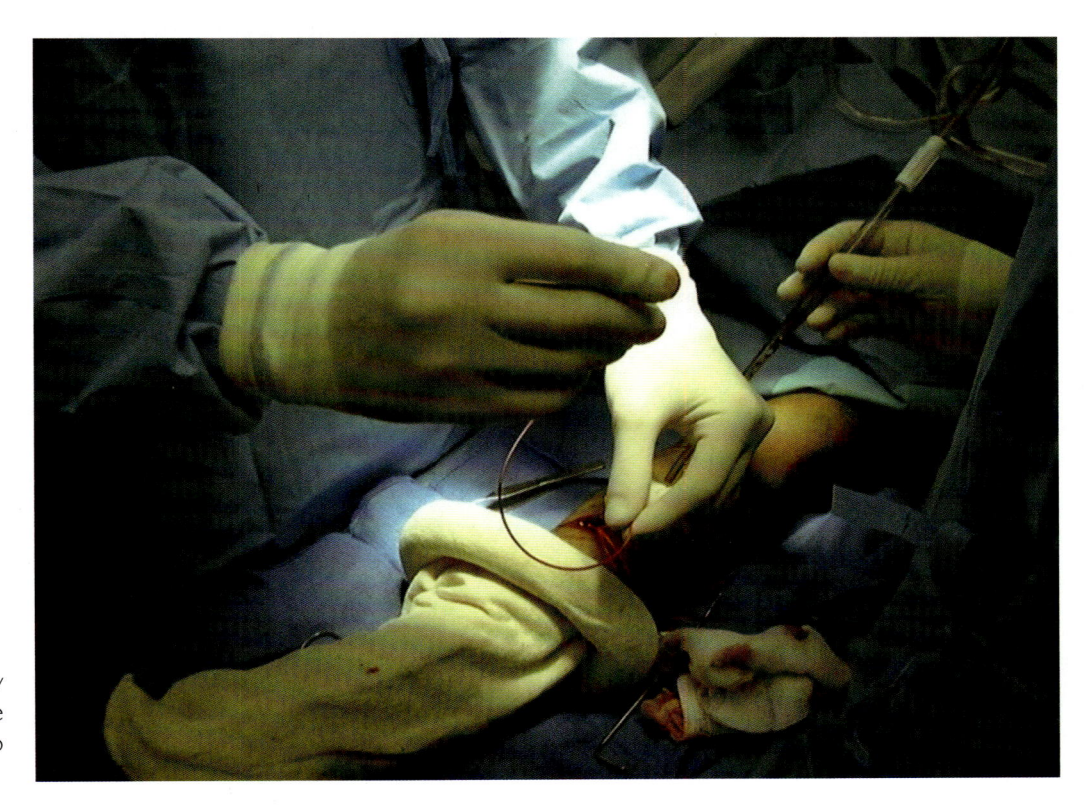

Figure 68-7. A Fogarty embolectomy catheter can be used to pull the arterial cap into the venous outflow.

to fragment residual thrombus and remove it. A portion of the thrombus inevitably embolizes into the pulmonary circulation, but clinical sequelae are exceedingly rare.

CLOSURE

At the conclusion of the procedure, a mattress suture of 4-0 absorbable monofilament is used to close each of the sheath sites to avoid delayed bleeding during subsequent dialysis.

Hybrid Interventions for Arteriovenous Graft Thrombosis

Although endovascular management may reduce the likelihood of access loss, open thrombectomy affords complete clot removal with minimal risk of distal embolization. Thus some practitioners have advocated the use of a hybrid technique that involves open exposure of the arteriovenous access with proximal and distal control (Fig. 68-8), followed by complete thrombectomy of the arterial and venous segments of the graft (Fig. 68-9). Once thrombectomy is complete, imaging and endovascular treatment complete the procedure.

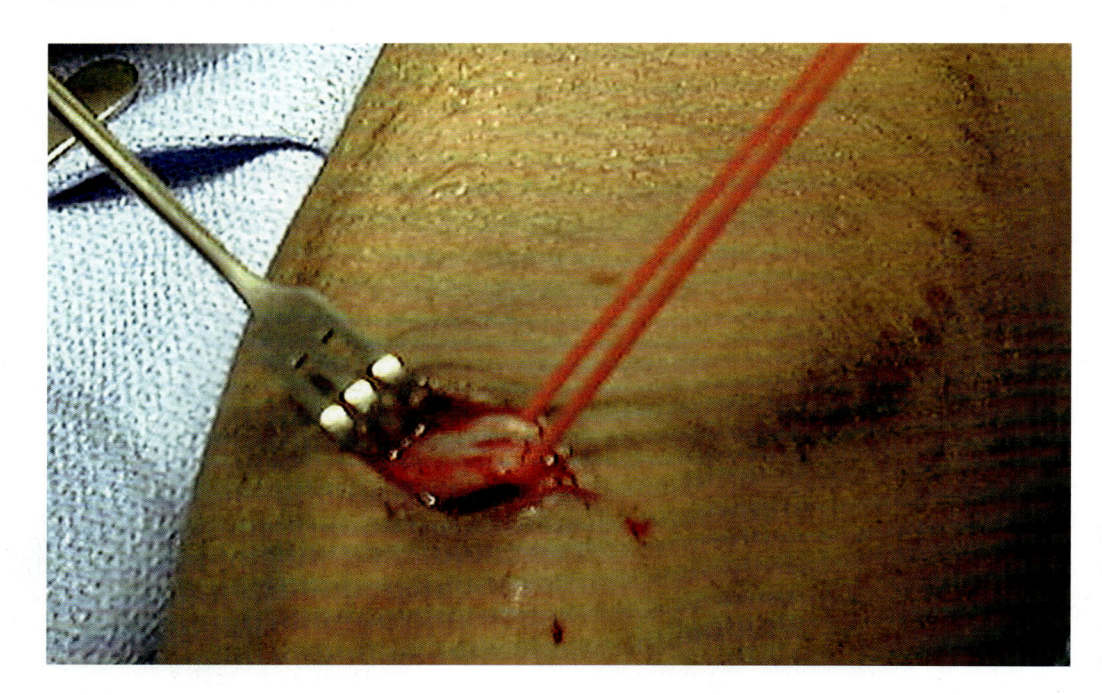

Figure 68-8. Surgical exposure of the arteriovenous graft is usually performed at an area remote from the sites of previous intervention.

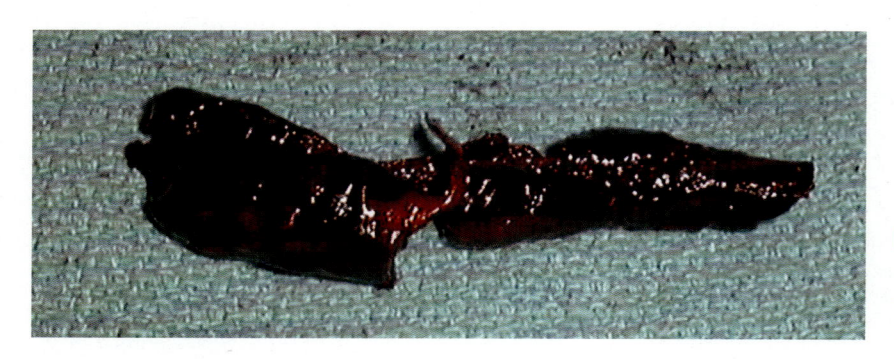

Figure 68-9. Thrombus removed after open thrombectomy. With percutaneous procedures, this thrombus is at risk for embolization to the pulmonary circulation.

Operative Strategy

In addition to standard skin preparation, the application of topical rifampin to exposed prosthetic material may help reduce the incidence of secondary graft infection. A complete thrombectomy is first performed through an open graft incision to avoid embolization to the pulmonary circulation. Thorough angiographic visualization of the arterial inflow and venous outflow, including central veins, is then performed. Endovascular treatment of the underlying lesions is performed, and the graft incision then closed.

Operative Technique

INCISION

Under local anesthesia with or without intravenous sedation, a transverse incision is made over a segment of the graft without significant scarring. Using blunt dissection with a hemostat, the graft is encircled and adequate length is exposed to allow proximal and distal clamping. A total of 3000 units of heparin are administered intravenously, and heparin flush is used liberally throughout the procedure.

THROMBECTOMY

Because the graft is occluded, a transverse arteriotomy is made in a convenient segment. Care should be taken to ensure that adequate length for clamping exists

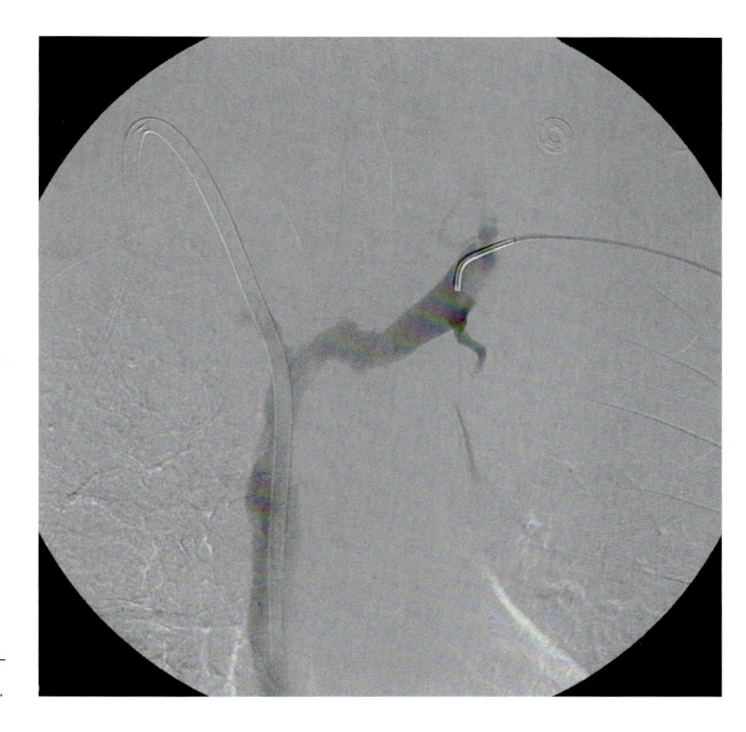

Figure 68-10. A selective venogram through a Berenstein-type catheter is used to visualize the central venous circulation.

on both sides of the graft incision. Vessel loops are used on either end and are double looped to provide hemostatic control once flow is reestablished. The venous end thrombectomy is performed first. A 4-Fr Fogarty embolectomy catheter is passed sequentially down the venous limb. If backbleeding is present, then a 9- or 10-Fr sheath is placed into the distal limb and controlled with a vessel loop. After flushing with heparinized saline, dye is injected to visualize the venous outflow. Although initial injections can be performed through the sheath, a Berenstein-type catheter is often needed to visualize the central circulation (Fig. 68-10). A venous anastomotic stenosis is usually present, but additional areas of stenosis or occlusive lesions may be noted.

ENDOVASCULAR INTERVENTION

A stenosis is treated using a high-pressure venous balloon with prolonged inflation lasting 2 to 3 minutes (Fig. 68-11). Contrast is injected to document treatment of the stenosis. Once the venous end is treated, attention is directed to the arterial end. Using the same 4-Fr Fogarty catheter, thrombectomy of the arterial end is performed by sequential passage of the catheter, in 5- to 10-cm lengths, to draw the arterial plug into the proximal graft. Once the arterial plug is delivered, proximal control of the graft is achieved by compression. If intervention is anticipated on the arterial end, an 8- or 10-Fr sheath is placed through the arteriotomy. If only a diagnostic arteriogram is planned, then an olive tip needle clamped by a Fogarty Hydragrip clamp allows infusion of contrast with proximal control. Once the arterial anastomosis and proximal arterial tree are visualized, the proximal graft is flushed with heparinized saline solution and clamped.

CLOSURE

The graft incision is closed with running or interrupted polypropylene sutures. Closure of subcutaneous tissue and skin is performed with absorbable sutures. If a thrill is not palpable, the graft should be accessed with a 19-Ga butterfly-type needle and contrast injected. If necessary, a micropuncture wire can be passed through the butterfly needle and a small sheath placed, which can be upsized, if necessary.

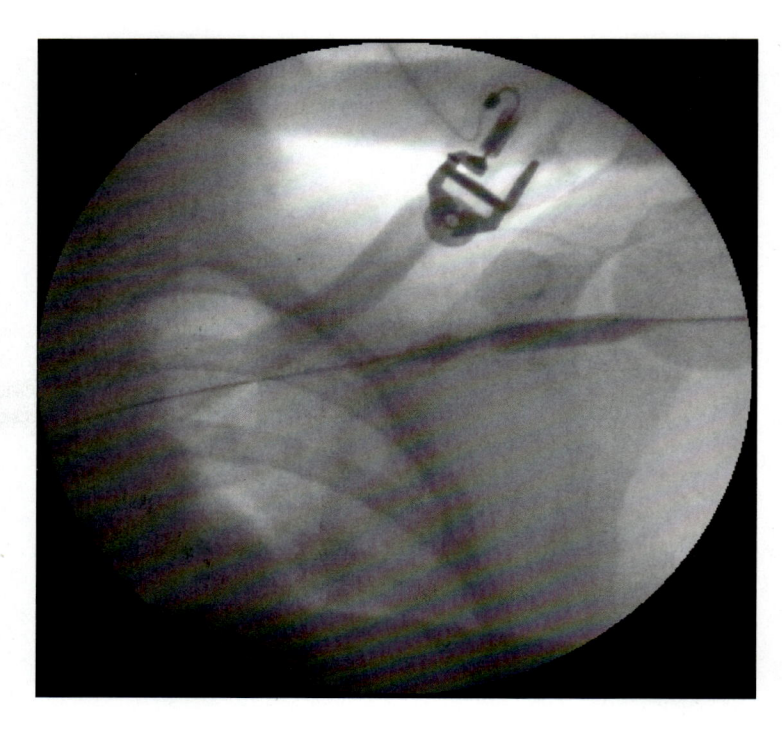

Figure 68-11. If a stenosis is identified, angioplasty should be performed with a high-pressure balloon.

Postoperative Care

- **Discharge instructions.** Patients are discharged the same day. Use of absorbable sutures for closure allows follow-up to be performed by the referring dialysis unit.
- **Initiation of dialysis.** The access graft can be used immediately as long as needle punctures are restricted to the area of previously incorporated graft material. Heparin during hemodialysis should be discouraged during the initial period after the surgical procedure.

Complications

- **Recurrent thrombosis.** The most common complication of graft thrombectomy and revision is recurrent thrombosis requiring further treatment.
- **Graft infection.** A local wound infection compromises healing and places the entire graft at risk. Meticulous surgical technique and appropriate use of prophylactic antibiotics cannot be overemphasized. Although the risk of thrombosis after an endovascular procedure is similar to that associated with an open procedure, the risk of infection is reduced because of limited graft exposure.
- **Hematoma.** Hematoma at the sheath insertion site is rare. In addition, should angioplasty of the graft-venous anastomosis be performed, a hematoma in this region is also infrequent due to low venous outflow pressures and inherent scarring around the access conduit.

REFERENCES

1. U.S. Renal Data System, USRDS: 2011 annual data report: Atlas of chronic kidney disease and end-stage renal disease in the United States, Bethesda, Md., 2011, National Institutes of Health, National Institute of Diabetes and Digestive and Kidney Diseases.
2. Hegstrom RM, Quinton WE, Dillard DH, et al: One year's experience with the use of indwelling Teflon cannulas and bypass, *Trans Am Soc Artif Intern Organs* 7:47-56, 1961.
3. Cimino JE, Brescia MJ: Simple venipuncture for hemodialysis, *N Engl J Med* 267:608-609, 1962.
4. Brescia MJ, Cimino JE, Appel K, et al: Chronic hemodialysis using venipuncture and a surgically created arteriovenous fistula, *N Engl J Med* 275:1089-1092, 1966.

5. Lemaitre P, Ackman CF, O'Regan S, et al: Polytetrafluoroethylene (PTFE) grafts for hemodialysis: 18 months' experience, *Clin Nephrol* 10:27-31, 1978.
6. Kootstra G: Secondary procedures for A-V fistula failure, *Proc Eur Dial Transplant Assoc* 19:99-105, 1983.
7. Criado E, Marston WA, Jaques PF, et al: Proximal venous outflow obstruction in patients with upper extremity arteriovenous dialysis access, *Ann Vasc Surg* 3:530-535, 1994.
8. Taber TE, Maikranz PS, Haag BW, et al: Maintenance of adequate hemodialysis access: Prevention of neointimal hyperplasia, *ASAIO J* 41:842-846, 1995.
9. Lazarides MK, Iatrou CE, Karanikas ID, et al: Factors affecting the lifespan of autologous and synthetic arteriovenous access routes for haemodialysis, *Eur J Surg* 162:297-301, 1996.
10. Bay WH, Henry ML, Lazarus JM, et al: Predicting hemodialysis access failure with color flow Doppler ultrasound, *Am J Nephrol* 18:296-304, 1998.
11. Brattich M: Vascular access thrombosis: Etiology and prevention, *ANNA J* 26:537-540, 1999.
12. Berman SS, Gentile AT: Impact of secondary procedures in autogenous arteriovenous fistula maturation and maintenance, *J Vasc Surg* 34:866-871, 2001.
13. Dember LM, Holmberg EF, Kaufman JS: Value of static venous pressure for predicting arteriovenous graft thrombosis, *Kidney Int* 61:1899-1904, 2002.
14. Sirken GR, Shah C, Raja R: Slow-flow venous pressure for detection of arteriovenous graft malfunction, *Kidney Int* 63:1894-1898, 2003.
15. Frinak S, Zasuwa G, Dunfee T, et al: Dynamic venous access pressure ratio test for hemodialysis access monitoring, *Am J Kidney Dis* 40:760-768, 2002.
16. Van Tricht I, De Wachter D, Vanhercke D, et al: Assessment of stenosis in vascular access grafts, *Artif Organs* 28:617-622, 2004.
17. Leon C, Asif A: Physical examination of arteriovenous fistulae by a renal fellow: Does it compare favorably to an experienced interventionalist? *Semin Dial* 21:557-560, 2008.
18. Paulson WD, Ram SJ, Zibari GB: Vascular access: Anatomy, examination, management, *Semin Nephrol* 22:183-194, 2002.
19. Sands JJ: A review of vascular access monitoring techniques: What works best? *Nephrol News Issues* 17:86-87, 2003.
20. Trerotola SO, Scheel PJ Jr, Powe NR, et al: Screening for dialysis access graft malfunction: Comparison of physical examination with US, *J Vasc Interv Radiol* 7:15-20, 1996.
21. Beathard GA: Fistula salvage by endovascular therapy, *Adv Chronic Kidney Dis* 16:339-351, 2009.
22. Nassar GM: Endovascular management of the "failing to mature" arteriovenous fistula, *Tech Vasc Interv Radiol* 11:175-180, 2008.
23. Manninen HI, Kaukanen E, Mäkinen K, et al: Endovascular salvage of nonmaturing autogenous hemodialysis fistulas: Comparison with endovascular therapy of failing mature fistulas, *J Vasc Interv Radiol* 19:870-876, 2008.
24. Greenberg JI, Suliman A, Angle N: Endovascular dialysis interventions in the era of DOQI, *Ann Vasc Surg* 22:657-662, 2008.
25. Kakkos SK, Haddad R, Haddad GK, et al: Results of aggressive graft surveillance and endovascular treatment on secondary patency rates of Vectra Vascular Access Grafts, *J Vasc Surg* 45:974-980, 2007.
26. Efstratiadis G, Platsas I, Koukoudis P, et al: Interventional nephrology: A new subspecialty of nephrology, *Hippokratia* 11:22-24, 2007.
27. Naoum JJ, Irwin C, Hunter GC: The use of covered nitinol stents to salvage dialysis grafts after multiple failures, *Vasc Endovascular Surg* 40:275-279, 2006.
28. Haskal ZJ, Trerotola S, Dolmatch B, et al: Stent graft versus balloon angioplasty for failing dialysis-access grafts, *N Engl J Med* 362:494-503, 2010.

Index

Note: Page numbers followed by *f* refer to figures, by *t* to tables, by *b* to boxes, and by *V* to videos.

A

Abdominal aorta
  average diameter of, 57t
  exposure in aortobifemoral bypass, 355
  exposure in total graft excision and extraanatomic repair of aortic graft infection, 414
Abdominal aortic aneurysm
  direct surgical repair of, 295–308
    adequate colonic perfusion in, 300
    aortocaval fistula and, 301
    assessment of infrarenal aortic neck in, 299–300
    balloon catheters for vascular control in, 300
    complications in, 307–308
    division of renal vein in, 299, 299f
    horseshoe kidney and, 301
    inflammatory aneurysm and, 300
    postoperative care in, 307
    preoperative preparation in, 296–297
    retroperitoneal exposure in, 298–299, 298b
    ruptured aneurysm and, 300
    site selection for distal exposure and control in, 300
    transperitoneal exposure in, 297–298, 298b
    transplanted kidney and, 301
    venous anomalies and, 301
  juxtarenal and pararenal, endovascular repair of, 344, 343–349
    branched grafts for, 344–346, 345f
    fenestrated grafts for, 343–344, 346
    hybrid surgical and endovascular approaches in, 347, 348f
    postoperative care in, 347–349
    postoperative complications in, 349
    preoperative preparation for, 343–344
    snorkel or chimney graft technique in, 346–347, 347f
  juxtarenal and pararenal, surgical repair of, 309–320
    control of supraceliac aorta in, 311
    control of suprarenal aorta in, 311
    iliac artery involvement in, 313–315, 314b
    indications for, 309
    postoperative care in, 318
    postoperative complications in, 318–319
    preoperative preparation in, 309–310
    retroperitoneal exposure in, 311–313, 312f
    selection of site for proximal control in, 310–311
Aberrant right subclavian artery, 159–160, 159f–160f
  Kommerell diverticulum and, 160
  surgical repair of, 165–166, 165f
    closure in, 166
    division and ligation of retroesophageal subclavian artery in, 166
    exposure of artery in, 165–166
    exposure of retroesophageal subclavian artery in, 166
    patient position and incision in, 165, 165f
    postoperative complications in, 169
    subclavian artery to carotid artery transposition in, 166

Above-knee amputation, 607–608, 607f
Above-knee femoral-popliteal bypass, 536–537
Above-knee popliteal bypass, 536–537
Access
  in carotid angioplasty and stenting, 90–91, 100
  in endovascular treatment
    of aortic arch vessels, 151–152, 152f
    of aortic dissection, 278
    of aortoiliac occlusive disease, 377–378, 379f
    of common carotid artery lesions, 150
    of descending thoracic aortic aneurysm, 258, 259f–261f
    of femoral-popliteal arterial occlusive disease, 580
    of infrapopliteal disease, 592, 593f
    of infrarenal aortic aneurysm, 324–325
    of mesenteric ischemia, 493–494, 495f
    of subclavian-axillary vein thrombosis, 208
    of tibial-peroneal arterial occlusive disease, 592, 593f, 594, 595f
    of traumatic thoracic artery disruption, 291
  in endovenous thermal ablation of saphenous and perforating veins, 699, 700f
  for hemodialysis. *See* Hemodialysis access
  in iliofemoral and femoral-popliteal deep vein thrombosis, 675
  in transjugular intrahepatic portosystemic shunt, 667
Access site management, 29–40
  activity restriction and, 37
  after endovascular treatment of mesenteric ischemia, 498
  anesthesia and, 31–32
  anticoagulation and, 36–37
  arterial bypass grafts and, 34
  arterial closure devices and, 37–38, 38f–39f
  axillary artery and, 34
  blood pressure and, 36, 36t
  brachial and basilic veins and, 35
  brachial artery and, 33–34, 35f
  calcification and, 36
  coagulation guidelines for, 30, 31t
  common femoral artery and, 32, 33f
  common femoral vein and, 34–35
  external compression devices and, 37, 37f
  indications for, 29–30
  internal jugular vein and, 34
  laboratory testing and, 30
  manual compression technique and, 36
  obesity and, 35
  patient positioning in, 31
  popliteal and posterior tibial veins and, 35
  pulselessness and, 36
  scarred groin and, 36
  ultrasound guidance in, 32, 33f
  vascular complications and, 38–40
  in vena cava filter placement, 638

Activase. *See* Alteplase
Activity
  after above- and below-knee amputation, 608
  after endovenous thermal ablation of saphenous and perforating veins, 705
  after femoral vein transposition, 756
  after surgical repair of aortic arch vessels, 136
  restriction after vascular access, 37
Acute limb compartment syndrome, 617
Acute lung injury after endovascular treatment of aortic dissection, 288
Acute mesenteric ischemia
  direct surgical repair of, 475–490
    antegrade bypass in, 482–485, 483f, 485f
    approach to superior mesenteric artery in, 480–481, 480f–481f
    complications in, 488–489
    indications for, 476–477
    ischemia secondary to embolization, in situ thrombosis, and dissection and, 478–479
    postoperative care in, 488
    preoperative preparation for, 477
    retrograde bypass in, 485–486, 486f
    selection of celiac artery outflow in, 479–480
    selection of conduit in, 481–482
    selection of inflow source in, 479
    superior mesenteric artery embolectomy in, 487–488, 487f
    surgical anatomy for, 478
  endovascular treatment of, 491–499
    complications in, 498
    indications for, 491–492
    pitfalls and danger points in, 493–495, 495f
    postoperative care in, 498
    preoperative preparation for, 492–493, 493f–494f
    strategy in, 495–496, 495f
    technique in, 496, 497f
Acute superior vena cava syndrome, 642
Acute tubular necrosis after direct surgical treatment of renovascular disease, 447
Adjunctive iliac angioplasty in endovascular repair of infrarenal aortic aneurysm, 323
AFX endograft, 330
Air embolism in reconstruction of inferior vena cava and iliofemoral venous system, 654
Allergic reaction
  to contrast media, 23, 24t
  to sclerosant solution, 722–723, 726
ALN Optional filter, 629t, 630f
Alteplase, 58
Ambulation
  after above- and below-knee amputation, 608
  after endovenous thermal ablation of saphenous and perforating veins, 705
  after femoral vein transposition, 756
Ambulatory phlebectomy, 691–692, 691f
Amplatzer II vascular plugs, 60t
Amputation in lower extremity arterial disease, 604–609
  above-knee amputation in, 607–608, 607f
  complications in, 608–609
  of forefoot, 610–616, 612f–615f
  indications for, 604
  long posterior flap below-knee amputation in, 605–607, 606f
  postoperative care in, 608
  preoperative preparation for, 604–605
Analgesia in vascular surgery, 17–18
Anastomosis, 8–12
  in arteriovenous graft thrombosis repair, 784, 784f
  in axillofemoral bypass, 365f–366f, 366–367
  beveled end-to-side, 8–10, 10f
  in brachial artery–axillary vein interposition graft, 740, 743, 744f

Anastomosis *(Continued)*
  in brachial vein transposition, 762, 762f
  in carotid body tumor surgery, 108, 108f
  in celiac axis and superior mesenteric artery occlusive disease
    antegrade bypass, 484, 485f
    retrograde bypass, 486
  in distal revascularization interval ligation, 774–778, 778f
  end-to-end, 11–12
  in femoral vein transposition, 753, 764V
  in femoral-femoral bypass, 364
  in forearm loop graft, 740, 742
  in hepatorenal bypass, 452, 453f–454f
  in HERO device procedure, 770
  of internal to common carotid artery in eversion endarterectomy, 80–82, 82f
  in juxtarenal abdominal aortic aneurysm surgery, 315
  in neoaortoiliac system procedure for aortic graft infection and, 422
  nonbeveled end-to-side, 10–11, 11f
  in popliteal artery aneurysm repair, 568
  in radial artery-cephalic vein arteriovenous fistula, 733–734
  in radiocephalic arteriovenous fistula, 733–734
  small vessel end-to-end, 12, 13f
  splenorenal, 454
  in superior vena cava syndrome reconstruction, 645–648, 647f
  in suprarenal aortic aneurysm surgery, 316–318, 319f
  in thoracofemoral bypass, 368–369
  in tibial-peroneal arterial occlusive disease, 546–547, 547f
Anastomotic stenosis in femoral-popliteal bypass, 529
Anesthesia
  in angioplasty, 51
  in arteriovenous graft thrombosis repair
    endovascular, 786
    surgical, 782–783
  in brachial vein transposition, 762
  in carotid angioplasty and stenting, 86
  in carotid endarterectomy, 67
  in catheter-based procedures, 31–32
  in distal revascularization interval ligation, 774
  in endovascular repair of infrarenal aortic aneurysm, 322
  in forefoot amputation, 611
  for HERO device procedure, 769
  in lower extremity vascular access for hemodialysis, 764
  in prosthetic chest wall vascular access for hemodialysis, 766
  in radial artery-cephalic vein arteriovenous fistula, 732
  in saphenous vein transposition, 763
  in subfascial endoscopic perforator surgery, 715
  in superior vena cava syndrome reconstruction, 644
  in transjugular intrahepatic portosystemic shunt, 666
  in varicose vein stripping, 688
  in vascular surgery, 17–18
Aneurysm repair
  of aortic arch aneurysm, 232–250
    anatomic considerations in, 234
    branch artery preservation in, 234–235
    choice of technique in, 235
    complications in, 243–244
    indications for, 232–233
    modular transcervical bifurcated stent graft in, 236–240, 237f–239f
    modular transfemoral multibranched stent graft in, 240–244, 241f
    patient selection for, 233
    preoperative preparation in, 233–234
  of descending thoracic aortic aneurysm, 251–273

Aneurysm repair *(Continued)*
    access in, 258, 259f–261f
    aortic tortuosity and, 261–262, 263f
    complications in, 271–272
    deployment of Gore TAG endograft in, 265–266, 265f–267f
    deployment of Medtronic vascular endograft in, 268–271, 269f–270f
    deployment of Zenith endograft in, 266–267, 268f–269f
    indications for, 252
    intraoperative imaging in, 263–264, 263f, 265f
    landing zones and, 262
    pitfalls and danger points in, 253–258, 256f–257f
    placement of stent graft in aortic arch in, 259
    postoperative care in, 271
    preoperative imaging in, 262
    preoperative preparation for, 252–253, 253f–254f
  of gastroduodenal artery aneurysm, 516, 518f–521f
  of hepatic artery aneurysm, 515–516, 517f
  of infrarenal aortic aneurysm, endovascular, 321–335
    adjunctive iliac angioplasty in, 323
    AFX endograft in, 330
    angiography in, 325–326, 325f–327f
    Aorfix endograft in, 330
    aortouniiliac graft in, 330–332, 331f
    arterial access in, 324–325
    arterial dissection during, 332
    device selection in, 322, 323f
    distal embolization in, 332
    Endurant device in, 329–330
    Excluder endograft in, 329
    external iliac to internal iliac artery bypass in, 333, 333f
    graft deployment and cannulation of contralateral gate in, 326–328, 328f–329f
    graft sizing in, 323
    hypogastric artery occlusion and, 333
    hypogastric embolization in, 338–340, 340f
    iliac artery conduit in, 324–325
    limb occlusion in, 332
    Ovation Prime endograft in, 330
    percutaneous deployment in, 323–325
    postoperative care in, 334
    postoperative complications in, 334
    PowerLink endograft in, 330
    preoperative preparation in, 321–322
    renal artery occlusion in, 332
    rupture of aorta or iliac vessels during, 332
    type I endoleak and, 336, 338, 339f
    type II endoleak and, 341–342
    unfavorable anatomy in, 336–337
    Zenith endograft in, 330
  of infrarenal aortic aneurysm, surgical, 295–308
    adequate colonic perfusion in, 300
    aortocaval fistula and, 301
    assessment of infrarenal aortic neck in, 299–300
    balloon catheters for vascular control in, 300
    complications in, 307–308
    division of renal vein in, 299, 299f
    horseshoe kidney and, 301
    inflammatory aneurysm and, 300
    postoperative care in, 307
    preoperative preparation in, 296–297
    retroperitoneal exposure in, 298–299, 298b
    ruptured aneurysm and, 300
    site selection for distal exposure and control in, 300
    transperitoneal exposure in, 297–298, 298b

Aneurysm repair (Continued)
  transplanted kidney and, 301
  venous anomalies and, 301
  of juxtarenal and pararenal aneurysms, endovascular, 344V, 343-349
    branched grafts for, 344-346, 345f
    fenestrated grafts for, 343-344, 346
    hybrid surgical and endovascular approaches in, 347, 348f
    postoperative care in, 347-349
    postoperative complications in, 349
    preoperative preparation for, 343-344
    snorkel or chimney graft technique in, 346-347, 347f
  of juxtarenal and pararenal aneurysms, surgical, 309-320
    control of supraceliac aorta in, 311
    control of suprarenal aorta in, 311
    iliac artery involvement in, 313-315, 314b
    indications for, 309
    postoperative care in, 318
    postoperative complications in, 318-319
    preoperative preparation in, 309-310
    retroperitoneal exposure in, 311-313, 312f
    selection of site for proximal control in, 310-311
    transperitoneal versus retroperitoneal exposure in, 310, 310b
  of pancreaticoduodenal artery aneurysm, 516, 518f-521f
  of popliteal artery aneurysm, 561-571
    acute thrombosis and, 566-567
    avoiding nerve injury in, 565f, 566
    avoiding venous injury in, 566
    conduit selection in, 565
    indications for, 561-562
    medial approach in, 567-568
    pitfalls and danger points in, 563-564, 563f-564f
    posterior approach in, 568-569, 570f
    preoperative preparation for, 562-563, 562f
    selection and assessment of inflow and distal outflow in, 566
    selection of approach in, 564-565
  of renal artery aneurysm, endovascular, 466-474, 468f
    complications in, 473
    deployment of bare stent in, 469
    deployment of stent graft in, 469-470, 469t
    embolization in, 470, 471f
    indications for, 466
    occlusion of renal artery in, 471, 472f-473f
    postoperative care in, 471-473
    preoperative preparation for, 466-467, 467f-468f
  of renal artery aneurysm, surgical, 439
    during branch repair using in situ and ex vivo techniques, 446-447
  of splenic artery aneurysm, 513-524
    access and guiding sheath placement in, 515
    angiographic imaging in, 515
    embolization in, 517-521
    indications for, 514
    postoperative care in, 523-524
    preoperative preparation for, 514
    stent-graft placement in, 521, 522f-523f
  of subclavian artery aneurysm, 162-165
    carotid-brachial artery bypass in, 164-165
    closure in, 165
    exposure of axillary artery in, 162-163, 164f
    exposure of supraclavicular subclavian artery in, 162, 163f
    interposition graft for, 161
    patient position and incision in, 162
    postoperative care in, 168-169

Aneurysm repair (Continued)
  postoperative complications in, 169
  preoperative preparation for, 157, 158f
  subclavian-axillary artery bypass in, 164
  of thoracoabdominal aortic aneurysm, endovascular, 232-250
    anatomic considerations in, 234
    branch artery preservation in, 234-235
    choice of technique in, 235
    complications in, 248-249
    indications for, 232-233
    modular transfemoral multibranched stent graft in, 244-249, 245f-246f, 248f
    patient selection for, 233
    preoperative preparation in, 233-234
  of thoracoabdominal aortic aneurysm, surgical, 215-231
    avoiding diaphragmatic paralysis in, 218, 219f
    avoiding embolization in, 218
    avoiding injuries to esophagus in, 219, 220f
    avoiding injuries to vagus nerve in, 218-219
    avoiding spinal cord ischemia in, 218
    avoiding visceral ischemia in, 218
    classification of aneurysms in, 217, 217f
    coagulopathy and, 218
    complications in, 228-229, 229f
    considerations in presence of chronic dissection in, 223
    descending thoracic aortic aneurysm and, 225V, 223-226, 225f
    distal aortic perfusion in, 221-222, 222f
    incision in, 221
    intraoperative corrective measures in, 220
    patient positioning for, 220-221, 221f
    postoperative care in, 228
    preoperative preparation in, 217
    retroperitoneal or transperitoneal thoracoabdominal exposure in, 221
    selection of site for distal control in, 222
    selection of site for proximal control in, 222, 223f
    somatosensory and motor-evoked potential monitoring in, 219-220
    type I aneurysm and, 226
    type II aneurysm andI, 226-228, 227f
    type III aneurysm and, 228
    type IV aneurysm and, 228
    use of balloon catheters for vascular control in, 218, 223, 224f
  of visceral artery aneurysms, 500-512
    celiac artery aneurysm in, 506, 508f-509f
    complications in, 511
    hepatic artery aneurysm in, 505-508, 507f
    indications for, 500-501
    operative strategy in, 502, 503f
    postoperative care in, 511
    preoperative preparation for, 501-502
    splenic artery aneurysm in, 502-505, 503f, 505f
Angiographic catheter, 45-46, 45f
Angiographic contrast media, 22-26
  carbon dioxide angiography and, 24-26, 25b, 25f-27f
  contrast media reactions and, 23, 24t
  renal dysfunction considerations and, 22-23, 22b, 23t
Angiography
  access site management in, 29-40
    activity restriction and, 37
    anesthesia and, 31-32
    anticoagulation and, 36-37
    arterial bypass grafts and, 34
    arterial closure devices and, 37-38, 38f-39f
    axillary artery and, 34
    blood pressure and, 36, 36t
    brachial and basilic veins and, 35
    brachial artery and, 33-34, 35f

Angiography (Continued)
  calcification and, 36
  coagulation guidelines for, 30, 31t
  common femoral artery and, 32, 33f
  common femoral vein and, 34-35
  external compression devices and, 37, 37f
  indications for, 29-30
  internal jugular vein and, 34
  laboratory testing and, 30
  manual compression technique and, 36
  obesity and, 35
  patient positioning in, 31
  popliteal and posterior tibial veins and, 35
  pulselessness and, 36
  scarred groin and, 36
  ultrasound guidance in, 32, 33f
  vascular complications and, 38-40
  in aortoiliac occlusive disease, 351
  carbon dioxide, 24-26, 25b, 25f-27f
  in carotid angioplasty and stenting
    anatomic considerations in, 87, 88t
    aortic arch, carotid, and cerebral circulation in, 92
  in carotid body tumor, 102
  before distal revascularization interval ligation, 773-774, 774f
  during endovascular treatment of aortoiliac occlusive disease, 376
  in femoral-popliteal arterial occlusive disease, 582
  in infrarenal aortic aneurysm, 325-326, 325f-327f
  in popliteal artery entrapment, 572
  in renal artery aneurysm, 467, 468f
  in renal artery stenosis, 457-458, 459f
  in splenic artery aneurysm repair, 523
  in subclavian-axillary vein thrombosis, 205-206, 206f-207f
  before supraclavicular approach to thoracic outlet syndrome, 173-174
  in thoracoabdominal aortic aneurysm, 234
  before vertebral artery surgery, 114, 115f
Angiojet device
  in acute femoral-popliteal artery occlusion, 586-587
  in subclavian-axillary vein thrombosis, 211-212, 211f
Angioplasty, 50-62
  anesthesia for, 51
  carotid, 86-101
    access in, 90-91
    angiographic anatomy and, 87, 88t
    angiographic technique in, 97V, 97-98
    angiography of aortic arch, carotid, and cerebral circulation in, 92
    aortic arch anatomy and, 88, 89f
    carotid lesions at risk for embolization and, 88
    catheterization of common carotid artery in, 91, 91f-92f
    cerebral protection devices and, 90
    completion studies in, 98
    crossing lesion and cerebral protection in, 95-97, 95f, 97f
    fibromuscular dysplasia and, 89-90
    indications for, 86, 87t
    kinks and coils of carotid artery and, 88
    management of arterial spasm, embolization, and acute occlusion in, 98-99
    neurorescue techniques in, 99-100
    occluded external carotid artery and, 88, 90f
    postoperative care in, 100
    postoperative complications in, 100-101
    preoperative care in, 86
    redo carotid angioplasty and, 90
    selection of stent for, 90
    severe stenosis and string sign and, 88-89
    sheath placement for planned intervention in, 92-95, 93f-94f

Angioplasty (Continued)
  stenting technique in, 98, 99f
    tandem lesions in common carotid artery and, 89
  in endovascular therapy for subclavian-axillary vein thrombosis, 212
  during endovascular treatment of aortoiliac occlusive disease
    of aorta, 386–387
    of common iliac artery, 387
    of external iliac artery, 389
  in femoral-popliteal arterial occlusive disease, 578–589
    access selection in, 580
    angiographic anatomy and common collateral pathways in, 580, 581f
    angiography of lower extremity in, 582
    complications in, 587
    femoral-popliteal artery occlusions and, 585–586
    femoral-popliteal artery stenosis and, 582–585, 583f–585f
    indications for, 578, 579b, 579t
    postoperative care in, 587
    preoperative preparation for, 578–579
    retrograde and antegrade approaches for arterial access in, 581–582
    stent selection in, 580–581
    thrombolysis of acute femoral-popliteal artery occlusions and, 586–587
    unfavorable anatomic features for, 580
  indications for, 50
  operative strategy in, 51
  operative technique in, 52–57, 52f, 53t, 56f
  patch, 5
    in carotid endarterectomy, 73, 73f
  postoperative care in, 60
  postoperative complications in, 60–61
  preoperative preparation for, 51
  in renal artery stenosis, 456–465
    angiographic anatomy for, 457–458, 459f
    antegrade versus retrograde access in, 463V, 459–460, 460f, 462
    branch vessel disease and, 458, 459f
    coaxial or monorail balloon catheter designs for, 460
    completion studies in, 464
    complications in, 464–465
    crossing lesions in, 463
    indications for, 456
    in situ physiologic assessment using Radi pressure wire in, 463
    postoperative care in, 464
    preoperative preparation for, 456–457
    recurrent stenosis and, 461–462, 462f
    role of balloon predilation in, 460
    selection of stent for, 461
    sheath placement in, 462–463
    solitary kidney and, 458–459
    stent placement in, 463–464
    unfavorable anatomic features for, 458
    use of embolic protection during, 461, 461f
  in subclavian-axillary vein thrombosis, 207
  in tibial-peroneal arterial occlusive disease, 592–594, 593f
  of vertebral artery, 153
Angioscope-assisted valvuloplasty, 712
Angio-Seal closure device, 38, 38f
Angled guidewire, 41, 43f, 44t
AnjioJet power pulse spray technique, 677–679, 678f
Ankle-brachial index
  in femoral-popliteal arterial occlusive disease, 527, 578–579
  in popliteal artery entrapment, 572
  in tibial-peroneal arterial occlusive disease, 591
Antegrade approach
  in crossing iliac artery lesion, 378
  in endovascular popliteal artery aneurysm repair, 600V, 599–600, 600f

Antegrade approach (Continued)
  in endovascular treatment of tibial-peroneal arterial occlusive disease, 592
  in femoral-popliteal arterial occlusive disease, 581–582
  in renal artery angioplasty and stenting, 463V, 459–460, 460f, 462
Antegrade bypass in mesenteric ischemia, 482–485
  distal anastomoses in, 484–485
  exposure of aorta in, 482
  exposure of celiac axis in, 482–483, 483f
  exposure of superior mesenteric artery in, 483–484
  incision for, 482
  patient position for, 482
  proximal aortic anastomosis in, 484, 485f
  tunneling of bypass graft in, 484
Anterior compartment, lower leg fasciotomy and, 620, 620f–621f
Anterior spine exposure, 392–402
  complications in, 400–401, 400t
  L2 to S1, 397–399, 398f–399f
  operative strategy in, 394–395
  pitfalls and danger points in, 393–394
  postoperative care in, 399–400
  preoperative preparation for, 392–393
  T12 to L2, 396–397
  thoracic, 395–396
Anterior tibial artery, angiographic anatomy of, 591
Anterolateral extensor compartment of thigh, 622
Anticoagulation
  in access site management, 36–37
  for deep vein thrombosis, 628
  in deep venous valve surgery, 710
  during extraanatomic repair of aortoiliac occlusive disease, 369
  in femoral vein transposition, 756
  in iliofemoral and femoral-popliteal deep vein thrombosis, 674, 681
  in reconstruction of inferior vena cava and iliofemoral venous system and, 662
  in subclavian-axillary vein thrombosis, 212
  in superior vena cava syndrome reconstruction, 648
  in surgical repair of popliteal artery aneurysm, 566
  in transaxillary rib resection for thoracic outlet syndrome, 195
Antiplatelet therapy
  in angioplasty and stenting, 60, 86
  in aortic arch vessels endovascular treatment, 149
  in aortoiliac occlusive disease endovascular repair, 375
  in carotid angioplasty and stenting, 86
  in carotid endarterectomy, 64
  in femoral-popliteal arterial occlusive disease, 527, 587
  in mesenteric ischemia, 498
  in popliteal artery aneurysm, 599, 602
  in renal artery stenosis endovascular repair, 375
  in tibial-peroneal arterial occlusive disease, 544, 595
Antithrombolytic prophylaxis, access site management and, 30, 31t
Aorfix endograft, 330
Aorta
  exposure of
    in antegrade bypass in mesenteric ischemia, 482
    in surgical repair of celiac artery aneurysm, 510
  infrarenal sympathetic nerves relationship to, 399f
  rupture during endovascular treatment of aortic dissection, 282–283, 283f

Aortic arch
  carotid angioplasty and stenting and, 88, 88t, 89f
  classification of, 89f
  endovascular treatment of descending thoracic aortic aneurysm and, 259
  surgical anatomy of, 128–129
  total debranching of, 284, 285f
Aortic arch aneurysm repair, 232–250
  anatomic considerations in, 234
  branch artery preservation in, 234–235
  choice of technique in, 235
  complications in, 243–244
  indications for, 232–233
  modular transcervical bifurcated stent graft in, 236–240, 237f–239f
  modular transfemoral multibranched stent graft in, 240–244, 241f
  patient selection for, 233
  preoperative preparation in, 233–234
Aortic arch vessels
  direct surgical repair of, 125–138
    ascending aorta-bilateral carotid artery bypass in, 134–135, 135f–137f
    ascending aorta-innominate artery bypass in, 132–134, 132f–134f
    assessment of aortic arch clamp site in, 129
    avoiding injury to anatomic structures in, 129
    avoiding intraoperative stroke in, 129
    closure in, 135
    complications in, 137
    dissection of arch vessels in, 130–132
    exposure of aortic arch in, 130, 131f
    incision in, 130, 131f
    indications for, 126–127
    postoperative care in, 135–137
    preoperative preparation for, 127–128
    special considerations for vasculitis in, 129–130
    surgical anatomy for, 128–129
  endovascular treatment of, 148–156
    access for common carotid artery lesions in, 150
    access for subclavian and innominate lesions in, 150, 150V
    access in, 151–152, 152f
    anatomic considerations in, 149–150, 151f
    angiographic anatomy and common collateral pathways in, 149
    common carotid artery stenting in, 155
    complications in, 155–156
    embolic protection devices and, 150
    imaging and selective catheterization in, 152–153
    indications for, 148–149
    innominate artery stenting in, 153, 153V, 775f
    Kommerell diverticulum and, 155
    lesion predilation in, 150
    postoperative care in, 155
    preoperative preparation for, 149
    protection of vertebral artery in, 150–151
    stent selection for, 150, 151f
    subclavian and axillary artery stenting in, 155
    vertebral artery angioplasty and stenting in, 153
  extraanatomic repair of, 139–147
    carotid-carotid artery bypass in, 144, 145f
    carotid-subclavian artery bypass in, 144, 145f
    carotid-subclavian artery transposition in, 142–143, 142f, 143V, 144f
    indications for, 139–140, 141f
    postoperative care in, 139–140
    postoperative complications in, 146–147
    preoperative preparation for, 140–141

Aortic arch vessels *(Continued)*
    surgical anatomy of common carotid and subclavian arteries and, 141, 142f
    subclavian and axillary artery surgery and, 157–170
        aberrant right subclavian artery and, 159–160, 159f–160f
        avoiding brachial plexus injuries in, 161
        avoiding injuries behind clavicle in, 161
        avoiding thoracic duct injuries in, 160–161
        avoiding vertebral artery injuries in, 161
        in Kommerell diverticulum repair, 167, 168f
        postoperative care in, 168–169
        postoperative complications in, 169
        preoperative preparation for, 157–158, 158f
        in repair of aberrant right subclavian artery, 165–166, 165f
        selection of conduit in, 161–162
        in subclavian artery aneurysm, 162–165, 163f–164f
        surgical anatomy in, 158–159

Aortic bifurcation
    aortoiliac occlusive disease and, 377
    endovascular repair of infrarenal aortic aneurysm and, 337

Aortic bifurcation disease, 380

Aortic dissection
    after endovascular treatment of descending thoracic aortic aneurysm, 272
    endovascular treatment of, 274–288
        after elephant trunk repair, 281, 281f
        aortic fenestration in, 285–286
        avoiding de novo type A dissection in, 278, 279f
        avoiding paraplegia in, 282
        avoiding rupture in, 282–283, 283f
        avoiding stroke in, 282
        avoiding visceral ischemia in, 283–284
        carotid-carotid and carotid-subclavian bypass in, 284–285, 285b, 286f
        complications in, 287–288
        defining extent of, 279–280, 280f, 281b
        differentiation of true and false thoracic aorta lumen and, 275–276, 277f
        endograft placement in, 286–287, 287f
        fenestration or endograft repair in, 281–282
        indications for, 274, 275b
        postoperative care in, 287
        preoperative imaging in, 278–279
        preoperative preparation for, 275
        total aortic arch debranching in, 284, 285f
        type A *versus* type B dissection and, 279
        visceral ischemia and, 275, 276f
    during endovascular treatment of aortoiliac occlusive disease, 385, 389–390

Aortic fenestration, 281–282, 285–286

Aortic graft infection
    neoaortoiliac system procedure for, 419–426
        complications in, 424–425
        construction of neoaortoiliac system in, 421–422, 423f
        distal anastomosis in, 422–423
        flap coverage in, 423–424, 424f
        harvesting femoral popliteal vein in, 420V, 420–421, 421f–422f
        postoperative care in, 424
        preoperative preparation for, 419–420
        proximal anastomosis in, 422
        selection of conduit for in situ repair in, 420
        staging of, 420
    total graft excision and extraanatomic repair of, 403–418
        avoiding ureteral injury in, 409
        choice of reconstruction in, 407–408
        closure of femoral arteries in, 416

Aortic graft infection *(Continued)*
        closure of proximal aortic stump and omental pedicle flap in, 414–415, 415f
        complications in, 417
        drains in, 416, 416f
        exposure of abdominal aorta in, 414
        exposure of common femoral, superficial femoral, and profunda femoris arteries in, 414
        graft excision in, 414
        historical background of, 404–405, 405f
        incision closure in, 416–417
        incision in, 413–414
        management of duodenal stump in, 415
        postoperative care in, 417
        preoperative preparation for, 405–407, 406f
        presence of aortoenteric fistula and, 409–412, 412f
        role of endovascular therapy in, 413, 413f
        sartorius muscle flap in, 416
        selection of extraanatomic bypass in, 409, 410f–411f
        staging of, 408–409
        underlying aneurysmal or occlusive disease and, 412

Aortic landing zones
    endovascular treatment of descending thoracic aortic aneurysm and, 262
    preoperative assessment of, 253, 254f

Aortic neck, endovascular repair of infrarenal aortic aneurysm and, 337

Aortic tortuosity
    endovascular treatment of aortic dissection and, 278
    endovascular treatment of descending thoracic aortic aneurysm and, 261–262, 263f

Aortobifemoral bypass, 355–356, 357f
Aortocarotid-subclavian artery bypass, 132–134, 133f
Aortocaval fistula, 301
Aortoenteric fistula, 409–412, 412f
Aortography in endovascular treatment of mesenteric ischemia, 495f, 496
Aortoiliac embolectomy, 369–371, 370f
Aortoiliac endarterectomy, 352–353, 353f
Aortoiliac occlusive disease
    direct surgical repair of, 350–361
        aortobifemoral bypass in, 355–356, 357f
        aortoiliac endarterectomy in, 352–353, 353f
        associated renal or visceral lesions in, 355
        classification of disease by pattern and, 351, 352f
        complications in, 358–361
        end-to-end *versus* end-to-side proximal anastomosis in, 351–352
        graft selection in, 353–354
        indications for, 350
        preoperative preparation for, 350–351
        proximal graft anastomosis in, 356–358, 357f, 359f
        simultaneous distal lower extremity bypass grafting in, 355
        thoracic aorta to femoral artery bypass in, 355
        totally occluded, calcified, and small aortas and, 354, 354f
    endovascular treatment of, 373–382
        adjunctive thrombolysis and percutaneous mechanical thrombectomy with, 384
        angioplasty and stenting in, 386–387, 389
        aortic bifurcation disease and, 380
        aortic occlusion in, 385–387, 386f
        arterial access in, 377–378, 379f
        assessing hemodynamic significance in, 376–377
        brachial artery access in, 35V, 378

Aortoiliac occlusive disease *(Continued)*
        calcification and, 377, 377f
        common iliac artery occlusion in, 387, 388f
        complications in, 390
        concomitant common femoral artery disease and, 377–378, 379f
        crossing iliac artery lesion in, 378, 385–386
        embolization, dissection, and rupture in, 385, 389–390
        external iliac artery occlusion in, 388–389, 389f
        indications for, 373, 374f, 375t
        initial intraoperative imaging in, 376
        lesions above aortic bifurcation and, 377
        outcomes in, 383, 384t
        postoperative care in, 382, 390
        preoperative preparation for, 375–376, 383–384
        reentry catheters and, 378–380, 381f
        selection of balloon stent dimensions in, 380–381
        unfavorable anatomic features in, 384
    extraanatomic repair of, 362–372
        aortoiliac embolectomy in, 369–371, 370f
        axillofemoral bypass in, 364–367, 365f–366f
        femoral-femoral bypass in, 363, 363f
        preoperative preparation for, 362
        thoracofemoral bypass in, 367–368, 368f
    spine exposure in, 392–402
        complications in, 400–401, 400t
        L2 to S1, 397–399, 398f–399f
        operative strategy in, 394–395
        pitfalls and danger points in, 393–394
        postoperative care in, 399–400
        preoperative preparation for, 392–393
        T12 to L2, 396–397
        thoracic, 395–396

Aortorenal bypass, 439–441, 440f
Aortouniiliac graft, 330–332, 331f, 341
Argon Option filter, 629t, 630f
Arm, fasciotomy of, 623, 623f
Arm claudication, 194
Arm edema
    after arteriovenous fistula, 737
    after arteriovenous graft, 745, 746f
Arm ischemia
    after endovascular treatment of descending thoracic artery aneurysm, 255
    after endovascular treatment of traumatic thoracic aortic disruption, 294
Arterial access
    in carotid angioplasty and stenting, 100
    in endovascular treatment
        of aortic dissection, 278
        of aortoiliac occlusive disease, 377–378, 379f
        of descending thoracic aortic aneurysm, 258, 259f–261f
        of infrarenal aortic aneurysm, 324–325
        of subclavian-axillary vein thrombosis, 208
        of traumatic thoracic artery disruption, 291
Arterial bypass graft
    carotid-carotid artery, 144, 145f
    carotid-subclavian artery, 144, 145f
    in endovascular treatment of aortic dissection, 284–285, 285b, 286f
    for vascular access, 34
    in vascular reconstruction, 5–6
Arterial closure device, 37–38, 38f–39f
Arterial dissection
    angioplasty-related, 51, 60
    during endovascular repair
        of femoral-popliteal arterial occlusive disease, 579
        of infrarenal aortic aneurysm, 332
        of tibial-peroneal arterial occlusive disease, 596

INDEX

Arterial injury
  in brachial artery-axillary vein interposition graft, 740
  in varicose vein stripping, 686–687, 692
Arterial lesion, popliteal artery entrapment and, 574
Arterial occlusion after sclerotherapy, 726
Arterial perforation in angioplasty, 61
Arterial puncture, ultrasound-guided, 20–22, 21f
Arterial spasm, carotid angioplasty and stenting and, 87, 98–99
Arterial steal syndrome
  after arteriovenous fistula, 737–738
  after arteriovenous graft, 745
Arterial thrombosis
  after vascular reconstruction, 15
  in endovascular treatment of femoral-popliteal arterial occlusive disease, 580
Arterial transposition, carotid-subclavian artery
  in aberrant right subclavian artery repair, 166
  in extraanatomic repair of aortic arch vessels, 139–140, 142–143, 143V, 143f–144f
Arteriography
  in popliteal artery aneurysm, 563, 566
  in visceral artery aneurysms, 501
Arteriolar occlusion after sclerotherapy, 726
Arteriotomy, 8, 9f
  in carotid endarterectomy, 70, 71f
  in distal revascularization interval ligation, 776–778, 777f–778f
Arteriovenous anastomosis
  in brachial vein transposition, 762, 762f
  in saphenous vein transposition, 764, 765f
Arteriovenous fistula
  after endovenous thermal ablation of saphenous and perforating veins, 706
  after percutaneous access, 40
  brachiocephalic, 734–735
    complications in, 736–738
    exposure of brachial artery in, 735, 736f
    exposure of cephalic vein in, 734–735
    incision in, 734, 735f
    postoperative care in, 736
  radial artery-cephalic vein, 729–738
    alternatives in absence of suitable cephalic vein and, 732
    anesthesia for, 732
    arteriovenous anastomosis in, 733–734
    confirmation of flow and closure in, 734, 734f
    exposure of cephalic vein in, 733
    exposure of radial artery in, 733
    heparinization in, 732
    incisions in, 732–733, 733f
    indications for, 730–731
    operative field in, 732
    preoperative preparation for, 731
    selection of fistula site for, 732
  in reconstruction of inferior vena cava and iliofemoral venous system, 653, 654f, 662
Arteriovenous graft
  brachial-axillary, 739–746
    anastomoses in, 743, 744f
    complications in, 744–746, 746f
    incision in, 742–743
    indications for, 739
    postoperative care in, 743–744
    preoperative preparation for, 739–740, 740f–741f
    selection of arteriovenous graft in, 741
    selection of sites for venous outflow and arterial inflow in, 741
  forearm loop, 739–746
    anastomoses in, 742
    complications in, 744–746, 746f
    confirmation of flow and closure in, 742
    incision in, 742
    indications for, 739

Arteriovenous graft (Continued)
  postoperative care in, 743–744
  preoperative preparation for, 739–740, 740f–741f
  selection of sites for venous outflow and arterial inflow in, 741
  tunneling of graft in, 742, 743f
Arteriovenous graft thrombosis, 745, 781–792
  complications in, 790
  endovascular treatment of, 784, 785f
    closure in, 787
    lyse-and-go technique in, 786
    preoperative preparation for, 784–785
    removal of residual clot in, 786–787, 787f
    sheath placement in, 785f, 786
    use of covered stents in, 786
  hybrid interventions for, 787, 787f–788f
    closure in, 789
    endovascular intervention in, 789, 789f
    incision in, 788
    thrombectomy in, 788–789, 788f
  postoperative care in, 790
  surgical intervention in, 781
    anesthesia and incision in, 782–783
    closure in, 784
    operative strategy for, 782, 783f
    preoperative preparation for, 781–782
    revision of distal venous anastomosis in, 784, 784f
    thrombectomy in, 783
Artery, average diameters of, 57t
Artificial valve implantation, 714–715
Ascending aorta-bilateral carotid artery bypass, 134–135, 135f–137f
Ascending aorta-innominate artery bypass, 132–134, 132f–134f
Ascites, transjugular intrahepatic portosystemic shunt and, 664, 671
Aspirin, preoperative
  in aortoiliac occlusive disease endovascular repair, 375
  in carotid angioplasty and stenting, 86
  in carotid endarterectomy, 64
  in mesenteric ischemia endovascular treatment, 498
  in subclavian and axillary artery endovascular treatment, 149
  in tibial-peroneal arterial occlusive disease, 544
Atherectomy device, 59, 59b
Atheroembolism, renal, 437, 447
Atheroma, embolization of, 14–15
Atherosclerosis
  of aortic arch vessels
    direct surgical repair of, 126
    endovascular treatment of, 148–149
    extraanatomic repair of, 139
  aortoiliac occlusive disease and, 350
  chronic mesenteric ischemia and, 491
  vertebral artery surgery for, 111
Atherosclerotic plaque, guidewire crossing of, 47–48, 47f–48f
Atherosclerotic waist, 55–56, 56f
Autogenous vein cuff in femoral-popliteal bypass, 533, 533f
Autologous neovalve construction, 713
Axial veins, endovenous thermal ablation of, 702–703
Axillary anastomosis in axillofemoral bypass, 366–367
Axillary artery
  access to, 34
  average diameter of, 57t
  exposure in subclavian artery aneurysm repair, 162–163, 164f
  injury in extraanatomic repair of aortoiliac occlusive disease, 362
  stenting of, 155
  surgical anatomy of, 158–159
Axillary artery surgery, 157–170
  aberrant right subclavian artery and, 159–160, 159f–160f
  avoiding brachial plexus injuries in, 161

Axillary artery surgery (Continued)
  avoiding injuries behind clavicle in, 161
  avoiding thoracic duct injuries in, 160–161
  avoiding vertebral artery injuries in, 161
  in Kommerell diverticulum repair, 167, 168f
  postoperative care in, 168–169
  postoperative complications in, 169
  preoperative preparation for, 157–158, 158f
  in repair of aberrant right subclavian artery, 165–166, 165f
  selection of conduit in, 161–162
  in subclavian artery aneurysm, 162–165, 163f–164f
  surgical anatomy in, 158–159
Axillary vein
  endovascular therapy for subclavian-axillary vein thrombosis and, 204–214, 205f
    access in, 208
    angiographic anatomy and collaterals in, 205–206, 206f–207f
    angioplasty and stenting in, 212
    completion studies in, 212
    complications in, 213
    postoperative care in, 212–213
    preoperative preparation for, 204–205
    sheath placement in, 208
    technique in, 208–212, 209f
    thrombolysis in, 209–212, 210f–211f
    timing of, 206–208, 208f
  injury in extraanatomic repair of aortoiliac occlusive disease, 362
Axillobifemoral extraanatomic bypass graft, 409, 410f
Axillofemoral bypass, 364–367, 365f–366f
Axillosuperficial femoral artery extraanatomic bypass graft, 409, 411f

B

Bair Hugger, 752
Balloon angioplasty, 52, 52f, 53t
  in tibial-peroneal arterial occlusive disease, 594
Balloon catheter
  in femoral-popliteal arterial occlusive disease, 582–583, 583f
  in renal artery stenosis repair, 460
  in thoracoabdominal aortic aneurysm surgery, 218, 223, 224f
  for vascular control in abdominal aortic aneurysm surgery, 300
Balloon stent, 58f
  in aortoiliac occlusive disease, 380–381
  in mesenteric ischemia, 496, 497f
  in renal artery stenosis repair, 461
Bard Eclipse filter, 629t, 630f
Bard Meridian filter, 629t, 630f
Bard Recovery G2 filter, 629t, 630f
Bard Simon Nitinol filter, 629t, 630f
Baroreflex failure after carotid body tumor surgery, 109
Basilic vein, 205, 206f
  access to, 35
  for femoral-popliteal bypass, 534–535
Basilic vein transposition, 747–757
  choice of one- or two-stage procedure in, 748, 749f
  complications in, 751
  harvest of basilic vein in, 748, 749f
  indications for, 747
  postoperative care in, 750–751
  preoperative preparation for, 747
  single-stage procedure in, 751
  steal syndrome and, 748
  superficialization of fistula in, 750
  two-stage procedure in, 748–750
  use of radial artery in, 750
Bedside transabdominal or intravascular ultrasound, percutaneous vena cava filter placement with, 635

Below-knee amputation, 605–607, 606f
Below-knee femoral-popliteal bypass, 537
Below-knee popliteal bypass, 537
Benign ileofemoral venous occlusion, 650
Beveled end-to-side anastomosis, 8–10, 10f
Bilateral axilloproximal superficial femoral artery extraanatomic bypass graft, 409, 410f
Bilateral venous reconstruction in superior vena cava syndrome, 644
Bipolar electrocautery of carotid body tumor, 104
Bird's Nest filter, 629t, 630f
Bladder injury in extraanatomic repair of aortoiliac occlusive disease, 363
Bleeding
  in aortic graft infection
    neoaortoiliac system procedure for, 424–425
    total graft excision and extraanatomic repair of, 407
  intraoperative
    in endovascular repair of infrarenal aortic aneurysm, 332
    in iliofemoral and femoral-popliteal deep vein thrombosis repair, 674
    in reconstruction of inferior vena cava and iliofemoral venous system, 653–654
    in superior vena cava syndrome reconstruction, 643
  postoperative
    in abdominal aortic aneurysm surgery, 307
    in aortoiliac occlusive disease, 358
    in femoral-popliteal bypass, 541
    in renal artery stenosis, 464
    in subclavian-axillary vein thrombosis, 213
    in thoracic outlet syndrome, 190
  risk in vascular access, 30
  vascular surgery-related, 15
Blood pressure
  access site management and, 36, 36t
  control in acute aortic dissection, 275
  control in traumatic thoracic aortic disruption, 290
Blood vessels
  angioplasty-related rupture of, 51
  exposure and control in vascular surgery, 6, 7f
Boston Scientific Greenfield filters, 629t, 630f
Botulinum toxin A for thoracic outlet syndrome, 194–195
Bowel injury in extraanatomic repair of aortoiliac occlusive disease, 363
Bowel ischemia in abdominal aortic aneurysm surgery, 297
Brachial artery
  access to, 33–34, 35f
    in endovascular treatment of aortoiliac occlusive disease, 378
  average diameter of, 57t
  distal revascularization interval ligation and, 772–780
    arteriotomy and bypass in, 776–778, 777f–778f
    choice of anesthesia for, 774
    closure in, 778, 778f
    complications in, 779
    conduit in, 774, 776
    dissection of the inflow vessel in, 775–776, 775f
    exposure of distal vessel in, 776, 777f
    historical background of, 772
    incision in, 775, 775f
    indications for, 772–773
    ligation of artery in, 778
    postoperative care in, 779
    preoperative preparation for, 773–774, 774f
    timing of, 774
    tunneling in, 776

Brachial artery-axillary vein interposition graft, 739–746
  anastomoses in, 743, 744f
  complications in, 744–746, 746f
  incision in, 742–743
  indications for, 739
  postoperative care in, 743–744
  preoperative preparation for, 739–740, 740f–741f
  selection of arteriovenous graft in, 741
  selection of sites for venous outflow and arterial inflow in, 741
Brachial plexus injury
  in extraanatomic repair of aortoiliac occlusive disease, 362
  in subclavian and axillary artery surgery, 161
  in supraclavicular approach to thoracic outlet syndrome, 177–178
  in surgical repair of subclavian and axillary arteries, 169
  in transaxillary rib resection for thoracic outlet syndrome, 195–196, 197f
Brachial plexus neurolysis in supraclavicular approach to thoracic outlet syndrome, 176, 185–186
Brachial vein access, 35
Brachial vein transposition, 759t, 760, 762–763, 762f–764f
Brachiocephalic arteriovenous fistula, 734–735
  complications in, 736–738
  exposure of brachial artery in, 735, 736f
  exposure of cephalic vein in, 734–735
  incision in, 734, 735f
  postoperative care in, 736
Brachiocephalic artery, average diameter of, 57t
Bradycardia
  during carotid angioplasty and stenting, 86
  carotid endarterectomy-related, 75
Branch artery preservation in endovascular repair of thoracoabdominal aortic aneurysm, 234–235
Branch vessel disease in renal artery stenosis, 458, 459f
Branched stent graft
  to innominate and left common carotid arteries, 135, 135f
  for repair of aneurysms of juxtarenal and pararenal aorta, 344–346, 345f
  for repair of aortic arch aneurysm, 235–244
  for repair of thoracoabdominal aortic aneurysm, 235
  to right subclavian and carotid arteries, 134, 134f
Braun Vena Tech LP filter, 629t, 630f
Bruising
  after endovenous thermal ablation of saphenous and perforating veins, 705
  after varicose vein stripping, 687–688
Buttock claudication after endovascular repair of infrarenal aortic aneurysm, 334
Bypass procedure
  aortocarotid-subclavian artery, 132–134, 133f
  carotid-brachial artery, 164–165
  carotid-carotid artery, 144, 145f
  carotid-subclavian artery, 144, 145f
  in celiac axis and superior mesenteric artery occlusive disease
    antegrade, 482, 483f, 485f
    retrograde, 485–486, 486f
  in direct surgical repair of aortoiliac occlusive disease
    aortobifemoral, 355–356, 357f
    iliofemoral, 358
    thoracic aorta to femoral artery, 355
  in direct surgical repair of renal artery aneurysm
    aortorenal, 439–441, 440f
    renal artery, 441, 442f

Bypass procedure (Continued)
  in distal revascularization interval ligation, 776–778, 777f–778f
  in endovascular treatment of aortic dissection
    carotid-carotid artery, 284–285, 285b, 286f
    carotid-subclavian artery, 284–285, 285b, 286f
  external iliac to internal iliac artery in repair of infrarenal aortic aneurysm, 333, 333f
  in extraanatomic repair of aortoiliac occlusive disease
    axillofemoral, 364–367, 365f–366f
    femoral-femoral, 363, 363f
    thoracofemoral, 367, 368f
  femoral-femoral venous, 658, 658f
  femoral-popliteal, 525–542
    above-knee, 536–537
    alternate inflow sources in, 538, 539f–540f
    below-knee, 537
    complications in, 541
    femoral-popliteal thromboembolectomy and, 538–539
    indications for, 526
    in situ or reversed great saphenous vein for, 534
    intraoperative assessment of, 537
    open vein harvest for, 534–536
    pitfalls and danger points in, 528–529, 528f
    postoperative care in, 540–541
    preoperative assessment of vein quality in, 533
    preoperative preparation for, 526–528
    selection and assessment of inflow in, 532
    selection and assessment of outflow in, 532
    selection of conduit for, 533–534, 533f
    surgical anatomy of femoral and popliteal arteries in, 529–531, 530f–532f
    wound closure in, 538
  hepatorenal, 450–452, 451f, 453f–454f
  mesenteric, 479
  in popliteal artery aneurysm, 569, 570f
  splenorenal, 453–454
  subclavian-axillary artery, 164
  in surgical repair of celiac artery aneurysm, 510
  in surgical repair of hepatic artery aneurysm, 506
  in tibial-peroneal arterial occlusive disease
    femoral distal artery-vein, 547–548
    femoral-anterior tibial artery, 552–554, 553f–554f
    femoral-peroneal artery, 555–558
    femoral-posterior tibial artery, 555, 557f
  in total graft excision and extraanatomic repair of aortic graft infection, 403–418
    avoiding ureteral injury in, 409
    choice of reconstruction in, 407–408
    closure of femoral arteries in, 416
    closure of proximal aortic stump and omental pedicle flap in, 414–415, 415f
    complications in, 417
    drains in, 416, 416f
    exposure of abdominal aorta in, 414
    exposure of common femoral, superficial femoral, and profunda femoris arteries in, 414
    graft excision in, 414
    historical background of, 404–405, 405f
    incision closure in, 416–417
    incision in, 413–414
    management of duodenal stump in, 415
    postoperative care in, 417
    preoperative preparation for, 405–407, 406f
    presence of aortoenteric fistula and, 409–412, 412f

INDEX

Bypass procedure *(Continued)*
  role of endovascular therapy in, 413, 413f
  sartorius muscle flap in, 416
  selection of extraanatomic bypass in, 409, 410f–411f
  staging of, 408–409
  underlying aneurysmal or occlusive disease and, 412
  in vascular reconstruction, 5–6
Bypass thrombosis after hepatic of celiac revascularization, 510

C

Calcified arteries
  access site management and, 36
  anterior spine exposure and, 393–394
  in aortoiliac occlusive disease, 377, 377f
  in mesenteric ischemia, 495
Cannulation of contralateral gate in endovascular repair of infrarenal aortic aneurysm, 326–328, 328f–329f
Carbon dioxide angiography, 24–26, 25b, 25f–27f
Carbon dioxide venography, 665, 666f, 667–668
Cardiac complications
  abdominal aortic aneurysm surgery-related, 307
  after endovascular repair of infrarenal aortic aneurysm, 334
  after juxtarenal and pararenal abdominal aortic aneurysms repair, 319
  carotid angioplasty and stenting-related, 100
  carotid endarterectomy-related, 74
Cardiac disease, direct surgical repair of aortic arch vessels and, 128
Cardiac evaluation, 4
  in aortoiliac occlusive disease, 351
  in descending thoracic artery aneurysm, 252
  in femoral-popliteal arterial occlusive disease, 527
  before reconstruction of inferior vena cava and iliofemoral venous system, 651
  in thoracoabdominal aortic aneurysm, 217
  in tibial-peroneal arterial occlusive disease, 543–544
  before transjugular intrahepatic portosystemic shunt, 664
Carotid angioplasty and stenting, 86–101
  access in, 90–91
  angiographic anatomy and, 87, 88t
  angiography of aortic arch, carotid, and cerebral circulation in, 92
  angioplasty technique in, 97V, 97–98
  aortic arch anatomy and, 88, 89f
  carotid lesions at risk for embolization and, 88
  catheterization of common carotid artery in, 91, 91f–92f
  cerebral protection devices and, 90
  completion studies in, 98
  crossing lesion and cerebral protection in, 95–97, 95f, 97f
  fibromuscular dysplasia and, 89–90
  indications for, 86, 87t
  kinks and coils of carotid artery and, 88
  management of arterial spasm, embolization, and acute occlusion in, 98–99
  neurorescue techniques in, 99–100
  occluded external carotid artery and, 88, 90f
  postoperative care in, 100
  postoperative complications in, 100–101
  preoperative care in, 86
  redo carotid angioplasty and, 90
  selection of stent for, 90
  severe stenosis and string sign and, 88–89
  sheath placement for planned intervention in, 92–95, 93f–94f
  stenting technique in, 98, 99f
  tandem lesions in common carotid artery and, 89

Carotid body tumor, 102–110
  avoiding cranial nerve injuries in, 103–104
  avoiding intraoperative stroke in, 104
  bipolar electrocautery in, 104
  classification and surgical anatomy of, 103, 103t
  exposure of carotid bifurcation in, 104–108, 105f
  incision for, 104, 105f
  postoperative care in, 108–109
  postoperative complications in, 109
  preoperative embolization in, 104
  preoperative preparation in, 102
  resection of Shamblin type I, 105, 106f
  resection of Shamblin type II/III, 107–108, 107f–108f
Carotid endarterectomy, 63–76
  anesthesia in, 67
  arteriotomy and shunt placement in, 70, 71f
  avoiding cranial nerve injuries in, 66–67
  avoiding intraoperative stroke in, 65–66
  closure in, 73–74
  complications in, 74–75
  concurrent with surgical repair of aortic arch vessels, 135, 136f–137f
  endarterectomy in, 70–73, 72f–73f
  exposure of common carotid artery in, 67, 69f
  exposure of distal internal carotid artery in, 70, 71f
  incision and position in, 67, 68f
  indications for, 64
  isolation of external carotid artery in, 68–70
  isolation of internal carotid artery in, 70
  mobilization of jugular vein and division of common facial vein in, 67, 69f
  mobilization of sternocleidomastoid muscle in, 67
  patch angioplasty in, 73, 73f
  postoperative care in, 74
  preoperative preparation in, 64–65
Carotid patch aneurysm, 85
Carotid patch infection, 85
Carotid shunt in carotid endarterectomy, 65
Carotid stenosis, carotid endarterectomy-related, 75
Carotid-brachial artery bypass, 164–165
Carotid-carotid artery bypass, 144, 145f, 284–285, 285b, 286f
Carotid-subclavian artery bypass, 144, 145f
  in endovascular treatment of aortic dissection, 279–280, 281b, 284–285, 285b, 286f
Carotid-subclavian artery transposition, 142–143, 142f, 143V, 144f
CAS. *See* Carotid angioplasty and stenting
Catheter manipulation in endovascular therapy, 41–49
  avoiding and managing subintimal guidewire in, 46
  catheter selection in, 43–46, 44t, 45f, 47f
  crossing of occlusion in, 47–48, 47f–48f
  crossing of stenosis in, 46
  guidewire handling and, 43, 44f
  guidewire selection and, 41–42, 42t, 43f
Catheter-directed thrombolysis in iliofemoral and femoral-popliteal deep vein thrombosis, 675–676
C-clamp type device, 37, 37f
CEAP classification of chronic venous disease, 694, 695f
Celect filter, 629t, 630f
Celiac artery
  anatomy of, 502, 503f
  endovascular treatment of aortic dissection and, 283
  endovascular treatment of descending thoracic artery aneurysm and, 256–257
Celiac artery aneurysm, 506, 508f–509f
Celiac axis
  arterial access to, 515
  surgical anatomy of, 478

Celiac axis occlusive disease, 475–490
  antegrade bypass in, 482–485, 483f, 485f
  approach to superior mesenteric artery in, 480–481, 480f–481f
  complications in, 488–489
  indications for, 476–477
  ischemia secondary to embolization, in situ thrombosis, and dissection and, 478–479
  postoperative care in, 488
  preoperative preparation for, 477
  retrograde bypass in, 485–486, 486f
  selection of celiac artery outflow in, 479–480
  selection of conduit in, 481–482
  selection of inflow source in, 479
  superior mesenteric artery embolectomy in, 487–488, 487f
  surgical anatomy for, 478
Celiac trunk, average diameter of, 57t
Central metatarsal ray resection, 612–613, 615f
Central venous catheter, vena cava filter placement and, 630
Central venous stenosis, brachial artery-axillary vein interposition graft-related, 740–741
Cephalic vein, 205, 206f
  brachiocephalic arteriovenous fistula and, 734–735
    complications in, 736–738
    exposure of brachial artery in, 735, 736f
    exposure of cephalic vein in, 734–735
    incision in, 734, 735f
    postoperative care in, 736
  for femoral-popliteal bypass, 534–535
  radial artery-cephalic vein arteriovenous fistula and, 729–738
    alternatives in absence of suitable cephalic vein and, 732
    anesthesia for, 732
    arteriovenous anastomosis in, 733–734
    confirmation of flow and closure in, 734, 734f
    exposure of cephalic vein in, 733
    exposure of radial artery in, 733
    heparinization in, 732
    incisions in, 732–733, 733f
    indications for, 730–731
    operative field in, 732
    preoperative preparation for, 731
    selection of fistula site for, 732
Cerebral hyperperfusion syndrome
  carotid angioplasty and stenting-related, 75
  carotid endarterectomy-related, 75
Cerebral protection
  in aortic arch vessels endovascular treatment, 150
  in carotid angioplasty and stenting, 90, 95–97, 95f, 97f
Cerebrospinal fluid pressure
  after endovascular treatment of aortic dissection, 287
  after thoracoabdominal aortic aneurysm surgery, 228
Cerebrovascular disease, extracranial
  carotid angioplasty and stenting in, 86–101
    access in, 90–91
    angiographic anatomy and, 87, 88t
    angiography of aortic arch, carotid, and cerebral circulation in, 92
    angioplasty technique in, 97V, 97–98
    aortic arch anatomy and, 88, 89f
    carotid lesions at risk for embolization and, 88
    catheterization of common carotid artery in, 91, 91f–92f
    cerebral protection devices and, 90
    completion studies in, 98
    crossing lesion and cerebral protection in, 95–97, 95f, 97f
    fibromuscular dysplasia and, 89–90
    indications for, 86, 87t

Cerebrovascular disease, extracranial *(Continued)*
    kinks and coils of carotid artery and, 88
    management of arterial spasm, embolization, and acute occlusion in, 98–99
    neurorescue techniques in, 99–100
    occluded external carotid artery and, 88, 90f
    postoperative care in, 100
    postoperative complications in, 100–101
    preoperative care in, 86
    redo carotid angioplasty and, 90
    selection of stent for, 90
    severe stenosis and string sign and, 88–89
    sheath placement for planned intervention in, 92–95, 93f–94f
    stenting technique in, 98, 99f
    tandem lesions in common carotid artery and, 89
  carotid body tumor and, 102–110
    avoiding cranial nerve injuries in, 103–104
    avoiding intraoperative stroke in, 104
    bipolar electrocautery in, 104
    classification and surgical anatomy of, 103, 103t
    exposure of carotid bifurcation in, 104–108, 105f
    incision for, 104, 105f
    postoperative care in, 108–109
    postoperative complications in, 109
    preoperative embolization in, 104
    preoperative preparation in, 102
    resection of Shamblin type I, 105, 106f
    resection of Shamblin type II/III, 107–108, 107f–108f
  carotid endarterectomy in, 63–76
    anesthesia in, 67
    arteriotomy and shunt placement in, 70, 71f
    avoiding cranial nerve injuries in, 66–67
    avoiding intraoperative stroke in, 65–66
    closure in, 73–74
    complications in, 74–75
    endarterectomy in, 70–73, 72f–73f
    exposure of common carotid artery in, 67, 69f
    exposure of distal internal carotid artery in, 70, 71f
    incision and position in, 67, 68f
    indications for, 64
    isolation of external carotid artery in, 68–70
    isolation of internal carotid artery in, 70
    mobilization of jugular vein and division of common facial vein in, 67, 69f
    mobilization of sternocleidomastoid muscle in, 67
    patch angioplasty in, 73, 73f
    postoperative care in, 74
    preoperative preparation in, 64–65
  eversion endarterectomy in, 77–85, 78V
    anastomosis of internal to common carotid artery in, 80–82, 82f
    in carotid patch aneurysm, 85
    complications in, 84
    endarterectomy of common carotid artery in, 80
    endarterectomy of internal carotid artery in, 80, 81f
    exposure of carotid artery in, 78–80, 79f, 81f
    in fibromuscular dysplasia, 84
    indications for, 77
    in infected carotid patch, 85
    for kinks and coils in internal carotid artery, 84
    operative strategy in, 78
    postoperative care in, 82–84
    preoperative preparation for, 77–78
    in recurrent carotid stenosis, 84–85
    shunting during, 82, 83f

Cerebrovascular disease, extracranial *(Continued)*
  vertebral artery surgery in, 111–112
    exposure and transposition of vertebral artery into common carotid artery in, 116–118, 117f, 118V, 119f
    exposure of V2 segment of vertebral artery in, 118–122, 120f–123f
    indications for, 111–112, 112b
    operative strategy in, 114
    postoperative care in, 122
    postoperative complications in, 122–124
    preoperative preparation for, 113f, 112–114, 113b, 113f, 115f
    surgical anatomy in, 114–116, 116f
    V3 exposure and distal vertebral artery reconstruction in, 118–122, 120f–123f
Cervical rib
  resection in supraclavicular approach to thoracic outlet syndrome, 176–177, 184–185, 185f
  subclavian artery aneurysm and, 162, 163f
  thoracic outlet syndrome and, 196
Chest radiography
  in superior vena cava syndrome, 642
  before supraclavicular approach to thoracic outlet syndrome, 172
  in traumatic thoracic aortic disruption, 290, 291t
Child, unconventional hemodialysis access and, 760
Child-Pugh score, 664
Chimney stent
  for aneurysms of juxtarenal and pararenal aorta, 346–347, 347f
  for thoracoabdominal aortic aneurysm, 235
Chronic mesenteric ischemia
  direct surgical repair for, 475–490
    antegrade bypass in, 482–485, 483f, 485f
    approach to superior mesenteric artery in, 480–481, 480f–481f
    complications in, 488–489
    indications for, 476–477
    ischemia secondary to embolization, in situ thrombosis, and dissection and, 478–479
    postoperative care in, 488
    preoperative preparation for, 477
    retrograde bypass in, 485–486, 486f
    selection of celiac artery outflow in, 479–480
    selection of conduit in, 481–482
    selection of inflow source in, 479
    superior mesenteric artery embolectomy in, 487–488, 487f
    surgical anatomy for, 478
  endovascular treatment of, 491–499
    complications in, 498
    indications for, 491–492
    pitfalls and danger points in, 493–495, 495f
    postoperative care in, 498
    preoperative preparation for, 492–493, 493f–494f
    strategy in, 495–496, 495f
    technique in, 496, 497f
Chronic venous disease
  after neoaortoiliac system procedure for aortic graft infection, 425
  deep venous valve surgery in, 708–720
    angioscope-assisted valvuloplasty in, 712
    artificial valve implantation in, 714–715
    autologous neovalve construction in, 713
    complications in, 719
    external banding valvuloplasty in, 712
    external valvuloplasty in, 711
    indications for, 708
    internal valvuloplasty in, 711, 712f
    operative strategy in, 710
    pitfalls and danger points in, 709–710
    postoperative care in, 718
    preoperative preparation for, 709
    transcommissural valvuloplasty in, 712

Chronic venous disease *(Continued)*
    vein segment transposition in, 713
    vein valve transplantation in, 708, 713–714
  endovenous thermal ablation of saphenous and perforating veins in, 694–707
    access in, 699, 700f
    complications in, 705–706, 706f
    confirmation of catheter tip position in, 701, 701f
    endovascular strategy in, 696–699, 698f
    endovenous laser in, 700
    indications for, 695f, 696
    patient positioning for, 699
    postoperative care in, 704–705
    preoperative preparation for, 696, 697f
    radiofrequency catheter in, 699–700, 700f
    treatment of axial veins in, 702–703
    treatment of perforator veins in, 703–704, 704f
    tumescent anesthesia in, 701, 702f
  inferior vena cava and iliofemoral venous system reconstruction surgery in, 650–663
    anatomy in, 656
    choice of incision for, 656–657, 657f
    complications in, 662–663
    femoral-femoral venous bypass in, 658, 658f
    ileocaval venous bypass in, 658–659, 659f
    indications for, 650, 651b
    inferior vena cava reconstruction in, 659–662, 660f
    pitfalls and danger points in, 653–656, 654f–656f
    postoperative care in, 662
    preoperative preparation for, 650–653, 652f–653f
    resection of suprarenal inferior vena cava in conjunction with major liver resection in, 657
  sclerotherapy in, 721–728
    complications in, 725–726
    foaming of sclerosant solution in, 724V, 724
    injection of target vein in, 724V, 724, 725f
    patient positioning for, 724
    postoperative care in, 724–725
    preoperative preparation for, 721–722
    selection of sclerosant solution in, 723, 723t
    sequence of treatment of superficial veins and, 723
  sequence of treatment of, 722
  subfascial endoscopic perforator surgery in, 708–720
    choice of anesthesia for, 715
    deep venous valve surgery in, 719
    distal ankle perforators and, 718
    exploration of subfascial space in, 716, 717f–718f
    incision in, 715–716, 715b, 715f
    indications for, 708
    operative strategy in, 710–711
    paratibial fasciotomy in, 716
    pitfalls and danger points in, 709–710
    port insertion in, 716, 716f
    postoperative care in, 718–719
    preoperative preparation for, 709
  superior vena cava syndrome reconstruction surgery in, 641–649
    anastomoses in, 645–648, 647f–648f
    anesthesia for, 644
    avoiding intraoperative bleeding in, 643
    avoiding pulmonary embolism in, 644
    closure of median sternotomy in, 648
    complications in, 648–649, 649t
    dissection of innominate veins and superior vena cava in, 645
    indications for, 641

Chronic venous disease *(Continued)*
  position and incision in, 645
  postoperative care in, 648
  preoperative preparation for, 641–643, 642f–643f
  selection of vascular conduit for, 644, 644t
  selection of venous inflow and outflow sites in, 644
  spiral vein graft in, 645, 646f
  unilateral *versus* bilateral, 644
Chylothorax
  after extraanatomic aortic arch vessel repair, 146
  after vertebral artery surgery, 123–124
  subclavian artery exposure and, 160–161
Cimino radiocephalic arteriovenous fistula, 732–734
  arteriovenous anastomosis in, 733–734
  confirmation of flow and closure in, 734, 734f
  exposure of cephalic vein in, 733
  exposure of radial artery in, 733
  incisions in, 732–733, 733f
CIN. *See* Contrast-induced nephropathy
Clavicle injury in subclavian and axillary artery surgery, 161
Clopidogrel
  in aortic arch vessels endovascular treatment, 149
  in aortoiliac occlusive disease endovascular repair, 375
  in carotid angioplasty and stenting, 86
  in carotid endarterectomy, 64
  in femoral-popliteal arterial occlusive disease, 587
  in mesenteric ischemia, 498
  in renal artery stenosis endovascular repair, 375
  in tibial-peroneal arterial occlusive disease, 544
Clot embolization in arteriovenous graft thrombosis treatment, 785
Coagulation, access site management and, 30, 31t
Coagulopathy
  after mesenteric revascularization, 488
  thoracoabdominal aortic aneurysm surgery and, 218
Coaxial balloon catheter, 52, 52f
  in repair of rental artery stenosis, 460
Cobra 2 catheter, 45f
Coil embolization, 59–60, 59f
  in endovascular repair
    of infrarenal aorta type II endoleak, 341
    of tibial-peroneal arterial occlusive disease, 596
  in hepatic artery aneurysm repair, 515–516
  in renal artery aneurysm repair, 470, 471f
  in splenic artery aneurysm repair, 517–521
Collateral vessels
  of aortic arch vessels, 149
  endovascular therapy for subclavian-axillary vein thrombosis and, 205–206, 206f–207f
  endovascular treatment of tibial-peroneal arterial occlusive disease and, 591
  varicose vein stripping and, 686–687, 687f
Colon ischemia
  abdominal aortic aneurysm surgery-related, 307
  after total graft excision and extraanatomic repair of aortic graft infection, 412
Colonic perfusion, abdominal aortic aneurysm surgery and, 300
Common carotid artery
  ascending aorta-bilateral carotid artery bypass and, 134–135, 135f–137f
  average diameter of, 57t
  carotid angioplasty and stenting and
    anatomic and pathologic conditions in, 88t
    catheterization of, 91, 91f–92f
    tandem lesions in, 89

Common carotid artery *(Continued)*
  carotid endarterectomy and, 67, 69f
  direct surgical repair of aortic arch vessels and, 127
  endovascular treatment of, 148–156
    access of lesions in, 150
    angiographic anatomy in, 149
    complications in, 155–156
    embolic protection devices in, 150
    imaging and selective catheterization in, 152–153
    lesion predilation in, 150
    postoperative care in, 155
    preoperative preparation for, 149
    protection of vertebral artery in, 150–151
    stent selection in, 150, 151f
    stenting in, 155
  eversion endarterectomy and, 78V, 80, 82f
  exposure and transposition of vertebral artery into, 116–118, 117f, 118V, 119f
  surgical anatomy for extraanatomic repair of aortic arch vessels, 141, 142f
Common facial vein, carotid endarterectomy and, 67, 69f
Common femoral artery
  for above-knee popliteal bypass, 536
  access to, 29, 32, 33f
    in carotid angioplasty and stenting, 90–91
  average diameter of, 57t
  endarterectomy of, 528–529, 532
  endovascular treatment of femoral-popliteal arterial occlusive disease and, 580, 581f
  exposure in total graft excision and extraanatomic repair of aortic graft infection, 414
  surgical anatomy of, 529–531, 530f
  surgical repair of tibial-peroneal arterial occlusive disease and, 548–551
Common femoral artery disease, aortoiliac occlusive disease with, 377–378, 379f
Common femoral vein
  access to, 34–35
  as inflow source in reconstruction of inferior vena cava and iliofemoral venous system, 653, 654f
  injury in varicose vein stripping, 686
Common hepatic artery, 502
  as outflow vessel in antegrade bypass in mesenteric ischemia, 479–480
Common iliac aneurysm, 338–340
Common iliac artery
  average diameter of, 57t
  exposure in retrograde bypass in mesenteric ischemia, 485
  occlusion during endovascular treatment of aortoiliac occlusive disease, 387, 388f
Common peroneal nerve, compartment syndrome and, 618
Common peroneal vein injury in varicose vein stripping, 686
Compartment syndrome
  after neoaortoiliac system procedure for aortic graft infection, 425
  after surgical repair of popliteal artery aneurysm, 567
  fasciotomy for, 617–626
    complications in, 624
    failure to release extremity compartments and, 618
    iatrogenic injury and, 618–619
    inadequate postoperative surveillance and, 619
    indications for, 617–618
    lower leg, 619, 619–621, 619f, 621f–622f
    postoperative care in, 624
    preoperative preparation for, 618
    thigh, 622–623
    unrecognized compartment syndrome and, 618
  femoral vein transposition and, 752, 755–756

Completion studies
  in carotid angioplasty and stenting, 98
  in endovascular therapy for subclavian-axillary vein thrombosis, 212
  in endovascular treatment of mesenteric ischemia, 496
  in popliteal artery aneurysm repair, 602
  in renal artery angioplasty and stenting, 464
  in splenic artery aneurysm repair, 523
  in transjugular intrahepatic portosystemic shunt, 669, 670f
Complex catheter-based vascular access for hemodialysis, 767–770, 768f–769f
CompressAR StrongArm device, 37, 37f
Compression and closure devices, 36–38
  activity restrictions and, 37
  anticoagulation and, 36–37
  blood pressure and, 36, 36t
  external, 37, 37f
  manual compression technique in, 36
Compression therapy
  after endovenous thermal ablation of saphenous and perforating veins, 705
  after reconstruction of inferior vena cava and iliofemoral venous system, 662
  after sclerotherapy, 725
Computed tomography
  in acute aortic dissection, 275
  of carotid body tumor, 102
  in descending thoracic aortic aneurysm, 262
  in descending thoracic artery aneurysm, 252–253, 253f
  in infrarenal aortic aneurysm, 321–322
  in popliteal artery entrapment, 572
  before reconstruction of inferior vena cava and iliofemoral venous system, 650–651, 652f
  in thoracoabdominal aortic aneurysm, 233–234
  before total graft excision and extraanatomic repair of aortic graft infection, 406, 406f
  in vena cava filter placement, 630–631
Computed tomography angiography
  before abdominal aortic aneurysm surgery, 296
  in aortic dissection, 278–279
  in aortoiliac occlusive disease, 351, 375
  in mesenteric ischemia, 493–495, 493f–494f
  in popliteal artery aneurysm, 562–563, 562f
  in renal artery aneurysm, 466–467, 467f–468f
  before spine exposure, 393
  in superior vena cava syndrome, 642, 643f
  in tibial-peroneal arterial occlusive disease, 591
  in traumatic thoracic aortic disruption, 289–290
  in visceral artery aneurysms, 501
Conduit
  covered stent graft or iliac limb as, 325
  in direct surgical repair for acute mesenteric ischemia, 481–482
  in distal revascularization interval ligation, 774, 776
  in endovascular repair of infrarenal aortic aneurysm, 324–325
  in extraanatomic repair in renovascular disease, 450
  in femoral-popliteal bypass, 533–534, 533f
  in reconstruction of inferior vena cava and iliofemoral venous system, 654
  in in situ repair of aortic graft infection, 420
  in subclavian and axillary artery surgery, 161–162
  in surgical repair of popliteal artery, 565
  in surgical repair of tibial-peroneal arterial occlusive disease, 544–545

Consent
  before anterior spine exposure, 393
  before endovascular popliteal artery aneurysm repair, 599
Contrast media, 22-26
  in carbon dioxide angiography, 24-26, 25b, 25f-27f
  injection techniques in fluoroscopy, 19, 19t
  reactions to, 23, 24t
  renal dysfunction considerations in, 22-23, 22b, 23t
Contrast venography in percutaneous vena cava filter placement, 632-633
Contrast-induced nephropathy, 22, 22b
  aortoiliac occlusive disease and, 376
Cook Medical Bird's Nest filter, 629t, 630f
Cook Medical Celect filter, 629t, 630f
Cook Medical Günther Tulip filter, 629t, 630f
Cordis OPTEASE filter, 629t, 630f
Coronary artery bypass, direct surgical repair of aortic arch vessels and, 128
Covered stent in arteriovenous graft thrombosis, 786
Cranial nerve injury
  during carotid body tumor surgery, 103-104
  during carotid endarterectomy, 66-67
Crawford classification of thoracoabdominal aortic aneurysms, 217, 217f
Critical ischemia of hand, 194
Critical limb ischemia
  direct surgical repair of tibial-peroneal arterial occlusive disease in, 543-560
    anastomotic technique in, 546-547, 547f
    complications in, 558-559
    femoral distal artery-vein bypass grafting in, 547-548
    femoral-anterior tibial artery bypass in, 552-554, 553f-554f
    femoral-peroneal artery bypass in, 555-558
    femoral-posterior tibial artery bypass in, 555, 557f
    indications for, 543
    inflow exposure at femoral and popliteal arteries in, 548-551, 549f-551f
    instrumentation and tunnelers for, 546
    lower extremity fasciotomy in, 558
    open ulcer and, 545-546
    pitfalls and danger points in, 544
    postoperative care in, 558
    preoperative preparation for, 543-544
    proximal and distal control in, 546
    selection and assessment of site for distal anastomosis in, 545
    selection and assessment of site for inflow in, 545
    selection of conduit for, 544-545
  endovascular treatment of femoral-popliteal arterial occlusive disease in, 578-589
    access selection in, 580
    angiographic anatomy and common collateral pathways in, 580, 581f
    angiography of lower extremity in, 582
    complications in, 587
    femoral-popliteal artery occlusions and, 585-586
    femoral-popliteal artery stenosis and, 582-585, 583f-585f
    indications for, 578, 579b, 579t
    postoperative care in, 587
    preoperative preparation for, 578-579
    retrograde and antegrade approaches for arterial access in, 581-582
    stent selection in, 580-581
    thrombolysis of acute femoral-popliteal artery occlusions and, 586-587
    unfavorable anatomic features for, 580
  open surgical bypass in femoral-popliteal arterial occlusive disease in, 525-542
    above-knee bypass in, 536-537

Critical limb ischemia (Continued)
    alternate inflow sources in, 538, 539f-540f
    below-knee bypass in, 537
    complications in, 541
    femoral-popliteal thromboembolectomy and, 538-539
    indications for, 526
    in situ or reversed great saphenous vein for, 534
    intraoperative assessment of, 537
    open vein harvest for, 534-536
    pitfalls and danger points in, 528-529, 528f
    postoperative care in, 540-541
    preoperative assessment of vein quality in, 533
    preoperative preparation for, 526-528
    selection and assessment of inflow in, 532
    selection and assessment of outflow in, 532
    selection of conduit for, 533-534, 533f
    surgical anatomy of femoral and popliteal arteries in, 529-531, 530f-532f
    wound closure in, 538
Crux Vena Cava Filter System, 629t, 630f
Cryoplasty balloon, 55
Cutting balloon, 55, 56f

D

De novo type A dissection, 278, 279f
Death
  in acute mesenteric ischemia, 488
  after endovascular treatment of descending thoracic aortic aneurysm, 271-272
  after endovascular treatment of mesenteric ischemia, 498
  after juxtarenal and pararenal abdominal aortic aneurysms repair, 318
  after renal artery bypass, 455
  after surgical repair of aortoiliac occlusive disease, 360
  after surgical repair of thoracoabdominal aortic aneurysm, 228
  after vena cava placement, 639
  in chronic mesenteric ischemia, 489
  in traumatic thoracic aortic disruption, 293
Decompression
  after supraclavicular approach to thoracic outlet syndrome, 175-177
  in subclavian-axillary vein thrombosis, 207
Deep vein thrombosis
  after endovenous thermal ablation of saphenous and perforating veins, 705, 706f
  after subfascial endoscopic perforator surgery, 719
  after superior vena cava syndrome reconstruction, 648, 649t
  benign ileofemoral venous occlusion and, 650
  iliofemoral and femoral-popliteal, 672-683
    access and crossing of lesion in, 675
    catheter-directed thrombolysis for, 675-676
    iliac vein stenosis in, 680, 682f
    inferior vena cava filters in, 675, 675f
    postoperative care in, 681-682
    postoperative complications in, 682
    preoperative preparation in, 673-674, 673f
    recalcitrant thrombus in, 680
    rheolytic thrombectomy: AnjioJet power pulse spray technique for, 677-679, 678f
    timing of intervention in, 674-675
    Trellis-8 peripheral infusion system for, 679, 680f-681f
    ultrasound-accelerated thrombolysis: Ekosonic endovascular system for, 676-677, 677f

Deep vein thrombosis (Continued)
  risk in deep venous valve surgery, 709, 719
  sclerotherapy and, 722
  vena cava filter placement in, 627-640
    avoiding inadvertent suprarenal filter placement and, 633, 634f
    complications in, 638-639
    contrast venography and ultrasound imaging in, 632-633
    historical background of, 628, 629t, 630f
    indications for, 628
    with intravascular ultrasound, 635-637, 637f
    percutaneous placement with venography bedside transabdominal or intravascular ultrasound in, 635
    percutaneous placement with venography in, 633
    percutaneous superior vena cava filter and, 637-638
    permanent versus retrievable filter in, 631-632, 632f
    postoperative care in, 638
    pregnant patient and, 633
    preoperative preparation for, 630-631, 632f
    retrieval of vena cava filter and, 638
    with transabdominal duplex ultrasound, 635, 635f-636f
Deep venous valve surgery, 708-720
  angioscope-assisted valvuloplasty in, 712
  anticoagulation in, 710
  artificial valve implantation in, 714-715
  autologous neovalve construction in, 713
  avoiding deep vein thrombosis at surgery site in, 710
  avoiding incompetent venous valve repair in, 710
  complications in, 719
  external banding valvuloplasty in, 712
  external valvuloplasty in, 711
  indications for, 708
  internal valvuloplasty in, 711, 712f
  pitfalls and danger points in, 709-710
  postoperative care in, 718
  preoperative preparation for, 709
  proximal venous obstruction and, 710
  selection of valve site for repair in, 710
  transcommissural valvuloplasty in, 712
  vein segment transposition in, 713
  vein valve transplantation in, 708, 713-714
Delayed paraplegia
  after endovascular treatment of aortic dissection, 287
  after surgical repair of thoracoabdominal aortic aneurysm, 229, 229f
Descending thoracic aortic aneurysm
  direct surgical repair of, 216-229
    avoiding diaphragmatic paralysis in, 218, 219f
    avoiding embolization in, 218
    avoiding injury to esophagus in, 219, 220f
    avoiding spinal cord ischemia in, 218
    avoiding vagus nerve injuries in, 218-219
    avoiding visceral ischemia in, 218
    classification of aneurysms and, 217, 217f
    closure in, 226
    coagulopathy and, 218
    distal anastomosis in, 225-226
    intraoperative corrective measures in, 220
    modified thoracoabdominal incision in, 223
    postoperative care in, 228
    preoperative preparation for, 217
    proximal anastomosis in, 225
    reimplantation of intercostal arteries in, 225, 225, 225f
    somatosensory and motor-evoked potential monitoring in, 219-220
    weaning from distal aortic perfusion in, 226
  endovascular repair of, 251-273

Descending thoracic aortic aneurysm (Continued)
  access in, 258, 259f–261f
  aortic tortuosity and, 261–262, 263f
  complications in, 271–272
  deployment of Gore TAG endograft in, 265–266, 265f–267f
  deployment of Medtronic vascular endograft in, 268–271, 269f–270f
  deployment of Zenith endograft in, 266–267, 268f–269f
  indications for, 252
  intraoperative imaging in, 263–264, 263f, 265f
  landing zones and, 262
  pitfalls and danger points in, 253–258, 256f–257f
  placement of stent graft in aortic arch in, 259
  postoperative care in, 271
  preoperative imaging in, 262
  preoperative preparation for, 252–253, 253f–254f
Diabetes mellitus
  forefoot amputation in, 610–616
    anesthesia in, 611
    complications in, 615
    digital or metatarsal ray resection in, 611–614, 614f–615f
    indications for, 610
    postoperative care in, 614–615
    preoperative preparation for, 610
    selection of amputation level in, 610–611
    transmetatarsal amputation in, 611, 612f–613f
  management in femoral-popliteal arterial occlusive disease, 527
Dialysis
  after femoral vein transposition, 756
  before arteriovenous graft thrombosis repair, 782
  before distal revascularization interval ligation, 774
Diaphragmatic paralysis after surgical repair of thoracoabdominal aortic aneurysm, 218, 219f
Diarrhea after mesenteric revascularization, 489
Digital ray resection, 611–614, 614f–615f
Digital subtraction angiography, 18–19
  in tibial-peroneal arterial occlusive disease, 544
Diphenhydramine for contrast media reaction, 23
Direct surgical repair of aortoiliac occlusive disease, 350–361
  aortobifemoral bypass in, 355–356, 357f
  aortoiliac endarterectomy in, 352–353, 353f
  associated renal or visceral lesions in, 355
  classification of disease by pattern and, 351, 352f
  complications in, 358–361
  end-to-end versus end-to-side proximal anastomosis in, 351–352
  graft selection in, 353–354
  indications for, 350
  preoperative preparation for, 350–351
  proximal graft anastomosis in, 356–358, 357f, 359f
  simultaneous distal lower extremity bypass grafting in, 355
  thoracic aorta to femoral artery bypass in, 355
  totally occluded, calcified, and small aortas and, 354, 354f
Direct surgical repair of thoracoabdominal aortic aneurysm
  classification of aneurysms in, 217, 217f
  complications in, 228–229, 229f
  considerations in presence of chronic dissection in, 223
  distal aortic perfusion in, 221–222, 222f

Direct surgical repair of thoracoabdominal aortic aneurysm (Continued)
  intraoperative corrective measures in, 220
  selection of site for distal control in, 222
  selection of site for proximal control in, 222, 223f
  type I aneurysm and, 226
  type II aneurysm andl, 226–228, 227f
  type III aneurysm and, 228
  type IV aneurysm and, 228
Direct valvular repair techniques, 711–715
  angioscope-assisted valvuloplasty in, 712
  artificial valve implantation in, 714–715
  autologous neovalve construction in, 713
  external banding valvuloplasty in, 712
  external valvuloplasty in, 711
  internal valvuloplasty in, 711, 712f
  transcommissural valvuloplasty in, 712
  vein segment transposition in, 713
  vein valve transplantation in, 708, 713–714
Directional atherectomy device, 59, 59b
Dissection
  acute mesenteric ischemia secondary to, 478–479
  angioplasty-related, 51, 60
Distal anastomosis
  in above-knee popliteal bypass, 537
  in antegrade bypass in mesenteric ischemia, 484, 485f
  in carotid body tumor repair, 108, 108f
  in extraanatomic repair for renovascular disease, 452, 453f
  in juxtarenal abdominal aortic aneurysm repair, 315
  in neoaortoiliac system, 422–423
  in pararenal or suprarenal abdominal aortic aneurysm repair, 318
  in repair of abdominal aortic aneurysm, 302–304
  in repair of celiac artery aneurysm, 510
  in repair of descending thoracic aortic aneurysm, 225–226
  in repair of hepatic artery aneurysm, 508
  in repair of tibial-peroneal arterial occlusive disease, 545–547
Distal ankle perforators, subfascial endoscopic surgery of, 718
Distal lower extremity bypass grafting
  in aortoiliac occlusive disease, 355
  in tibial-peroneal arterial occlusive disease, 557–558
Distal revascularization interval ligation procedure, 772–780
  for arterial steal syndrome, 737–738
  arteriotomy and bypass in, 776–778, 777f–778f
  choice of anesthesia for, 774
  closure in, 778, 778f
  complications in, 779
  conduit in, 774, 776
  dissection of the inflow vessel in, 775–776, 775f
  exposure of distal vessel in, 776, 777f
  historical background of, 772
  incision in, 775, 775f
  indications for, 772–773
  ligation of artery in, 778
  postoperative care in, 779
  preoperative preparation for, 773–774, 774f
  timing of, 774
  tunneling in, 776
Distal venous anastomosis in arteriovenous graft thrombosis repair, 784, 784f
Double-wall puncture needle, 33f
Drain in total graft excision and extraanatomic repair of aortic graft infection, 416, 416f
DRIL. See Distal revascularization interval ligation
Drug-coated balloon, 55
DSA. See Digital subtraction angiography

Dual venous access technique in percutaneous vena cava filter placement, 637
Duodenal stump in total graft excision and extraanatomic repair of aortic graft infection, 415
Duplex ultrasound
  in aortoiliac occlusive disease, 375
  before basilic vein transposition, 747
  before brachiocephalic and radiocephalic arteriovenous fistulas, 731
  in carotid body tumor, 102
  before distal revascularization interval ligation, 773
  before endovenous ablation of saphenous and perforating veins, 696
  before femoral vein transposition, 751–752
  in femoral-popliteal arterial occlusive disease, 579
  before femoral-popliteal bypass, 533
  in iliofemoral and femoral-popliteal deep vein thrombosis, 673–674, 673f
  in mesenteric ischemia, 492, 493f
  before reconstruction of inferior vena cava and iliofemoral venous system, 650–651
  before sclerotherapy, 721
  in subclavian-axillary vein thrombosis, 204
  in superior vena cava syndrome, 642
  during surgical repair of renovascular disease, 438–439
  in tibial-peroneal arterial occlusive disease, 591
  before transaxillary rib resection for thoracic outlet syndrome, 195
  before transjugular intrahepatic portosystemic shunt, 665
  before varicose vein stripping, 685
  in vena cava filter placement, 630–631, 635, 635f–636f
  before vertebral artery surgery, 113
DVT. See Deep vein thrombosis
Dysphagia lusoria, 157

E

Early graft thrombosis
  after direct surgical repair of tibial-peroneal arterial occlusive disease, 559
  after femoral-popliteal bypass, 538–539, 541
  after renal artery bypass, 455
Ecchymosis
  after endovenous thermal ablation of saphenous and perforating veins, 705
  after varicose vein stripping, 687–688
Echocardiography before femoral artery pseudoaneurysm repair, 427
Effort thrombosis, 194, 204–214, 205f
  access in, 208
  angiographic anatomy and collaterals in, 205–206, 206f–207f
  angioplasty and stenting in, 212
  completion studies in, 212
  complications in, 213
  postoperative care in, 212–213
  preoperative preparation for, 204–205
  sheath placement in, 208
  technique in, 208–212, 209f
  thrombolysis in, 209–212, 210f–211f
  timing of, 206–208, 208f
Ehlers-Danlos syndrome, 501
EkoSonic endovascular system
  in iliofemoral and femoral-popliteal deep vein thrombosis, 676–677, 677f
  in subclavian-axillary vein thrombosis, 212
Electromyography before supraclavicular approach to thoracic outlet syndrome, 172
Elephant trunk repair, 281, 281f
Elevated arm stress test, 194
Embolectomy
  aortoiliac, 369–371, 370f
  superior mesenteric artery, 487–488, 487f

Embolic protection device during aortic arch vessels endovascular treatment, 150
Embolism
  after direct surgical repair of tibial-peroneal arterial occlusive disease, 543–559
  contraindication to endovascular repair of thoracoabdominal aortic aneurysm, 248
  pulmonary
    after endovascular therapy for subclavian-axillary vein thrombosis, 213
    after superior vena cava syndrome reconstruction, 644, 648, 649t
    after vena cava placement, 639
    in reconstruction of inferior vena cava and iliofemoral venous system, 654, 655f
  renal, 437, 447
Embolization
  in abdominal aortic aneurysm surgery, 297
  acute mesenteric ischemia secondary to, 478–479
  after percutaneous access, 40
  angioplasty-related, 51, 60–61
  of atheroma or thrombus, 14–15
  carotid angioplasty and stenting and
    carotid lesions at risk in, 88
    management of, 98–99
  in carotid body tumor, 104
  in endovascular repair
    of aortoiliac occlusive disease, 385, 389–390
    of arteriovenous graft thrombosis, 785
    of femoral-popliteal arterial occlusive disease, 579
    of gastroduodenal and pancreaticoduodenal artery aneurysms, 516, 518f–521f
    of hepatic artery aneurysm, 515–516
    of infrarenal aortic aneurysm, 332, 338–340, 340f
    of mesenteric ischemia, 498
    of renal artery aneurysm, 470, 471f
    of splenic artery aneurysm, 517–521
    of tibial-peroneal arterial occlusive disease, 596
  of internal iliac artery, 324
  of renal artery before reconstruction of inferior vena cava and iliofemoral venous system, 653, 653f
  therapeutic, 59–60, 59f, 60t
  in thoracoabdominal aortic aneurysm surgery, 218
Embolization tools, 53t
Endarterectomy, 5
  aortoiliac, 350–353
  carotid, 63–76, 72f–73f
    anesthesia in, 67
    arteriotomy and shunt placement in, 70, 71f
    avoiding cranial nerve injuries in, 66–67
    avoiding intraoperative stroke in, 65–66
    closure in, 73–74
    complications in, 74–75
    exposure of common carotid artery in, 67, 69f
    exposure of distal internal carotid artery in, 70, 71f
    incision and position in, 67, 68f
    indications for, 64
    isolation of external carotid artery in, 68–70
    isolation of internal carotid artery in, 70
    mobilization of jugular vein and division of common facial vein in, 67, 69f
    mobilization of sternocleidomastoid muscle in, 67
    patch angioplasty in, 73, 73f
    postoperative care in, 74
    preoperative preparation in, 64–65
  common femoral artery and profunda femoris artery, 528–529, 532
  eversion, 77–85

Endarterectomy (Continued)
    anastomosis of internal to common carotid artery in, 80–82, 82f
    in carotid patch aneurysm, 85
    complications in, 84
    endarterectomy of common carotid artery in, 80
    endarterectomy of internal carotid artery in, 80, 81f
    exposure of carotid artery in, 78–80, 79f, 81f
    in fibromuscular dysplasia, 84
    indications for, 77
    in infected carotid patch, 85
    for kinks and coils in internal carotid artery, 84
    operative strategy in, 78
    postoperative care in, 82–84
    preoperative preparation for, 77–78
    in recurrent carotid stenosis, 84–85
    shunting during, 82, 83f
  renal artery, 442–444
    exposure of pararenal aorta in, 442, 443f
    transaortic, 442–444, 444f, 446f
End-hole catheter, 44t, 45–46
Endograft
  Gore, 265–266, 265f–267f
  Medtronic, 268–271, 269f–270f
  Viabahn, 599, 601–602, 602f
  Zenith, 266–267, 268f–269f
Endoleak
  after descending thoracic artery aneurysm repair, 255, 256f–257f, 272
  after infrarenal aortic aneurysm repair, 322
  after popliteal artery aneurysm repair, 603
  after repair of juxtarenal and pararenal aneurysms, 349
  of infrarenal aortic aneurysm, 336, 338, 339f, 341–342
End-organ ischemia, vascular surgery-related, 15
Endovascular aneurysm repair
  of descending thoracic aortic aneurysm, 251–273
    access in, 258, 259f–261f
    aortic tortuosity and, 261–262, 263f
    complications in, 271–272
    deployment of Gore TAG endograft in, 265–266, 265f–267f
    deployment of Medtronic vascular endograft in, 268–271, 269f–270f
    deployment of Zenith endograft in, 266–267, 268f–269f
    indications for, 252
    intraoperative imaging in, 263–264, 263f, 265f
    landing zones and, 262
    pitfalls and danger points in, 253–258, 256f–257f
    placement of stent graft in aortic arch in, 259
    postoperative care in, 271
    preoperative imaging in, 262
    preoperative preparation for, 252–253, 253f–254f
  of infrarenal aortic aneurysm, 321–335
    adjunctive iliac angioplasty in, 323
    angiography in, 325–326, 325f–327f
    aortouniiliac graft in, 330–332, 331f
    arterial access in, 324–325
    arterial dissection during, 332
    device selection in, 322, 323f
    distal embolization in, 332
    Endurant device in, 329–330
    Excluder endograft in, 329
    external iliac to internal iliac artery bypass in, 333, 333f
    graft deployment and cannulation of contralateral gate in, 326–328, 328f–329f
    graft sizing in, 323
    hypogastric artery occlusion and, 333
    hypogastric embolization in, 338–340, 340f

Endovascular aneurysm repair (Continued)
    iliac artery conduit in, 324–325
    limb occlusion in, 332
    percutaneous deployment in, 323–325
    postoperative care in, 334
    postoperative complications in, 334
    PowerLink endograft in, 330
    preoperative preparation in, 321–322
    renal artery occlusion in, 332
    rupture of aorta or iliac vessels during, 332
    type I endoleak and, 336, 338, 339f
    type II endoleak and, 341–342
    unfavorable anatomy in, 336–337
    Zenith endograft in, 330
  of juxtarenal and pararenal aortic aneurysms, 344V, 343–349
    branched grafts for, 344–346, 345f
    fenestrated grafts for, 343–344, 346
    hybrid surgical and endovascular approaches in, 347, 348f
    postoperative care in, 347–349
    postoperative complications in, 349
    preoperative preparation for, 343–344
    snorkel or chimney graft technique in, 346–347, 347f
  of popliteal artery aneurysm, 598–603
    antegrade approach in, 600V, 600
    completion imaging studies in, 602
    complications in, 603
    endograft deployment in, 601–602, 602f
    indications for, 598–599
    intraoperative imaging in, 600–601
    postoperative care in, 602–603
    preoperative preparation for, 599
    selection of access site for, 598–599
    selection of endograft for, 599–600
    sheath placement in, 601, 601f
  of renal artery aneurysm, 466–474, 468f
    complications in, 473
    deployment of bare stent in, 469
    deployment of stent graft in, 469–470, 469t
    embolization in, 470, 471f
    indications for, 466
    occlusion of renal artery in, 471, 472f–473f
    postoperative care in, 471–473
    preoperative preparation for, 466–467, 467f–468f
  of thoracoabdominal aortic aneurysm, 232–250
    anatomic considerations in, 234
    branch artery preservation in, 234–235
    choice of technique in, 235
    complications in, 248–249
    indications for, 232–233
    modular transfemoral multibranched stent graft in, 244–249, 245f–246f, 248f
    patient selection for, 233
    preoperative preparation in, 233–234
Endovascular therapy
  access site management in, 29–40
    activity restriction and, 37
    anesthesia and, 31–32
    anticoagulation and, 36–37
    arterial bypass grafts and, 34
    arterial closure devices and, 37–38, 38f–39f
    axillary artery and, 34
    blood pressure and, 36, 36t
    brachial and basilic veins and, 35
    brachial artery and, 33–34, 35f
    calcification and, 36
    coagulation guidelines for, 30, 31t
    common femoral artery and, 32, 33f
    common femoral vein and, 34–35
    external compression devices and, 37, 37f
    indications for, 29–30
    internal jugular vein and, 34
    laboratory testing and, 30

Endovascular therapy (Continued)
  manual compression technique and, 36
  obesity and, 35
  patient positioning in, 31
  popliteal and posterior tibial veins and, 35
  pulselessness and, 36
  scarred groin and, 36
  ultrasound guidance in, 32, 33f
  vascular complications and, 38–40
 angioplasty in, 50–62
  anesthesia for, 51
  indications for, 50
  operative strategy in, 51
  operative technique in, 52–57, 52f, 53t, 56f
  postoperative care in, 60
  postoperative complications in, 60–61
  preoperative preparation for, 51
 fluoroscopic principles in, 18–22
  contrast injection techniques in, 19, 19t
  image acquisition in, 18–19
  radiation exposure and safety in, 19–20, 20b
  ultrasound-guided arterial puncture and, 20–22, 20V, 21f
 guidewire and catheter manipulation in, 41–49
  avoiding and managing subintimal guidewire in, 46
  catheter handling in, 46
  catheter selection in, 43–46, 44t, 45f, 47f
  crossing of occlusion in, 47–48, 47f–48f
  crossing of stenosis in, 46
  guidewire handling in, 43, 44f
  guidewire selection in, 41–42, 42t, 43f
 recanalization in, 58–59, 59b
 role in total graft excision and extraanatomic repair of aortic graft infection, 413, 413f
 stenting in, 57–58, 57t, 58f
  indications for, 50
  postoperative care in, 60
  postoperative complications in, 60–61
  preoperative preparation for, 51
 therapeutic embolization in, 59–60, 59f, 60t
Endovascular thrombolysis and thrombectomy in iliofemoral and femoral-popliteal deep vein thrombosis, 672–683
 access and crossing of lesion in, 675
 catheter-directed thrombolysis for, 675–676
 iliac vein stenosis in, 680, 682f
 inferior vena cava filters in, 675, 675f
 postoperative care in, 681–682
 postoperative complications in, 682
 preoperative preparation in, 673–674, 673f
 recalcitrant thrombus in, 680
 rheolytic thrombectomy: AnjioJet power pulse spray technique for, 677–679, 678f
 timing of intervention in, 674–675
 Trellis-8 peripheral infusion system for, 679, 680f–681f
 ultrasound-accelerated thrombolysis: Ekosonic endovascular system for, 676–677, 677f
Endovenous laser ablation
 of axial veins, 700, 703
 of perforator veins, 704
Endovenous thermal ablation of saphenous and perforating veins, 694–707
 access in, 699, 700f
 catheter placement in, 699–701
  confirmation of catheter tip position in, 701, 701f
  endovenous laser and, 700
  radiofrequency catheter and, 699–700, 700f
  tumescent anesthesia and, 701, 702f
 complications in, 705–706, 706f
 endovascular strategy in, 696–699, 698f
 indications for, 695f, 696

Endovenous thermal ablation of saphenous and perforating veins (Continued)
 patient positioning for, 699
 postoperative care in, 704–705
 preoperative preparation for, 696, 697f
 treatment of axial veins in, 702–703
  laser ablation in, 703
  radiofrequency energy in, 702–703
 treatment of perforator veins in, 703–704
  laser ablation in, 704
  radiofrequency ablation in, 704, 704f
End-to-end anastomosis, 11–12
 in distal revascularization interval ligation, 778, 778f
 small vessel, 12, 13f
 in surgical repair of aortoiliac occlusive disease, 351–352, 356, 357f
 in vascular reconstruction, 6
End-to-side anastomosis
 beveled, 8–10, 10f
 in bypass procedure, 6
 in distal revascularization interval ligation, 777f, 778
 in HERO device, 770
 nonbeveled, 10–11, 11f
 in surgical repair of aortoiliac occlusive disease, 351–352, 356–358, 359f
Endurant device, 329–330
Esophageal compression, aberrant right subclavian artery-related, 159, 160f
Esophageal injury in surgical repair of thoracoabdominal aortic aneurysm, 219, 220f
Ethylene vinyl alcohol copolymer in renal artery aneurysm repair, 470
EVAR. See Endovascular aneurysm repair
Eversion endarterectomy, 78V, 77–85
 anastomosis of internal to common carotid artery in, 80–82, 82f
 in carotid patch aneurysm, 85
 complications in, 84
 endarterectomy of common carotid artery in, 80
 endarterectomy of internal carotid artery in, 80, 81f
 exposure of carotid artery in, 78–80, 79f, 81f
 in fibromuscular dysplasia, 84
 indications for, 77
 in infected carotid patch, 85
 for kinks and coils in internal carotid artery, 84
 operative strategy in, 78
 postoperative care in, 82–84
 preoperative preparation for, 77–78
 in recurrent carotid stenosis, 84–85
 shunting during, 82, 83f
Excluder endograft in repair of infrarenal aortic aneurysm, 329
Extensor compartment of arm, 623
External banding valvuloplasty, 712
External carotid artery
 average diameter of, 57t
 carotid angioplasty and stenting and, 86–100, 90f
 carotid endarterectomy and, 68–70
External compression device, access site management and, 37, 37f
External iliac artery
 average diameter of, 57t
 endovascular treatment of aortoiliac occlusive disease and, 388–389, 389f
External iliac to internal iliac artery bypass, 333, 333f, 340
External valvuloplasty, 711
Extraanatomic repair
 of aortic arch vessels, 139–147
  carotid-carotid artery bypass in, 144, 145f
  carotid-subclavian artery bypass in, 144, 145f
  carotid-subclavian artery transposition in, 142–143, 142f, 143V, 144f
  indications for, 139–140, 141f
  postoperative care in, 139–140

Extraanatomic repair (Continued)
  postoperative complications in, 146–147
  preoperative preparation for, 140–141
  surgical anatomy of common carotid and subclavian arteries and, 141, 142f
 of aortic graft infection, 403–418
  avoiding ureteral injury in, 409
  choice of reconstruction in, 407–408
  closure of femoral arteries in, 416
  closure of proximal aortic stump and omental pedicle flap in, 414–415, 415f
  complications in, 417
  drains in, 416, 416f
  exposure of abdominal aorta in, 414
  exposure of common femoral, superficial femoral, and profunda femoris arteries in, 414
  graft excision in, 414
  historical background of, 404–405, 405f
  incision closure in, 416–417
  incision in, 413–414
  management of duodenal stump in, 415
  postoperative care in, 417
  preoperative preparation for, 405–407, 406f
  presence of aortoenteric fistula and, 409–412, 412f
  role of endovascular therapy in, 413, 413f
  sartorius muscle flap in, 416
  selection of extraanatomic bypass in, 409, 410f–411f
  staging of, 408–409
  underlying aneurysmal or occlusive disease and, 412
 of aortoiliac occlusive disease, 362–372
  aortoiliac embolectomy in, 369–371, 370f
  axillofemoral bypass in, 364–367, 365f–366f
  femoral-femoral bypass in, 363, 363f
  preoperative preparation for, 362
  thoracofemoral bypass in, 367–368, 368f
 of renovascular disease, 449–455
  complications in, 455
  conduit selection in, 450
  hepatorenal bypass in, 450–452, 451f, 453f–454f
  preoperative preparation for, 449
  splenorenal bypass in, 453–454
  surgical anatomy of hepatic and splenic arteries and, 450, 451f
Extracranial cerebrovascular disease
 carotid angioplasty and stenting in, 86–101
  access in, 90–91
  angiographic anatomy and, 87, 88t
  angiography of aortic arch, carotid, and cerebral circulation in, 92
  angioplasty technique in, 97V, 97–98
  aortic arch anatomy and, 88, 89f
  carotid lesions at risk for embolization and, 88
  catheterization of common carotid artery in, 91, 91f–92f
  cerebral protection devices and, 90
  completion studies in, 98
  crossing lesion and cerebral protection in, 95–97, 95f, 97f
  fibromuscular dysplasia and, 89–90
  indications for, 86, 87t
  kinks and coils of carotid artery and, 88
  management of arterial spasm, embolization, and acute occlusion in, 98–99
  neurorescue techniques in, 99–100
  occluded external carotid artery and, 88, 90f
  postoperative care in, 100
  postoperative complications in, 100–101
  preoperative care in, 86
  redo carotid angioplasty and, 90
  selection of stent for, 90
  severe stenosis and string sign and, 88–89
  sheath placement for planned intervention in, 92–95, 93f–94f

Extracranial cerebrovascular disease *(Continued)*
    stenting technique in, 98, 99f
    tandem lesions in common carotid artery and, 89
  carotid body tumor and, 102–110
    avoiding cranial nerve injuries in, 103–104
    avoiding intraoperative stroke in, 104
    bipolar electrocautery in, 104
    classification and surgical anatomy of, 103, 103t
    exposure of carotid bifurcation in, 104–108, 105f
    incision for, 104, 105f
    postoperative care in, 108–109
    postoperative complications in, 109
    preoperative embolization in, 104
    preoperative preparation in, 102
    resection of Shamblin type I, 105, 106f
    resection of Shamblin type II/III, 107–108, 107f–108f
  carotid endarterectomy in, 63–76
    anesthesia in, 67
    arteriotomy and shunt placement in, 70, 71f
    avoiding cranial nerve injuries in, 66–67
    avoiding intraoperative stroke in, 65–66
    closure in, 73–74
    complications in, 74–75
    endarterectomy in, 70–73, 72f–73f
    exposure of common carotid artery in, 67, 69f
    exposure of distal internal carotid artery in, 70, 71f
    incision and position in, 67, 68f
    indications for, 64
    isolation of external carotid artery in, 68–70
    isolation of internal carotid artery in, 70
    mobilization of jugular vein and division of common facial vein in, 67, 69f
    mobilization of sternocleidomastoid muscle in, 67
    patch angioplasty in, 73, 73f
    postoperative care in, 74
    preoperative preparation in, 64–65
  eversion endarterectomy in, 77–85
    anastomosis of internal to common carotid artery in, 80–82, 82f
    in carotid patch aneurysm, 85
    complications in, 84
    endarterectomy of common carotid artery in, 80
    endarterectomy of internal carotid artery in, 80, 81f
    exposure of carotid artery in, 78–80, 79f, 81f
    in fibromuscular dysplasia, 84
    indications for, 77
    in infected carotid patch, 85
    for kinks and coils in internal carotid artery, 84
    operative strategy in, 78
    postoperative care in, 82–84
    preoperative preparation for, 77–78
    in recurrent carotid stenosis, 84–85
    shunting during, 82, 83f
  vertebral artery surgery in, 111–112
    exposure and transposition of vertebral artery into common carotid artery in, 116–118, 117f, 118V, 119f
    exposure of V2 segment of vertebral artery in, 118–122, 120f–123f
    indications for, 111–112, 112b
    operative strategy in, 114
    postoperative care in, 122
    postoperative complications in, 122–124
    preoperative preparation for, 112–114, 113b, 113f, 115f
    surgical anatomy in, 114–116, 116f
    V3 exposure and distal vertebral artery reconstruction in, 118–122, 120f–123f

F

Facial nerve injury
  during carotid body tumor surgery, 103
  during carotid endarterectomy, 70
Fasciotomy, 617–626
  in aortoiliac occlusive disease, 371
  complications in, 624
  failure to release extremity compartments in, 618
  iatrogenic injury and, 618–619
  inadequate postoperative surveillance in, 619
  indications for, 617–618
  lower leg, 619, 619–621, 619f, 621f–622f
  paratibial, 716
  postoperative care in, 624
  preoperative preparation for, 618
  thigh, 622–623
  unrecognized compartment syndrome and, 618
Femoral anastomosis
  in aortoiliac occlusive disease repair, 358, 359f
  in axillofemoral bypass, 365f–366f, 367
Femoral arteriotomy and embolectomy, 369, 369–371
Femoral artery
  access to, 29, 32, 33f
  average diameter of, 57t
  direct surgical repair of tibial-peroneal arterial occlusive disease and, 548–551
  endovascular treatment of femoral-popliteal arterial occlusive disease and, 580, 581f
  injury in endovascular repair of infrarenal aortic aneurysm, 322
  surgical anatomy of, 529–531, 530f–532f
  thoracic aorta bypass to, 355
  total graft excision and extraanatomic repair of aortic graft infection and
    closure of, 416
    exposure in, 414
Femoral artery pseudoaneurysm, 427–434
  endovascular options and, 432
  iatrogenic pseudoaneurysm and, 432–433
  indications for, 427
  infected pseudoaneurysm and, 429–432, 430f–431f
  noninfected anastomotic pseudoaneurysm and, 428–429, 429f
  postoperative care in, 433
  preoperative preparation for, 427–428
Femoral distal artery-vein bypass grafting, 547–548
Femoral triangle, 529–531, 530f
Femoral vein
  access to, 34–35
  neoaortoiliac system procedure for aortic graft infection and, 420V, 420–421, 421f–422f
Femoral vein graft in superior vena cava syndrome reconstruction, 644
Femoral vein transposition, 751, 759t, 764V
  arteriovenous anastomosis in, 753, 754f
  avoiding wound complications in, 752
  complications in, 756–757
  exposure of distal femoral and popliteal vein in, 753
  exposure of femoral vein in, 752–753
  incision in, 752
  indications for, 751
  loop composite polytetrafluoroethylene-femoral vein arteriovenous access and, 755, 755f
  mobilization of proximal femoral vein in, 753
  postoperative care in, 755–756
  preoperative preparation in, 751–752
  steal syndrome and, 752
  transposition procedure in, 753, 754f
Femoral vessels exposure in aortobifemoral bypass, 356, 357f

Femoral-anterior tibial artery bypass, 552–554, 553f–554f
Femoral-femoral bypass, 363, 363f
Femoral-femoral venous bypass, 658, 658f
Femoral-peroneal artery bypass, 555–558
Femoral-popliteal arterial occlusive disease
  endovascular treatment of, 578–589
    access selection in, 580
    angiographic anatomy and common collateral pathways in, 580, 581f
    angiography of lower extremity in, 582
    complications in, 587
    femoral-popliteal artery occlusions and, 585–586
    femoral-popliteal artery stenosis and, 582–585, 583f–585f
    indications for, 578, 579b, 579t
    postoperative care in, 587
    preoperative preparation for, 578–579
    retrograde and antegrade approaches for arterial access in, 581–582
    stent selection in, 580–581
    thrombolysis of acute femoral-popliteal artery occlusions and, 586–587
    unfavorable anatomic features for, 580
  open surgical femoral-popliteal bypass in, 525–542
    above-knee bypass in, 536–537
    alternate inflow sources in, 538, 539f–540f
    below-knee bypass in, 537
    complications in, 541
    femoral-popliteal thromboembolectomy and, 538–539
    indications for, 526
    in situ or reversed great saphenous vein for, 534
    intraoperative assessment of, 537
    open vein harvest for, 534–536
    pitfalls and danger points in, 528–529, 528f
    postoperative care in, 540–541
    preoperative assessment of vein quality in, 533
    preoperative preparation for, 526–528
    selection and assessment of inflow in, 532
    selection and assessment of outflow in, 532
    selection of conduit for, 533–534, 533f
    surgical anatomy of femoral and popliteal arteries in, 529–531, 530f–532f
    wound closure in, 538
Femoral-popliteal bypass, 525–542
  above-knee bypass in, 536–537
  alternate inflow sources in, 538, 539f–540f
  below-knee bypass in, 537
  complications in, 541
  femoral-popliteal thromboembolectomy and, 538–539
  indications for, 526
  in situ or reversed great saphenous vein for, 534
  intraoperative assessment of, 537
  open vein harvest for, 534–536
  pitfalls and danger points in, 528–529, 528f
  postoperative care in, 540–541
  preoperative assessment of vein quality in, 533
  preoperative preparation for, 526–528
  selection and assessment of inflow in, 532
  selection and assessment of outflow in, 532
  selection of conduit for, 533–534, 533f
  surgical anatomy of femoral and popliteal arteries in, 529–531, 530f–532f
  wound closure in, 538
Femoral-popliteal deep vein thrombosis, 672–683
  access and crossing of lesion in, 675
  catheter-directed thrombolysis for, 675–676
  iliac vein stenosis in, 680, 682f
  inferior vena cava filters in, 675, 675f

Femoral-popliteal deep vein thrombosis (*Continued*)
- postoperative care in, 681–682
- postoperative complications in, 682
- preoperative preparation in, 673–674, 673f
- recalcitrant thrombus in, 680
- rheolytic thrombectomy: AngioJet power pulse spray technique for, 677–679, 678f
- timing of intervention in, 674–675
- Trellis-8 peripheral infusion system for, 679, 680f–681f
- ultrasound-accelerated thrombolysis: Ekosonic endovascular system for, 676–677, 677f

Femoral-popliteal artery occlusions, 585–586
Femoral-popliteal artery stenosis, 582–585, 583f–585f
Femoral-popliteal thromboembolectomy, 538–539
Femoral-posterior tibial artery bypass, 555, 557f
FemoStop Gold compression assist device, 37, 37f
Femur, above-knee amputation and, 607
Fenestrated stent graft
- for aneurysms of juxtarenal and pararenal aorta, 343–344, 346
- for thoracoabdominal aortic aneurysm, 234

Fenestration in aortic dissection, 281–282, 285–286
Fentanyl, 18
Fibromuscular dysplasia
- carotid angioplasty and stenting and, 89–90
- eversion endarterectomy in, 84

Fibula, long posterior flap below-knee amputation and, 605
Filter placement in carotid angioplasty and stenting, 95–96, 95f
First bite syndrome after carotid body tumor surgery, 109
First intercostal nerve injury in supraclavicular approach to thoracic outlet syndrome, 178
First rib bypass collaterals, 206, 207f
First rib resection
- complications after, 213
- in supraclavicular approach to thoracic outlet syndrome, 174, 176–177, 181–185, 184f–185f
- in transaxillary rib resection for thoracic outlet syndrome, 193–203
  - avoiding injury to brachial plexus in, 196, 197f
  - closure in, 200–201
  - exposure in, 198–199, 199f–200f
  - incision in, 198
  - indications for, 193–194
  - postoperative care in, 202
  - postoperative complications in, 202–203
  - preoperative preparation for, 194–195
  - rib resection in, 200, 201f
  - surgical anatomy of thoracic outlet and, 195–196, 196V, 197f

Fistula, arteriovenous. *See* Arteriovenous fistula
Fistula thrombosis, 738
- basilic vein transposition and, 751

Flap coverage
- in extraanatomic repair of aortic graft infection, 416
- in neoaortoiliac system procedure for aortic graft infection, 423–424

Flexor compartments of arm, 623
Fluency endograft for infrarenal aortic aneurysm, 340
Fluid resuscitation before fasciotomy, 618
Flumazenil, 18
Fluoroscopy, 18–22
- contrast injection techniques in, 19, 19t
- image acquisition in, 18–19
- radiation exposure and safety in, 19–20, 20b
- ultrasound-guided arterial puncture and, 20–22, 20V, 21f

Flush catheter, 45–46, 45f
FMD. *See* Fibromuscular dysplasia
Foot surgery after surgical repair of tibial-peroneal arterial occlusive disease, 558
Forearm fasciotomy, 623, 623f
Forearm loop graft, 739–746
- anastomoses in, 742
- complications in, 744–746, 746f
- confirmation of flow and closure in, 742
- incision in, 742
- indications for, 739
- postoperative care in, 743–744
- preoperative preparation for, 739–740, 740f–741f
- selection of sites for venous outflow and arterial inflow in, 741
- tunneling of graft in, 742, 743f

Forefoot amputation, 610–616
- anesthesia in, 611
- complications in, 615
- digital or metatarsal ray resection in, 611–614, 614f–615f
- indications for, 610
- postoperative care in, 614–615
- preoperative preparation for, 610
- selection of amputation level in, 610–611
- transmetatarsal amputation in, 611, 612f–613f

G

Gas embolization after sclerotherapy, 725–726
Gastrocnemius muscle, popliteal artery entrapment and, 573, 574f
Gastrocnemius vein, varicose vein stripping and, 685–686
Gastroduodenal artery aneurysm, 513–524, 518f–521f
- access and guiding sheath placement in, 515
- angiographic imaging in, 515
- indications for, 514
- postoperative care in, 523–524
- preoperative preparation for, 514

Gastroduodenoscopy before total graft excision and extraanatomic repair of aortic graft infection, 405, 406f
Gastrointestinal complications
- after juxtarenal and pararenal abdominal aortic aneurysms repair, 319
- after surgical repair of thoracoabdominal aortic aneurysm, 229

Gastrointestinal hemorrhage in aortic graft infection, 405
General anesthesia, 18
Giant Palmaz stent in type I endoleak, 338, 339f
Glossopharyngeal nerve injury
- during carotid body tumor surgery, 103–104
- during carotid endarterectomy, 66

Glycerin as sclerosant, 723
Gore endograft
- for descending thoracic aortic aneurysm, 265–266, 265f–267f
- for infrarenal aortic aneurysm, 340

Graft excision in total graft excision and extraanatomic repair of aortic graft infection, 414
Graft failure
- after direct surgical repair of tibial-peroneal arterial occlusive disease, 559
- after femoral-popliteal bypass, 538–539, 541
- after renal artery bypass, 455
- after surgical repair of aortoiliac occlusive disease, 360–361
- after unconventional vascular access for hemodialysis, 770

Graft infection
- after arteriovenous graft thrombosis treatment, 790
- after reconstruction of inferior vena cava and iliofemoral venous system and, 655
- after transjugular intrahepatic portosystemic shunt, 671

Graft thrombosis, 781–792
- after arteriovenous graft, 745
- after renal artery bypass, 455
- after superior vena cava syndrome reconstruction, 643
- complications in, 790
- endovascular treatment of, 784, 785f
  - closure in, 787
  - lyse-and-go technique in, 786
  - preoperative preparation for, 784–785
  - removal of residual clot in, 786–787, 787f
  - sheath placement in, 785f, 786
  - use of covered stents in, 786
- in femoral-popliteal bypass, 538–539, 541
- hybrid interventions for, 787, 787f–788f
  - closure in, 789
  - endovascular intervention in, 789, 789f
  - incision in, 788
  - thrombectomy in, 788–789, 788f
- postoperative care in, 790
- surgical intervention in, 781
  - anesthesia and incision in, 782–783
  - closure in, 784
  - operative strategy for, 782, 783f
  - preoperative preparation for, 781–782
  - revision of distal venous anastomosis in, 784, 784f
  - thrombectomy in, 783

Great saphenous vein, 697, 698f
- distal revascularization interval ligation and, 775
- for femoral-popliteal bypass, 534
  - endoscopic harvest of, 535
  - in situ or reversed technique in, 534
  - open harvest of, 534–536
  - small-caliber vein and, 528, 528f
  - surgical anatomy of, 529–531, 530f
- injury in surgical repair of popliteal artery aneurysm, 566
- injury in surgical repair of popliteal artery entrapment, 574
- ligation and stripping of, 688–690, 689f–690f
- for superior vena cava syndrome reconstruction, 645, 646f–648f
- for surgical repair of tibial-peroneal arterial occlusive disease, 544, 547f, 548

Greenfield filter, 629t, 630f, 675f
Guidewire manipulation in endovascular therapy, 41–49, 44f
- avoiding and managing subintimal guidewire in, 46
- catheter handling and, 46
- catheter selection and, 43–46, 44t, 45f, 47f
- crossing of occlusion in, 47–48, 47f–48f
- crossing of stenosis in, 46
- guidewire selection in, 41–42, 42t, 43f

Guillotine amputation, 604
Günther Tulip filter, 629t, 630f, 675f

H

Hand, critical ischemia of, 194
Headhunter 1 catheter, 45f
Heart, left ventricular perforation during modular transcervical bifurcated stent graft, 239
Heart disease, direct surgical repair of aortic arch vessels and, 128
Hematoma
- after above- and below-knee amputation, 608
- after arteriovenous graft, 745

Hematoma (Continued)
    after arteriovenous graft thrombosis treatment, 790
    after carotid body tumor surgery, 109
    after carotid endarterectomy, 75
    after deep venous valve surgery, 719
    after percutaneous access, 38–40
    after sclerotherapy, 725
    after subfascial endoscopic perforator surgery, 719
    after varicose vein stripping, 687–688
    vascular surgery-related, 15
Hemodialysis access
    basilic vein transposition for, 747–757
        choice of one- or two-stage procedure in, 748, 749f
        complications in, 751
        harvest of basilic vein in, 748, 749f
        indications for, 747
        postoperative care in, 750–751
        preoperative preparation for, 747
        single-stage procedure in, 751
        steal syndrome and, 748
        superficialization of fistula in, 750
        two-stage procedure in, 748–750
        use of radial artery in, 750
    brachial artery-axillary vein interposition graft for, 739–746
        anastomoses in, 743, 744f
        complications in, 744–746, 746f
        incision in, 742–743
        indications for, 739
        postoperative care in, 743–744
        preoperative preparation for, 739–740, 740f–741f
        selection of arteriovenous graft in, 741
        selection of sites for venous outflow and arterial inflow in, 741
    brachiocephalic arteriovenous fistula for, 734–735
        complications in, 736–738
        exposure of brachial artery in, 735, 736f
        exposure of cephalic vein in, 734–735
        incision in, 734, 735f
        postoperative care in, 736
    distal revascularization interval ligation procedure for, 772–780
        arteriotomy and bypass in, 776–778, 777f–778f
        choice of anesthesia for, 774
        closure in, 778, 778f
        complications in, 779
        conduit in, 774, 776
        dissection of the inflow vessel in, 775–776, 775f
        exposure of distal vessel in, 776, 777f
        historical background of, 772
        incision in, 775, 775f
        indications for, 772–773
        ligation of artery in, 778
        postoperative care in, 779
        preoperative preparation for, 773–774, 774f
        timing of, 774
        tunneling in, 776
    femoral vein transposition for, 751
        arteriovenous anastomosis in, 753, 754f
        avoiding wound complications in, 752
        complications in, 756–757
        exposure of distal femoral and popliteal vein in, 753
        exposure of femoral vein in, 752–753
        incision in, 752
        indications for, 751
        loop composite polytetrafluoroethylene-femoral vein arteriovenous access and, 755, 755f
        mobilization of proximal femoral vein in, 753
        postoperative care in, 755–756
        preoperative preparation in, 751–752
        steal syndrome and, 752
        transposition procedure in, 753, 754f

Hemodialysis access (Continued)
    forearm loop graft for, 739–746
        anastomoses in, 742
        complications in, 744–746, 746f
        confirmation of flow and closure in, 742
        incision in, 742
        indications for, 739
        postoperative care in, 743–744
        preoperative preparation for, 739–740, 740f–741f
        selection of sites for venous outflow and arterial inflow in, 741
        tunneling of graft in, 742, 743f
    radial artery-cephalic vein arteriovenous fistula for, 729–738
        alternatives in absence of suitable cephalic vein and, 732
        anesthesia for, 732
        arteriovenous anastomosis in, 733–734
        complications in, 736–738
        confirmation of flow and closure in, 734, 734f
        exposure of cephalic vein in, 733
        exposure of radial artery in, 733
        heparinization in, 732
        incisions in, 732–733, 733f
        indications for, 730–731
        operative field in, 732
        postoperative care in, 736
        preoperative preparation for, 731
        selection of fistula site for, 732
    unconventional, 758–771
        assessment of remaining options for upper extremity access and, 760
        brachial vein transposition in, 760, 762–763, 762f–764f
        complex catheter-based vascular access in, 767–770, 768f–769f
        complications in, 770
        hemodialysis reliable outflow vascular access device placement in, 761
        indications for, 758, 759t
        options for temporary dialysis access and, 759–760
        pediatric patient and, 760
        postoperative care in, 770
        preoperative preparation for, 758–759
        prosthetic chest wall vascular access in, 761, 765–767, 767f
        prosthetic lower extremity vascular access in, 760–761, 764–765, 766f
        saphenous vein transposition in, 760, 763–764, 765f
        transthoracic cuffed dialysis catheter placement in, 761
Hemodialysis reliable outflow vascular access device placement, 761, 769, 769f
Hemodynamic monitoring
    after endovascular treatment of aortic dissection, 287
    after surgical repair of aortic arch vessels, 136
    after transjugular intrahepatic portosystemic shunt, 670
    during endovascular treatment of aortoiliac occlusive disease, 376–377
Hemorrhage
    in aortic graft infection
        neoaortoiliac system procedure for, 424–425
        total graft excision and extraanatomic repair of, 407
    in iliofemoral and femoral-popliteal deep vein thrombosis repair, 674
    postoperative
        in abdominal aortic aneurysm surgery, 307
        in aortoiliac occlusive disease, 358
        in femoral-popliteal bypass, 541
        in renal artery stenosis, 464
        in subclavian-axillary vein thrombosis, 213
        in thoracic outlet syndrome, 190

Hemorrhage (Continued)
    in transjugular intrahepatic portosystemic shunt, 670
    in reconstruction of inferior vena cava and iliofemoral venous system, 653–654
    risk in vascular access, 30
    during superior vena cava syndrome reconstruction, 643
    vascular surgery-related, 15
Hemothorax
    after extraanatomic aortic arch vessel repair, 146
    after surgical repair of subclavian and axillary arteries, 169
Heparin
    after reconstruction of inferior vena cava and iliofemoral venous system and, 662
    in deep venous valve surgery, 710
    during endovascular treatment of mesenteric ischemia, 496
    before endovenous thermal ablation of saphenous and perforating veins, 696
    radial artery-cephalic vein arteriovenous fistula and, 732
    for subclavian-axillary vein thrombosis, 210
Hepatic artery
    average diameter of, 57t
    hepatorenal bypass and, 452
    surgical anatomy of, 450, 451f, 502, 503f
Hepatic artery aneurysm
    direct surgical repair of, 505–508, 507f
    endovascular treatment of, 513–524
        access and guiding sheath placement in, 515
        angiographic imaging in, 515
        embolization in, 515–516
        indications for, 514
        postoperative care in, 523–524
        preoperative preparation for, 514
        stent placement in, 516, 517f
Hepatic encephalopathy, transjugular intrahepatic portosystemic shunt and, 665–666, 670–671
Hepatic ischemia
    after hepatic or celiac revascularization, 510
    after renal artery bypass, 455
Hepatic vein torsion, 654–655, 656f
Hepatic venography, 667
Hepatorenal bypass, 450–452, 451f, 453f–454f
HERO device, 759t, 769, 769f
Horner syndrome
    after carotid body tumor surgery, 109
    after extraanatomic aortic arch vessel repair, 146
    after vertebral artery surgery, 123
Horseshoe kidney, abdominal aortic aneurysm surgery and, 301
Hybrid interventions for arteriovenous graft thrombosis, 787, 787f–788f
    closure in, 789
    endovascular intervention in, 789, 789f
    incision in, 788
    thrombectomy in, 788–789, 788f
Hybrid surgical and endovascular approaches in juxtarenal and pararenal aneurysms, 347, 348f
Hydralazine, 36t
Hydration
    control in acute aortic dissection, 275
    for renal protection, 22–23, 23t
Hydrocortisone for contrast media reaction, 23
Hydrophilic guidewire, 41
Hyperperfusion syndrome
    carotid angioplasty and stenting-related, 75
    carotid endarterectomy-related, 75
Hyperpigmentation after sclerotherapy, 726
Hypertonic saline as sclerosant, 723
Hypogastric artery occlusion in endovascular repair of infrarenal aortic aneurysm, 333

Hypogastric embolization in endovascular repair of infrarenal aortic aneurysm, 338–340, 340f
Hypoglossal nerve injury
 during carotid body tumor surgery, 103
 during carotid endarterectomy, 66
Hypotension during carotid angioplasty and stenting, 86–100

I

Iatrogenic femoral artery pseudoaneurysm, 432–433
Iatrogenic injury, compartment syndrome and, 618–619
Iliac aneurysm repair, 304–305, 306f
Iliac angioplasty, 323
Iliac artery
 as conduit in repair of infrarenal aortic aneurysm, 324–325
 exposure in infrarenal aortic aneurysm repair, 302
 infrarenal sympathetic nerves relationship to, 399f
 involvement in juxtarenal abdominal aortic aneurysm, 313–315, 314b
Iliac artery injury
 in abdominal aortic aneurysm surgery, 297
 in endovascular repair of infrarenal aortic aneurysm, 322
Iliac artery pseudoaneurysm, 278
Iliac vein
 stenosis of, 680, 682f
 surgical anatomy of, 656
Iliocaval conduit, 654
Iliocaval graft thrombosis and stenosis, 654
Iliocaval venous bypass, 658–659, 659f
Iliofemoral bypass, 358
Iliofemoral deep vein thrombosis, 672–683
 access and crossing of lesion in, 675
 catheter-directed thrombolysis for, 675–676
 iliac vein stenosis in, 680, 682f
 inferior vena cava filters in, 675, 675f
 postoperative care in, 681–682
 postoperative complications in, 682
 preoperative preparation in, 673–674, 673f
 recalcitrant thrombus in, 680
 rheolytic thrombectomy: AnjioJet power pulse spray technique for, 677–679, 678f
 timing of intervention in, 674–675
 Trellis-8 peripheral infusion system for, 679, 680f–681f
 ultrasound-accelerated thrombolysis: Ekosonic endovascular system for, 676–677, 677f
Iliofemoral venous system reconstruction surgery, 650–663
 anatomy in, 656
 choice of incision for, 656–657, 657f
 complications in, 662–663
 femoral-femoral venous bypass in, 658, 658f
 ileocaval venous bypass in, 658–659, 659f
 indications for, 650, 651b
 inferior vena cava reconstruction in, 659–662, 660f
 pitfalls and danger points in, 653–656, 654f–656f
 postoperative care in, 662
 preoperative preparation for, 650–653, 652f–653f
 resection of suprarenal inferior vena cava in conjunction with major liver resection in, 657
Image acquisition in fluoroscopy, 18–19
Imaging studies
 in aortic dissection, 275, 278–279
 in aortic graft infection, 405, 406f, 419–420
 in aortoiliac occlusive disease, 351, 376
 before basilic vein transposition, 747

Imaging studies *(Continued)*
 before brachial artery-axillary vein interposition graft, 740, 741f
 of carotid body tumor, 102
 of descending thoracic aortic aneurysm, 263–264, 263f, 265f
 in endovenous thermal ablation of saphenous and perforating veins, 694–696, 697f
 of femoral artery pseudoaneurysm, 428
 before femoral vein transposition, 751–752
 in femoral-popliteal arterial occlusive disease, 527
 before forearm loop graft, 740, 741f
 in iliofemoral and femoral-popliteal deep vein thrombosis, 673–674, 673f
 of infrarenal aortic aneurysm, 321–322
 of popliteal artery aneurysm, 599–601
 of renal artery aneurysm, 466–467
 in spine exposure, 393
 in superior vena cava syndrome, 642, 643f, 648
 in surgical repair of aortic arch vessels, 127
 in tibial-peroneal arterial occlusive disease, 544, 591, 594
 before unconventional venous access for hemodialysis, 758
 in vena cava filter placement, 632–633, 638
 in vertebral artery surgery, 113–114, 113f
Impotence
 after abdominal aortic aneurysm surgery, 297, 308
 after repair of aortoiliac occlusive disease, 360
In situ valve lysis in femoral-popliteal bypass, 535–536
Incision
 in aberrant right subclavian artery repair, 165, 165f
 in above-knee amputation, 607, 607f
 in antegrade bypass in mesenteric ischemia, 482
 in anterior spine exposure, 393
 in aortic arch vessels repair, 130, 131f
 in aortobifemoral bypass, 355
 in aortoiliac embolectomy, 369
 in aortorenal bypass, 439, 440f
 in arteriovenous fistula
  brachiocephalic, 734, 735f
  radiocephalic, 732–733, 733f
 in arteriovenous graft thrombosis repair
  hybrid intervention and, 788
  surgical intervention and, 782–783
 in axillofemoral bypass, 366
 in brachial artery-axillary vein interposition graft, 742–743
 in carotid body tumor, 104, 105f
 in carotid endarterectomy, 67, 68f
 in celiac artery aneurysm, 509
 in descending thoracic aortic aneurysm, 223
 in distal revascularization interval ligation, 775, 775f
 in femoral artery pseudoaneurysm
  of infected pseudoaneurysm, 429–430, 430f
  of noninfected pseudoaneurysm, 428, 429f
 in femoral vein transposition, 752
 in femoral-femoral bypass, 363, 363
 in forearm loop graft, 742
 in forefoot amputation, 611
  in digital or metatarsal ray resection, 611
  transmetatarsal, 610–611, 612f–613f
 in hepatic artery aneurysm, 504, 506
 in hepatorenal bypass, 450, 451f
 in infrarenal aortic aneurysm, 301–302, 303f
 in juxtarenal abdominal aortic aneurysm, 311–313, 312f
 in juxtarenal abdominal aortic aneurysm with iliac artery involvement, 313–315
 in Kommerell diverticulum, 167

Incision *(Continued)*
 in long posterior flap below-knee amputation, 605, 606f
 in lower leg fasciotomy
  anterior compartment and, 620, 620f–621f
  lateral compartment and, 620, 621f
  superficial and deep posterior compartments and, 620–621, 622f
 in neoaortoiliac system procedure for aortic graft infection, 420–421, 421f
 in pararenal abdominal aortic aneurysm, 313, 315–318
 in popliteal artery aneurysm, 563, 563f–564f
  medial approach, 567
  posterior approach, 568–569
 in popliteal artery entrapment, 573–574
 in reconstruction of inferior vena cava and iliofemoral venous system and, 656–657, 657f
 in splenorenal bypass, 453
 in stab avulsion, 691–692, 691f
 in subclavian artery aneurysm, 162
 in subfascial endoscopic perforator surgery, 715–716, 715b, 715f
 in superior vena cava syndrome reconstruction, 645
 in supraclavicular approach to thoracic outlet syndrome, 179–180, 179f
 in suprarenal aortic aneurysm, 315–316, 315V, 317f
 in thigh fasciotomy, 622
 in thoracoabdominal aortic aneurysm, 221
 in thoracofemoral bypass, 367, 368f
 in tibial-peroneal arterial occlusive disease, 548, 549f
 in total graft excision and extraanatomic repair of aortic graft infection, 413–414
 in transaxillary rib resection for thoracic outlet syndrome, 198
 in type II thoracoabdominal aortic aneurysm, 226–227
 in type IV thoracoabdominal aortic aneurysm, 228
 in volar fasciotomy, 623, 623f
Incompetent deep venous valves, 708–720
 deep venous valve surgery in
  angioscope-assisted valvuloplasty in, 712
  artificial valve implantation in, 714–715
  autologous neovalve construction in, 713
  complications in, 719
  external banding valvuloplasty in, 712
  external valvuloplasty in, 711
  indications for, 708
  internal valvuloplasty in, 711, 712f
  operative strategy in, 710
  pitfalls and danger points in, 709–710
  postoperative care in, 718
  preoperative preparation for, 709
  transcommissural valvuloplasty in, 712
  vein segment transposition in, 713
  vein valve transplantation in, 708, 713–714
 subfascial endoscopic perforator surgery in
  choice of anesthesia for, 715
  deep venous valve surgery in, 719
  distal ankle perforators and, 718
  exploration of subfascial space in, 716, 717f–718f
  incision in, 715–716, 715b, 715f
  indications for, 708
  operative strategy in, 710–711
  paratibial fasciotomy in, 716
  pitfalls and danger points in, 709–710
  port insertion in, 716, 716f
  postoperative care in, 718–719
  preoperative preparation for, 709
Infarction, mesenteric, 488
Infected femoral artery pseudoaneurysm, 429–432, 430f–431f

Infection
- after arteriovenous graft, 744-745
- after fasciotomy, 624
- after femoral-popliteal bypass, 541
- after forefoot amputation, 615
- after transjugular intrahepatic portosystemic shunt, 671
- eversion endarterectomy-related, 84
- vascular surgery-related, 16

Inferior mesenteric artery, infrarenal aortic aneurysm repair and, 304

Inferior vena cava
- filter placement in, 627-640
  - avoiding inadvertent suprarenal filter placement and, 633, 634f
  - complications in, 638-639
  - contrast venography and ultrasound imaging in, 632-633
  - historical background of, 628, 629t, 630f
  - in iliofemoral and femoral-popliteal deep vein thrombosis, 675, 675f
  - indications for, 628
  - with intravascular ultrasound, 635-637, 637f
  - percutaneous placement with venography bedside transabdominal or intravascular ultrasound in, 635
  - percutaneous placement with venography in, 633
  - percutaneous superior vena cava filter and, 637-638
  - permanent *versus* retrievable filter in, 631-632, 632f
  - postoperative care in, 638
  - pregnant patient and, 633
  - preoperative preparation for, 630-631, 632f
  - retrieval of vena cava filter and, 638
  - with transabdominal duplex ultrasound, 635, 635f-636f
- reconstruction surgery of, 650-663
  - anatomy in, 656
  - choice of incision for, 656-657, 657f
  - complications in, 662-663
  - femoral-femoral venous bypass in, 658, 658f
  - ileocaval venous bypass in, 658-659, 659f
  - indications for, 650, 651b
  - pitfalls and danger points in, 653-656, 654f-656f
  - postoperative care in, 662
  - preoperative preparation for, 650-653, 652f-653f
  - resection of suprarenal inferior vena cava inconjunction with major liver resection in, 657
  - technique in, 659-662, 660f

Inflammatory abdominal aortic aneurysm, 300

Infrapopliteal disease
- direct surgical repair of, 543-560
  - anastomotic technique in, 546-547, 547f
  - complications in, 558-559
  - femoral distal artery-vein bypass grafting in, 547-548
  - femoral-anterior tibial artery bypass in, 552-554, 553f-554f
  - femoral-peroneal artery bypass in, 555-558
  - femoral-posterior tibial artery bypass in, 555, 557f
  - indications for, 543
  - inflow exposure at femoral and popliteal arteries in, 548-551, 549f-551f
  - instrumentation and tunnelers for, 546
  - lower extremity fasciotomy in, 558
  - open ulcer and, 545-546
  - pitfalls and danger points in, 544
  - postoperative care in, 558
  - preoperative preparation for, 543-544
  - proximal and distal control in, 546
  - selection and assessment of site for distal anastomosis in, 545

Infrapopliteal disease *(Continued)*
- selection and assessment of site for inflow in, 545
- selection of conduit for, 544-545
- endovascular treatment of, 590-597
  - angiographic anatomy and common collateral pathways in, 591
  - complications in, 596-597
  - indications for, 590
  - postoperative care in, 595-596
  - preoperative preparation for, 590-591
  - selection of antegrade or retrograde access in, 592
  - selection of stent for, 592
  - tibial artery angioplasty and stenting in, 592-594, 593f
  - tibial artery laser angioplasty and stenting in, 595
  - tibial artery subintimal angioplasty and stenting in, 594-595, 595f-596f
  - unfavorable anatomic and physiologic features for interventions in, 592

Infrapopliteal percutaneous angioplasty, 592-594, 593f

Infrarenal aortic aneurysm
- direct surgical repair of, 301-304
  - aortic incision in, 302, 303f
  - closure in, 304
  - complications in, 307-308
  - distal anastomosis in, 302-304, 305f
  - exposure of abdominal aorta in, 301-302, 303f
  - exposure of iliac arteries in, 302
  - graft coverage in, 304
  - incision in, 301
  - postoperative care in, 307
  - proximal anastomosis in, 302
  - proximal and distal control in, 302
  - reimplantation of inferior mesenteric or accessory renal artery in, 304
- endovascular repair of, 321-335
  - access in unfavorable anatomy in, 336-337
  - adjunctive iliac angioplasty in, 323
  - AFX endograft in, 330
  - angiography in, 325-326, 325f-327f
  - Aorfix endograft in, 330
  - aortouniiliac graft in, 330-332, 331f
  - arterial access in, 324-325
  - arterial dissection during, 332
  - distal embolization in, 332
  - Endurant device in, 329-330
  - Excluder endograft in, 329
  - external iliac to internal iliac artery bypass in, 333, 333f
  - graft deployment and cannulation of contralateral gate in, 326-328, 328f-329f
  - graft sizing and selection in, 322-323, 323f, 337
  - hypogastric artery occlusion and, 333
  - hypogastric embolization in, 338-340, 340f
  - iliac artery conduit in, 324-325
  - limb occlusion in, 332
  - Ovation Prime endograft in, 330
  - percutaneous deployment in, 323-325
  - postoperative care in, 334, 342
  - postoperative complications in, 334
  - PowerLink endograft in, 330
  - preoperative preparation in, 321-322, 336
  - renal artery occlusion in, 332
  - rupture of aorta or iliac vessels during, 332
  - type I endoleak and, 336, 338, 339f
  - type II endoleak and, 341-342
  - unfavorable anatomy in, 336-337
  - Zenith endograft in, 330

Infrarenal sympathetic nerves, 399f

Inherited thrombophilia, 674

Injury to adjacent structures in vascular surgery, 13-14

Innominate artery, ascending aorta-innominate artery bypass and, 132-134, 132f-134f

Innominate artery endovascular treatment, 148-156
- access in, 150V, 150-152, 152f-154f
- angiographic anatomy in, 149
- complications in, 155-156
- embolic protection devices in, 150
- imaging and selective catheterization in, 152-153
- lesion predilation in, 150
- postoperative care in, 155
- preoperative preparation for, 149
- protection of vertebral artery in, 150-151
- stent selection in, 150, 151f
- stenting in, 152f, 153

Innominate veins, superior vena cava syndrome reconstruction and, 645

In-stent stenosis
- after transjugular intrahepatic portosystemic shunt, 666, 671
- during carotid angioplasty and stenting, 86-100

Instruments for vascular surgery, 12, 14f

Intercostal arteries reimplantation in repair of descending thoracic aortic aneurysm, 225, 225V, 225f

Intermittent pneumatic compression after reconstruction of inferior vena cava and iliofemoral venous system, 662

Internal carotid artery
- average diameter of, 57t
- carotid angioplasty and stenting and anatomic and pathologic conditions and, 88t
- spasm during, 87
- carotid endarterectomy and, 70, 71f
- eversion endarterectomy and, 78V, 79f, 80, 81f, 84

Internal iliac artery, average diameter of, 57t

Internal iliac artery aneurysm repair
- embolization in, 324
- preservation of flow in, 324-325

Internal iliac artery to external iliac artery bypass, 333, 333f, 340

Internal jugular vein
- for access in transjugular intrahepatic portosystemic shunt, 667
- access to, 34

Internal valvuloplasty, 711, 712f

Interposition vein graft
- in arteriovenous graft thrombosis, 784
- in popliteal artery aneurysm repair, 569, 570f
- in subclavian artery aneurysm repair, 161

Intestinal injury in abdominal aortic aneurysm surgery, 297

Intestinal ischemia after surgical repair of aortoiliac occlusive disease, 360

Intraarterial thrombolysis in popliteal artery aneurysm, 567

Intraoperative imaging
- in endovascular popliteal artery aneurysm repair, 600-601
- in endovascular treatment of aortoiliac occlusive disease, 376
- in endovascular treatment of descending thoracic aortic aneurysm, 263-264, 263f, 265f

Intraoperative stroke
- during carotid angioplasty and stenting, 87
- during carotid body tumor surgery, 104
- during carotid endarterectomy, 65-66
- during surgical repair of aortic arch vessels, 129

Intraperitoneal hemorrhage in transjugular intrahepatic portosystemic shunt, 665-666, 666f

Intravascular ultrasound, 26–27, 27f
  before endovascular repair of thoracoabdominal aortic aneurysm, 234
  percutaneous vena cava filter placement with, 635–637
    bedside, 635
    dual venous access technique in, 637
    preprocedural imaging in, 636, 637f
    single venous access technique in, 636–637
    ultrasound system and filter choice in, 635–636
Iodixanol, 22
Iohexol, 22

J

J-shaped guidewire, 41, 43f
Jugular vein
  carotid endarterectomy and, 67, 69f
  injury in surgical repair of aortic arch vessels, 129
Juxtarenal abdominal aortic aneurysm
  direct surgical repair of, 309–320
    control of supraceliac aorta in, 311
    control of suprarenal aorta in, 311
    iliac artery involvement in, 313–315, 314b
    indications for, 309
    postoperative care in, 318
    postoperative complications in, 318–319
    preoperative preparation in, 309–310
    retroperitoneal exposure in, 311–313, 312f
    selection of site for proximal control in, 310–311
  endovascular repair of, 344V, 343–349
    branched grafts for, 344–346, 345f
    fenestrated grafts for, 343–344, 346
    hybrid surgical and endovascular approaches in, 347, 348f
    postoperative care in, 347–349
    postoperative complications in, 349
    preoperative preparation for, 343–344
    snorkel or chimney graft technique in, 346–347, 347f

K

Kissing balloon technique in aortoiliac occlusive disease, 380
Knee contracture after above- and below-knee amputation, 608–609
Kocher maneuver in direct surgical repair of renal artery aneurysm, 439–441, 441f
Kommerell diverticulum, 155
  aberrant right subclavian artery and, 160
  surgical repair of, 167, 168f
    closure in, 168
    distal exposure in, 167
    patient position and incision in, 167
    postoperative care in, 169
    postoperative complications in, 169
    thoracic exposure in, 167, 168f
Kumpe catheter, 45f

L

L2 to S1 exposure, 397–399, 398f–399f
Labetalol, 36t
Laboratory testing
  access site management and, 30
  in femoral-popliteal arterial occlusive disease, 527
  preoperative, 3
Laser angioplasty and stenting in tibial-peroneal arterial occlusive disease, 595
Late graft thrombosis in femoral-popliteal bypass, 541
Lateral compartment, lower leg fasciotomy and, 620, 621f
Lateral compartment of arm, 623
Lateral tunneling in femoral-anterior tibial artery bypass, 554
Lazy S-shaped incision in popliteal artery aneurysm repair, 563, 563f–564f
Left ventricular perforation during modular transcervical bifurcated stent graft, 239
Leg. *See also* Lower extremity arterial disease.
  edema after repair of tibial-peroneal arterial occlusive disease, 558
  lower leg fasciotomy and, 619–621, 619f
    anterior compartment and, 620, 620f–621f
    lateral compartment and, 620, 621f
    superficial and deep posterior compartments and, 620–621, 622f
Ligation
  of popliteal artery aneurysm, 568
  of splenic artery aneurysm, 504–505, 505f
Limb ischemia
  after neoaortoiliac system procedure for aortic graft infection, 425
  after surgical repair in aortoiliac occlusive disease, 359–360
  in popliteal artery aneurysm, 561
Limb occlusion in endovascular repair of infrarenal aortic aneurysm, 332
Liver
  ischemia after reconstruction of inferior vena cava and iliofemoral venous system, 655
  transjugular intrahepatic portosystemic shunt and, 664–671
    accessing portal vein in, 665–666, 668, 669f
    anesthesia in, 666
    completion portosystemic gradient measurement and portography in, 669, 670f
    complications in, 670–671
    localizing catheter tip in right hepatic vein in, 665
    mapping portal venous system in, 665, 666f, 667–668
    parenchymal tract in, 666, 668–669
    patient positioning and venous access in, 667
    portosystemic gradient measurements in, 666
    portosystemic pressure gradient measurement in, 667
    postoperative care in, 670
    preoperative preparation for, 664–665
    selection and deployment of stent in, 666, 669
    selective hepatic venography in, 667
    stent deployment in, 669
    target portosystemic gradient in, 666
Liver function tests after reconstruction of inferior vena cava and iliofemoral venous system and, 662
Liver resection, resection of inferior vena cava in conjunction with, 657
Local anesthesia
  in carotid angioplasty and stenting, 86
  in endovascular repair of arteriovenous graft thrombosis, 786
Long posterior flap below-knee amputation, 605–607, 606f
Long thoracic nerve
  injury in supraclavicular approach to thoracic outlet syndrome, 178, 191
  within thoracic outlet, 196
Loop composite polytetrafluorethylene-femoral vein arteriovenous access, 755, 755f
Lower extremity arterial disease
  amputation in, 604–609
    above-knee amputation in, 607–608, 607f
    complications in, 608–609
    of forefoot, 610–616, 612f–615f

Lower extremity arterial disease *(Continued)*
    indications for, 604
    long posterior flap below-knee amputation in, 605–607, 606f
    postoperative care in, 608
    preoperative preparation for, 604–605
  endovascular treatment of femoral-popliteal occlusive disease in, 578–589
    access selection in, 580
    angiographic anatomy and common collateral pathways in, 580, 581f
    angiography of lower extremity in, 582
    complications in, 587
    femoral-popliteal artery occlusions and, 585–586
    femoral-popliteal artery stenosis and, 582–585, 583f–585f
    indications for, 578, 579b, 579t
    postoperative care in, 587
    preoperative preparation for, 578–579
    retrograde and antegrade approaches for arterial access in, 581–582
    stent selection in, 580–581
    thrombolysis of acute femoral-popliteal artery occlusions and, 586–587
    unfavorable anatomic features for, 580
  femoral-popliteal bypass for, 525–542
    above-knee bypass in, 536–537
    alternate inflow sources in, 538, 539f–540f
    below-knee bypass in, 537
    complications in, 541
    femoral-popliteal thromboembolectomy and, 538–539
    indications for, 526
    in situ or reversed great saphenous vein for, 534
    intraoperative assessment of, 537
    open vein harvest for, 534–536
    pitfalls and danger points in, 528–529, 528f
    postoperative care in, 540–541
    preoperative assessment of vein quality in, 533
    preoperative preparation for, 526–528
    selection and assessment of inflow in, 532
    selection and assessment of outflow in, 532
    selection of conduit for, 533–534, 533f
    surgical anatomy of femoral and popliteal arteries in, 529–531, 530f–532f
    wound closure in, 538
  politeal artery entrapment in, 572–577
    avoiding nerve injury in, 573
    avoiding venous injury in, 574
    complications in, 576–577
    division of fascial and muscular bands in, 575–576
    exposure of popliteal artery in, 575f, 575, 576f
    incision for, 573–574
    preoperative preparation for, 572–573, 574f
    presence of arterial lesion and, 574
    surgical anatomy of posterior popliteal fossa and, 573
  popliteal artery aneurysm, direct surgical repair of, 561–571
    acute thrombosis and, 566–567
    avoiding nerve injury in, 565f, 566
    avoiding venous injury in, 566
    conduit selection in, 565
    indications for, 561–562
    medial approach in, 567–568
    pitfalls and danger points in, 563–564, 563f–564f
    posterior approach in, 568–569, 570f
    preoperative preparation for, 562–563, 562f
    selection and assessment of inflow and distal outflow in, 566
    selection of approach in, 564–565

Lower extremity arterial disease (Continued)
  popliteal artery aneurysm, endovascular treatment of, 598–603
    antegrade approach in, 600V, 600
    completion imaging studies in, 602
    complications in, 603
    endograft deployment in, 601–602, 602f
    indications for, 598–599
    intraoperative imaging in, 600–601
    postoperative care in, 602–603
    preoperative preparation for, 599
    selection of access site for, 598–599
    selection of endograft for, 599–600
    sheath placement in, 601, 601f
  tibial-peroneal arterial occlusive disease, direct surgical repair of, 543–560
    anastomotic technique in, 546–547, 547f
    complications in, 558–559
    femoral distal artery-vein bypass grafting in, 547–548
    femoral-anterior tibial artery bypass in, 552–554, 553f–554f
    femoral-peroneal artery bypass in, 555–558
    femoral-posterior tibial artery bypass in, 555, 557f
    indications for, 543
    inflow exposure at femoral and popliteal arteries in, 548–551, 549f–551f
    instrumentation and tunnelers for, 546
    lower extremity fasciotomy in, 558
    open ulcer and, 545–546
    pitfalls and danger points in, 544
    postoperative care in, 558
    preoperative preparation for, 543–544
    proximal and distal control in, 546
    selection and assessment of site for distal anastomosis in, 545
    selection and assessment of site for inflow in, 545
    selection of conduit for, 544–545
  tibial-peroneal arterial occlusive disease, endovascular treatment of, 590–597
    angiographic anatomy and common collateral pathways in, 591
    complications in, 596–597
    indications for, 590
    postoperative care in, 595–596
    preoperative preparation for, 590–591
    selection of antegrade or retrograde access in, 592
    selection of stent for, 592
    tibial artery angioplasty and stenting in, 592–594, 593f
    tibial artery laser angioplasty and stenting in, 595
    tibial artery subintimal angioplasty and stenting in, 594–595, 595f–596f
    unfavorable anatomic and physiologic features for interventions in, 592
Lower extremity bypass grafting in repair of aortoiliac occlusive disease, 355
Lower extremity deep and perforator vein incompetence, 708–720
  deep venous valve surgery in
    angioscope-assisted valvuloplasty in, 712
    artificial valve implantation in, 714–715
    autologous neovalve construction in, 713
    complications in, 719
    external banding valvuloplasty in, 712
    external valvuloplasty in, 711
    indications for, 708
    internal valvuloplasty in, 711, 712f
    operative strategy in, 710
    pitfalls and danger points in, 709–710
    postoperative care in, 718
    preoperative preparation for, 709
    transcommissural valvuloplasty in, 712
    vein segment transposition in, 713
    vein valve transplantation in, 708, 713–714
  subfascial endoscopic perforator surgery in
    choice of anesthesia for, 715

Lower extremity deep and perforator vein incompetence (Continued)
    deep venous valve surgery in, 719
    distal ankle perforators and, 718
    exploration of subfascial space in, 716, 717f–718f
    incision in, 715–716, 715b, 715f
    indications for, 708
    operative strategy in, 710–711
    paratibial fasciotomy in, 716
    pitfalls and danger points in, 709–710
    port insertion in, 716, 716f
    postoperative care in, 718–719
    preoperative preparation for, 709
Lower extremity fasciotomy, 617–626
  complications in, 624
  failure to release extremity compartments and, 618
  iatrogenic injury and, 618–619
  inadequate postoperative surveillance and, 619
  indications for, 617–618
  lower leg, 619, 619–621, 619f, 621f–622f
  postoperative care in, 624
  preoperative preparation for, 618
  thigh, 622–623
  in tibial-peroneal arterial occlusive disease, 558
  unrecognized compartment syndrome and, 618
Lower extremity ischemia
  abdominal aortic aneurysm surgery-related, 308
  after neoaortoiliac system procedure for aortic graft infection, 425
  after surgical repair in aortoiliac occlusive disease, 359–360
Lower extremity perfusion assessment, 407
Lower extremity vascular access for hemodialysis, 764–765
Lower extremity venous anatomy, 697, 698f
Lower leg fasciotomy, 619–621, 619f
  anterior compartment and, 620, 620f–621f
  lateral compartment and, 620, 621f
  superficial and deep posterior compartments and, 620–621, 622f
Low-molecular-weight heparin
  access site management and, 31t
  before endovenous thermal ablation of saphenous and perforating veins, 696
Lumbosacral spine exposure, 397–399, 398f–399f
Lymph node dissection in carotid body tumor surgery, 104
Lymphatic leak
  after extraanatomic aortic arch vessel repair, 146
  after femoral-popliteal bypass, 541
  after supraclavicular approach to thoracic outlet syndrome, 190
  after surgical repair of subclavian and axillary arteries, 169
  after vertebral artery surgery, 123–124
Lymphocele
  after extraanatomic aortic arch vessel repair, 146
  after femoral vein transposition, 756
  after femoral-popliteal bypass, 541
  after vertebral artery surgery, 123–124
  vascular surgery-related, 15
Lyse-and-go technique in endovascular treatment of arteriovenous graft thrombosis, 786

M

MAC. See Monitored anesthesia care
Magnetic resonance angiography
  in aortic dissection, 278–279
  in aortoiliac occlusive disease, 351, 375
  in popliteal artery aneurysm, 562–563
  in renal artery aneurysm, 466–467, 468f

Magnetic resonance angiography (Continued)
  before sclerotherapy, 721
  in superior vena cava syndrome, 642
  in tibial-peroneal arterial occlusive disease, 591
  before vertebral artery surgery, 113–114, 113f
  in visceral artery aneurysms, 501
Magnetic resonance imaging
  of carotid body tumor, 102
  in popliteal artery entrapment, 572
  before reconstruction of inferior vena cava and iliofemoral venous system, 650–651
  in thoracoabdominal aortic aneurysm, 234
Malignancy, superior vena cava syndrome secondary to, 642
Malignant ileofemoral venous occlusion, 650, 651b
Malpositioned stent, 61
Manual compression technique, access site management and, 36
Matting after sclerotherapy, 726
May-Thurner syndrome, 680, 682f
Mechanical thrombectomy, 586–587, 783
Medial adductor compartment of thigh, 622–623
Medial approach in popliteal artery aneurysm repair, 567–568
Medial cutaneous sural nerve injury in repair of popliteal artery aneurysm, 566
Median nerve, compartment syndrome and, 618
Median sternotomy
  in direct surgical repair of aortic arch vessels, 128
  in superior vena cava syndrome reconstruction, 648
Mediastinal hematoma after superior vena cava syndrome reconstruction, 649
Mediastinal tube after surgical repair of aortic arch vessels, 136
Medical therapy in vascular disease, 3
Medtronic vascular endograft for descending thoracic aortic aneurysm, 268–271, 269f–270f
MELD score, 664
Mesenteric bypass, 479
Mesenteric infarction, 488
Mesenteric ischemia
  direct surgical repair for, 475–490
    antegrade bypass in, 482–485, 483f, 485f
    approach to superior mesenteric artery in, 480–481, 480f–481f
    complications in, 488–489
    indications for, 476–477
    ischemia secondary to embolization, in situ thrombosis, and dissection and, 478–479
    postoperative care in, 488
    preoperative preparation for, 477
    retrograde bypass in, 485–486, 486f
    selection of celiac artery outflow in, 479–480
    selection of conduit in, 481–482
    selection of inflow source in, 479
    superior mesenteric artery embolectomy in, 487–488, 487f
    surgical anatomy for, 478
  endovascular treatment of, 491–499
    complications in, 498
    indications for, 491–492
    pitfalls and danger points in, 493–495, 495f
    postoperative care in, 498
    preoperative preparation for, 492–493, 493f–494f
    strategy in, 495–496, 495f
    technique in, 496, 497f
Metatarsal ray resection, 611–614, 614f–615f
Methicillin-resistant Staphylococcus aureus in aortic graft infection, 405

INDEX

Methylprednisolone for contrast media reaction, 23
Micropuncture kit, 33-34, 35f
Midazolam, 18
Midthigh prosthetic access for hemodialysis, 765, 766f
Miller vein cuff in femoral-popliteal bypass, 533-534, 533f
Mobile wad compartments of arm, 623
Model for end-stage liver disease score, 664
Modified Crawford classification of thoracoabdominal aortic aneurysms, 217, 217f
Modular branched repair of aortic arch aneurysm, 235-244
    modular transcervical bifurcated stent graft in, 233, 236-240, 237f-239f
    modular transfemoral multibranched stent graft in, 240-244, 241f
Modular transfemoral multibranched stent graft
    for aortic arch aneurysm, 240-244, 241f
    for thoracoabdominal aortic aneurysm, 244-249, 245f-246f, 248f
Monitored anesthesia care, 18
Monomelic neuropathy after arteriovenous graft, 745
Monorail balloon catheter, 52, 52f, 460
Motor-evoked potential monitoring, 219-220
MRI. *See* Magnetic resonance imaging

N

N-acetylcysteine
    before endovascular treatment of aortoiliac occlusive disease, 376
    for renal protection, 22-23
NAIS. *See* Neoaortoiliac system procedure
Naloxone hydrochloride, 18
Negative pressure wound therapy after fasciotomy, 624
Neoaortoiliac system procedure for aortic graft infection, 419-426
    complications in, 424-425
    construction of neoaortoiliac system in, 421-422, 423f
    distal anastomosis in, 422-423
    flap coverage in, 423-424, 424f
    harvesting femoral popliteal vein in, 420V, 420-421, 421f-422f
    postoperative care in, 424
    preoperative preparation for, 419-420
    proximal anastomosis in, 422
    selection of conduit for in situ repair in, 420
    staging of, 420
Nephropathy, contrast-induced, 22, 22b, 376
Nerve conduction studies
    before supraclavicular approach to thoracic outlet syndrome, 172
    before transaxillary rib resection for thoracic outlet syndrome, 195
Nerve injury
    in basilic vein transposition, 747
    in brachial artery-axillary vein interposition graft, 740
    in carotid body tumor surgery, 109
    carotid endarterectomy-related, 75
    in subfascial endoscopic perforator surgery, 719
    in supraclavicular approach to thoracic outlet syndrome, 177-178
    in surgical repair of aortic arch vessels, 128
    in surgical repair of popliteal artery aneurysm, 565f, 566
    in surgical repair of popliteal artery entrapment, 573
    in transaxillary rib resection for thoracic outlet syndrome, 202
    in varicose vein stripping, 686-687, 692
    in vertebral artery surgery, 123

Neuromonitoring
    in endovascular treatment of aortic dissection, 287
    in surgical repair of thoracoabdominal aortic aneurysm, 219-220
    in transjugular intrahepatic portosystemic shunt, 670
Neuropathic pain
    after arteriovenous fistula procedure, 738
    after arteriovenous graft, 745
    after neoaortoiliac system procedure for aortic graft infection, 425
Neurorescue techniques in carotid angioplasty and stenting, 99-100
Nitroglycerin for periprocedural blood pressure control, 36t
Nonbeveled end-to-side anastomosis, 10-11, 11f
Noninfected anastomotic femoral artery pseudoaneurysm, 428-429, 429f
Nonrecurrent right laryngeal nerve, aberrant right subclavian artery and, 160
Nonselective angiographic catheter, 45-46, 45f
Nutritional assessment
    before surgical repair of thoracoabdominal aortic aneurysm, 217
    before total graft excision and extraanatomic repair of aortic graft infection, 407

O

Obesity
    access site management and, 35
    anterior spine exposure and, 393
    difficult access of fistulas and, 737
Occlusion
    aortic, 385-387, 386f
    in carotid angioplasty and stenting, 98-99
    femoral-popliteal artery, 585-586
    guidewire crossing of, 47-48, 47f-48f
    hypogastric artery, 333
    ileofemoral venous
        benign, 650
        malignant, 650, 651b
    in renal artery aneurysm, 471, 472f-473f
    vascular, 6-7, 8f
Occlusive femoral-popliteal arterial disease
    endovascular treatment of, 578-589
        access selection in, 580
        angiographic anatomy and common collateral pathways in, 580, 581f
        angiography of lower extremity in, 582
        complications in, 587
        femoral-popliteal artery occlusions and, 585-586
        femoral-popliteal artery stenosis and, 582-585, 583f-585f
        indications for, 578, 579b, 579t
        postoperative care in, 587
        preoperative preparation for, 578-579
        retrograde and antegrade approaches for arterial access in, 581-582
        stent selection in, 580-581
        thrombolysis of acute femoral-popliteal artery occlusions and, 586-587
        unfavorable anatomic features for, 580
    open surgical femoral-popliteal bypass for, 525-542
        above-knee, 536-537
        alternate inflow sources in, 538, 539f-540f
        below-knee, 537
        complications in, 541
        femoral-popliteal thromboembolectomy and, 538-539
        indications for, 526
        in situ or reversed great saphenous vein for, 534
        intraoperative assessment of, 537
        open vein harvest for, 534-536
        pitfalls and danger points in, 528-529, 528f
        postoperative care in, 540-541

Occlusive femoral-popliteal arterial disease *(Continued)*
        preoperative assessment of vein quality in, 533
        preoperative preparation for, 526-528
        selection and assessment of inflow in, 532
        selection and assessment of outflow in, 532
        selection of conduit for, 533-534, 533f
        surgical anatomy of femoral and popliteal arteries in, 529-531, 530f-532f
        wound closure in, 538
Occlusive superior mesenteric artery disease
    direct surgical repair for, 475-490
        antegrade bypass in, 482-485, 483f, 485f
        approach to superior mesenteric artery in, 480-481, 480f-481f
        complications in, 488-489
        indications for, 476-477
        ischemia secondary to embolization, in situ thrombosis, and dissection and, 478-479
        postoperative care in, 488
        preoperative preparation for, 477
        retrograde bypass in, 485-486, 486f
        selection of celiac artery outflow in, 479-480
        selection of conduit in, 481-482
        selection of inflow source in, 479
        superior mesenteric artery embolectomy in, 487-488, 487f
        surgical anatomy for, 478
    endovascular treatment of, 491-499
        complications in, 498
        indications for, 491-492
        pitfalls and danger points in, 493-495, 495f
        postoperative care in, 498
        preoperative preparation for, 492-493, 493f-494f
        strategy in, 495-496, 495f
        technique in, 496, 497f
Occlusive tibial-peroneal arterial disease
    direct surgical repair of, 543-560
        anastomotic technique in, 546-547, 547f
        complications in, 558-559
        femoral distal artery-vein bypass grafting in, 547-548
        femoral-anterior tibial artery bypass in, 552-554, 553f-554f
        femoral-peroneal artery bypass in, 555-558
        femoral-posterior tibial artery bypass in, 555, 557f
        indications for, 543
        inflow exposure at femoral and popliteal arteries in, 548-551, 549f-551f
        instrumentation and tunnelers for, 546
        lower extremity fasciotomy in, 558
        open ulcer and, 545-546
        pitfalls and danger points in, 544
        postoperative care in, 558
        preoperative preparation for, 543-544
        proximal and distal control in, 546
        selection and assessment of site for distal anastomosis in, 545
        selection and assessment of site for inflow in, 545
        selection of conduit for, 544-545
    endovascular treatment of, 590-597
        angiographic anatomy and common collateral pathways in, 591
        complications in, 596-597
        indications for, 590
        postoperative care in, 595-596
        preoperative preparation for, 590-591
        selection of antegrade or retrograde access in, 592
        selection of stent for, 592

Occlusive tibial-peroneal arterial disease *(Continued)*
  tibial artery angioplasty and stenting in, 592-594, 593f
  tibial artery laser angioplasty and stenting in, 595
  tibial artery subintimal angioplasty and stenting in, 594-595, 595f-596f
  unfavorable anatomic and physiologic features for interventions in, 592
Olcott torque device, 44f
Omental pedicle flap in aortic graft infection
  neoaortoiliac system procedure for, 423
  total graft excision and extraanatomic repair of, 414-415
Omni flush diagnostic catheter, 45f, 582
Omnipaque. *See* Iohexol
Open femoral artery exposure in endovascular repair of infrarenal aortic aneurysm, 324
Operating room preparation in vascular surgery, 4-5
OptEase filter, 629t, 630f, 675f
Ovation Prime endograft, 330
Oversedation, 18

P

PAD. *See* Peripheral artery disease
Paget-Schroetter syndrome, 194, 204-214, 205f
  access in, 208
  angiographic anatomy and collaterals in, 205-206, 206f-207f
  angioplasty and stenting in, 212
  completion studies in, 212
  complications in, 213
  postoperative care in, 212-213
  preoperative preparation for, 204-205
  sheath placement in, 208
  technique in, 208-212, 209f
  thrombolysis in, 209-212, 210f-211f
  timing of, 206-208, 208f
Pain
  in acute aortic dissection, 275
  after arteriovenous fistula procedure, 738
  after arteriovenous graft, 745
  after endovenous thermal ablation of saphenous and perforating veins, 705
  after varicose vein stripping, 687-688
  in compartment syndrome, 617-618
Pancreaticoduodenal artery aneurysm, 513-524, 518f-521f
  access and guiding sheath placement in, 515
  angiographic imaging in, 515
  indications for, 514
  postoperative care in, 523-524
  preoperative preparation for, 514
Pancreatitis after splenic artery aneurysm repair, 511
Parachuting technique in beveled end-to-side anastomosis, 8-9
Paraplegia
  after endovascular treatment of aortic dissection, 282
  after endovascular treatment of descending thoracic artery aneurysm, 254, 271-272
  after endovascular treatment of traumatic thoracic aortic disruption, 293
  after surgical repair of thoracoabdominal aortic aneurysm, 229, 229f
Pararenal abdominal aortic aneurysm repair, 315V, 315-318
  control of supraceliac aorta in, 311
  control of suprarenal aorta in, 311
  incision for, 313, 315-316
  indications for, 309
  postoperative care in, 318
  preoperative preparation in, 309-310
  selection of site for proximal control in, 310-311
  transperitoneal *versus* retroperitoneal exposure in, 310, 310b

Pararenal aorta exposure
  in aortorenal bypass, 439, 440f
  in direct surgical repair of renovascular disease, 438
  in renal artery endarterectomy, 442, 443f
Paratibial fasciotomy, 716
Parenchymal tract in transjugular intrahepatic portosystemic shunt, 668-669
Patch angioplasty, 5
  in arteriovenous graft thrombosis, 784
  in carotid endarterectomy, 73, 73f
Patent foramen ovale, sclerotherapy and, 722
Patient positioning
  in aberrant right subclavian artery repair, 165, 165f
  access site management and, 31
  in brachial vein transposition, 762
  in carotid endarterectomy, 67, 68f
  in endovascular treatment of infrapopliteal disease, 592
  in endovenous thermal ablation of saphenous and perforating veins, 699
  in femoral distal artery-vein bypass grafting, 547-548
  in hepatorenal bypass, 450, 451f
  for HERO device, 769
  in internal jugular vein access, 34
  in Kommerell diverticulum repair, 167
  in lower extremity vascular access for hemodialysis, 764
  in popliteal artery aneurysm repair
    medial approach, 567
    posterior approach, 568-569
  for prosthetic chest wall vascular access for hemodialysis, 766
  in saphenous vein transposition, 763
  in sclerotherapy, 724
  in subclavian artery aneurysm repair, 162
  in superior vena cava syndrome reconstruction, 645
  in supraclavicular approach to thoracic outlet syndrome, 179-180, 179f
  in surgical repair of aortic arch vessels, 130, 131f
  in surgical repair of thoracoabdominal aortic aneurysm, 220-221, 221f
  in transaxillary rib resection for thoracic outlet syndrome, 196, 197f
  in transjugular intrahepatic portosystemic shunt, 667
  in vascular surgery, 5
Pectoralis minor tenotomy, 177, 186, 186f
Pediatric patient, unconventional hemodialysis access and, 760
Perclose closure device, 39f, 39f
Percutaneous access in endovascular repair of infrarenal aortic aneurysm, 324-325
Percutaneous filter placement with venography, 633
Percutaneous mechanical thrombectomy, 384
Percutaneous mesenteric revascularization, 491-499
  complications in, 498
  indications for, 491-492
  pitfalls and danger points in, 493-495, 495f
  postoperative care in, 498
  preoperative preparation for, 492-493, 493f-494f
  strategy in, 495-496, 495f
  technique in, 496, 497f
Percutaneous superior vena cava filter placement, 637-638
Percutaneous transluminal angioplasty
  balloons for, 53t
  indications for, 50
  in tibial-peroneal arterial occlusive disease, 592
Percutaneous vena cava filter placement with bedside transabdominal or intravascular ultrasound, 635

Perforator veins
  endovenous thermal ablation of, 694-707
    access in, 699, 700f
    complications in, 705-706, 706f
    confirmation of catheter tip position in, 701, 701f
    endovascular strategy in, 696-699, 698f
    endovenous laser in, 700
    indications for, 695f, 696
    patient positioning for, 699
    postoperative care in, 704-705
    preoperative preparation for, 696, 697f
    radiofrequency catheter in, 699-700, 700f
    treatment of axial veins in, 702-703
    tumescent anesthesia in, 701, 702f
  subfascial endoscopic surgery of, 708-720
    choice of anesthesia for, 715
    deep venous valve surgery in, 719
    distal ankle perforators and, 718
    exploration of subfascial space in, 716, 717f-718f
    incision in, 715-716, 715b, 715f
    indications for, 708
    operative strategy in, 710-711
    paratibial fasciotomy in, 716
    pitfalls and danger points in, 709-710
    port insertion in, 716, 716f
    postoperative care in, 718-719
    preoperative preparation for, 709
Periarteritis nodosa, visceral aneurysms in, 501
Pericardial effusion, 649
Periincisional hypesthesia, carotid endarterectomy-related, 75
Peripheral artery disease
  amputation in, 604-609
    above-knee amputation in, 607-608, 607f
    complications in, 608-609
    of forefoot, 610-616, 612f-615f
    indications for, 604
    long posterior flap below-knee amputation in, 605-607, 606f
    postoperative care in, 608
    preoperative preparation for, 604-605
  endovascular treatment of femoral-popliteal occlusive disease in, 578-589
    access selection in, 580
    angiographic anatomy and common collateral pathways in, 580, 581f
    angiography of lower extremity in, 582
    complications in, 587
    femoral-popliteal artery occlusions and, 585-586
    femoral-popliteal artery stenosis and, 582-585, 583f-585f
    indications for, 578, 579b, 579t
    postoperative care in, 587
    preoperative preparation for, 578-579
    retrograde and antegrade approaches for arterial access in, 581-582
    stent selection in, 580-581
    thrombolysis of acute femoral-popliteal artery occlusions and, 586-587
    unfavorable anatomic features for, 580
  femoral-popliteal bypass for, 525-542
    above-knee bypass in, 536-537
    alternate inflow sources in, 538, 539f-540f
    below-knee bypass in, 537
    complications in, 541
    femoral-popliteal thromboembolectomy and, 538-539
    indications for, 526
    in situ or reversed great saphenous vein for, 534
    intraoperative assessment of, 537
    open vein harvest for, 534-536
    pitfalls and danger points in, 528-529, 528f
    postoperative care in, 540-541
    preoperative assessment of vein quality in, 533
    preoperative preparation for, 526-528

Peripheral artery disease *(Continued)*
  selection and assessment of inflow in, 532
  selection and assessment of outflow in, 532
  selection of conduit for, 533-534, 533f
  surgical anatomy of femoral and popliteal arteries in, 529-531, 530f-532f
  wound closure in, 538
popliteal artery aneurysm, direct surgical repair of, 561-571
  acute thrombosis and, 566-567
  avoiding nerve injury in, 565f, 566
  avoiding venous injury in, 566
  conduit selection in, 565
  indications for, 561-562
  medial approach in, 567-568
  pitfalls and danger points in, 563-564, 563f-564f
  posterior approach in, 568-569, 570f
  preoperative preparation for, 562-563, 562f
  selection and assessment of inflow and distal outflow in, 566
  selection of approach in, 564-565
popliteal artery aneurysm, endovascular treatment of, 598-603
  antegrade approach in, 600V, 600
  completion imaging studies in, 602
  complications in, 603
  endograft deployment in, 601-602, 602f
  indications for, 598-599
  intraoperative imaging in, 600-601
  postoperative care in, 602-603
  preoperative preparation for, 599
  selection of access site for, 598-599
  selection of endograft for, 599-600
  sheath placement in, 601, 601f
popliteal artery entrapment in, 572-577
  avoiding nerve injury in, 573
  avoiding venous injury in, 574
  complications in, 576-577
  division of fascial and muscular bands in, 575-576
  exposure of popliteal artery in, 576f, 575, 576f
  incision for, 573-574
  preoperative preparation for, 572-573, 574f
  presence of arterial lesion and, 574
  surgical anatomy of posterior popliteal fossa and, 573
tibial-peroneal arterial occlusive disease, direct surgical repair of, 543-560
  anastomotic technique in, 546-547, 547f
  complications in, 558-559
  femoral distal artery-vein bypass grafting in, 547-548
  femoral-anterior tibial artery bypass in, 552-554, 553f-554f
  femoral-peroneal artery bypass in, 555-558
  femoral-posterior tibial artery bypass in, 555, 557f
  indications for, 543
  inflow exposure at femoral and popliteal arteries in, 548-551, 549f-551f
  instrumentation and tunnelers for, 546
  lower extremity fasciotomy in, 558
  open ulcer and, 545-546
  pitfalls and danger points in, 544
  postoperative care in, 558
  preoperative preparation for, 543-544
  proximal and distal control in, 546
  selection and assessment of site for distal anastomosis in, 545
  selection and assessment of site for inflow in, 545
  selection of conduit for, 544-545
tibial-peroneal arterial occlusive disease, endovascular treatment of, 590-597

Peripheral artery disease *(Continued)*
  angiographic anatomy and common collateral pathways in, 591
  complications in, 596-597
  indications for, 590
  postoperative care in, 595-596
  preoperative preparation for, 590-591
  selection of antegrade or retrograde access in, 592
  selection of stent for, 592
  tibial artery angioplasty and stenting in, 592-594, 593f
  tibial artery laser angioplasty and stenting in, 595
  tibial artery subintimal angioplasty and stenting in, 594-595, 595f-596f
  unfavorable anatomic and physiologic features for interventions in, 592
Peripheral vascular examination before spine exposure, 393
Peroneal artery
  angiographic anatomy of, 591
  femoral-peroneal artery bypass and, 555-558
Peroneal nerve
  injury in surgical repair of popliteal artery aneurysm, 566
  posterior myocutaneous flap and, 605-607
Pharmacomechanical thrombolysis in subclavian-axillary vein thrombosis, 211-212, 211f
Phlebitis after endovenous thermal ablation of saphenous and perforating veins, 705
Phrenic nerve, 196
Phrenic nerve injury
  in extraanatomic aortic arch vessel repair, 146
  in supraclavicular approach to thoracic outlet syndrome, 178, 190-191
  in surgical repair of subclavian and axillary arteries, 169
Physical activity
  after above- and below-knee amputation, 608
  after endovenous thermal ablation of saphenous and perforating veins, 705
  after femoral vein transposition, 756
  after surgical repair of aortic arch vessels, 136
  restriction after vascular access, 37
Physical examination
  in aortoiliac occlusive disease, 350, 383
  before brachial artery-axillary vein interposition graft, 739, 740f
  before brachiocephalic and radiocephalic arteriovenous fistulas, 731
  before distal revascularization interval ligation, 773
  before fasciotomy, 618
  in femoral-popliteal arterial occlusive disease, 526
  before forearm loop graft, 739, 740f
  in infrarenal aortic aneurysm, 321
  before sclerotherapy, 721
  before surgical repair of aortic arch vessels, 127
  before transaxillary rib resection for thoracic outlet syndrome, 193-194
  before varicose vein stripping, 685
Pigtail catheter, 44t, 45f
Pin vise, 44f
Plavix. *See* clopidogrel
Pneumothorax
  after extraanatomic aortic arch vessel repair, 146
  after surgical repair of subclavian and axillary arteries, 169
  after transaxillary rib resection for thoracic outlet syndrome, 202-203
Popliteal artery
  angiographic anatomy of, 591
  average diameter of, 57t
  direct surgical repair of tibial-peroneal arterial occlusive disease and, 548-551

Popliteal artery *(Continued)*
  above-knee, 551, 551f
  below-knee, 551, 552f
  exposure in surgical repair of popliteal artery entrapment, 575f, 575, 576f
  surgical anatomy of, 529-531, 530f-532f
Popliteal artery aneurysm
  direct surgical repair of, 561-571
    acute thrombosis and, 566-567
    avoiding nerve injury in, 565f, 566
    avoiding venous injury in, 566
    conduit selection in, 565
    indications for, 561-562
    medial approach in, 567-568
    pitfalls and danger points in, 563-564, 563f-564f
    posterior approach in, 568-569, 570f
    preoperative preparation for, 562-563, 562f
    selection and assessment of inflow and distal outflow in, 566
    selection of approach in, 564-565
  endovascular treatment of, 598-603
    antegrade approach in, 600V, 600
    completion imaging studies in, 602
    complications in, 603
    endograft deployment in, 601-602, 602f
    indications for, 598-599
    intraoperative imaging in, 600-601
    postoperative care in, 602-603
    preoperative preparation for, 599
    selection of access site for, 598-599
    selection of endograft for, 599-600
    sheath placement in, 601, 601f
Popliteal artery entrapment, 572-577
  avoiding nerve injury in, 573
  avoiding venous injury in, 574
  complications in, 576-577
  division of fascial and muscular bands in, 575-576
  exposure of popliteal artery in, 576f, 575, 576f
  incision for, 573-574
  preoperative preparation for, 572-573, 574f
  presence of arterial lesion and, 574
  surgical anatomy of posterior popliteal fossa and, 573
Popliteal fossa
  surgical anatomy of, 529, 531f-532f, 573
  varicose vein stripping and, 685-686
Popliteal vein
  access to, 35
  femoral vein transposition and, 751
  injury in surgical repair of popliteal artery aneurysm, 566
  neoaortoiliac system procedure for aortic graft infection and, 420V, 420-421, 421f-422f
Portal vein
  access in transjugular intrahepatic portosystemic shunt, 665-666, 668, 669f
  thrombosis after transjugular intrahepatic portosystemic shunt, 671
Portography in transjugular intrahepatic portosystemic shunt, 669, 670f
Portosystemic gradient measurements, 666-667
Positioning of patient. *See* Patient positioning
Posterior approach
  in popliteal artery aneurysm repair, 568-569, 570f
  in popliteal artery entrapment, 573
Posterior myocutaneous flap, 605-607
Posterior tibial artery
  angiographic anatomy of, 591
  compartment syndrome and, 618
  femoral-posterior tibial artery bypass and, 555, 557f
  injury in varicose vein stripping, 686
Posterior tibial nerve injury in repair of popliteal artery entrapment, 573
Posterior tibial vein access, 35
Posterolateral flexor compartment of thigh, 622

Postoperative bleeding
  in aortoiliac occlusive disease, 358
  in femoral-popliteal arterial occlusive disease, 587
  in femoral-popliteal bypass, 541
  in renal artery stenosis, 464
  in subclavian-axillary vein thrombosis, 213
  in thoracic outlet syndrome, 190
Postoperative care
  in abdominal aortic aneurysms, 307
  in above- and below-knee amputation, 608
  in angioplasty and stenting, 60
  in anterior spine exposure, 399-400
  in aortic arch vessels surgery, 135-137, 139-140
  in aortic dissection repair, 287
  in aortic graft infection, 417, 424
  in aortoiliac occlusive disease, 382, 390
  in arteriovenous graft thrombosis, 790
  in basilic vein transposition, 750-751
  in brachial artery-axillary vein interposition graft, 743-744
  in brachiocephalic arteriovenous fistula, 736
  in carotid angioplasty and stenting, 100
  in carotid body tumor, 108-109
  in carotid endarterectomy, 74
  in celiac axis and superior mesenteric artery occlusive disease, 488
  in deep venous valve surgery, 718
  in descending thoracic aortic aneurysm, 271
  in distal revascularization interval ligation procedure, 779
  in endovenous thermal ablation of saphenous and perforating veins, 704-705
  in eversion endarterectomy, 82-84
  in fasciotomy, 624
  in femoral artery pseudoaneurysm repair, 433
  in femoral vein transposition, 753
  in femoral-popliteal arterial occlusive disease, 587
  in femoral-popliteal bypass, 540-541
  in forearm loop graft, 743-744
  in forefoot amputation, 614-615
  in iliofemoral and femoral-popliteal deep vein thrombosis, 681-682
  in infrarenal aortic aneurysm, 307, 334
  in juxtarenal and pararenal aortic aneurysms, 318, 347-349
  in Kommerell diverticulum repair, 169
  in mesenteric ischemia, 498
  in popliteal artery aneurysm repair, 602-603
  in radiocephalic arteriovenous fistula, 736
  in reconstruction of inferior vena cava and iliofemoral venous system and, 662
  in renal artery aneurysm repair, 471-473
  in renal artery stenosis endovascular repair, 464
  in renovascular disease, 447
  in sclerotherapy, 724-725
  in subclavian and axillary artery surgery, 168-169
  in subclavian artery aneurysm repair, 168-169
  in subclavian-axillary vein thrombosis, 212-213
  in subfascial endoscopic perforator surgery, 718-719
  in superior vena cava syndrome reconstruction, 648
  in thoracic outlet syndrome, 189-190, 202
  in thoracoabdominal aortic aneurysm, 228
  in tibial-peroneal arterial occlusive disease, 558, 595-596
  in transjugular intrahepatic portosystemic shunt, 670
  in traumatic thoracic aortic disruption, 292-293
  in unconventional hemodialysis access, 770
  in varicose vein stripping, 692
  in vena cava filter placement, 638
  in visceral artery aneurysms, 511
PowerLink endograft in repair of infrarenal aortic aneurysm, 330
Predilation in aortic arch vessels endovascular treatment, 150
Prednisone for contrast media reaction, 23
Pregnant patient
  sclerotherapy and, 723
  vena cava filter placement in, 633
Preoperative assessment, 4
Preoperative embolization of carotid body tumor, 104
Preoperative marking for varicose vein stripping, 686
Preoperative preparation
  in abdominal aortic aneurysm surgery, 296-297
  in above- and below-knee amputation, 604-605
  for anterior spine exposure, 392-393
  in aortic arch vessels surgical repair, 127-128
  in aortic graft infection
    neoaortoiliac system procedure for, 419-420
    total graft excision and extraanatomic repair of, 405-407, 406f
  in aortoiliac occlusive disease, 350-351
  in arteriovenous graft thrombosis repair
    endovascular, 784-785
    surgical, 781-782
  for basilic vein transposition, 747
  in brachial artery-axillary vein interposition graft, 739-740, 740f-741f
  in carotid angioplasty and stenting, 86-87
  in carotid body tumor resection, 102
  in carotid endarterectomy, 64-65
  in deep venous valve surgery, 709
  in distal revascularization interval ligation, 773-774, 774f
  in endovascular repair
    of aneurysms of juxtarenal and pararenal aorta, 343-344
    of aortic dissection, 275
    of aortoiliac occlusive disease, 375-376
    of descending thoracic aortic aneurysm, 252-253, 253f-254f
    of femoral-popliteal arterial occlusive disease, 578-579
    of infrarenal aortic aneurysm, 321-322
    of renal artery stenosis, 456-457
    of subclavian-axillary vein thrombosis, 204-205
    of traumatic thoracic aortic disruption, 289-290, 291t
  in endovenous thermal ablation of saphenous and perforating veins, 696, 697f
  in eversion endarterectomy, 77-78
  in extraanatomic repair
    of aortic arch vessels, 140-141
    of aortoiliac occlusive disease, 362
  for fasciotomy, 618
  in femoral artery pseudoaneurysm repair, 427-428
  for femoral-popliteal bypass, 526-528
  in forearm loop graft, 739-740, 740f-741f
  in iliofemoral and femoral-popliteal deep vein thrombosis, 673-674, 673f
  for mesenteric ischemia
    endovascular treatment of, 492-493, 493f-494f
    surgical repair of, 477
  in popliteal artery aneurysm repair
    direct surgical repair of, 562-563, 562f
    endovascular repair of, 599
  for popliteal artery entrapment, 572-573, 574f
  in radial artery-cephalic vein arteriovenous fistula, 731
  for reconstruction of inferior vena cava and iliofemoral venous system, 650-653, 652f-653f
  in renal artery aneurysm repair, 466-467, 467f-468f
Preoperative preparation (Continued)
  for renovascular disease
    direct surgical repair of, 437
    extraanatomic repair of, 449
  in sclerotherapy, 721-722
  in subclavian and axillary artery surgery, 157-158, 158f
  in subclavian artery aneurysm repair, 157, 158f
  in subfascial endoscopic perforator surgery, 709
  in superior vena cava syndrome, 641-643, 642f-643f
  in thoracic outlet syndrome
    supraclavicular approach to, 172-174, 173b
    transaxillary rib resection for, 194-195
  in thoracoabdominal aortic aneurysm
    direct surgical repair of, 217
    endovascular repair of, 233-234
  in tibial-peroneal arterial occlusive disease
    direct surgical repair of, 543-544
    endovascular treatment of, 590-591
  for transjugular intrahepatic portosystemic shunt, 664-665
  in unconventional hemodialysis access, 758-759
  for varicose vein stripping, 685-686
  for vena cava filter placement, 630-631, 632f
  in vertebral artery surgery, 115, 112-114, 113b, 113f, 115f
  in visceral artery aneurysms, 501-502
Profunda femoris artery
  average diameter of, 57t
  direct surgical repair of tibial-peroneal arterial occlusive disease and, 549-550, 549f-550f
  endarterectomy of, 528-529
  exposure in total graft excision and extraanatomic repair of aortic graft infection, 414
  in femoral-popliteal bypass, 538
Profundaplasty in aortobifemoral bypass, 356
Proper hepatic artery, 502
Prophylactic antibiotics, 5
  after tibial-peroneal arterial occlusive disease surgery, 558
  before arteriovenous graft thrombosis repair, 782, 784
  before distal revascularization interval ligation, 774
  before transjugular intrahepatic portosystemic shunt, 665
Prophylactic fasciotomy, 617
Prosthetic axillary-axillary loop access for hemodialysis, 766-767, 767f
Prosthetic axillary-axillary straight (necklace) access for hemodialysis, 767
Prosthetic chest wall vascular access for hemodialysis, 759t, 761, 765-767, 767f
Prosthetic lower extremity vascular access for hemodialysis, 759t, 760-761, 764-765, 766f
Proximal anastomosis
  in abdominal aortic aneurysm repair, 302
  in above-knee popliteal bypass, 536-537
  in antegrade bypass in mesenteric ischemia, 484, 485f
  in carotid body tumor repair, 108, 108f
  in celiac artery aneurysm repair, 510
  in descending thoracic aortic aneurysm repair, 225
  in direct surgical repair of aortoiliac occlusive disease, 356-358, 357f, 359f
  in distal revascularization interval ligation, 776, 777f
  in Type I thoracoabdominal aortic aneurysm repair, 226
  in extraanatomic repair for renovascular disease, 452, 454f
  in hepatic artery aneurysm repair, 507
  in juxtarenal abdominal aortic aneurysm repair, 315

INDEX

Proximal anastomosis (Continued)
   in neoaortoiliac system, 422
   in pararenal or suprarenal abdominal aortic aneurysm repair, 316-318, 319f
Proximal aortic stump closure in total graft excision and extraanatomic repair of aortic graft infection, 414-415, 415f
Proximal pelvic veins, 699
Proximal prosthetic thigh access for hemodialysis, 759t, 765, 766f
Pseudoaneurysm
   after percutaneous access, 40
   femoral artery, 427-434
      endovascular options for, 432
      iatrogenic, 432-433
      indications for surgical treatment of, 427
      infected, 429-432, 430f-431f
      noninfected anastomotic, 428-429, 429f
      postoperative care in, 433
      preoperative preparation for surgical treatment of, 427-428
   iliac artery, 278
Pulmonary complications
   after distal revascularization interval ligation procedure, 773
   after surgical repair of thoracoabdominal aortic aneurysm, 229
Pulmonary embolism
   after endovascular therapy for subclavian-axillary vein thrombosis, 213
   after vena cava placement, 639
   in reconstruction of inferior vena cava and iliofemoral venous system, 654
   superior vena cava syndrome reconstruction and, 644, 648, 649t
Pulmonary function tests, 4
   before reconstruction of inferior vena cava and iliofemoral venous system, 653
   before surgical repair of thoracoabdominal aortic aneurysm, 217
Pulse volume recordings in arterial steal syndrome, 737-738
Pulselessness, access site management and, 36

R

Radi pressure wire in renal artery stenosis, 463
Radial artery
   average diameter of, 57t
   basilic vein transposition and, 750
Radial artery-cephalic vein arteriovenous fistula, 729-738
   alternatives in absence of suitable cephalic vein and, 732
   anesthesia for, 732
   arteriovenous anastomosis in, 733-734
   complications in, 736-738
   confirmation of flow and closure in, 734, 734f
   exposure of cephalic vein in, 733
   exposure of radial artery in, 733
   heparinization in, 732
   incisions in, 732-733, 733f
   indications for, 730-731
   operative field in, 732
   postoperative care in, 736
   preoperative preparation for, 731
   selection of fistula site for, 732
Radiation exposure in fluoroscopy, 19-20, 20b
Radiation-induced arteritis, 126-127
Radiofrequency ablation of perforator veins, 704, 704f
Radiofrequency catheter in endovenous thermal ablation of saphenous and perforating veins, 699-700, 700f
Recanalization, 58-59, 59b
Reconstruction surgery
   of inferior vena cava and iliofemoral venous system, 650-663
      anatomy in, 656
      choice of incision for, 656-657, 657f
      complications in, 662-663

Reconstruction surgery (Continued)
      femoral-femoral venous bypass in, 658, 658f
      ileocaval venous bypass in, 658-659, 659f
      indications for, 650, 651b
      inferior vena cava reconstruction in, 659-662, 660f
      pitfalls and danger points in, 653-656, 654f-656f
      postoperative care in, 662
      preoperative preparation for, 650-653, 652f-653f
      resection of suprarenal inferior vena cava inconjunction with major liver resection in, 657
   in superior vena cava syndrome, 641-649
      anastomoses in, 645-648, 647f-648f
      anesthesia for, 644
      avoiding intraoperative bleeding in, 643
      avoiding pulmonary embolism in, 644
      closure of median sternotomy in, 648
      complications in, 648-649, 649t
      dissection of innominate veins and superior vena cava in, 645
      indications for, 641
      position and incision in, 645
      postoperative care in, 648
      preoperative preparation for, 641-643, 642f-643f
      selection of vascular conduit for, 644, 644t
      selection of venous inflow and outflow sites in, 644
      spiral vein graft in, 645, 646f
      unilateral versus bilateral, 644
Recovery G2 filter, 630f
Recurrence of thoracic outlet syndrome
   after supraclavicular approach to, 175-177
   after transaxillary rib resection, 203
Recurrent carotid stenosis, eversion endarterectomy for, 84-85
Recurrent dysphagia after repair of subclavian and axillary arteries, 169
Recurrent laryngeal nerve injury in surgical repair of aortic arch vessels, 129
Recurrent stenosis
   after endovascular treatment of mesenteric ischemia, 498
   complication during renal artery stenosis repair, 461-462, 462f
Redo surgery
   anterior spine exposure in, 393
   carotid
      carotid angioplasty and stenting in, 90
      eversion endarterectomy in, 84-85
   in femoral-popliteal bypass, 529
Reentry catheter in endovascular treatment of aortoiliac occlusive disease, 378-380, 381f
Renal artery
   anatomy of, 438
   average diameter of, 57t
   branch repair using in situ and ex vivo techniques, 445V, 445-447
   embolization before reconstruction of inferior vena cava and iliofemoral venous system, 653, 653f
   endovascular repair of thoracoabdominal aortic aneurysm and, 249
   endovascular treatment of aortic dissection and, 283
   hepatorenal bypass and, 450-452
   infrarenal aortic aneurysm repair and, 304
   occlusion in renal artery aneurysm, 471
   splenorenal bypass and, 453
   unilateral or bilateral repair of, 437
Renal artery aneurysm
   direct surgical repair of, 439
   endovascular treatment of, 466-474, 468f
      complications in, 473
      deployment of bare stent in, 469
      deployment of stent graft in, 469-470, 469t

Renal artery aneurysm (Continued)
      embolization in, 470, 471f
      indications for, 466
      occlusion of renal artery in, 471, 472f-473f
      postoperative care in, 471-473
      preoperative preparation for, 466-467, 467f-468f
   repair during branch repair using in situ and ex vivo techniques, 446-447
Renal artery angioplasty and stenting, 456-465
   angiographic anatomy for, 457-458, 459f
   antegrade versus retrograde access in, 459-460, 460f, 462, 463V
   branch vessel disease and, 458, 459f
   coaxial or monorail balloon catheter designs for, 460
   completion studies in, 464
   complications in, 464-465
   crossing lesions in, 463
   indications for, 456
   in situ physiologic assessment using Radi pressure wire in, 463
   postoperative care in, 464
   preoperative preparation for, 456-457
   recurrent stenosis and, 461-462, 462f
   role of balloon predilation in, 460
   selection of stent for, 461
   sheath placement in, 462-463
   solitary kidney and, 458-459
   stent placement in, 463-464
   unfavorable anatomic features for, 458
   use of embolic protection during, 461, 461f
Renal artery bypass
   in direct surgical repair of renal artery aneurysm, 441, 442f
   for renovascular disease, 449-455
      complications in, 455
      conduit selection in, 450
      hepatorenal bypass in, 450-452, 451f, 453f-454f
      preoperative preparation for, 449
      splenorenal bypass in, 453-454
      surgical anatomy of hepatic and splenic arteries and, 450, 451f
Renal artery endarterectomy, 442-444
   criteria for, 437
   exposure of pararenal aorta in, 442, 443f
   transaortic, 442-444, 444f, 446f
Renal artery occlusion during endovascular repair of infrarenal aortic aneurysm, 332
Renal artery stenosis, 456-465
   angiographic anatomy for, 457-458, 459f
   angioplasty in, 463
   angioplasty versus primary stenting in, 460
   antegrade versus retrograde access in, 459-460, 460f, 462, 463V
   branch vessel disease and, 458, 459f
   coaxial or monorail balloon catheter designs for, 460
   completion studies in, 464
   complications in, 464-465
   crossing lesions in, 463
   indications for, 456
   in situ physiologic assessment using Radi pressure wire in, 463
   postoperative care in, 464
   preoperative preparation for, 456-457
   recurrent stenosis and, 461-462, 462f
   role of balloon predilation in, 460
   selection of stent for, 461
   sheath placement in, 462-463
   solitary kidney and, 458-459
   stent placement in, 463-464
   unfavorable anatomic features for, 458
   use of embolic protection during, 461, 461f
Renal atheroembolism, 437, 447
Renal duplex sonography during surgical repair of renovascular disease, 438-439

Renal failure
  abdominal aortic aneurysm surgery-related, 307–308
  in aortoiliac occlusive disease
    endovascular treatment and, 390
    surgical repair and, 360
  in contrast induced-nephropathy, 24
  endovascular treatment of aortic dissection-related, 288
  juxtarenal and pararenal abdominal aortic aneurysms repair-related, 318
  thoracoabdominal aortic aneurysm surgery-related, 229
Renal function
  after renal artery bypass, 455
  after transjugular intrahepatic portosystemic shunt, 670
  angiographic contrast media and, 22–23, 22b, 23t
  preoperative assessment of, 4
    in endovascular repair of splenic artery aneurysm, 514
    in surgical repair of thoracoabdominal aortic aneurysm, 217
Renal lesions, direct surgical repair of aortoiliac occlusive disease and, 355
Renal vein division in abdominal aortic aneurysm surgery, 299, 299f
  with iliac artery involvement, 313–314
Renal vein retractors, 394
Renovascular disease
  direct surgical repair of, 435–448
    aortorenal bypass in, 439–441, 440f–441f
    branch repair using in situ and ex vivo techniques in, 445V, 445–447
    complications in, 447–448
    exposure of pararenal aorta in, 438
    indications of, 436–437
    intraoperative assessment of, 438–439
    postoperative care in, 447
    preoperative preparation for, 437
    renal artery anatomy and, 438
    renal artery aneurysm and, 439
    renal artery bypass in, 441, 442f
    renal artery endarterectomy in, 442–444, 444f, 446f
    selection of method for, 438
    source of inflow in, 438
    unilateral versus bilateral renal artery repair in, 437
  extraanatomic repair for, 449–455
    complications in, 455
    conduit selection in, 450
    hepatorenal bypass in, 450–452, 451f, 453f–454f
    preoperative preparation for, 449
    splenorenal bypass in, 453–454
    surgical anatomy of hepatic and splenic arteries and, 450, 451f
Resection of carotid body tumor
  Shamblin type I, 105, 106f
  Shamblin type II/III, 107–108, 107f–108f
Respiratory complications
  after distal revascularization interval ligation procedure, 772–779
  after surgical repair of thoracoabdominal aortic aneurysm, 229
Restenosis
  after aortic arch vessels endovascular treatment, 156
  after neoaortoiliac system procedure for aortic graft infection, 425
  carotid angioplasty and stenting and, 86, 100
Reteplase for recanalization, 58
Reticular veins, 699
Retraction injury in abdominal aortic aneurysm surgery, 297
Retrievable filter
  in iliofemoral and femoral-popliteal deep vein thrombosis, 675, 675f
  permanent versus, 631–632, 632f

Retrieval of vena cava filter, 638
Retroesophageal subclavian artery, aberrant right subclavian artery repair and, 166
Retrograde approach
  in crossing iliac artery lesion, 378
  in endovascular popliteal artery aneurysm repair, 599
  in endovascular treatment of mesenteric ischemia, 496, 497f
  in endovascular treatment of tibial-peroneal arterial occlusive disease, 592
  in femoral-popliteal arterial occlusive disease, 581–582
  in renal artery angioplasty and stenting, 459–460, 460f, 462
Retrograde bypass in mesenteric ischemia, 485–486, 486f
Retrograde ejaculation
  after abdominal aortic aneurysm surgery, 297, 308
  after surgical repair of aortoiliac occlusive disease, 360
Retroperitoneal exposure
  in abdominal aortic aneurysm surgery, 298–299, 298b
    juxtarenal and pararenal aneurysms and, 310, 310b, 312f
    in infrarenal aortic aneurysm repair, 305–306, 306f
    in thoracoabdominal aortic aneurysm surgery, 221
Rheolytic thrombectomy in iliofemoral and femoral-popliteal deep vein thrombosis, 677–679, 678f
Rib resection in thoracic outlet syndrome surgery, 200, 201f
Right hepatic vein, transjugular intrahepatic portosystemic shunt and, 665
Right-sided discectomy, 394
Risk factor modification
  in femoral-popliteal arterial occlusive disease, 527
  in tibial-peroneal arterial occlusive disease, 544, 558
Road mapping, 18–19
Romazicon. See Flumazenil
Rupture
  of abdominal aortic aneurysm, 300
  during endovascular repair
    of aortic dissection, 282–283, 283f
    of aortoiliac occlusive disease, 385, 389–390
    of femoral-popliteal arterial occlusive disease, 587
    of infrarenal aortic aneurysm, 332
    of tibial-peroneal arterial occlusive disease, 596
  in traumatic thoracic aortic disruption, 289, 290f
  of visceral artery aneurysm, 501

S

St. Mary's vein cuff in femoral-popliteal bypass, 533–534, 533f
Saphenofemoral junction, 694, 698f
Saphenous nerve injury
  in surgical repair of popliteal artery aneurysm, 566
  in varicose vein stripping, 686
Saphenous vein(s)
  endovascular thermal ablation of, 694–707
    access in, 699, 700f
    complications in, 705–706, 706f
    confirmation of catheter tip position in, 701, 701f
    endovascular strategy in, 696–699, 698f
    endovenous laser in, 700
    indications for, 695f, 696
    patient positioning for, 699
    postoperative care in, 704–705
    preoperative preparation for, 696, 697f

Saphenous vein(s) (Continued)
    radiofrequency catheter in, 699–700, 700f
    treatment of axial veins in, 702–703
    treatment of perforator veins in, 703–704, 704f
    tumescent anesthesia in, 701, 702f
  mapping before reconstruction of inferior vena cava and iliofemoral venous system, 651
Saphenous vein graft in superior vena cava syndrome reconstruction, 644
Saphenous vein transposition, 759t, 760, 763–764, 765f
Sartorius muscle flap for aortic graft infection
  neoaortoiliac system procedure for, 424, 424f
  total graft excision and extraanatomic repair of, 416
Scalene block in transaxillary rib resection for thoracic outlet syndrome, 194–195
Scalenectomy in supraclavicular approach to thoracic outlet syndrome, 175–176, 180–181, 181f–183f
Scarred groin, access site management and, 36
Sciatic nerve injury in varicose vein stripping, 686
Sclerosant solution
  allergic reaction to, 722–723
  foaming of, 724V, 724
  selection of, 723, 723t
Sclerotherapy, 721–728
  complications in, 725–726
  foaming of sclerosant solution in, 724V, 724
  injection of target vein in, 724V, 724, 725f
  patient positioning for, 724
  postoperative care in, 724–725
  preoperative preparation for, 721–722
  selection of sclerosant solution in, 723, 723t
  sequence of treatment of superficial veins and, 723
Sedation in vascular surgery, 17–18
Selective angiographic catheter, 45–46, 45f
Selective hepatic venography in transjugular intrahepatic portosystemic shunt, 667
Self-expanding stent, 53t, 58f
  in carotid angioplasty and stenting, 98, 99f
  in endovascular treatment of femoral-popliteal arterial occlusive disease, 580–581, 583f
  in endovascular treatment of mesenteric ischemia, 496, 497f
  in renal artery stenosis repair, 461
Self-retaining renal vein retractors, 394
Sexual function impairment, abdominal aortic aneurysm surgery-related, 308
Shamblin classification system for carotid body tumor, 103, 103t
Sheath placement
  in arteriovenous graft thrombosis, 785f, 786
  in carotid angioplasty and stenting, 92–95, 93f–94f
  in popliteal artery aneurysm, 601, 601f
  in renal artery stenosis, 462–463
  in subclavian-axillary vein thrombosis, 208
Shunting
  in carotid endarterectomy, 70, 71f
  during eversion endarterectomy, 82, 83f
Sidewinder 2 catheter, 45f
Simon Nitinol filter, 629t, 630f, 675f
Single venous access technique in percutaneous vena cava filter placement, 636–637
Single-wall puncture needle, 33f
Small saphenous veins, 698, 698f
  for femoral-popliteal bypass, open vein harvest of, 534–536
  injury in surgical repair of popliteal artery aneurysm, 566
  injury in surgical repair of popliteal artery entrapment, 574
  ligation and stripping of, 690–691

Small vessel end-to-end anastomosis, 12, 13f
Snorkel stent
 for aneurysms of juxtarenal and pararenal aorta, 346–347, 347f
 for thoracoabdominal aortic aneurysm, 235
Sodium nitroprusside, 36t
Sodium tetradecyl sulfate, 723, 723t
Solitary kidney, renal artery stenosis repair and, 458–459
Somatosensory-evoked potential monitoring in surgical repair of thoracoabdominal aortic aneurysm, 219–220
Spinal accessory nerve injury
 during carotid body tumor surgery, 103–104
 during vertebral artery surgery, 123
Spinal anesthesia, 18
Spinal cord ischemia
 after endovascular treatment of aortic dissection, 282
 after endovascular treatment of descending thoracic artery aneurysm, 254, 271–272
 after endovascular treatment of traumatic thoracic aortic disruption, 293
 thoracoabdominal aortic aneurysm-related
  after direct surgical repair, 218
  after endovascular repair, 248
Spine exposure, 392–402
 complications in, 400–401, 400t
 L2 to S1, 397–399, 398f–399f
 operative strategy in, 394–395
 pitfalls and danger points in, 393–394
 postoperative care in, 399–400
 preoperative preparation for, 392–393
 T12 to L2, 396–397
 thoracic, 395–396
Spiral saphenous vein graft in superior vena cava syndrome reconstruction, 645, 646f–648f
Splenic artery
 anatomy of, 502, 503f
 average diameter of, 57t
 splenorenal bypass and, 453
 surgical anatomy of, 450, 451f
Splenic artery aneurysm
 direct surgical repair of, 502–505, 503f, 505f
 endovascular treatment of, 517V, 513–524
  access and guiding sheath placement in, 515
  angiographic imaging in, 515
  embolization in, 517–521
  indications for, 514
  postoperative care in, 523–524
  preoperative preparation for, 514
  stent-graft placement in, 521, 522f–523f
Splenic ischemia after renal artery bypass, 455
Splenorenal anastomosis, 454
Splenorenal bypass, 453–454
Spliced vein conduits in femoral-popliteal bypass, 535
S-shaped incision
 in popliteal artery aneurysm repair, 563, 563f–564f
 in popliteal artery entrapment, 574, 575f
Stab avulsion, 691–692, 691f
StarClose closure device, 39f, 38
Steal syndrome
 after arteriovenous fistula, 737–738
 after arteriovenous graft, 745
 basilic vein transposition and, 748, 751
 femoral vein transposition and, 752, 756
 goals for treatment of, 772
Steel coil for therapeutic embolization, 59–60, 59f
Stenosis
 crossing with guidewire, 46
 iliac vein, 680, 682f
 iliocaval graft, 654
 renal artery, 456–465
  angiographic anatomy for, 457–458, 459f

Stenosis *(Continued)*
 angioplasty in, 463
 angioplasty *versus* primary stenting in, 460
 antegrade *versus* retrograde access in, 459–460, 460f, 462, 463V
 branch vessel disease and, 458, 459f
 coaxial or monorail balloon catheter designs for, 460
 completion studies in, 464
 complications in, 464–465
 crossing lesions in, 463
 indications for, 456
 in situ physiologic assessment using Radi pressure wire in, 463
 postoperative care in, 464
 preoperative preparation for, 456–457
 recurrent stenosis and, 461–462, 462f
 role of balloon predilation in, 460
 selection of stent for, 461
 sheath placement in, 462–463
 solitary kidney and, 458–459
 stent placement in, 463–464
 unfavorable anatomic features for, 458
 use of embolic protection during, 461, 461f
Stent fracture
 after renal artery aneurysm repair, 473
 in aortic arch vessels endovascular treatment, 151f, 156
Stent graft, 53t
 in arteriovenous graft thrombosis repair, 786
 in femoral artery pseudoaneurysm repair, 432
 in gastroduodenal and pancreaticoduodenal artery aneurysms, 516, 517f
 in hepatic artery aneurysm repair, 516, 517f
 in renal artery aneurysm repair, 469–470, 469t
 in splenic artery aneurysm repair, 521, 522f–523f
Stent migration, 61
 of modular transcervical bifurcated stent graft, 240
Stenting, 57–58, 57t, 58f
 of aortic arch vessels, 155
  common carotid and, 155
  innominate artery and, 153
  selection of stent for, 150
  vertebral artery and, 153
 balloons for, 53t
 carotid angioplasty and, 86–101
  access in, 90–91
  angiographic anatomy and, 87, 88t
  angiography of aortic arch, carotid, and cerebral circulation in, 92
  angioplasty technique in, 97V, 97–98
  aortic arch anatomy and, 88, 89f
  carotid lesions at risk for embolization and, 88
  catheterization of common carotid artery in, 91, 91f–92f
  cerebral protection devices and, 90
  completion studies in, 98
  crossing lesion and cerebral protection in, 95–97, 95f, 97f
  fibromuscular dysplasia and, 89–90
  indications for, 86, 87t
  kinks and coils of carotid artery and, 88
  management of arterial spasm, embolization, and acute occlusion in, 98–99
  neurorescue techniques in, 99–100
  occluded external carotid artery and, 88, 90f
  postoperative care in, 100
  postoperative complications in, 100–101
  preoperative care in, 86
  redo carotid angioplasty and, 90
  selection of stent for, 90

Stenting *(Continued)*
 severe stenosis and string sign and, 88–89
 sheath placement for planned intervention in, 92–95, 93f–94f
 stenting technique in, 98, 99f
 tandem lesions in common carotid artery and, 89
 in endovascular therapy for subclavian-axillary vein thrombosis, 212
 during endovascular treatment of aortoiliac occlusive disease, 377, 377f
 of aorta, 386–387
 of common iliac artery, 387
 of external iliac artery, 389
 indications for, 50
 postoperative care in, 60
 postoperative complications in, 60–61
 preoperative preparation for, 51
 in renal artery aneurysm, 469, 469t
 in renal artery stenosis, 456–465
  angiographic anatomy for, 457–458, 459f
  antegrade *versus* retrograde access in, 459–460, 460f, 462, 463V
  branch vessel disease and, 458, 459f
  coaxial or monorail balloon catheter designs for, 460
  completion studies in, 464
  complications in, 464–465
  crossing lesions in, 463
  indications for, 456
  in situ physiologic assessment using Radi pressure wire in, 463
  postoperative care in, 464
  preoperative preparation for, 456–457
  recurrent stenosis and, 461–462, 462f
  role of balloon predilation in, 460
  selection of stent for, 461
  sheath placement in, 462–463
  solitary kidney and, 458–459
  stent placement in, 463–464
  unfavorable anatomic features for, 458
  use of embolic protection during, 461, 461f
 in subclavian-axillary vein thrombosis, 205–207
 tibial artery angioplasty and, 592–594, 593f
  laser, 595
  subintimal, 594–595, 595f–596f
Sternocleidomastoid muscle
 carotid body tumor surgery and, 104
 carotid endarterectomy and, 67
Sternotomy in superior vena cava syndrome reconstruction, 645
Straight catheter, 45f, 47f
Straight guidewire, 41, 43f, 44t
String sign, 88–89
Stroke
 intraoperative
  in carotid angioplasty and stenting, 87
  in carotid endarterectomy, 65–66, 74
  in endovascular treatment of aortic dissection, 282
  in modular transcervical bifurcated stent graft, 239
  in surgical repair of aortic arch vessels, 129
 postoperative
  in aortic arch vessels endovascular treatment, 155
  in carotid body tumor surgery, 109
  in carotid endarterectomy, 74
  in endovascular treatment of aortic dissection, 288
  in endovascular treatment of descending thoracic aortic aneurysm, 271–272
  in endovascular treatment of descending thoracic artery aneurysm, 253
  in traumatic thoracic aortic disruption, 293
  in vertebral artery surgery, 122

Stump ischemia after above- and below-knee amputation, 608
Subclavian artery
  average diameter of, 57t
  endovascular treatment of, 148–156
    access of lesions in, 150
    angiographic anatomy in, 149
    complications in, 155–156
    embolic protection devices in, 150
    imaging and selective catheterization in, 152–153
    lesion predilation in, 150
    postoperative care in, 155
    preoperative preparation for, 149
    protection of vertebral artery in, 150–151
    stent selection in, 150, 151f
    stenting in, 155
  injury during extraanatomic repair of aortoiliac occlusive disease, 362
  supraclavicular approach to thoracic outlet syndrome and, 178, 186–187
  surgical anatomy of, 158–159
  within thoracic outlet, 196
Subclavian artery aneurysm repair, 162–165
  carotid-brachial artery bypass in, 164–165
  closure in, 165
  exposure of axillary artery in, 162–163, 164f
  exposure of supraclavicular subclavian artery in, 162, 163f
  interposition graft for, 161
  patient position and incision in, 162
  postoperative care in, 168–169
  postoperative complications in, 169
  preoperative preparation for, 157, 158f
  subclavian-axillary artery bypass in, 164
Subclavian artery compression syndrome, 157
Subclavian artery surgery, 157–170
  aberrant right subclavian artery and, 159–160, 159f–160f
  avoiding brachial plexus injuries in, 161
  avoiding injuries behind clavicle in, 161
  avoiding thoracic duct injuries in, 160–161
  avoiding vertebral artery injuries in, 161
  in Kommerell diverticulum repair, 167, 168f
  postoperative care in, 168–169
  postoperative complications in, 169
  preoperative preparation for, 157–158, 158f
  in repair of aberrant right subclavian artery, 165–166, 165f
  selection of conduit in, 161–162
  surgical anatomy in, 158–159
Subclavian steal syndrome, 140, 141f
Subclavian vein, 205, 206f
  injury during surgical repair of aortic arch vessels, 129
  injury in supraclavicular approach to thoracic outlet syndrome, 178
  within thoracic outlet, 196
Subclavian-axillary artery bypass, 164
Subclavian-axillary vein thrombosis, 204–214, 205f
  access in, 208
  angiographic anatomy and collaterals in, 205–206, 206f–207f
  angioplasty and stenting in, 212
  completion studies in, 212
  complications in, 213
  postoperative care in, 212–213
  preoperative preparation for, 204–205
  sheath placement in, 208
  technique in, 208–212, 209f
  thrombolysis in, 209–212, 210f–211f
  timing of, 206–208, 208f
Subfascial endoscopic perforator surgery, 708–720
  choice of anesthesia for, 715
  deep venous valve surgery in, 719
  distal ankle perforators and, 718
  exploration of subfascial space in, 716, 717f–718f

Subfascial endoscopic perforator surgery (Continued)
  incision in, 715–716, 715b, 715f
  indications for, 708
  operative strategy in, 710–711
  paratibial fasciotomy in, 716
  pitfalls and danger points in, 709–710
  port insertion in, 716, 716f
  postoperative care in, 718–719
  preoperative preparation for, 709
Subintimal guidewire, 46
Subintimal technique in femoral-popliteal artery occlusion, 586
Subintimal tibial artery angioplasty and stenting, 594–595, 595f–596f
Superficial and deep compartments of arm, 623
Superficial and deep posterior compartments of leg, lower leg fasciotomy and, 620–621, 622f
Superficial femoral artery
  average diameter of, 57t
  direct surgical repair of tibial-peroneal arterial occlusive disease and, 551, 551f
  endovascular treatment of femoral-popliteal arterial occlusive disease and, 581f, 580, 584f–585f
  exposure in total graft excision and extraanatomic repair of aortic graft infection, 414
  in femoral-popliteal bypass, 538
  surgical anatomy of, 529–531, 530f
Superficial venous system, ultrasound evaluation of, 694–696, 697f
Superior laryngeal nerve injury during carotid endarterectomy, 66
Superior mesenteric artery
  average diameter of, 57t
  endovascular treatment of aortic dissection and, 283
  endovascular treatment of descending thoracic artery aneurysm and, 256–257
  surgical anatomy of, 478
Superior mesenteric artery embolectomy, 487–488, 487f
Superior mesenteric artery occlusive disease
  direct surgical repair for, 475–490
    antegrade bypass in, 482–485, 483f, 485f
    approach to superior mesenteric artery in, 480–481, 480f–481f
    complications in, 488–489
    indications for, 476–477
    ischemia secondary to embolization, in situ thrombosis, and dissection and, 478–479
    postoperative care in, 488
    preoperative preparation for, 477
    retrograde bypass in, 485–486, 486f
    selection of celiac artery outflow in, 479–480
    selection of conduit in, 481–482
    selection of inflow source in, 479
    superior mesenteric artery embolectomy in, 487–488, 487f
    surgical anatomy for, 478
  endovascular treatment of, 491–499
    complications in, 498
    indications for, 491–492
    pitfalls and danger points in, 493–495, 495f
    postoperative care in, 498
    preoperative preparation for, 492–493, 493f–494f
    strategy in, 495–496, 495f
    technique in, 496, 497f
Superior vena cava filter placement, 637
Superior vena cava syndrome reconstruction, 641–649
  anastomoses in, 645–648, 647f–648f
  anesthesia for, 644
  avoiding intraoperative bleeding in, 643
  avoiding pulmonary embolism in, 644
  closure of median sternotomy in, 648

Superior vena cava syndrome reconstruction (Continued)
  complications in, 648–649, 649t
  dissection of innominate veins and superior vena cava in, 645
  indications for, 641
  position and incision in, 645
  postoperative care in, 648
  preoperative preparation for, 641–643, 642f–643f
  selection of vascular conduit for, 644, 644t
  selection of venous inflow and outflow sites in, 644
  spiral vein graft in, 645, 646f
  unilateral versus bilateral, 644
Supraceliac aorta, juxtarenal and pararenal aneurysms and, 311
Supraclavicular approach to thoracic outlet syndrome, 171–192
  associated subclavian artery aneurysm management in, 186–187
  associated subclavian vein stenosis or occlusion management in, 187–188
  avoiding inadequate decompression and recurrence in, 175–177
  avoiding nerve injury in, 177–178
  avoiding vascular and lymphatic injury in, 178–179
  brachial plexus neurolysis in, 185–186
  closure in, 188–189, 189f
  exposure in, 180, 180f
  first rib resection in, 181–185, 184f–185f
  patient position and incision in, 179–180, 179f
  pectoralis minor tenotomy in, 186, 186f
  postoperative care in, 189–190
  postoperative complications in, 190–191
  preoperative preparation in, 172–174, 173b
  scalenectomy in, 180–181, 181f–183f
  surgical anatomy of thoracic outlet in, 174–175, 175f, 176b
Supraclavicular subclavian artery, exposure in subclavian artery aneurysm repair, 162, 163f
Suprarenal aorta, juxtarenal and pararenal aneurysms and, 311
Suprarenal aortic aneurysm, 315V, 315–318, 317f
Suprarenal filter placement, inadvertent, 633, 634f
Sural nerve injury
  in surgical repair of popliteal artery aneurysm, 566
  in surgical repair of popliteal artery entrapment, 573
  in varicose vein stripping, 686
Surgical exposure in vascular surgery, 5
Surgical history before spine exposure, 393
Synthetic obturator bypass graft, 409, 411f

T

T12 to L2 exposure, 396–397
Takayasu arteritis, 126, 129–130
Talent thoracic stent-graft system for descending thoracic aortic aneurysm, 268–271, 269f–270f
TASC classification of aortoiliac lesions, 373, 374f, 375t, 579b, 579t
Taylor vein patch in femoral-popliteal bypass, 533–534, 533f
TEE. See Transesophageal echocardiography
Telangiectasia, sclerotherapy for, 724
Temporary dialysis access, 759–760
Tenecteplase for recanalization, 58
Tessari method of foaming sclerosant solution, 724V, 724
TEVAR. See Thoracic endovascular aortic repair
Therapeutic embolization, 59–60, 59f, 60t
Therapeutic infusion catheters, 53t
Thigh access for hemodialysis, 759t, 765, 766f

Thigh fasciotomy, 622–623
Thoracic aorta
  average diameter of, 57t
  endovascular treatment of dissection of, 274–288
    after elephant trunk repair, 281, 281f
    aortic fenestration in, 285–286
    avoiding de novo type A dissection in, 278, 279f
    avoiding paraplegia in, 282
    avoiding rupture in, 282–283, 283f
    avoiding stroke in, 282
    avoiding visceral ischemia in, 283–284
    carotid-carotid and carotid-subclavian bypass in, 284–285, 285b, 286f
    complications in, 287–288
    defining extent of, 279–280, 280f, 281b
    differentiation of true and false thoracic aorta lumen and, 275–276, 277f
    endograft placement in, 286–287, 287f
    fenestration or endograft repair in, 281–282
    indications for, 274, 275b
    postoperative care in, 287
    preoperative imaging in, 278–279
    preoperative preparation for, 275
    total aortic arch debranching in, 284, 285f
    type A versus type B dissection and, 279
    visceral ischemia and, 275, 276f
  endovascular treatment of traumatic disruption of, 289–294
    complications in, 293–294
    extent of repair in, 291
    indications for, 289, 290f
    postoperative care in, 292–293
    preoperative preparation for, 289–290, 291t
    sizing of endovascular graft for, 290–291
    technique in, 291–292, 292f–293f
Thoracic aorta to femoral artery bypass, 355
Thoracic duct
  aberrant right subclavian artery and, 160
  injury of
    in subclavian and axillary artery surgery, 160–161
    in supraclavicular approach to thoracic outlet syndrome, 178–179
    in surgical repair of aortic arch vessels, 128
  key anatomic features in, 164–165
Thoracic endovascular aortic repair, 274–288
  after elephant trunk repair, 281, 281f
  aortic fenestration in, 285–286
  avoiding de novo type A dissection in, 278, 279f
  avoiding paraplegia in, 282
  avoiding rupture in, 282–283, 283f
  avoiding stroke in, 282
  avoiding visceral ischemia in, 283–284
  carotid-carotid and carotid-subclavian bypass in, 284–285, 285b, 286f
  complications in, 287–288
  defining extent of, 279–280, 280f, 281b
  differentiation of true and false thoracic aorta lumen and, 275–276, 277f
  endograft placement in, 286–287, 287f
  fenestration or endograft repair in, 281–282
  indications for, 274, 275b
  postoperative care in, 287
  preoperative imaging in, 278–279
  preoperative preparation for, 275
  total aortic arch debranching in, 284, 285f
  type A versus type B dissection and, 279
  visceral ischemia and, 275, 276f
Thoracic outlet, surgical anatomy of, 174–175, 175f, 176b, 195–196, 196V, 197f
Thoracic outlet syndrome
  supraclavicular approach to, 171–192
    associated subclavian artery aneurysm management in, 186–187
    associated subclavian vein stenosis or occlusion management in, 187–188

Thoracic outlet syndrome (Continued)
    avoiding inadequate decompression and recurrence in, 175–177
    avoiding nerve injury in, 177–178
    avoiding vascular and lymphatic injury in, 178–179
    brachial plexus neurolysis in, 185–186
    closure in, 188–189, 189f
    exposure in, 180, 180f
    first rib resection in, 181–185, 184f–185f
    patient position and incision in, 179–180, 179f
    pectoralis minor tenotomy in, 186, 186f
    postoperative care in, 189–190
    postoperative complications in, 190–191
    preoperative preparation in, 172–174, 173b
    scalenectomy in, 180–181, 181f–183f
    surgical anatomy of thoracic outlet in, 174–175, 175f, 176b
  transaxillary rib resection for, 193–203
    avoiding injury to brachial plexus in, 196, 197f
    closure in, 200–201
    exposure in, 198–199, 199f–200f
    incision in, 198
    indications for, 193–194
    postoperative care in, 202
    postoperative complications in, 202–203
    preoperative preparation for, 194–195
    rib resection in, 200, 201f
    surgical anatomy of thoracic outlet and, 195–196, 196V, 197f
Thoracic spine exposure, 395–396
Thoracoabdominal aortic aneurysm
  direct surgical repair of, 215–231
    avoiding diaphragmatic paralysis in, 218, 219f
    avoiding embolization in, 218
    avoiding injuries to esophagus in, 219, 220f
    avoiding injuries to vagus nerve in, 218–219
    avoiding spinal cord ischemia in, 218
    avoiding visceral ischemia in, 218
    classification of aneurysms in, 217, 217f
    coagulopathy and, 218
    complications in, 228–229, 229f
    considerations in presence of chronic dissection in, 223
    descending thoracic aortic aneurysm and, 223–226, 225V, 225f
    distal aortic perfusion in, 221–222, 222f
    incision in, 221
    intraoperative corrective measures in, 220
    patient positioning for, 220–221, 221f
    postoperative care in, 228
    preoperative preparation in, 217
    retroperitoneal or transperitoneal thoracoabdominal exposure in, 221
    selection of site for distal control in, 222
    selection of site for proximal control in, 222, 223f
    somatosensory and motor-evoked potential monitoring in, 219–220
    type I aneurysm and, 226
    type II aneurysm andl, 226–228, 227f
    type III aneurysm and, 228
    type IV aneurysm and, 228
    use of balloon catheters for vascular control in, 218, 223, 224f
  endovascular repair of, 232–250
    anatomic considerations in, 234
    branch artery preservation in, 234–235
    choice of technique in, 235
    complications in, 248–249
    indications for, 232–233
    modular transfemoral multibranched stent graft in, 244–249, 245f–246f, 248f
    patient selection for, 233
    preoperative preparation in, 233–234

Thoracofemoral bypass, 367–369, 368f
Thoracolumbar spine exposure, 396–397
Thrombectomy
  in acute femoral-popliteal artery occlusion, 586–587
  anesthesia and incision in, 782–783
  in arteriovenous graft thrombosis repair
    hybrid intervention and, 788–789, 788f
    surgical intervention and, 783
  in endovascular treatment of aortoiliac occlusive disease, 384
  in iliofemoral and femoral-popliteal deep vein thrombosis, 674
Thrombin injection for femoral artery pseudoaneurysm, 432–433
Thromboembolectomy
  femoral-popliteal, 538–539
  in popliteal artery aneurysm, 567
Thromboembolism
  after direct surgical repair of tibial-peroneal arterial occlusive disease, 543–559
  in reconstruction of inferior vena cava and iliofemoral venous system, 654, 655f
Thrombolysis
  in arteriovenous graft thrombosis, 786–787
  in femoral-popliteal artery occlusions, 586–587
  in iliofemoral and femoral-popliteal deep vein thrombosis, 674
  in popliteal artery aneurysm, 567
  in subclavian-axillary vein thrombosis, 209–212, 210f–211f
Thrombolytic therapy
  before endovascular treatment of aortoiliac occlusive disease, 384
  recanalization and, 58
  for subclavian-axillary vein thrombosis, 206, 209–212, 210f–211f
  before surgical repair of popliteal artery aneurysm, 567
Thrombophilia evaluation
  in iliofemoral and femoral-popliteal deep vein thrombosis, 674
  before sclerotherapy, 722
Thrombosis
  embolization of, 14–15
  in endovenous thermal ablation of saphenous and perforating veins, 696
  eversion endarterectomy and, 82
  fistula, 738
  graft. See Graft thrombosis
  guidewire crossing of, 47–48, 47f–48f
  postoperative
    in aortic arch vessels endovascular treatment, 155
    in basilic vein transposition, 751
    in endovascular treatment of mesenteric ischemia, 498
    in femoral vein transposition, 756
    in femoral-popliteal arterial occlusive disease, 580
    in femoral-popliteal bypass, 538–539, 541
    in percutaneous access, 40
    in popliteal artery aneurysm repair, 566–567, 603
    in renal artery aneurysm repair, 473
    in renal artery bypass, 455
    in sclerotherapy, 725
    in superior vena cava syndrome reconstruction, 643
    in tibial-peroneal arterial occlusive disease endovascular repair, 596
    in transjugular intrahepatic portosystemic shunt, 671
    in vascular reconstruction, 15
    in vena cava filter placement, 639
  postoperative care in, 790
  in reconstruction of inferior vena cava and iliofemoral venous system, 654
  subclavian-axillary vein, 204–214, 205f
    access in, 208

Thrombosis (Continued)
    angiographic anatomy and collaterals in, 205–206, 206f–207f
    angioplasty and stenting in, 212
    completion studies in, 212
    complications in, 213
    postoperative care in, 212–213
    preoperative preparation for, 204–205
    sheath placement in, 208
    technique in, 208–212, 209f
    thrombolysis in, 209–212, 210f–211f
    timing of, 206–208, 208f
  surgical intervention in, 781
    anesthesia and incision in, 782–783
    closure in, 784
    operative strategy for, 782, 783f
    preoperative preparation for, 781–782
    revision of distal venous anastomosis in, 784, 784f
    thrombectomy in, 783
  in vascular access, 30, 31t
Tibia, long posterior flap below-knee amputation and, 605
Tibial artery angioplasty and stenting, 592–594, 593f
  laser, 595
  subintimal, 594–595, 595f–596f
Tibial nerve
  injury of
    in surgical repair of popliteal artery aneurysm, 566
    in varicose vein stripping, 686
  posterior myocutaneous flap and, 605–607
Tibialis artery, 57t
Tibial-peroneal arterial occlusive disease
  direct surgical repair of, 543–560
    anastomotic technique in, 546–547, 547f
    complications in, 558–559
    femoral distal artery-vein bypass grafting in, 547–548
    femoral-anterior tibial artery bypass in, 552–554, 553f–554f
    femoral-peroneal artery bypass in, 555–558
    femoral-posterior tibial artery bypass in, 555, 557f
    indications for, 543
    inflow exposure at femoral and popliteal arteries in, 548–551, 549f–551f
    instrumentation and tunnelers for, 546
    lower extremity fasciotomy in, 558
    open ulcer and, 545–546
    pitfalls and danger points in, 544
    postoperative care in, 558
    preoperative preparation for, 543–544
    proximal and distal control in, 546
    selection and assessment of site for distal anastomosis in, 545
    selection and assessment of site for inflow in, 545
    selection of conduit for, 544–545
  endovascular treatment of, 590–597
    angiographic anatomy and common collateral pathways in, 591
    complications in, 596–597
    indications for, 590
    postoperative care in, 595–596
    preoperative preparation for, 590–591
    selection of antegrade or retrograde access in, 592
    selection of stent for, 592
    tibial artery angioplasty and stenting in, 592–594, 593f
    tibial artery laser angioplasty and stenting in, 595
    tibial artery subintimal angioplasty and stenting in, 594–595, 595f–596f
    unfavorable anatomic and physiologic features for interventions in, 592
TIPS. See Transjugular intrahepatic portosystemic shunt

Tissue plasminogen activator
  for recanalization, 58
  for subclavian-axillary vein thrombosis, 210
TNKase. See Tenecteplase
Torque device, 43, 44f
TOS. See Thoracic outlet syndrome
Total aortic arch debranching, 284, 285f
Total graft excision and extraanatomic repair of aortic graft infection, 403–418
  avoiding ureteral injury in, 409
  choice of reconstruction in, 407–408
  closure of femoral arteries in, 416
  closure of proximal aortic stump and omental pedicle flap in, 414–415, 415f
  complications in, 417
  drains in, 416, 416f
  exposure of abdominal aorta in, 414
  exposure of common femoral, superficial femoral, and profunda femoris arteries in, 414
  graft excision in, 414
  historical background of, 404–405, 405f
  incision closure in, 416–417
  incision in, 413–414
  management of duodenal stump in, 415
  postoperative care in, 417
  preoperative preparation for, 405–407, 406f
  presence of aortoenteric fistula and, 409–412, 412f
  role of endovascular therapy in, 413, 413f
  sartorius muscle flap in, 416
  selection of extraanatomic bypass in, 409, 410f–411f
  staging of, 408–409
  underlying aneurysmal or occlusive disease and, 412
tPA. See Tissue plasminogen activator
Transabdominal ultrasound
  before abdominal aortic aneurysm surgery, 296
  percutaneous vena cava filter placement with, 635, 635f–636f
Transaortic renal artery endarterectomy, 442–444, 444f, 446f
Transarterial catheter embolization in gastroduodenal and pancreaticoduodenal artery aneurysms, 516, 518f–521f
Transarterial selective coil embolization in endovascular repair of type II endoleak, 341
Trans-Atlantic Inter-Society Consensus classification of aortoiliac lesions, 373, 374f, 375t, 579b, 579t
Transaxillary rib resection for thoracic outlet syndrome, 193–203
  avoiding injury to brachial plexus in, 196, 197f
  closure in, 200–201
  exposure in, 198–199, 199f–200f
  incision in, 198
  indications for, 193–194
  postoperative care in, 202
  postoperative complications in, 202–203
  preoperative preparation for, 194–195
  rib resection in, 200, 201f
  surgical anatomy of thoracic outlet and, 195–196, 196V, 197f
Transcommissural valvuloplasty, 712
Transesophageal echocardiography
  before extraanatomic repair of aortic arch vessels, 140
  before reconstruction of inferior vena cava and iliofemoral venous system, 651
Transient ischemic attack, vertebral artery surgery for, 111, 112b
Transjugular intrahepatic portosystemic shunt, 664–671
  accessing portal vein in, 665–666, 668, 669f
  anesthesia in, 666
  completion portosystemic gradient measurement and portography in, 669, 670f

Transjugular intrahepatic portosystemic shunt (Continued)
  complications in, 670–671
  localizing catheter tip in right hepatic vein in, 665
  mapping portal venous system in, 665, 666f, 667–668
  parenchymal tract in, 666, 668–669
  patient positioning and venous access in, 667
  portosystemic pressure gradient measurement in, 666–667
  postoperative care in, 670
  preoperative preparation for, 664–665
  selection and deployment of stent in, 666, 669
  selective hepatic venography in, 667
  stent deployment in, 669
  target portosystemic gradient in, 666
Translumbar glue in endovascular repair of type II endoleak, 341
Transmetatarsal amputation, 611, 612f–613f
Transperitoneal exposure
  in abdominal aortic aneurysm surgery, 297–298, 298b
  in thoracoabdominal aortic aneurysm surgery, 221
Transplantation, vein valve, 713–714, 714f
Transplanted kidney, abdominal aortic aneurysm surgery and, 301
Transthoracic cuffed dialysis catheter placement, 759t, 761, 768, 768f
Traumatic thoracic aortic disruption, 289–294
  complications in, 293–294
  extent of repair in, 291
  indications for, 289, 290f
  postoperative care in, 292–293
  preoperative preparation for, 289–290, 291t
  sizing of endovascular graft for, 290–291
  technique in, 291–292, 292f–293f
Treatment planning, 3
Trellis-8 peripheral infusion system, 679, 680f–681f
Tumescent anesthesia in endovenous thermal ablation of saphenous and perforating veins, 701, 702f
Tumor
  carotid body, 102–110
    avoiding cranial nerve injuries in, 103–104
    avoiding intraoperative stroke in, 104
    bipolar electrocautery in, 104
    classification and surgical anatomy of, 103, 103t
    exposure of carotid bifurcation in, 104–108, 105f
    incision for, 104, 105f
    postoperative care in, 108–109
    postoperative complications in, 109
    preoperative embolization in, 104
    preoperative preparation in, 102
    resection of Shamblin type I, 105, 106f
    resection of Shamblin type II/III, 107–108, 107f–108f
  inferior vena cava, 650, 651b
Tunneling
  in aortobifemoral bypass, 356
  in axillofemoral bypass, 366
  in distal revascularization interval ligation, 776
  in femoral-anterior tibial artery bypass, 553–554, 554f
  in femoral-femoral bypass, 364
  in femoral-popliteal bypass, 529
  in forearm loop graft, 740, 742, 743f
  in popliteal artery aneurysm repair, 568
  in saphenous vein transposition, 764, 765f
  in thoracofemoral bypass, 367–368
Two-suture technique in beveled end-to-side anastomosis, 8–9
Type A versus type B aortic dissection, 279

Type I endoleak
  of descending thoracic aneurysm, 255, 256f–257f
  of infrarenal aortic aneurysm, 336, 338, 339f
  of juxtarenal and pararenal aneurysms, 349
Type II endoleak
  of descending thoracic aneurysm, 256
  of infrarenal aortic aneurysm, 341–342
  of juxtarenal and pararenal aneurysms, 349

U

UCAP. *See* Ultrasound-guided arterial puncture
Ulcer, tibial-peroneal arterial occlusive disease repair and, 545–546
Ulnar artery, 57t
Ultrasound
  in aortoiliac occlusive disease, 375
  before brachial artery-axillary vein interposition graft, 740, 741f
  before brachiocephalic and radiocephalic arteriovenous fistulas, 731
  in carotid body tumor, 102
  before distal revascularization interval ligation, 773
  before endovascular repair of infrarenal aortic aneurysm, 321
  before endovenous ablation of saphenous and perforating veins, 696
  before endovenous thermal ablation of saphenous and perforating veins, 694–696, 697f
  in femoral-popliteal arterial occlusive disease, 579
  before femoral-popliteal bypass, 533
  before forearm loop graft, 740, 741f
  in iliofemoral and femoral-popliteal deep vein thrombosis, 673–674, 673f
  intravascular, 26–27, 27f
  in mesenteric ischemia, 492, 493f
  before reconstruction of inferior vena cava and iliofemoral venous system, 650–651
  before sclerotherapy, 721
  in subclavian-axillary vein thrombosis, 204
  in superior vena cava syndrome, 642
  during surgical repair of renovascular disease, 438–439
  in tibial-peroneal arterial occlusive disease, 591
  before transaxillary rib resection for thoracic outlet syndrome, 195
  before transjugular intrahepatic portosystemic shunt, 665
  before varicose vein stripping, 685
  in vena cava filter placement, 630–633, 635, 635f–636f
  before vertebral artery surgery, 113
Ultrasound guidance
  access site management and, 32, 33f
  in percutaneous endovascular aneurysm repair, 323
  in percutaneous vena cava filter placement, 631
Ultrasound-accelerated thrombolysis
  in iliofemoral and femoral-popliteal deep vein thrombosis, 676–677, 677f
  in subclavian-axillary vein thrombosis, 212
Ultrasound-guided arterial puncture, 20–22, 20V, 21f
Unconventional venous access for chronic hemodialysis, 758–771
  assessment of remaining options for upper extremity access and, 760
  brachial vein transposition in, 760, 762–763, 762f–764f
  complex catheter-based vascular access in, 767–770, 768f–769f
  complications in, 770
  hemodialysis reliable outflow vascular access device placement in, 761

Unconventional venous access for chronic hemodialysis *(Continued)*
  indications for, 758, 759t
  options for temporary dialysis access and, 759–760
  pediatric patient and, 760
  postoperative care in, 770
  preoperative preparation for, 758–759
  prosthetic chest wall vascular access in, 761, 765–767, 767f
  prosthetic lower extremity vascular access in, 760–761, 764–765, 766f
  saphenous vein transposition in, 760, 763–764, 765f
  transthoracic cuffed dialysis catheter placement in, 761
Unilateral venous reconstruction in superior vena cava syndrome, 644
Upper extremity access for hemodialysis, 760
Upper extremity deep vein thrombosis, percutaneous superior vena cava filter placement for, 637
Upper extremity fasciotomy, 623, 623f
Upper extremity vascular disease
  endovascular therapy for subclavian-axillary vein thrombosis in, 204–214, 205f
    access in, 208
    angiographic anatomy and collaterals in, 205–206, 206f–207f
    angioplasty and stenting in, 212
    completion studies in, 212
    complications in, 213
    postoperative care in, 212–213
    preoperative preparation for, 204–205
    sheath placement in, 208
    technique in, 208–212, 209f
    thrombolysis in, 209–212, 210f–211f
    timing of, 206–208, 208f
  supraclavicular approach to thoracic outlet syndrome in, 171–192
    associated subclavian artery aneurysm management in, 186–187
    associated subclavian vein stenosis or occlusion management in, 187–188
    avoiding inadequate decompression and recurrence in, 175–177
    avoiding nerve injury in, 177–178
    avoiding vascular and lymphatic injury in, 178–179
    brachial plexus neurolysis in, 185–186
    closure in, 188–189, 189f
    exposure in, 180, 180f
    first rib resection in, 181–185, 184f–185f
    patient position and incision in, 179–180, 179f
    pectoralis minor tenotomy in, 186, 186f
    postoperative care in, 189–190
    postoperative complications in, 190–191
    preoperative preparation in, 172–174, 173b
    scalenectomy in, 180–181, 181f–183f
    surgical anatomy of thoracic outlet in, 174–175, 175f, 176b
  transaxillary rib resection for thoracic outlet syndrome in, 193–203
    avoiding injury to brachial plexus in, 196, 197f
    closure in, 200–201
    exposure in, 198–199, 199f–200f
    incision in, 198
    indications for, 193–194
    postoperative care in, 202
    postoperative complications in, 202–203
    preoperative preparation for, 194–195
    rib resection in, 200, 201f
    surgical anatomy of thoracic outlet and, 195–196, 196V, 197f
Upper extremity venography
  in subclavian-axillary vein thrombosis, 207f–208f, 209, 210f
  before supraclavicular approach to thoracic outlet syndrome, 174

Upper gastrointestinal endoscopy before total graft excision and extraanatomic repair of aortic graft infection, 405, 406f
Upper limb tension test, 194
Ureteral injury
  in abdominal aortic aneurysm surgery, 297
  in surgical repair of aortoiliac occlusive disease, 360
  in total graft excision and extraanatomic repair of aortic graft infection, 409

V

Vagus nerve injury
  in aortic arch vessels endovascular treatment, 156
  during carotid body tumor surgery, 103
  during carotid endarterectomy, 66
  in extraanatomic aortic arch vessel repair, 146
  in surgical repair of aortic arch vessels, 129
  in surgical repair of thoracoabdominal aortic aneurysm, 218–219
  during vertebral artery surgery, 123
Valiant thoracic stent-graft system for descending thoracic aortic aneurysm, 271
Valvular repair techniques, 711–715
  angioscope-assisted valvuloplasty in, 712
  artificial valve implantation in, 714–715
  autologous neovalve construction in, 713
  external banding valvuloplasty in, 712
  external valvuloplasty in, 711
  internal valvuloplasty in, 711, 712f
  transcommissural valvuloplasty in, 712
  vein segment transposition in, 713
  vein valve transplantation in, 708, 713–714
Valvuloplasty
  angioscope-assisted, 712
  external banding, 712
  internal, 711, 712f
  transcommissural, 712
Variceal bleeding after transjugular intrahepatic portosystemic shunt, 671
Varicose veins
  endovenous thermal ablation of saphenous and perforating veins in, 694–707
    access in, 699, 700f
    complications in, 705–706, 706f
    confirmation of catheter tip position in, 701, 701f
    endovascular strategy in, 696–699, 698f
    endovenous laser in, 700
    indications for, 695f, 696
    patient positioning for, 699
    postoperative care in, 704–705
    preoperative preparation for, 696, 697f
    radiofrequency catheter in, 699–700, 700f
    treatment of axial veins in, 702–703
    treatment of perforator veins in, 703–704, 704f
    tumescent anesthesia in, 701, 702f
  sclerotherapy for, 721–728
    complications in, 725–726
    foaming of sclerosant solution in, 724V, 724
    injection of target vein in, 724V, 724, 725f
    patient positioning for, 724
    postoperative care in, 724–725
    preoperative preparation for, 721–722
    selection of sclerosant solution in, 723, 723t
    sequence of treatment of superficial veins and, 723
  stripping of, 684–693
    anesthesia for, 688
    complications in, 692
    great saphenous vein, 688–690, 689f–690f
    indications for, 684–685, 685b
    operative strategy in, 686–688, 687f

Varicose veins *(Continued)*
    postoperative care in, 692
    preoperative preparation for, 685–686
    small saphenous vein, 690–691
    stab or ambulatory phlebectomy and, 691–692, 691f
Vascular conduit
    in direct surgical repair for acute mesenteric ischemia, 481–482
    in endovascular repair of infrarenal aortic aneurysm, 324–325
    in extraanatomic repair in renovascular disease, 450
    in femoral-popliteal bypass, 533–534, 533f
    in in situ repair of aortic graft infection, 420
    in subclavian and axillary artery surgery, 161–162
    in superior vena cava syndrome reconstruction, 644, 644t
    in surgical repair of popliteal artery, 565
    in surgical repair of tibial-peroneal arterial occlusive disease, 544–545
Vascular disease
    diagnosis of, 2–3
    planning treatment of, 3
    preoperative assessment in, 4
    presentation and natural history of, 2
Vascular injury
    in abdominal aortic aneurysm surgery, 297
    in anterior spine exposure, 394
    in endovascular repair of infrarenal aortic aneurysm, 322
    in surgical repair of popliteal artery aneurysm, 566
    in surgical repair of popliteal artery entrapment, 574
    in transaxillary rib resection for thoracic outlet syndrome, 202
Vascular occlusion, 6–7, 8f
Vascular reconstruction, 5–6
    arterial thrombosis after, 15
    bypass procedure in, 5–6
    in femoral artery pseudoaneurysm repair, 428–429
Vascular surgery
    anastomosis technique in, 8–12
        beveled end-to-side anastomosis in, 8–10, 10f
        end-to-end anastomosis in, 11–12, 12t
        nonbeveled end-to-side anastomosis in, 10–11, 11f
        small vessel end-to-end anastomosis in, 12, 13f
    angiographic contrast media in, 22–26
        carbon dioxide angiography and, 24–26, 25b, 25f-27f
        contrast media reactions in, 23, 24t
        renal dysfunction considerations and, 22–23, 22b, 23t
    arteriotomy in, 8, 9f
    common problems associated with, 13–16
        arterial thrombosis after vascular reconstruction in, 15
        bleeding, hematomas, lymphoceles in, 15
        embolization of atheroma or thrombus in, 14–15
        end-organ ischemia in, 15
        infection in, 16
        injury to adjacent structures in, 13–14
    diagnosis of vascular disease and, 2–3
    exposure and control of blood vessels in, 6, 7f
    fluoroscopic principles in, 18–22
        contrast injection techniques in, 19, 19t
        image acquisition in, 18–19
        radiation exposure and safety in, 19–20, 20b
        ultrasound-guided arterial puncture in, 20–22, 20V, 21f
    intravascular ultrasound in, 26–27, 27f
    planning treatment in, 3
    positioning and prepping of patient in, 5

Vascular surgery *(Continued)*
    preoperative assessment in, 4
    preparation in operating room in, 4–5
    presentation and natural history of vascular diseases and, 2
    sedation, analgesia, and anesthesia in, 17–18
    surgical exposure in, 5
    vascular occlusion in, 6–7, 8f
    vascular reconstructions in, 5–6
    visualization of operative field in, 6
Vasculitis, 129–130
Vein conduit
    in popliteal artery aneurysm repair, 565
    in popliteal artery entrapment, 573
    in reconstruction of inferior vena cava and iliofemoral venous system, 654
Vein graft
    in carotid body tumor surgery, 107
    in superior vena cava syndrome reconstruction, 645, 646f-648f
Vein mapping
    before brachial artery-axillary vein interposition graft, 740, 741f
    in endovenous thermal ablation of saphenous and perforating veins, 696
    before femoral-popliteal bypass, 533
    before forearm loop graft, 740, 741f
    before popliteal artery aneurysm repair, 563
    before reconstruction of inferior vena cava and iliofemoral venous system, 651
    before transjugular intrahepatic portosystemic shunt, 665, 666f
Vein segment transposition, 713
Vein transposition for hemodialysis access
    basilic, 747–757
        choice of one- or two-stage procedure in, 748, 749f
        complications in, 751
        harvest of basilic vein in, 748, 749f
        indications for, 747
        postoperative care in, 750–751
        preoperative preparation for, 747
        single-stage procedure in, 751
        steal syndrome and, 748
        superficialization of fistula in, 750
        two-stage procedure in, 748–750
        use of radial artery in, 750
    brachial, 760, 762–763, 762f-764f
    femoral, 751, 764V
        arteriovenous anastomosis in, 753, 754f
        avoiding wound complications in, 752
        complications in, 756–757
        exposure of distal femoral and popliteal vein in, 753
        exposure of femoral vein in, 752–753
        incision in, 752
        indications for, 751
        loop composite polytetrafluorethylene-femoral vein arteriovenous access and, 755, 755f
        mobilization of proximal femoral vein in, 753
        postoperative care in, 755–756
        preoperative preparation in, 751–752
        steal syndrome and, 752
        transposition procedure in, 753, 754f
    saphenous, 760, 763–764, 765f
Vein valve transplantation, 708, 713–714
Vena cava filter placement, 627–640
    after reconstruction of inferior vena cava and iliofemoral venous system and, 662
    avoiding inadvertent suprarenal filter placement and, 633, 634f
    complications in, 638–639
    contrast venography and ultrasound imaging in, 632–633
    historical background of, 628, 629t, 630f
    indications for, 628
    with intravascular ultrasound, 635–637, 637f
    percutaneous placement with venography bedside transabdominal or intravascular ultrasound, 635

Vena cava filter placement *(Continued)*
    percutaneous placement with venography in, 633
    percutaneous superior vena cava filter and, 637–638
    permanent *versus* retrievable filter in, 631–632, 632f
    postoperative care in, 638
    pregnant patient and, 633
    preoperative preparation for, 630–631, 632f
    retrieval of vena cava filter and, 638
    with transabdominal duplex ultrasound, 635, 635f-636f
Vena cava thrombosis after vena cava filter placement, 639
Vena Tech LP filter, 629t, 630f
Venography
    in iliofemoral and femoral-popliteal deep vein thrombosis, 673–674, 673f
    percutaneous vena cava filter placement with, 633
    before reconstruction of inferior vena cava and iliofemoral venous system, 651
    in superior vena cava syndrome, 642
    in transjugular intrahepatic portosystemic shunt, 665, 666f, 667–668
    upper extremity
        in subclavian-axillary vein thrombosis, 207f-208f, 209, 210f
        before supraclavicular approach to thoracic outlet syndrome, 174
Venous anomalies
    abdominal aortic aneurysm surgery and, 301
    basilic vein transposition and, 747
Venous bypass
    femoral-femoral, 658, 658f
    iliocaval, 658–659, 659f
    in reconstruction of inferior vena cava and iliofemoral venous system and, 655
Venous disease
    deep venous valve surgery in, 708–720
        angioscope-assisted valvuloplasty in, 712
        artificial valve implantation in, 714–715
        autologous neovalve construction in, 713
        complications in, 719
        external banding valvuloplasty in, 712
        external valvuloplasty in, 711
        indications for, 708
        internal valvuloplasty in, 711, 712f
        operative strategy in, 710
        pitfalls and danger points in, 709–710
        postoperative care in, 718
        preoperative preparation for, 709
        transcommissural valvuloplasty in, 712
        vein segment transposition in, 713
        vein valve transplantation in, 708, 713–714
    endovenous thermal ablation of saphenous and perforating veins in, 694–707
        access in, 699, 700f
        complications in, 705–706, 706f
        confirmation of catheter tip position in, 701, 701f
        endovascular strategy in, 696–699, 698f
        endovenous laser in, 700
        indications for, 695f, 696
        patient positioning for, 699
        postoperative care in, 704–705
        preoperative preparation for, 696, 697f
        radiofrequency catheter in, 699–700, 700f
        treatment of axial veins in, 702–703
        treatment of perforator veins in, 703–704, 704f
        tumescent anesthesia in, 701, 702f
    iliofemoral and femoral-popliteal deep vein thrombosis in, 672–683
        access and crossing of lesion in, 675
        catheter-directed thrombolysis for, 675–676
        iliac vein stenosis in, 680, 682f
        inferior vena cava filters in, 675, 675f
        postoperative care in, 681–682
        postoperative complications in, 682
        preoperative preparation in, 673–674, 673f

Venous disease (Continued)
    recalcitrant thrombus in, 680
    rheolytic thrombectomy: AnjioJet power pulse spray technique for, 677–679, 678f
    timing of intervention in, 674–675
    Trellis-8 peripheral infusion system for, 679, 680f–681f
    ultrasound-accelerated thrombolysis: Ekosonic endovascular system for, 676–677, 677f
  sclerotherapy in, 721–728
    complications in, 725–726
    foaming of sclerosant solution in, 724V, 724
    injection of target vein in, 724V, 724, 725f
    patient positioning for, 724
    postoperative care in, 724–725
    preoperative preparation for, 721–722
    selection of sclerosant solution in, 723, 723t
    sequence of treatment of superficial veins and, 723
  subfascial endoscopic perforator surgery in
    choice of anesthesia for, 715
    deep venous valve surgery in, 719
    distal ankle perforators and, 718
    exploration of subfascial space in, 716, 717f–718f
    incision in, 715–716, 715b, 715f
    indications for, 708
    operative strategy in, 710–711
    paratibial fasciotomy in, 716
    pitfalls and danger points in, 709–710
    port insertion in, 716, 716f
    postoperative care in, 718–719
    preoperative preparation for, 709
  superior vena cava syndrome reconstruction in, 641–649
    anastomoses in, 645–648, 647f–648f
    anesthesia for, 644
    avoiding intraoperative bleeding in, 643
    avoiding pulmonary embolism in, 644
    closure of median sternotomy in, 648
    complications in, 648–649, 649t
    dissection of innominate veins and superior vena cava in, 645
    indications for, 641
    position and incision in, 645
    postoperative care in, 648
    preoperative preparation for, 641–643, 642f–643f
    selection of vascular conduit for, 644, 644t
    selection of venous inflow and outflow sites in, 644
    spiral vein graft in, 645, 646f
    unilateral versus bilateral, 644
  surgical reconstruction of inferior vena cava and iliofemoral venous system in, 650–663
    anatomy in, 656
    choice of incision for, 656–657, 657f
    complications in, 662–663
    femoral-femoral venous bypass in, 658, 658f
    ileocaval venous bypass in, 658–659, 659f
    indications for, 650, 651b
    inferior vena cava reconstruction in, 659–662, 660f
    pitfalls and danger points in, 653–656, 654f–656f
    postoperative care in, 662
    preoperative preparation for, 650–653, 652f–653f
    resection of suprarenal inferior vena cava inconjunction with major liver resection in, 657
  transjugular intrahepatic portosystemic shunt in, 664–671
    accessing portal vein in, 665–666, 668, 669f
    anesthesia in, 666

Venous disease (Continued)
    completion portosystemic gradient measurement and portography in, 669, 670f
    complications in, 670–671
    localizing catheter tip in right hepatic vein in, 665
    mapping portal venous system in, 665, 666f, 667–668
    parenchymal tract in, 666, 668–669
    patient positioning and venous access in, 667
    portosystemic gradient measurements in, 666
    portosystemic pressure gradient measurement in, 667
    postoperative care in, 670
    preoperative preparation for, 664–665
    selection and deployment of stent in, 666, 669
    selective hepatic venography in, 667
    stent deployment in, 669
    target portosystemic gradient in, 666
  varicose vein stripping in, 684–693
    anesthesia for, 688
    complications in, 692
    great saphenous vein, 688–690, 689f–690f
    indications for, 684–685, 685b
    operative strategy in, 686–688, 687f
    postoperative care in, 692
    preoperative preparation for, 685–686
    small saphenous vein, 690–691
    stab or ambulatory phlebectomy and, 691–692, 691f
  vena cava filter placement in, 627–640
    avoiding inadvertent suprarenal filter placement and, 633, 634f
    complications in, 638–639
    contrast venography and ultrasound imaging in, 632–633
    historical background of, 628, 629t, 630f
    indications for, 628
    with intravascular ultrasound, 635–637, 637f
    percutaneous placement with venography bedside transabdominal or intravascular ultrasound in, 635
    percutaneous placement with venography in, 633
    percutaneous superior vena cava filter and, 637–638
    permanent versus retrievable filter in, 631–632, 632f
    postoperative care in, 638
    pregnant patient and, 633
    preoperative preparation for, 630–631, 632f
    retrieval of vena cava filter and, 638
    with transabdominal duplex ultrasound, 635, 635f–636f
Venous injury
  in surgical repair of popliteal artery aneurysm, 566
  in surgical repair of popliteal artery entrapment, 574
  in varicose vein stripping, 686–687, 692
Venous outflow obstruction after arteriovenous graft, 745
Venous plethysmography before reconstruction of inferior vena cava and iliofemoral venous system, 650–651
Venous thromboembolism
  after direct surgical repair of tibial-peroneal arterial occlusive disease, 543–559
  in reconstruction of inferior vena cava and iliofemoral venous system, 654, 655f
Venovenous bypass in reconstruction of inferior vena cava and iliofemoral venous system and, 655
Vertebral artery
  angioplasty and stenting of, 153
  average diameter of, 57t

Vertebral artery (Continued)
  injury in subclavian and axillary artery surgery, 161
  surgical anatomy of, 114–116, 116f
Vertebral artery surgery, 111–112
  exposure and transposition of vertebral artery into common carotid artery in, 116–118, 117f, 118V, 119f
  exposure of V2 segment of vertebral artery in, 118–122
  indications for, 111–112, 112b
  operative strategy in, 114
  postoperative care in, 122
  postoperative complications in, 122–124
  preoperative preparation for, 113f, 112–114, 113b, 113f, 115f
  surgical anatomy in, 114–116, 116f
Vertebrobasilar transient ischemic attack, 111, 112b
Vessel rupture, angioplasty-related, 51
Viabahn endograft, 599
Visceral arteries reimplantation in Type II thoracoabdominal aortic aneurysm repair, 227, 227f
Visceral artery aneurysms repair, 500–512
  of celiac artery aneurysm, 506, 508f–509f
  complications in, 511
  of hepatic artery aneurysm, 505–508, 507f
  indications for, 500–501
  operative strategy in, 502, 503f
  postoperative care in, 511
  preoperative preparation for, 501–502
  of splenic artery aneurysm, 502–505, 503f, 505f
Visceral ischemia
  after endovascular treatment of aortic dissection, 275, 276f, 283–284, 288
  after endovascular treatment of descending thoracic artery aneurysm, 256–257
after surgical repair of thoracoabdominal aortic aneurysm, 218
Visceral lesions, direct surgical repair of aortoiliac occlusive disease and, 355
Visceral vessel stenosis after endovascular repair of juxtarenal and pararenal aneurysms, 349
Visipaque. See Iodixanol
Visualization of operative field, 6
Volar fasciotomy incision of forearm, 623, 623f

W

Warfarin
  access site management and, 30, 31t
  hold before endovascular treatment of renal artery stenosis, 456
  before transaxillary rib resection for thoracic outlet syndrome, 195
Wedged carbon dioxide venography, 665, 666f, 667–668
Wound infection
  after above- and below-knee amputation, 608
  after direct surgical repair of tibial-peroneal arterial occlusive disease, 559
  after eversion endarterectomy, 84
  after fasciotomy, 624
  after femoral vein transposition, 756
  after forefoot amputation, 615
  after subfascial endoscopic perforator surgery, 719

Z

Zenith endograft
  for descending thoracic aortic aneurysm, 266–267, 268f–269f
  for infrarenal aortic aneurysm, 330, 341